PHILIP L. HILLSMAN, M.D.

Comprehensive Handbook of Drug and Alcohol Addiction

Comprehensive Handbook of Drug and Alcohol Addiction

edited by

Norman S. Miller

Cornell University Medical College
The New York Hospital–Cornell Medical Center
White Plains, New York

Marcel Dekker, Inc.   **New York • Basel • Hong Kong**

Library of Congress Cataloging-in-Publication Data

Comprehensive handbook of drug and alcohol addiction/edited by
   Norman S. Miller.
      p.   cm.
      Includes bibliographical references and index.
      ISBN: 0-8247-8474-X (alk. paper)
      1. Substance abuse.   2. Alcoholism.   I. Miller, Norman S.
      [DNLM: 1. Alcohol Ethyl-handbooks.   2. Narcotics-handbooks.
   3. Substance Dependence-handbooks.   WM 34 C737]
   RC564.C652   1991
   616.86–dc20
   DLC
   for Library of Congress

This book is printed on acid-free paper.

MARCEL DEKKER, INC.
270 Madison Avenue, New York, New York 10016

Current printing (last digit):
10 9 8 7 6 5 4 3

PRINTED IN THE UNITED STATES OF AMERICA

To residents and students who inspire energy and to colleagues who provide knowledge to drive the creation of this book

Foreword

In writing this foreword, it is important to put this book and the field of addiction treatment in context. At present, there are literally millions of people receiving help through self-help, outpatient, rehabilitation, hospital, and other public and private treatment programs in their recovery from drug and alcohol addiction. To assist these recovering addicts, thousands of treatment providers have chosen the career of an addiction healthcare provider.

Have they made the wrong choice? After all, many statistics and news reports assure us that the drug epidemic is over. In reality, the addiction treatment professionals have *not* made the wrong choice. On the contrary, we need these professionals to treat the millions of alcohol and drug addicts. A closer examination of important findings reveals that while we no longer have an epidemic of drug use and experimentation, we do have an epidemic of drug *addiction*. What studies support this conclusion?

First the good news. According to the National Institute of Drug Abuse's (NIDA) 1990 National Household Survey on Drug Abuse, drug and alcohol use among those age 12 and older has been in steady decline since 1985:

In 1985 some 23 million people, 12 percent of the population, were drug users. That number fell in 1988 to 14.5 million regular users, and in 1990 it fell to 13 million users.

There has been an astounding 72 percent decrease in the number of current users of cocaine since 1985, when an estimated 5.8 million people were considered current users. In 1990, the number declined to 1.6 million users.

Use of cigarettes has also been in decline. In 1985, 32 percent of the population smoked cigarettes. In 1988 it was estimated that 29 percent of the population smoked, and that figure fell further to 27 percent in 1990. Overall this represents a decrease of 6.7 million smokers.

The number of people consuming alcohol has been in decline. In 1985 there were an estimated 113.1 million drinkers in this country (59 percent of the population). In 1988, there were 105.8 million drinkers, and in 1990 that number declined to 102.9 million.

The number of people in this country who have used cocaine in the past year has significantly dropped since 1985. Among those age 12 to 17 the rate dropped from a high of 4 percent in 1985 to 2.2 percent in 1990, and for those 18 to 25, use dropped from 16.3 percent in 1985 to 7.5 percent in 1990.

While these statistics are highly encouraging, the fight against drug and alcohol use is far from over. We still have a widespread drug problem. Consider these statistics:

Over 74 million people, 37 percent of the population, have tried marijuana, cocaine, or some other illicit drug in their lifetime, and almost 27 million of these people have used them within the past year.

Among youths age 12 to 17, almost 16 percent had used drugs or alcohol in the past year, and over 8 percent had used them within the past month.

Among those 18 to 25, over 28 percent had used drugs or alcohol in the past year, and almost 15 percent had used them within the past month.

Among 18- to 34-year-old Americans who are employed full-time, 24.4 percent, nearly one-quarter of the young-adult population, had used drugs in the past year, and over 10 percent had used them within the past month.

While it is true that the number of occasional users (those who used cocaine within the past year and past month) has dropped considerably since 1985, frequent or more intense use has not. Simply put, *use* is down, but *addiction* is up.

In fact, there are now more people using cocaine on a weekly or daily basis than ever before. In 1985, an estimated 647,000 used the drug weekly, and 246,000 used cocaine daily. In 1990, 662,000 people had used cocaine weekly and another 336,000 used it daily.

As bad as these figures may seem, they may actually be worse. According to the 1990 Senate Judiciary Committee report released by Senator Joseph Biden, Jr. (D–Delaware), the figures reported by the NIDA may be too *low*. According to Senator Biden, a whopping 2.4 million Americans use cocaine once a week, a significantly higher number than the 662,000 cited in the NIDA survey. In either case, first-time use is down, but addiction and the consequences of frequent cocaine use are up.

What can be done about the rise in addiction? Is there something we have overlooked that has led to this? I believe that in the future we must take full advantage of the technological breakthroughs in drug testing that have been made recently, and we must vigorously pursue education as a resource in our efforts to curb the rising incidence of addiction.

In the field of addiction health care we debate a wide range of drug-related issues, from the merits of drug testing (and its constitutionality) to drug legalization. Recent advances made in laboratory testing technologies, including rapid laboratory turnaround time and heightened testing sensitivity and specificity, have sparked a heated debate about the limitations there should, or should not, be on the use of drug testing. Where do we, as clinicians, fit in this debate? As clinicians I feel we should focus our attention on understanding what these new technologies and advances can do for our patients and programs, rather than involve ourselves in the public debate surrounding drug testing. Whether these new technologies are used to simply monitor an identified drug-using patient during and after treatment or are employed to help diagnose supposedly psychiatric syndromes accurately, we should actively partake of these recent breakthroughs in our treatment of addiction. These advances can only aid in our fight against drug abuse, which should be our first and foremost concern.

In addition to these new technologies, I believe that education is one of the most powerful and useful tools we have available in battling drug and alcohol abuse. I believe that in the future, education will lead the way in the addiction treatment process, and rather than minimize or belittle the effectiveness of parent's groups such as PRIDE (National Parents

Resource Institute for Drug Education), educational materials produced by groups like the American Council for Drug Education, or messages produced by the Media Partnership for a Drug Free America and NIDA, we should learn more about these and other recent initiatives, which have gone a long way to prove that education is powerful medical treatment.

Education can help stop people—especially children—from taking that first step toward alcohol and drug abuse. Through education, we can wipe away the myths surrounding drugs and alcohol and point out the real dangers. I think of education as one of our most important tools in the treatment and prevention of drug and alcohol abuse. And just as we did in the war on cigarette smoking, health care professionals have an important front-line responsibility to educate their patients about the dangers of drugs and alcohol.

I feel that education in the generalist's or pediatrician's office should begin with a history and examination and end with a urinalysis and a series of specific questions regarding drugs, alcohol, and lifestyle. When making a diagnosis we need to be medical sleuths, on the one hand, and at the same time we must be fully aware of the part that denial and deception play in drug and alcohol addiction. We need to take histories not only from the patient but also from friends and family who know the patient and are witnesses to the patient's self-destructive habits. We need to ask many questions, but we also must be prepared not to take a patient at his word, and not to take it personally if the patient's version of reality and the reality of a positive blood or urine test cannot be reconciled.

For this very reason we must be experienced clinicians and clinical toxicologists. We must know the latest laboratory methods. We must know how to choose the right body fluid and the right laboratory method to make or confirm a diagnosis. And above all, we need to know our place and the place of the patients and family in addiction treatment. We have to understand and put to good use the many treatment options available—day programs, night programs, rehabs, self-help groups, inpatient treatment, psychotherapy, antagonist pharmacotherapy, and so on. We must fight the tendency to see these options as competing or mutually exclusive and make every effort to work together as one in our efforts to curb addiction, because we cannot ask our patients to fight our treatment ideology battles with their abstinence. As President Reagan said of Soviet leader Mikhail S. Gorbachev, we must "trust but verify."

It is of the utmost importance that we make every effort to prevent relapse and limit the impact of a slip or relapse once it occurs. All the while we must keep the nature of addictive disease in mind and not take it personally when the patient fails the treatment program we have prescribed. Unfortunately, we are better at designing and administrating treatment programs than in prognosticating who will succeed or fail in which program. Treatment options available to a person can only mean that more people will become abstinent and stay in treatment. We must understand the power of group support and the traditions of Alcoholics Anonymous. We must treat the identified patient and their family. Finally, we must understand the differences between rehabilitation and habilitation and try to find new ways to help those who have missed normal development, education, and job training while learning firsthand the important lessons in this text.

At this time, we appear ready to discard the prejudices and myths surrounding drugs and drug abuse and look at the facts generated by the exhaustive clinical and basic research that has been done by those in the addiction treatment field. All too often in the past, so-called experts have blindly claimed that certain drugs were safe, and with a virtual absence of scientific data could often convince others of their belief. In the process we aided the drug user's denial and prolonged our own suspension of reality. I am glad to say the days of ignorance, lack of research, and "blind" following are over.

Much of the research that led to the decline of cocaine and alcohol use can be applied to other drug addictions. However I feel it is important for clinicians to have a firm grasp on *all* of the available data concerning drug and alcohol neuropharmacology, and that we *not* pursue the current trend of having specialized experts (alcohol experts, marijuana experts, cocaine experts, etc.). Why not specialize? After all, are not most physicians specialists nowadays? While this may be true for other disciplines, the unfortunate fact is that most drug and alcohol abusers rarely follow so rigid an agenda, and most users are addicted to more than one drug.

This book is evidence in itself to the complexity and importance of this new medical field and to the depth and richness of available research and clinical data. As physicians we need to use our experience and expertise in identifying the consequences of drug and alcohol use and make every effort to cure the patient, or, at the very least, minimize its effects on the patient's life after abstinence.

We have a demanding and ever-changing task that above all else demands extreme caring and self-education. Self-education is essential because it provides a sound basis for understanding and treating addiction, and for educating our patients and communities. This text provides that information, with state-of-the-art data detailing the complex associations between the body, brain, person, society, and drugs and alcohol. I am aware of how much I still do not know about this vast medical field, and I am grateful to the authors for providing a timely, well-written, comprehensive single source for my use.

Mark S. Gold

Preface

Three objectives have determined the structure of this book. My major purpose was to conceptualize and implement these objectives for a wide audience of prospective readers.

First, the book is intended to be useful and comprehensive in its approach and content. The reader should expect to be able to have this book serve as a single reference for the field of drug and alcohol addiciton. It has been the goal to include all clinically relevant areas for perspective and depth, and provide adequate bibliographies for more intensive review. The reader is encouraged to use the book as a coherent discussion of drug and alcohol addiction or select chapters in any sequence as desired.

Second, the book is robust in its presentation of reliable and tested knowledge of past and current research in the field of drug and alcohol addiction. The attempt was made to synthesize for the reader the useful theoretical and practical implications of the research. The theme of addiction provides a framework for critical questions to be posed and presentation of essential data, which are summarized in many of the chapters.

Third, the editor purposely selected authors who would furnish chapters in order to construct a coherent and cogent literary work of the field of drug and alcohol addiction. These contributing authors are leaders in the field, and have demonstrated the capacity to correlate clinically useful practices with current research information. These are minimum standards shared by the editor and authors as demonstrated throughout the book.

The book may fall short of achieving these objectives in full, and in no way does it represent the final statement in this rapidly changing field. However, the book in its present form is not duplicated anywhere else and contains chapters that are not found in other sources. In the sense that the book brings together apparently divergent poles—clinical and research, pharmacological and nonpharmacological, applied and theoretical—it is an original contribution. In the estimation of the editor, no other single book contains this breadth and depth of information.

The greater purpose of this edition is to stimulate new ideas and practices by clinicians, students, and researchers for the ultimate benefit of those who suffer from drug and alcohol addiction. The field of drug and alcohol addiction has grown to assume a stature comparable with that of other medical specialties. The science of addiction no longer must rely on other disciplines to define it. These are exciting and inspiring times, especially for those who are contemplating or beginning a career in this field. We dedicate this book to them.

Finally, the title of the book contains the term *addiction* purposely to highlight our focus. As in other medical specialties, the proper definition of concepts is critical for consistent communication with others within and outside the field of drug and alcohol addiction. As the editor, I have endeavored to provide a consistent and reliable text for instruction and reference by selecting the term addiction and using it in concert with the contributing authors. However, because of tradition, the terms alcoholism and dependence may be used interchangeably with alcohol and drug addiction.

Norman S. Miller

Contents

II. Special Populations

III. Adolescents

IV. Diagnosis

V. Pharmacology of Drugs/Alcohol

VI. Medical Implications

VII. Behavior

VIII. Psychiatric Implications

IX. Genetics

X. Neurochemistry

XI. Education

XII. Laboratory Testing for Drugs

XIII. Family

Contributors

James C. Anthony, Ph.D.   The Johns Hopkins University, School of Hygiene and Public Health, Baltimore, Maryland

Heather Ashton, D.M., F.R.C.P.   The University of Newcastle upon Tyne, Newcastle upon Tyne, England

Beth M. Belkin, M.D., Ph.D.   Cornell University Medical College, The New York Hospital–Cornell Medical Center, White Plains, New York

David G. Benzer, D.O.   Milwaukee Psychiatric Hospital, Wauwatosa, Wisconsin

Sheila B. Blume, M.D.   South Oaks Hospital, Amityville, New York

Kirk J. Brower, M.D.   University of Michigan School of Medicine, and Alcohol Research Center, Ann Arbor, Michigan

Audrey Burnam, Ph.D.   The Rand Corporation, Santa Monica, California

Giovanni Caracci, M.D.   Cornell University Medical College, The New York Hospital–Cornell Medical Center, White Plains, New York

Arthur W. K. Chan, Ph.D.   Research Institute on Alcoholism, Buffalo, New York

John N. Chappel, M.D.   University of Nevada School of Medicine, and Truckee Meadows Hospital, Reno, Nevada

Ira J. Chasnoff, M.D.   Northwestern University Medical School, Chicago, Illinois

J. Calvin Chatlos, M.D.   St. Mary Hospital, Hoboken, New Jersey

Paula J. Clayton, M.D.   Washington University School of Medicine, St. Louis, Missouri

C. Robert Cloninger, M.D.   Washington University School of Medicine, St. Louis, Missouri

James Cocores, M.D.   Fair Oaks Hospital, Summit, New Jersey

Gregory B. Collins, M.D.   Cleveland Clinic Foundation, Cleveland, Ohio

Dennis Cozzens, M.D.   Cleveland Clinic Foundation, Cleveland, Ohio

Dorynne Czechowicz, M.D.   National Institute on Drug Abuse, Rockville, Maryland

Charles A. Dackis, M.D.   Hampton Hospital, Westampton, New Jersey

Ronald I. Dozoretz, M.D.   First Hospital Corporation, Norfolk, Virginia

Elke D. Eckert, M.D.   University of Minnesota Hospital and Clinic, Minneapolis, Minnesota

Charles J. Engel, M.D.   Milwaukee Psychiatric Hospital, Wauwatosa, Wisconsin

Marc Galanter, M.D.   New York University School of Medicine, New York, New York

Anne Geller, M.D.   Smithers Alcohol Treatment Center, New York, New York

A. James Giannini, M.D., F.C.P.   Ohio State University, Columbus, Ohio

Mark S. Gold, M.D.   Fair Oaks Hospital, Summit, New Jersey, and Delray Beach, Florida

Samuel B. Guze, M.D.   Washington University School of Medicine, St. Louis, Missouri

Katherine Halmi, M.D.   Cornell University Medical College, The New York Hospital–Cornell Medical Center, White Plains, New York

Patricia Ann Harrison, Ph.D.*   Ramsey Clinic, St. Paul, Minnesota

John E. Helzer, M.D.   University of Vermont, College of Medicine, Burlington, Vermont

Lawrence E. Hoeschen, M.D., Ph.D.   University of Manitoba, Winnipeg, Manitoba, Canada

Lynne Hoffman, M.D.   Cornell University Medical College, The New York Hospital–Cornell Medical Center, White Plains, New York

Normam G. Hoffmann, Ph.D.[†]   Ramsey Clinic, St. Paul, Minnesota

John E. Imhof, Ph.D.   North Shore University Hospital–Cornell University Medical College, Manhasset, New York

Joseph W. Janesz, M.Ed.   Cleveland Clinic Foundation, Cleveland, Ohio

Edward Kaufman, M.D.   University of California, Irvine, California

Hiten Kisnad, M.D.   Cornell University Medical College, The New York Hospital–Cornell Medical Center, White Plains, New York

Therese A. Kosten, Ph.D.   Yale University School of Medicine, New Haven, Connecticut

Thomas R. Kosten, M.D.   Yale University School of Medicine, New Haven, Connecticut

Margaret Kotz, D.O.   Cleveland Clinic Foundation, Cleveland, Ohio

Nathan M. Kravis, M.D.   Cornell University Medical College, New York, New York

---

Current affiliations:
*Minnesota Department of Human Services Chemical Dependency Division, St. Paul, Minnesota.
†CATOR/New Standards, Inc., St. Paul, Minnesota.

Karol L. Kumpfer, Ph.D.   University of Utah, Salt Lake City, Utah

Malcolm Lader, D.Sc., Ph.D., M.D., F.R.C.   Institute of Psychiatry, University of London, London, England

David C. Lewis, M.D.   Brown University, Providence, Rhode Island

George A. Mann, M.D.   St. Mary's Hospital, Minneapolis, Minnesota

Arthur Margolin, Ph.D.   Yale University School of Medicine, New Haven, Connecticut

David M. Martin, Ph.D.   FirstLab at Horsham Clinic, Ambler, Pennsylvania

Ronald Martin, M.D.   Washington University School of Medicine, St. Louis, Missouri

Steven D. Martin, M.D.   Parkview Episcopal Medical Center, Pueblo, Colorado

Richard A. Meisch, M.D., Ph.D.   Substance Abuse Research Center, University of Texas Health Sciences Center at Houston, Houston, Texas

David J. Mersy, M.D.   St. Paul–Ramsey Medical Center/Ramsey Clinic, St. Paul, Minnesota

Norman S. Miller, M.D.   Cornell University Medical College, The New York Hospital–Cornell Medical Center, White Plains, New York

Steven M. Mirin, M.D.   McLean Hospital, Belmont Massachusetts, and Harvard Medical School, Boston, Massachusetts

James E. Mitchell, M.D.   University of Minnesota Hospital and Clinic, Minneapolis, Minnesota

David J. Nyman, Ph.D.   Fair Oaks Hospital, Summit, New Jersey

Charles P. O'Brien, M.D.   Philadelphia Veterans Affairs Medical Center, and University of Pennsylvania, Philadelphia, Pennsylvania

Joseph M. Palumbo, M.D.   Stony Lodge Hospital, Briarcliff Manor, New York

Samuel W. Perry, M.D.   Cornell University Medical College, New York, New York

A. Carter Pottash, M.D.   Fair Oaks Hospital, Summit, New Jersey, and Delray Beach, Florida

Richard L. Pyle, M.D.   University of Minnesota Hospital and Clinic, Minneapolis, Minnesota

Joseph P. Reoux, M.D.*   University of California, Irvine, Medical Center, Orange, California

John D. Roache, Ph.D.   Substance Abuse Research Center, University of Texas Health Sciences Center at Houston, Houston, Texas

Marc A. Schuckit, M.D.   Veterans Affairs Medical Center, and University of California, San Diego, California

---

Current affiliation: Public Health Service Commissioned Officer, Indian Health Service, Sitka, Alaska

Terry K. Schultz, M.D.   Walter Reed Army Medical Center, Washington, D.C.

Jerome E. Schulz, M.D.   University of California, San Francisco, California

Richard B. Seymour, M.A.   Haight Ashbury Free Clinics, Inc., San Francisco, California

Andrew E. Slaby, M.D., Ph.D., M.P.H.   Fair Oaks Hospital, Summit, New Jersey; The Regent Hospital, and New York University, New York, New York

David E. Smith, M.D.   Haight Ashbury Free Clinics, Inc., San Francisco, California

Sheila Specker, M.D.   University of Minnesota Hospital and Clinic, Minneapolis, Minnesota

David E. Sternberg, M.D.   The Kansas Institute, Olathe, Kansas, and Yale University School of Medicine, New Haven, Connecticut

Susan G. Streed, B.A.   Ramsey Clinic, St. Paul, Minnesota

Jan Thrope, M.A.   Cleveland Clinic Foundation, Cleveland, Ohio

Karl Verebey, Ph.D., DABFT   Bureau of Laboratories, New York City Department of Health, New York, New York

Matthew E. Weinstein   First Hospital Corporation, Norfolk, Virginia

Carol J. Weiss, M.D. Cornell University Medical College, New York, New York

Kathleen Weiss, R.N., M.S.N.   Cleveland Clinic Foundation, Cleveland, Ohio

Roger D. Weiss, M.D.   McLean Hospital, Belmont, Massachusetts, and Harvard Medical School, Boston, Massachusetts

Joseph Westermeyer, M.D., Ph.D., M.P.H.   University of Oklahoma, Oklahoma City, Oklahoma

George E. Woody, M.D.   Philadelphia Veterans Affairs Medical Center, and University of Pennsylvania, Philadelphia, Pennsylvania

Donna Yi, M.D.   Cornell University Medical College, The New York Hospital–Cornell Medical Center, White Plains, New York

Comprehensive Handbook of Drug and Alcohol Addiction

Introduction

Norman S. Miller
Cornell University Medical College, The New York Hospital–Cornell Medical Center, White Plains, New York

I. DEFINITIONS

The term *addiction* is used in the title of this book and throughout the work for reasons that will become apparent as one reads further. It defines a set of behaviors that describes a specific clinical entity that cannot be confused with any other. Addiction to drugs and alcohol is defined as a preoccupation with acquiring these agents, their compulsive use, and a pattern of recurrent relapse to drugs and alcohol. Preoccupation, compulsivity, and relapse are indicative of the pervasive loss of control that is evident in drug and alcohol addiction. These three specific behaviors directed at drugs and alcohol are necessary and sufficient to establish an independent clincial entity that does require further justification.

Drug and alcohol addiction has no known cause, and in this way shares etiological characteristics with cancer as well as other well-established diseases. Although drug and alcohol addiction is defined in behavioral terms, it must have a neurological substrate that underlies preoccupation, compulsivity, and relapse. The direct interaction of a chemical and the brain provides a clear model for drug- or alcohol-induced neurological disorders, which are with psychiatric manifestations. Pharmacological models exist to formulate specific locations in the brain that appear to be responsible for addictive behavior associated with alcohol and drugs.

George Vaillant points out in *The Natural History of Alcoholism* that diseases such as coronary artery disease and hypertension share many similar characteristics with alcoholism. The parallelism between these medical diseases, including alcoholism, continues from pathogenesis through pathophysiology. The etiology is not known for either coronary artery disease or hypertension, and the known risk factors are considered "lifestyle" issues as is alcoholism; i.e., diet, weight, stress, cigarette smoking, and others. Further research is needed to investigate if in fact these lifestyle behaviors that are considered under the personal control of the individual are clearly psychological choices and not biologically driven by genetic and physiological determinants themselves.

II. AN OVERVIEW

A. Epidemiology of Drug and Alcohol Addiction

The organization of this book follows a traditional format, more or less, and begins with a detailed and current presentation of the epidemiological data for drug and alcohol addiction (see Chaps. 1–6). The uniqueness of these data is that the prevalence of drug and alcohol addiction was determined by structured interviews, using established diagnostic criteria. Heretofore, prevalence rates had been estimates based on alcohol and drug consumption or medical consequences. The data presented in this book are instead based on actual diagnoses obtained by examining the subject. The data were also collected from different geographical areas of the country for a representative sample of the United States.

The results of the study are alarming. The high rate of alcoholism, over one-quarter of the male population, is a statement of the magnitude of the health problem of alcoholism. Drug addiction also has a high prevalence rate with its consequent morbidity and mortality. These data are helpful in defining the scope of the problem.

The patterns of use have changed dramatically in the recent decades in several major ways. The use of multiple drugs by alcoholics and drug addicts as well as alcohol by drug addicts has become the rule (see Chap. 3). The vast majority of alcoholics are drug addicts and the reverse also is true: Most drug addicts are alcoholics. Furthermore, there has been a proliferation of prescription medications to which various populations have become addicted. Also, the use of new routes of administration for old drugs has accentuated the addictive potential and increased the number of addictive users of these drugs.

B. Special Populations

Indeed, special populations do have particular consequences from drug and alcohol addiction. Investigations and individualized assessments and interventions are needed to protect the unborn. Women have long been a neglected population in that there has been a concerted denial that a drug and alcohol problem exists for them (see Chaps. 7 and 8). Studies clearly show that women have peculiar patterns of use and manifestations of drug and alcohol addiction. The elderly population is one that needs intensive review and specialized attention (see Chap. 9). Eating disorders and other addictive behaviors are serious complicating factors for drug and alcohol addiction and problems in their own right (see Chap. 10).

C. Adolescents

Longitudinal studies clearly show that drug and alcohol addiction are youthful disorders that have their origin in early adolescence (see Chaps. 11–13). The myth that alcoholism is a habit of old age has never been more clearly refuted by today's practices by adolescents. Over 90% of senior high school students have used alcohol, many weekly and monthly. This would be significant alone for the fact that high school seniors usually do not meet the legal age of drinking, which in most states is 21 years of age. However, it is further complicated by noting that over 60% of them have used marijuana and other illicit drugs. The rate of alcohol and drug addiction for adolescents is equal to the adult population.

D. Diagnosis

No misconception is greater than drug and alcohol addiction cannot be diagnosed (see Chaps. 14–18). High rates of agreement exist for identifying the behaviors of addiction. Furthermore, ample data exist, as will be presented in many chapters, that the addiction syndrome can be clearly defined and readily applied.

Alcoholism and drug addiction as medical disorders are unequivocally supported by studies from a diverse array of specialties. It is useless and counterproductive to continue a moral debate over whether or not alcoholism and drug addiction are diseases. It only delays providing the needed assessment and intervention, as well as the research that will open new avenues for clinical application.

E. Pharmacology of Drugs/Alcohol

The individual drugs are discussed to amplify their peculiar pharmacological characteristics and properties. The drugs have typical manifestations of acute and chronic intoxication, tolerance, and dependence, and psychiatric and medical complications derived from their chemical actions. The history and other clinically useful aspects of the drugs are presented in detail in Chapters 19–30.

F. Medical Implications

The medical and neurological complications from drug and alcohol addiction are well known and documented (see Chaps. 31 and 33). The neurological complications are also equally as important and have grown in number with the advent of more extensive and exotic drugs and patterns of drug use. Although medical and neurological complications affect only a minority of the population of drug addicts and alcoholics, the combined morbidity and mortality are substantial. Physicians particularly are responsible for the diagnosis and treatment of the drug- and alcohol-related disorders. The chapters on these subjects are especially detailed and informative, and are written by physicians who practice wholly in addiction medicine.

G. Behavior

Drug self-administration studies are particulary revealing in describing the addictive process (see Chap. 34). Observations in animals and humans have yielded specific knowledge regarding addictive behaviors. These studies more than any others have confirmed the powerful reinforcing effects of drugs and alcohol on modifying and controlling drug-seeking behavior. The opportunity exists in these types of studies to define parameters of addictive behaviors, and isolate the critical factors in addiction to drugs and alcohol.

H. Psychiatric Implications

Psychiatric syndromes are linked to drug and alcohol addiction (see Chaps. 35 and 38). The pharmacological effects of drugs and alcohol on brain function is to induce psychiatric syndromes, which tend to resolve with abstinence. Exclusionary status for drug and alcohol addiction is required before making an additional psychiatric diagnosis. Because of the effects of addiction on the mind and behavior, it is often necessary to withhold the diagnosis of an additional psychiatric disorder until a period of abstinence and specific treatment of addiction have been instituted. Furthermore, genetic and family studies demonstrate that the categories of disorders are separate.

However, psychiatric disorders do occur in the setting of drug and alcohol addiction, It is particularly challenging to the clinician to differentiate the two categories of disorders and implement effective treatment strategies. The two disorders must be treated concurrently for an optimal prognosis for both categories of disorders.

I. Genetics

Perhaps the greatest evidence other than clinical observation that alcoholism is a disease is the recent genetic studies that have demonstrated inheritance factors in the development of alcoholism (see Chaps. 38 and 39). Twin, adoption, familial, and high-risk studies have provided the data to support alcoholism as an inherited disorder. By establishing a genetic predisposition, investigations can be undertaken to find the biological factors responsible for alcoholism. Similar studies need to be performed for drug addiction.

J. Neurochemistry

Genetic studies have emphasized the biological vulnerability to alcoholism, and the importance of conceptualizing it as having a physical basis. The limbic system is a likely candidate for the neurosubstrate for the behaviors of addiction. Within this ancient portion of the brain lies the neurochemical apparatus for the preoccupation with, compulsivity to use, and relapse potential to drugs and addiction.

The pharmacokinetics and pharmacodynamic characteristics of a drug determine its addictive potential as well as the tendency to develop tolerance and dependence. The receptors and the neurotransmitters that act on them may play a role in the addictive process, tolerance, and dependence (see Chaps. 40 and 41).

K. Education

The answer to the urgent clinical needs of the alcoholic and drug addict ultimately lies in the education of clinicians and researchers. As with other medical conditions, information about current methods for diagnosis and treatment and continued research rests with one professional passing it on to another. Drug and alcohol addiction require specialized training for professionals at all levels (see Chaps. 42 and 43).

L. Laboratory Testing for Drugs

The intelligent and informed use of the laboratory is an important aspect of the diagnosis and treatment of drug and alcohol addiction. Because alcohol and drugs can produce virtually any psychiatric syndrome, it is important to have drug testing as a clinical tool to differentiate drug-induced psychiatric disorders from other causes. Although the methodology is complex, effective use of the laboratory is possible once a basic understanding is achieved. Also, controversy surrounding the practices and legalities of drug testing exists. We have included chapters that clarify these aspects of drug testing (see Chaps. 44 and 45).

M. Family

The family is an important ingredient in the devleoment of drug and alcohol addiction as well as its maintenance. Coaddiction is an important clinical phenomenon based on the addiction model. It is important to diagnose and treat coaddiction as a disorder by itself and in order to successfully manage the drug addict and alcoholic as well. Also, because alcoholism and drug addiction have such a strong familial tendency, a comprehensive evaluation of the family members should always be done (see Chaps. 46 and 47).

N. Special Topics

This is an inadequate title for these critically important areas that are books in themselves (see Chaps. 48–54). Acquired immunodeficiency syndrome (AIDS) as a consequence of drug and alcohol addiction is one of our most pressing health problems. Protracted withdrawal syndromes are unrecognized and poorly characterized clinical states that probably have a significant impact on the recovery of the addict. Countertransference is perhaps the most important obstacle to understanding and treating the addict. Drug and alcohol addiction among physicians is a major health problem for physicians themselves. And gambling addiction is another underdiagnosed problem among alcoholics.

O. Prevention

The area of prevention of drug and alcoholic addiction is not traditionally highlighted in a textbook of medicine. Prevention as an outgrowth of epidemiology is based on eliminating those risk factors for the development of a malady. In the case of drug and alcohol addiction, prevention is considered the responsibility of the individual and not the health care professional. This attitude has not been effective in reducing many health problems, and shows little promise for drug and alcohol addiction. This chapter will illustrate this conclusion as well as provide concrete suggestions for remedies (see Chap. 56).

P. Interventions

An important new development in the delivery of effective treatment of drug and alcohol addiction has been the introduction of the technique of intervention. Intervention is an initiation of the treatment process that overcomes many of the inherent obstacles in the addictive mode such as denial and resistance to treatment. The techniques of intervention are new and require an understanding of the dynamics of addiction before proper and full implementation is possible. This chapter provides an in-depth analysis and step-by-step approach for instituting and executing interventions (see Chap. 57).

The physician is a potent source for intervention for the drug and alcohol addict. He or she is commonly faced with diagnosing and treating drug and alcohol addiction. A working knowledge of Alcoholics Anonymous (AA) and Narcotics Anonymous (NA) by the physician is critically important. Studies have shown that 25–50% of a general medical practice and 50–75% of a general psychiatric practice is composed of drug addicts and alcoholics. A chapter for the physician in this regard has been included (see Chap. 58).

Q. Pharmacological Treatment

The physician must be familiar and adept at the use of pharmacological agents for the detoxification from drugs and alcohol (see Chaps. 59–62). Detoxification is almost a subspecialty in itself, and requires a high degree of skill in clinical assessment and administration of therapeutic agents. The physician needs to understand as well as gain clinical experience in the use of the wide variety of complex detoxification schedules. Also, newer pharmacological agents are being tested in the treatment of the addictive behaviors. A review of the state of the art of pharmacologic research for cocaine addiction has been included.

R. Treatment Outcome

It is not well appreciated that effective treatments exist for drug and alcohol addiction. Many outcome studies have documented high abstinence rates for alcoholics and multiple drug addicts in traditional addiction-oriented treatment centers from a wide geographic distribution, both private and public, and staffed by physicians and nonphysicians. The essential factors that are correlated with a positive treatment outcome are reviewed in the chapter on treatment outcome (see Chap. 63).

A thorough comparison is made between inpatient and outpatient forms of treatment for drug and alcohol addiction. A case is made that the view to decide "between" the two is not productive, rather there are different indications for both forms of treatment. Moreover, innovative combinations of inpatient and outpatient forms of treatment show definite promise to meet the needs of the drug addict and alcoholic.

Outpatient Treatment

This is undoubteldy a legitimate and effective form of treatment for drug and alcohol addiction. Many forms of outpatient treatment have been based on successful models of inpatient treatment. However, newer strategies have been devised to meet the special needs of the outpatient. This form of treatment will continue to grow in popularity in the foreseeable future (see Chaps. 64 and 65).

We have also included a chapter on diagnosis and treatment in the office practice, as this constitutes a common form of practice in drug and alcohol addiction. The chapter provides specific recommendations and guidelines for the office practice.

The psychotherapy of drug and alcohol addiction is an important chapter because of the need present in the addict as well as for the treatment provider who administers psychotherapy as a common form of treatment for the drug and alcohol addict. Also, many addicts have additional psychiatric and personality disturbances that are amenable to intensive short-term and long-term psychotherapy.

Inpatient Treatment

This has been the paradigm of treatment for the drug and alcohol addict in recent decades. Inpatient treatment programs utilizing the 12-step philosophy of Alcoholics Anonymous have revolutionized the treatment of drug and alcohol addiction. The treatment approach is based on accurate diagnosis, current methods for detoxification, and formalized treatment concepts that are pragmatic and effectively applied. Physician and nonphysician involvement in a cooperative effort is required for full implementation.

Chapters on the history and structure of treatment have been included to provide the reader with an unusual perspective that is not available in standard textbooks, and rarely found in this degree of professional form in other sources. The authors of these chapters know treatment of addiction first hand and have introduced important advances themselves (see Chaps. 66 and 67).

S. Long-Term Recovery

A complete presentation of the 12-step program in recovery is provided and is written by a physician (see Chap. 68). This particular chapter was written with the professional in mind who is not actively engaged in the specialty of drug and alcohol addiction. It provides a complete and informative discussion of the 12-step programs for the addict and coaddict, as well as for those who wish to learn more about the long-term treatment of drug and alcohol addiction.

T. Interactions Between Drugs and Alcohol and Psychiatric Symptoms: Origin and Course

It is critically important to establish that the addiction disorders have a primary place and independent status and are not defined by other disorders. Self medication for drug and alcohol addiction is not a viable explanation for addictive use. Drug and alcohol addiction produces virtually all known psychiatric symptoms, and the resultant psychiatric syndromes can be clinically indistinguishable from psychiatric disorders from other causes. The overall course and prognosis of addiction are predictable and unique and drug and alcohol addictions are primary disorders.

I
Prevalence and Patterns of Use

1

Epidemiology of Alcohol Addiction: United States

John E. Helzer
University of Vermont, College of Medicine, Burlington, Vermont

Audrey Burnam
The Rand Corporation, Santa Monica, California

I. THE DIAGNOSIS OF ALCOHOLISM

A clear understanding of the prevalence and nature of alcoholism in the U.S. population has been frustrated by disagreement among researchers and clinicians as to how the variety of patterns of alcohol involvement should be classified and labeled. Broadly, these patterns are composed of three types of behaviors (Polich and Kaelber, 1985): (1) excessive consumption of alcohol, (2) the social and health problems that are a consequence of excessive consumption, and (3) alcohol dependence, characterized by impaired ability to regulate drinking and the development of physical tolerance and/or dependence. Alcohol dependence is central to many of the definitions of alcoholism (e.g., Edwards et al., 1977). However, other definitions accept alcohol-related social and health problems as alternative indicators of alcoholism (Davies, 1976). Many practicing physicians use a variety of indicators in addition to dependence (Filstead et al., 1976).

The definition of alcoholism provided by DSM-III (see American Psychiatric Association, 1980) recognizes both dependence and negative social consequences as significant indicators of disorder. Two diagnoses are specified: Alcohol abuse requires a pattern of pathological (excessive or uncontrolled) alcohol use *plus* impairment in social or occupational functioning due to alcohol use. Alcohol dependence diagnosis requires *either* a pattern of pathological use *or* impairment in social or occupational functioning *plus* evidence of tolerance or withdrawal (physical dependence). Specific behaviors indicative of each of these criteria are given in DSM-III, and a summary of these criteria and symptoms as they are

This work was supported by United States Public Health Service grants MH 31302, DA 04001, Research Scientist Development Award MH 00617 (Dr. Helzer), and the MacArthur Foundation Risk Factor Network.
"Alcohol Abuse and Dependence" by John E. Helzer and Audrey Burnam. In *Psychiatric Disorders in America*, Lee N. Robins and Darrel A. Regier, Eds. Copyright 1990 by Lee N. Robins and Darrell A. Regier. Reprinted by Permission of the Free Press, a Division of MacMillan, Inc.

queried in the Diagnostic Interview Schedule (DIS) is shown below in Table 14. According to DSM-III, abuse and dependence are independent; it is possible to diagnose abuse without dependence, dependence without abuse, or both dependence and abuse.

One advantage of the DSM-III criteria is that the focus is on specified patterns of behavior. Definitions that emphasize underlying constructs, such as the dependence syndrome (Edwards and Gross, 1976), are more difficult to utilize because the condition is not directly observable, nor easily inferred from observable behaviors. Perhaps as a result of this emphasis on specific behavior, the DSM-III definition of alcoholism has demonstrated a remarkably high degree of reliability and validity (Robins, 1982). Theoretical disagreements about the nature of alcoholism as a disorder have not been resolved. But DSM-III does provide a standard that can be used to identify, relatively consistently, those persons whose patterns of alcohol involvement are cause for concern.

The recently revised DSM-III criteria (DSM-III-R; see American Psychiatric Association, 1987) include modifications in the alcohol diagnoses. According to these revisions, the central diagnosis is dependence, and alcohol abuse without dependence is defined only as a residual category; i.e., evidence of continuing, but below threshold, problems with alcohol. These revisions reflect previous theoretical work and clinical experience suggesting that dependence represents a more severe stage of the disorder, preceded by abuse. The DSM-III-R revisions retain the emphasis on objective symptoms of pathological use, tolerance, and withdrawal, but change the emphasis on impairment in social/occupational functioning to continued use despite such impairment.

II. PREVIOUS EPIDEMIOLOGICAL STUDIES

Most of what we know about the epidemiology of alcoholism in the United States from previous studies is based on rates of cirrhosis mortality, volume of alcohol beverage sales, and population surveys of drinking patterns. These studies, however, have provided information which is "fragmented, ambiguous, and often imprecise" with respect to the prevalence and incidence of alcoholism (Warheit and Auth, 1985).

A formula to estimate the number of alcoholics in the population from cirrhosis death rates (Jellinek, 1959) is inexact, both because of inaccuracies in recorded causes of death, and because there is no fixed ratio of alcoholism to liver cirrhosis, as the formula must assume. Alcohol beverage sales records can be used to calculate average per capita consumption of a population. But per capita consumption does not necessarily tell us about the prevalence of alcoholism. A given per capita level, for example, could be associated with low rates of alcoholism in a population with a high proportion of moderate drinkers, or conversely with high rates of alcoholism in a population with a high proportion of abstainers.

Cirrhosis death rates and per capita consumption have another limitation. They are aggregate statistics, which can be used only to estimate overall rates in large populations. Aggregate statistics tell us nothing about the structure of alcoholism in the population, such as its severity, frequency of occurrence, or relationships among its component symptoms. Aggregate statistics are also uninformative about personal characteristics associated with alcoholism or its risk factors such as age, sex, or the presence of other disorders. Such knowledge is obviously crucial to ultimately understanding causation, and can inform efforts to develop appropriate health policies for prevention and treatment.

Given the weaknesses of such secondary indicators, the preferred, albeit more costly, way to study the epidemiology of a disorder has been to personally examine representative samples of the general population. Several epidemiological surveys of alcohol use have been conducted in the United States. Typically, these surveys focus on drinking patterns (usually frequency of drinking and volume consumed per occasion), and on any number of a variety of alcohol-related problems or consequences. Most, however, have not attempted to define or assess prevalence of alcoholism as a specific disorder. This is perhaps not surprising given the predominant trend in this country since the early 1940s to characterize alcoholism as an underlying disease construct that eludes reliable measurement (Rohan, 1982).

Warheit and Auth (1985) have reviewed 12 of the most important of these surveys, all of which used samples representative of the national population. Taken together, they suggest that between 7 and 12% of adult, household residents are current heavy drinkers. Definitions of heavy drinking are necessarily arbitrary, but include levels of drinking that are less than what is generally associated with alcoholism in clinical contexts (e.g., having five drinks twice a month). The studies also suggest that between 5 and 10% of respondents currently have one or more alcohol-related problems, although the findings in this regard have been quite variable, ranging from 2 to 37% depending on the study.

The Epidemiological Catchment Area (ECA) contributes in a number of ways to the wealth of information that has been collected in prior surveys on drinking patterns and problems. Most important is that the ECA is the first survey to assess alcoholism as a disorder in a large general population, using objective definitions that have been agreed upon for use in research and clinical practice by a significant portion of the medical community. Thus, this study represents an important link between what we know about alcoholism from our experience in treatment settings and the distribution of the disorder in the general population. Second, the study tells us much about the structure of alcoholism in the general population, including the frequency of specific symptoms and age of onset, and its distribution among particular subsamples. Finally, the study permits us to examine associated risk factors and the relationship of alcoholism or alcohol problems to the occurrence of other psychiatric disorders.

As we will see, DSM-III–defined alcohol disorder is one of the most prevalent of the lifetime disorders ascertained in the ECA survey. Alcoholism (a term of convenience we will henceforth use synonymously with alcohol abuse and/or dependence) is a major public health problem, both in the number of persons affected and in the damage it causes to the individual, his or her family, and society at large. In this chapter, we will discuss the prominence of alcohol disorders in the country as a whole, which symptoms are the most and lease common, the age at which alcoholism begins, in which social groups it is most common, and inferences about its causes and consequences.

III. PREVALENCE FROM THE ECA

Prevalence is the proportion of persons who reported enough alcohol symptoms on the DIS (Robins et al., 1981) to meet the DSM-III requirements for an alcohol diagnosis. Lifetime prevalence counts symptoms occurring at any time in the individual's life, and for the DSM-III alcoholism criteria, symptoms need not be overlapping in time. The definition of current prevalence rates in the DIS (1 year, 1 month) varies with the diagnostic category, but for the alcohol disorders the last appearance of at least one symptom defines whether the diagnosis is current, given that full criteria were met at some time.

Lifetime prevalence in the total ECA sample is 13.8% (Table 1); i.e., one out of every 7 persons meets criteria. Lifetime prevalence for men is even more dramatic, with almost one-quarter (23.8%) meeting criteria. The rate for women is much lower, 4.6%. Alcoholism is clearly a predominantly male disorder with a male:female ratio of over 5:1.

The huge lifetime prevalence for men strains credibility, but it is important to recognize what this represents. The DIS adheres strictly to the DSM-III criteria. For some disorders, like major depression and mania, DSM-III requires that the diagnosis be based on a cluster of symptoms occurring together. But for the alcohol disorders, a minimum of two symptoms

Table 1 Alcohol Abuse and/or Dependence: Prevalence of Alcoholism by Sex and Ethnicity (weighted to national demographic distribution)

	Prevalence			Remission
	1 month (%±SE)	1 year (%±SE)	lifetime (%± SE)	lifetime—one year lifetime (%)
Total	3.29±0.18	6.80±0.26	13.76±0.36	51
Ethnicity				
Whites	3.17±0.20	6.69±0.28	13.58±0.39	51
Blacks	3.77±0.61	6.59±0.80	13.76±1.11	52
Hispanics	4.21±0.89	9.08±1.28	16.70±1.66	46
Men	5.74±0.35	11.90±0.49	23.83±0.64	50
White	5.49±0.37	11.69±0.53	23.44±0.69	50
Blacks	6.68±1.19	11.51±1.53	23.71±2.03	51
Hispanics	7.39±1.66	15.97±2.33	30.02±2.91	47
Women	1.06±0.15	2.16±0.21	4.57±0.30	53
Whites	1.03±0.16	2.11±0.23	4.52±0.33	53
Blacks	1.35±0.50	2.50±0.68	5.47±0.99	54
Hispanics	1.17±0.67	2.46±0.97	3.85±1.20	36

is necessary, and there is no requirement that they occur at about the same time. Therefore, a respondent can qualify for this diagnosis with one symptom during youth and one during middle years or old age. The occurrence at any time in the respondent's life of one symptom of pathological alcohol use and one of social or occupational impairment is sufficient for a DSM-III lifetime diagnosis of alcohol abuse. A minimum of one symptom of either of these along with some evidence of either tolerance or withdrawal is sufficient for a diagnosis of dependence. However, few of those given the diagnosis of alcoholism have only the minimum number of symptoms.

Almost 7% of the total sample both met lifetime criteria and had at least one alcohol symptom during the past year, and about 3% have had a symptom in the past month (Table 1). The 1-year: lifetime prevalence ratio (6.80/13.76) for the total sample is 0.49; i.e., half of those who have ever met DSM-III criteria for alcoholism have had an alcohol-related problem in the past year. Similarly, a quarter (24%) of the lifetime cases report a problem in the last 30 days; 48% with a problem in the past year have had one in the past month.

It is generally assumed that alcoholism is a chronic disorder; i.e., those who have had serious difficulties with alcohol at some point in their lives are likely to continue having them. However, those impressions about the chronicity and persistence of alcoholism are based largely on clinical samples—alcoholics who come to treatment for the disorder. Previous studies in the general population show turnover and recovery (Clark, 1976) consistent with our findings, suggesting that the disorder is not necessarily continuous. Even in samples drawn from treatment settings, alcoholism is known for remissions and relapse, "going on and off the wagon." At any one point in time, a large proportion of alcoholics can be expected to be sober. In our sample, 63% of those who met lifetime criteria for alcoholism and had been especially heavy consumers at some point in their lives (seven or more drinks daily for 2 weeks or more) told us that they had not had a period of drinking that heavily at any time in the past year.

There are few differences in rates between blacks and whites, either overall or by sex (Table 1). Blacks have only a slightly higher 1-month prevalence than whites, and rates

Table 2 Alcohol Abuse and/or Dependence: Site Differences (weighted to local population)

	Prevalence			Remission
	1 month (%±SE)	1 year (%±SE)	lifetime (%±SE)	lifetime—1 year lifetime (%)
New Haven	3.16±0.33	6.07±0.45	11.34±0.60	46
Baltimore	4.73±0.41	7.73±0.53	15.23±0.72	49
St. Louis	2.50±0.38	7.51±0.64	15.88±0.89	53
Durham	2.72±0.34	5.07±0.46	10.72±0.64	53
Los Angeles	3.71±0.38	6.98±0.51	14.96±0.72	53

for lifetime and 1-year prevalences are even more similar. (Recall that the "whites" category includes a few Orientals and American Indians. Since these ethnic groups other than blacks and Hispanics combined constitute only 2.5% of the total population, the category of "whites" is dominated by non-Hispanic caucasians.)

Lifetime, 1-year, and 1-month prevalence rates for Hispanic men are higher than for the other two ethnic groups, although not significantly so, while rates for Hispanic women are more similar to rates for other ethnic groups but generally lower. Thus, the sex differential for Hispanics is particularly great.

Remission rates (defined as the proportion of lifetime cases that have had no alcohol problems in the past year) are quite consistent across the sex and ethnic groups. They are nearly identical for men and women and for blacks and whites. Remission rates are lower for Hispanics, especially Hispanic women, but again the difference is not statistically significant.

There is a significant variation in the lifetime prevalence rates among the five study sites (Table 2). Baltimore, Maryland, St. Louis, Missouri, and Los Angeles, California, are similar to one another but have higher lifetime rates than New Haven, Connecticut, and Durham, North Carolina. This pattern also holds for 1-year prevalence, although Baltimore replaces St. Louis as the site having the highest rate. Remission rates at every site are in the range of 45–55%.

IV. PREVALENCE BY AGE, SEX, AND ETHNICITY

Lifetime prevalence rates are significantly higher among men and women under the age of 45 than among those older. For men, lifetime prevalence in the youngest age group (18–29 years) is 27%. This rises in those aged 30–44, but falls in those aged 45–64, and is lowest of all (14%) in those 65 years and older (Table 3). Among women, the highest prevalence rate (7%) is found in the youngest age group, and falls steadily to just over 1% in those 65 years and older. Possible reasons for this fall in lifetime prevalence with age include artifact of recall, low survival rates among alcoholics, and response style (as discussed in Chapter 2), but we cannot dismiss the possibility that this is a reflection of a true cohort effect; i.e., that alcoholism is more prevalent in younger generations of Americans. There has been a steady increase in per capita alcohol consumption in the United States since at least 1950 that has only begun to level off since 1981 (National Institute of Alcoholism and Alcohol Abuse, 1985), about the time the first ECA interviews were being conducted. In fact, in some areas, per capita alcohol consumption has almost doubled in the last 30 years (Wattis, 1983). Changes in societal drinking habits that might lead to increased rates of alcoholism are likely to affect younger adults more than older ones. As we will see below, alcoholism tends to

Table 3 Prevalence of Alcoholism by Age, Sex, and Ethnicity: Combined 5-Site ECA Data (weighted to national demograhic distribution)

	Men				Women				Male to Female Ratio		
	1 month (%±SE)	1 year (%±S)	lifetime (%±SE)	remission 1Y-LT/LT (%)	1 month (%±SE)	1 year (%±SE)	lifetime (%±SE)	remission 1Y-LT/LT (%)	1 month (M/F)	1 year (M/F)	lifetime (M/F)
Total	5.74±0.35	11.90±0.49	23.83±0.64	50	1.60±0.15	2.16±0.21	4.75±0.30	53	5.4	5.5	5.2
Age											
18–29	7.16±0.67	17.03±0.98	26.63±1.16	36	2.03±0.37	4.14±0.53	6.89±0.67	40	3.5	4.1	3.9
30–44	7.29±0.75	14.10±1.10	27.91±1.29	49	1.14±0.30	2.12±0.40	5.50±0.64	61	6.4	6.7	5.1
45–64	4.34±0.58	7.85±0.77	21.15±1.17	63	0.33±0.16	1.04±0.28	3.06±0.47	66	13.2	7.5	6.9
65+	1.93±0.58	3.10±0.73	13.52±1.45	77	0.40±0.22	0.46±0.24	1.49±0.43	69	4.8	6.7	9.1
Whites											
18–29	7.63±0.78	18.10±1.13	28.31±1.32	36	2.22±0.44	4.54±0.62	7.50±0.78	39	3.4	4.0	3.8
30–44	6.46±0.78	13.52±1.08	27.00±1.40	50	1.04±0.31	1.96±0.43	5.47±0.70	64	6.2	6.9	4.9
45–64	4.02±0.61	7.20±0.80	19.75±1.23	64	0.20±0.13	0.81±0.27	2.60±0.47	69	20.1	8.9	7.6
65+	1.74±0.59	2.85±0.75	12.53±1.49	77	0.42±0.24	0.47±0.25	1.46±0.45	68	4.1	6.1	8.6
Blacks											
18–29	4.03±1.53	7.92±2.11	12.61±2.59	37	1.11±0.77	2.37±1.12	4.19±1.48	44	3.6	3.3	3.0
30–44	11.04±2.80	16.30±3.30	31.33±4.15	48	2.08±1.18	3.37±1.49	6.88±2.09	51	5.3	4.8	4.6
45–64	8.17±2.68	15.24±3.52	32.99±4.61	54	1.34±1.01	2.56±1.39	7.33±2.99	65	6.1	6.0	4.5
65+	0.82±1.36	2.93±2.55	21.63±6.21	86	0.34±0.72	0.60±0.96	2.20±1.82	73	2.4	4.9	9.8
Hispanics											
18–29	6.06±2.30	19.29±3.81	29.76±4.41	35	1.90±1.38	3.59±1.87	4.90±2.17	27	3.2	5.4	6.1
30–44	12.24±3.86	19.16±4.63	35.91±5.65	47	0.97±1.10	1.84±1.51	3.67±2.11	50	12.6	10.4	9.8
45–64	3.86±2.65	7.69±3.67	25.97±6.03	70	0.81±1.20	2.65±2.15	3.46±2.44	23	4.8	2.9	7.5
65+	5.47±5.79	6.57±6.31	18.10±9.81	64	0.00	—	0.79±1.88	100	—	—	22.9

have a youthful onset. Older persons were already beyond the major period of risk when recent changes in societal drinking patterns occurred.

Ethnic groups show strikingly different patterns of age-related lifetime rates of alcoholism (Table 3 and Fig. 1). First, we contrast blacks and whites. Among the youngest men (aged 18–29), the lifetime prevalence rate of alcoholism in whites is over twice what it is in blacks. In the next age group, the rates are more similar, with a slight predominance in blacks. The black predominance in men becomes greater in men aged 45–64, and in the oldest group (65 and over), the rates of black to white rates are the reverse of what they were among the youngest group; i.e., nearly twice as high in blacks compared to whites. The pattern for black and white women is similar to that for men.

In the two younger age groups, lifetime prevalence rates are higher for Hispanic men than for either black or white men, and Hispanics are intermediate in the older two groups. Hispanic men's rates exceed white men's in every age group, whereas Hispanic women exceed whites only in the 45–64 age group. Rates for elderly Hispanic women are the lowest found for any ethnic age group; less than 1%. None of these differences is statistically significant.

One-year prevalence rates are highest in the youngest ages and fall in each successive older group (Table 3). Further, at each successive age group, the current rates are a smaller proportion of the lifetime rates. Thus, not only have older persons had less alcoholism, but older alcoholics less often have recent problems. This is demonstrated by the remission rates, which rise consistently with age. The high rate of remission in the elderly is particularly notable in blacks. While elderly black men have rates of lifetime alcoholism almost double that in elderly whites, their 1-year prevalence rates are about the same, and their 1-month rate is less than half of that in whites. Only 14% of blacks aged 65 and older who have a lifetime diagnosis of alcoholism have had any problems in the last year, and less than 4%

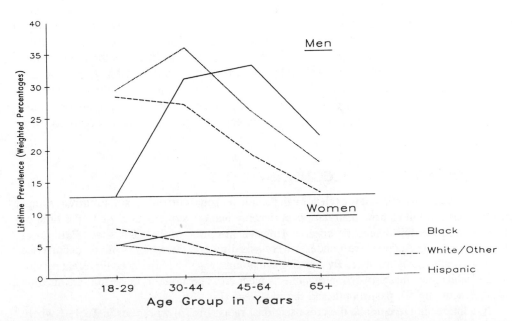

Figure 1 Alcohol abuse and/or dependence Prevalence by age, sex, and ethnicity. (combined 5-site ECA data adjusted to adult U.S. population).

in the last month. The corresponding figures for elderly whites are 23% in the last year and 14% in the last month.

While alcoholism is obviously a disorder predominant among males, there is evidence of convergence in the rates between sexes in the younger age groups. With only one exception, the male to female ratios in Table 3 are lowest in the 18- to 29-year-olds for all prevalence periods and ethnic groups. Thus, alcoholism has become more prevalent in younger age groups for both men and women, but the increase is particularly great for young women.

V. SUBTYPES OF ALCOHOLISM

According to DSM-III, an individual can simultaneously meet DSM-III criteria for alcohol abuse and dependence. Of the total ECA sample, 1.6% met criteria for alcohol dependence but not abuse; 5.8% for abuse but not dependence, and 6.4% met criteria for both abuse and dependence. We will group together those who met criteria for dependence, with and without abuse in addition, transforming alcohol abuse into a residual category as it is in DSM-III-R. Alcoholism, as we use the term here, is the sum of the abuse only and dependence (with or without abuse) subgroups (columns 1 + 4, Table 4).

For the entire sample, the lifetime prevalence of total alcoholism is 13.8%, and 7.9% have been dependent. The proportion of alcoholics who have been dependent rises with age (Table 4). Among men, 46% of those in the youngest age group met criteria for dependence; this rises steadily to 82% in those aged 65 and over. Among women, this rise is from 51% in the youngest group to 76% in the oldest. The increase with age in the proportion of alcoholics who have been dependent is consistent across ethnic groups. This indicates either that the relatively few older persons who have warranted a diagnosis of alcoholism are more likely than younger persons to have had the more serious form of the disorder, or perhaps this low rate is partly explained by poor recall for the less serious form that did not progress to dependency.

As we might expect, the symptom level for abusers (without dependence) is much lower than for those dependent, though criteria for either disorder requires only two symptoms. There is a wide range of severity, as measured by the number of reported lifetime symptoms, among those meeting criteria for either alcohol abuse or dependence (Fig. 2). However, among those with abuse only, the modal number of lifetime symptoms is the minimum of 2, and the mean number of symptoms is only 3.3. Among those diagnosed as alcohol dependent, the mode is 6, and the mean is 6.4. Despite their lower number of lifetime symptoms, abusers are slightly *more* likely than those dependent to have experienced a symptom in the past year (54 vs 47%), showing that abuse is an early (or perhaps easily forgotten) form of the disorder.

VI. CROSS-SECTIONAL ALCOHOLISM RATES

Since our measure of current prevalence can include persons with only a single current symptom, it does not tell us how many are experiencing enough symptoms close to the time of interview to meet full diagnostic criteria. However, in three of the ECA sites—Baltimore, Durham, and Los Angeles—respondents were asked to date the recency of last occurrence of every symptom they reported. By counting symptoms present within a specific recent period, we can determine what proportion of subjects meet cross-sectional criteria for various time frames, including the past month and the past year (Fig. 3).

It is interesting to contrast the cross-sectional rates (Fig. 3) with rates in Table 1 where "current" prevalence requires the presence of only a single symptom. The latter are greater, but not strikingly so. One-month prevalence for the total sample is 3.29% versus 2.17%

Table 4 Prevalences of Alcohol Abuse and/or Dependence (weighted to national demographic distribution)

	Men					Women				
	Abuse only (% ± SE)	Dependence only (% ± SE)	Abuse plus dependence (% ± SE)	Dependence with/without abuse (% ± SE)	Proportion of all alcoholics who have been dependent (%)	Abuse only (% ± SE)	Dependence only (% ± SE)	Abuse plus dependence (% ± SE)	Dependence with/without abuse (% ± SE)	Proportion of all alcoholics who have been dependent (%)
Total	10.30±0.46	2.69±0.24	10.84±0.47	13.53±0.51	57	1.76±0.19	0.51±0.10	2.31±0.22	2.82±0.24	62
Age										
18–29	14.41±0.92	2.16±0.38	10.05±0.79	12.21±0.86	46	3.35±0.47	0.41±0.17	3.12±0.46	3.53±0.49	51
30–44	13.27±0.97	2.82±0.48	11.82±0.93	14.64±1.02	52	1.73±0.36	0.67±0.23	3.09±0.48	3.76±0.53	68
45–64	6.03±0.68	2.87±0.48	12.25±0.94	15.12±1.03	72	0.90±0.26	0.47±0.19	1.69±0.35	2.16±0.40	70
65+	2.43±0.65	3.42±0.77	7.66±1.13	11.09±1.33	82	0.36±0.21	0.48±0.24	0.66±0.29	1.14±0.37	76
Whites										
18–29	15.66±1.06	2.09±0.42	10.56±0.90	12.65±0.97	45	3.76±0.56	0.31±0.16	3.43±0.54	3.74±0.56	50
30–44	14.10±1.10	2.76±0.52	10.13±0.95	12.90±1.06	48	1.76±0.41	0.63±0.24	3.08±0.53	3.71±0.58	68
45–64	5.61±0.71	2.56±0.49	11.58±0.99	14.14±1.08	72	0.73±0.25	0.38±0.18	1.49±0.36	1.87±0.40	72
65+	2.18±0.66	3.01±0.77	7.34±1.17	10.35±1.37	83	0.38±0.23	0.47±0.26	0.61±0.29	1.08±0.39	74
Blacks										
18–29	5.33±1.75	2.05±1.10	5.23±1.74	7.28±2.03	58	1.19±0.80	0.75±0.63	2.25±1.09	3.00±1.26	72
30–44	8.64±2.51	3.33±1.60	19.37±3.53	22.69±3.75	72	1.92±1.13	1.41±0.97	3.55±1.53	4.96±1.79	72
45–64	9.09±2.82	5.75±2.28	18.16±3.78	23.91±4.18	72	2.37±1.33	1.26±0.98	3.70±1.66	4.96±1.91	68
65+	3.85±2.90	5.24±3.36	12.54±5.00	17.78±5.77	82	0.19±0.54	0.71±1.04	1.30±1.41	2.01±1.74	91
Hispanics										
18–29	15.73±3.51	3.52±1.78	10.51±2.96	14.03±3.35	47	3.14±1.75	1.04±1.02	0.72±0.85	1.76±1.32	36
30–44	11.05±3.69	3.04±2.02	21.81±4.86	24.86±5.09	69	1.27±1.26	0.04±0.22	2.36±1.70	2.39±1.71	65
45–64	8.58±3.85	1.80±1.83	15.59±4.99	17.39±5.22	70	1.31±1.52	0.66±1.08	1.50±1.62	2.15±1.94	62
65+	7.28±6.62	3.90±4.94	6.92±6.47	10.83±7.92	60	0.11±0.71	0.00 —	0.68±1.74	0.68±1.74	86

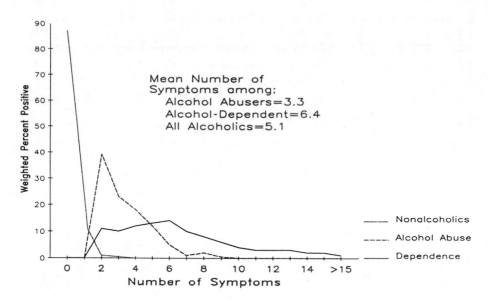

Figure 2   Number of alcoholic symptoms in alcoholics and nonalcoholics (combined 5-site ECA data weighted to national demographic distribution).

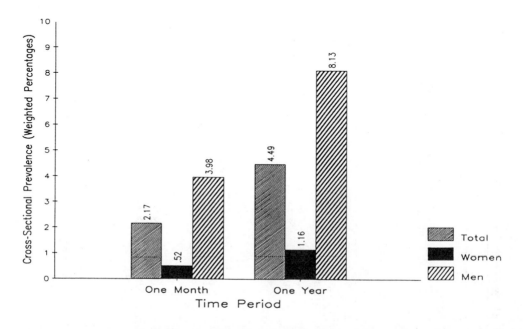

Figure 3   Cross-sectional prevalence of alcohol abuse and/or dependence (data from 3 ECA sites—Baltimore, Durham, Los Angeles, weighted to national demographic distribution).

for the 1-month cross-sectional diagnosis, and the comparable 1-year figures are 6.80% compared to 4.49% for the cross-sectional diagnosis. By either estimate, alcoholism is a major problem, with 4.5–7.0% of the population being actively symptomatic in the past year, and 2–3% in the past month. The sex ratio heavily favors males for both 1-month (7.7) and 1-year (7.0) cross-sectional findings.

VII. DRINKING PATTERNS

So far, we have been looking only at DSM-III–defined alcohol disorders. But substance use is unique among the psychiatric disorders in that substance exposure is a prerequisite for illness development. Since differences in exposure will affect the frequency of disorder, it is interesting to examine alcohol consumption patterns by ECA site (Fig. 4). The first category is those who have never taken a drink of alcohol; i.e. lifelong abstention. Next are social drinkers, those who do not deny drinking but do deny both heavy consumption and all of the alcohol-related problems we asked about. Heavy/problem drinkers are those who report consumption of seven or more drinks at least 1 evening a week for several months (or daily for 2 or more weeks) and/or one or more lifetime drinking problems, but fail to meet DSM-III criteria for alcohol abuse or dependence. It is clear that the vast majority of people included in this survey have consumed alcohol in their lives; only 10% of the aggregate ECA sample are classified as life-long abstainers.

More than two-thirds of those who have been exposed to alcohol are social drinkers, while one out of six have enough problems to be considered alcoholic. But these rates vary by ECA site. New Haven and Durham, which have the lowest lifetime prevalence rates of alcoholism, also have the lowest rates of heavy/problem drinking; apart from this similarity, however, the drinking patterns in these two sites differ. New Haven has the lowest rate of abstinence, and the highest rate of social drinking. For Durham, a more rural region lying

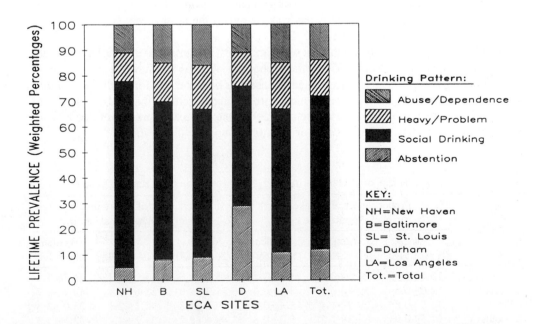

Figure 4 Lifetime drinking patterns by ECA site (site data weighted to local population; total weighted to national demographic distribution).

in the Bible Belt, the opposite is the case. Here, nearly a third (28%) of the population abstains from alcohol, and a correspondingly smaller proportion drinks socially.

We can calculate the lifetime prevalence rate of abuse and/or dependence among those who are at risk for alcoholism because they have at least tried an alcoholic drink. Lifetime prevalence of alcoholism among drinkers is highest in St. Louis and lowest in New Haven (Table 5). Durham is near the average. This challenges a long-held theory; i.e., that within environments that are relatively abstinent, those who do drink are more likely to be alcoholic.

Lifetime prevalence of alcoholism among all drinkers is 15.4% compared to 13.8% in the total population, including abstainers. Removing abstainers from the denominator has a greater impact on female than male prevalences, since more women (15.4%) are abstainers than men (4.8%). Overall, the lifetime prevalence of alcoholism among female drinkers is 5.4% compared to 4.6% for all women, still far below the male rate. Thus, women's lower rate is only trivially explained by their having a disproportionate number of abstainers.

One of the theories about the male predominance among alcoholics is that many women drinkers are never exposed to enough alcohol to be at risk, either because of social custom or because women more often than men have negative physiological reactions after drinking small amounts. If this is the case, then women's advantage should disappear when only heavy drinkers are considered. Across the five sites, there were over 3700 men who were heavy drinkers and about 1300 women. Among heavy drinkers, the alcoholism prevalence rate for men is 53% and for women 35% (Table 5). The male/female prevalence ratio drops to 1.5:1.0 as compared to 5:1 in the total population. Thus, it is clear that heavy-drinking women are much like their male counterparts in their rate of alcoholism. This would seem to support the idea that social and biological factors influencing exposure to alcohol are important contributors to the sex differential in rates.

VIII. AGE OF RISK

The ECA defined the age of onset of alcohol-associated disorders as the age at which the first symptom was experienced, and recency as the age of the most recent symptom. Duration is the period between these two.

Alcoholism is a disorder of youthful onset. Almost 40% of those who ever had the disorder had a symptom between 15 and 19, and the proportion of cases that have begun by age 30 is more than 80% (Fig. 5). Furthermore, early onset has been the rule for all the generations alive in the 1980s (Fig. 6). (For the youngest group, not yet out of their 20s, onset is, of course, entirely before 30, and mostly before 25.) However, there continues to be a small but measurable incidence of new cases of alcoholism up into the 1970s.

Table 5 Lifetime Prevalence of Alcoholism Among All Drinkers and All Heavy Drinkers

	Proportion of all drinkers who are alcoholic			Proportion of heavy/problem drinkers who are alcoholic		
	Total (N=16,518)	Men (N=7,821)	Women (N=8,697)	Total (N=5,087)	Men (N=3,719)	Women (N=1,368)
Total	15.4±0.4	25.1±0.7	5.4±0.4	48.5±1.0	53.0±1.1	34.7±1.9
New Haven	12.0±0.6	19.4±0.1	5.1±0.6	51.3±2.0	55.6±2.4	40.4±3.7
Baltimore	16.5±0.8	29.0±1.4	5.4±0.6	49.8±1.8	55.8±2.1	33.0±3.3
St. Louis	17.5±0.9	30.3±1.7	5.0±0.8	49.4±2.2	54.2±2.4	32.5±4.3
Durham	15.1±0.9	23.4±1.4	4.8±0.8	45.3±2.1	49.5±2.4	30.0±4.2
Los Angeles	16.8±0.8	25.6±1.3	7.1±0.8	46.7±1.8	50.3±2.1	36.2±3.4

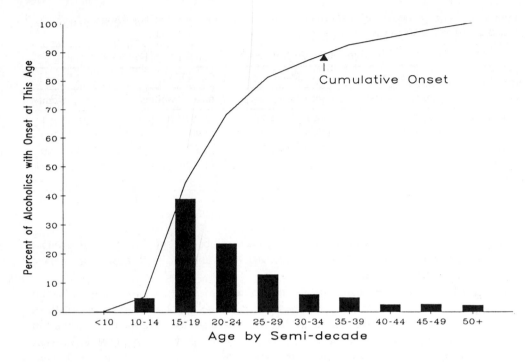

Figure 5 Age of onset of first alcoholic symptoms among those with alcoholism. (weighted to national demographic distribution).

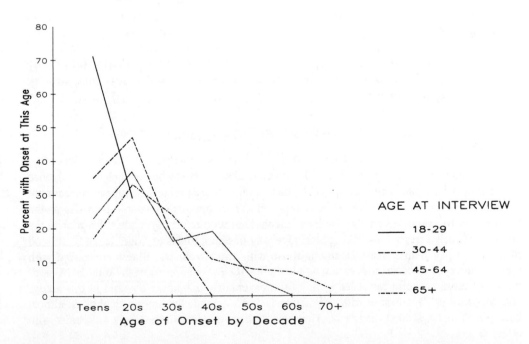

Figure 6 Age of onset of alcoholism by age group at interview. (weighted to national demographic distribution).

Table 6 Cumulative Rates (/100) of Alcoholism by Age of Onset, Sex, and Age Group at Interview: Combined 5-Site ECA Data (weighted to national demographic distribution)

Age of onset	Cumulative proportion (%) of indicated age/sex group							
	18–29		30–44		45–64		65+	
	men	women	men	women	men	women	men	women
< 18 years	12.2	3.0	6.4	0.7	2.8	0.1	1.0	0.1
18–29	26.6	6.9	23.6	3.7	13.6	1.1	6.8	0.5
30–44			27.9	5.5	18.5	2.2	10.8	1.0
45–64					21.1	3.1	13.3	1.4
65+							13.5	1.5

Among men, at least half of all onsets have occurred before age 30 for all age groups; among women, this is true only for those under age 45 (Table 6). At all ages, women have a later age of onset than men.

Having found that alcoholism typically begins early and that the probability of having had a symptom in the current year decreases with age, we might surmise that alcoholism has a natural history of a fixed duration. Of course, we can estimate its duration only in persons no longer actively alcoholic. It is clear from clinical studies that even a full year without alcohol problems is no guarantee that remission will continue indefinitely (Vaillant, 1983). Nonetheless, we will require only 1 year free of symptoms when we examine duration so as to make our definition of remission consistent with that used for the other disorders discussed in this volume; as a result, we may be including some cases who will in fact relapse later. Most (54%) remitted cases give dates for their first and last symptoms less than 5 years apart, suggesting a short duration of the disorder. In almost three-quarters, the estimated duration is less than 11 years (Fig. 7). These results are very different from those seen in patients who frequently come to treatment for the first time only after many years of alcohol problems. Our findings may help to explain why so few persons with alcohol problems in the general population seek care. Many appear to be able to reduce their drinking sufficiently to terminate their difficulties quite early in the course of their disorder. It is those who try and fail who appear for treatment.

IX. ALCOHOLISM AND OTHER PSYCHIATRIC DISORDERS

There is evidence from clinical samples that alcoholism and other psychiatric disorders often occur together, but what is difficult to tell from clinical samples is whether such co-occurrence might simply be a sampling bias. It may be that alcoholics are unlikely to appear in treatment settings unless some other disorder is also present. This population sample provides us the opportunity to examine the comorbidity of alcoholism with other psychiatric disorder in the absence of such a treatment-seeking bias. One way of doing this is to examine the likelihood of a second psychiatric disorder among those with any psychiatric illness contrasted with the likelihood of a second illness among alcoholics. One-third (35%) of the total ECA sample met lifetime criteria for at least one of the psychiatric diagnoses covered in this study, and one-third (32%) of those with one diagnosis had a second. But among alcoholics, almost half (47%) had a second diagnosis. Thus, alcoholism is particularly likely to coexist with other diagnoses.

Much of this comorbidity is accounted for by drug abuse and dependence. Among those who do not meet lifetime criteria for alcohol abuse or dependence, 3.8% have a positive drug

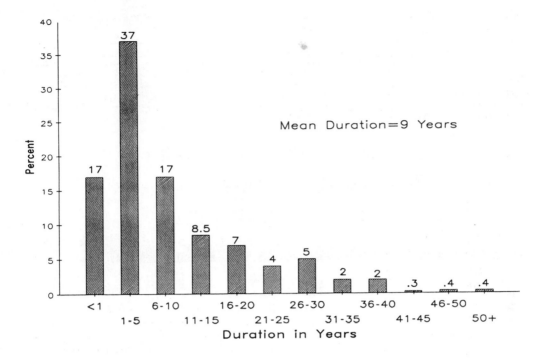

Figure 7 Duration of alcoholism among those in remission twelve months or more (weighted to national demographic distribution).

diagnosis, and for two-thirds, this is only abuse of cannabis (marijuana and its derivatives). Among those with alcohol abuse or dependence, the likelihood of a drug diagnosis is much greater (22%) and abuse is limited to cannabis for only half of those affected.

Conversely, among those using only cannabis, the lifetime prevalence rate of alcoholism is about one-third (36%) (Fig. 8). Among users of harder drugs, the alcoholism rate is much higher, ranging from a low of 62% in users of stimulants to a dramatic high of 84% in cocaine users. In this general population sample, alcoholism occurs in a majority of those using "hard" drugs.

Other diagnoses with which alcoholism is highly associated are antisocial personality, mania, and schizophrenia (Table 7). Antisocial personality is even more strongly associated with alcoholism than is drug abuse. This is consistent for every age group, and at all five of the ECA sites. The diagnosis most often reported in the clinical literature among alcoholics is depression (Hesselbrock et al., 1985), a diagnosis only moderately elevated among alcoholics in this general population. However, our findings are not inconsistent with the clinical experience. It seems likely that the occurrence of depression motivates alcoholics to seek treatment more often than do drug abuse or antisocial personality, diagnoses with low rates of treatment. Mania and schizophrenia have high rates of treatment, but since these disorders are so infrequent compared with depression, chance alone dictates that alcoholics are more likely to show depression than either mania or schizophrenia.

Comorbidity of alcoholism with other disorders is more common in women than men. While 44% of the male alcoholics have a second diagnosis, 65% of the female alcoholics do. This higher rate is in part because women are more likely than men to have the common diagnoses of depression and phobia. But the more important reason seems to be the fact that alcoholism is so much more deviant in women than men, as indicated by a male/female

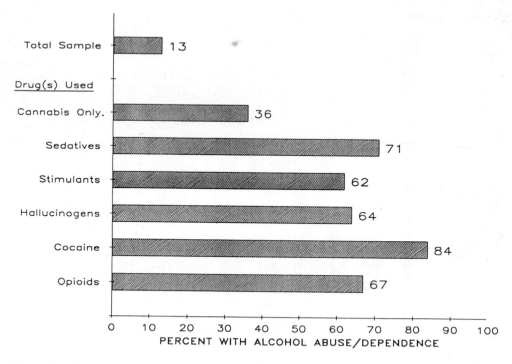

Figure 8 Lifetime prevalence of alcohol abuse/dependence among users of specific drugs.

prevalence ratio of over 5 (see Table 3). For every disorder except cognitive impairment, which is not elevated in alcoholics of either sex, comorbidity rates are higher for female than male alcoholics. Nonetheless, female and male alcoholics have the highest comorbidity ratios with the same diagnoses: antisocial personality, drug abuse, mania, and schizophrenia.

A. Which Comes First

When two disorders are associatd, the one that occurs first might be a risk factor for the other. Overall, alcoholism precedes the onset of depression in the majority of cases (78%). However, among women, depression is usually antecedent (66%). (We dropped from these analyses alcoholics with diagnoses of antisocial personality disorder, drug abuse/dependence, or schizophrenia, since these disorders are themselves associated with depression and alcoholism, and might have explained the relationship between depression and alcoholism.) In both sexes, alcoholism is slightly less severe when depression is the antecedent diagnosis.

By definition, antisocial personality has its onset before age 15. Therefore, it necessarily virtually always precedes alcoholism. However, it has the effect of lowering the age of onset of alcoholism. Consistent with findings in clinical samples that antisocial alcoholics have exceptionally early onsets, the mean age of onset for antisocial alcoholics is only 20 versus 24 in alcoholics without antisocial personality. Antisocial alcoholics also have a higher lifetime alcohol symptom count and a longer duration of alcoholism. In fact, the severity (based on symptom counts) of the two disorders is positively related, with a correlation of 0.37 for women and 0.57 for men. The association of these two disorders is stronger in older respondents than in younger ones. This suggests that in the past alcoholism was closely associated with other forms of social deviance, but that as alcoholism has become more prevalent, less antisocial portions of the population have been affected by it.

Table 7 Comorbidity of Alcoholism and Other Psychiatric Disorders (weighted to national demographic distribution)

Psychiatric Diagnosis	Risk ratios (prevalence in alcoholics divided by prevalence in nonalcoholics)		
	total	men	women
Antisocial personality	19.6	12.0	29.6
Mania	5.4	6.5	9.3
Drug abuse/dependence	5.7	4.8	8.8
Schizophrenia	3.4	4.6	5.6
Panic disorder	2.6	4.2	4.4
Obsessive compulsive	2.0	3.0	2.1
Dysthymia	1.7	2.5	2.2
Major depression	1.6	2.4	2.7
Phobic disorders	1.4	1.8	2.1
Cognitive impairment	1.1	1.2	0.7
Any core diagnosis	2.0	2.4	2.2

X. OTHER ASSOCIATED FACTORS

A. Education

Overall, there is a downward trend in lifetime prevalence with higher levels of education (Fig. 9). What is more interesting is the sawtooth shape of this curve. Regardless of final level of attainment, those who finish an educational program and go no farther have lower rates of alcoholism than those who begin the next higher level but drop out. Thus, those with an eighth grade education have lower rates of alcoholism not only than those with less education, but also lower rates than those who begin but drop out of high school or college. (We include as high school dropouts those whose highest degree is the graduate equivalency [GED], available to dropouts who later pass an equivalency test.) Similarly, high school graduates who do not enter college have a lower prevalence of alcoholism than those who begin but do not complete college as well as lower than high school dropouts. College graduates have the lowest prevalence, but it is only slightly lower than that of eighth grade graduates who never entered high school.

Age is a confounding factor because young people have had more years of schooling than older people. For example, many of those with only an eighth grade education are older people who went as far in school as they were expected to at the time they were growing up, and, as we have shown, older people have a low lifetime prevalence of alcoholism. Looking at specific age groups disrupts the consistency of the relationship between alcoholism and education only for the youngest age group, many of whom have not yet completed their education. The pattern shown in Figure 9 is quite consistent for every other age group, with one exception: For those 65 and older, prevalence of alcoholism is as low among those with some college education as it is in college graduates, but relatively few in this age group have attended college, let alone graduated.

B. Marital Status

Marital history is distinctly related to lifetime prevalence of alcohol abuse and/or dependence (Fig. 10). Those with a stable marriage have the lowest lifetime prevalence (9%), the never married who have not cohabited for a year or more are next, then less stable marriages,

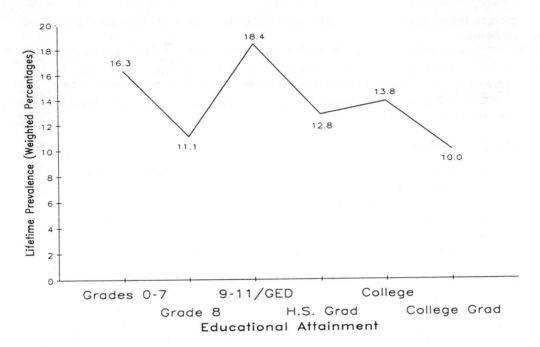

Figure 9 Lifetime prevalence of alcoholism by educational attainment (weighted to national demographic distribution).

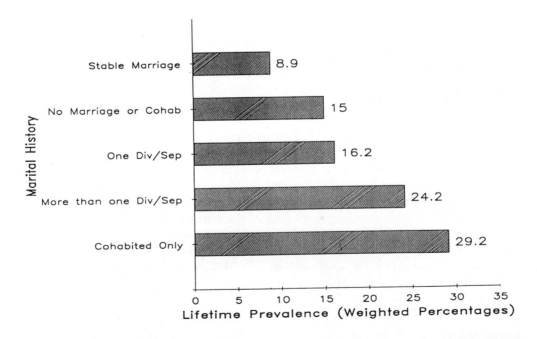

Figure 10 Lifetime prevalence of alcoholism by marital history (weighted to national demographic distribution)

and finally highest rates (nearly 30%) occur among those who have cohabited without ever marrying.

Current marital status (as opposed to marital history) shows similar results with a 1-year alcoholism prevalence among those who have never been married of 9.7%. This falls between that of the currently married (4.2%) and currently separated or divorced (9.9%), but is closer to the latter. Those currently widowed, a group largely made up of older women, have the lowest prevalences (2.3%).

C. Occupation

The lowest 1-year rates of alcoholism are found among professionals and managers and the highest rates among laborers (Fig. 11). The higher rate in skilled compared with unskilled laborers is due only to the fact that women are particularly uncommon among skilled workers. Alcoholism is inversely related to occupational status for men (Table 8). Results are less consistent for women, perhaps because their status depends as much on their spouse's as their own occupation.

D. Underemployment

We asked about employment status both as of the time of interview and over the last 5 years. Those currently unemployed may be either temporarily out of work or out of the work force because they are students, housewives, retired, or incapacitated. Their current status may be long lived or brief. Because of those problems, we will use a measure we have labeled "underemployment," defined as a total of 6 months or more out of the 5 years prior to interview when expected to work, i.e., excluding periods when one was not in the work force for the reason listed above. About 13% of the total sample met this definition, with under-

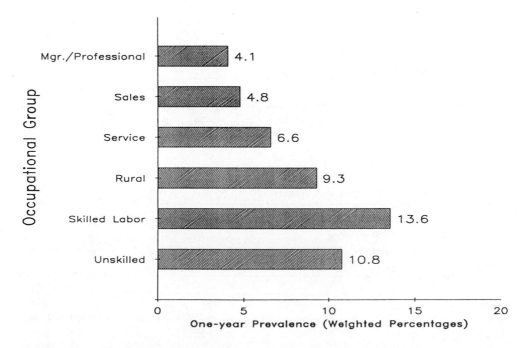

Figure 11 One-year prevalence of alcoholism by type of occupation at time of interview (weighted to National Demographic Distribution).

Table 8 Occupation and Alcoholism (weighted to national demographic distribution)

Occupation at time of interview	Current (1 year) prevalence	
	men (% ±SE)	women (% ±SE)
Unskilled labor	13.92±1.46	2.76±1.12
Skilled labor	14.79±1.47	0.93±1.31
Farm/rural	10.57±3.89	0.00 —
Service occupations	10.35±2.03	3.35±1.12
Sales/support	9.15±1.19	1.86±0.46
Management/professional	5.97±0.81	1.16±0.46

employment twice as common in blacks as whites (Table 9). The underemployed have a 1-year prevalence of alcoholism of 12% compared to only 5% among those not underemployed. Although the rate of underemployment is highest in blacks, the difference in alcoholism prevalence between the underemployed and others is lower than in other ethnic groups, indicating that most black unemployment has other explanations.

E. Income

The higher the current income in those holding full-time jobs at the time of interview, the lower the 1-year prevalence of alcoholism (Table 11). In other words, there are fewer current alcoholics among the well paid. The only exception is among women earning more than $50,000, a very small group, as reflected by their high standard error.

   This negative association of alcoholism and income holds for all age groups. It is weakest in the youngest group, where recent entry into the labor market means low incomes generally, but even among the young there is a significant negative correlation (-0.21). For all the other age groups this correlation is a startling -0.80 or better.

F. Household Size

The modal household size was two persons, and 32% of households fell into this category. Household size was not associated with the prevalence of alcoholism—those from small households were no more or less likely to be alcoholic than those from large ones.

Table 9 Employment Status and Prevalence of Alcoholism: Data from 3 ECA Sites (weighted to national demographic distribution)

Ethnicity	Proportion underemployed (%)	Current (1 year) prevalence	
		underemployed (% ±SE)	not underemployed[a] (% ±SE)
		(N=1673)	(N=8458)
Whites	12	12.03±1.55	4.85±0.38
Blacks	23	6.71±2.45	4.15±1.08
Hispanics	18	16.80±5.72	5.88±1.67
Total	13	11.52±1.31	4.80±0.35

[a]Includes students, retirees, and others not currently in the labor market.

Table 10 Alcoholism and Welfare Assistance (weighted to national demographic distribution)

		Men	
	receiving welfare assistance	current (1 year) alcohol prevalence	
Ethnicity	(%)	on assistance (N=981)	not on assistance (N=6935)
Blacks	17	15.93±4.40	9.33±1.56
Hispanics	13	10.32±5.57	15.04±2.52
Whites	8	12.56±1.96	10.10±0.53
		Women	
		(N=1726)	(N=9072)
Blacks	27	3.68±1.59	1.65±0.66
Hispanics	19	3.26±2.60	1.76±0.93
Whites	7	2.99±1.00	1.82±0.22

G. Rural-Urban Residence

Of the five ECA sites, only two, St. Louis and Durham, included rural areas. In the St. Louis site, 6% of the sample was drawn from two rural counties contiguous to the metropolitan area. In the Durham site, there were four rural counties contiguous to its much smaller central city. In St. Louis, the rural counties are virtually all white, whereas in Durham, they are approximately half black. Whether it is because of the discrepancy in the size of the central city, or whether rural residence has a different significance for blacks and whites, or for other reasons, the association between rural-urban residence and alcoholism differs in the two sites, and therefore will be presented separately. The 1-year prevalence of alcoholism is higher in urban dwellers in St. Louis and in rural dwellers in Durham, but neither difference is statistically significant. Since there are likely to be other demographic differences between urban and rural dwellers, we examined area of residence, controlling for age, race, and sex, showing the cross-site comparison for whites only in Table 12, and then blacks in Durham separately. (Numbers in age groups are low for the St. Louis rural sample, ranging from 12 to 28. Standard errors are correspondingly high.)

In St. Louis, the urban predominance mentioned above for the total sample holds for both sexes and for all age groups, with the exception of 30- to 44-year-old women (Table 12). Across all age groups, this difference is significant for men but not for women.

Among white men in the Durham sample, that urban predominance is not seen; in fact, there is a slightly (nonsignificant) higher rate in rural white males. Urban white women in the Durham sample are about twice as likely to have a lifetime diagnosis of alcoholism compared to female rural dwellers; thus their pattern is consistent with that of women in the St. Louis site. However, in neither site are the differences for women statistically significant.

For blacks in the Durham area, lifetime rates were higher for male rural dwellers ($p < 0.01$), whereas for women, they were nonsignificantly higher for the urban dwellers (Table 13). Blazer et al. (1987) also examined these differences and suggested a number of possible explanations, including consanguinity, extreme poverty, and "reverse drift" from urban to rural areas among established black male alcoholics.

Table 11 Current Annual Income and Prevalence of Alcoholism Among Those Fully Employed at Time of Interview (weighted to national demographic distribution)

Current annual income ($)	Lifetime prevalence		Current (1 year) prevalence	
	men (%±SE)	women (%±SE)	men (%±SE)	women (%±SE)
Less than 5,000	23.41±3.10	6.82±1.63	15.68±2.72	3.76±1.23
5,000– 9,999	31.86±2.76	4.62±0.90	18.90±2.35	2.03±0.63
10,000–14,999	23.89±1.94	6.11±1.09	11.59±1.49	2.62±0.73
15,000–19,999	23.38±1.90	6.03±1.55	9.22±1.32	0.82±0.59
20,000–24,999	19.49±1.91	4.86±2.05	6.10±1.17	1.10±0.99
25,000–34,999	18.74±1.97	4.40±2.17	9.56±1.50	0.94±1.03
35,000–49,999	12.77±2.50	3.17±2.93	5.28±1.68	0.00 —
50,000+	14.34±3.0	5.08±6.93	1.72±1.13	5.08±6.93
Rank order correlation (income group, lowest to highest, and prevalence rate)	−0.86	−0.59	−0.91	−0.10

H. The Institutional Sample

At each of the ECA sites, representative samples of those in long-term institutions were interviewed, either personally or by proxy when necessary. The institutional sample was then weighted so that they represented their true proportion in the community sampled at each site. Up to this point, we have been presenting household and institutional data together so that the sample is representative of the full community. As a group, institutionalized subjects have a higher 1-year prevalence of alcoholism than do household residents, but there is sharp

Table 12 Prevalence of Alcoholism by Urban vs Rural Residence (white, household dwellers only, weighted to local population)

	St. Louis		Durham	
	current (1 year) prevalence		current (1 year) prevalence	
	rural (N=159)	urban (N=1597)	rural (N=1148)	urban (N=1270)
Males Age				
18–29	14.64±7.30	20.29±3.17	13.47±4.68	11.60±2.71
30–44	10.65±9.13	17.87±3.20	8.21±3.35	7.18±2.25
45–64	0.00 —	7.03±2.03	10.05±3.62	6.60±2.23
65+	2.14±3.37	3.67±2.35	1.45±1.96	1.36±1.79
Totals	6.76±2.91	13.61±1.49	8.90±1.89	7.88±1.29
Females Age				
18–29	0.00 —	3.75±1.43	2.06±1.67	2.80±1.41
30–44	4.83±5.64	0.49±0.54	0.00 —	1.30±1.04
45–64	0.00 —	0.44±0.51	0.00 —	0.20±0.40
65+	0.00 —	0.82±0.85	0.00 —	0.00 —
Totals	0.94±1.12	1.45±0.48	0.48±0.39	1.25±0.52

Table 13 Prevalence of Alcoholism in Blacks: Durham vs Surrounding Rural Areas (black, household dwellers only, weighted to local population)

	Males			Females		
	current (1 year) prevalence			current (1 year) prevalence		
	rural (N=280)	urban (N=196)		rural (N=494)	urban (N=377)	
Age						
18–29	8.11±3.20	1.11±1.37		1.21±1.24	1.24±1.22	
30–44	13.47±4.67	8.00±4.67		0.30±0.69	0.75±1.11	
45–64	20.37±5.66	6.29±4.16		3.94±2.28	0.00 —	
65+	2.92±3.62	1.75±2.90		0.00 —	1.09±1.96	
Totals	12.12±2.32	3.99±1.62	<0.01	1.57±0.78	0.81±0.61	NS

variation depending on the type of institution (Fig. 12), with high rates among those in prison and mental hospitals, but rates even lower than the household population's in nursing homes and other chronic care settings that serve the elderly.

I. Treatment

Alcohol problems in the past year are highly associated with recent use of mental health services, about which we have self-report information for outpatient care in the past 6 months and inpatient care for the past year. One-year prevalence is almost twice as high among those who have had any outpatient mental health treatment in the past 6 months as among those who have not (10.4 vs 5.6%). This proportion more than quadruples to 26.8% among those who have had any inpatient mental health treatment in the past year.

We have also examined the relationship to treatment controlling for sex, since women are more likely to receive outpatient mental health services than men. (Men and women are equally likely to have received inpatient mental health care.) The association of alcoholism with treatment is found for both men and women.

The elevated rates of alcoholism found in persons who have received mental health treatment is not found among those receiving medical (non–mental health–related) outpatient care (5.9% for those with care vs 6.0% for those without). A different picture was seen for those who had been hospitalized. Unlike medical outpatients, the 1-year prevalence of alcoholism was significantly higher among those who had had a medical hospitalization in the past year (8.1%) than in those not recently hospitalized (5.6%). This confirms the impression that alcoholism is a frequent, and perhaps frequently undetected, disorder among general medical inpatients.

Our findings of a high rate of alcoholism among those receiving mental health treatment or medical hospitalization do not necessarily suggest that these patients were being seen for their alcoholism or for medical problems it caused. We did, however, ask about specific alcohol-related contact with the health care system by asking whether the respondent had ever told a physician about an alcohol problem. In the four sites where this question was asked, only 12% of those with alcoholism had talked to a doctor about a drinking problem. This rate was considerably higher for those with alcohol dependence (27%) than among those with abuse only (8%). Among those with neither diagnosis but at least one problem or heavy drinking, only 3% had discussed their drinking with a physician. This low frequency among those with no diagnosis suggests that the DSM-III diagnostic threshold for alcoholism misses few cases who see themselves as requiring medical services.

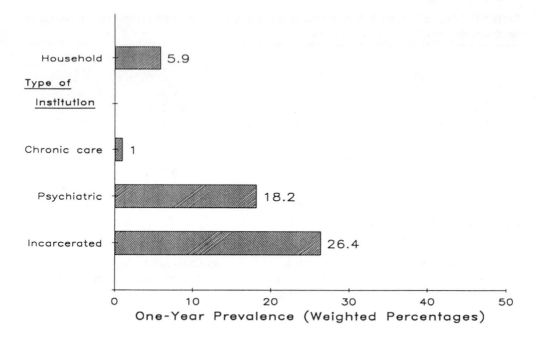

Figure 12 Prevalence of alcoholism by type of institutional residence. (weighted to national demographic distribution).

XI. CRITERIA AND SYMPTOMS OF ALCOHOL DISORDERS

The relative frequency of specific alcohol symptoms is highly consistent across the five ECA sites. If we arrange symptoms in order of frequency of occurrence in the total sample at each site, the rank order correlations between pairs of sites range from 0.71 to 0.97. In fact, the only correlations below 0.90 are with Yale, where a few of the symptoms used in other sites were not available. Despite differences in the prevalence rates of alcoholism among sites, the symptomatic expression of the disorder is highly consistent.

The DSM-III diagnosis of alcohol abuse requires evidence of pathological drinking plus impairment in social or occupational function due to alcohol. Each of the specific DSM-III symptoms for pathological drinking and impairment contributes to the diagnosis of alcoholism, as shown by the fact that each is more common in those with a diagnosis than in other drinkers (Table 14). Among both alcoholics and other drinkers, the most common symptom of a pathological pattern was drinking a fifth or more in 1 day. Objections by family members is the most common of the social and occupational impairment symptoms.

A diagnosis of dependence in DSM-III requires at least one symptom of a pathological pattern or social impairment plus evidence for either tolerance or withdrawal. In the DIS, tolerance was scored positive if the person drank heavily every day for 2 weeks or more. Withdrawal was positive if the person drank first thing on waking—presumably to treat withdawal symptoms—or reported any of the classic alcohol withdrawal symptoms when stopping or cutting down, including the shakes, seizures, delirium tremens (DTs), or hallucinations. Tolerance was more common than withdrawal symptoms, occurring in 7% of the total population.

As we noted earlier, while it is possible to have a diagnosis of either alcohol abuse or dependence with only two symptoms, persons with these diagnoses usually had many more

Table 14 Lifetime Prevalence Rates of Specific Alcohol Symptoms (weighted to national demographic distribution)

DIS item no.	Abbreviated question	Total sample	% ever experiencing this symptom among all who have ever had		
			any alcohol consumption (N=16,518)	alcohol abuse only (N=892)	alcohol dependence (with/without abuse) (N=1,738)
A. Pattern of pathological alcohol use					
152.	Drank fifth (or equivalent) in 1 day	14	15	72	74
166.	Blackouts	7	8	55	59
165B.	Alcohol binges or benders	4	4	12	39
157.	Wanted to stop but could not	4	4	9	25
158.	Set rules to control drinking	3	4	11	21
169.	Drank despite serious health problem	1	2	6	19
170.	Could not do daily work without alcohol	1	1	2	18
Proportion with at least one of these symptoms		17	19	100[a]	92
B. Impairment in social or occupational functioning due to alcohol					
150.	Family objects that respondent drinks too much	11	13	54	61
164.	Physical fights while drinking	10	12	50	46
162.	Trouble driving due to drinking	7	8	30	32
163.	Arrested for drinking	6	7	23	32
156.	Friends, doctor, clergyman, or other professionals said drinking too much	5	6	20	32
160.	Job or school troubles from drinking	2	3	4	20
161.	Lost job (or expelled) due to drinking	1	1	2	10
Proportion with at least one of these symptoms		19	21	100[a]	88
C. Symptoms of alcohol tolerance or withdrawal					
153.	Period of daily heavy drinking	7	8	0	80
167.	Any severe withdrawal symptoms (shakes, seizures, DTs, or hallucinations)	3	4	0	45
159.	Drinking before breakfast	3	4	0	33
Proportion with at least one of these symptoms		9	10	0[a]	100[a]

continued

Table 14 *Continued*

DIS item no.	Abbreviated question	Total sample	% ever experiencing this symptom among all who have ever had		
			any alcohol consumption (N = 16,518)	alcohol abuse only (N = 892)	alcohol dependence (with/without abuse) (N = 1,738)
D. Other (non–DSM-III) symptoms					
154.	Period of weekly heavy drinking	16	18	52	90
151.	Thought self excessive drinker	10	11	36	64
168.	Severe health problems (liver disease, vomiting blood, paresthesias, memory loss, or pancreatitis)	3	3	10	30
155.	Told doctor about drinking problem	3	4	8	27

[a]By definition.
Not ascertained: Nonbeverage alcohol

than the minimum. Symptoms that occurred in a majority of those diagnosed as having abuse included drinking a fifth in 1 day, having blackouts, suffering family complaints about their drinking, and being in fights they attributed to their drinking. Symptoms that occurred in most people diagnosed as dependent included all the symptoms common among abusers except for fighting. In addition, they were almost all tolerant to alcohol as indicated by daily heavy drinking. A very rare symptom, even among those with a positive diagnosis, was losing a job because of drinking. This was reported by 10% of the dependent and 7% of the abusers.

Alcohol symptoms generally require heavy drinking (Table 15). None of the alcohol symptoms occurred in as many as 10% of persons who did not meet our criteria for weekly heavy drinking. And daily heavy drinking was virtually required to meet criteria for withdrawal or tolerance.

Those who had had a period of daily heavy drinking (seven or more drinks per day) had elevated rates of every symptom, including binge drinking. In fact, about 70% of those who have had alcoholic binges had also drunk heavily on a daily basis. This calls into question the claim that there are two types of alcoholics: binge drinkers, who never drink steadily, and steady drinkers.

XII. CONCLUSIONS

Alcoholism is one of the most common lifetime psychiatric disorders in America. Over their lifetimes, nearly 14% of adults have met DSM-III criteria for lifetime abuse and/or dependence, and half of these had had at least one active symptom in the past year. There is variation in the prevalence by region, but even in the Durham area, it was a common disorder.

Men are about five times as likely as women to suffer from alcoholism. But the fact that the difference is least in the youngest age group suggests that women may be catching up.

Lifetime rates of alcoholism are higher in younger than in older respondents, suggesting that the illness rate has been increasing over time for both sexes, albeit more rapidly in women.

Table 15 Lifetime Prevalence Rates of DSM-III Alcohol Symptoms in Nonheavy vs Heavy Drinkers (weighted to national demographic distribution)

DIS item no.	Abbreviated question	% experiencing this symptom among		
		nonheavy drinkers (N=13,704)	weekly heavy drinkers only (N=1357)	daily heavy drinkers (N=1457)
A. Pattern of pathological alcohol use				
152.	Drank fifth (or equivalent) in 1 day	7	41	72
166.	Blackouts	2	27	53
165B.	Alcohol binges or benders	<0.5	8	37
157.	Wanted to stop but could not	1	6	23
158.	Set rules to control drinking	1	8	19
169.	Drank despite serious health problem	<0.5	3	19
170.	Could not do daily work without alcohol	<0.5	1	18
	Proportion with at least one symptom	9	56	85
B. Impairment in social or occupational functioning due to alcohol				
150.	Family objects that respondent drinks too much	7	31	54
164.	Physical fights while drinking	5	27	43
162.	Trouble driving due to drinking	3	18	29
163.	Arrested for drinking	2	15	29
156.	Friends, doctor, clergyman, or other professionals said drinking too much	2	14	42
160.	Job (or school) troubles from drinking	<0.5	4	19
161.	Lost job (or expelled) due to drinking	<0.5	1	79
	Proportion with at least one symptom	11	56	79
C. Symptoms of alcohol tolerance or withdrawal				
153.	Period of daily heavy drinking	—	—	100[a]
167.	Any severe withdrawal symptoms (shakes, seizures, DTs, or hallucinations)	1	8	34
159.	Drinking before breakfast	1	4	27
	Proportion with at least one symptom	1	10	100[a]
Proportions meeting DSM-III criteria for:				
	Abuse only	3.9	33	0
	Dependence with or without abuse	1.0	9.7	91

[a]By definition
Not ascertained: Nonbeverage alcohol

Obviously, the prevalence of a disorder depends on its definition, and some would argue that the DSM-III definitions are too inclusive. A diagnosis of either alcohol abuse or dependence can be made in the presence of only two symptoms, and even these need not have been present at the same time. Most of those with four or more symptoms meet criteria.

But one of the strengths of the DIS inverview is that it ascertains a symptom profile rather than terminating an inquiry once a diagnosis can be assigned or definitely excluded. Therefore, rather than simply wonder at the high rates of alcoholism with the DSM-III thresholds as defined, we can estimate what the rates would have been had the thresholds been different.

Figure 2 is informative here. About 40% of those defined as alcohol abusers had the minimum of two positive lifetime symptoms—the corollary is that the majority of abusers were above the minimum threshold and the mean number of lifetime symptoms was 3.3, more than one symptom above the minimum. Only 10% of those with a diagnosis of dependence had the minimum of two symptoms, and the mean number of lifetime symptoms in them was six and four-tenths. Thus, if the symptom threshold were raised by one, rates of alcohol abuse and/or dependence would fall but not dramatically, and the ratio of those dependent to those with abuse only would increase.

We examine the threshold issue in a slightly different way in Figure 13. Here we have plotted the number of positive alcohol symptoms for the total sample, and by sex, to see if there is a plateau in symptom frequency. Such a plateau might suggest a natural threshold for the diagnosis; i.e., a place to "carve nature at the joints," as Kendell has put it (1975). We have deleted from the illustration the data points for no symptoms. The minimum threshold for the diagnosis of alcoholism in DSM-III is two symptoms and the particular symptoms positive determine whether a case meets criteria and the subtype of alcoholism (abuse, dependence, or both). It is clear from the graph that for women there is a relative threshold at two symptoms; the downward slope of the curve tends to flatten at that point. For men and for the total sample there is an even more distinct change in the slope at three symptoms. This might suggest that the minimum threshold, at least for men, should be raised, or that there be a second diagnostic threshold at three symptoms. In fact, DSM-III-R now specifies a minimum of three symptoms for alcohol dependence, with fewer symptoms for the now residual alcohol abuse. Since DSM-III-R's criterion symptoms have been altered significantly from DSM-III's, it is difficult to judge from our data what impact the revision will have on the prevalence rates of alcoholism. But on the basis of the numbers of symptoms, there appears to be some justification for this change, at least for men. Additionally our findings suggest that a lower threshold for women might be appropriate.

Past debates about the definition of alcoholism have involved more than questions about the appropriate number of symptoms. Another issue has been the types of symptoms; i.e., whether the definition should be based on the personal and social consequences of drinking, as in DSM-III, versus a definition based on the quantity and frequency of alcohol intake. Since the DIS is based on DSM-III, it contains relatively few quantity/frequency questions, but it appears that with groups selected based on quantity and frequency would largely overlap with groups selected based on personal and social consequences. We found that 80% of those who meet criteria for alcohol dependence have been heavy drinkers on a daily basis (see Table 14). Conversely, 91% of daily heavy drinkers met the DSM-III criteria for alcohol dependence (see Table 15).

While alcoholism is approximately equally common in the three ethnic groups studied, there is an increase in the black/white ratio of lifetime prevalence with increasing age. This suggests that at least some of the fall in lifetime prevalence with age observed in the total sample is due to a true cohort effect because if it were entirely a failure of recall in older cohorts, we would have to assume blacks have enormously better recall than whites. Second, it suggests that whites have contributed more than blacks to the increase in per capita alcohol consumption that has been seen in this country for the past 2 decades.

This increase in per capita consumption coupled with the finding reported here of a higher lifetime prevalence of alcoholism in younger groups is cause for considerable concern. However, other findings mitigate this concern. First, per capita consumption appears to be tapering off since about 1980 (National Institute of Alcoholism and Alcohol Abuse, 1985). Second, we have shown that a lower proportion of the younger alcoholics are dependent (see Table 4). Presumably this is at least partialy because they have had fewer years in which to become dependent, but coupled with this is the fact that the association between alcoholism

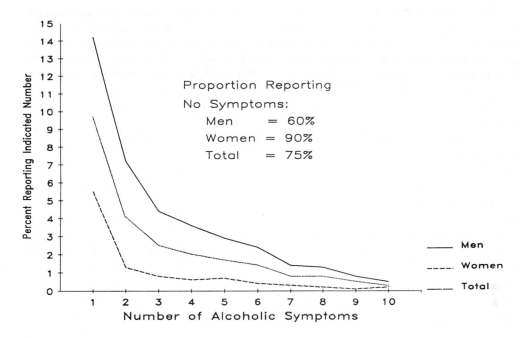

Figure 13 Distribution of positive alcoholic symptoms among those with any. (weighted to national demographic distribution).

and antisocial personality disorder is not as strong in younger drinkers. Only further follow-up will tell us if alcoholism in the younger age groups is indeed less virulent, but these findings give us some hope that is the case.

Certainly, self-recognition of excessive drinking appears to be prominent. In fact, for dependent drinkers such self-recognition is slightly more prevalent than objections by family members (see Table 14). Many alcoholics recognize that they are consuming more than they should, even if they often seem reluctant to admit it in the context of a treatment setting. Perhaps we can make increasing use of this self-recognition to design even better treatments so as to reduce what is one of the most prevalent psychiatric disorders in America.

REFERENCES

American Psychiatric Association (1980). *Diagnostic and Statistical Manual of Mental Disorder*, 3rd ed. (DSM-III). American Psychiatry Association, Washington, D.C.

American Psychiatric Association (1987). *Diagnostic and Statistical Manual of Mental Disorders*, 3rd ed., Revised (DSM-IIIR). American Psychiatric Association, Washington, D.C.

Blazer, D., Crowell, B.A., and George, L.K. (1987). Alcohol abuse and dependence in the rural south. *Arch. Gen. Psychiatry 44*:736–747.

Clark, W.B., and Cahalan, D. (1976). Changes in problem drinking over a four-year span. *Addict. Behav. 1*:251–259.

Davies, D.L. (1976). Definition issues in alcoholism, *Alcoholism: Interdisciplinary Approaches to an Enduring Problems* (R.E. Tarter, and A.A. Sugarman (eds.). Addison-Wesley, Reading, Massachusetts.

Edwards, G., and Gross, M.M. (1976). Alcohol dependence: Provisional description of a clinical syndrome. *Br. Med. J. 1*:1058–1061.

Edwards, G., Gross, M.M., Keller, M., Moser, J., and Room, R. (1977). Alcohol-related disabilities. Offset Publication Number 32, World Health Organization, Geneva.

Filstead, W.J., Goby, M.J., and Bradley, N.J. (1976). Critical elements in the diagnosis of alcoholism: A national survey of physicians. *J.A.M.A. 236*:2767-2769.

Hesselbrock, M.N., Meyer, R.E., and Keener, J.J. (1985). Psychopathology in hospitalizd alcoholics. *Arch. Gen. Psychiatry 42*:1050-1055.

Jellinek, E.M. (1959). Estimating the prevalence of alcoholism: Modified values in the Jellinek formula and an alternative approach. *Qu. J. Stud. Alcohol 20*:261-269.

Kendell, R.E. (1975). *The Role of Diagnosis in Psychiatry*. Blackwell, London.

National Institute of Alcoholism and Alcohol Abuse (September 1985). *U.S. Alcohol Epidemiological Data Reference Manual*, Vol. 1.

Polich, J.M., and Kaelber, C.T. (1985). Sample survey and the epidemiology of alcoholism, *Alcohol Patterns and Problems. Series in Psychosocial Epidemiology* Vol. 5 (M.A. Schuckit and A.E. Slaby, Rutgers University Press, New Brunswick, New Jersey.

Robins, L.N. (1982). The diagnosis of alcoholism after DSM-III, *Encyclopedic Handbook of Alcoholism* (E.M. Pattison and E. Kaufman, eds.). Gardner Press, New York.

Robins, L.N., Helzer, J.E., Croughan, J., and Ratcliff, K.S. (1981). National Institute of Mental Health Diagnostic Interview Schedule: Its history, characteristics, and validity. *Arch. Gen. Psychiatry 38*:381-189.

Rohan, W.P. (1982). The concept of alcoholism: Assumptions and issues, *Encyclopedic Handbook of Alcoholism*, (E.M. Pattison and E. Kaufman, eds.). Gardner Press, New York.

Warheit, G.J., and Auth, J.B. (1985). Epidemiology of alcohol abuse in adulthood, *Psychiatry*, Vol. 3, (J.O. Cavenar, ed.).

Wattis, J.P. (1983). Alcohol and old people. *Br. J. Psychiatry 143*:306-307.

Vaillant, G.E. (1983). *The Natural History of Alcoholism*. Harvard University Press, Cambridge, Massachusetts.

2

Epidemiology of Alcohol Addiction: International

John E. Helzer
University of Vermont, College of Medicine, Burlington, Vermont

I. INTRODUCTION

A basic difficulty in conceptualizing the epidemiology of alcoholism lays in deciding what constitutes the disorder or if, in fact, there is a "disorder." There is considerable disagreement about what the essential features of alcoholism are. It can be broadly defined as "the repetitive intake of alcoholic beverages to a degree that harms the drinker in health or socially or economically, with indication of inability consistently to control the occasion or amount of drinking" (Keller, McCormick, and Efron, 1982, p 20). But this definition is not precise enough for research purposes because the terms *harm* and *inability to control* are not specific enough for investigators to agree on individual cases.

Several more specific definitions have been proposed. Some of these are based on the amount of harm caused (American Psychiatric Association [APA], 1980; Feighner et al., 1972), the loss of the ability to control alcohol intake (Jellinek, 1960), a core syndrome of alcohol dependence (Edwards, 1977), and the number and type of alcohol problems (Cahalan, 1970). The major definitions, and some definitional dilemmas, have recently been reviewed by Pattison and Kaufman (1982). Rohan (1982) summarized these issues by pointing out that if the term *alcoholism* is used to imply an underlying disease essence that can account for the observed self-destructive behavior of the alcohol abuser, we are left with conceptual difficulties. "Rather, the focus is on observation and description of drinking behavior and how it becomes problematic. The term 'alcoholism' should be limited to being a convenient reference label for selected sequences of harmful ingestion activity. . . . Alcoholism may be defined in terms of patterns of behavior" (Rohan, 1982, p. 33).

Despite conceptual problems, a definable and consistent label is essential, not only for epidemiology but also for meaningful communication (Helzer et al., 1977; Kendell, 1975). The definition currently used by many mental health workers in this country is provided by the *Diagnostic and Statistical Manual of Mental Disorders* (DSM-III; APA, 1980), which follows Rohan's (1982) recommendation and bases the label of alcoholism on behaviors. This is a robust definition, having both high interrater reliability and considerable predictive utility.

> It is remarkable, given logical difficulties, the assembling of symptoms from grossly different conceptual grounds, and the reported unreliability of alcoholics as historians, that the diagnosis of alcoholism by symptom self-report is repeatedly found to be one of the most valid and reliable of the psychiatric diagnoses. There seems little doubt that . . . a sturdy entity is being tapped with counting social, medical, and psychological alcohol problems (L.N. Robins, 1982, p. 53).

II. MEASUREMENT OF ALCOHOLISM IN THE GENERAL POPULATION

Both for health planning on a national level and for the discovery of etiology, it is of obvious interest to know how many cases of a disorder there are in the total population. Because it is not practical to examine every member of the general population, secondary indicators of number of cases are often sought. Several such indicators are available for estimating alcoholism. Because the legal production and sale of alcohol are taxed, one estimator of per capita alcohol consumption is available from federal departments of revenue. There are some problems with this estimate, in that illegal production is not ascertained and no account is taken of the relative volume of unsold stocks of liquor before and after the period of study. But, as Kreitman (1977) pointed out, despite these difficulties, estimates of per capita consumption based on revenue are probably fairly accurate because there is a financial incentive for accuracy. These estimates are also available for nearly every country and can thus be compared cross-nationally. But how relevant is per capita consumption to alcoholism or problem drinking?

Ledermann (1956) proposed that there is a direct relation between the alcohol consumption of a country and the proportion of heavy users in that population. He reviewed distribution curves of consumption and observed that their shape (lognormal) was similar from one country to the next and that the dispersion differed little (Schmidt, 1977). Ledermann hypothesized that drinking is a type of social contagion; that is, personal attitudes and behavior regarding alcohol are heavily influenced by societal attitudes and behaviors.

Ledermann's (1956) hypothesis has been widely debated (Duffy, 1980; Skog, 1980). One major criticism is that Ledermann's work assumes rather than proves that dispersions between populations with similar levels of per capita consumption are small. But the relation between per capita consumption and other indicators of alcoholism, such as liver cirrhosis rates and alcohol-related traffic offenses and deaths, seems to provide supportive evidence (Davies, 1982). For example, in the United Kingdom, annual figures from 1970–1979 showed a considerable rise in per capita alcohol consumption and a 0.95 correlation between this variable and deaths from liver cirrhosis, deaths which are presumably alcohol related. Kendell (1984) found supportive evidence in his examination of a recent slight fall in per capita consumption in the United Kingdom, whereas deLint found "no evidence which is inconsistent with the theory that overall levels of consumption rise and fall with rates of excessive use" (deLint, 1978, p. 78).

If Ledermann's hypothesis is correct, there is cause for concern because there has been a worldwide trend toward increasing levels of consumption in recent decades. Table 1 (deLint, 1978, p. 78) compares consumption levels for 25 countries from 1960 to 1973. All but 1

Table 1 Alcohol Consumption in Liters of Absolute Alcohol per Capita for Those Aged 15 Years and Older

Country	1960	1973	Change[a]
France	27.3	24.1	−12
Italy	19.1	21.1	10
Spain	11.9	18.5	55
Luxembourg	13.8	18.5	34
West Germany	10.2	16.8	65
Portugal	15.3	17.9	17
Russia	10.4	14.7	41
Switzerland	12.5	19.3	54
Austria	10.9	16.0	47
Belgium	11.7	14.5	24
Hungary	9.2	13.2	43
Australia	9.5	12.2	28
New Zealand	9.3	11.7	26
East Germany	7.8	12.3	58
Yugoslavia	8.0	10.5	31
United States	7.8	10.6	36
Denmark	6.1	11.0	80
Canada	7.8	11.1	42
Great Britain	6.8	10.0	47
Sweden	5.9	8.0	36
Netherlands	3.8	10.1	166
Poland	6.2	9.2	48
Republic of Ireland	4.9	9.0	84
Finland	3.9	7.8	100
Norway	3.6	5.4	50

[a]1960 = 100

Source: deLint, J. (1978). Alcohol consumption and alcohol problems from an epidemiological perspective. *Br. J. Alcohol Alcohol., 13*:75–85. Copyright 1978 by Pergamon Press, reprinted with permission.

of these countries show an increase, and for most the increase is considerable. Ledermann's model also has important public health implications. If per capita consumption can be reduced by raising minimum drinking ages, restricting the number of retail outlets, or increasing alcohol taxes, these methods may successfully reduce the number of alcoholics (Colon, Cutter, and Jones, 1982). deLint (1978) felt that the gradual weakening of social control measures due to increasing public acceptance of alcohol accounted for the increases in overall consumption.

Another indicator often used to estimate the magnitude of alcoholism in a population is the liver cirrhosis mortality rate. Schmidt (1977) listed several reasons in support of this as a uniquely suitable index of alcoholism. First, cirrhosis is not an uncommon cause of death and is a leading cause among alcoholics. Second, there is no doubt about the etiological importance of alcohol in the development of a prominent form of cirrhosis. Third, the mortality rate from cirrhosis among drinkers is stable over time, and cirrhosis mortality due to factors other than alcohol has changed little. Jellinek (1960) proposed a formula for estimating the prevalence of alcoholism on the basis of cirrhosis deaths: $A = P \times D/K$, where A = alcoholics with physical consequences; P = percent of cirrhosis cases attributable to alcoholism; D = total cases of cirrhosis at autopsy; and K = a constant based on the mortality of cirrhotic alcoholics.

There is debate about this method of estimating prevalence (Warheit and Auth, 1985). Cooper and Morgan (1973) suggested that, when using the best available general population survey data as a comparison standard, the formula appears to overestimate the population prevalence. However, Popham (1970) concluded that, although imperfect, the formula produces estimates that are in rough agreement with most survey estimates of the prevalence of alcoholism. Furthermore, cirrhosis death rates and per capita alcohol consumption are correlated. Figure 1 (Schmidt, 1977, p. 25) shows a correlation of 0.94 between these variables. Decreases in the availability of alcohol are correlated with a fall in cirrhosis rates. Figure 2 (Schmidt, 1977, p. 29) shows the results of the natural experiment that occurred during the two world wars. There was a precipitous fall in cirrhosis death rates during the war years when alcohol was in short supply and an equally dramatic rise when alcohol became freely available again.

Death rates from cirrhosis provide convergent evidence for concern about a recent secular trend toward increasing rates of alcoholism. Both overall rates of cirrhosis and the proportion of cirrhosis deaths due to alcohol have risen steadily in the second half of this century (Schmidt, 1977). There is also evidence of a differential increase in some countries of alcoholism among women. Using hospital admissions for alcoholism from 1957 to 1975 as an indirect indicator, Sclare (1978) found a sixfold increase for men and an 11-fold increase for women.

III. PERSONAL INTERVIEW SURVEYS

A. Methodological Issues

Secondary indicators of a disorder are useful epidemiologically for a number of reasons. Because they are usually available on both a regional and a national level, they can be used to make comparisons between regions of the same country or between countries that may differ in relevant social variables such as religion or alcohol production and to make comparisons within or between countries over time to look for secular trends. Despite their relative accessibility, there are difficulties in using secondary indicators. One problem is accuracy. As mentioned, department of revenue statistics on alcohol production suffer from various types of error, and these errors are likely to vary depending on the country.

Another difficulty is the fact that they are only secondary indicators. The alcohol production rate is not identical to the consumption rate, and even the latter is only arguably correlated with alcoholism. Thus, production is twice removed from the true variable of interest. Furthermore, because of national differences in the way production is measured, cross-national comparisons are probably less dependable than estimates of secular trends within a country (Kreitman, 1977).

The most serious problem is that, regardless of their quality and consistency, national indicators can rarely be used to examine differences in demographic subsegments of the population and can never be used to test the relevance of personal characteristics to a specific disorder. For this latter goal, personal interview data are necessary (Mulford, 1982). For many reasons, personal interview data are preferable for epidemiological estimates; however, problems of ascertainment do exist (Edwards, 1973). Overcoming or minimizing these difficulties is at the heart of contemporary epidemiology in the mental health field.

One difficulty in the use of personal interview data is its expense. Most disorders are relatively rare in the general population; thus, to have stable estimates, it is necessary to examine large numbers of people. If interview-based estimates are to be referred back to the population from which they came, subjects have to be sampled systematically. This implies prior enumeration so that a meaningful sample can be drawn. Enumeration of large

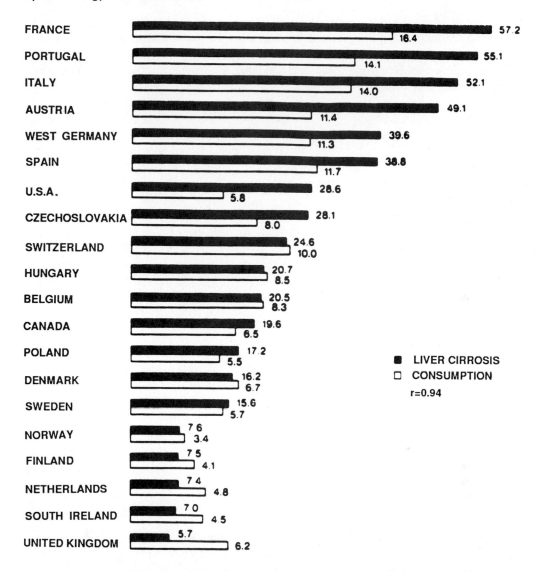

Figure 1 Cirrhosis mortality per 100,000 population 25 years of age and older and alcohol consumption per capita. (Death rates for the United States and Belgium are for 1971; all other death rates are for 1972. Consumption figures are the 1968–1970 averages. (From Schmidt, W. (1977). Cirrhosis and alcohol consumption: An epidemiological perspective, G. Edwards and M. Grant (eds.), *Alcoholism: New Knowledge and New Responses*. Croom Helm London, pp. 15–47. Reprinted by permission.)

populations is costly. Once identified, subjects may be difficult to contact or may be reluctant to participate; considerable effort may be required to complete an interview. Obviously, this degree of effort is usually impractical for pursuing large segments of the general populations; thus, it is often necessary to estimate rates based on personal examination of relatively few subjects and even fewer positive cases.

Another difficulty in the use of personal interview data is its dependence on the ability and willingness of respondents to give accurate self-reports. There is evidence that people forget rather quickly even important personal events such as hohspitalization and surgery

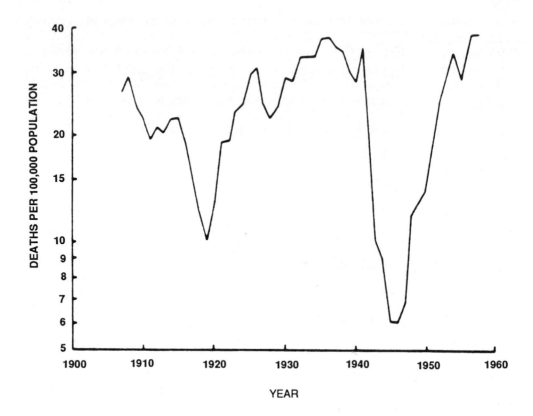

Figure 2   Cirrhosis mortality rates for Paris, 1907–1956. (Based on data in Ledermann, 1964. (From Schmidt, W. (1977). Cirrhosis and alcohol consumption: An epidemiological perspective, G. Edwards and M. Grant (eds.), *Alcoholism: New Knowledge and New Responses*. Croom Helm, London, pp. 15–47. Reprinted by permission.)

(Cannell, 1977). Furthermore, even in typically anonymous survey interviews, respondents may be reluctant to admit excessive use of alcohol and its consequences.

The estimation of lifetime alcoholism rates may be thwarted by a systematic cohort effect on accuracy in older respondents. For example, older people lived much of their adult lives during a period when this society was less psychologically minded than it is now. Thus, older persons may be less likely to recognize or acknowledge emotional symptoms like depression or anxiety for what they are and more likely to attribute them to vague physical disorders. This may have less impact on the reports of the behavioral problems associated with abuse of alcohol, but other systematic errors can also occur with the passage of time. Because problems related to drinking are more likely to occur in the teens and 20s, older respondents may be less likely to recall lifetime symptoms than those who are closer to that period in their lives.

A third difficulty has been the development of survey interview instruments that are diagnostic specific, cover a broad range of diagnoses, minimize examination variance, and do not require administration by experienced clinicians. It is also important that survey instruments cover a broad range of psychopathology. Until the past few years, survey interviews tended to focus on individual symptoms or scales of impairment rather than on specified constellations of symptoms or diagnoses. The greatest disadvantage of this was that population survey results were not consonant with data from clinical research, which was typically diagnostically oriented. Thus, examination of comorbidities and risk factors that had first been observed in clinical populations could not be pursued in relatively unbiased (Berkson, 1946) samples from the general population. However, the expense of utilizing experienced clinicians as interviewers seemed to preclude the possibility of ascertaining diagnostic-specific rates in surveys. Within the past few years, survey instruments have been developed that cover a broad range of diagnoses, minimize examination variance by being highly structured, and can be administered by lay examiners (Helzer, 1983; Robins et al., 1981).

B. Results

There have been many personal interview surveys of alcoholism or alcohol problems over the past years. A comprehensive review of this work may be found elsewhere (Auth and Warheit, 1982/1983; Warheit and Auth, 1985). I will present a brief overview of these results and will discuss in more detail a large multicenter general population survey being conducted now in the United States, the Epidemiologic Catchment Area (ECA) survey.

Although most population surveys utilize a sample of the population of interest, there have been a few notable efforts in which entire populations have been assessed. One of these, by Fremming (1951), gathered interview or record data on all persons born on the Danish island of Bornholm between 1883 and 1887 who survived at least to the age of 10 years. Only 3.2% of those who survived to adulthood were not personally interviewed, and record data were available for most of them. The lifetime expectancy of alcoholism was estimated at 3.5% for men and 0.1% for women.

A similar heroic effort was made by Helgason (1964) in Iceland. His sample included all persons born between 1895 and 1897 who were still living in 1910. Helgason obtained information from doctors, relatives, acquaintainces, clergy, and local officials and from health records. He sent questionnaires to those without other sources of information and obtained sufficient data on 99.4% of his target population. His lifetime expectancy estimates for alcoholism were 9.8% for men and 0.5% for women.

A third notable effort was headed by Essen-Möller (Essen-Möller, et al., 1956) in Lunby, a rural area of southern Sweden. Four psychiatrists examined the area's 2550 residents in 8 weeks, missing only 30 persons. Information was also obtained from official records and family physicians. A follow-up study of the survivors was conducted in 1972–1974, again with almost 100% participation (Ojesjö, Hagnell, and Lanke, 1982). The latter investigators estimated the lifetime risk of developing alcoholism among men to be 19.3%.

Warheit and Auth (1985) reviewed 12 United States surveys conducted between 1946 and 1982. Together, these surveys indicated that 20–25% of men and about 40% of women abstain from alcohol, that 12–33% of men and 2–5% of women drink heavily, and that 10% or more of men and 2–3% of women have experienced alcohol-related problems. The rates vary widely depending on the method of ascertainment, the definitions used, and the demographic composition of the samples.

What is perhaps the largest comprehensive epidemiological survey ever done in the field of mental health, the Epidemiologic Catchment Area (ECA) survey, is currently in progress in the United States, and some of the early data from this study have been reported. The ECA is a multicenter survey funded by the National Institute of Mental Health (Regier et al., 1984). Approximately 20,000 respondents are being personally interviewed at two times in order to estimate lifetime and current prevalence and 1-year incidence of major mental disorders, utilization of health services, barriers to utilization, and other relevant issues. Clinical data are being gathered with the Diagnostic Interview Schedule (DIS), which ascertains lifetime occurrence of symptoms from three diagnostic systems (a system designed by Feighner et al.,

1972; Research Diagnostic Criteria; DSM-III) and can be administered by lay examiners (Helzer et al., 1985; L.N. Robins et al., 1981). Subjects are sampled from both the general household population and from representative institutions such as nursing homes, chronic hospitals, and prisons. Interviewed subjects at each of the field sites are weighted to reflect the demographic composition of the catchment areas from which they were drawn (Holzer et al., 1985).

Table 2 shows results from the ECA survey (Myers et al., 1984; Robins et al., 1984) for lifetime and current (6-month) prevalence rates of alcohol abuse and dependence as defined by DSM-III diagnostic criteria (APA, 1980). These figures represent three of the five ECA field sites. Current prevalence rates have been published more recently from a fourth site at Durham, North Carolina (Blazer et al., 1985). As shown, the rates for current prevalence are comparable to those estimated for problem drinking by Warheit and Auth (1985) on the basis of their review. Estimates for lifetime prevalence are higher, ranging up to more than 28% for men. It is important to recognize that these latter estimates are based on the occurrence of problems at any time, problems that need not be temporally overlapping. Nonetheless, a remarkably high proportion of the male population endorsed at least some serious problems related to alcohol as occurring at some time in their lives. Alcohol abuse and dependence was the most commonly diagnosed disorder in men up until the age of 65, and even in older men, it was third most common. Among women, alcoholism was not among the most common diagnoses except in the youngest age group, 18–24 years old (Myers et al., 1984), which may provide more suggestive evidence that alcoholism is becoming more prevalent among females.

IV. RISK FACTORS FOR ALCOHOLISM

Risk factors are variables that are associated with an increased risk of a disorder, and even though an association does not imply a causal relation, these factors help to identify groups who are at relatively high risk for developing a condition and may provide clues concerning its etiology.

Apart from sex, perhaps the greatest risk factor for alcoholism is family history. Alcoholism clearly runs in families, and whereas increased familial risk can be due to either environmental or genetic factors, there is little doubt that at least some of this familial tendency is genetic. Disaggregating genetic from environmental influences in a research design is difficult, but one method involves examining probands born of alcoholic parents but adopted by nonalcoholic foster parents in an early age. The offspring are then followed to see how their prevalence of alcoholism in adulthood compares with that of children both born and raised in alcoholic families (evidence of genetic inheritance) or with that of those born and raised in nonalcoholic families (evidence of environmental influence). Further elaborations of this research include cross-fostering (Wender, Rosenthal, Kety, Schulsinger, and Welner, 1974) and half-sibling studies (Schuckit, Goodwin, and Winokur, 1972), in which various combinations of genotype and environment are studied.

The results of contemporary adoption and cross-fostering studies are reasonably consistent and have been summarized by Goodwin (1985). Findings for daughters are equivocal, but the biological sons of alcoholic parents are three to four times more likely than the sons of nonalcoholics to develop alcoholism, whether they are raised by their biological parents or not. Furthermore, sons of alcoholics are not at higher risk for developing other adult psychiatric disorders. However, there is evidence of a gene × environment interaction in the development of alcoholism, and it appears that as many as one-third or more of alcoholics have no evidence of any family history of alcoholism (Schuckit, 1983).

Studies of twins are also used to disaggregate nature and nuture. Adoption designs can

Table 2 Lifetime and Current Prevalence of DSM-III-Estimated Alcohol Abuse and Dependence

ECA site	N	6-month prevalence (%)		Lifetime prevalence (%)	
		men	women	men	women
New Haven, CT	3,058	8.2	1.9	19.1	4.8
Baltimore, MD	3,481	10.4	1.7	24.9	4.2
St. Louis, MO	3,004	8.5	1.0	28.9	4.3

Note. Table contains weighted household Diagnostic Interview Schedule data from three Epidemiologic Catchment Area sites.

be conceived of as an examination of the impact of varying environments in those with similar genetic backgrounds. In twins studies, the aim is to compare illness concordance rates in monozygotic versus dizygotic co-twins. Thus, the impact is compared of differing degrees of genetic similarity (all genes in common versus only half in common) in two persons raised in a similar environment. As with adoption studies, much of the twins research has been done in Scandinavia, where national records of medical contacts, twinship, and temperance board registrations are relatively accessible for research investigation.

Results of twins studies have not been as consistently supportive of a genetic component in the etiology of alcoholism. The most supportive study is that by Kaij (1960), which used temperance board registrations. The concordance rate for alcoholism was 54% for monozygotic cotwins and 28% for dizygotic cotwins, a statistically significant difference consistent with a genetic contribution. A study using records from the U.S. Veterans Administration also showed a higher concordance rate for alcoholism among monozygotic versus digygotic male twins (Hrubec and Omenn, 1981). There are two other large studies of twins and alcoholism. One from the United Kingdom was negative: There was no difference in concordance between monozygotic and dizygotic twins (Murray, Clifford, and Gurlin, 1983). Another from Finland showed equivocal results (Partanen, Bruun, and Markkanen, 1966).

It is reasonable to conclude that there are genetic determinants in alcoholism but that environmental determinants are also powerfully involved. This brings us to the search for other risk factors, one of which is sex. Alcoholism is clearly a male-predominant disorder. Although alcohol-related problems may be increasing in women, they are considerably more common in men in virtually every culture. This may partially reflect a lower tolerance for alcohol among women (Goodwin, 1985) or the existence of societal constraints. One study (Cloninger, et al., 1978) suggested that the difference in prevalence by sex is accounted for by nonfamilial environmental factors, such as social constraints against heavy drinking in women, but that women who do drink heavily have the same risk for becoming alcoholic as do heavy drinking men.

Another risk factor for alcoholism is the presence of other mental disorders. For example, there is considerable evidence of an association between alcoholism and depression, and these two disorders often run in families (Winokur, 1979). However, current evidence suggests that these disorders are independently transmitted but that there may be a familial clustering of social risk factors related to their development (Merikangas et al., 1985). There is also a strong association between alcoholism and early behavioral problems, especially school problems, in children (Robins, 1966) and antisocial personality disorder in adults (Lewis et al., 1983). Using population data gathered from surveys in four countries, Helzer et al. (in press) showed that the relative risk of many other psychiatric disorders is increased in alcoholic versus nonalcoholics but that these relative risks tend to be even higher in countries with a low population prevalence of alcoholism. This was true of many of the other risk factors for alcoholism as well.

In adults, other mental disorders may be antecedent to or may follow alcoholism, but there is evidence of a sex differential. Dahlgren (1981) found in his Swedish sample that 80% of the alcoholic women had some antecedent psychiatric disorder, whereas this was found in only 50% of the alcoholic men. Finally, there is a strong association between alcoholism and suicide. Robins (1981) found in a study of 134 completed suicides 25% of the cases had a diagnosis of alcoholism. The frequency of this diagnosis was second only to affective disorders.

Age is another risk factor. Alcoholism typically begins early in life, although there is some evidence that the age of onset tends to be somewhat later in women than in men. Ojesjö et al. (1982) provided a table of annual incidence from their followup examination of the Essen-Möller (Essen-Möller et al., 1956) Lundby sample. For men, the incidence rate of alcohol dependence was highest in the 20–29 years cohort. They found that 61% of the probability of developing alcoholism was manifested before age 30 and 78% before age 40.

There is some evidence of social class differences in alcoholism, although these may have more to do with the expression or ascertainment of the disorder than with its rate of occurrence. Halldin (1985) found that the social consequences of drinking were more apparent in the lower social classes but that high levels of alcohol consumption were more apparent in the upper classes. It has also been claimed that upper-class abusers are more likely to show negative medical consequences from drinking (Bjurulf, Sternby, and Wistedt, 1971).

Prevalence differences by race are equivocal. In the initial report from the first three ECA survey sites, lifetime prevalence rates were higher in Blacks at the first site, about the same at the second site, and higher in non-Blacks at the third site (Robins et al., 1984). Prevalence differences by urban versus rural residence are also equivocal. The ECA survey should provide useful new data on this issue, especially from the sites in Durham, North Carolina and St. Louis, Missouri, where substantial portions of the respondents live in rural areas. In their initial report from the Durham site, Blazer et al. (1985) found alcoholism to be more prevalent among rural residents but also found that this may have been related to differences in demographic composition between the urban and rural samples. At present, there is no unequivocal evidence that area of residence is causally or consistently related to the development of alcoholism.

Finally, possible protective factors require a brief comment. Alcoholics often say that they suffer few of the immediate adverse consequences of drinking (e.g., the hangover) and sometimes complain that if alcohol were harder on them in the short run, they might have fewer problems with it in the long run. There may be some truth in that complaint. Women tend to be less tolerant of alcohol than men, and perhaps there are fewer alcoholic women because many cannot drink large enough amounts to become dependent. The best example of a possible consumption-related protective factor in alcoholism is the oriental flushing phenomenon. A majority of Asians experience an unpleasant facial flush after drinking small amounts of alcohol, a phenomenon which may be related to metabolic enzymes (Harada, Agarwah, and Goedde, 1981). This may be enough of a deterrent to regular drinking to help account for the very low rates of alcoholism in most Asian countries (Goodwin, 1985). The relative absence of an acute flushing phenomenon is also thought to be consistent with the relatively high rate of alcoholism in Korea (Park et al., 1984).

V. EPIDEMIOLOGY IN THE TREATMENT AND PREVENTION OF ALCOHOLISM

The treatment of alcoholism is discussed elsewhere in this book, but a few words are appropriate here on how epidemiology can be informative regarding treatment. Epidemiological data are often used to gain a better understanding of the natural history of a disorder, which in turn has utility both in providing treatment suggestions and as a benchmark against which to evaluate treatment outcome. In his book on the natural history of alcoholism, Vaillant (1983) noted that, at any given time, a majority of alcoholics can be expected to be in a period of sobriety. One of the hallmarks of alcoholism is that it is characterized, in the majority of cases, by frequent relapses and remissions. Recognizing that relapse is a part of the natural history of the disorder may reduce the likelihood that the treating clinician will blame the patient or himself when it occurs.

Another important aspect of the natural history of alcoholism is the occurrence of spontaneous remission with age. It was noted by Åmark (1951) in his Scandinavian sample that many alcoholics underwent a tapering-off of problems in their fifties. Accelerated mortality and the institutionalization of deteriorated alcoholics could account for some of this decline, but Drew (1968) felt that these factors would not sufficiently account for the fall-off of older alcoholics in treatment. It is not clear whether spontaneous remission occurs only in those who have mild cases of alcoholism (Taylor and Helzer, 1983).

Additional studies that examine prevention are urgently needed. It has been claimed that alcoholism is the third most serious public health problem in the United States, after cardiovascular disease and cancer (Selzer, 1980). In a study of middle-aged men, Halldin (1985) found that 29% of all inpatient days were a result of alcohol-related or influenced conditions, and 31% of all deaths in this age group were estimated to be alcohol-related. The ECA survey has demonstrated the high prevalence of alcoholism relative to other mental disorders.

One method of prevention that does not seem to hold much promise is the restriction of alcohol advertising. Ogborne and Smart (1980) found only a weak relation between consumption and advertising regulations in the United States. Furthermore, in the period after restrictions on beer advertising in Manitoba, Canada, beer consumption continued to rise at a similar rate as in the control province of Alberta. In an econometric analysis, Duffy (1981) examined the effect of income, price, and advertising on alcohol consumption. He found that income and price did have an effect on the consumption of wine and spirits but had little effect on beer consumption. There was an advertising effect on demand for spirits and beer, but it was small and shortlived. No effect was detected for wine. Duffy concluded that the main effect of advertising was to influence the market share for a particular product but that there was little effect on overall consumption and no long-term effect of any kind.

The way alcohol use and abuse is distributed in the population, clearly an epidemiological issue, has important implications for prevention. I have discussed the single distribution model of alcohol consumption, that is, that per capita consumption is continuous, unimodal, and positively skewed and that the proportion of heavy drinkers is predictable from the per capita consumption. The competing model is one in which the distribution curve is bimodal, with normal drinkers forming one consumption curve and alcoholics forming another. In the first model, any measure that reduces per capita consumption, such as laws that restrict access to alcohol, would also lower the rate of alcoholism, and measures that increase per capita consumption would have the opposite effect. The biomodal model would imply that measures that produce a change in the consumption level of normal drinkers would have little or no effect on alcoholics (Robinson, 1977). The accuracy of these two models is still under debate, but considerable evidence does seem to support the single-distribution model. Obviously, model selection has profound implications both for the understanding and prevention of alcoholism.

ACKNOWLEDGMENTS

This research was supported by the Epidemiological Catchment Area Program (ECA). The ECA is a series of five epidemiologic research studies performed by independent research teams in collaboration with staff of the Division of Biometry and Epidemiology of the National Institute of Mental Health (NIMH). The NIMH principal collaborators are Darrel A. Regier, Ben Z. Locke, and Jack D. Burke, Jr.; the NIMH project officer is Carl A. Taube. The principal investigators and coinvestigators from the five sites are: Yale University (Grant UO1 MH 34224), Jerome K. Myers, Myrna M. Weissman, and Gary L. Tischler; Johns Hopkins University (Grant UO1 MH33870), Morton Kramer and Sam Shapiro; Washington University, St. Louis (Grant UO1 MH 33883), Lee N. Robins and John E. Helzer; Duke University (Grant UO1 MH 35386), Dan G. Blazer and Linda George; University of California, Los Angeles (Grant UO1 MH 35865), Marvin Karno, Richard L. Hough, Javier I. Escobar, and M. Audrey Burnam. This research was also supported by United States Public Health Service Grants AA 03539, MH00617, and MH-31302 and by the MacArthur Foundation Risk Factor Network.

REFERENCES

Åmark, C. (1951). A study in alcoholism: Clinical, social-psychiatric, and genetic investigations. *Acta Psychiatr. et Neurolo. Scand.* (Suppl. 70), 1–283.

American Psychiatric Association. (1980). *Diagnostic and Statistical Manual of Mental Disorders* (3rd ed.). Washington, D.C.

Auth, J.B., and Warheit, G.J. (1982/1983). Estimating the prevalence of problem drinking and alcoholism in the general population: An overview of epidemiological studies. *Alcohol Health Res. World, 7*:10–21.

Berkson, J. (1946). Limitations of the application of fourfold table analysis to hospital data. *Biomet. Bull., 1*:47–53.

Bjurulf, P., Sternby, N.H., and Wistedt, B. (1971). Definitions of alcoholism: Relevance of liver disease and temperance board registrations in Sweden. *Qu. J. Stud. on Alcohol, 32*:393–405.

Blazer, D., George, L.K., Landerman, R., Pennybacker, M., Melville, M.L., Woodbury, M., Manton, K.G., Jordan, K., and Locke, B. (1985). Psychiatric disorders: A rural/urban comparison. *Arch. Gen. Psychiatry, 42*:651–656.

Cahalan, D. (1970). *Problem Drinkers: A National Survey.* Jossey-Bass, San Francisco.

Cannell, C.F. (1977). *A Summary of Studies of Interviewing Methodology* (Pub. No. [HRA] 77-1343). Department of Health, Education, and Welfare, Washington, D.C.

Cloninger, C.R., Christiansen, K.O., Reich, T., and Gottesman, I.I. (1978). Implications of sex differences in the prevalences of antisocial personality, alcoholism, and criminality for familial transmission. *Arch. Gen. Psychiatry, 35*:941–951.

Colon, I., Cutter, H.S.G., and Jones, W.C. (1982). Prediction of alcoholism from alcohol availability, alcohol consumption and demographic data. *J. Stud. Alcohol, 43*:1199–1213.

Cooper, B., and Morgan, H.G. (1973). *Epidemiological Psychiatry.* Thomas, Springfield, Illinois.

Dahlgren, L. (1981). Kvinnor och alkohol—missbruket okar [Women and alcohol abuse]. *Lakartidningen, 78*:786–788.

Davies, P. (1982). Some empirical grounds for controlling consumption. *Br. J. Alcohol Alcohol., 17*:109–116.

deLint, J. (1978). Alcohol consumption and alcohol problems from an epidemiological perspective. *Br. J. Alcohol Alcohol., 13*:75–85.

Drew, L.R.H. (1968). Alcoholism as a self-limiting disease. *Q. J. of Stud. Alcohol, 29*:956–967.

Duffy, J.C. (1980). The association between per capita consumption of alcohol in the proportion of excessive consumers: A reply to Skog. *Br. J. Addic. 75*:147–151.

Duffy, M. (1981). The influence of prices, consumer incomes, and advertising on the demand for alcoholic drink in the United Kingdom. *Br. J. Alcohol Alcohol. 16*:200–208.

Edwards, G. (1973). Epidemiology applied to alcoholism. *Q. J. Stud. Alcohol, 34*:28–56.

Edwards, G. (1977). The alchol dependence syndrome: Usefulness of an idea, G. Edwards and M. Grant (eds.), *Alcoholism: New Knowledge and New Responses.* Croom Helm, London, pp. 136–156.

Essen-Möller, E., Larsson, H., Uddenberg, C-E., and White G. (1956). Individual traits and morbidity in a Swedish rural population. *Acta Psychiatr. Neurol. Scand.* (Suppl. 100):1–160.

Feighner, J.P., Robins, E., Guze, S.B., Woodruff, R.A., Winokur, G., and Munoz, R. (1972). Diagnostic criteria for use in psychiatric research. *Arch. Gen. Psychiatry, 26*:57–63.

Fremming, K.H. (1951). *The Expectation of Mental Infirmity in a Sample of the Danish Population: Occasional Papers on Eugenics* (No. 7). Cassell, London.

Goodwin, D.W. (1985). Alcoholism and genetics. *Arch. Gen. Psychiatry, 42*:171–174.

Halldin, J. (1985). Alcohol consumption and alcoholism in an urban population in central Sweden. *Acta Psychiatr. Scand., 71*:128–140.

Harada, S., Agarwah, D.P., and Goedde, H.W. (1981). Aldehyde dehydrogenase deficiency as cause of facial flushing reaction to alcohol in Japanese. *Lancet, 1*, 982.

Helgason, T. (1964). Epidemiology of mental disorders in Iceland. *Acta Psychiatri. Scand., 40* (Suppl. 173):1–258.

Helzer, J.E. (1983). Standardized interviews in psychiatry. *Psychiatric Developments, 2*:161–178.

Helzer, J.E., Clayton, P.J., Pambakian, R., Reich, T., Woodruff, R.A., Jr., and Reveley, M.A. (1977). Reliability of psychiatric diagnosis: II. The test/retest reliability of diagnostic classification. *Arch. Gen. Psychiatry, 34*:136–141.

Helzer, J.E., Stolzman, R.K., Farmer, A., Brockington, I.F., Plesons, D., Singerman, B., and Works, J. (1985). Comparing the DIS with a DIS/DSM-III-based physician reevaluation, W.W. Eaton and L.G. Kessler (eds.), *Epidemiologic Field Methods in Psychiatry: The NIMH Epidemiologic Catchment Area Program.* Academic Press, New York, pp. 285–308.

Helzer, J.E., Canino, G.J., Hwu, H-G., Bland, R.C., Newman, S., and Yeh, E-K. Alcoholism: A cross-national comparison of population surveys with the DIS, R.M. Rose and J. Barrett (Eds.), *Alcoholism: A Medical Disorder.* New York: Raven Press.

Holzer, C.E. III, Spitznagel, E., Jordan, K.B., Timbers, D.M., Kessler, L.G., and Anthony, J.C. (1985). Sampling the household population, W.W. Eaton and L.G. Kesler (eds.), *Epidemiologic Field Methods in Psychiatry: The NIMH Epidemiologic Catchment Area Program.* Academic Press, New York, pp. 23–48.

Hrubec, Z., and Omenn, G.S. (1981). Evidence of genetic predisposition to alcoholic cirrhosis and psychosis: Twin concordances flism from alcohol availability, alcohol consumption and demographic data. *J. Stud. Alcohol, 43*:1199–1213.

Jellinek, E.aM. (1960). *The Disease Concept of Alcoholism.* Hillhouse Press, New Brunswich, New Jersey.

Kaij, L. (1960). *Studies on the Etiology and Sequels of Alcohol Abuse.* University of Lund, Lund, Sweden.

Keller, M., McCormick, M., and Efron, V. (1982). *A Dictionary of Words About Alcohol* (2nd ed.). Rutgers University, Center of Alcohol Studies, New Brunswick, New Jersey.

Kendell, R.E. (1975). *The Role of Diagnosis in Psychiatry.* Blackwell, London.

Kendell, R.E. (1984). The beneficial consequences of the United Kingdom's declining per capita consumption of alcohol in 1979–1982. *Alcohol Alcohol., 19*:271–276.

Kreitman, N. (1977). Three themes in the epidemiology of alcoholism, G. Edwards and M. Grant (eds.), *Alcoholism: New Knowledge and New Responses.* Croom Helm, London, pp. 48–59.

Ledermann, S. (1956). *Alcool, Alcoolisme, Alcoolisation: Données Scientifiques de Caractère Physiologique Economique et Social* [Alcohol, Alcoholism, Alcoholization: Scientific Data of Economic and Social Psychological Character]. (Institut National d'Etudes Demographiques, Travaux et Documents; Cahier No. 29). Presses Universitaires de France, Paris.

Lewis, C.E., Rice, J., and Helzer, J.E. (1983). Diagnostic interactions: Alcoholism and antisocial personality. *J. Nerv. Ment. Dis., 171*:105–113.

Merikangas, K.R., Leckman, J.F., Prusoff, B.A., Pauls, D.L., and Weissman, M.M. (1985). Familial transmission of depression and alcoholism. *Arch. Gen. Psychiatry, 42*:367–372.

Mulford, H.A. (1982). The epidemiology of alcoholism and its implications, E.M. Pattison and E. Kaufman (eds.), *Encyclopedic Handbook of Alcoholism.* Gardner Press, New York, pp. 441–457.

Murray, R.M., Clifford, C., and Gurlin, H.M. (1983). Twin and adoption studies: How good is the evidence for a genetic role? M. Galanter (ed.), *Recent Developments in Alcoholism*, Vol. 1. Gardner Press, New York, pp. 25–48.

Myers, J.K., Weissman, M.M., Tischler, G.L., Holzer, C.E. III, Leaf, P.J., Orvaschel, H., Anthony, J.C., Boyd, J.H., Burke, J.D., Jr., Kramer, M., and Stoltzman, R. (1984). Six-month prevalence of psychiatric disorders in three communities. *Arch. Gen. Psychiatry, 41*:959–970.

Ogborne, A.C., and Smart, R.G. (1980). Will restrictions on alcohol advertising reduce alcohol consumption? *Br. J. Addic., 75*:293–296.

Öjesjö, L. Hagnell, O., and Lanke, J. (1982). Incidence of alcoholism among men in the Lundby community cohort: Sweden, 1957–1972. *J. Stud. Alcohol, 43*:1190–1198.

Park, J.Y., Huang, Y-H., Nagoshi, C.T., Yuen, S., Johnson, R.C., Ching, C.A., and Bowman, K.S. (1984). The flushing response to alcohol use among Koreans and Taiwanese. *J. Stud. on Alcohol, 45*:481–485.

Partanen, J., Bruun, K., and Markkanen, T. (1966). *Inheritance of Drinking Behavior.* Helsinki; Finnish Foundation for Alcohol Studies.

Pattison, E.M., and Kaufman, E. (1982). The alcoholism syndrome: Definitions and models, in E.M. Pattison and E. Kaufman (eds.), *Encyclopedic Handbook of Alcoholism.* Gardner Press, New York, pp. 3–30.

Popham, R.E. (1970). Indirect methods of alcoholism prevalence estimation: A critical evaluation R.E. Popham (ed.), *Alcohol and Alcoholism.* University of Toronto Press, Toronto, Ontario, Canada, pp. 294–306.

Regier, D.A., Myers, J.K., Kramer, M., Robins, L.N., Blazer, D.G., Hough, R.L., Eaton, W.W., and Locke, B.Z. (1984). The NIMH Epidemiologic Catchment Area program. *Arch. Gen. Psychiatry, 41*:934–941.

Robins, L.N. (1966). *Deviant Children Grown Up.* Williams and Wilkins, Baltimore, Maryland.

Robins, E. (1981). *The Final Months.* Oxford University Press, New York.

Robins, L.N. (1982). The diagnosis of alcoholism after DSM-III, E.M. Pattison and E. Kaufman (eds.), *Encyclopedic Handbook of Alcoholism.* Gardner Press, New York, pp. 40–54.

Robins, L.N., Helzer, J.E., Croughan, J., and Ratcliff, K.S. (1981). National Institute of Mental Health Diagnostic Interview Schedule: Its history, characteristics, and validity. *Arch. Gen. Psychiatry, 38*:381–389.

Robins, L.N., Helzer, J.E., Weissman, M, Orvaschel, H., Gruenberg, E., Burke, J.D., and Regier, D. (1984). Lifetime prevalence of specific psychiatric disorders in three sites. *Arch. Gen. Psychiatry, 41*:949–958.

Robinson, D. (1977). Factors influencing alcohol consumption, G. Edwards and M. Grant (eds.), *Alcoholism: New Knowledge and New Responses.* Croom Helm, London, pp. 60–70.

Rohan, W.P. (1982). The concept of alcoholism: Assumptions and issues, E.M. Pattison and E. Kaufman (eds.), *Encyclopedic Handbook of Alcoholism.* Gardner Press, New York, pp. 31–39.

Schmidt, W. (1977). Cirrhosis and alcohol consumption: An epidemiologic perspective, G. Edwards and M. Grant (eds.), *Alcoholism: New Knowledge and New Responses.* Croom Helm, London, pp. 15–47.

Schuckit, M.A. (1983). Alcoholic men with no alcoholic first-degree relatives. *Am. J. Psychiatry, 140*:439–443.

Schuckit, M.A., Goodwin, D.W., and Winokur, G. (1972). A half-sibling study of alcoholism. *Am. J. Psychiatry, 128*:1132–1136.

Sclare, A.B. (1978). The epidemiology of alcoholism. *Br. J. Alcohol Alcohol., 13*:86–92.

Selzer, M.L. (1980). Alcoholism and a coholic psychoses (3rd ed.), H.J. Kaplan, A.M. Freedman, and B.J. Sadock (eds.), *Comprehensive Textbook of Psychiatry* Vol. 2. Williams and Wilkins, Baltimore, Maryland, pp. 1629–1645.

Skog, O-J. (1980). Total alcohol consumption and rates of excessive use: A rejoiner to Duffy and Cohen. *Br. J. Addic., 75*:133–145.

Taymor, J.R., and Helzer, J.E. (1983). The natural history of alcoholism, B. Kissin and H. Begleiter (eds.), *The Biology of Alcoholism*: Vol. 6. *The Pathogenesis of Alcoholism: Psychosocial Factors*. Plenum Press, New York, pp. 17–65.

Vaillant, G.E. (1983). *The Natural History of Alcoholism*. Harvard University Press, Cambridge, Massachusetts.

Warheit, G.J., and Auth, J.B. (1985). Epidemiology of alcohol abuse in adulthood, J.O. Cavenar (ed.), *Psychiatry*, Vol. 3. Lippincott, Philadelphia, pp. 1–18.

Wender, P.H., Rosenthal, D., Kety, S, Schulsinger, F., and Welner, J. (1974). Cross-fostering. *Arch. Gen. Psychiatry, 30*:121–128.

Winokur, G. (1979). Alcoholism and depression in the same family, D.W. Goodwin and C.K. Erikson, *Alcoholism and Affective Disorders: Clinical, Genetic, and Biochemical Studies*. SP Medical and Scientific Books, New York, pp. 49–56.

3

The Epidemiology of Drug Addiction

James C. Anthony
The Johns Hopkins University, School of Hygiene and Public Health, Baltimore, Maryland

I. INTRODUCTION

A. Main Use of Epidemiology

Morris has argued cogently that the main use of epidemiology is to search for the causes of health and illness, with prevention as a primary goal. This search often starts with a test for specific agents, features of the environment, and host characteristics that are associated with the risk of acquiring an illness. With time, the search moves toward full evaluation of suspected causal associations. For a more complete search, the evaluation sometimes includes full-scale field experiments to test the causal significance of observed associations and to evaluate prevention strategies based on the observed associations [1,2].

B. Importance of Careful Clinical Observations

The point of departure in an epidemiological search for causes often has been a careful and orderly observation of patients, as recorded by one or more attending clinicians. These careful clinical observations can spawn imaginative thinking about what accounts for frankly disturbed human functioning, including pathological changes that give rise to clinically observable signs and symptoms. Careful clinical observations also can point toward distal causes or conditions that are more or less favorable to the genesis and maintenance of pathology or disturbed functioning. This pathway from clinical observation to causal hypotheses can be seen in many successful epidemiological studies of causes where the original paving stones were the carefully observed and recorded facts about patients, laid down by responsible clinicians [1,3].

It is reasonable to ask whether epidemiology has to be brought into the picture at all. One might imagine that the clinical observations about causes stand on their own merits. Sometimes they can.

Much has been written on issues of interdependence between the clinical sciences and epidemiology (e.g., see Refs. 1 and 3). It has become apparent that some classes of suspected causal associations do not require epidemiological study. For example, within the realm of drug addiction there would seem to be little need for an epidemiological study of whether naloxone can cause an opioid withdrawal syndrome among daily users of heroin. In fact, the key scientific questions about the causal association between withdrawal syndromes and opioid agonist-antagonists can be answered through clinical and laboratory studies, with no need for information from epidemiological studies.

On the other hand, there are many suspected causal associations that cannot be fully evaluated without epidemiological studies that look beyond the clinical case material at hand to the population experience out of which the cases arose. To illustrate, for almost a century, clinicians treating opioid-dependent patients have observed that some of these patients—but certainly not all of them—carry histories of marginal social adjustment, if not delinquency, prior to drug usage. In 1925, Kolb codified this observation as part of a careful clinical study of 230 patients with drug addiction [4]. He grouped his patients into five categories:

1. People of normal nervous constitution accidentally or necessarily addicted through medication in the course of illness;
2. Care-free individuals, devoted to pleasure, seeking new excitements and sensations, and usually having some ill-defined instability of personality that often expresses itself in mild infractions of social customs;
3. Cases with definite neuroses not falling into classes 2, 4, or 5;
4. Habitual criminals, always psychopathic;
5. Inebriates.

The patients with marginal social adjustment or outright maladjustment were assigned to categories 2 and 4, respectively (K-2 and K-4, by the Lexington Hospital classification). In later clinical studies, it was shown that a majority of drug addicts remanded for federal incarceration at the Lexington Hospital in Lexington, Kentucky, could be assigned to either one or the other of these two categories: Kolb and Ossenfort [5] assigned 51.5% to groups 2 and 4; Pescor's result was 67.9% [6].

These percentages look large, but the excellent clinical research of Kolb and Pescor could not reveal whether they were in excess of expected values. These percentages might be no different from those obtained by drawing a control group without addiction, or by drawing a representative sample of individuals from the free-living populations that gave rise to the patients. Moreover, it might be the case that social maladjustment and drug addiction co-occur more frequently among federally incarcerated patients than in a less-restricted population sample of cases with drug addiction. Clearly, this is a situation in which an epidemiological study is needed to supply a satisfactory expected value for comparison with the value observed by studying patients. Parenthetically, it should be noted that within the samples of federally incarcerated drug addiction cases seen by Kolb and Pescor, there were many who were not classified with a premorbid history of social maladjustment. This evidence strongly indicates that development of drug addiction does not presuppose a background of social maladjustment.

C. Introduction to Observational Strategies in Epidemiology

Within this framework, the suspected causal association between early social maladjustment and development of drug addiction can be laid out in relation to a fourfold table: early social maladjustment (present/absent) defining the two rows of the table; drug addiction (present/absent) defining the two columns. As depicted in Table 1, the clinical study of patients can provide an estimate for no more than two of the four cells of the table. The values belonging

Table 1 Fourfold Table for Estimation of the Relative Odds, an Index of the Degree of Association Between Clinical Case Status, and a Suspected Cause or Noncausal Risk Indicator

History of social maladaptation	Clinical case status	
	Cases	Noncases
Present	A^a	B^b
Absent	C^a	D^b

[a]These cell values might be obtained from a clinical case series.
[b]These cell values require information from noncases, preferably candidates for future casehood, drawn from the population out of which the cases arose.

in the other two cells can be estimated only by considering the characteristics of persons who were candidates for drug addiction, but have not become cases: those without addiction. Furthermore, once values for all four cells have been estimated validly, it is possible to quantify the degree of association between early social maladjustment and drug addiction.

This quantified association can be estimated in several ways, for example, via the relative odds (synonymous with odds ratio and in fourfold tables, the cross-product ratio). For example, the odds of drug addiction among those with early social maladjustment can be contrasted with the odds of drug addiction among those without early social maladjustment.

The relative odds estimate by itself is an extremely useful estimate for the degree of association between variables, when at least one variable is dichotomous; for example, drug addiction: present/absent [7]. Moreover, under certain conditions, the relative odds estimate serves well to estimate whether a suspected causal characteristic is associated with increased risk of acquiring an illness. When study samples are large enough, relative odds estimates can be "adjusted" for other suspected causes and confounding variables. That is, through stratified analyses or multivariable modeling, these extraneous variables can be held constant to increase the validity of any given relative odds estimate. Under such conditions, a properly derived relative odds value can serve as an especially useful estimate of relative risk [8].

Against this background, it may be seen that one of the central challenges in epidemiological research on drug addiction is to augment clinical studies in the direction of more valid estimates for the magnitude of suspected causal associations involving cases of drug addiction. Through these studies, it is possible to probe the causal significance of observed associations in greater detail than clinical studies generally allow.

Epidemiological studies to quantify and probe suspected causal associations can make use of the epidemiological case-control strategy, where relative odds are estimated by comparing newly developed cases of drug addiction with suitable clinical or population controls. This strategy, discussed in detail elsewhere (e.g., see Refs. 8 and 9), is illustrated in drug addiction studies by Gerard and Cornetsky [10] and by Chein et al. [11]. A related alternative approach involves the epidemiological case-base strategy, described by Miettinen [8], and illustrated in a study of intravenous drug use by Tomas et al. [12].

A general concern about case-control studies and the more generic case-base strategy is that the observed associations might be biased as a result of too-heavy reliance upon measurements made after the drug addiction has developed. For example, the degree of association between drug addiction and early social maladjustment might be magnified if drug-addicted cases or informants for these cases were to exaggerate their preaddiction maladjustment.

Epidemiological studies by Robins [13] and Kellam et al. [14] illustrate how a prospective strategy can be used to overcome concern about measurements of the type relied upon in case-control and case-base studies. For example, Robins used a nonconcurrent prospective design to discover generally higher cumulative occurrence of illicit drug use and addiction among grown-ups who as children were identified as deviant via child guidance clinic assessments, compared to corresponding occurrence rates among adults not identified as deviant children [13]. The Woodlawn study group, led by Kellam, used a concurrent prospective design to find higher cumulative occurrence of heavy drug use among teenagers, especially males, who as children were identified as socially maladaptive by their first-grade teachers, compared to teenagers not identified as socially maladaptive in first grade [14]. Thus, major strengths of these prospective studies stem from reduced reliance upon measurements taken after drug use or drug addiction had developed. These strengths offered a major probing look at the suspected associations, adding new evidence that early social maladjustment, maladaptation, or deviance might be causally linked to later occurrence of illicit drug use or drug addiction.

A general concern about all epidemiological studies of suspected causal associations is that the causal model is misspecified. A specific instance of a misspecified causal model involves uncontrolled confounding variables that function to create spurious associations. If these confounding variables are known, they can be controlled through matching at the stage of sample selection, or through stratification and multivariable modeling at the stage of data analysis. Nonetheless, in many instances, confounding variables are unknown or cannot be measured well enough for control via design or analysis techniques.

In the case of early social maladjustment and later drug addiction, it is conceivable that a vulnerability to drug addiction develops very early in life, perhaps at the time of conception. Further, it might be that early social maladjustment represents an early developmental expression of this vulnerability, with drug addiction as an expression of vulnerability later in development; early temperamental characteristics of preschoolers (e.g., lack of ego resilience) might be an extremely early developmental expression of the vulnerability [15]. By extension, it is possible that maladaptation during early school years (e.g., as rated in a child guidance clinic or by first-grade teachers) is an intermediary variable linking a vulnerability acquired quite early with later drug addiction, but is not an important causal condition antedating drug addiction.

However important such a hypothesized vulnerability might be, it would be difficult to know whether vulnerability was well measured in any observational study. As a result, observational studies are subject to the misspecification errors just mentioned.

D. Prevention Research as Experimental Epidemiology

The field experiment with randomization is one of the few epidemiological strategies that can limit misspecification errors of this type in efforts to probe suspected causal associations. To some extent, the strength of the field experiment rests upon a capacity of randomization to create balanced distributions of both known and unknown confounding variables and alternative causal conditions in preventive intervention and control groups. Further, it is possible to randomly assign children to experimental interventions that are designed to prevent or reduce social maladjustment (even though it is impossible to randomly allocate different levels of social maladjustment). If the results of such an experiment were to show reduced occurrence of illicit drug use, drug addiction, or related conditions in a successfully treated intervention group, this would be evidence favoring social maladjustment as more than just a noncausal intermediary step in an unfolding developmental path. Rather, the new evidence would strengthen the chain of causal inference linking early social maladjustment with later drug addiction; the program to prevent or reduce early social maladjustment would have apparent benefits in relation to prevention of drug addiction as well [16].

At present, there are at least two on-going field experiments that represent contemporary efforts to probe the suspected causal association between early social maladjustment and later development of illicit drug use and conditions related to drug addiction [17,18]. In each of these field trials, epidemiological samples of elementary school children have been assigned to preventive interventions directed toward early social maladjustment and other suspected causal conditions. The impact of the elementary school interventions now is being tested via periodic follow-up assessments of the children as they mature into the ages of initial drug self-administration and beyond. Thus, these prevention experiments are the most recent epidemiological probes into the suspected causal significance of the original clinical and epidemiological observations about early social maladjustment and later drug involvement.

Needless to say, not all suspected causal hypotheses about drug addiction are being worked up as carefully or thoroughly as the hypotheses about early social maladjustment. Indeed, the bulk of contemporary epidemiological and prevention research on drug abuse is not directed toward drug addiction or other clinical syndromes requiring drug dependence treatment. Rather, for the past 2 decades, the focus in this research generally has been surveillance of illicit drug use or other precursors of the clinical syndromes. The result is a mountain of epidemiological data on illicit drug use, but a meagre supply of epidemiological evidence on the clinical syndromes associated with drug addiction.

This situation might be remedied with a more deliberate integration of clinical, epidemiological, and prevention research [16]. Indeed, to some extent, the clinical treatment of drug dependence and other syndromes related to drug addiction represents a potential strengthening of family characteristics that might have a bearing on whether children of the treated patients go on to develop these syndromes in their later years. Thus, efforts to treat child-rearing patients with these syndromes, and especially experimental treatment evaluations, represent an opportunity for important epidemiological and prevention research; i.e., to test whether treatment of a child-rearing parent reduces occurrence of illicit drug use and related syndromes in the next generation. Well-organized clinical and prevention trials along these lines might play a key role in discovering mechanisms for familial aggregation of these syndromes.

What follows is a selective review of case definitions, case-ascertainment methods, and recently available epidemiological evidence on clinically defined syndromes related to drug addiction, with some concluding remarks on how to bring about a greater convergence of clinical, social, behavioral, and epidemiological research on drug dependence syndromes. Where the evidence concerns drug addiction specifically, this is noted with a comment. Otherwise, the evidence concerns the less specific clinical syndromes of drug abuse and drug dependence, or the nonspecific conglomerate of drug problems defined operationally in the next sections of this chapter.

II. RECENT CASE DEFINITIONS FOR CLINICAL SYNDROMES RELATED TO DRUG ADDICTION

A. DSM-III Drug Abuse and Dependence Syndromes

The third edition of the American Psychiatric Association's *Diagnostic and Statistical Manual of Mental Disorders* (DSM-III) offered case definitions and a conceptual framework that divides the psychiatric symptoms and behavioral changes due to illicit drug use into four main groups: (a) tolerance to drug effects; (b) withdrawal symptoms; (c) pathological use; and (d) impairments in social or occupational functioning due to drug use [19]. DSM-III case definitions for drug abuse and dependence syndromes are based on these symptom groups, singly or in combination.

In general, the DSM-III case definitions for abuse of a psychoactive drug call for evidence of a pattern of pathological use and also impaired functioning due to drug use. As a rule, DSM-III case definitions for dependence on a psychoactive drug call for signs of either tolerance or withdrawal, nothing more. Alcohol dependence and cannabis dependence are two of the exceptions: either pathological use *or* impaired functioning are required in addition to tolerance or withdrawal. The case definitions also require persistence of drug-related disturbances for at least 1 month. Short-lived syndromes due to psychoactive drug use might qualify for diagnosis as an intoxication or some other organic mental disorder, but not as drug abuse or dependence [19].

DSM-III provides separate drug abuse and drug dependence case definitions for each major class of psychoactive drugs, such as alcohol, cannabis, cocaine, and opioids. Nevertheless, in some epidemiological studies, these categories have been grouped under a broad heading of drug-use disorders, or substance-use disorders, or drug abuse/dependence syndromes. In this chapter, drug abuse/dependence refers to the presence of either drug abuse or drug dependence, or both, where the drug involved is an internationally or federally controlled substance such as marijuana, cocaine, heroin, lysergic acid diethylamide (LSD), diazepam, secobarbital, or the amphetamines. Alcohol abuse/dependence refers to the presence of either alcohol abuse or alcohol dependence, or both.

B. DSM-III-R Psychoactive Substance Dependence and Abuse

The DSM-III-R (DSM-III-Revised, 1987) psychoactive substance dependence and abuse case definitions are discussed in detail in Chapter 15 and elsewhere (e.g., see Ref. 20). In brief, under DSM-III-R, drug dependence is redefined along the lines of the Edwards-Gross alcohol dependence syndrome concept [21]. Thus, the case definition gives increased emphasis to salience of drug taking, compulsion to take drugs, avoidance of withdrawal symptoms, and liability for reinstatement of drug taking after cessation. There is continuing emphasis on the appearance of pharmacological tolerance and also withdrawal symptoms. The DSM-III-R case definition does not stress social consequences due to drug use (e.g., impaired functioning) unless these consequences appear as manifestations of salience or compulsion to take drugs. Finally, the Edwards-Gross alcohol dependence syndrome originally was described as a continuum. In contrast, DSM-III-R imposes a cut point, presumably as an aid to clinical decision making: drug-takers must meet three or more of the listed diagnostic criteria in order to qualify as cases.

Under DSM-III, a drug taker might qualify for both drug dependence and also for drug abuse. By comparison, DSM-III-R specifies that drug abuse is a residual category for drug takers who present with features of pathological drug use or impaired functioning due to drug use, but who never have qualified for the drug dependence diagnosis.

C. Draft Revision of the International Classification of Diseases—1987

The published draft of clinical guidelines and case definitions for diagnosis of drug abuse/dependence under the International Classification of Diseases—Tenth Revision (ICD-10) also stresses a dependence syndrome concept along the lines of the Edwards-Gross concept and the DSM-III-R case definition [22]. However, there is no prescribed cut point or threshold for clinical decision making as in DSM-III-R. Moreover, the DSM-III and DSM-III-R drug abuse categories do not appear in the ICD-10 draft. In their place are two new categories: harmful drug use and hazardous drug use. Harmful drug use refers to drug taking in which actual harms or losses have been actualized, whereas hazardous drug use refers to drug taking thought to be associated with increased risk of loss or harm (even though no loss or harm has occurred).

The innovative category of harmful drug use offers an alternative designation for the nonspecific category of drug problems that sometimes appears in the epidemiological literature (e.g., see Ref. 23). However, the term *drug problems* typically has referred to a conglomerate that includes any problem attributed to drug use, including tolerance and withdrawal symptoms. It sometimes has encompassed presumptively hazardous patterns of drug use, such as sustained use of a drug on a daily basis (e.g., for 2 weeks or more).

This chapter uses the term drug problem in the sense of this conglomerate, without specificity, except that there is a restriction to harmful or hazardous experiences involving federally controlled substances, as discussed in relation to drug abuse/dependence syndromes. As a practical matter, much of the available epidemiological evidence pertain to the DSM-III case definitions for drug abuse/dependence. Several large-scale prevalence surveys based on DSM-III-R criteria are underway: published results are expected to appear in the early 1990s.

III. METHODS FOR ASCERTAINING CASES OF DRUG ADDICTION IN EPIDEMIOLOGICAL FIELD STUDIES

A. Clinical Case-Ascertainment Methods

One area of progress in the last 3 decades of research on drug addiction has been the development of standardized clinical methods to identify individuals meeting the criteria stated in case definitions for drug abuse and dependence. Assembled in the form of a more or less scheduled sequence of standard questions or ratings, these clinical case-ascertainment methods often require high-level technical skills associated with clinical experience and training. These methods sometimes incorporate evidence from clinical or laboratory studies to determine the presence of neuroadaptive responses to drug exposure (e.g., response to opioid agonist-antagonist administration). Most allow evidence from informants other than the cases themselves. Kosten and Kosten (Chap. 15) describe the SADS/RDC, the Structured Clinical Interview for DSM-III-R (SCID), the Addiction Severity Index, and other clinical methods of this type.

B. Other Epidemiological Case-Ascertainment Methods

Many epidemiological studies of drug addiction and related clinical syndromes have been carried out on a large scale and under conditions otherwise not conducive to application of clinical methods for case-ascertainment. In an effort to approximate the standardized diagnoses that can be made by clinicians, epidemiologists often have turned to semistructured or completely structured schedules of interview questions that can be administered by study personnel without the credentials of clinical training or experience. One of the first such studies was Robins' pioneering prospective study of early deviance, later illicit drug use and drug addiction [13].

In another centrally important epidemiological study of drug addiction, Helzer (with Robins and others) hired and trained lay interviewers without clinical credentials to conduct interviews with U.S. Army enlisted men who had returned to the United States in September 1971 after serving in Vietnam, as well as with nonveteran control subjects. The interview covered behavioral, educational, and drug-use variables prior to and after serving in Vietnam, as well as questions about parental adjustment and demographic characteristics during the respondent's early years. The method of ascertaining narcotics addiction was this self-report interview conducted by the lay interviewers, with questions on feelings of dependence, as well as the classic withdrawal symptoms that might have been experienced after cutting down on opioid usage. Although the interview was about the lifetime history of addiction, the men were asked to provide urine samples that would allow testing of recent drug use. Virtually all of the men provided a urine sample, and the results were largely congruent with interview reports about recent illicit drug use [24].

Encouraged by an accumulation of positive experiences in field studies without clinical personnel, a Washington University research group led by Robins and Helzer developed the Diagnostic Interview Schedule (DIS) for the National Institute of Mental Health (NIMH). With a section for each of several specific categories of DSM-III mental disorders and including coverage of DSM-III drug abuse and dependence syndromes, the DIS was intended to produce diagnoses comparable to those obtained by clinicians, though it was to be administered by lay interviewers without clinical credentials [25]. DIS covers DSM-III abuse and dependence categories for most of the major drug classes, and also provides for measurement of the more general and less specific drug problem category. This is accomplished by having the interviewer ask a fixed schedule of standardized questions on the types of drug experiences and problems listed as examples under the DSM-III case definitions for drug abuse and dependence [23].

For the most part, DIS lifetime diagnoses for drug abuse and dependence that are obtained by lay interviewers compare favorably with DIS lifetime diagnoses obtained by psychiatrists and other experienced clinicians (e.g., see Refs. 25 and 26). In studies in which the clinical diagnoses have been based on other methods of case-ascertainment, the congruence with lay DIS diagnoses is less substantial, as might be expected due to the methods difference (e.g., see Ref. 27). The differences in these diagnoses, when observed, often have related to variation in methods of making the DSM-III criteria operational, or in methods of dating when abuse or dependence was most recently present [27].

In recent years, several methods have been developed as refinements of the DIS approach to case-ascertainment (e.g., the Composite International Diagnostic Interview), and as extensions to self-administered questionnaires (e.g., Skinner's alcohol and drug dependence inventories). These methods also are discussed in Chapter 15.

C. Context for the Use of These Methods

The earliest epidemiological studies of drug addiction were based on the patients treated in clinical settings, addicts known to informed health practitioners such as doctors and pharmacists, and addicts known to law enforcement officials [28,29]. The dominance of this tradition continued into the 1960s, when population surveys began to hold sway. Even so, as late as 1970, a major monograph entitled *The Epidemiology of Opiate Addiction in the United States* was based almost entirely upon evidence gathered from cases seen and treated in U.S. Public Health Service hospitals in Lexington, Kentucky, and Fort Worth, Texas, or appearing in the New York City registry of known narcotics addicts, or known as active addicts to the U.S. Bureau of Narcotics [30].

Between 1970 and 1980, there was an increasing number of epidemiologically oriented population surveys focused on illicit drug use per se. Epidemiological studies based on samples of treated patients with clinically defined drug addiction or dependence fell from favor, it seems, just as enthusiasm was growing for population surveys of drug use. Nevertheless, particularly since 1980, there have been several major epidemiological studies of syndromes related to drug addiction that have used clinical or quasi-clinical case-ascertainment methods (e.g., see Ref. 31). Moreover, as will be mentioned in the concluding sections of this chapter, some evidence indicates that the decline in number of epidemiological studies focused on drug dependence syndromes has been reversed. In part, the impression of a reversal is due to application of the clinically oriented DIS in the NIMH Epidemiologic Catchment Area (ECA) population surveys.

D. The NIMH Epidemiologic Catchment Area Program

Because the bulk of available epidemiological data on DSM-III drug abuse/dependence syndromes has come from the ECA population surveys, there is reason for an overview of ECA methods. In brief, the ECA Program was a multisite collaborative study of the prevalence and incidence of mental disorders and related conditions in the United States. Subjects for the study were more than 20,000 adults aged 18 years and older. Collaborators at each site selected these subjects between 1980 and 1984 by drawing probability samples from a combined total of 35,793 sampled households and separate probability samples of adult institutional residents in each of five metropolitan areas: New Haven, Connecticut; Baltimore, Maryland; St. Louis, Missouri; Durham-Piedmont, North Carolina; and Los Angeles, California. To assess lifetime history and occurrence of psychiatric conditions over time, the lay interviewing staff administered the DIS soon after sampling, and again at follow-up roughly 1 year later. The mean household survey participation rate was 76% at baseline; substantially higher values were obtained for the institutional survey. The mean interview completion rate for the reinterview after 1 year was close to 80%.

Data from the baseline DIS have been used to identify currently active cases of drug abuse/dependence syndromes, as well as no longer active cases with a prior history of drug abuse/dependence. Numerators for prevalence of currently active drug abuse/dependence consist of the currently active cases. Numerators for lifetime prevalence of drug abuse/dependence consist of both currently active and formerly active cases of drug abuse/dependence. Denominators for these prevalence estimates consist of all persons participating in the study or subsets of these participants.

In contrast, numerators for the estimated incidence (average risk) of becoming a case of drug abuse/dependence consist of persons who did not qualify as current or former drug abuse/dependence cases at baseline, but whose DIS reinterviews showed evidence of active drug abuse/dependence during the follow-up: these were subjects who started the interval as candidates for future occurrence of drug abuse/dependence, and who ended the interval qualifying for the DIS/DSM-III diagnosis. Denominators for estimated incidence (average risk) of becoming a case of drug abuse/dependence are based on the experience of all participants who started the interval as candidates for future occurrence of drug abuse/dependence, without regard for abuse/dependence status at follow-up: the experience of subjects whose baseline DIS showed either a currently active drug/dependence syndrome or a past history is counted in neither the numerators nor the denominators for these incidence estimates.

These methods of estimating current prevalence, lifetime prevalence, and cumulative incidence are consistent with broadly accepted epidemiological practices. Because the data are based on survey samples and on self-report interviews, there are a variety of cautions associated with the resulting estimates. These issues are the subject of separate reports on methods used in the ECA Program [23,25,32]. Two published monographs describe additional details about the methods and results of the ECA surveys [33,34].

IV. THE RISK AND PREVALENCE OF DRUG ADDICTION AND RELATED CLINICAL SYNDROMES

A. Risk Estimates for Drug Abuse/Dependence Syndromes

The risk of drug addiction and related clinical syndromes is determined by (1) the presence of conditions that are more or less favorable to drug exposure, and (2) the presence of conditions that are more or less favorable to development of a clinical syndrome once exposure takes place. This formulation happens to be congruent with Frost's statement of epidemiological theory as applied to infectious diseases [35]; others have arrived at related formulations independently (e.g., see Refs. 11, 36, 37).

According to the best available evidence, the only individuals who are not at risk of becoming a new case of drug addiction and related clinical syndromes are those who already have become cases. At the level of the individual, we now have no way of knowing who will be spared and who will become a case of drug addiction. As far as we can tell, there is no individual whose level of risk is zero. For the time being, the set defined by the presence of "invulnerability" to drug addiction remains an empty set.

Even though the zero-risk set is empty, individual differences in the risk of drug addiction can be inferred from a nonrandom distribution of the incidence of drug abuse/dependence syndromes in human populations. For example, Eaton et al. recently published age-specific annual incidence estimates for drug abuse/dependence, separately for the adult males and females who were studied prospectively for the ECA surveys [38]. At the population level, these annual incidence estimates are a statistical summary of the individual risks of developing drug abuse/dependence for the first time during adult life, *among individuals who have survived into adulthood with no prior history of drug abuse/dependence*. Stated differently, these incidence estimates express the average probability of becoming a case of drug abuse/dependence for the first time during a year of adult life, among the adult candidates for first-time occurrence of drug abuse/dependence. Thus, these estimates of average risk at the population level express the dynamic occurrence of drug abuse/dependence in adulthood.

It is important to recognize that annual incidence estimates are fundamentally different from lifetime prevalence estimates discussed later in this chapter. Unlike annual incidence, which reflects the average risk of developing drug abuse/dependence for the first time during some stated period of time, a lifetime prevalence proportion is an estimate of ever having been a case of drug abuse/dependence among persons who have survived to be studied at some particular point in time [39].

Based on ECA incidence data, the estimated average risk of becoming a new case of drug abuse/dependence in adulthood is 1.09%/year. As an indication of nonrandom distribution at the population level, the estimated annual incidence for adult males is 1.66%/year; for adult females, it is 0.66%/year [38]. Of course, this sex difference in annual incidence relates back to possible differences in risk at the individual level, to be discussed in Section VI.

The nonrandom distribution of drug abuse/dependence also is apparent in age-specific annual incidence estimates based on ECA survey data. Whereas the average risk of becoming a new case of drug abuse/dependence was 1.09%/year for adults of all ages, it was 2.84%/year for young adults aged 18–29 years old (SE = 0.53%); 0.69%/year for those 30–44 years old (SE = 0.18%); and less than 0.05%/year for adults age 45 years and older [38].

The pattern of strong age-dependent variation in annual incidence of drug abuse/dependence can be seen clearly in smoothed curves based on regression modeling, as depicted in Figure 1. On the left is the smoothed age-specific incidence curve for adult males, which shows sharply declining values from age 18 to near-zero values after age 44. On the right, the smoothed curve for females also shows sharply declining values with increasing age, though it should be noted that the peak predicted annual incidence for females is 2.75%/year (at age 18), as compared to a corresponding peak value close to 8.0%/year for 18-year-old males.

The smoothed curves also serve as a reminder that the incidence of drug addiction and related conditions does not begin at age 18. Rather, first illicit drug use and initial drug problems often are experiences of adolescence. This is apparent in the age of onset distributions shown in Figure 2. The data for these distributions were obtained by asking adult ECA subjects with a DIS-identified lifetime history of drug abuse/dependence to tell their ages of

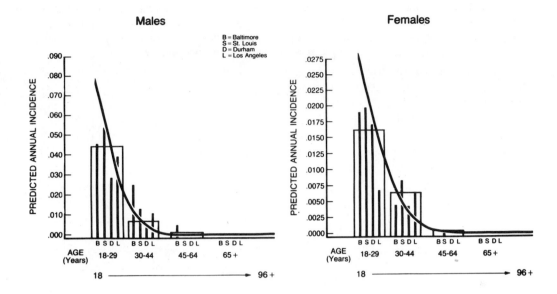

Figure 1 Estimated annual incidence of DIS/DSM-III drug abuse/dependence, separately for males and females, based on prospective data from four sites of the NIMH Epidemiologic Catchment Area Program: Baltimore (MD), St. Louis (MO), Durham-Piedmont (NC), and Los Angeles (CA), 1981–85. All values shown are percentages (per year). The smoothed curve is based on regression modeling of the association between age and the probability of becoming a drug abuse/dependence case. The histogram blocks show estimates for the following age groups: 18–29, 30–44, 45–64, and 65 years and older. Within the histogram blocks, the vertical bars show estimates for each of the four ECA sites represented in these age-specific estimates. Placement of the bars along the abscissa is approximate. (From Ref. 38, used with permission.)

initial drug use and drug problems. While many of these cases reported initiation during adult years, a large proportion already had experienced at least one drug problem by age 18. The question of age-specific incidence for adolescent drug abuse/dependence should be answered within the next decade, as soon as child-oriented ECA studies have been completed.

B. Prevalence Estimates for Drug Abuse/Dependence Syndromes

At any point in time, the number of currently active drug abuse/dependence cases in the population consists of long-standing cases plus recently developed cases. It follows that the prevalence of currently active drug abuse/dependence is determined not only by the incidence or risk of drug problems, but also by the duration of previously developed cases [39,40]. In theory, one of the most potent determinants of duration in drug abuse/dependence is availability and effectiveness of treatment. Another key determinant is mortality; i.e., whether death terminates an active case. Of course, neither treatment of cases nor their mortality influences the incidence or risk of drug abuse/dependence in any direct manner [39].

For reasons such as these, prevalence analyses bear uncertain value in the search for causes or other factors associated with risk of drug abuse/dependence (i.e., risk factors and risk indicators). This is true for analyses of lifetime prevalence data, which are especially dependent upon selective survivorship, mortality, and out-migration, and also for analysis of prevalence data on currently active cases. The basic problem is not knowing whether

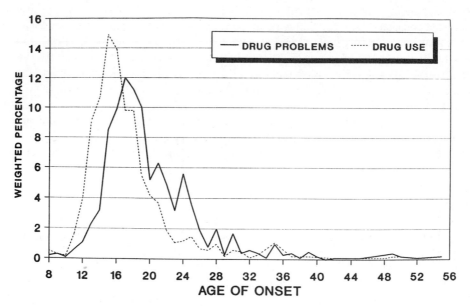

Figure 2 Estimated percentage distribution of cases qualifying for the DIS/DSM-III lifetime diagnosis of drug abuse/dependence, separately for age of onset of illicit drug use and for age of onset of the initial problem attributed to illicit drug use. Baseline data from the NIMH Epidemiologic Catchment Area surveys in New Haven (CT), Baltimore (MD), St. Louis (MO), Durham-Piedmont (NC), and Los Angeles (CA), 1980–84. The percentages are based on a weighting procedure that compensates for varying sample segment selection probabilities, with a poststratification adjustment to make the total estimated population distribution for cases and noncases balanced with the age-sex-race distributions for the U.S. population in 1980. (From Ref. 23, used with permission.)

prevalence variation is determined by differential survivorship among cases, by differences in access to effective treatment, or by other conditions that influence duration of drug abuse/dependence and thereby its prevalence [39,40].

Despite these weaknesses, prevalence estimates do have some valuable uses. For example, in planning for intervention and treatment services, there is need for estimates of present caseloads; these can be derived by knowing the prevalence of currently active cases [40]. It also should be mentioned that lifetime prevalence analyses sometimes have pointed in the right direction, even though they yield information of uncertain value in the search for causes or risk factors. To illustrate, lifetime prevalence analyses have implicated sex and age as indicators of the risk of drug abuse/dependence [41]. As shown in Figure 1, these implications were borne out in the estimates for incidence and risk of drug abuse/dependence [38].

Based on ECA data for the United States, an estimated 2.67% of the adult population qualifies as a currently active case of drug abuse/dependence, with at least one drug problem in the year prior to ascertainment (SE = 0.22%). This proportion might double in size if currently active drug abuse/dependence were defined in terms of recent illicit drug use and did not require persistence of a drug problem [23].

Among adult men, the prevalence of currently active drug abuse/dependence was estimated as 4.0% (SE =0.38%). For adult women, the corresponding estimate was 1.37% (SE = 0.21%). As in the incidence estimates, prevalence declined sharply with age [23].

Because former cases are included, the lifetime prevalence of drug abuse/dependence almost always will be greater than prevalence of currently active cases. For all adults, the ECA lifetime prevalence estimate was 6.19% (SE = 0.25%); for adult men, it was 7.72%

(SE = 0.40%), and for adult women, it was 4.78% (SE = 0.31%). Again, age-specific estimates varied considerably, reflecting not only recent conditions of adulthood in American society, but also long-standing cohort, period, and age differences in the population's experience with illicit drug use. At ages 18–29, the lifetime prevalence for both sexes was an estimated 13.46% (SE = 0.63%); for men aged 18–29, it was 15.96% (SE = 0.96%), and for women aged 18–29, it was 10.92% (SE = 0.82%). Estimates for older age groups were one-half those values or lower [23].

To provide a comparison with these values for lifetime prevalence of clinically defined syndromes of drug abuse and dependence, the ECA surveys also produced estimates for lifetime prevalence of illicit drug use. For all adults, the estimate was 30.48%; for adult men it was 36%, and for adult women it was 25%. Thus, overall, roughly one-fifth of adults reporting a history of illicit drug use (on one or more occasion) also qualified as currently active or former cases of drug abuse/dependence.

The ECA lifetime prevalence estimates for illicit drug use were roughly comparable to corresponding estimates from recent National Institute of Drug Abuse (NIDA) surveys of the household population (e.g., see Ref. 42), though they were somewhat on the low side. This was true even though the ECA samples included residents of prisons, mental hospitals, and other institutions. Prison residents especially were a high prevalence group. Over 55% of male prison residents and more than 70% of female prison residents qualified as currently active or former cases of drug abuse/dependence. Even so, because the number of adults living in institutions is small relative to the number of adults living in households, inclusion of these high-prevalence groups generally had little impact on prevalence estimation. For example, as compared with the lifetime prevalence estimate of 7.72% for all adult men, the estimate based solely upon the ECA household sample was 7.58%. Corresponding values for women were 4.78% and 4.79% [23,43].

The homeless represent a segment of the general population not frequently sampled in drug abuse surveys, and not included in the multisite collaborative study plan for the ECA Program. However, a special survey of homeless adults was conducted in several ECA sites, including Baltimore, Maryland. Results from this survey showed the homeless also to be a generally high-prevalence group for drug abuse/dependence, often complicated by the presence of alcohol abuse/dependence and other psychiatric conditions [44]. Nonetheless, even though the homeless became a large and growing segment of the population during the 1980s, this segment still is quite small relative to the household population. As a result, inclusion of data on the homeless would not be expected to increase the reported drug abuse/dependence prevalence estimates to any great extent.

In a final note on these lifetime prevalence estimates, it should be mentioned that a small difference in a prevalence estimate can make a large difference in caseloads for outreach, intervention, treatment, and aftercare programs. This is because a prevalence estimate is a proportion that is multiplied by the number in the population to yield an estimated number of cases. In the United States, the number of adults is well over 150 million. Thus, even a small difference in a prevalence estimate of the type reported here is translated into a large difference in number of cases to be cared for. This note of caution should be borne in mind while considering the topic of special populations such as the homeless, the imprisoned, and others in group quarters, who typically are ignored in epidemiological surveys of the so-called "general" population.

C. Prevalence Estimates for Drug Addiction

While an estimated 7.72% of adult men have a DIS-identified lifetime history of either drug abuse or drug dependence or both, an estimated 4.55% qualified for the DIS/DSM-III drug dependence diagnosis (with or without abuse). The drug dependence estimate for men aged 18–29 was 9.04%; for men aged 30–44 it was 5.14%, and for men aged 45–64 it was 0.83%. Among elderly men aged 65 years and older, the lifetime prevalence of drug dependence was 0.12%, with a standard error at least as large as the estimate itself [23]. Because DSM drug dependence criteria conform generally to accepted concepts of drug addiction, these values might serve well as approximations for the lifetime prevalence of drug addiction among adult men.

The lifetime prevalence of DIS/DSM-III drug dependence among adult women (with or without drug abuse) was an estimated 2.64%. The drug dependence estimate for women aged 18–29 was 5.51%; for women aged 30–44 it was 3.03%, and for women aged 45–64 it was 0.77%. Among elderly women aged 65 years and older, the lifetime prevalence of drug dependence was 0.05%, also with a large standard error [23].

V. CHARACTERISTICS OF PERSONS WITH A LIFETIME HISTORY OF DRUG ABUSE/DEPENDENCE

It should be understood that the DIS-identified cases with a lifetime history of drug abuse/ dependence for the most part were individuals who qualified for DIS/DSM-III diagnoses of cannabis abuse, cannabis dependence, or both. This can be seen in Table 2, which shows characteristics of these 1316 drug abuse/dependence cases. In constructing this table, no hierarchical plan was followed. Thus, one individual might be counted as a case of heroin dependence and also as a case of cannabis abuse or dependence. Further, the 2630 cases of alcohol abuse/ dependence have been included in Table 2 for comparison. These alcohol abuse/dependence cases were not counted in the group of 1316 drug abuse/dependence cases unless abuse/ dependence involving federally controlled drugs was diagnosed as well. An estimated 21% of DIS-identified alcohol abuse/dependence cases also qualify for at least one DIS/DSM-III drug abuse/dependence diagnosis (see Table 2).

In Table 2, columns 1 and 2 present unweighted numbers and proportions corresponding to the characteristics of drug abuse/dependence cases in the ECA sample. The remaining columns give the unweighted number of cases for each drug-specific category of abuse/ dependence syndromes, along with weighted proportions to indicate characteristics of these cases, where the weighting scheme was designed to compensate for variable sample selection probabilities and to yield age-sex-race distributions comparable to the U.S. population in 1980. The rationale and nature of this weighting procedure are described elsewhere [34].

Considering all DIS-identified cases of drug abuse/dependence in the sample, a total of 876 (67%) were living in households at the time of sampling (see Table 2, columns 1 and 2). However, because household residents were undersampled with respect to residents of prisons and other institutions, this proportion does not give an accurate portrayal of where drug abuse/dependence cases are located in the general population. The weighting procedure takes this difference in sample selection probabilities into account. As shown in column 3 of Table 2, after weighting, an estimated 98% of adult drug abuse/dependence cases reside in households, with fewer than 1% in prison or jail, and the remainder in treatment programs, mental hospitals, and other group quarters.

Each of the columns of Table 2 shows that the preceding general statement about residential locations of drug abuse/dependence cases is true mainly for cases of abuse/dependence involving cannabis, amphetamine-like stimulants, sedative-hypnotic-anxiolytic drugs, hallucinogens, and alcohol. This generality is not so true for abuse/dependence cases involving heroin and associated opioids or cocaine. An estimated 7% of cases with lifetime diagnoses for an opioid and/or cocaine syndrome were residing in jails or prisons.

Table 2 Characteristics of Individuals with a History of Currently Active or Past DSM/DSM-III Drug and Alcohol Abuse/Dependence Syndromes.[a,b]

Selected characteristics	Characteristics of cases with a DIS/DSM diagnosis for drug abuse/dependence (all drug groups)			Characteristics of cases who qualified for the DIS/DSM-III lifetime diagnosis of drug abuse/dependence, specific for individual drug groups (weighted percentages)						Weighted % of alcohol abuse/dependence cases (n=2630)
	Unweighted number of cases (n=1316)	Unweighted percentage of cases (n=1316)	Weighted percentage of cases (n=1316)	Cannabis group (n=837)	Heroin-opioid group (n=364)	Amphetamine stimulant group (n=314)	Sedative-hypnotic-anxiolytic group (n=289)	Cocaine group (n=101)	Hallucinogen group (n=97)	
Currently living in a household	876	67	98	99	92	98	97	91	96	99
Currently living in a prison/jail	—	—	<1	1	7	2	2	7	3	<1
Male	854	65	60	63	64	59	54	55	70	83
Black (self-designated)	367	29	9	11	15	2	3	3	<1	10
Hispanic (self-designated)	163	13	4	4	5	4	5	6	8	7
Current age:										
18–29 years	832	63	67	74	54	58	61	59	78	38
30–44 years	436	33	29	25	41	37	29	35	19	32
45–64 years	43	3	3	<1	6	5	9	6	3	23
65 years or older	5	<1	<1	<1	0	<1	0	0	0	7
With a college degree	172	13	18	21	8	12	9	5	10	11
Some college, no degree	340	26	33	32	28	36	31	38	35	21
High school diploma, no college	287	22	25	26	24	24	20	18	8	26
Some high school, no diploma	415	32	20	19	33	22	34	34	34	24
Currently married	325	25	35	31	32	43	37	25	34	50
Now separated or divorced	278	21	15	13	21	24	24	34	11	16
Never married	700	53	48	56	46	31	37	41	55	30
Lived as if married (never married)	305	23	14	15	19	12	13	21	17	7
Currently working for pay	551	72	74	74	82	72	72	88	79	74
Among those now working for pay:										
Managerial or professional job	139	25	24	25	16	22	16	16	7	20
Unskilled labor job	95	17	17	17	26	21	18	10	18	24

continued

Table 2 *(Continued)*

Selected characteristics	Characteristics of cases with a DIS/DSM diagnosis for drug abuse/dependence (all drug groups)			Characteristics of cases who qualified for the DIS/DSM-III lifetime diagnosis of drug abuse/dependence, specific for individual drug groups (weighted percentages)						
	Unweighted number of cases (n=1316)	Unweighted percentage of cases (n=1316)	Weighted percentage of cases (n=1316)	Cannabis group (n=837)	Heroin-opioid group (n=364)	Amphetamine stimulant group (n=314)	Sedative-hypnotic-anxiolytic group (n=289)	Cocaine group (n=101)	Hallucinogen group (n=97)	Weighted % of alcohol abuse/dependence cases (n=2630)
Earning less than $5000/year	55	13	15	16	0	13	12	17	37	9
Earning more than $50,000/year	7	2	2	1	2	4	1	4	3	3
Now receiving unemployment, disability, or welfare benefits	175	14	10	8	20	10	12	10	9	14
Qualifying for DIS/DSM lifetime diagnosis involving:										
Cannabis (e.g., marijuana)	837	64	72	100	45	43	46	42	67	15
Heroin or opioid analgesics	364	28	11	7	100	17	25	34	17	3
Amphetamine-like stimulants	314	24	27	16	42	100	52	41	47	7
Sedatives, hypnotics, anxiolytics	289	22	20	13	44	38	100	48	42	6
Cocaine	101	8	3	2	10	5	8	100	18	1
Hallucinogens (e.g., LSD)	97	7	6	5	9	10	12	31	100	2
Only one of the above drug groups	935	71	77	76	37	39	30	33	22	14
Two or more drug groups	381	29	23	24	63	31	70	67	78	7
Three or more drug groups	179	14	10	11	46	32	44	55	55	4
Five or more drug groups	82	6	4	6	27	16	22	37	34	2
All of the listed drug groups	14	1	<1	<1	5	2	3	15	9	<1
Qualifying for DIS/DSM lifetime diagnosis of alcohol abuse/dependence	656	50	48	46	69	62	71	85	64	100

[a]Cross-sectional survey data from the NIMH Epidemiologic Catchment Area Surveys conducted in New Haven (CT), Baltimore (MD), St. Louis (MO), Durham-Piedmont (NC), and Los Angeles (CA), 1980–1984.

[b]Except for numbers given within parentheses and in columns 1 & 2, all values in this table are estimated percentages, weighted to compensate for varying sample segment selection probabilities, and with poststratification factors to make the total estimated population distributions (cases and noncases combined) comparable to those of the U.S. population in 1980, with respect to age, sex, and race.

An estimated 60% of drug abuse/dependence cases were male (see Table 2, Row 3). The male-female ratio was more nearly equal for cases of abuse/dependence involving cocaine (55%) or sedative-hypnotic-anxiolytic drugs (54%); it was more pronounced for cases of hallucinogen abuse (70%) and also for the alcohol abuse/dependence syndromes (83%).

Overall, an estimated 9% of DIS-identified drug abuse-dependence cases were self-designated as black–not Hispanic; 4% were designated as Hispanic (see Table 2, rows 4 and 5). A somewhat greater proportion of heroin-opioid abuse/dependence cases were black (15%). As compared to all cases, blacks were to some extent underrepresented among abuse/dependence cases involving amphetamine stimulants, sedative-hypnotic-anxiolytic drugs, cocaine, and hallucinogens; Hispanics seemed to be somewhat overrepresented in the last two of these groups.

In a separate analysis of prospective data from the ECA Program, Ritter and Anthony have found that blacks and Hispanics were at essentially equal risk of initiating or progressing into repeat-occasion cocaine use during the ECA follow-up interval, as compared to other population groups, including those self-designated as white–not Hispanic [45]. We are not certain if this situation has changed since ECA data gathering in the early 1980s, perhaps as part of the epidemic of "crack" cocaine smoking in the United States after 1986.

The proportional distribution of drug abuse/dependence cases by age conforms with the age-specific lifetime prevalence estimates reported in the prior section of this chapter (see Table 2, rows 6–9). Younger adults aged 18–29 predominate (67%), whereas elderly cases were rare (<1%). By comparison, cases of cannabis abuse/dependence and hallucinogen abuse were more frequently in the younger adult group (74 and 78%, respectively); cases of heroin-opioid abuse/dependence were not (54%). With respect to age, it is notable that only 38% of the alcohol abuse/dependence cases were aged 18–29, whereas 7% were aged 65 years and older (see Table 2, last column).

The educational levels of drug abuse/dependence cases varied considerably across types of drug abuse/dependence. At one extreme, only 5% of the cocaine abuse cases held a college degree (see Table 2, row 10); heroin-opioid cases also were not likely to have earned college degrees (8%). At the other extreme, 21% of the cannabis abuse/dependence cases were degreed.

There also were some apparent differences between cases involving marital status and living arrangements (see Table 2, rows 14–17). Overall, 35% of the drug abuse/dependence cases were currently married, as compared to only 25% of the cocaine abuse cases and 50% of the alcohol abuse/dependence cases. The cocaine abuse cases were more likely to be currently separated or divorced (34%), or never married but living with a partner as if married (21%). Among the cases, those with abuse/dependence syndromes involving either cannabis or hallucinogens were most likely never to have been married (56 and 55%, respectively, as compared to 48% among all cases).

Almost three-quarters of the drug abuse/dependence cases were employed and working for pay, either part time or full time (see Table 2, row 18). More than 80% of the heroin-opioid cases and almost 90% of the cocaine abuse cases were working for pay. However, managerial and professional specialty jobs were underrepresented among the currently working heroin-opioid and cocaine cases, as compared to all currently employed drug abuse/dependence cases (16 vs 25%); unskilled labor jobs were overrepresented among employed heroin-opioid cases (26%), but underrepresented among employed cocaine cases (10%), as compared to all cases currently working for pay (17%).

With respect to earnings, an estimated 15% of all employed drug abuse/dependence cases had an annual income of under $5000; an estimated 2% had a reported annual income in excess of $50,000 (see Table 2, rows 21–22). By comparison, none of the employed heroin-opioid cases had a reported annual income under $5000, but 37% of the employed hallucinogen abuse cases did so. There was little variability across drug diagnosis groups in the proportion earning more than \$50,000/year, though it is of note that 4% of the workers in the cocaine group and in the amphetamine-like stimulant group were in this category (vs the mean value of 2% for all currently employed cases).

A total of 10% of the drug abuse/dependence cases were current recipients of unemployment, disability, or welfare benefits, based on ECA self-report interview data (see Table 2, row 23). Among drug diagnosis groups, the cases of cannabis abuse/dependence were least likely to be receiving these benefits (8%), whereas the heroin-opioid abuse/dependence cases were most likely (20%).

The remainder of Table 2 gives some indication of the extent to which individual cases qualified for more than one DIS lifetime diagnosis for drug abuse/dependence syndromes. Overall, 72% of the DIS/DSM-III drug abuse/dependence cases qualified as cases of cannabis abuse/dependence (see Table 2, row 24). In addition, the cannabis abuse/dependence diagnosis was assigned to 67% of the hallucinogen abuse cases. However, only 15% of alcohol abuse/dependence cases qualified for the cannabis abuse/dependence diagnosis, and the other groups were intermediate, with values ranging from 42 to 46%.

Abuse/dependence syndromes involving heroin and other opioids were characteristic of 11% of all drug abuse/dependence cases and 3% of alcohol abuse/dependence cases. In contrast, 34% of the cocaine abuse cases also had heroin-opioid abuse/dependence, as did 25% of cases affected by abuse/dependence syndromes involving sedative, hypnotic, or anxiolytic drugs.

On average, 27% of the drug abuse/dependence cases qualified for abuse/dependence diagnoses involving amphetamine-like stimulant drugs. This was true for 16% of the cannabis abuse/dependence cases, and only 7% of the alcohol abuse/dependence cases. By comparison, 52% of cases with sedative-hypnotic-anxiolytic abuse/dependence syndromes and 47% with hallucinogen abuse also qualified for a stimulant abuse/dependence diagnosis. Corresponding values for heroin-opioid cases and for cocaine abuse cases were 42 and 41%, respectively.

The estimated proportion of drug abuse/dependence cases with abuse or dependence involving sedative, hypnotic, or anxiolytic drugs was 20%. Estimates for the specific drug diagnosis groups ranged from a low of 6% among cases with alcohol abuse/dependence to a high of 48% among the cocaine abuse cases.

Whereas 42% of the cocaine abuse cases also qualified for heroin-opioid abuse/dependence, 10% of the heroin-opioid cases qualified for the cocaine abuse diagnosis, as compared with 2% of the cannabis abuse/dependence cases. The hallucinogen abuse cases had an exceptionally high prevalence of DIS-identified cocaine abuse (18%), whereas a surprising low value was obtained for persons diagnosed with abuse/dependence on amphetamine-like stimulants (5%).

Another reflection of co-occurrence involving cocaine abuse and hallucinogen abuse was the high prevalence of hallucinogen abuse among those with cocaine abuse (31%), as compared with only 5% among cannabis abuse/dependence cases and 2% of alcohol abuse/dependence cases. Intermediate estimates were obtained for the other diagnostic groups.

A different impression of co-occurring drug and alcohol abuse/dependence syndromes can be found in the estimates for the number of lifetime diagnoses assigned by the DIS. As shown in Table 2, row 30, a total of 77% of the drug abuse/dependence cases qualified for only one abuse/dependence diagnosis involving controlled drugs; 23% qualified for two or more drug diagnoses; 10% qualified for three or more drug diagnoses, and 4% qualified for five or more drug diagnoses. The values for the cannabis abuse/dependence cases are quite similar to these values for all cases.

At one extreme, it was found that 22% of the hallucinogen abuse cases qualified for hallucinogen abuse and nothing else. Fully 78% of the hallucinogen abuse cases also qualified for an additional drug diagnosis: often cocaine abuse or cannabis abuse/dependence. A total of 55% of these cases qualified for three or more drug diagnoses (including hallucinogen abuse), and 34% qualified for five or more drug diagnoses.

At another extreme, just 14% of the alcohol abuse/dependence cases qualified for only one DIS abuse/dependence diagnosis involving controlled drugs. An additional 7% qualified for two or more drug diagnoses, so that an estimated 21% of the alcohol abuse/dependence cases qualified for at least one drug abuse/dependence diagnosis. An estimated 2% of the alcohol abuse/dependence cases qualified for five or more drug diagnoses.

What is notable about the intermediate groups of cases is the frequency with which individuals qualified for three or more drug diagnoses. Only for cannabis abuse/dependence and alcohol abuse/dependence did this frequency fall below 30%.

Finally, one of the most important findings of the ECA surveys on drug abuse/dependence concerned how frequently drug abuse/dependence cases also qualified for other DIS diagnoses. For example, as shown in Table 3, among the drug diagnosis groups, the lowest frequency of alcohol abuse/dependence was found among cases of cannabis abuse/dependence (46%). That is, almost one-half of the DIS-identified cases of cannabis abuse/dependence also qualified for the DIS/DSM-III diagnosis of alcohol abuse/dependence. Among DIS-identified cases of DSM-III cocaine abuse, an estimated 85% qualified as currently active or former cases of DIS/DSM-III alcohol abuse/dependence (see Table 3).

In a separate analysis of age at onset data from the ECA Program, Anthony and Helzer have found that alcohol intoxication preceded illicit drug use for an estimated 64% of the individuals who received at least one DIS drug diagnosis and also the DIS alcohol abuse/dependence diagnosis. Alcohol intoxication clearly came after illicit drug use for 13.7% of these cases. Further, the first alcohol problem came in advance of the first illicit drug problem for 43%; the problem involving illicit drugs clearly came first for 36% [23].

The degree of co-occurrence between the lifetime diagnosis of drug abuse/dependence and the lifetime diagnosis of alcohol abuse/dependence can be conveyed by an estimated ratio of lifetime prevalence for the alcohol disorders among persons with and without the other drug disorders. Estimated from ECA lifetime prevalence values for alcohol abuse/dependence, this ratio is 4.1 [23].

Corresponding non-zero ratios indicating co-occurrence of drug abuse/dependence with DIS diagnoses for other disorders were in a range from 1.9 (phobic disorders) to more than 10.0 (antisocial personality; manic episode). The intermediate ratios generally were between 3.0 and 4.0: these ratios indicated co-occurrence of DIS/DSM-III drug abuse/dependence with DIS-identified major depression, dysthymia, obsessive-compulsive disorder, and panic disorder [31]. The validity of these co-occurrence ratios is unknown. For example, they might be spuriously high, owing to shared methods co-variation (i.e., reliance upon the DIS self-report method for making both the drug diagnoses and the other diagnoses).

VI. A STUDY OF SUSPECTED CAUSES AND RISK FACTORS FOR THE DRUG ABUSE/DEPENDENCE SYNDROMES
(James C. Anthony and Vivien T. Chen)

A. Introduction

As explained in the introduction to this chapter and in Section IV, short of a field experiment, epidemiological analyses of prospectively gathered data generally can give the least clouded view of suspected causes of drug addiction and related syndromes. Prospectively gathered data can limit measurement errors that sometimes contaminate cross-sectional and

Table 3 Estimated Prevalence of DIS/DSM-III Alcohol Abuse-Dependence Among Currently Active and Former Cases of DIS/DSM-III Drug Abuse/Dependence Syndromes[a]

Type of drug abuse/dependence	Number of cases	Estimated[b] prevalence of DIS/DSM-III alcohol abuse/dependence (%)
Cannabis	837	46
Heroin-opioid	364	69
Amphetamine-like stimulant	314	62
Sedatives, hypnotics, anxiolytics	289	71
Cocaine	101	85
Hallucinogens	97	64
All drug abuse/dependence cases	1316	48

[a]Cross-sectional data from the NIMH Epidemiologic Catchment Area survey samples in New Haven (CT), Baltimore (MD), St. Louis (MO), Durham-Piedmont (NC), and Los Angeles (CA), 1980–1984.
[b]Weighted to compensate for varying sample segment selection probabilities, and with poststratification factors to make the total estimated population distributions (cases and noncases combined) comparable to those of the U.S. population in 1980, with respect to age, sex, and race.

retrospective data. Moreover, they can constrain the influence of factors that affect duration of drug abuse/dependence, while focusing attention on factors associated with higher or lower levels of risk. Finally, to the extent that prospective analyses include data on noncases or control subjects as well as newly developed cases of drug abuse/dependence, these analyses actually can yield quantitative estimates for the magnitude of these associations (e.g., via the relative odds). For these reasons, it has seemed important to augment the basic incidence estimates, the prevalence analyses, and the comparison of drug abuse/dependence case characteristics derived from epidemiological samples drawn for the ECA Program. Thus, before concluding this review of epidemiological evidence on drug addiction, some preliminary results from risk factor analyses of prospectively gathered ECA data are presented. These results extend analyses of data on lifetime prevalence, 6-month prevalence, and 1-month prevalence that have been published elsewhere in the scientific literature [41,46–51) and edited books [23,43]. The new analyses that produced these preliminary results were conducted in an attempt to clarify some of the plausible causal associations that were suggested in the prior work on lifetime prevalence of drug abuse/dependence and the characteristics of drug abuse/dependence cases identified via ECA surveys.

In particular, these new analyses have been guided by a central concern about co-occurrence of psychiatric conditions with drug abuse/dependence, especially co-occurrence of alcohol abuse/dependence. For many reasons, including the evidence reported in Section V, it seemed likely that characteristics of alcohol abuse/dependence cases might put them at increased risk of drug abuse/dependence in adult life. Because of progress in early intervention and treatment programs for alcoholism, we thought it important to probe this suspected causal association linking alcohol abuse/dependence with later occurrence of drug abuse/dependence [23].

The foundation of prior epidemiological research upon which these analyses were based included the seminal investigation of Vietnam veterans, discussed in Section III of this chapter and described in detail by Helzer [24]. Helzer's study had a focus on use of and addiction to narcotics (heroin and other opioid drugs), with a distinction drawn between predictors of narcotics exposure (making narcotics use more likely) and predictors of narcotic addiction (among those using narcotics). The analysis strategy implicated alcohol abuse as a predictor of both narcotics use and narcotics addiction, and also identified other personal sociodemographic, behavioral, and psychiatric characteristics of veterans that were associated with occurrence of narcotics use and addiction after they had returned from Vietnam. These predictors, including city size, age, race, education, employment, marital status, job level, and depression, also have been taken into account in the present study [24].

B. Methods

In brief, data from the ECA baseline interviews were used to group adult household respondents into risk sets defined in terms of the census tract of residence and the age of the respondents (18–19, 20–24, 25–29 years, etc.). Risk of drug abuse/dependence in relation to age already had been studied [38], and risk sets defined by age provided control over age-related variables without necessitating multiple polytomous age terms at the stage of data analysis. By defining risk sets in terms of census tract, it was possible to focus the study on personal and behavioral characteristics of individuals that might be associated with increased risk of drug abuse/dependence, while constraining the influence of environmental or macrosocial characteristics (e.g., drug availability, local customs, city size, urban-rural differences). At the same time, residence-defined risk sets also allowed control over potential intersite methodological differences that otherwise might influence the study results. This approach to ECA analyses via residence-defined and age-defined risk sets has been used and explained in detail as part of prior studies, including published work on suspected causal associations between cocaine use and psychiatric disturbances, as well as risk factors for depression and suicide attempts (e.g., see Refs. 52–56).

The ECA subjects whose baseline interviews showed currently or formerly active DIS/DSM-III drug abuse/dependence were excluded from these risk sets because they no longer were at risk of developing drug abuse/dependence for the first time (see Sec. IV). Subsequently, follow-up data obtained by readministering the DIS after 1 year was used to identify incident cases of drug/dependence. Apparent new cases whose follow-up data indicated no active drug problem during the follow-up interval were excluded from the analysis, as in Eaton et al. [38]; the remaining incident cases were those with evidence of active drug problems during the follow-up interval.

In the analysis of data from the risk sets, multiple regression modeling was used to identify associations between the risk of drug abuse/dependence and suspected causes or risk factors that had been measured at baseline, including the lifetime history of psychiatric conditions such as alcohol abuse/dependence and sociodemographic characteristics found to be important by Helzer or others (e.g. 24). Owing to the grouping of subjects into risk sets, the underlying model was that of conditional logistic regression [57]; the computing software was PECAN.

As a practical matter, although the number of risk sets defined by census tracts and age was large, most of these risk sets did not include newly incident cases of drug abuse/dependence; thus, they made no contribution of information during data analysis. The total number of incident cases of drug abuse/dependence was 101. These cases belonged to 99 risk sets, each including from one to 19 candidates for future occurrence of drug abuse/dependence for a total of 342 candidates. Typically, the age of each case was within 4 years of the age of all noncase candidates in his or her risk set. For a small number of cases, it was necessary to combine adjacent age-defined sets within individual census tracts in order to avoid excluding these otherwise informative cases from the analysis.

To sharpen the focus of the study on conditions associated with increased risk of drug abuse/dependence once exposure to illicit drug use has occurred, subsidiary models were constructed after eliminating risk set members with no pre-baseline history of illicit drug use. That is, in these subsidiary vulnerability analyses, all cases and noncase candidates were individuals who had a baseline history of illicit drug use (but not drug abuse/dependence). The total number of risk sets for the vulnerability analyses was 56; there were 148 noncase candidates and 57 incident cases distributed across the risk sets. It turned out that virtually all of the cases had a pre-baseline history of illicit drug use; the exclusion of risk sets came about when noncases were eliminated because they had never engaged in illicit drug use. The result was a large number of risk sets in which a singleton case was grouped with no noncase candidates. Thus, the consequence of sharpening the focus on conditions of vulnerability after drug exposure was a loss of statistical power in the analyses. This should be borne in mind when considering the p-values from the vulnerability analyses. Here, as in most contexts, the p-values should be regarded as aids to interpretation of observed associations, not as arbitrary designators of what is important and what is not.

C. Results

Table 4 presents the results from the initial analyses based on all available cases and noncases in the 99 risk sets, as well as results from the subsidiary vulnerability analyses restricted to 56 risk sets and subjects who had a pre-baseline history of illicit drug use. The results are expressed in the form of relative odds estimates, based on conditional logistic regression models that take into account the risk set grouping factors of residence and age. Unless mentioned explicitly, these are not multiple regression models where advanced statistics are used to hold constant one or more variables while estimating the relative odds; uncontrolled confounding might be present [57].

Sex/Gender

Being female was associated with a reduced risk of becoming a new case of drug abuse/ dependence in adulthood, as shown in Table 4. This inverse risk factor association was observed in the initial analysis in which the odds of developing drug abuse/dependence among women was an estimated 0.44 times the corresponding odds for men (p = 0.001). The inverse association also was observed in the vulnerability analysis, but it was of reduced magnitude (relative odds, RO = 0.62) and precision of the estimate was compromised owing to the smaller number of observations (p = 0.156). The difference between a relative odds of 0.44 and one of 0.62 is not entirely insubstantial; it would seem to indicate that some of the male-female difference in risk of drug abuse/dependence can be explained by males being more likely to take illicit drugs in the first place.

Education

As compared to persons with neither a high school diploma, nor a General Equivalency Diploma (GED), nor a higher degree, those with a higher degree (e.g., B.S., A.A., M.D., Ph.D.) had lower odds of becoming a case of drug abuse/dependence (RO = 0.50; p = 0.091) in adult life (see Table 4). In the vulnerability analysis restricted to those with a history of illicit drug use, the degree of inverse association between holding a higher degree and the odds of drug abuse/dependence became even stronger (RO = 0.21) and the estimate was suitably precise (p = 0.009).

   The difference between the initial analysis and the vulnerability analysis might become clearer if the inverse of the relative odds estimates were calculated and interpreted. Taking the inverse of RO = 0.50, we have 2.0, which can be interpreted as conveying that the odds of becoming a new case of drug abuse/dependence are twice as great for persons without a high school diploma or GED, compared to persons holding any higher degrees. Taking the inverse of RO = 0.21, we obtain a value of 4.8, interpreted as showing that the odds of drug abuse/dependence are almost five times greater for persons without a diploma or GED, compared to those with the higher degree, among illicit drug users.

Table 4 Estimated Relative Risk of DIS/DSM-III Drug Abuse/Dependence Syndromes Among Adults, in Relation to Suspected Causes and Risk Factors[a]

Suspected risk factors	Reference category	Risk factor analyses based on all cases and noncases in 99 risk sets		Vulnerability analyses with a focus on the illicit drug users in 56 risk sets	
		Estimated relative odds	p-value	Estimated relative odds	p-value
Being female	Male	0.44	0.001	0.62	0.156
Educational level:	No diploma/degree				
high school diploma, GED		1.35	0.309	1.61	0.204
higher degree		0.50	0.091	0.21	0.009
Now working for pay	Not working	0.96	0.882	1.01	0.977
Job prestige ranking:	Lowest quartile				
2nd quartile		1.36	0.286	1.17	0.710
3rd quartile		0.99	0.977	0.78	0.640
Top quartile		0.64	0.341	0.26	0.042
Marital status:	Married				
never married		2.06	0.030	1.01	0.973
formerly married		1.61	0.283	0.88	0.804
Race/ethnicity:	White–not Hispanic				
Hispanic		0.84	0.787	1.79	0.499
black		2.02	0.095	1.49	0.510
other minority		0.67	0.577	0.97	0.975
History of DIS/DSM disorder:					
any DIS/DSM disorder	None	4.02	<0.001	2.82	0.003
antisocial personality disorder (ASP)	No ASP	5.25	0.009	3.41	0.066
alcohol abuse/dependence	No alcohol disorder	4.80	<0.001	4.01	<0.001
any affective disorder	No affective disorder	2.62	0.012	1.08	0.890
major depression	No major depression	2.70	0.028	0.99	0.992
dysthymic disorder	No dysthymia	4.13	0.013	2.01	0.313
bipolar disorder	No bipolar disorder	5.23	0.099	[b]	
schizophrenia	No schizophrenia	3.06	0.113	3.25	0.338
obsessive-compulsive disorder (OC)	No OC disorder	2.24	0.205	[b]	
any phobic disorder	No phobic disorder	1.04	0.918	0.99	0.979
agoraphobia	No agoraphobia	2.57	0.012	2.09	0.168

[a]Data from 101 incident cases and 342 noncases in residence-matched and age-matched risk sets drawn from the NIMH Epidemiologic Catchment Area household samples in New Haven (CT), Baltimore (MD), St. Louis (MO), Durham-Piedmont (NC), and Los Angeles (CA), 1980–1985.
[b]The observations were too sparsely distributed to yield a useful estimate.

Although Helzer did not find educational attainment to be a predictor of narcotics use or addiction among male Vietnam veterans, many drug abuse/dependence cases in treatment have a limited educational attainment [24]. Moreover, Clayton has suggested that failure to achieve expected goals in education might be a psychosocial risk factor for intensification of drug use and possible for drug problems [58]. The vulnerability analysis in particular offered evidence congruent with this hypothesis.

In this regard, it also should be noted that the anlyses did not coincide fully with a speculation voiced after a prior analysis of ECA lifetime prevalence data. Specifically, the lifetime prevalence analyses led us to consider that initiating but failing to complete an educational landmark might be associated with relatively higher rates of drug abuse/dependence [23]. The present, more probing analyses of incidence data have shown that the odds of developing drug abuse/dependence during adult life were not unusually different and possibly were lower for persons who did not complete high school, as compared to those who received a diploma or GED. This is indicated by a relative odds values of 1.35 (p = 0.309) and 1.61 (p = 0.204), which suggests that the diplomates might be a group at higher risk (see Table 4). Alternatively, it is conceivable that educational failure is most important as a risk factor for drug abuse/dependence that arises during adolescence, or that the present analyses did not codify educational attainment so as to draw out the "failures" in the educational process.

Employment

Being currently employed for pay was not strongly associated with the odds of developing drug abuse/dependence in adult life either via the first analysis with all available risk sets (RO = 0.96) or via the vulnerability analysis, as shown in Table 4 (RO = 1.01). Further, in the initial analysis, these odds did not seem to vary considerably in relation to a job prestige ranking according to quartiles. Nevertheless, in the vulnerability analysis, an apparently important and strong degree of association emerged in relation to job prestige. Specifically, as compared to persons working at jobs in the lowest quartile of job prestige, those working at the highest prestige jobs appeared to be at substantially lower risk of developing drug abuse/dependence (RO = 0.26; p = 0.042). Again, by taking the inverse, we can re-express these results in a different way: the risk of drug abuse/dependence was an estimated 3.8 times greater for workers in the lowest prestige jobs, as compared to workers in the highest prestige jobs. In both analyses, there was an apparent gradient in the relative odds: those in the 2nd quartile of job prestige appeared to be the least well off, since the corresponding relative odds estimates were in excess of 1 (though not reliably different from 1.0 when the p-values are taken into account).

Although Helzer did not find job level (classified as blue collar or white collar) to be an important predictor of narcotics use or addiction among male Vietnam veterans, there is a clinical literature on treated cases of drug abuse and dependence that is congruent with the results on job prestige that emerged from the present analyses. In addition, Helzer found a trend toward both greater exposure and more vulnerability for those with poorer jobs [24].

We note also that these results are not consistent with Helzer's discovery that unemployment was a predictor of vulnerability to narcotics addiction among narcotics users [24]. The relative odds estimates from the present analysis indicate virtually identical risk of drug abuse/dependence for both the unemployed and the currently employed (see Table 4).

Marital Status

Considering the evidence on both illicit drug users and those with no history of illicit drug use, it appears that the never married are at increased risk of becoming new cases of drug abuse/dependence, as compared to married persons. Shown in Table 4, the relative odds estimate for the never married versus the married was 2.06 (p = 0.030).

In the vulnerability analysis, there was essentially no difference in the odds for the never married versus the married (RO = 1.01; p = 0.973). This suggests that one reason for the originally observed difference might be a greater likelihood among the never married to use illicit drugs. However, once illicit drug use has occurred, it appears that being married has not been protective against development of drug abuse/dependence in adult life. The marital status analysis also showed that the formerly married (predominately separated or divorced persons, with a few widows) might be at increased risk of developing drug abuse/dependence. However, the degree of association with neither strong (RO = 1.61), nor was the estimate reliably different from 1.0 (p = 0.283). Moreover, in the vulnerability analysis, there was an inverse association (RO = 0.88).

To examine this association in greater detail, we tested for an interaction of sex and marital status, hypothesizing that formerly married men and formerly married women might differ in their risks of drug abuse/dependence as compared to the married. The results indicated that formerly married men were an estimated three times more likely to develop drug abuse/dependence as compared to married and never married men (RO = 3.22; p = 0.038). With the same married and never married men as a reference group, women were at lower risk of developing drug abuse/dependence: For formerly married women, the relative odds estimate was 0.17 (p = 0.032), and for the married and never married women, it was 0.54 (p = 0.028). The vulnerability analyses showed the same tendencies, but none of the estimated associations was statistically significant with a p value less than 0.05 (data not shown in a table).

Race/Ethnicity

Race/ethnicity did not appear to be a risk factor of major importance in relation to drug abuse/dependence syndromes developing during adulthood. As compared to those self-desginated as white–not Hispanic, the relative odds for black adults were 1.49–2.02 times as great (see Table 4). However, these estimates were not precise, and the reduced degree of association that can be observed in the vulnerability analysis suggests that important differences might be understood in relation to whether illicit drug use occurs. Based on his analyses of the Vietnam veteran data, Helzer reported that being black was a predictor of exposure to narcotics use, but not a predictor of vulnerability to narcotics addiction [24].

History of DIS/DSM Disorders

Turning our analyses toward pre-existing psychiatric conditions as potential causes or risk factors for drug abuse/dependence, we observed that persons with a history of any DIS-identified mental disorder (not including drug abuse/dependence) were at greater risk than those with no such history (see Table 4). This association was apparent in the vulnerability analysis (RO = 2.82; p = 0.003), and also in the analysis based on all available observations (RO = 4.02; p < 0.001).

Consistent with the long-standing literature on social maladjustment and drug addiction, adults with a history of DIS/DSM-III antisocial personality disorder also were at increased risk of drug abuse/dependence (see Table 4). In the vulnerability analysis, the estimated level of increased risk was 3.41 (p = 0.066); in the risk factor analysis that included nonusers as well as illicit drug users, the estimated level of increased risk was 5.25 (p = 0.009). Both relative odds estimates indicated a consistently elevated relative risk; the p-value in the vulnerability analysis should be understood in relation to the limited number of observations available for study, as mentioned in Section VI.B.

Because we had selected alcoholism for special focus in our continuing analyses, we were interested to find that both analyses indicated four to five times greater risk of developing drug abuse/dependence in adult life for persons with a history of alcohol abuse/dependence syndromes as compared to persons with no such history (see Table 4). Consistent with these results, Helzer found alcohol abuse since returning from Vietnam to be a predictor of exposure to narcotics use and also a predictor of vulnerability to narcotics addiction among users [24]. These results also jibe with prior evidence from lifetime prevalence analyses (e.g., see Table 3 and Ref. 31; also Chap. 1), and also with a separate literature on developmental sequencing of problem behavior [59].

In brief, virtually all of the DIS/DSM-III affective disorders were associated with risk of drug abuse/dependence in the initial risk factor analyses for this study (see Table 4, left-hand columns). However, the estimated relative odds dropped in magnitude and none were statistically significant at the p = 0.05 level in the vulnerability analyses (see Table 4, right-hand columns). The apparent conclusion is that major depression, dysthymia, and the other affective disorders identified by the DIS are not strongly associated with substantially increased risk of drug abuse/dependence once illicit drug use has occurred. However, this conclusion is contradicted by Helzer's study in which the presence of the depressive syndrome since Vietnam was a predictor of vulnerability to narcotics addiction, but not exposure to narcotic use. It is conceivable that the association found in Helzer's study is specific to opioid addiction, but not to the more generic diagnostic category marked off by DIS/DSM-III drug abuse/dependence.

DIS-identified schizophrenia and obsessive-compulsive disorder had some degree of association with risk of drug abuse/dependence. However, the estimates were not statistically reliable and in the case of obsessive-compulsive disorder the observations were too sparsely distributed to provide for useful estimation of the relative odds in the vulnerability analyses (see Table 4).

Although DIS-identified phobic disorders had essentially no association with risk of drug abuse/dependence, a specific phobic disorder in the form of agoraphobia showed a potentially important association (see Table 4). In the initial analysis, adults with a history of agoraphobia were found to be an estimated 2.57 times more likely to develop drug abuse/dependence, as compared to persons without agoraphobia (p = 0.012). In the vulnerability analysis, the associated p-value was 0.168, but there was little more than a slight reduction in the estimated degree of association (RO = 2.07). This indicates that agoraphobia might be important in the progression to drug/dependence syndromes once illicit drug use has occurred, with a possibility of additional influence at earlier stages in the developmental sequence toward drug abuse/dependence.

Continuing analyses of the association involving agoraphobia have indicated a possibly important interaction between agoraphobia and alcohol abuse/dependence. In these analyses, the agoraphobia cases with no history of alcohol abuse/dependence have emerged as an important subgroup in relation to risk of drug abuse/dependence. Further, it appears that the estimated association becomes stronger in multiple regression models that include a term to hold constant the presence of other phobic disorders. Results from these analyses and a more complete multiple regression modelling of these data will be the subject of future papers (e.g., see Refs. 60 and 61).

D. Discussion and Summary

Before summarizing these preliminary results, there are several sources of bias and possible limitations to be mentioned, including the somewhat limited nature of the ECA follow-up sample, which provided only 101 incident cases of drug abuse/dependence. A potentially important source of bias stems from use of the self-report interview method to ascertain cases and also to measure the suspected causes and risk factors. Even though the latter were measured at baseline, and the incidence of drug abuse/dependence was determined at follow-up, it is possible that reliance upon self-report interview data in this study has led to spuriously high estimates of the relative odds. This might be particularly true for the variables relating the DIS-identified psychiatric conditions, e.g., bias arising via shared methods co-variation.

Despite limitations such as these, the study represents one of the few opportunities to examine suspected causes and risk factors for drug abuse/dependence in a prospective epidemiological study of adults. The number of incident cases of drug abuse/dependence in this analysis, though limited, is without precedent in prior epidemiological field studies of drug addiction and related conditions, though some clinical samples and prevalence survey samples have been larger. The measurement of suspected causes and risk factors at baseline, with follow-up ascertainment of incident cases, represents an additional strength not often seen in studies of drug abuse/dependence.

Notwithstanding the preliminary nature of the regression models and the need for more exacting analyses, a few conclusions may be warranted. Specifically, neither race/ethnicity nor current employment status had strong or statistically reliable associations in relation to risk of drug abuse/dependence. On the other hand, characteristics associated with being female, having completed a higher degree after the high school diploma or GED, and job prestige ranking were inversely associated with risk of drug abuse/dependence. In part, it seemed that being female was associated with reduced risk as a result of conditions influencing whether illicit drug use occurs. By comparison, the inverse associations between educational attainment and job prestige were stronger when studying risks of drug abuse/dependence among illicit drug users than when studying these risks among all persons without regard to history of illicit drug use.

Marital status also appeared to be associated with risk of developing drug abuse/dependence in adult life. As was true with being female, having never married seemed important in relation to the conditions that influence whether illicit drug use occurs, but not necessarily in relation to occurrence of drug abuse/dependence among illicit drug users. In contrast, an exploratory analysis showed the estimated odds of drug abuse/dependence to be greater among formerly married men as compared to married or never married men; women had lower odds, whether formerly married or not. This pattern of associations held in analyses based on all persons and also in analyses searching for conditions of vulnerability to drug abuse/dependence among illicit drug users.

Finally, a history of alcohol abuse/dependence, a history of antisocial personality, and a history of agoraphobia, in separate analyses, were found to be associated with increased risk of drug abuse/dependence. The evidence indicated the importance of these conditions in relation to drug abuse/dependence vulnerability once illicit drug use has occurred, and also possibly in relation to earlier stages of development toward drug abuse/dependence. In contrast, major depression and other affective disorders appeared to have greatest importance at the earlier stage of abuse/dependence, but were of less or little importance as conditions of vulnerability among illicit drug users.

E. What Was Not Studied

A number of suspected causal associations were not studied in the course of these analyses of prospectively gathered data from the ECA Program. Macrosocial characteristics necessarily were constrained in order to provide sharper focus on personal and behavioral characteristics thought to influence occurrence of drug abuse/dependence; moreover, many of these macrosocial characteristics simply were not measured in the ECA collaborative study (e.g., drug availability; local attitudes toward illicit drug use). It also should be noted that the ECA surveys were conducted in the early 1980s; major determinants of drug abuse/dependence are likely to have remained the same since that time. Nonetheless, there is recent evidence of changing risk factor patterns over relatively short spans of time (e.g., see Refs. 11, 30, and 58).

In addition to the conditions of place and time that might have causally significant associations with the occurrence of drug addiction and related clinical syndromes, in future studies it would be important to consider family characteristics that might qualify as causes or risk factors. These characteristics include family history of alcohol and other drug abuse/dependence (e.g., see Refs. 62, and 63), which might be important in relation to biologically inherited genetic material, exposures during fetal development or during later development, and also family learning environments (e.g., see Refs. 64 and 65). Commensurate attention to the peer group, especially opportunities for exposure made available by peers [11], would be important as well. These family and peer characteristics also were not part of the ECA measurement plan.

Finally, it should be noted that this chapter has given little or no attention to the potential influence of government action and regulatory decisions on occurrence of drug addiction, nor to results from microsocial investigations of the spread of intravenous drug use or illicit drug use. These factors surely deserve consideration in any comprehensive conceptual model for the epidemiology of drug addiction (e.g., see Ref. 66). Combining investigation of macrosocial and microsocial influences and investigation of individual, personal characteristics within a single epidemiological study of clinically defined drug addiction would seem, in theory, to be an achievable goal.

VII. CONCLUSIONS

This chapter began with an introduction to the epidemiological study of drug addiction and related clinical syndromes. By intention, the introduction was written with a deliberate focus on the bridges between clinical practice, clinical research, epidemiology, and prevention research that are required for a full evaluation of suspected causal associations involving drug syndromes. This intentional focus resulted in a clear imbalance during the chapter's coverage of epidemiological methods and evidence concerning suspected causes and risk factors for clinically defined drug abuse/dependence syndromes.

Given this emphasis on the study of associations with potential causal significance for drug addiction, this chapter necessarily attended less to what has become a more dominant activity for epidemiologically minded researchers interested in drug abuse: namely, surveillance of the prevalence and occurrence of illicit drug use, and miscellaneous consequences of illicit drug taking. Readers are referred elsewhere for reviews of the surveillance material, which has more to do with illicit drug use and drug overdose than with clinically defined syndromes related to drug addiction [67].

Over the past 2 decades, the pendulum has swung away from clinico-epidemiological research on drug addiction in favor of the surveillance activities just mentioned. There is a need for the pendulum to swing in the other direction without swinging so far that the now-strong tradition of surveillance activities is undermined.

This can be accomplished by more deliberate bridging across the clinical sciences and other disciplines more closely aligned with epidemiological or field research on illicit drug use: sociology, psychology, social psychology, and the other social and behavioral sciences. To some extent, these bridges can be built by using the strongest clinical case-ascertainment methods in the planned and on-going field studies now carried out in the name of surveillance, social and behavioral science research (e.g., on deviance), and prevention research. However, because the clinically significant drug syndromes occur rather infrequently, there also is a requirement for bridges developed via greater use by clinical scientists of the hospital- or clinic-based epidemiological case-control strategy. If this bridge building is to be successful, there must be a greater tolerance for the study of cases coming to clinical attention. Fortunately, recent studies suggest that this greater tolerance would not produce major errors with respect to many characteristics of clinical cases (e.g., see Ref. 31). An on-going program of research with alternating or sequential clinical and population-based samples could provide mid-course corrections, even if temporarily misleading results were to arise owing to study of cases seeking treatment.

Along these lines, some of the best possible clinico-epidemiological research on the drug syndromes can be completed if three conditions are fulfilled. First, clinical scientists must arrange to have their clinical cases measured by the field survey methods used to assess these syndromes and their suspected causes and risk factors, in addition to the clinical case-ascertainment methods they might use for other purposes. Second, epidemiologists and field researchers must arrange to have their field survey participants measured in the same fashion, including, when possible, the best possible clinical case-ascertainment methods; for example, via two-stage designs (e.g., see Ref. 27). Three, a means must be created for bridging the clinical and field samples and using the information from each in the most sensible fashion; for example, via the epidemiologic case-base strategy described by Miettinen [8]. Recent NIDA initiatives for collaborative treatment research units and also ECA-like intensive metropolitan area population surveys would seem to offer a great deal of potential in this direction, provided these clinical and epidemiological efforts are coordinated with one another, as illustrated in recent research [e.g., 12].

Unlike studies restricted to clinical case series, strategies of this type lend themselves toward valid comparison of characteristics seen in clinical cases to characteristics of the population out of which the cases arise. If the population characteristics were to be based upon a nationally representative sample, and the clinical cases were to come from a more local aggregation of clinical facilities, the resulting comparison could represent an important step in the right direction. Eventually, the science should progress toward greater alignment of the cases and the source population for those cases, with resulting improvements in evaluation of suspected causes and risk factors. The coordination of NIDA-sponsored treatment research units and NIDA-sponsored metropolitan area surveys within a single conurbation will make this happen sooner rather than later.

In conclusion, over the past 20 years there has been a remarkable strengthening of epidemiology as a way of learning about the suspected causes of drug addiction and related clinical syndromes. During the same interval, the clinical, social, and behavioral sciences also have gained much-increased capacities for studying these causes. Nevertheless, key questions about the nature and suspected causes of the drug syndromes remain unanswered. Progress during the next 10 years and beyond may depend to a large extent upon our success in bridging these strengths and capacities, and managing to work together as each discipline moves forward.

ACKNOWLEDGMENTS

Supported in part by research grants to the author, made by the National Institute of Drug Abuse (DA03992, DA04392). The National Institute of Mental Health (NIMH) Epidemiologic Catchment Area Program was a series of five epidemiological research studies performed by independent research teams in collaboration with staff of the Division of Biometry and Epidemiology of the NIMH. The NIMH principal collaborators were Darrel A. Regier, Ben Z. Locke, and William Eaton. The Project Officers with William Eaton and Carl A. Taube. The principal investigators from the five sites and their grant numbers were as follows: New Haven (J.K. Myers; U01 MH 34224); Baltimore (M. Kramer; U01 MH 33870); St. Louis (L.N. Robins; U01 MH 33883); Durham-Piedmont (D. Blazer, L. George; U01 MH 35386); Los Angeles (R. Hough, M. Karno; U01 MH 35865). Section VI was co-authored by James C. Anthony and Vivien T. Chen. We are grateful to Jean Lavelle for word processing the manuscript and tables, and to John Harbold for drawing Figure 1.

REFERENCES

1. Morris, J.N. *Uses of Epidemiology.* 3rd ed. New York, Churchill Livingstone, 1975.
2. Lilienfeld, A.M., and Lilienfeld, D.E. *Foundations of Epidemiology.* Boston, Little, Brown, 1980.
3. Feinstein, A.R. *Clinical Epidemiology: The Architecture of Clinical Research.* Philadelphia, Saunders, 1985.
4. Kolb, L. (1925). Types and characteristics of drug addicts. *Ment. Hyg. 9:*300–313.
5. Kolb, L., and Ossenfort, W.F. (1938). The treatment of addicts at the Lexington Hospital. *South. Med. J. 31:*914–920.
6. Pescor, M.J. (1939). The Kolb classification of drug addicts. *Public Health Rep.* (Suppl.) No. 155.
7. Bishop, Y., et al. *Discrete Multivariate Analysis.* Cambridge, Massachusetts, MIT Press, 1975.
8. Miettinen, O.S. *Theoretical Epidemiology: Principles of Occurrence Research in Medicine.* New York, Wiley, 1985.
9. Breslow, N., and Day, N. *Statistical Methods in Cancer Research*, Lyon, International Agency for Research on Cancer, 1980.
10. Gerard, D.L., and Cornetsky, C. (1957). Adolescent opiate addiction: A study of control and addict subjects. *Psychiatr. A. 29:*457–486.
11. Chein, I., Gerard, D.L., Lee, R.S., Rosenfeld, E., and Wilner, D.M. *The Road to H.* New York, Basic Books, 1964.
12. Tomas, J.M., Vlahov, D., and Anthony, J.C. (1990). Association between intravenous drug use and early misbehavior. *Drug Alcohol Depend. 25:*79–89.
13. Robins, L.N. *Deviant Children Grown Up.* Baltimore, Williams & Wilkins, 1966.
14. Kellam, S.G., Brown, C.H., Rubin, B.R., et al. Paths leading to teenage psychiatric symptoms and substance use: Developmental epidemiological studies in Woodlawn, *Childhood Psychopathology and Development* (S.B. Guze, F.J. Earls, and J.E. Barrett, eds.). New York, Raven Press, pp. 17–47, 1983.
15. Block, J., Block, J.H., and Keyes, S. (1988). Longitudinally foretelling drug usage in adolescence: Early childhood personality and environmental precursors. *Child Devel. 59:*336–355.
16. Kellam, S.G., Anthony, J.C., Brown, C.H., et al. Prevention research and early risk behaviors in cross-cultural studies, *Needs and Prospects of Child and Adolescent Psychiatry* (M.H. Schmidt and H. Remschmidt, eds.). Toronto, Hans Huber Verlag, pp. 241–254, 1989.
17. Kellam, S.G., Werthamer-Larsson, L., Dolan, L., et al. *Developmental Epidemiologically-Based Preventive Trials: Baseline Modelling of Early Target Behaviors and Depressive Symptoms.* Baltimore, Maryland, The Johns Hopkins Prevention Research Center, submitted.
18. Hawkins, J.D., and Weis, J.G. (1985). The social development model: An integrated approach to delinquency prevention. *J. Primary Prevent. 6:*73–97.
19. American Psychiatric Association. *Diagnostic and Statistical Manual of Mental Disorders.* Washington, D.C., 1980.
20. Kosten, T.R., Rounsaville, B.J., Babor, T.F., Spitzer, R.L., Williams, J.B. (1987). Substance-use disorders in DSM-III-R. Evidence for the dependence syndrome across different psychoactive substances. *Br. J. Psychiatry 151:*834–843.
21. Edwards, G., Gross, M.M. (1976). Alcohol dependence: Provisional description of a clinical syndrome. *Br. Med. J. 1:*1058–1061.
22. World Health Organization. *Mental, Behavioural and Developmental Disorders: Clinical Descriptions and Diagnostic Guidelines.* I.C.D.—10, 1987 Draft of Chapter V, Categories F00-F99. WHO, Division of Mental Health, Geneva, 1987.
23. Anthony, J.C., and Helzer, J.E. Syndromes of drug abuse and dependence, *Psychiatric Disorders in America* (L.N. Robins and D.A. Regier, eds.). New York, Free Press, 1990.
24. Helzer, J.E. Specification of predictors of narcotic use versus addiction, *Studying Drug Abuse* (L.N. Robins, ed.). New Brunswick, New Jersey, Rutgers University Press, pp. 173–205, 1985.
25. Robins, L.N., Helzer, J.E., Croughan, J., and Ratcliff, K.S. (1981). National Institute of Mental Health Diagnostic Interview Schedule: Its history, characteristics, and validity. *Arch. Gen. Psychiatry 38:*381–389.

26. Helzer, J.E., Robins, L.N., McEvoy, L.T., et al. (1985). A comparison of clinical and diagnostic interview schedule diagnoses: Physician re-examination of lay-interviewed cases in the general population. *Arch. Gen. Psychiatry 42*:657–666.

27. Anthony, J.C., Folstein, M.F., Romanoski, A.J., et al. (1985). Comparison of the lay Diagnostic Interview Schedule and a standardized psychiatric diagnosis: Experience in Eastern Baltimore. *Arch. Gen. Psychiatry 42*:667–675.

28. Terry, C.E., and Pellens, M. *The Opium Problem*. New York, Bureau of Social Hygiene, 1928.

29. Morgan, H.W. (ed.). *Yesterday's Addicts: American Society and Drug Abuse: 1865–1920*. Norman, Oklahoma, University of Oklahoma Press, 1974.

30. Ball, J.C., and Chambers, C.D. (eds.). *The Epidemiology of Opiate Addiction in the United States*. Springfield, Illinois, Thomas, 1970.

31. Rounsaville, B.J., and Kleber, H.D. (1985). Untreated opiate addicts: How do they differ from those seeking treatment? *Arch. Gen. Psychiatry 42*:1072–1077.

32. Eaton, W.W., Holzer, C.E., Von Korff, M.R., Anthony, J.C., et al. (1984). The design of the ECA surveys: The control and measurement of error. *Arch. Gen. Psychiatry 41*:942–948.

33. Eaton, W.W., Kessler, L.G. (eds.). *Epidemiological Field Methods in Psychiatry: The NIMH Epidemiologic Catchment Area Program*. Orlando, Florida, Academic Press, 1985.

34. Robins, L.N., Regier, D.A. (eds.). *Psychiatric Disorders in America*. New York, Free Press, 1990.

35. Frost, W.H. Epidemiology, Chapter 7, Nelson Loose-Leaf System. *Public Health-Preventive Medicine*, Vol. 2. New York, Thos. Nelson & Sons, 1927, pp. 163–190. Reprinted in: Maxcy, K.F. (ed.). *Papers of Wade Hampton Frost, M.D.* New York, Commonwealth Fund, 1941, pp. 493–542.

36. Robins, L.N. The epidemiology of drug use and abuse: Where are we now?, *Studying Drug Abuse* (L.N. Robins, ed.). New Brunswick, New Jersey, Rutgers University Press, 1985, pp. 1–23.

37. de Alarcon, R. The uses of clinical epidemiology, *Studying Drug Abuse* (L.N. Robins, ed.). New Brunswick, New Jersey, Rutgers University Press, 1985, pp. 25–45.

38. Eaton, W.W., Kramer, M., Anthony, J.C., Dryman, A., Shapiro, S., and Locke, B.Z. (1989). The incidence of specific DIS/DSM-III mental disorders: Data from the NIMH Epidemiologic Catchment Area Program. *Acta Psychiatr. Scand. 79*:163–178.

39. Kramer, M., Von Korff, M., and Kessler, L. (1980). The lifetime prevalence of mental disorders: estimation, uses and limitations. *Psychol. Med. 10*:429–435.

40. Kramer, M. (1957). A discussion of the concepts of incidence and prevalence as related to epidemiologic studies of mental disorders. *Am. J. Public Health 47*:826–840.

41. Robins, L.N., Helzer, J.E., Weissman, M.M., Orvaschel, H., Gruenberg, E., Burke, J.D., and Regier, D.A. (1984). Lifetime prevalence of specific psychiatric disorders in three sites. *Arch. Gen. Psychiatry 41*:949–958.

42. National Institute on Drug Abuse. *National Household Survey On Drug Abuse: Population Estimates 1985*. Department of Health And Human Services Publication No. (ADM) 87-1539. Rockville, Maryland, 1987.

43. Anthony, J.C., and Trinkoff, A.M. United States epidemiologic data on drug use and abuse: How are they relevant to testing abuse liability of drugs?, *Testing of Abuse Liability of Drugs in Humans* (M. Fischman and N. Mello, eds.). National Institute on Drug Abuse Research Monograph No. 92, Rockville, Maryland, 1989, pp. 241–266.

44. Fischer, P., Shapiro, S., Breakey, W., Anthony, J.C., and Kramer, M. (1986). Mental health and social characteristics of the homeless: A survey of mission users. *Am. J. Public Health 76*:519–524.

45. Ritter, C., Anthony J.C. Factors influencing cocaine use among adults: Findings from the Epidemiologic Catchment Area program, *The Epidemiology of Cocaine Use and Abuse* (C. Schade and S. Schober, eds.). National Institute on Drug Abuse, Research Monograph, Rockville, Maryland, in press.

46. Regier, D.A., Boyd, J.H., Burke, J.D., Rae, D.S., Myers, J.K., Kramer, M., Robins, L.N., George, L.K., Karno, M., and Locke, B.Z. (1988). One-month prevalence of mental disorders in the United States: Based on five epidemiologic catchment area sites. *Arch. Gen. Psychiatry 45*:977–986.

47. Myers, J.K., Weissman, M.M., Tischler, G.L., Holzer, C.E., Leaf, P.J., Orvaschel, H., Anthony, J.C., Boyd, J.H., Burke, J.D., Kramer, M., and Stoltzman, R. (1984). Six-month prevalence of psychiatric disorders in three communities: 1980–1982. *Arch. Gen. Psychiatry 41*:959–970.
48. Blazer, D., George, G.K., Landerman, R., and Pennybacker, M., Melville, M.L., Woodbury, M., Manton, K.G., Jordan, K., and Locke, B. (1985). Psychiatric disorders: A rural/urban comparison. *Arch. Gen. Psychiatry 42*:651–656.
49. Karno, M., Hough, R.L., Burnam, M.A., Escobar, J.I., Timbers, D.M., Santana, F., and Boyd, J.H. (1987). Lifetime prevalence of specific psychiatric disorders among Mexican Americans and non-Hispanic whites in Los Angeles. *Arch. Gen. Psychiatry 44*:695–701.
50. Burnam, M.A., Hough, R.L., Escobar, J.I., Karno, M., Timbers, D.M., Telles, C.T., and Locke, B.Z. (1987). Six-month prevalence of specific psychiatric disorders among Mexican Americans and non-Hispanic whites in Los Angeles. *Arch. Gen. Psychiatry 44*:687–694.
51. Kessler, L.G., Burns, B.J., Shapiro, S., Tischler, G.L., George, L.K., Hough R.L., Bodison, D., and Miller, R.H. (1987). Psychiatric diagnoses of medical service users: Evidence from the Epidemiologic Catchment Area Program. *Am. J. Public Health 77*:18–24.
52. Anthony, J.C., Petronis, K. Epidemiologic evidence on suspected causal associations between cocaine use and psychiatric disturbances, *The Epidemiology of Cocaine Use and Abuse* (C. Schade and S. Schober, eds.). National Institute on Drug Abuse, Research Monograph, Rockville, Maryland, in press.
53. Anthony, J.C., Tien, A.Y., and Petronis, K.R. (1989). Epidemiologic evidence on cocaine use and panic attacks. *Am. J. Epidemiol. 129*:543–549.
54. Tien, A.Y., and Anthony, J.C. Epidemiological analysis of alcohol and drug use as risk factors for psychotic experiences. *J. Nerv. Ment. Dis*, in press.
55. Anthony, J.C., and Petronis, K.R. Epidemiologic study of suspected risk factors for depression among adults 18–44 years old. *Epidemiology*, in press.
56. Petronis, K.R., Samuels, J.F., Moscicki, E.K., Anthony, J.C. An epidemiologic investigation of potential risk factors for suicide attempts. *Soc. Psychiatry Psychiatr. Epidemiol*, in press.
57. Breslow, N., Day, N., Halvorsen, K., Prentice, R., and Sabai, C. (1978). Estimation of multiple relative risk functions in matched case-control studies. *Am. J. Epidemiol. 108*:299–307.
58. Clayton, R.R. Cocaine use in the United States: In a blizzard or just being snowed? Paper presented at National Institute on Drug Abuse Technical Review, *Cocaine Use in America: Epidemiologic and Clinical Perspectives*, Bethesda, Maryland, July 11–13, 1984.
59. Donovan, J.E., and Jessor, R. (1983). Problem drinking and the dimension of involvement with drugs: A Guttman scalogram analysis of adolescent drug use. *Am. J. Public Health 73*:543–552.
60. Chen, V. "Factors Associated with Adult-Onset Drug Abuse and Dependence Syndromes." Baltimore, The Johns Hopkins University, (1990). Unpublished doctoral thesis.
61. Chen, V., and Anthony, J.C. (1990). Alcoholism and other suspected risk factors for adult-onset drug abuse and dependence syndromes. Manuscript in preparation.
62. Pickens, R.W., and Svikis, D.S. Genetic vulnerability to drug abuse, *Biological Vulnerability to Drug Abuse*, (R.W. Pickens and D.S. Svikis, eds.). Rockville, Maryland, National Institute on Drug Abuse, 1988, pp. 1–8.
63. Cadoret, R.J., Troughton, E., O'Gorman, T.W., and Heywood, E. (1986). An adoption study of genetic and environmental factors in drug abuse. *Arch. Gen. Psychiatry 43*:1131–1136.
64. Rounsaville, B.J. The role of psychopathology in the familial transmission of drug abuse, *Biological Vulnerability to Drug Abuse* (R.W. Pickens and D.S. Svikis, eds.). Rockville, Maryland, National Institute on Drug Abuse, 1988, pp. 108–119.
65. Dishion, T.J., Patterson, G.R., and Reid, J.B. Parent and peer factors associated with early adolescent drug use: Implications for treatment, *Adolescent Drug Abuse: Analyses of Treatment Research* (E.R. Rahdert and J. Grabowski, eds.). Rockville, Maryland, National Institute on Drug Abuse, 1988, pp. 69–93.
66. Anthony, J.C. The regulation of dangerous psychoactive drugs, *Society and Medication: Conflicting Signals for Prescribers and Patients* Lexington, Kentucky, Heath (Lexington Books), (J.P. Morgan and D.V. Kagan, eds.). pp. 163–180, 1983.
67. Kozel, N.J., and Adams, E.H. (1986). Epidemiology of drug abuse: an overview. *Science 234*:970–974.

4

Multiple Drug Use in Drug and Alcohol Addiction

Arthur W. K. Chan
Research Institute on Alcoholism, Buffalo, New York

I. INTRODUCTION

Multiple drug use and addiction have been an ongoing phenomenon for many decades [24,25,60]. The recent proliferation and availability of a large number of drugs coupled with the prevalence of heavy alcohol intake and alcoholism have stimulated much awareness of the medical and social problems associated with multiple drug use and addiction. The traditional categorizations of drug users as alcoholic, "pothead," "cokehead," "pillhead," and the like, are no longer consistent with contemporary patterns of drug use and abuse, especially for people below the age of 40 [23,38]. The prevalent trend is for drug users to have a primary drug by preference, and also to use (concurrently or sequentially) a variety of other drugs depending on factors such as availability, peer group influence, desired pharmacological effects, price, and environments [38]. The majority of persons entering drug treatment facilities all over the country are multiple drug users. Alcohol is the most frequently used drug for multiple drug addicts, and is often combined with marijuana, heroin, cocaine, amphetamines, or tranquilizers [23,25,120]. Several reasons for simultaneous multiple drug use have been suggested [38,41]: (1) To enhance the effects of the primary drug; e.g., the combination of alcohol with sedatives or tranquilizers. (2) To counteract the effects of the primary drug; e.g., the use of alcohol to reduce the jittery feeling caused by the use of amphetamines. (3) To substitute for the preferred drug that is not available; e.g., an individual may use alcohol, marijuana, or other drugs, either alone or in combinations, addictively, to substitute for heroin. Substitution with another drug(s) may also be a means to self-medicate withdrawal symptoms. (4) To conform to what are considered normative ways of using drugs; e.g., the high prevalence of alcohol and marijuana renders the combined use of these drugs "normative." There is a small portion of the drug-using population that engages in an indiscriminate ingestion of an array of drugs for the sake of multiple drug use, a practice which has been called the "garbage head" syndrome [38,41].

The objectives of this chapter are: (1) To highlight the methodological issues pertaining to epidemiological studies of multiple drug use in alcoholics and drug addicts. (2) To review research data on the prevalence and patterns of multiple drug use in alcoholics and drug addicts. Readers are referred to other publications which review epidemiological studies of drug use in the general population [38,39,93,125]. (3) To discuss factors such as age, sex, race, and familial alcoholism, which can influence the prevalence of multiple drug use. (4) To summarize research findings concerning the stages of drug use, with special emphasis on the "gateway" drug theory. (5) To discuss the consequences of multiple drug use. (6) To discuss the policy implications of multiple drug use. (7) To recommend future research.

II. METHODOLOGICAL ISSUES

The following highlights some of the important and complex issues relating to epidemiological studies of multiple drug use [38,50,143].

1. Since much of the data on multiple drug use in alcoholics or drug addicts is derived from patients' self-reports or questionnaires conducted during interviews, one major concern is the reliability of the information elicited [50]. Apart from the limitation imposed by the inability of a patient to recall accurately patterns, quantities, and frequencies of taking drugs, there may be underreporting or overreporting of drug intake depending on the circumstances. The inability to give an accurate drug history may be partly accentuated by alcohol or drug-induced cognitive deficits [120]. Because of the traditional separation of treatment for "alcoholics" and "drug addicts," a client's complete drug use/abuse history may be inaccurately obtained and/or evaluated by personnel not properly trained to deal with polydrug addicts [2,23]. This may lead to inaccurate statistics concerning the epidemiology of drug abuse patterns [23]. There is also a tendency for drug addicts to emphasize their drug of choice and minimize their involvement with other drugs [120]. Likewise, fear of being excluded from alcoholism treatment centers may prompt alcoholics who are also multiple drug abusers to underreport or lie about the use of other drugs [44]. Thus, low correspondence between self-reported drug use and results of analysis of urine drug levels has been reported [25,44,132]. Moreover, some of those who tested positive in urine drug analyses might not be the same persons who reported using drugs. On the other hand, some of the so-called alcoholics or drug addicts might fake the problems of abusing multiple drugs to gain access to facilities which offer free lodging and meals [132]. It should be noted that under research conditions in which cnfidentiality is guaranteed and there is no fear of exclusion from treatment or punitive actions, self-reports of alcohol intake [43,58,79,154,162,172] and use of other drugs [6,111] have been shown to be valid. However, it has been suggested that self-report by itself is not a valid method for measuring treatment outcome in alcoholism treatment studies [61,133]. Among strategies to improve the validity of self-reported data are: establishing rapport with the clients, checking records and informing subjects of intent, soliciting corroborative information from others such as friends or family, urine monitoring and making subjects aware of the intent, concentrating on recent events, and making questions less specific [75,129]. The "bogus pipeline" method is one of convincing subjects that researchers do have a measure of their drug use, even though they do not have such a means [50]. This method may increase the reporting of illicit drug use.

There is a tendency for subjects to exaggerate socially positive behavior and to underreport socially negative behavior [75]. Miller [115] has summarized some of the novel survey-based estimation techniques which have been devised to encourage deviant respondents to report truthfully. Among these are: (1) the randomized response method, in which the respondent can avoid complete disclosure by secretly choosing to answer yes or no on one of two questions, one soliciting sensitive information about drug use, the other being innocuous. By combining the results for all respondents and based on prior knowledge of the prevalence of the innocuous behavior as well as the probability of choosing the question about the deviant behavior, it is possible to estimate the overall prevalence of the deviant behavior [115]; (2) the aggregated response method, in which the subject adds a random number to his/her quantitative answer; (3) the "item-count/paired lists" method, in which one subsample of respondents is asked how many categories of a list of behavioral items (including the deviant behavior) apply to them; another subsample is shown the same list except that the deviant item is omitted; (4) the nominative technique was developed expressedly for the study of heroin use [115]. It is based on the premise that if each member of the population reports the number of close friends who have used heroin, then, with appropriate correction for duplication, it is possible to estimate the number of heroin users in the population.

2. One limitation of urine screening for illicit or licit drugs is that positive findings only suggest recent drug use; they do not provide any indication whether the individuals involved are tolerant to or addicted to the drugs detected. In many instances, the test data are at best semiquantitative, or they indicate just presence or absence of drugs [66]. In fact, sometimes a positive screen for marijuana does not necessarily indicate recent use of the drug. This is because long-term heavy users of marijuana may have considerable stores of cannabinoids in fatty tissues which may be steadily released into the blood for days even though the person is not currently using the drug [156]. On the other hand, because of the rapid metabolism of cocaine, a positive test for this drug is a reliable indicator of recent use, but a negative test does not necessarily rule out frequent (but not recent) usage.

3. It is important to provide clear definition of "use" and "abuse," of drugs. The latter term has been used with a wide range of meaning, e.g., to denote nonmedical use of prescription drugs, use (with or without specification on quantity or frequency) of any illicit drugs, or use of any drugs to a degree that can lead to psychosocial or medical problems. Established guidelines, e.g., the DSM III-R (the *Diagnostic and Statistical Manual of Mental Disorders*, 3rd Edition–Revised, American Psychiatric Association, Washington, D.C., 1987) criteria for dependence (addiction), need to be adopted by all researchers to facilitate meaningful comparisons of data in different studies. Likewise, unambiguous definitions of "regular" use and "occasional" use are also needed. Some investigators define "regular" use as daily use for 1 month, whereas others define it as multiple weekly use [95]. The "ever" use category will be more meaningful if a time period is specified.

Information on the quantity of drug intake can be elicited more easily for alcohol than for other drugs, especially illicit ones. This is because alcohol researchers rely heavily on the quasi uniform definition of "a drink"—4.0 oz of wine, 12.0 oz of beer, and 1.25 oz of liquor—to establish data on the quantity and frequency of alcohol consumption. However, imprecise estimation of the amount of alcohol in a drink can still occur because bartenders and the like do not uniformly dispense the same amount of alcohol in mixed drinks; heavy drinkers are more likely to mix larger drinks than are light drinkers [50]. Another source of error is not adjusting for the alcohol content in light beer and wine coolers. Theoretically, the amount of prescription drugs consumed can be determined with some degree of certainty if drug names and dosages are known, and if patients follow the prescribed schedule of taking drugs. The same is not true for illicit drugs because the nature and concentrations of various ingredients are by no means uniform. Moreover, some street drugs may have ingredients which have addictive properties not known to the persons taking the drugs [50,138]. At times, drug users may have problems with the terminology of drugs; e.g., what have been reported as "sleeping pills" or "pain killers" might actually be benzodiazepines [132]. With the recent proliferation of "crack" and "ice crystals," these terms need to be included when drug users are questioned about their drug intake.

4. Comparisons across studies are sometimes difficult because of different subject pools and different methods of recruiting subjects. Most studies of drug use in alcoholics and drug addicts have, by necessity or practical constraints, used subjects in treatment programs or

those in prisons. These samples are not necessarily representative of the total population of drug abusers. In fact, the prevalence of multiple drug use in household populations is lower than that of those who are jailed or homeless [126]. Most investigations have been cross-sectional and retrospective. There is a need for more longitudinal studies so that the causes and factors affecting the progression to multiple drug use can be better understood.

5. Theoretically, many combinations are possible for the multiple use of just several drugs. Thus, Simpson [152] identified 28 different patterns of the use for a set of eight drug classes in clients from the Drug Abuse Reporting Program (DARP). Based primarily on self-reports, investigators are faced with the problems of extracting meaningful information concerning the developmental patterns of onset of drug use, how and when the various drugs are used, the possible influence using one drug may have on the use of another, the frequency and quantity of use, and the consequences of multiple drug use. Clayton [38] has summarized the investigative approaches to assess multiple drug use, and concluded that a comprehensive composite index of multiple drug use is yet to be developed.

III. PREVALENCE

Several national data systems provide some information on the prevalence of multiple drug use in alcoholics or drug addicts, even though none was designed specifically to investigate multiple drug users/abusers per se [25]. These include: the Drug Abuse Reporting System (DARP), a data base for treatment outcome evaluation research; the Client Oriented Data Acquisition Process (CODAP), which collects data on clients in federally funded drug treatment programs; the Drug Abuse Warning Network (DAWN), which has available data on drug abuse from 24 standard metropolitan statistical areas in the United States; and the National Alcoholism Program Information System (NAPIS), which collects data on a large number of alcoholics receiving treatment in designated alcoholism centers. Another program, the National Drug/Alcohol Collaborative Project (NDACP) consists of a series of special demonstration programs designed to reach and treat multiple-drug addicts. The Treatment Outcome Prospective Study (TOPS) elicited detailed drug use histories of 11,750 clients entering 41 detoxification, methadone, residential, and outpatient drug-free treatment programs in 10 cities from 1979 to 1981 [86]. Other data sources include review articles dealing with multiple drug use [24,25,28,38,60,70,127], and individual research studies (cited below) which either have their own subject pools or utilized data from one of the national data systems. Since alcohol is the most frequently used drug for multiple-drug addicts, it is convenient to categorize multiple-drug users into two broad groups; namely, alcoholics who use or abuse other drugs, and drug addicts who use or abuse alcohol.

However, it should be stressed that although labels such as alcohol/opiate or alcohol/barbiturate addicts are often used to denote primary drug combinations, these addicts may also use other drugs; e.g., marijuana, amphetamines, and tranquilizers. Likewise, labels such as heroin addicts with alcoholism do not preclude the use and addiction to other drugs; e.g., in a randomly selected sample of 140 patients in a treatment center in the NDACP, all but three of them reported multiple drug use, and the mean number of drugs abused was 4.9 [26]. One of the most frequent patterns was alcohol, cocaine, heroin, and methadone.

A. Use of Other Drugs in Alcoholics

Freed's [60] review actually did not focus exclusively on drug abuse by alcoholics, but rather summarized studies up to 1972 on the combined use and abuse of alcohol and other drugs. He concluded that about 20% of addicts used both alcohol and other addictive drugs. In the review by Carroll et al. [24], only studies on subjects officially diagnosed as alcoholics and/or problem drinkers were included. The authors also included data from the NDACP. They estimated that the prevalence of drug abuse by alcoholics and problem drinkers lay between 60 and 80%, being somewhat higher for those under age 40. Because "abuse" was defined in the review as the use of an illicit (e.g., heroin) or licit drug (e.g., a medically prescribed sedative) in a nonmedically prescribed manner, the alcoholics or problem drinkers who were considered abusers of other drugs might not necessarily be physically dependent on these drugs. In contrast, in a later review by the same authors [25], the conclusion was that a relatively small percentage of alcoholics abused other drugs. These authors emphasized that self-reports of drug abuse by alcoholics likely led to considerable underestimation of the true prevalence. They cited residual intoxication with alcohol and/or drugs (which might interfere with memory) and distrust of the admitting institution as two frequently encountered factors militating against valid self-reports. According to clinicians interviewed in a study of alcoholism treatment programs, funded by the National Institute of Drug Abuse (NIDA), about 15–30% of all clients were thought to be abusing other drugs [165]. In a NIDA-funded investigation, about 11% of individuals who presented themselves for alcoholism treatment also reported using significant amounts of nonopiate drugs [127,171]. An unpublished retrospective review of clinical records in a treatment center revealed that in 1982, 25% of the patients there showed addiction to some other drugs in addition to alcohol. By 1986, this figure of other-drug addiction was increased to 45%, owing largely to cocaine addiction [167].

Table 1 summarizes data from studies published since 1981. These are primarily investigations of individual alcoholism treatment centers, and while the list is not meant to be exhaustive, it serves to illustrate the magnitude of drug addiction in alcoholics. It also demonstrates some of the methodological limitations (as outlined in Sec. II) of these investigations. Thus, most studies (except Refs. 14 and 119) reported recent use or addiction to drugs without any indications of whether the subjects were dependent on the drugs. Among the few investigations which had included urine analyses of commonly addicting drugs [22,44,99,132,145], there was only low or medium concordance (7–53%) between positive urine tests and self-reports of drug use. Exceptions are two studies dealing with the intake of benzodiazepines (BZDs) in alcoholics which found reasonably good concordance between positive BZD urine tests and self-reports of BZD use [22,145]. In contrast, Ogborne et al. [132] found that the majority (75%) of the discrepancies between self-reports and urine analyses were due to the underreporting of the use of BZDs. Likewise, Crane et al. [44] reported that 82% of their subjects denied use of BZDs to all interviewers even though the urine samples tested positive for BZDs. They suggested that these patients might have been self-medicating their withdrawal with BZDs and barbiturates and did not consider this worth mentioning to the interviewers. Virtually all the studies summarized in Table 1 lack information concerning the quantity and frequency of drug (other than alcohol) use, as well as the temporal relationship between alcohol consumption and intake of other drugs.

Data from some of the studies shown in Table 1 indicate that in alcoholics BZDs are one of the more often addictively used class of drugs [14,22,44,132,158]. Ciraulo et al. [37] have reviewed literature over the past 2 decades dealing with the abuse potential of BZDs among alcoholics. They conclude that while the data suggest that the prevalence of BZD use among alcoholics (3–41%) is greater than that in the general population (9.6–16%) and comparable to use by psychiatric patients, no firm conclusion can be reached concerning whether there is a greater liability for addiction to BZDs in alcoholics. However, another study by Ciraulo et al. [36] suggests that alcoholics may be at high risk for the addiction to alprazolam because it has a positive mood effect not seen in nonalcoholics.

Investigations of other population groups also provide some useful information concerning the prevalence of multiple drug use/abuse, despite the lack of the diagnosis of alcoholism in most of the subjects under study. In a randomized study of trauma patients in an urban

Table 1 Prevalence of Drug Use and Addiction by Alcoholics

Ref. no.	Subjects	Findings
157	1,340 male and female alcoholics in 17 NY alcoholism rehabilitaton units	46% had used other psychoactive drugs in the month before entering treatment; 20% reported using two or more drugs plus alcohol
89	163 consecutive alcoholics in a VA Medical Center	29% gave histories of misuse of drugs other than alcohol or marijuana
11	Urinalysis on 154 clients admitted to a drug and alcohol treatment program	30% had a positive urine screen for cannabinoids; of these clients, 75% admitted using marijuana prior to their interview
22	261 consecutive alcoholic outpatients with urine screens for drugs	One-third of the patients tested positive for BZDs. The predictive value of self-reported BZD use was high for positive and negative allegations
99	112 alcoholic outpatients with urine tests for commonly abused drugs	Ten (8.9%) tested positive for psychoactive drugs, six for marijuana, and four for BZD
80	231 male and 90 female outpatient alcoholics	Lifetime prevalence of drug abuse was 45% for men and 38% for women, with current diagnosis of drug abuse being 8 and 13%, respectively. For both sexes, sedatives were the most abused drug, followed by marijuana and stimulants
174	107 alcoholic inpatients had urine tests for licit drugs and completed a medication questionnaire	76% took some drugs in the 2 weeks prior to admission; of these, 86% had taken alcohol with their drugs; 44% had taken BZDs
180	Alcoholics in a 30-day detoxification and treatment unit	Only three out of 258 abused alcohol without using other drugs. No details on statistics of drug use
148	507 consecutive inpatient male alcoholics	9.2% were alcoholics with primary drug abuse and 8.3% were primary alcoholics who used drugs intravenously, but did not meet criteria for drug abuse. Among these two groups 55% used marijuana and between 2 and 30% used cocaine, opiates, amphetamines, depressants, or hallucinogens. 12% of those who did not belong to the above two groups used marijuana
14	100 abstinent alcoholic women physicians (96) and medical students (5) reporting in a face-to-face structured interview	40% reported alcoholism only. Addiction to other drugs included marijuana (12%), narcotics (13%), and cocaine (10%). Higher prevalence of other drugs use was reported; e.g., amphetamines (31%), BZDs (28%). Some reported addiction to more than one drug
132	111 consecutive inpatient male alcoholics	50% had traces of drugs other than alcohol in their urine. 53% concordance between positive urine tests and self-reports of drug use. BZDs were the most frequently detected drugs (32%), followed by cannabinoids (10%) and barbiturates (7%)

continued

Table 1 *Continued*

Ref. no.	Subjects	Findings
145	282 alcoholics in a special unit of a psychiatric hospital	Based on questionnaire and urinalysis, 25.5% were found to have taken BZDs before hospital admission. Higher dosages of BZDs were found in those alcoholics who had mentioned taking them
44	266 alcoholics consecutively admitted for detoxification	52% had one or more types of drugs in urine, with BZDs (27%), cocaine (22%), and tetrahydrocannabinol (THC) (10%) topping the list. Concordance between self-reports of drug use and positive urine tests ranges 10 (barbiturates) to 52% (cocaine)
141	229 male and 198 female Canadian alcoholics	44% of both sexes had lifetime drug disorders and 29–30% were abusing or dependent upon them at admission. Prominent drug disorders for both sexes include those for sedatives, (20–34%), stimulants (28–32%), and cannabis (23–35%)
119	1627 male and female patients admitted to a primary rehabilitation program	Based on DSM-III-R criteria, 28% diagnosed as dependent on alcohol and drugs other than cocaine; 29% diagnosed as dependent on alcohol, cocaine, and other drugs; 2% diagnosed as alcohol and cocaine dependent
158	906 male and female German alcoholics in a university hospital	Clinical examination and medical history suggested 41.3% had additional drug abuse. BZDs were detected in 78.4% of 231 patients with urinary drug analysis

trauma center [109], 24.3% had toxicological screens positive for two or more drugs and 28.4% were screened positive for alcohol and at least one illicit drug. In this patient sample, the drugs most commonly found were cocaine (54.4%) and cannabinoids (37.2%). Cocaine was present in 97.7% of patients who tested positive for alcohol and drugs, or two or more drugs. Other studies of traumatized patients include one [163] reporting that 5.5% of the patients were screened positive for both alcohol and other drugs, and another [156] finding that 16.5% of the patients used alcohol and marijuana in combination. Based on medical examiner data between 1981 and 1984 in New Jersey's Essex County, Haberman and Natarajan [73] determined trends in alcoholism and narcotics abuse in those who had died of violent and unnatural deaths. They found that 5% of the decedents could be classified as both alcoholics and narcotic abusers according to the following criteria: case record report of drinking problems or narcotic abuse, alcoholism or narcotic addiction indicated in the manner or cause of death, or autopsy findings of liver damage due to alcoholism or toxicology findings of narcotics. Drug abuse itself was the manner of death for alcoholics and most of those classified as alcoholics/narcotic addicts.

Gallegos et al. [62] surveyed drug addiction in impaired physicians (impairment defined as an inability to practice medicine with reasonable skill and safety to patients by reason of physical or mental illness, including alcoholism or drug dependence), and found that about 60% of over 1000 such physicians had previous psychiatric and/or alcohol and drug addiction treatment. Depending on their specialties, between 45 and 50% of the impaired physicians used addictively alcohol and other drugs; the five most frequently used drugs were alcohol, fentanyl citrate, meperidine hydrochloride, diazepam, and cocaine. In a study of 35 bulimic women [20], 48.6% had the diagnosis of alcohol abuse and 22.9% were alcohol dependent according to DSM-III criteria. Similarly, drug abuse and drug dependence were diagnosed in 25.7 and 34.3%, respectively. Ten of the women suffered from both alcohol and drug use disorders, but no information was provided about the types of drugs used. A survey of alcohol and drug problems in incarcerated offenders [108] found that 40% of the inmates reported having used both drugs and alcohol on the day of committing the criminal offense for which they were convicted. Among the inmates surveyed, 20.8 and 33.9% described themselves as alcoholic and heavy drinkers, respectively. Based on the inmates' scores on the Drug Abuse Screening Test, 13% were in the "severe range" and 25% in the "substantial range" of drug abuse. Worldwide surveys of U.S. military personnel indicated that between 11.9 and 14% of those surveyed could be classified as heavy drinkers (drink at least once a week and five or more drinks per occasion) and about 25% as moderate/heavy drinkers [18]. Between 0.4 and 8.9% of these personnel reported use of nonmedical drugs, especially marijuana, during the past 30 days. The prevalence of multiple drug use was not determined in this study, but it can be assumed that such a practice exists in a significant degree.

B. Use of Alcohol and Other Drugs in Drug Addicts

Many studies (e.g., see Refs. 70,103,118,126,144,151,168) have shown that there is a relatively high prevalence of alcoholism and alcohol abuse among drug addicts. In a national survey of adolescent polydrug users [144], 15–30% were found to be daily users of alcohol with the most frequently used drugs being marijuana (86%), amphetamines (40%), hashish (42%), barbiturates (40%), and hallucinogens as well as phencyclidine (PCP) (32%) [120]. In the 1982 National Household Survey on drug abuse, 14% of men and 6% of women reported having used both alcohol and marijuana in the month preceding the survey [126]. Among these respondents, 79% of the men and 67% of the women reported occasional or more frequent use of alcohol and marijuana together. These data may underestimate the true prevalence of marijuana/alcohol use or abuse because certain groups such as the homeless and those in jails were not included; these latter populations are known to have a higher prevalence of heavy alcohol and other drug use.

The following summarizes data on multiple drug use, particularly alcohol, in those who had identifiable primary drug addiction. It should be emphasized that the designation of primary drug addiction was probably arbitrary or circumstantial, dependent largely on the type of treatment facility that each client chose to be involved with or was referred to. Thus, a so-called narcotic addict could well be labeled as an alcoholic who uses addictively narcotic drugs if he/she was treated in an alcoholism clinic.

Opiate Addicts

Green and Jaffe [70] reviewed the literature prior to 1977 pertaining to alcohol use among opiate addicts. They concluded the following: (1) prior to beginning narcotic use, rates of excessive drinking might be as high as 65%; (2) although alcohol use apparently diminished during the addictive phase to narcotics, 10–20% of the opiate users still had problems related to excessive alcohol intake; (3) during treatment in methadone maintenance programs, 7–27% of the patients drank excessively. Another review [10] cited the prevalence of problematic alcohol use by opiate addicts to be 10–50%. Comparable prevalence has also been reported in more recent studies. For example, Kosten et al. [101] reported that 35% of their opiate addict probands were alcoholics. Other estimates of prevalence of alcohol abuse or problem drinkers in narcotic addicts ranged from 16 to 53% [5,8,9,45,76,87,94,161,168].

Using data from the NDACP, Chambers [27] found that of 1544 clients in the project, 40.5% reported the prior use of both alcohol and opiates. Within this group, heroin was the opiate of choice (99.4%), and 43.7% regularly used both heroin and alcohol (nearly every day for at least a month). The same investigator found that the prevalence for regular users of both heroin and alcohol was 47.9% in subjects from four drug treatment centers in South Florida [107]. There were some differences in the characteristics of these two samples (NDACP vs Florida) of heroin/alcohol abusers, with 34.8% of the Florida subjects reporting they had at some time been psychologically dependent on alcohol, compared to 20.5% of the NDACP subjects. Similarly, 13% of the Florida sample reported they had at some time been physically addicted to alcohol, compared to 20.5% reported by the NDACP clients. One report of CODAP indicated that about 18% of the 55,120 heroin addicts had some kind of alcohol problem, but in another CODAP report of 34,135 patients, only 3.3% listed alcohol as a secondary drug of abuse [159]. It should be noted that CODAP was designed primarily to report admissions of heroin addicts, and therefore the prevalence of alcohol use in these clients might have been underestimated. Using the Research Diagnostic Criteria for alcoholism, Rounsaville et al. [142] found that the overall lifetime and current rates of alcoholism in opiate addicts were 13.7 and 34.5%, respectively. Between 53 and 75% of two different California samples of male heroin addicts in treatment reported having ever been arrested for alcohol-related offenses, and between 4 and 11% had ever been hospitalized for alcoholism [2]. Data from the TOPS indicated that 46.8% of the outpatient methadone clients reported weekly or more frequent use of alcohol in the year before treatment intake [86]. Higher prevalence for the same period (62–64%) was reported by clients in outpatient drug-free or residential treatment programs.

There is much debate about whether methadone clients increase their alcohol intake while in treatment, and whether any increased drinking was the result of methadone treatment [2,70,87]. Several studies (reviewed in Ref. 87) have suggested that rates of alcoholism increased in heroin addicts after methadone treatment. However, the so-called changes in rates of "alcohol abuse" or "alcoholism," terms not uniformly defined, might have been confounded by some of the methodological problems discussed in Section II; in particular, underreporting by clients at treatment admission for fear of repercussions. Given the fact that many narcotic addicts began extensive use of alcohol in their early teens [2,71,87,159] and had alcohol problems prior to developing addiction to other drugs [142], a plausible explanation to the apparent increase in alcohol use or addiction in methadone clients is that it is simply the resurfacing of an old problem [2,87]. By examining the relationship between the patterns of use of alcohol and heroin by narcotic addicts, Anglin et al. [2] concluded that alcohol and heroin consumption were inversely related throughout the addicts' careers, encompassing the addiction, treatment, and postdischarge stages. In other words, use of alcohol during methadone treatment reflects a lifetime pattern of increased alcohol consumption which follows any decline in heroin intake. This finding agrees with the conclusion of Rounsaville et al. [142] that alcohol addiction in methadone patients occurred in those who had a history of alcohol problems. Likewise, DeLeon [51] found that use of alcohol and/or marijuana increased significantly in abstinent opioid addicts.

Stimmel et al. [160] reported that of the 789 persons enrolled in a methadone program, 15% had a positive urinalysis for one psychotropic drug, and 48% had evidence of using two or more drugs. Of these, cocaine was the most common (45%), followed by amitriptyline (20%), barbiturates (17%), and diazepam (12%). Self-reports by methadone clients of other drug use (excluding alcohol) at least once in the week prior to interview in one study [87] included illicit methadone (10%), cocaine (35%), tranquilizers/sedatives (31%), marijuana (53%), barbiturates (6%), and amphetamines (4%). Similar prevalence rates were reported by those methadone clients who were also considered abusive pattern drinkers.

Drug addicts admitted to the different treatment programs in the TOPS reported weekly or more frequent use of the following drugs (besides heroin, methadone and alcohol) in the year before treatment intake: marijuana (57–66%), cocaine (16–28%), BZDs (17–24%), other narcotics (16–29%), amphetamines (10–28%), and sedatives (5–16%) [86]. Heroin addicts in a methadone maintenance program in Pennsylvania also reported frequent (8–22 days per month) use of the following drugs during the first addiction period (at least 4 days per week or at least 16 days per month of regular opiate use); other opiates (35.2%), cocaine (21.9%), amphetamines (29.5%), alcohol (20%), barbiturates (10.5%), diazepam (Valium) (18.1%), marijuana (44.8%), and other nonopiates (15.2%) [5]. Thus, marijuana appears to be the most prevalence nonopiate drug used by heroin addicts. During the nonaddiction period (less frequent use than that defined above), the frequency of using marijuana and alcohol remained the same as in the addiction period, but the number of days spent in using heroin and other opiates were reduced by about 75% [5]. Hartman et al. [76] reported that marijuana use was nearly ubiquitous in a population of youthful (mean age about 19 years) methadone patients, and that other drug use was found in 75% of those who had high alcohol intake.

According to Hartog and Tusel [77], the proportion of methadone maintenance clients using or abusing Valium remains relatively constant at most clinics, despite the wide range (4–65%) of prevalence having been reported for some clinics [145]. In Hartog and Tusel's study [77], the use of Valium was determined by three randomly administered urine tests within a 6-month period. Only those clients who tested positive three times were considered Valium users. Of those tested, 18% fit the criteria of Valium users, with 46% testing positive in one or two such tests and the rest never testing positive. Among the Valium users and nonusers, 67 and 50%, respectively, were also alcohol addicts.

Cocaine Addicts

The large overlap in alcohol and cocaine dependence is known clinically but is not well recognized in the literature [17,119,153]. Gold [65] indicated that 87% of cocaine addicts also use and are addicted to other psychoactive drugs, with alcohol being the most common. Miller et al. [119] reported that 94% of those addicts with the diagnosis of cocaine dependence were also diagnosed as being dependent on alcohol and other drugs. Only 5% of the cocaine addicts were addicted to another drug (other than alcohol), and only 1% was addicted to cocaine alone. A lower rate (50%) of alcoholism was found in 94 cocaine abusers admitted to a drug dependence unit in Belmont, Massachusetts [168].

Other Drug Addicts

Weiss et al. [168] reported that drug (other than opioids and cocaine) addicts in a drug dependence treatment unit had high rates of alcoholism; e.g., 48.1% of the depressant abusers (N=52), 66.7% of the amphetamine abusers (N=6), 50% of the phencyclidine abusers (N=2), and 87.5% of the marijuana abusers (N=8). Almost one-fifth of the drug addicts in a therapeutic community and whose primary drug of addiction was marijuana reported daily use of alcohol before and 2 years after treatment [51]. Roffman et al. [140] remarked on the paucity of data on the treatment of marijuana dependence, and suggested that one of the reasons might be the assumption that marijuana dependence rarely occurs without concurrent abuse of alcohol or other drugs. In a pilot study conducted by Roffman and Barnhart [139] in which they used an anonymous telephone survey to assess the potential current need for marijuana treatment services in Seattle, the investigators classified 73.8% of the respondents as being currently adversely involved with only marijuana, and 18.2% of the sample as being current multiple-drug abusers. A subsequent study of 110 marijuana abusers or addicts (used marijuana at least 50 times in the past 90 days) revealed that 63% had used alcohol and 22% had used cocaine in the past 90 days, and 18 and 22% were ever dependent on alcohol and cocaine, respectively [140].

Hubbard et al. [86] described seven drug-use patterns among the clients in the TOPS; the alcohol/marijuana group constituted about 16% of the clients, with 36.1 and 24.3% of them reporting daily use of marijuana and alcohol, respectively. The "single nonnarcotic" group had weekly or more frequent use of one nonnarcotic drug in addition to daily use of marijuana (38.3%), alcohol (25.1%), or amphetamines (15.3%); others of the same group reported weekly use of marijuana (30.1%), alcohol (38.7%), cocaine (18.0%), and amphetamines (20.9%). Within the "multiple nonnarcotics" group (weekly or greater use of at least two nonnarcotics in addition to marijuana and alcohol use), daily use of the following drugs was reported: marijuana (53.8%), alcohol (35.6%), barbiturates/sedatives (22.9%), cocaine (16.3%), amphetamines (27.8%), and tranquilizers (21.5%). Between 26 and 43% of the same group reported weekly use of these drugs.

Judd et al. [95] found that among the NDACP clients, the most frequent abusers of multiple drugs were those subjects categorized in the barbiturate group (used this drug regularly) and the barbiturate/alcohol (used both drugs regularly). These two groups accounted for about 6% of the clients. The majority of the clients could be categorized as belonging to the alcohol group (used alcohol regularly; 52%) or the "neither" group (used neither alcohol nor barbiturates regularly; 42%). Marijuana and heroin were the most frequently used drugs in the four groups, especially by the barbiturate and barbiturate/alcohol groups (marijuana, 52.5 and 58.7%, respectively, for the two groups; similarly for heroin, 42.5 and 23.9%, respectively). Other drugs frequently (11–39%) abused by the two groups were other opiates, amphetamines, cocaine, and tranquilizers. The same investigators also categorized addicts in the San Diego Polydrug Study Unit (SDPSU) (95) into the same four groups, and marijuana remained the most frequently used drug by the barbiturate (50%) and barbiturate/alcohol (79%) groups, whereas heroin use was reported by 6.3% of the barbiturate group, and by 42.9% of the barbiturate/alcohol group. It should be noted that primary abusers of opiates and those dependent on opiates were not included in the study. This might have contributed to the low prevalence of heroin use in one of the groups. Use of other drugs in the SDPSU sample was similar to that described above for clients in the NDACP.

Because of the widespread use of BZDs and the demonstration that chronic administration of these drugs, not only for high doses but also for therapeutic doses, could lead to the development of physical dependence [176], there are legitimate concerns about multiple drug use in BZD addicts. However, literature dealing with this topic is not plentiful, probably because few treatment facilities have specific programs and treatment protocols for BZD addicts. Rather, most BZD addicts are probably treated for addiction to another drug, particularly alcoholism, and the BZD abuse or addiction is treated as secondary. In a study of mortality in patients dependent on BZDs, it was found that only 18% of the 384 patients used BZDs alone; the majority combined BZDs with alcohol and/or other legal or illegal drugs [136]. Busto et al. [21] found that among 176 Canadian BZD users seen in the Addiction Research Foundation Clinical Institute for assessment of BZD abuse and/or dependence, 56% used only BZDs (median daily dose: 15 mg diazepam or equivalent) and 44% used BZDs (median daily dose: 40 mg of diazepam or equivalent) and the context of multiple drug abuse. In 32% of the latter group of multiple-drug abusers, BZDs were the primary drugs of abuse. The other abused drugs were ethanol (47%), barbiturates (27%), opiates (27%), analgesics (27%), and cannabis (4%). These BZD addicts reported a mean of 1.2 drugs abused concurrently with BZDs in the last month. Other investigators also found a high prevalence of alcoholism (30–75%) in BZD addicts [48,56]. In case reports of five female BZD addicts, three had histories of and/or recent alcoholism [19].

IV. FACTORS AFFECTING PREVALENCE

A. Age

Because of the growing incidence of multiple drug use and abuse among adolescents and young adults [39,76,90,93,137], it is not surprising that the prevalence of other drug use and addiction in alcoholics appears to be more widespread for those under age 30 [41,120]. For example, Novick et al. [128] and Carroll et al. [26] have reported that the mean age of abusers of alcohol only was significantly higher than that of multiple-drug addicts. As Vaillant [166] has suggested, alcohol use tends to occur at younger ages in those who later abuse alcohol and/or other drugs. A typical pattern is the use of alcohol beginning at age 13–15 or younger and progressing to addictive use by age 16 [27,87,120]. Intake of other drugs begins about 2 years after the onset of alcohol use, and in many cases these are consumed in conjunction with alcohol. Thus, the triad of alcohol, marijuana, and cocaine dependence is frequently encountered in young alcoholics seen in inpatient and outpatient facilities [120]. Data from the 1982 National Household Survey on Drug Abuse [126] indicate that of those who reported using alcohol and marijuana in combination, the highest percentage (24% for men and 12% for women) was in the 18- to 25-year-old group, followed by the 26- to 34-year-old group. Using data from the National Youth Survey, Menard and Huizinga [114] found that for polydrug use in those aged 11–24, there was a nonlinear age effect with a peak at about age 20. The same applies to the use of alcohol and marijuana.

B. Sex

Gender differences in the manifestations of alcoholism or alcohol related problems have often been reported in the literature [141]. Therefore, it is not unreasonable to assume that such sex differences may be extended to multiple-drug users or addicts, particularly those who combine alcohol with other drugs. Sex differences in narcotic addiction have been reported with reference to initiation of use [84], becoming addicted [4], period of addiction [83], and treatment [3]. Most of these differences appeared to be related to traditional sex role expectations. Some specific sex differences related to prevalence are: (1) Unlike men, the initial use of heroin by women was highly influenced by a man, especially by a sex partner who is often a daily heroin user [84]. (2) More women than men became addicted to heroin within 1 month after initial use [83]. About 25% of the heroin addicts (both sexes) fell into this category. (3) Narcotic addiction careers for women were shorter than those for men, and women entered treatment earlier. In contrast to most studies of opioid addicts and alcoholics, Griffin et al. [72] found that female cocaine abusers initiated drug use at a younger age than their male counterparts. The women cocaine addicts also entered treatment at a younger age, following a shorter period of cocaine use [72]. Since these addicts were treated in a private psychiatric hospital, they may not be representative of all cocaine abusers. Several studies [53,97] have found that teenage males reported more use of drugs (except cigarettes), particularly alcohol and marijuana, than females. The fact that more males than females use and/or abuse alcohol and other drugs explains why most investigations of alcoholics or drug addicts reported male to female ratios of between 2 and 5 (e.g., see Refs. 27, 87, and 119).

Although it has been stated that women alcoholics in treatment are more likely than their male counterparts to present with drug abuse problems [16,67], research data on this topic are scant [141]. Curlee [46] has reported that alcoholic women used and abused more tranquilizers and sedatives than alcoholic men, probably a reflection that women generally use or are prescribed more of these drugs than men [28,141]. Ross [141] recently confirmed Curlee's finding, but noted that, in terms of the overall prevalence of lifetime abuse of other drugs, there is no sex difference because it is offset by men having more abuse of cannabis and tobacco. Similarly, in a study of detoxified alcoholics and healthy nonalcoholics, Glenn et al. [64] found that alcoholics reported greater use of a variety of drugs, but there were no significant interactions for sex differences. In the NDACP sample of alcohol/opiate users, men outnumbered women by almost 5–1, but sex was not seen as a variable distinguishing between levels of abuse [27].

C. Race

Differences in the racial composition of the clientele of different drug treatment facilities are largely dependent on the specific locations of the facilities. Thus, there will be a substantial difference in the racial composition of clients in a treatment center located in a mostly white neighborhood compared to another which is situated in a predominantly black neighborhood. These differences may lead to erroneous interpretations of apparent racial differences in the prevalence of multiple drug use in alcoholics or other drug addicts. Many other factors can contribute to the apparent racial differences in multiple drug use; e.g., peer group and family influences, availability of drugs in neighborhoods, income or purchasing power, drug culture, psychosocial factors, and so forth. Therefore, unless representative populations of each racial group are studied, generalizations of racial differences in multiple drug use may not be valid. The paucity of information about racial differences in multiple drug use is likely due to our incomplete knowledge concerning epidemiological aspects of multiple drug use and addiction [38]. In fact, most studies only listed the racial compositions of their subjects as part of the statistical data on demographics, but there were no in-depth analyses of racial differences in the patterns of multiple drug use in alcoholics or drug addicts.

Using data from NDACP (a nationally representative sample of multiple drug users in treatment), Chambers [27] found that blacks were significantly more involved in the regular use of both heroin/alcohol than were nonblacks (66.3 vs 29.3%). In contrast, there were no differences between black and white drug addicts in two treatment facilities in South Florida with respect to regular alcohol/opiate use and other measures such as arrests and incarcerations [27]. However, white alcohol/opiate addicts in this study reported more use of alcohol as a temporary substitute to eliminate pain and anxiety when heroin was not available than black addicts; the white addicts also reported more use of alcohol as a means to kick the drug habit without entering a treatment program. In a study of four methadone maintenance clinics in three states, Hunt et al. [87] reported that more black opiate addicts were heavy drinkers than white addicts. Among the NDACP clients categorized on patterns of regular alcohol/sedative use for 3 months prior to treatment, more American blacks were in the group of regular alcohol users, but Hispanics were most frequent in the group of regular barbiturate users and least frequent in the regular use of barbiturates and alcohol together, and more American whites were in the group of regular users of both alcohol and barbiturates [95]. Anglin et al. [2] reported that both American white and Chicano narcotic addicts showed the inverse relationship between alcohol and heroin consumption throughout their addiction careers.

The foregoing examples illustrate that there are no consistent patterns of racial differences in multiple drug use in alcoholics or drug addicts.

D. Familial Alcoholism or Other Drug Addiction

Research has convincingly shown that alcoholism is a genetically influenced disorder [68]. Although much research has been focused on the familial transmission (the term familial is not synonymous with hereditary; the former is used to imply association rather than causation) of alcoholism, there have been only limited investigations on the influence of familial alcoholism on the development of other drug addictions in the children of alcoholics. Even less explored is the question of whether children of drug (other than alcohol) addicts are more likely to become drug addicts than children of non–drug addicts. The paucity of data is probably due to the ubiquitous occurrence of alcohol misuse or alcoholism in drug addicts [122], which confounds the clear distinction between a family history of alcoholism and a family history of addiction to other drugs. Meller et al. [113] have summarized the limited data which suggest that specific familial transmission of drug abuse does occur. For example, there was a high correlation between tranquilizer use in parents and the use and abuse of tranquilizers as well as marijuana by their college-age children. However, at present there is no hard evidence for a specific genetic vulnerability to specific psychotropic drugs other than alcohol. Fisher et al. [57] found that among a sample of college students, the use of drugs by men was relatively independent of perceived parental drug use, whereas the use of drugs by women was strongly related to perceived parental usage.

Parental alcoholism may impart a general proclivity for the excessive use of or addiction to other drugs in children of alcoholics. Glenn et al. [64] have shown that male and female subjects with a positive history of familial alcoholism, regardless of whether they were alcoholics or nonalcoholics, reported the use of more barbiturates, opiates, analgesics, and street drugs than subjects with a negative history of familial alcoholism. Ciraulo et al. [35] found that nine of 12 men with a family history of alcoholism but only two of 12 control subjects had euphoric responses to alprazolam, and they concluded that sons of alcoholics may be at high risk to abuse this BZD. Based mostly on direct interviews, Weiss et al. [168] reported that the first-degree relatives of alcoholic drug addicts had significantly more alcoholism than the first-degree relatives of nonalcoholic drug addicts. However, there was no difference in polydrug abuse between the alcoholic and nonalcoholic drug addicts. In a study of male inpatients admitted to a Veterans Administration alcohol treatment program, 68% of those who were alcoholics/primary drug abusers had a familial history of alcoholism, compared to 49% of those who were primary alcoholics, but neither met other diagnostic criteria for drug abuse nor had taken drugs intravenously [148]. However, this finding may not be generalizable to other populations because of the special patient groups used in the study.

A high prevalence of familial alcoholism was found among probands with cocaine dependence or cocaine and other drug (alcohol and/or marijuana) dependence [116,117,119]; for example, for those diagnosed as being dependent on cocaine, 47% of the male and 65% of the female clients had family histories of alcohol dependence; for those dependent on cocaine and alcohol, 46% of the males and 90% of the females had familial alcoholism. The skewed male and female ratio was due to the much smaller number of females. Using the family history method, Kosten et al. [101] examined the relationship of parental alcoholism to alcoholism, depression, and antisocial personality disorder among more than 600 opioid addicts. They concluded that opioid addicts with parental alcoholism were more frequently concurrent alcoholics, and more often had severe problems of alcohol abuse, depression, and antisocial personality disorder than addicts without parental alcoholism. The data implied that alcoholic opioid addicts with parental alcoholism may need more intensive intervention than other addicts. Mirin et al. [122] also reported higher rates of familial alcoholism in a group of male and female drug addicts comprising those addicted to opiates (57%); stimulants, primarily cocaine, 22%; and depressants (20%). In contrast, Schuckit and Sweeney [149] did not find a close relationship between familial alcoholism and personal drug abuse in a population of young adult males. However, their subject selection criteria excluded those with severe early life problems such as antisocial personality disorder. Nevertheless, these investigators suggested that a heightened risk for drug use and minor alcohol-related problems is associated with familial alcoholism.

V. THE GATEWAY DRUG THEORY

Ever since the development of the "stages of drug use" model by Kandel [96], there have been ample investigations confirming that among adolescents, alcohol use constitutes a necessary stage in the sequence of the use of and addiction to other drugs [57,78,85,92, 98,130,131,169,173,177,178]. Thus, adolescents are unlikely to use marijuana unless they have used alcohol first; likewise, marijuana is a necessary intermediate for the transition to using "hard" drugs, such as heroin or cocaine. Therefore, alcohol serves as the "gateway" drug to other drug use. Based on data from a survey of alcohol and other drug use in over 27,000 seventh- through twelfth-grade students in New York State, the following order of drug use by white, black, and Hispanic students has been suggested: alcohol, marijuana, pills and hard drugs [169]. Among the 4600 students who reported having used hard drugs, only 40 reported use of hard drugs without having used alcohol. Data from the same study also indicate that cigarette smoking constitutes an important step between alcohol and marijuana use for younger students, especially for females, supporting the earlier finding of Yamaguchi and Kandel [177,178]. However, using principal components analysis as a scaling technique, Fisher et al. [57] suggested that tobacco use was not related to either marijuana or cocaine use in a small sample of college students. For black and Hispanic students, pills are not as important a transition between marijuana and hard drugs as they are for whites [169]. Investigations involving adult multiple-drug addicts also support the notion that alcohol use predates use of hard drugs (e.g., see Refs. 27,70,87,119,121).

Although the stages involved in the gateway drug theory are relatively invariant for a particular social trend [38], the order of the stages can change due to an emergence of cultural shift. Thus, Fisher et al. [57] have shown that the Guttman scaling position of cocaine varied depending on the years that studies of stages of drug use were conducted, probably reflecting the cultural shift toward increased cocaine use. The stage progression model is not intended to suggest that anyone who uses alcohol will necessarily proceed through the ensuing stages of drug use, nor does it preclude the simultaneous use of more than one drug (e.g., alcohol plus marijuana or cocaine) during each succeeding stage [38,173]. In fact, drugs used in the early stages are usually "carried forward" into the later stages of drug use, often with increased intensity and frequency [39]. This is consistent with the suggestion of Donovan and Jessor [52] that problem drinking may be a stage subsequent to marijuana use and prior to use of heroin and cocaine. Adolescents who have gone through all the stages of drug use and who use hard drugs with high frequency are also likely to report a higher incidence of problems both at home and in the classroom [7].

As a further refinement of the gateway drug theory, Windle et al. [173] used statistical causal models to investigate the stages of drug use in selected groups of the above New York State adolescent student sample; namely, male and female (analyzed separately) white high school adolescents aged 15 and older. The selection was to minimize possible heterogeneous influences associated with age, racial, and ethnic group differences. The results suggested that the best-fit model for either sex is a four-variable simplex model, in which alcohol use predicted marijuana use, and marijuana use predicted "enhancer" (e.g., amphetamines, cocaine, hallucinogens) as well as "dampener" (e.g., barbiturates, tranquilizers) hard drug use [173]. This finding supports previous research indicating the adequacy of the simplex model of stages of drug use (e.g., see Refs. 85,96,98,169,177,178). The simplex model also suggests that marijuana use predicts the use of enhancer drugs better than it predicts that of dampener drugs for both male and female adolescents [78,173]. However, it does not mean that the developmental pathways leading to substance use and abuse are necessarily the same with regard to other psychosocial factors for both male and female adolescents [173].

VI. CONSEQUENCES OF MULTIPLE DRUG USE

It is not the intent of this chapter to review the individual metabolic and physiological effects or the psychosocial and medical consequences of intake of each addictive drug. But it suffices to emphasize that no doubt these effects and consequences are ever present, perhaps in certain instances in a more than additive fashion, in those who use or abuse multiple drugs. The consequences of multiple drug use have been reviewed [26,38,49,103,147]. Major ones include drug interactions, medical complications, mortality, traffic accidents, and delinquency or criminal activities.

A. Drug Interactions

One of the complications of using two or more psychotropic drugs concurrently is the interaction that each drug may have on another. The interactions may be additive, more than additive, or antagonistic. Awareness of these interactions is essential for the treatment and possible prevention of polydrug toxicity, and for the management and counseling of multiple-drug addicts. By far the more common interactions are those involving alcohol and other sedative/depressant drugs, e.g., BZDs and barbiturates, and these have been reviewed by several investigators [28,41,47,81,82,146,147,150]. In general, acute combinations of alcohol and other sedatives produce additive or more than additive sedative effects [47,147]. In extreme cases such interactions can lead to coma and death owing to severe respiratory and cardiac depressions [28]. Fatal respiratory depression can also result from the simultaneous intravenous administration of cocaine plus heroin [103]. According to Kreek [102], alcohol played a prominent role in over 50% of the so-called overdoses involving heroin or methadone. Misra et al. [123] recently reported that cocaine potentiated the hypothermic and hypnotic effects of barbiturates and ethanol in rats. The acute combination of alcohol and another sedative, e.g., a BZD, such as diazepam or chlordiazepoxide, can result in the suppression of BZD metabolism by alcohol. This may account partly for the enhanced psychomotor impairment following combined alcohol/BZD intake, but pharmacodynamic interactions may also play a significant role [28,81,147]. Chronic alcohol intake causes induction of the hepatic drug-metabolizing system, and can result in the acceleration of metabolism of other drugs. There has been no animal study which examines the effects of chronic administration of both alcohol and another drug on drug metabolism or other long-term effects. The induction of cocaine metabolism as a result of chronic alcohol exposure can enhance the production of metabolites which are hepatotoxic, and can thus augment the hepatotoxic effect of alcohol [81,103]. On the other hand, alcoholics with impaired liver function will also have a diminished capacity to metabolize other drugs, and the concurrent intake of alcohol and other drugs will have detrimental effects. Recently, McAllister et al. [112] reported that chronic cocaine injection in rats caused an increase in BZD receptor densities in several brain regions. The combined central nervous system effects of cocaine and BZD have not been investigated.

Kreek [102,104] has reviewed the opioid interactions with alcohol. Both human and animal studies have shown that high blood levels of ethanol can inhibit methadone metabolism, but during subsequent periods of ethanol withdrawal methadone metabolism may be accelerated. This biphasic effect of ethanol can jeopardize the maintenance of steady methadone levels in methadone patients who abuse alcohol. The combination of alcohol and heroin can cause profound disruptions of several endocrine and neuroendocrine systems [103,104].

It is not clear how the concurrent use of multiple drugs affects the phenomena of tolerance to and physical dependence on each drug, as well as the processes of cross tolerance and cross dependence. Cross tolerance is the state in which tolerance to one drug has the effect of causing tolerance to another drug of the same or a different chemical type [135]. Cross dependence is the ability of one drug to suppress the manifestations of physical dependence produced by another and to maintain the physically dependent state [88]. These two phenomena are defined here because there have been misconceptions about their meanings. It is a common misconception that a drug is cross dependent or cross tolerant with ethanol simply because it can alleviate alcohol withdrawal signs. Many drugs can suppress alcohol withdrawal because of their sedative, anticonvulsant, or antianxiety properties, rather than their being fully substitutable with ethanol. In these cases, the other criterion of cross dependence (i.e., maintenance of the dependent state) is not met. Even drugs that have similar pharmacological actions may not necessarily be fully cross tolerant or cross dependent on one another. Thus, data from one human study [59] and one animal study [179] indicate that alcohol is a partial substitute for barbiturates in patients and animals chronically exposed to barbiturates. Likewise, partial cross dependence on ethanol in mice dependent on the BZD chlordiazepoxide has been reported [31]. Although it is a generally accepted notion that drugs with similar pharmacological actions are cross tolerant to one another, cross tolerance among ethanol, barbiturates, and other depressants has not always been observed, depending on the test to measure tolerance [100]. On the other hand, ethanol and opioids, which belong to different pharmacological classes, have been shown to be cross tolerant under certain conditions [100]. Le et al. [107] found that chronic treatment of rats with chlordiazepoxide conferred full cross tolerance to ethanol and pentobarbital; however, prior treatment with ethanol only conferred partial cross tolerance to chlordiazepoxide. Chan et al. [32] reported that the degree of equivalence between tolerance to ethanol and cross tolerance to chlordiazepoxide in ethanol-dependent mice varied with the behavioral tests to assess tolerance. Therefore, the statement that "any drugs that demonstrate cross-tolerance and cross-dependence with one another have a similar mechanism for the development of dependence" [26a] is not based on firm experimental support. Nevertheless, one can speculate that a drug addict who uses multiple drugs may because of the phenomenon of cross tolerance need higher doses of these drugs to achieve the desired pharmacological effects. This would tend to facilitate drug abuse or the development of physical dependence which in turn triggers more drug usage.

Women who use or abuse multiple drugs during pregnancy may risk damaging the fetuses [1]. Zuckerman et al. [181] reported that the use of marijuana or cocaine during pregnancy is associated with impaired fetal growth. One study has shown that there are dose-dependent effects of cocaine on maternal weight gain, maternal food and water consumption, fetal weight, fetal fatalities, and so forth [34]. The combined alcohol/cocaine use may pose a greater risk to fetal health than the use of either drug alone [33]. Prenatal exposure to both alcohol and BZDs can impact subtle behavioral changes or it may affect mental development in the growing child, but more research is needed in this area [28].

B. Medical Complications and Mortality

Alcoholics with the diagnosis of additional drug abuse (predominantly BZDs) have been shown to have significantly more seizures during withdrawal than alcoholics without other drug abuse [158]. However, the criteria for the diagnosis of other drug abuse were not defined in this study. Cushman and Benzer [48] reported that the risk of major withdrawal symptoms was about 50% for patients categorized as "high BZD–heavy alcohol" users. This withdrawal syndrome was atypical for alcoholics in that the onset was later (2–10 days after withdrawal), and was characterized by more psychomotor and fewer autonomic nervous system signs. Over 60% of parenteral abusers of heroin or cocaine in New York City were tested positive for the human T-cell leukemia/lymphoma virus/lymphadenopathy-associated virus (HTLVIII/LAV) antibody as a marker of acquired immunodeficiency syndrome (AIDS) in 1984–1985 [103]. Although the possible role of the combined use of alcohol and other drugs in the

development of AIDS infection is not known, alcohol abuse may lead to significant alteration of endocrine and immunological functions [103].

Multiple-drug addicts may be at greater risk for myocardial injury and cardiac arrhythmias
because drugs such as cocaine, heroin, and amphetamines are known to be associated with
acute myocardial damage, and because alcohol is also toxic to the heart [103,106]. It has
been suggested that acute myocardial injury associated with polydrug abuse is far more common than recognized [106]. A case of fatal malignant hyperthermia after recreational cocaine and ethanol abuse has been reported [110]. Sexual dysfunction was found in 62% of
male cocaine/alcohol abusers admitted to a drug disorder treatment unit [40]. The recent
availability of crack cocaine has led to a great increase in neurological complications associated
with the use of this drug [124]. These complications included seizures, lateral medullary syndrome, transient ischemic attacks, infarction of the spinal cord and brain, and others. It should
be noted that these cases involved patients who had also consumed a considerable amount
of alcohol before taking crack, or they had histories of alcoholism. Young multiple drug
abusers tended to have more neuropsychological impairments than young alcoholics [69].
However, this finding needs to be confirmed because of the small number of drug addicts
studied, and because the investigators could not rule out preexisting neuropsychological
disorders in the subjects.

Two-thirds of the drug-related emergency room episodes in 1982 as reported by the
DAWN involved multiple drug abuse [38]. "Alcohol-in-combination" is the largest category
with respect to multiple drug use in emergency cases [38]. A leading cause of death in
methadone maintenance patients is alcoholism and alcohol-related factors, accounting for
18–60% of all mortalities [12,94,102]. Likewise, Sells and Simpson [151] found that the
mortality rate of narcotic addicts between the sixth and twelfth years following treatment
was almost seven times greater than the rate for the general population, and heavy alcohol
intake was the strongest predictor of mortality risk. Most of the addict deaths were attributed
to overdose and other drug effects (48%), or violence (29%) [151]. These statistics agree
with the earlier conclusion by Green and Jaffe [70] that persons with dual drug addictions
have higher mortality rates and increased morbidity than those who abuse only one drug.
For those aged 15–24 years, there is a very significant contribution of alcohol and drug abuse
to traffic accidents, trauma, suicide, and homicide, which account for almost three-quarters
of all mortality in this population [49]. A Danish study [105] of deaths among drug addicts
found that between 1968 and 1986 there had been increases of the percentages of addicts
with an abuse of alcohol.

C. Traffic Accidents

Data from numerous investigations of the relationship between alcohol and traffic safety
strongly implicate alcohol as a problem for road safety [29]. Many other studies have also
shown that a significant percentage of those involved in motor vehicle accidents had taken
psychotropic drugs, frequently in combination with alcohol (e.g., see Refs. 15, 55, 63, 155).
The two drugs most often found, either alone or in combination with alcohol, are marijuana
and a BZD (particularly diazepam) [29]. However, much remains unknown about the
mechanisms by which alcohol or alcohol combined with other drugs contributes to traffic
accidents. Chan [29] has reviewed the factors which can interact with alcohol in the drinking
driver. It should be stressed that statistical data on the association between multiple drug
use and traffic accidents do not necessarily reflect the actual incidences of driving after consuming alcohol and other drugs because data are not available on those who were neither
caught for impaired or drunk driving nor involved in car accidents.

D. Delinquency or Criminal Activities

Clayton [38] has stressed that much of the criminality attributed to "heroin" use by drug addicts is actually a function of chronic heavy use of many drugs, especially alcohol. Likewise, Hammersley and Morrison [74] concluded that the use of other drugs, particularly alcohol and depressants, influenced both heroin and crime. Based on the analysis of data from the National Youth Survey, Clayton [38] has shown that youths (15–21 years old) who were multiple drug users accounted for a disproportionate share of all the criminal acts reported by the sample. Therefore, multiple drug use is a rather potent predictor of the probability of involvement in criminal activities, not only in alcoholics or drug addicts but also in the general population.

VII. POLICY IMPLICATIONS AND FUTURE RESEARCH

There is no doubt that multiple drug use is a huge, growing, and costly public health problem. Despite our incomplete knowledge of many facets of multiple drug use, several policy implications are obvious and they beckon a concerted effort of professionals as well as policy and law makers to devise effective, realistic, and creative programs on prevention and treatment. Prevention efforts should emphasize the developmental nature of multiple drug use and addiction. Thus, the "war on drugs" should include widespread educational coverages of the so-called gateway drugs, especially the important message that alcohol is a drug and its role in the development of multiple drug use. The young generation needs to be taught that the best way never to begin using hard drugs is never to begin using alcohol or other gateway drugs. In this context, the philosophy of teaching "responsible" or "social" drinking can be criticized for opening the gate to the use of other drugs [169]. Clayton [38] suggests that the health promotion and disease prevention approach may be the most efficacious prevention policy to reduce the use of alcohol, cigarettes, and other drugs. Educational efforts need to integrate programs involving the school, home, community, and workplace. Pentz et al. [134] have recently reported on the effectiveness of multicommunity approach for primary prevention of adolescent drug abuse.

Another major policy implication concerns how best to treat multiple-drug addicts. The traditional segregation of treatment programs for alcoholics and those for other drug addicts ignores the prevalent trend of multiple drug use in these addicts. In order that the treatment for multiple-drug addicts be completely effective, the problems associated with the addiction to each drug need to be taken care of, preferably under the same treatment setting. It does not make sense to just concentrate on the perceived "primary" drug of abuse and ignore problems associated with the abuse or addiction to other drugs. Several investigators have discussed the pros and cons of the combined treatment of multiple-drug addicts and some of the recent innovations [12,13,23,38,42,51,54,140,153,164]. Carroll [23] has stressed that although treatment regimens in a combined-treatment facility may vary to meet differing individual addiction and clinical problems, treatment does not differ simply on the basis of which drugs have been abused, except that methods of detoxification may vary. The ideal treatment goal is abstinence from all addictive drugs. The successful implementation of any program to treat multiple-drug addicts depends heavily on the types of training that the staff receive and the attitudes of the staff about the combined-treatment philosophy. Experts recommend integrating Alcoholics Anonymous with Narcotics Anonymous, and providing ancillary services such as family therapy, remedial education, and psychiatric, psychological, or legal services [23]. Urine screening for psychotropic drugs should be an integral part of the admission procedure.

Some recommendations for future research are listed below:

1. In terms of treatment research, there is a need to determine the matching of various treatment approaches to client types, and to develop more effective methods of treating multiple-drug addicts. For example, Bickel et al. [12] have suggested a combined behavioral and pharmacological treatment for alcoholic methadone patients.

2. Methods of detoxifications which have been used for "single-drug" addicts may not be efficacious or appropriate for multiple-drug addicts, particularly those methods involving the use of pharmacological agents; e.g., the use of BZDs to treat alcohol/BZD addicts. Likewise, the length of treatment may need to be optimized for those who are addicted to more than one drug.

3. Although investigations of the stages of drug use have provided important information about the gateway drugs, more research is needed to identify patterns of multiple drug use in adolescents and young adults. More longitudinal studies are called for to determine salient factors which can influence the development and maintenance of multiple drug use.

4. Animal studies to investigate the molecular mechanisms of individual drug actions will pave the way to our eventual understanding of the complex interactions arising from the concurrent intake of two or more drugs. Other investigations should focus on the molecular mechanism of tolerance, dependence, cross tolerance, and cross dependence. Long-term behavioral and biochemical changes resulting from acute or chronic multiple drug use have yet to be investigated.

5. We need more reliable and accurate methods of detection of multiple-drug addiction. The continued search for biochemical markers for alcoholism and/or other drug addiction will hopefully provide new techniques to identify multiple-drug addiction. These should be combined with existing diagnostic interview schedules.

ACKNOWLEDGMENTS

I thank Joyce Ulinski and Carol Tixier for skillful typing and Donna Schanley for proofreading and collating some of the references.

REFERENCES

1. Abel, E., and Dintcheff, B.A. (1986). Increased marijuana-induced fetotoxicity by a low dose of concomitant alcohol administration, *J. Stud. Alcohol, 47*:440.
2. Anglin, M.D., Almog, I.J., Fisher, D.G., and Peters, K.R. (1989). Alcohol use by heroin addicts: Evidence for an inverse relationship, *Am. J. Drug Alcohol Abuse, 15*:191.
3. Anglin, M.D., Hser, Y.I., and Booth, M.W. (1987). Sex differences in addict careers. 4. Treatment, *Am. J. Drug Alcohol Abuse, 13*:253.
4. Anglin, M.D., Hser, Y.I., and McGlothlin, W.H. (1987). Sex differences in addict careers. 2. Becoming addicted, *Am. J. Drug Alcohol Abuse, 13*:59.
5. Ball, J.C., Corty, E., Erdlen, D.L., and Nurco, D.N. (1986). Major patterns of polydrug abuse among heroin addicts, *NIDA Research Monograph Series, No. 67*, p. 256.
6. Barnea, Z., Rahav, G., and Teichman, M. (1987). The reliability and consistency of self-reports on substance use in a longitudinal study, *Br. J. Addict., 82*:891.
7. Barnes, G.M, and Welte, J.W. (1986). Adolescent alcohol abuse: Subgroup differences and relationships to other problem behaviors, *J. Adolesc. Res., 1*:79.
8. Barr, H.L., and Cohen, A. (1980). The problem drinking drug addict, *National Drug/Alcohol Collaborative Project: Issues in Multiple Substance Abuse* (S.E. Gardener, ed.), U.S. Government Printing Office, Washington, D.C., p. 78.
9. Barr, H.L., and Cohen, A. (1987). Abusers of alcohol and narcotics: Who are they?, *Int. J. Addict., 22*:525.

10. Belenko, S. (1979). Alcohol abuse by heroin addicts: Review of research findings and issues, *Int. J. Addict., 14*:965.
11. Benzer, D., and Cushman, P. (1983). Marijuana use in alcoholism: Demographic characteristics and effects on therapy, *Adv. Alcohol Subs. Abuse, 2*:53.
12. Bickel, W.K., Marion, I., and Lowinson, J.H. (1987). The treatment of alcoholic methadone patients: A review, *J. Subst. Abuse Treat., 4*:15.
13. Bickel, W.K., Rizzuto, P., Zielony, R.D., Klobas, J., Pangiosonlis, P., Mernit, R., and Knight, W.F. (1989). Combined behavioral and pharmacological treatment of alcoholic methadone patients, *J. Subst. Abuse, 1*:161.
14. Bissell, L.C., and Skorina, J.K. (1987). One hundred alcoholic women in medicine: An interview study, *J.A.M.A., 257*:2939.
15. Bjorneboe, A., Bjorneboe, G.-E.A.A., Gjerde, H., Bugge, A., Drevon, C.A., and Morland, J. (1987). A retrospective study of drugged driving in Norway, *Forensic Sci. Int. 33*:243.
16. Blume, S.B. (1986). Women and alcohol: A review, *J.A.M.A., 256*:1467.
17. Blume, S.B. (1987). Alcohol problems in cocaine abusers, *Cocaine. A Clinician's Handbook* (A.M. Washton and M.S. Gold, eds.), Guilford Press, New York, p. 202.
18. Bray, R.M., Marsden, M.E., Guess, L.L., and Herbold, J.R. (1989). Prevalence, trends, and correlates of alcohol use, nonmedical drug use, and tobacco use among U.S. military personnel, *Milit. Med., 154*:1.
19. Brenner, P.M., Wolf, B., Grohmann, R., and Ruther, E. (1988). Benzodiazepine dependence— Aetiological factors, time course, consequences and withdrawal symptomatology: A study of five cases, *Drug Alcohol Depend., 22*:253.
20. Bulik, C.M. (1987). Drug and alcohol abuse by bulimic women and their families, *Am. J. Psychiatry, 144*:1604.
21. Busto, U., Sellers, E.M., Naranjo, C., Cappell, H.D., Sanchez-Craig, M., and Simpkins, J. (1986). Patterns of benzodiazepine abuse and dependence, *Br. J. Addict., 81*:87.
22. Busto, U., Simpkins, J., Sellers, E.M., Sisson, B., and Segal, R. (1983). Objective determination of benzodiazepine use and abuse in alcoholics, *Brit. J. Addict., 78*:429.
23. Carroll, J.F.X. (1986). Treating multiple substance abuse clients, *Recent Developments in Alcoholism*, Vol. 4 (M. Galanter, ed.), Plenum Press, New York, p. 85.
24. Carroll, J.F.X., Malloy, T.E. and Kendrick, F.M. (1977). Drug abuse by alcoholics and problem drinkers: A literature review and evaluation, *Am. J. Drug Alcohol Abuse, 4*:317.
25. Carroll, J.F.X., Malloy, T.E. and Kendrick, F.M. (1980). Multiple substance abuse: A review of the literature, *National Drug/Alcohol Collaborative Project: Issues in Multiple Substance Abuse* (S.E. Gardener, ed.), U.S. Government Printing Office, Washington, D.C., p. 9.
26. Carroll, J.F.X., Santo, Y., and Hannigan, P.C. (1980). Description of the total client sample, analysis of substance use patterns, and individual program description, *National Drug/Alcohol Collaborative Project: Issues in Multiple Substance Abuse* (S.E. Gardner, ed.), U.S. Government Printing Office, Washington, D.C. p. 25.
27. Chambers, C.D. (1981). Characteristics of combined opiate and alcohol abusers, *Drug and Alcohol Abuse: Implications for Treatment. NIDA Treatment Research Monograph Series* (S.E. Gardner, ed.), U.S. Department of Health and Human Services, Rockville, Maryland, p. 131.
28. Chan, A.W.K. (1984). Effects of combined alcohol and benzodiazepine: A review, *Drug Alcohol Depend., 13*:315.
29. Chan, A.W.K. (1987). Factors affecting the drinking driver, *Drug Alcohol Depend., 19*:99.
30. Chan, A.W.K. (1990). Biochemical markers for alcoholism, *Children of Alcoholics: Critical Perspectives* (M. Windle and J.S. Searles, eds.), Guilford Press, New York, p. 39.
31. Chan, A.W.K., Langan, M.C., Leong, F.W., Penetrante, M.L., and Schanley, D.L. (1990). Partial cross-dependence on ethanol in mice dependent on chlordiazepoxide, *Pharmacol. Biochem. Behav., 35*:379.
32. Chan, A.W.K., Langan, M.C., Leong, F.W., Schanley, D.L., and Penetrante, M.L. (1988). Does chronic ethanol intake confer full cross-tolerance to chlordiazepoxide? *Pharmacol. Biochem. Behav., 30*:385.

33. Church, M.W., Dintcheff, B.A., and Gessner, P.K. (1987). Alcohol, cocaine and pregnancy in the rat: II. Fetal data, *Alcoholism: Clin. Exp. Res., 11*:196.

34. Church, M.W., Dintcheff, B.A., and Gessner, P.K. (1988). Dose-dependent consequences of cocaine on pregnancy outcome in the Long-Evans rat, *Neurotoxicol. Teratol., 10*:51.

35. Ciraulo, D.A., Barnhill, J.G., Ciraulo, A.M., Greenblatt, D.J., and Shader, R.I. (1989). Parental alcoholism as a risk factor in benzodiazepine abuse: A pilot study, *Am. J. Psychiatry, 146*:1333.

36. Ciraulo, D.A., Barnhill, J.G., Greenblatt, D.J., Shader, R.I., Ciraulo, A.M., Tarmey, M.F., Molloy, M.A., and Foti, M.E. (1988). Abuse liability and clinical pharmacokinetics of alprazolam in alcoholic men, *J. Clin. Psychiatry, 49*:333.

37. Ciraulo, D.A., Sands, B.F., and Shader, R.I. (1988). Critical review of liability for benzodiazepines abuse among alcoholics, *Am. J. Psychiatry, 145*:1501.

38. Clayton, R.R. (1986). Multiple drug use: Epidemiology, correlates, and consequences, *Recent Dev. Alcohol., 4*:7.

39. Clayton, R.R., and Ritter, C. (1985). The epidemiology of alcohol and drug abuse among adolescents, *Adv. Alcohol Subst. Abuse, 4*:69.

40. Cocores, J.A., Miller, N.S., Pottash, A.C., and Gold, M.S. (1988). Sexual dysfunction in abusers of cocaine and alcohol, *Am. J. Drug Alcohol Abuse, 14*:169.

41. Cohen, S. (1981). The effects of combined alcohol/drug abuse on human behavior, *Drug and Alcohol Abuse: Implications for Treatment. NIDA Treatment Research Monograph Series* (S.E. Gardner, ed.), U.S. Department of Health and Human Services, Rockville, Maryland, p. 5.

42. Cole, S.G., Cole, E.A., Lehman, W., and Jones, A. (1981). The combined treatment of drug and alcohol abusers: An overview, *J. Drug Issues, 11*:109.

43. Cooper, A.M., Sobell, M.B., Sobell, L.C., and Maisto, S.A. (1981). Validity of alcoholics; self-reports: Duration data, *Int. J. Addict., 16*:401.

44. Crane, M., Sereny, G., and Gordis, E. (1988). Drug use among alcoholism detoxification patients: Prevalence and impact on alcoholism treatment, *Drug Alcohol Depend., 22*:33.

45. Croughlin, J.L., Miller, J.P., Whitman, B.Y., and Schober, J.G. (1981). Alcoholism and alcohol dependence in narcotic addicts: A retrospective study with five years' follow up, *Am. J. Drug Alcohol Abuse, 8*:85.

46. Curlee, J. (1970). A comparison of male and female patients at an alcoholism treatment center, *J. Psychol., 74*:239.

47. Cushman, P. (1986). Sedative drug interactions of clinical importance, *Recent Developments in Alcoholism*, Vol. 4 (M. Galanter, ed.), Plenum Press, New York, p. 61.

48. Cushman, P., and Benzer, D. (1980). Benzodiazepines and drug abuse: Clinical observations in chemically dependent persons before and during abstinence, *Drug Alcohol Depend., 6*:365.

49. Czechowicz, D. (1988). Adolescent alcohol and drug abuse and its consequences—An overview, *Am. J. Drug Alcohol Abuse, 14*:189.

50. Day, N.L., and Robles, N. (1989). Methodological issues in the measurement of substance use, *Ann. N.Y. Acad. Sci., 562*:8.

51. De Leon, G. (1987). Alcohol use among drug abusers: Treatment outcomes in a therapeutic community, *Alcoholism, 11*:430.

52. Donovan, J.E., and Jessor, R. (1983). Problem drinking and the dimension of involvement with drugs: A Guttman scalogram analysis, *Am. J. Public Health, 73*:543.

53. Ensminger, M.E., Brown, C.H., and Kellam, S.G. (1982). Sex differences in antecedents of substance use among adolescents, *J. Soc. Issues, 38*:25.

54. Feigelman, W., Hyman, M.M., and Amann, K. (1988). Day-care treatment for youth multiple drug abuse: A six-year follow-up study, *J. Psychoactive Drugs, 20*:385.

55. Ferrara, S.D. (1987). Alcohol, drugs and traffic safety, *Br. J. Addict., 82*:871.

56. Fialip, J., Aumaitre, O., Eschalier, A., Maradeix, B., Dordain, G., and Lavarenne, J. (1987). Benzodiazepine withdrawal seizures: Analysis of 48 case reports, *Clin. Neuropharmacol., 10*:538.

57. Fisher, D.G., MacKinnon, D.P., Anglin, M.D., and Thompson, J.P. (1987). Parental influences on substance use: Gender differences and stage theory, *J. Drug Ed., 17*:69.

58. Fox, N.L., Sexton, M., Hebel, J.R., and Thompson, B. (1989). The reliability of self-reports of smoking and alcohol consumption by pregnant women, *Addict. Behav., 14*:187.

59. Fraser, H.F., Wickler, A., Isbell, H., and Johnson, N.K. (1957). Partial equivalence of chronic alcohol and barbiturate intoxications, *Q. J. Stud. Alcohol, 18*:541.

60. Freed, E.X. (1973). Drug abuse by alcoholics: A review, *Int. J. Addict., 8*:451.

61. Fuller, R.K., Lee, K.K., and Gordis, E. (1988). Validity of self-report in alcoholism research: Results of a Veterans Administration cooperative study, *Alcohol. Clin. Exp. Res., 12*:201.

62. Gallegos, K.V., Browne, C.H., Veit, F.W., and Talbott, G.D. (1988). Addiction in anesthesiologists: Drug access and patterns of substance abuse, *Q.R.B., 14*:116.

63. Girre, C., Facy, F., Lagier, G., and Dally, S. (1988). Detection of blood benzodiazepines in injured people. Relationship with alcoholism, *Drug Alcohol Depend., 21*:61.

64. Glenn, S.W., Parsons, O.A., and Stevens, L. (1989). Effects of alcohol abuse and familial alcoholism on physical health in men and women, *Health Psychol., 8*:325.

65. Gold, M.S. (1984). *800-Cocaine*, Bantam Books, New York.

66. Gold M.S., Verebey, K., and Dackis, C.A. (1985). Diagnosis of drug abuse, drug intoxication and withdrawal states, *Psychiatry Lett., 3*:23.

67. Gomberg, E.S. (1976). Alcoholism in women, *Social Aspects of Alcoholism* (B. Kissin and H. Begleiter, eds.), Plenum Press, New York.

68. Goodwin, D.W. (1987). Genetic influences in alcoholism, *Adv. Intern. Med., 32*:283.

69. Grant, I., Reed, R., Adams, K., and Carlin, A. (1979). Neuropsychological function in young alcoholics and polydrug abusers, *J. Clin. Neuropsychol., 1*:39.

70. Green, J., and Jaffe, J.H. (1977). Alcohol and opiate dependence: A review, *J. Stud. Alcohol, 38*:1274.

71. Green, J., Jaffe, J.H., Carlisi, J.A., and Zaks, A. (1978). Alcohol use in the opiate use cycle of the heroin addict, *Intr. J. Addict., 13*:1021.

72. Griffin, M.L., Weiss, R.D., Mirin, S.M., and Lange, U. (1989). A comparison of male and female cocaine abusers, *Arch. Gen. Psychiatry, 46*:122.

73. Haberman, P.W.,and Natarajan, G. (1986). Trends in alcoholism and narcotics abuse from medical examiner data, *J. Stud. Alcohol, 47*:316.

74. Hammersley, R., and Morrison, V. (1987). Effects of polydrug use on the criminal activities of heroin-users, *Br. J. Addict., 82*:899.

75. Harrel, A.V. (1985). Validation of self-report: The research record, *Self-Report Methods of Estimating Drug Use: Meeting Current Challenges to Validity* (B.A. Rouse, N.J. Kozel, and L.G. Richards, eds.), U.S. Government Printing Office, Washington, D.C., p. 12.

76. Hartman, N., Kreek, M.J., Ross, A., Khuri, E., Millman, R.B. and Rodriquez, R. (1983). Alcohol use in youthful methadone-maintained former heroin addicts: Liver impairment and treatment outcome, *Alcoholism Clin. Exp. Res., 7*:316.

77. Hartog, J., and Tusel, D.J. (1987). Valium use and abuse by methadone maintenance clients, *Int. J. Addict., 22*:1147.

78. Hays, R.D., Widaman, K.F., DiMatteo, M.R., and Stacey, A.W. (1987). Structural-equation models of current drug use: Are appropriate models so simple?, *J. Pers. Soc. Psychol., 52*:134.

79. Hesselbrock, M., Babor, T.F., Hesselbrock, V., Mayer, R.E., and Workman, K. (1983). "Never believe an alcoholic"? On the validity of self-report measures of alcohol dependence and related constructs, *Int. J. Addict., 18*:593.

80. Hesselbrock, M.N., Meyer, R.E., Keener, J.J. (1985). Psychopathology in hospitalized alcoholics, *Arch. Gen. Psychiatry, 42*:1050.

81. Hoyumpa, A.M., Jr. (1984). Alcohol interactions with benzodiazepines and cocaine, *Adv. Alcohol Subst. Abuse, 3*:21.

82. Hoyumpa, A.M., and Schenker, S. (1982). Major drug interactions: Effect of liver disease, alcohol, and malnutrition, *Ann. Rev. Med., 33*:113.

83. Hser, Y.I., Anglin, M.D., and Booth, M.W. (1987). Sex differences in addict careers. 3. Addiction, *Am. J. Drug Alcohol Abuse, 13*:231.

84. Hser, Y.I., Anglin, M.D., and McGlothlin, W. (1987). Sex differences in addict careers. 1. Initiation of use, *Am. J. Drug Alcohol Abuse., 13*:33.

85. Huba, G.J., Wingard, J.A., and Bentler, P.M. (1981). A comparison of two latent variable causal models for adolescent drug use, *J. Pers. Soc. Psychol., 40*:180.

86. Hubbard, R.L., Bray, R.M., Craddock, S.G., Cavanaugh, E.R., Schlenger, W.E., and Rachal, J.V. (1986). Issues in the assessment of multiple drug use among drug treatment clients, *Strategies for Research on the Interactions of Drugs of Abuse: NIDA Research Monograph Series, No. 68* (M.C. Braude and H.M. Ginzburg, eds.), U.S. Department of Health and Human Services, Rockville, Maryland, p. 15.

87. Hunt, D.E., Strug, D.L., Goldsmith, D.S., Lipton, D.S., Robertson, K., and Truitt, L. (1986). Alcohol use and abuse: Heavy drinking among methadone clients, *Am. J. Drug Alcohol Abuse, 12*:147.

88. Jaffe, J.H. (1985). Drug addiction and drug abuse, *The Pharmacological Basis of Therapeutics,* 7th Ed. (A.G. Gilman, L.S. Goodman, T.W. Rall, and F. Murad, eds.), Macmillan, New York, p. 532.

89. Jaffe, L., and Schuckit, M.A. (1981). The importance of drug use histories in a series of alcoholics. *J. Clin. Psychiary, 42*:224.

90. Jekel, J.F., and Allen, D.F. (1987). Trends in drug abuse in the mid-1980s, *Yale J. Biol. Med., 60*:45.

91. Johnson, B.D. (1973). *Marijuana Users and Drug Subcultures,* p. 90.

92. Johnston, L. (1973). *Drug and American Youth: A Report from the Youth in Transition Project,* Institute for Social Research, University of Michigan, Ann Arbor.

93. Johnston, L.D., O'Malley, P.M., and Bachman, J.G. (1987). Psychotherapeutic, licit, and illicit use of drugs among adolescents: An epidemiological perspective, *J. Adolesc. Health Care, 8*:36.

94. Joseph, H., and Appel, P. (1985). Alcoholism and methadone treatment: Consequences for the patient and program, *Am. J. Drug Alcohol Abuse, 11*:37.

95. Judd, L.L., Gerstein, D.R., Lee, W.G., Riney, W.B., and Takahashi, K.I. (1981). The role and significance of alcohol and sedative use in the multisubstance abuser: An investigation of two patient samples, *Drug and Alcohol Abuse: Implications for Treatment. NIDA Treatment Research Monograph Series* (S.E. Gardner, ed.), U.S. Department of Health and Human Services, Rockville, Maryland, p. 75.

96. Kandel, D.B. (1975). Stages in adolescent involvement in drug use, *Science, 190*:912.

97. Kandel, D.B. (1980). Drug and drinking behavior among youth, *Ann. Rev. Sociology, 6*:235.

98. Kandel, D.B., and Faust, R. (1975). Sequence and stages in patterns of adolescent drug use, *Arch. Gen. Psychiatry, 32*:923.

99. Kania, J., and Kofoed, L. (1984). Drug use by alcoholics in outpatient treatment, *Am. J. Drug Alcohol Abuse, 10*:529.

100. Khanna, J., and Mayer, J.M. (1982). An analysis of cross-tolerance among ethanol, other general depressants and opioids, *Subst. Alcohol Actions/Misuse, 3*:243.

101. Kosten, T.R., Rounsaville, B.J., and Kleber, H.D. (1985). Parental alcoholism in opioid addicts, *J. Nerv. Ment. Dis., 173*:461.

102. Kreek, M.J. (1984). Opioid interactions with alcohol, *Adv. Alcohol Subst. Abuse, 3*:35.

103. Kreek, M.J. (1987). Multiple drug abuse patterns and medical consequences, *Psychopharmacology: The Third Generation of Progress* (H.Y. Meltzer, ed.), Raven Press, New York, p. 1597.

104. Kreek, M.J. (1988). Opiate-ethanol interactions: Implications for the biological basis and treatment of combined addictive diseases, *Problems of Drug Dependence 1987: NIDA Monograph Series, No. 81* (L.S. Harris, ed.), U.S. Department of Health and Human Services, Rockville, Maryland, p. 428.

105. Kringsholm, B. (1988). Deaths among drug addicts in Denmark in 1968–1986, *Forensic Sci. Int., 38*:139.

106. Lam, D., and Goldschlager N. (1988). Myocardial injury associated with polysubstance abuse, *Am. Heart J., 115*:675.

107. Le, A.D., Khanna, J.M., Kalant, H., and Grossi, F. (1986). Tolerance to and cross-tolerance among ethanol, pentobarbital and chlordiazepoxide, *Pharmacol. Biochem. Behav., 24*:93.

108. Lightfoot, L.O., and Hodgins, D. (1988). A survey of alcohol and drug problems in incarcerated offenders, *Int. J. Addict., 23*:687.

109. Lindenbaum, G.A., Carroll, S.F., Daskal, I., and Kapusnick, R. (1989). Patterns of alcohol

and drug abuse in an urban trauma center: The increasing role of cocaine abuse, *J. Trauma,* 29:1658.

110. Loghmanee, F., and Tobak, M. (1986). Fatal malignant hyperthermia associated with recreational cocaine and ethanol abuse, *Am. J. Forensic Med. Pathol.,* 7:246.

111. Martin, G.W., Wildinson, D.A., and Kapur, B.M. (1988). Validation of self-reported cannabis use by urine analysis, *Addict. Behav., 13*:147.

112. McAllister, K., Goeders, N., and Dworkin, S. (1988). Chronic cocaine modifies brain benzodiazepine receptor densities, *Problems of Drug Dependence, 1987* (L.S. Harris, ed.), NIDA Research Monograph 81, Rockville, Maryland, p. 101.

113. Meller, W.H., Rinehart, R., Cadoret, R.J., and Troughton, E. (1988). Specific familial transmission in substance abuse, *Int. J. Addict., 23*:1029.

114. Menard, S., and Huizinga, D. (1989). Age, period, and cohort size effects on self-reported alcohol, marijuana, and polydrug use: Results from the national youth survey, *Social Sci. Res., 18*:174.

115. Miller, J.D. (1985). The nominative technique: A new method of estimating heroin prevalence, *Self-Report Methods of Estimating Drug Use: Meeting Current Challenges to Validity* (B.A. Rouse, N.J. Kozel, and L.G. Richards, eds.), U.S. Government Printing Office, Washington, D.C., p. 104.

116. Miller, N.S., and Gold, M.S. (1988). Cocaine and alcoholism: Distinct or part of a spectrum, *Psychiatry Ann., 18*:538.

117. Miller, N.S., Gold, M.S., Belkin, B.M., and Klahr, A.L. (1989). Family History and Diagnosis of Alcohol dependence in cocaine dependence, *Psychiatry Res., 29*:113.

118. Miller, N.S., Gold, M.S., Klahr, A.L., Sweeney, K., and Sweeney, D.R. (1988). Alcohol use in cocaine addicts, *Subst. Abuse, 9*:216.

119. Miller, N.S., Millman, R.B., and Keskinen, S. (1989). The diagnosis of alcohol, cocaine, and other drug dependence in an inpatient treatment population, *J. Subst. Abuse Treat., 6*:37.

120. Miller, N.S., and Mirin, S.M. (1989). Multiple drug use in alcoholics: Practical and theoretical implications, *Psychiatry Ann., 19*:248.

121. Miller, S.I., Frances, R.J., and Holmes, D.J. (1988). Use of psychotropic drugs in alcoholism treatment: A summary, *Hosp. Community Psychiatry, 39*:1252.

122. Mirin, S.M., Weiss, R.D., Sollogub, A., and Michael J. (1984). Psychopathology in the families of drug abusers, *Substance Abuse Psychopathology* (S.M. Mirin, ed.), American Psychiatric Press, Washington, D.C., p. 80.

123. Misra, A.L., Pontani, R.B., and Vadlamani, N.L. (1989). Interactions of cocaine with barbital, pentobarbital and ethanol, *Arch. Int. Pharmacodyn., 299*:44.

124. Mody, C.K., Miller, B.L., McIntyre, H.B., Cobb, S.K., and Goldberg, M.A. (1988). Neurologic complications of cocaine abuse, *Neurology, 38*:1189.

125. National Institute on Drug Abuse (1986). *Highlights of the 1985 National Household Surveys on Drug Abuse.* National Institute on Drug Abuse, Rockville, Maryland.

126. Norton, R., and Colliver, J. (1988). Prevalence and patterns of combined alcohol and marijuana use, *J. Stud. Alcohol, 49*:378.

127. Norton, R., and Noble, J. (1987). Combined alcohol and other drug use and abuse; A status report, *Alcohol Health Res. World, 16*:78.

128. Novick, D.M., Senie, R.T., Kreek, M.J., and Yancovitz, S.R. (1987). Clinical and demographic features of patients admitted to a new chemical dependency program in New York City, *Drug Alcohol Depend., 20*:271.

129. Nurco, D.N. (1985). A discussion of validity, *Self-Report Methods of Estimating Drug Use: Meeting Current Challenges to Validity* (B.A. Rouse, N.J. Kozel, and L.G. Richards, eds.), U.S. Government Printing Office, Washington, D.C., p. 4.

130. O'Donnell, J.A. (1979). Determinants of early marijuana use, *Youth Drug Abuse: Problems, Issues, and Treatment* (G.M. Bescher and A.S. Friedman, ed.), D.C. Heath, Lexington, Massachusetts.

131. O'Donnell, J.A., and Clayton, R.R. (1982). Determinants of early marijuana use, *Youth Drug Abuse: Problems, Issues, and Treatment,* (G.M. Beschner and A.S. Friedman, eds.), D.C. Heath, Lexington, Massachusetts.

132. Ogborne, A.C., and Kapur, B.M. (1987). Drug use among a sample of males admitted to an alcohol detoxication center, *Alcoholism, 11*:183.

133. Orrego, H., Blendis, L.M., Blake, J.E., Kapur, B.M., and Israel, Y. (1979). Reliability of assessment of alcohol intake based on personal interviews in a liver clinic, *Lancet, 2*:1354.

134. Pentz, M.A., Dwyer, J.H., Mackinnon, D.P., Flay, B.R., Hansen, W.B., Wang, E.Y., and Johnson, C.A. (1989). A multicommunity trial for primary prevention of adolescent drug abuse. Effects on drug use prevalence. *J.A.M.A., 261*:3259.

135. Petursson, H., and Lader, M. (1984). *Dependence on Tranquilizers*, Oxford University Press, New York.

136. Piesiur-Strehlow, B., Strehlow, U., and Poser, W. (1986). Mortality of patients dependent on benzodiazepines, *Acta Psychiatr. Scand., 73*:330.

137. Radosevich, M., Lanza-Kaduce, L., Akers, R., and Krohn, M. (1979). The sociology of adolescent drug and drinking behavior, a review of the state of the field, part 1, *Deviant Behav., 1*:15.

138. Renfroe, C.L. and Messinger, T.A. (1985). Street drug analysis: An eleven year perspective on illicit drug alteration, *Semin. Adolesc. Med., 1*:247.

139. Roffman, R.A., and Barnhart, R. (1987). Assessing need for marijuana dependence treatment through an anonymous telephone interview, *Int. J. Addict., 22*:639.

140. Roffman, R.A., Stephens, R.S., Simpson, E.E., and Whitaker, D.L. (1988). Treatment of marijuana dependence: Preliminary results, *J. Psychoactive Drugs, 20*:129.

141. Ross, H.E. (1989). Alcohol and drug abuse in treated alcoholics: A comparison of men and women, *Alcoholism Clin. Expr. Res., 13*:810.

142. Rounsaville, B.J., Weissman, M.M., and Kleber, H.D. (1982). The significance of alcoholism in treated opiate addicts, *J. Nerv. Ment. Dis., 170*:479.

143. Sadava, S.W. (1985). Research approaches in illicit drug use: A critical review, *Genet. Psychol. Monogr., 91*:3.

144. Santo, Y., Farley, E.C., and Griedman, A.S. (1980). Highlights from the national youth polydrug study, *Drug Abuse Patterns Among Young Polydrug Abusers and Urban Appalachian Youths*, U.S. Department of Health and Human Services, Washington, D.C., p. 1.

145. Schmidt, L.G., Muller-Oerlinghausen, B., Schlunder, M., Seidel, M., and Platz, W.E. (1987). Benzodiazepines and barbiturates in chronic alcoholics and opiate addicts: An epidemiological study of hospitalized addicts, *Dtsch. Med. Wochenschr., 112*:1849.

146. Schoener, E.P. (1986). Mechanisms of depressant drug action/interaction, *Recent Development in Alcoholism*. Vol. 4 (M. Galanter, ed.), Plenum Press, New York, p. 39.

147. Schuckit, M.A. (1987). Alcohol and drug interactions with antianxiety medications, *Am. J. Med., 82*:27.

148. Schuckit, M.A., and Bogard, B. (1986). Intravenous drug use in alcoholics, *J. Clin. Psychiatry, 47*:551.

149. Schuckit, M.A., and Sweeney, S. (1987). Substance use and mental health problems among sons of alcoholics and controls, *J. Stud. Alcohol, 48*:528.

150. Sellers, E.M., and Busto, V. (1982). Benzodiazepine and ethanol: Assessment of the effects and consequences of psychotropic drug interactions, *J. Clin. Psychopharmacol, 2*:249.

151. Sells, S.B. and Simpson, D.D. (1987). Role of alcohol use by narcotic addicts as revealed in the DARP research on evaluation of treatment for drug abuse, *Alcoholism Clin. Exp. Res., 11*:437.

152. Simpson, D.D. (1974). Patterns of multiple drug abuse, *The Effectiveness of Drug Abuse Treatment* Vol. 1 (S.B. Sells, ed.), Ballinger, Cambridge, Massachusetts.

153. Smith, D.E. (1986). Cocaine-alcohol abuse: Epidemiological, diagnostic and treatment considerations, *J. Psychoactive Drugs, 18*:117.

154. Sobell, L.C., Sobell, M.B., Riley, D.M., Schuller, R., Pavan, S.S., Cancilla, A., Klajner, F., and Leo, G.I. (1988). The reliability of alcohol abusers' self-reports of drinking and life events that occurred in the distant past, *J. Stud. Alcohol, 49*:225.

155. Soderstrom, C.A., and Carson, S.L. (1988). Update: Alcohol and other drug use among vehicular crash victims, *Md. Med. J., 37*:541.

156. Soderstrom, C.A., Trifillis, A.L., Shankar, B.S., Clark, W.E., and Cowley, R.A. (1988). Marijuana and alcohol use among 1023 trauma patients: A prospective study, *Arch. Surg., 123*:733.

157. Sokolow, L., Welte, J., Hynes, G., and Lyons, J. (1981). Multiple substance abuse by alcoholics, *Br. J. Addict.*, *76*:147.

158. Soyka, M., Lutz, W., Kauert, G., and Schwarz, A. (1989). Epileptic seizures and alcohol withdrawal: Significance of additional use (and misuse) of drugs and electroencephalographic findings, *J. Epilepsy*, *2*:109.

159. Stimmel, B. (1981). Methadone maintenance and alcohol use, *Drug and Alcohol Abuse: Implications for Treatment. NIDA Treatment Research Monograph Series* (S.E. Gardner, ed.), U.S. Department of Health and Human Services, Rockville, Maryland, p. 57.

160. Stimmel, B., Cohen, M., and Hanbury, R. (1978). Alcoholism and polydrug abuse in persons on methadone maintenance, *Ann. N.Y. Acad. Sci.*, *311*:99.

161. Stimmel, B., Hanbury, R., Sturiano, V., Korts, D., Jackson, G., and Cohen, M. (1982). Alcoholism as a risk factor in methadone maintenance, A randomized controlled trial, *Am. J. Med.*, *73*:631.

162. Strecher, V.J., Becker, M.H., Clark, N.M., Prasada-Rao, P. (1989). Using patient's descriptions of alcohol consumption, diet, medication compliance, and cigarette smoking: The validity of self-reports in research and practice, *J. Gen. Inter. Med.*, *4*:160.

163. Thal, E.R., Bost, R.O. and Anderson, R.J. (1985). Effects of alcohol and other drugs on traumatized patients, *Arch. Surg.*, *120*:708.

164. Thorpe, G.L., Parker, J.D., Bush, M.J., and Magill, S.A. (1987). Alcohol and cocaine abuse treatment in Maine, *Alcohol Health Res. World, Summer*:28.

165. Tuchfield, B.S., McLeroy, K.R., Waterhouse, G.J., Guess, L.L., and Williams, J.R. (1975). *Multiple Drug Abuse Among Persons with Alcohol-Related Problems,* Research Triangle Institute, Research Triangle Park, North Carolina.

166. Vaillant, G.E. (1970). The natural history of narcotic drug addiction, *Semin. Psychiatry*, *2*:486.

167. Wallace, J. (1986). The other problems of alcoholics, *J. Subst. Abuse Treat.*, *3*:163.

168. Weiss, R.D., Mirin, S.M., Griffin, M.L., and Michael, J.L. (1988). A comparison of alcoholic and nonalcoholic drug abusers, *J. Stud. Alcohol*, *49*:510.

169. Welte, J.W., and Barnes, G.M. (1985). Alcohol: The gateway to other drug use among secondary-school students, *J. Youth Adolesc.*, *14*:487.

170. Welte, J.W., and Barnes, G.M. (1987). Youthful smoking: Patterns and relationships to alcohol and other drug use, *J. Adolesc.*, *10*:327.

171. Wesson, D.R., Carlin, A.S., Adams, K.M., and Beschner, G. (1978). *Polydrug Abuse: The Results of a National Collaborative Study.* Academic Press, New York.

172. Williams, G.D., Aitken, S.S., and Malin, H. (1985). Reliability of self-reported alcohol consumption in a general population survey, *J. Stud. Alcohol*, *46*:223.

173. Windle, M., Barnes, G.M., and Welte, J. (1989). Causal models of adolescent substance use: An examination of gender differences using distribution-free estimators, *J. Pers. Soc. Psychol.*, *56*:132.

174. Wiseman, S.M., and Spencer-Peet, J. (1985). Prescribing for alcoholics: A survey of drugs taken prior to admission to an alcoholism unit, *Practitioner*, *229*:88.

175. Wolf, B., Grohmann, R., Biber, D., Brenner, P.M., and Ruther, E. (1989). Benzodiazepine abuse and dependence in psychiatric inpatients, *Pharmacopsychiatry*, *22*:54.

176. Woods, J.H., Katz, J.L., and Winger, G. (1987). Abuse liability of benzodiazepines, *Pharmacol. Rev.*, *39*:251.

177. Yamaguchi, K., and Kandel, D.B. (1984). Patterns of drug use from adolescence to young adulthood: III. Predictors of progression, *Am. J. Public Health*, *74*:673.

178. Yamaguchi, K., and Kandel, D.B. (1984). Patterns of drug use from adolescence to young adulthood: II. Sequence of progression, *Am. J. Public Health*, *74*:668.

179. Yanaura, S., and Suzuki, T. (1977). Cross-dependence between phenobarbital and alcohol in rats, *Jpn. J. Pharmacol.*, *27*:751.

180. Zeiner, A.R., Stanitis, T., Spurgeon, M. and Nichols, N. (1985). Treatment of alcoholism and concomitant drugs of abuse, *Alcohol*, *2*:555.

181. Zuckerman, B., Frank, D.A., Hingson, R., Amaro, H., Levenson, S.M., Kayne, H., Parker, S., Vinci, R., Aboagye, K., Fried, L.E., Cabral, H., Timperi, R., and Bauchner, H. (1989). Effects of maternal marijuana and cocaine use on fetal growth, *N. Engl. J. Med.*, *320*:762.

5

History of Benzodiazepine Dependence

Malcolm Lader
Institute of Psychiatry, University of London, London, England

I. INTRODUCTION

The benzodiazepines (BZDs) were first developed in the 1950s and many were introduced in the 1960s. Many of the people involved in the story of the BZDs are still active in psychopharmacology and psychiatry. Any attempt at a history of one particular aspect of the BZDs must inevitably be impressionistic because many issues are still unresolved and the contributions of various individuals to the topic too recent and even current to be assessed dispassionately. This historical approach is even more difficult for a medical scientist like myself who has worked continuously on the BZDs for 30 years. During the latter half of that time, my views on the BZDs became increasingly maverick, although in the United Kingdom at least the consensus has moved close to my viewpoint.

This chapter, therefore, must be seen within the context of looking back at events well within a single professional lifetime, within the geographical limitations of concentrating on one country, the U.K., and within the biases inescapable in one so long involved in controversy. I have attempted to give a balanced account; the reader must judge if I have succeeded.

II. BEFORE THE BENZODIAZEPINES

"And Noah. . . . . . planted a vineyard: and he drank of the wine, and was drunken . . . ." Despite this the Bible tells us that Noah survived for many years. The use of alcohol goes back about 8000 years, and it is possible that it originally had a mostly religious and highly controlled role in primitive societies. Later it became used medicinally, often as an anxiolytic, and was abused by some. When the Arabs introduced the science of distilling into Europe in the Middle Ages, the alchemist and his customers hailed alcohol as the long-sought elixir of life. The Gaelic term *usquebaugh*, meaning water of life, the term for whisky, was regarded as a panacea. But by the eighteenth century with the introduction of cheap gin, the curses of alcohol had become apparent.

Opium also has a history of extending over thousands of years, and was regarded by Sydenham in 1680 as the most universal and efficacious of "the remedies which it has pleased Almighty God to give to man to relieve his sufferings." Like alcohol, opium and its derivatives were also taken to relieve anxiety. Also, like alcohol, its addictive properties became increasingly apparent. During the nineteenth century, De Quincey, a habitué, dubbed it "dread agent of unimaginable pleasure and pain."

The nineteenth century also witnessed the effects of the Industrial Revolution transforming alchemy into chemistry and old wives' nostrums into pharmaceutical remedies. Nitrous oxide was introduced as a dental and surgical anaesthetic, as were ether and chloroform. The first psychotropic drug to institute the noble tradition of introduction by mistake was bromide. Because potassium bromide was believed to lessen sexual urges and because epilepsy was thought to be a consequence of masturbation, bromides were introduced by Locock for the treatment of epilepsy, apparently with gratifying results! By the 1870s bromides were used very widely as sedatives, and, again, the dependence potential eventually became apparent.

Two organic chemicals were synthesized and introduced as sedatives. Chloral hydrate has retained some usage in its solid derivative forms in the elderly; paraldehyde, however, is obsolete: both are associated with abuse and dependence.

The most widely used synthetics were the barbiturates. Barbituric acid was prepared by Adolf von Baeyer working in Kekulé's laboratory. The first hypnotic barbiturate, barbital (Veronal), was introduced by Fischer and von Mering in 1903, followed by phenobarbital (Luminal) in 1912. Amobarbital came on the market in 1923. About 2500 barbiturate compounds were synthesized over the succeeding years, and about 50 were marketed, of which a dozen or so survive. The dependence-producing potential of these compounds became increasingly apparent, and together with alarm over the dangers in overdose led to campaigns in the 1970s to replace the barbiturates with the BZDs. Other compounds with similar pharmacological properties were introduced, but they met a similar fate as their dependence potential and toxicity became apparent. They include ethchlorvynol, ethinamate, carbromal, glutethimide, methyprylon, and methaqualone.

The story of meprobamate in retrospect seems like a dress rehearsal for that of the BZDs. This story begins with the discovery of mephenesin in 1946 by Berger and Bradley (Berger, 1970). Mephenesin is a muscle relaxant with too short a duration of action for clinical use in anxiety disorders. Meprobamate (Miltown, Equanil) was developed in 1950 as a longer-acting compound. It was widely promoted and widely prescribed as an anxiolytic, but it was found to have an alarming dependence potential. By 1964, there existed "ample evidence that it could induce physical dependence in man" (Essig, 1964). Although meprobamate is still available, and indeed quite widely used in some countries because it is inexpensive (as are the barbiturates), it has largely been supplanted by the BZDs.

III. INTRODUCTION OF THE BENZODIAZEPINES

The story of the BZDs begins in Cracow in Poland in the mid-1930s. Leo Sternbach was working on a chemical grouping called the heptoxdiazines (Sternbach, 1980). He went to the United States and resumed work on these compounds in the Chemical Research Department of Hoffmann–La Roche, USA in Nutley, New Jersey. The heptoxdiazines seemed biologically inactive. However, one, Ro 5-0690, was investigated further, and in 1957 it was found to have hypnotic, sedative and antistrychnine effects, similar to those of meprobamate (Cohen, 1970). To the surprise of the chemists, this compound was found to have undergone a molecular rearrangement to become a 1:4-benzodiazepine.

The first clinical tests nearly led to the drug (now called methaminodiazepoxide, and later chlordiazepoxide) being discarded because it was given in too large a dose to geriatric patients, resulting in dysarthria and ataxia. Eventually, the clinical effectiveness of chlordiazepoxide was established and it was introduced in 1960. Its even more successful congener, diazepam, followed in 1963.

Many other compounds were introduced either as daytime anxiolytics ("tranquilizers"), or night-time hypnotics, or both. The most successful have been nitrazepam, flurazepam, temazepam, and triazolam as hypnotics, and diazepam, lorazepam, and alprazolam as tranquilizers. The last is the current market leader in terms of value. The dates of introduction in the United Kingdom of various benzodiazepines in terms of dosage forms are shown in Table 1. The anxiolytic market is currently worth $2 billion worldwide, and that for hypnotics $650 million.

IV. GROWTH OF BENZODIAZEPINE USAGE

There is no doubt that the usage of BZDs increased dramatically during the 1960s and early 1970s. This gave rise to the perception that the widespread use of anxiolytics and hypnotics is a new phenomenon, reflecting the latter half of the twentieth century as an "age of anxiety." Nothing could be further from the truth. The growth in BZD usage has been almost entirely at the expense of older products, notably the barbiturates. This change was encouraged by the pharmaceutical industry as newer more profitable BZDs replaced the older barbiturates.

In 1975, the year in which BZD sales peaked in the United States, total anxiolytic and hypnotic sales accounted for about 10% of all prescriptions, only a percent or so higher for those in the 1950s and 1960s. From 1975 to about 1981, sales of anxiolytics declined and have since risen slightly. In the United Kingdom, prescriptions are mostly dispensed under the National Health Service. About 15% of all prescriptions are for hypnotics and anxiolytics. Again, this figure has hardly changed in the past decades. Prescriptions for anxiolytic benzodiazepines in the United Kingdom have fallen considerably since 1975, but those for

Table 1 Year of Introduction of Benzodiazepines to U.K.

Generic name	Brand (manufacturer)	Sold since
Chlordiazepoxide	Librium (Roche), etc.	1960
Diazepam	Valium, etc.	1963
Nitrazepam	Mogadon (Roche), etc.	1965
Oxazepam	Serenid (Wyeth)	1966
Medazepam	Nobrium (Roche)	1971
Lorazepam	Ativan (Wyeth), etc.	1972
Clorazepate	Tranxene (Boehringer)	1973
Flurazepam	Dalmane (Roche)	1974
Temazepam	Euhypnos (FCE)	1977
	Normison (Wyeth)	1977
Triazolam	Halcion (Upjohn)	1979
Clobazam	Frisium (Hoechst)	1979
Ketazolam	Anxon (Beecham)	1980
Lormetazepam	Noctamid (Schering)	1981
Flunitrazepam	Rohypnol (Sauter)	1982
Bromazepam	Lexotan (Roche)	1982
Prazepam	Centrax (Warner)	1982
Alprazolam	Xanax (Upjohn)	1983

hypnotics have remained steady. Indeed, now more prescriptions are written for hypnotics than for anxiolytics.

Nevertheless, such replacement of one group of sedative/hypnotics for another is no reason for complacency. First, the use of medicines generally has been increasing, partly but not entirely as a result of a changing demography with an increasing proportion of elderly in the population. Therefore, the absolute amount of anxiolytic and hypnotic use has been increasing in many Western countries. Second, much of the usage of sedatives and hypnotics may always have been excessive and inappropriate, perhaps based on habituation and dependence.

V. ABUSE AND DEPENDENCE

The confusions and controversies which have attended the history of BZD dependence reflect those more generally in the addiction field (Lader, 1988). The lack of consensus among experts concerning the dependence potential of the BZDs hinges on the establishment or not to each expert's satisfaction of the reality of normal therapeutic dose physical dependence. Until recently, dosage escalation was regarded as a cardinal and essential feature of dependence; i.e., tolerance was inextricably linked to dependence and abuse.

It is helpful, consequently, to distinguish however arbitrarily between three main conditions:

1. *Drug abuse* with regular or intermittent self-administration of large doses of benzodiazepines, outside the medical context. Drug-seeking behavior is the rule.
2. *Drug misuse* with regular oral ingestion of large amounts of BZDs, sometimes but not always obtained by prescription. Such usage typically starts within the medical context, but the dosage is increased beyond normal therapeutic levels. If supplies are restricted, drug-seeking behavior ensues.
3. *Physical dependence* at normal therapeutic doses as manifested by a withdrawal syndrome of the sedative/alcohol type on discontinuation, abrupt or tapered. Drug-seeking behavior will occur if injudicious attempts are made to restrict the supply.

Too often, data obtained concerning one type of problem has been used injudiciously to support a viewpoint concerning another type of dependence.

VI. ABUSE OF BENZODIAZEPINES

The scientific literature contains many instances of BZD abuse. Marks collected 151 cases worldwide of benzodiazepine dependence within the framework of multiple-drug abuse or alcoholism, plus 250 less definite cases (Marks, 1978). As he points out, assigning individual cases to the "abuse" or "therapeutic" groups is difficult. It is unclear how many people become dependent within the clinical situation, and then resort to the black market for excess illicit supplies. Furthermore, the nature and degree of possible benzodiazepine dependence in people who are currently dependent on other drugs and/or alcohol is difficult to estimate.

According to Cooperstock and Hill (1982), polydrug use was a common pattern among some BZD users. One common pattern which emerged in the 1970s was for opioid abusers to use oral BZDs to "come down" from the "high." However, in the 1980s in the United Kingdom, a more serious abuse emerged. Temazepam is available in liquid-filled capsules and abusers were extracting the fluid and injecting it intravenously. The burgeoning problem was contained by reformulating the capsules to contain a solid but rapidly absorbed form of temazepam.

In many countries, abuse of benzodiazepines gave rise to alarm and was instrumental in the World Health Organization recommending the scheduling of BZDs in the early 1980s. Signatories to the 1971 Convention on Psychotropic Substances have brought in Scheduling Regulations, usually of a fairly mild nature.

VII. HIGH-DOSE DEPENDENCE

Two studies carried out in the early 1960s established the potential of the benzodiazepines to induce a physical dependence state when the drug was given in a high dose for several weeks. The first involved 36 chronically ill psychiatric patients who were administered 300–600 mg/day of chlordiazepoxide for 2–6 months (Hollister et al., 1961). These doses are several times the usual recommended clinical dose but the patients tolerated them. The drug was abruptly discontinued in 11 patients with single-blind placebo substitution, but because of the long elimination half-lives of some of the active metabolites of chlordiazepoxide, bodily concentrations presumably took some time to dissipate. Depression supervened in six patients and aggravation of the psychoses in five. Insomnia, agitation, and loss of appetite developed in other patients and major convulsions supervened in three. Symptoms started about 2 days after cessation of the BZD, became severe between the fourth and eighth days, and had largely waned by day 10. Parallel data were obtained in the second study involving high doses of diazepam (Hollister et al., 1963).

Thus, the existence of physical dependence in patients taking high doses of BZDs was established right from the initiation of BZD use. However, as Hollister was to emphasize later, these studies involved very artificial conditions of forced high dose use for several months. What such studies cannot tell us is how many patients started on therapeutic courses of BZDs escalate their doses to such high levels that physical dependence is inevitable.

Throughout the 1960s and 1970s, the scientific literature is peppered with case reports of patients who had escalated their dose of tranquilizer to above the upper recommended therapeutic limit. For example, Peters and Boeters (1970) described eight cases of physical dependence on diazepam, average dose 60–80 mg/day. In another study of two patients, withdrawal from 60 and 120 mg, respectively, was accompanied by convulsions and confusional states (Venzlaff, 1972). Woody and his colleagues (1975) described two patients taking 100–150 mg of diazepam daily who developed insomnia, tremor, and grand mal seizures on stopping the medication. Bliding (1978) encountered four cases of withdrawal reactions from oxazepam, the most prominent symptoms being anxiety, tension, tremor, and palpitations. Patients within the high-dose category have typically taken 2–5 times the recommended therapeutic doses of the various BZDs.

However, little notice was taken of these reports. Part of the problem was the widespread perception of the safety of the BZDs. During the 1960s the medical profession realized that the BZDs were surprisingly safe in overdosage compared with their predecessors the barbiturates. This awareness coincided with a pandemic of suicidal attempts, particularly in young women. So impressed were the British doctors that they mounted a campaign under the auspices of the British Medical Association to phase out the barbiturates. Implicit in that initiative in the mid-1970s was acquiescence in the growth in use of the BZDs.

Coupled with many reports of the safety of BZDs was the paucity of reports on abuse and misuse, with escalation of dosage. Despite the several hundred reports in the literature, Marks (1978) claimed that only 118 of those published up to mid-1977 contained fully verified cases of physical dependence with a definite withdrawal syndrome or carefully documented cases of psychological dependence. He concluded reassuringly:

> Dependence on benzodiazepines occurs rarely under conditions of clinical use and then usually only after prolonged administration at above average dosage. Clinically it resembles that described as "barbiturate" or "alcohol-barbiturate" type. . . . (p. 1)

The dependence risk with benzodiazepines is very low and is estimated to be approximately one case per 5 million patient months "at risk" for all recorded cases and probably less than one case per 50 million months in therapeutic use. . . . (p. 2)

This anodyne conclusion was almost entirely based on patients who had escalated their dose beyond therapeutic levels, that being the way they had come to medical notice. Although there was criticism of Marks' conclusion at the time, pointing out that case reports are a useless epidemiological reference frame (Editorial, 1979), most prescribers accepted it as consistent with their clinical experience: patients did stay on the same dose indefinitely, tolerance was uncommon, and therefore dependence unlikely.

About this time, the U.K. Regulatory Authorities became concerned about the extensive long-term use of BZDs. Following the lead of the Institute of Medicine (USA) and the conclusions of the White House Office of Drug Policy and the National Institute of Drug Abuse (USA), the Committee on Review of Medicines (1980) concluded that there was little evidence that hypnotics retained their sleep-promoting properties within 3–14 days of continuous use, nor that anxiolytics were effective beyond 4 months. However, in the absence of proper epidemiological surveys, they concurred with Marks' low estimate of dependence risk. They were particularly concerned, however, with the question of withdrawal symptoms and urged gradual withdrawal even after short courses of BZDs at therapeutic doses.

By the middle of 1981, the number of publications on benzodiazepines had risen substantially and the tally of cases had doubled, and Marks (1983) partly recanted.

VIII. NORMAL-DOSE DEPENDENCE

The extensive usage of the BZDs was beginning to raise doubt in a few clinician's minds by the early 1970s. Astute observers noted an increasing cohort of long-term users. The oft-repeated assertion that this just reflected the chronic nature of anxiety disorders failed to reassure some. But the alternative explanation—that patients could become physically dependent at therapeutic doses—was so dissonant with accepted teachings on dependence to be dismissed by almost all authorities.

However, one study was consistent with this view, that of Covi and his colleagues (1973). In this study, and a preceding one (1969), a minor withdrawal syndrome was found in anxious patients discontinuing chlordiazepoxide after 20 weeks' use. None of the patients took more than the prescribed dose. The authors also raised the possibility that patients who persist with BZD treatment may represent an "addictive personality type," although they had no data to support this speculation. These studies, both prospective, should have received more attention. However, Covi and his colleagues stressed the minor nature of the symptoms, did not design their studies specifically to evaluate withdrawal, and wrote up their results in a complex and confusing way. Furthermore, the patients had been treated with other psychotropic drugs, such as phenobarbital. The study failed to make an impact.

Another publication comprised a review of the literature on diazepam dependence and then a survey of 50 diazepam users (Maletzky and Klotter, 1976). The review of literature is admirably critical and points out that none of the studies reviewed used controls sufficient to disprove the possibility that diazepam induced dependence. Their own study comprised an interview of 50 patients taking diazepam. The data show clearly that patients tended to increase their dosage, had difficulty discontinuing, experiencing anxiety, tremor, insomnia, and other symptoms. The authors argue cogently that this constitutes a withdrawal syndrome because sometimes the patient had been free of anxiety when the drug was initially prescribed or the initial anxiety had resolved. Also, many of the patients (17/24 who had attempted discontinuation) complained of new symptoms. There were no predictors of drug use or dependence. This study should have had a major influence, setting the alarm bells ringing among the medical profession. It did not. The authors themselves state:

> The retrospective, uncontrolled nature of most of the data reported herein makes this study merely suggestive. (p. 111)

The authors point out the need for a prospective systematic study, affirmed their intention to do so, but never did. Finally, the report was published in a specialist journal in the addiction field, and did not come to general attention.

Two clinicians in the United Kingdom continued their jeremiad. I wrote a paper entitled "Benzodiazepines—The opium of the masses?" (Lader, 1978), and Tyrer drew attention to the "Benzodiazepine bonanza." Almost simultaneously we instituted studies to explore the possibility that long-term BZD users might be physically dependent and undergo definite withdrawal reactions of the sedative/hypnotic type, similar to those associated with barbiturate and alcohol use. Tyrer conducted his studies within a clinical context substituting placebo (or propranolol) for diazepam or lorazepam (Tyrer et al., 1981). My own studies were laboratory-based (Petursson and Lader, 1984). These studies established unequivocally that normal dose dependence as manifested by a physical withdrawal syndrome was a real entity and supervened even if the dosage was tapered off. Tolerance with escalation of dosage was not a prerequisite for physical dependence. Indeed, one of our studies compared the withdrawal syndromes in small groups of patients withdrawing from high- or low-dose usage: the syndromes were identical (Hallstrom and Lader, 1981).

It became accepted that normal-dose BZD could occur, but controversy raged as to whether this was a common feature. Certainly, the patients I studied were in a way self-selected; that is, they had tried to stop their medication, had withdrawal symptoms, reinstituted their drug, and sought my help. It was impossible to know whether this was the tip of a very large iceberg or whether these patients were uncommon. More recent studies, such as that by Busto et al. (1986), have established that about 15–25% of long-term (over 12 months) users undergo a definite withdrawal syndrome. Only a few percent experience major distress. However, no large-scale prospective studies have been carried out to establish with any precision the precise parameters of the epidemiology of benzodiazepine withdrawal.

A further development has been the realization that withdrawal may be prolonged (Ashton, 1984) or associated with major depressive disorder (Olajide and Lader, 1984).

Recently, appreciation of the hazards of long-term BZD usage has led to parallel guidelines being issued by the U.K. Committee on Safety of Medicines and the Royal College of Psychiatrists. These guidelines restrict benzodiazepines to short-term use, stress the need to establish a definite indication, and warn against abrupt withdrawal. In similar vein, in the United States (Schweizer et al., 1989) have averred "we have unpublished data which demonstrate that many patients, once they have been withdrawn from their maintenance benzodiazepines, show more improvement on clinical measures of anxiety and depression than they did during their chronically medicated state."

The widespread usage of the benzodiazepines has inevitably led to thousands of people becoming dependent, perhaps 500,000 in the United Kingdom, twice that number in the United States where long-term use is less common. Patients who have become dependent and have either been unable to withdraw or have only done so with great symptomatic distress justifiably feel aggrieved against their doctors and the BZD manufacturers for not warning them about the risk. In the United Kingdom, about 2000 people have started legal proceedings, coordinated by about 300 firms of lawyers. It is the largest civil action ever.

It is interesting to examine the different attitudes toward BZD use between the United Kingdom and United States. The United States has also seemed more concerned about abuse and high-dose use of BZDs, reflecting the much greater drug addiction problem in general there (American Psychiatric Association, 1990). The United Kingdom has concentrated its attention on normal-dose BZD dependence, partly because most of the early and original research was carried out in the United Kingdom and was effectively publicized, and partly because chronic usage is high. Yet, other countries where usage is even higher, such as Belgium and France, seem blissfully unaware of the problem.

The situation in the United States will change. The leading BZD there is now alprazolam, which like lorazepam is highly potent and appears to be associated with more dependence problems than, say, diazepam. Usage of alprazolam in high dosage for long periods in the management of panic disorders must inevitably lead to a dependence problem of major proportions. Severe reactions such as seizures and delirium may follow abrupt discontinuation (Breier et al., 1984; Levy, 1984; Noyes et al. 1986). In one interesting account, withdrawal delirium from alprazolam was unresponsive to diazepam and the alprazolam itself had to be reinstituted (Zipursky et al., 1985).

In clinical studies, withdrawal from alprazolam needs careful management. In one study 15/17 patients had recurrent or increased panic attacks and nine had significant new withdrawal symptoms (Fyer et al., 1987). Rebound anxiety was noted in 22% of patients undergoing a four-week taper from alprazolam; in 28% rebound panics occurred. Four out of 33 patients had three or more significant withdrawal symptoms (Pecknold and Swinson, 1986). In a large-scale multicenter alprazolam/placebo comparison, a subset of 126 patients was carefully studied during and after a four-week taper period (Pecknold et al., 1988). Of the 60 alprazolam-treated patients, 16 (27%) experienced rebound panic attacks and 21 (35%) had some form of withdrawal syndrome although it was marked in only six.

Along with withdrawal and rebound at the end of alprazolam treatment, attention has been drawn to daytime interdose symptom recurrence with an increasingly short period of drug effectiveness, so-called "clock watching." Presumably tolerance with rebound occurs after each dose: this is characteristic of shorter-acting BZDs. Related to this is early morning "rebound"—patients wake feeling anxious and shaky until they take their first dose of the day.

Will history repeat itself with alprazolam and the last decade of the 20th century see a major dependence problem in the United States and elsewhere? Let us hope that this time we are sufficiently forewarned to limit the duration and the dosage of alprazolam to the minima.

REFERENCES

American Psychiatric Association. *Task Force Report on Benzodiazepine Dependence, Toxicity, and Abuse*. Washington, D.C., American Psychiatric Association, in press.

Anon. (1990). Cost of neurosis. *Lancet, i*:23.

Ashton, H. (1984). Benzodiazepine withdrawal: An unfinished story. *Br. Med. J., 288*:1135–1140.

Berger, F.M. (1970). Anxiety and the discovery of tranquilizers. In F.J. Ayd and B. Blackwell (eds.), *Discoveries in Biological Psychiatry*, Lippincott, Philadelphia, pp. 115–129.

Bliding, A. (1978). The abuse potential of benzodiazepines with special reference to oxazepam. *Acta Psychiat. Scand. (Suppl.) 274*:111–16.

Breier, A. Charney, D.S., Nelson, J.C. (1984). Seizures induced by abrupt discontinuation of alprazolam. *Am. J. Psychiatry, 141*:1606–1607.

Busto, U., Sellers, E.M., Naranjo, C.A., Cappell, H.D., Sanchez, C.M., and Simpkins, J. (1986). Patterns of benzodiazepine abuse and dependence. *Br. J. Addict., 81*:87–94.

Cohen, I.M. (1970). The benzodiazepines. In F.J. Ayd and B. Blackwell (eds.), *Discoveries in Biological Psychiatry* Lippincott, Philadelphia, pp. 130–141.

Committee on Review of Medicines (UK) (1980). Systematic review of the benzodiazepines. *Br. Med. J., 2*:719–720.

Cooperstock, R., and Hill, J. (1982). *The Effects of Tranquillization: Benzodiazepine Use in Canada*. Ministry of National Health and Welfare, Toronto.

Covi, L., Lipman, R.S., Patterson, J.H., Derogatis, L.R., and Uhlenhuth, E.H. (1973). Length of treatment with anxiolytic sedatives and response to their sudden withdrawal. *Acta Psychiat. Scand.,* *49*:51–64.

Covi, L., Park, L.C., Lipman, R.S., Uhlenhuth, E.H., and Rickels, K. (1969). Factors affecting withdrawal response to certain minor tranquilizers. In J. Cole and J. Wittenborn (eds.), *Drug Abuse: Social and Psychopharmacological Aspects*, pp. 93–108.

Editorial (1979). Benzodiazepine withdrawal. *Lancet, 1*:196.

Essig, C.F. (1964). Addiction to nonbarbiturate sedative and tranquillizing drugs. *Clin. Pharmacol. Therapeut. 5*:334–343.

Fyer, A.J., Liebowitz, M.R., Gorman, J.M., Campeas, R., Levin, A., Davies, S.O., Goetz, D., and Klein, D.F. (1987). Discontinuation of alprazolam treatment in panic patients. *Am. J. Psychiatry, 144*:303–308.

Hallstrom, C., and Lader, M.H. (1981). Benzodiazepine withdrawal phenomena. *Int. Pharmaco-psychiatry, 16*:235–44.

Hollister, L.E., Bennett, J.L., Kimbell, I., Savage, C., and Overall, J.E. (1963). Diazepam in newly admitted schizophrenics. *Dis. Nerv. System, 24*:746–750.

Hollister, L.E., Motzenbecker, F.P., and Degan, R.O. (1961). Withdrawal reactions from chlordiazepoxide ("Librium"). *Psychopharmacologia, 2*:63–68.

Lader, M.H. (1978). Benzodiazepines—The opium of the masses? *Neuroscience, 3*:159–165.

Lader, M.H. (ed.) (1988). *The Psychopharmacology of Addiction.* Oxford Medical Publications, Oxford, England.

Levy, A.B. 1984). Delirium and seizures due to abrupt alprazolam withdrawal: case report. *J. Clinical Psychiatry, 45*:38–39.

Maletzky, B.M., and Klotter, J. (1976). Addiction to diazepam. *Int. J. Addict., 11*:95–115.

Marks, J. (1978). *The Benzodiazepines. Use, Overuse, Misuse, Abuse.* MTP, Lancaster, England.

Marks, J. (1983). The benzodiazepines—for good or evil. *Neuropsychobiology, 10*:115–126.

Noyes, R., Perry, P.J., Crowe, R.R., Coryell, W.H., Clancy, J., Yamada, T., and Gabel, J. (1986). Seizures following the withdrawal of alprazolam. *J. Nervous & Mental Disorders, 174*:50–52.

Olajide, D., and Lader, M.H. (1984). Depression following withdrawal from long-term benzodiazepines use: A report of four cases. *Psychol. Med., 14*:937–940.

Pecknold, J.C., and Swinson, R.P. (1986). Taper withdrawal studies with alprazolam in patients with panic disorder and agoraphobia. *Psychopharmacology Bulletin, 22*:173–176.

Pecknold, J.C., Swinson, R.P., Kuch, K., and Lewis, C.P. (1988). Alprazolam in panic disorder and agoraphobia: results from a multicenter trial. III. Discontinuation effects. *Archives of General Psychiatry, 45*:429–436.

Peters, U.H., and Boeters, U. (1970). Valium-Sucht. Eine Analyse anhand von 8 Fällen. *Pharmaco-psychiat. Neuropsychopharmacol., 3*:339–48.

Petursson, H., and Lader, M. (1984). *Dependence on Tranquillizers.* Oxford University Press, Oxford, England.

Schweizer, E., Case, W.G., and Rickels, K. (1989). Dr. Schweizer and associates reply. *Am. J. Psychiatry, 146*:1242.

Sternbach, L.H. (1980). *The Benzodiazepine Story.* Editiones Roche, Basel.

Tyrer, P., Rutherford, D., and Huggett, T. (1981). Benzodiazepine withdrawal symptoms and propranolol. *Lancet, 1*:520–522.

Venzlaff, V. (1972). Valiumsucht. *Internist. Praxis, 12*:349.

Woody, G.E., O'Brien, C.P., and Greenstein, R. (1975). Misuse and abuse of diazepam: An increasingly common medical problem. *Int. J. Addict., 10*:843–848.

Zipursky, R.B., Baker, R.W., and Zimmer, B. (1985). Alprazolam withdrawal delirium unresponsive to diazepam: case report. *J. Clinical Psychiatry, 46*:344–345.

6

Cocaine: Epidemiology

Joseph M. Palumbo
Stony Lodge Hospital, Briarcliff Manor, New York

Mark S. Gold and A. Carter Pottash
Fair Oaks Hospital, Summit, New Jersey, and Delray Beach, Florida

I. SOURCES AND DISTRIBUTION

Cocaine is nearly ubiquitous in this country. It is consumed in all types of environments, urban and rural, and by all strata of the socioeconomic ladder. In 1989, the United States Drug Enforcement Administration (DEA) reported that while wholesale and retail prices for cocaine declined, purity levels of the drug at the wholesale level remained consistently better than 90%. At the street level, a "gram" of cocaine was 25% pure in 1981, but 70% pure by 1988 and cost $100 to purchase. A tenth of a gram of "crack" costs $10 [1].

In 1988, 60,000 kg of cocaine was confiscated by the DEA, fewer than 200 kg was seized in 1977 [3]. Crude forms of cocaine are often smuggled from Peru and Bolivia to laboratories in Colombia, Ecuador, Central America, and South Florida for conversion to cocaine hydrochloride. Distribution is achieved through organized crime gangs, "possees," and other agents. The smuggling of cocaine is complex, especially well organized, and often performed by women who act as couriers, and who conceal the drug in luggage, "presents," and body cavities [1]. Indiscriminate violence, conversion of legitimate businesses, false identities, and high-powered weapons are used routinely in assuring delivery of their product to eager consumers [1]. In New York City, some groups have confederated to sell cocaine and crack. Those individuals declining to join the confederation are frequently the victims of homicides as turf wars begin.

Crack has been distributed wholesale in chunks or in prefilled vials. Each vial contains an average of 65–135 mg of crack. Vials are often sold from heavily fortified apartments in which the buyer passes money through a small slot in the door, and receives the vials through the slot [1]. At $5–$20 per vial, an ounce of cocaine can be retailed as crack for approximately $3700, or about $2000 more than it would sell for in the hydrochloride form [1]. Trafficking cocaine has become so lucrative that children as young as 10 years of age are making up to $500 per week selling crack [1].

II. PREVALENCE

Recent surveys [2] suggest cocaine use has spread into the work place, with 73% of the responders to a 1985 "hotline" survey claiming that they abuse cocaine while on the job. Overall, approximately 60% of users are males and over 60% are white. The average user is 27 years old, makes over $25,000 a year, uses better than a gram of cocaine per day, and employs other drugs to combat the side effects of cocaine. Half of the users "snort" the drug, a third "freebase," and about 20% inject the drug intravenously. The typical user spends better than $500 per week on cocaine, but might spend over $3000 on a binge—using cocaine continuously, often without sleep and little or no food, for days at a time until money, the supply of the drug, or their physical evidence is exhausted [3]. In 1989, the 800-COCAINE telephone Helpline reported that crack users were a particularly "addicted" group, with 97% of the users reporting daily use of the drug. They are also a particularly violent group, with over one-fourth of the users self-reporting that they have been involved in a violent crime while on crack [4].

Also, in 1989, the Gordon S. Black Corporation reported the results of interviews conducted in 1987 with 7325 respondents across the United States. It described considerable prevalence of cocaine abuse in teenagers, high school seniors, college students, and young adults. By age 17, 13.5% of all teens have tried cocaine, with 8.4% claiming use in the past 30 days. Eighteen percent of high school seniors have tried cocaine, with 13.7% expressing their use of the drug in the past month. Fourteen percent of college students have taken cocaine in the last 12 months. By age twenty-seven, 38.8% of all young adults have tried cocaine, with 20% admitting to cocaine use in the past year [9].

Additional trends are alarming. Sixteen percent of children aged 9–12 have already been approached to buy drugs. Nearly 40% of these children claim that it is both hard to say "no" to drugs and that drug users are "popular." By the age of 13, 4–5% of teenagers have tried cocaine. It appears that the single factor chiefly responsible for all drug use among teens is peers who abuse drugs. If a child has friends who abuse drugs, then he or she probably does as well [5]. And, the earlier a child begins to use drugs, the more likely he or she is to increase the frequency of drug abuse currently, and the less likely that the child will reduce the abuse in the future [5]. Overall, women are nearly identical to men in their use of cocaine, but blacks and Hispanics are more likely to abuse drugs than whites. By age 12, 27% of black children have been offered drugs, and fully 29% of black teens perceive no risk in using cocaine. Likewise, Hispanics are also less inclined to view drugs as harmful. Both affluence and poverty are related to higher levels of drug use, whereas regular church attendance predicts lower levels of drug abuse [5].

Additional problems of great concern arise when specific sectors of the population are sampled. Women addicted to crack may have few financial resources. Frequently, female addicts barter sex for cocaine, and may become literal slaves to a dealer or "crack house" to feed their addictions [6]. Marked increases in the incidence rates of syphilis has been linked to crack [7]. Twenty-three percent of all pregnant adolescents in a Boston University Study were cocaine users [8]. In Dallas, a sample of 102 pregnant women revealed that approximately 10% of these women were abusing cocaine while pregnant [9]. A similar study in Boston revealed that 17% of pregnant women used cocaine during the pregnancy, but that 24% of the women involved denied cocaine use [10].

The use of cocaine in the armed services continues to be an active problem [11]. In 1988, 2.15% of all Navy recruits had positive urine toxicology results for cocaine [12]. This percentage is very significant, but dwarfed by the prevalence of cocaine use in a "post-military" group. An anonymous survey of Veterans Administration patients in a metropolitan area demonstrated that 46% of all patients had tried cocaine, with 23% admitting to current use [13].

In Los Angeles County, automobile drivers who were fatally injured in accidents between May 1987 and May 1988 were screened for cocaine in their blood or urine. Eight percent of these drivers demonstrated detectable amounts of cocaine when toxicology results were studied. A preliminary study from 1985 to 1986 revealed that 9.8% of similar fatalities tested positive for cocaine [14]. When all overdose and drug-related deaths in Los Angeles County were examined in 1985, cocaine was implicated in 279 of 1923 cases, or 14.5% of all cases. By 1987, the number had soared to 818 cases, although percentages had not yet been reported [14].

In December, 1986 a group of 359 tractor trailer drivers in Tennessee were asked to participate in a voluntary health survey for which they would be paid $30 for their participation. Of this group, 317 provided usable samples of blood or urine. Two percent of this group tested positive for cocaine, and half of the positive group was also positive for marijuana [15].

The use of cocaine in the workplace by individuals in positions of responsibility has not spared the "professions." In 1986, 589 of 1427 senior medical students at 13 medical schools returned a questionnaire pertaining to drug use. Thirty-six percent of the students reported ever having used cocaine. Seventeen percent reported use in the past year, with 7% having used cocaine within the last month [16,17]. A similar study looked at physicians' use of cocaine in a New England state in 1984–1985, and 9% of the responding physicians admitted to current or past cocaine use. The same study revealed that 39% of that state's medical students had ever used cocaine [18].

REFERENCES

1. Featherly, J.W., and Hill, E.B. (1989). *Crack/Cocaine Overview*. Drug Enforcement Administration of the U.S. Department of Justice.
2. Washton, A.M., and Gold, M.S. (1987). Recent trends in cocaine abuse: A view from the national hotline, 800-COCAINE. *Cocaine: Pharmacology, Addiction and Therapy*, Haworth Press, pp. 3147.
3. Roehrich, H., and Gold, M.S. (1988). 800-Cocaine: Origin, significance and findings. *Yale J. Biol. Med. 61*:149–155.
4. Gold, M.S., and Palumbo, J.M. (in preparation). Characteristics of the user of crack cocaine.
5. Black, G.S. (1989). *The Attitudinal Basis of Drug Use—1987 and Changing Attitudes Toward Drug Use—1988*. Reports from The Media-Advertising Partnership for a Drug-free America, Inc. Gordon S. Black Corporation. Rochester, New York.
6. Guinan, M.E. (1989). Women and crack addiction. *J. Am. Med. Women's Assoc. 44*:129.
7. Syphilis and congential syphilis—United States, 1985–1988. *M.M.W.R. 37*:486–489.
8. Amaro, H., et al. (1989). Drug use among adolescent mothers: Profile of risk. *Pediatrics 84*(1):144–150.
9. Little, B.B., et al. (1988). Cocaine use in pregnant women in a large public hospital. *Am. J. Perinatol. 5*(3):206–207.
10. Frank, D.A., et al. (1988). Cocaine use during pregnancy: Prevalence and correlates. *Pediatrics 82*(6):888–894.
11. Needleman, S.B., and Romberg, R.W. (1989). Comparison of drug abuse in different military populations. *J. Forensic Sci. 34*:848–857.
12. Prevalence of drug use among applicants for military service—United States, June—December, 1988. *M.M.W.R. 38*(33):580–583.
13. Brower, K.J., et al. (1989). Recent trends in cocaine abuse in a VA psychiatric population. *Hosp. Commun. Psychiatry 37*(12):1229–1234.
14. Budd, R.D., et al. (1989). Drugs of abuse found in fatally injured drivers in Los Angeles county. *Drug Alcohol Depend. 23*:153–158.
15. Lund, A.K., et al. (1988). Drug use by tractor-trailer drivers. *J. Forensic Sci. 33*(3):648–661.

16. Conrad, S., et al. (1989). Cocaine use by senior medical students. *Am. J. Psychiatry* *146*(3):382–383.
17. Conrad, S., et al. (1988). Substance use by fourth-year students at 13 U.S. medical schools. *J. Med. Ed.* *63*:747–758.
18. McAuliffe, W.E., et al. (1986). Psychoactive drug use among practicing physicians and medical students. *New Engl. J. Med.* *315*(13):805–810.

II

Special Populations

7

Drug and Alcohol Effects on Pregnancy and the Newborn

Ira J. Chasnoff
Northwestern University Medical School, Chicago, Illinois

I. EPIDEMIOLOGY

Since the early 1970s with the full description of the fetal alcohol syndrome by Jones and Smith in the United States [1], there has been increasing recognition of the importance of the use of licit and illicit drugs by pregnant women. In 1988, a survey of 36 hospitals in the United States [2] found that 11% of pregnant women delivering in those hospitals had used an illegal drug at some time during the pregnancy. This finding was supported by the most recent National Institute on Drug Abuse (NIDA) Household Survey [3], in which approximately 9% of women of child-bearing age admitted to having used an illegal drug in the 1 month prior to the completion of the questionnaire.

The problems of alcohol and other drug use and addiction in pregnancy cross all racial and socioeconomic lines. In a population-based survey of 715 women entering prenatal care over a period of 6 months in Pinellas County, Florida, 14.8% of the women had a positive urine toxicology for cocaine, marijuana, alcohol, or heroin [4]. Women enrolled in the public health care system had an overall prevalence rate of 16%, whereas 13% of women in private obstetric care had a positive urine toxicology. There was no difference in rates of positive toxicologies when analyzed along racial lines: 14.1% of black women and 15.4% of white women were positive. The most common drugs found in the urine of this population of women were marijuana and cocaine.

The impact of these high rates of alcohol and other drug use and addiction by pregnant women has had a profound effect on fetal and neonatal outcome. Intensive care nurseries are stretching their capacities to care for infants affected by maternal cocaine use. Foster care systems are overburdened with abandoned and medically high-risk infants. In a survey conducted by the Child Abuse Prevention Program, Department of Health Services in Los Angeles, California, of a total of 5973 cases of child abuse reported in 1985, 538 cases (9%) involved neonatal withdrawal owing to maternal drug use in pregnancy. In the first 6 months of 1986, 403 of 4299 cases (9.4%) of child abuse were due to maternal addiction during pregnancy. The patterns of drug use in this population showed a shift toward an even higher frequency of cocaine use among the reported cases in the first 6 months of 1986 as compared to 1985 [5].

In Illinois in FY1989, over 2300 infants were reported to the Department of Children and Family Services because they were born with cocaine in their urine. Thus, the societal costs of these infants continue to mount.

II. PHARMACOLOGY OF ILLICIT DRUGS IN PREGNANCY

It is a common belief that the placenta acts as a barrier protecting the fetus from various toxic substances. However, this is not so. Numerous reviews of drug use during pregnancy show that the placenta is freely crossed by most drugs taken by the mother during pregnancy. Drugs which act on the central nervous system are usually lipophilic and are of relatively low molecular weight, characteristics that facilitate the crossing of the substance from the maternal to the fetal circulation. For many sedative-hypnotic medications, there is rapid equilibration of free drug between the maternal and the fetal circulation. Although the exact distribution of drug between the maternal and the fetal circulation is difficult to determine, it is reasonable to say that drugs with high abuse potential (opiates, cocaine, sedative-hypnotics, alcohol, and stimulants) are found at significant levels in the fetus if the mother is using or abusing these drugs.

Some drugs which accumulate in the fetus can be metabolized by the fetal liver and the placenta. Frequently, the metabolites are water soluble, which hinders the passage of the metabolite back across the placenta to the maternal circulation where it can be excreted. Because the fetal liver is not fully developed, it is frequently difficult to anticipate the exact fate of a specific drug in the fetus. The majority of drugs that have been studied have a longer half-life in the fetus than in the adult. This is also true in the neonate, since the enzymes involved in the metabolic process of glucoronidation and oxidation are not fully developed in the fetus. In addition, the immature renal function of the newborn may delay the excretion of drugs which have been metabolized to an excretable form.

III. IDENTIFICATION OF THE DRUG ABUSE/ADDICTED PREGNANT WOMAN

Medical personnel have an excellent opportunity to thoroughly evaluate the pregnant woman for drug abuse/addiction. The clinical assessment should include an evaluation of the physical appearance, a medical and obstetrical history, and a substance abuse interview (Table 1).

It is important to always bear in mind that the drug addict/alcoholic, whether pregnant or not, usually denies, minimizes, or rationalizes drug/alcohol use, abuse, or addiction. Awareness of this and skillful history taking and persistent diagnostic approaches will improve the opportunity to detect drug/alcohol use during pregnancy. A disregard of the insidiousness of the denial will result in a lost opportunity for intervention to arrest drug/alcohol use and addiction in order to treat the mother and prevent damage to the fetus.

A. Medical History

In the medical history, a positive history for cirrhosis, hepatitis, bacterial endocarditis, cellulitis, pneumonia, or pancreatitis should call attention to a possibility of substance abuse.

In a general medical unit, 25–40% of the admissions are due to the effects of chemical dependence [6]. Medical personnel must be willing to explore specific questions regarding

Table 1   Identifying the Drug Addict

Medical history	Obstetric history	Physical Appearance and demeanor
AIDS	In prior pregnancies, history of:	Patient looks physically exhausted/malnourished
Cellulitis	Abruptio placentae	
Cirrhosis	Fetal death	Evidence of trauma
Endocarditis	Low–birth weight infant	Pupils are extremely dilated or constricted
Hepatitis	Meconium staining	
Pancreatitis	Premature labor	Appearance of pregnancy fails to coincide with stated gestational age
Pneumonia	Premature rupture of membranes	
Anemia	Spontaneous abortion	
Gastrointestinal hemorrhage	In current pregnancy, history of evidence of:	Track marks, abscesses, or edema are visible in upper or lower extremities
Syncope/seizures		
Trauma	Early contractions	
	Inactive or hyperactive fetus	Nasal mucosae are inflamed or indurated
	Poor weight gain	
	Sexually transmitted disease	
	Spotting or vaginal bleeding	

prior hospitalization. A drug addict will volunteer little information; if past medical history appears negative, the pregnant woman's obstetrical history may be more revealing.

The physical appearance of the patient may give subtle or overt clues to alert the interviewer to possible drug use. The following areas of concern should be noted:

Is the patient well-oriented?
Does the patient appear physically exhausted?
Are the patient's pupils extremely dilated or constricted?
Does the appearance of the patient's pregnancy coincide with the stated gestational age?
Are there signs of track marks, abscesses or edema in the upper or lower extremities?

The physical appearance and signs of chemical dependence are especially helpful in diagnosing the intravenous drug addict. These women, owing to their ambivalence toward the pregnancy coupled with their denial of drug use, frequently delay medical intervention until late in gestation. Medical staff often find no history or prior obstetrical care.

Some pregnant nonnarcotic and alcohol-addicted women may seek obstetrical care earlier in gestation, but since these women have less overt physical signs of drug and alcohol addiction, a very careful medical and obstetrical assessment is necessary.

B.   Obstetrical History

As the interview proceeds to the obstetrical history, the physician, regardless of the patient's self-disclosure may discover prior complications due to perinatal drug addiction. These prior complications of pregnancy, labor, or delivery require further exploration, and a request for past obstetrical records is indicated. Complications associated with drug use in previous pregnancies may include spontaneous abortion, premature labor, premature rupture of membranes, abruptio placentae, fetal death, meconium-stained amniotic fluid, or a low–birth weight infant [7].

Pertinent findings in regard to the present pregnancy may include poor weight gain, spotting or vaginal bleeding, an inactive fetus, reports of early contractions, or a hyperactive fetus.

The obstetrical history also provides the interviewer with an opportunity to discuss the patient's emotional response to the current pregnancy. An inconsistent pattern of prenatal care may indicate apathy or ambivalence regarding the pregnancy. On the other hand, frequent emergency room visits may reveal extreme anxiety regarding the physical well-being of the fetus, and in this setting, the interviewer can explore the patient's coping mechanisms. A good question to introduce the drug history would be one asking how the woman handles stress. Questions about medications and other drugs are a natural extension to discussing stress.

Drug use is explored in a nonjudgmental manner while identifying early drug abuse patterns. The patient's drug use history should begin with the earliest exposure to cigarettes, over-the-counter medications, prescribed medications, alcohol, marijuana, and other illicit drugs and continue along a time continuum to the present.

C. Drug Abuse/Addiction During Past Pregnancies

It is important to look at the substance abuse patterns during past pregnancies. Some women abstain from drugs during pregnancy, whereas others curb drug use but return to drugs immediately postpartum. There are also women who have binges of drug abuse, and others who are addicted to drugs regardless of their pregnancy. Some questions to be explored regarding past pregnancies are:

Did the patient experience any complications with the pregnancy, labor, or delivery?
Did the patient's pediatrician notice any physical or behavioral problems with the newborn?
How is the child doing now? Does the patient notice any differences in behavior or growth patterns?

D. Current Pregnancy

The current drug abuse/addiction history should begin at least 1 month prior to the last normal menstrual period. Many drug-using women do not have a regular menstrual cycle, and they often are unaware of a pregnancy until relatively late in gestation.

E. Drug/Alcohol History

All prenatal evaluations should include questions pertaining to drugs used during pregnancy. Beginning a drug-use history with cigarettes and proceeding to over-the-counter drugs, prescribed drugs, alcohol, marijuana, and other illicit drugs appears less threatening to the patient. A positive drug abuse/addiction history requires immediate intervention by the medical staff.

IV. INTERVENTION PROCEDURES

A medical intervention procedure can include patient confrontation, education, inpatient or community referral to drug/alcohol treatment, or referral to a social worker or clinical nurse specialist for in-depth interview and/or follow-up for treatment.

Urine toxicological examination can be used as an adjunct to evaluation and intervention. The physician should be certain as to what compounds are included in a screening toxicology, and specifically request those drugs or metabolites not routinely included. Urine toxicology can be used as part of the evaluation for drug addiction, but it should never replace a thorough history and physical examination as part of the screening procedure. Regardless of the type of evaluation and intervention procedure used, any woman with a history or evidence of drug use or addiction during the current pregnancy should be immediately referred for treatment, as any illicit drug use during pregnancy can have major ramifications for the unborn child.

A. Clinical Management

Care during pregnancy of a woman who uses drugs requires a multidisciplinary team. The group should include an obstetrician practiced in identifying and treating the medical problems frequently encountered among addicted women—anemia, vaginitis, sexually transmitted disease (STD), and other infectious complications. Also invaluable are a psychologist or psychiatrist experienced in caring for persons addicted to drugs and a specially trained nurse or social worker qualified to provide guidance and support. Although members of the team often function individually, their efforts must be integrated and directed toward common goals that extend beyond the pregnancy.

B. Laboratory Evaluation

Adequate care begins with a thorough medical evaluation and appropriate laboratory studies (Table 2). For the woman with evidence of drug use, maternal urine should be obtained and screened for the presence of drugs. Any maternal or fetal infection—especially urinary tract infections, vaginitis, and sexually transmitted disease—demands aggressive treatment. Recent information from the Centers for Disease Control shows that while the incidence of all STDs in this country is continuing to rise, chlamydial infections are showing the most rapid rate of increase.

Serial ultrasound examination to measure the biparietal diameter, head and abdominal circumferences, and fetal femur lengths are advised. Ideally, these should be obtained between 14 and 20, 20 and 26, 30 and 32, and 36 and 38 weeks to establish gestational age and the fetal growth pattern. Because menstrual irregularity is common in drug users (addicts, obtaining the growth-adjusted sonar age is valuable. Nonstress testing may be advisable weekly from the thirty-second week of gestation if intrauterine growth retardation is suspected.

C. Delivery

Prenatal care of patients who use substances should include plans for delivery. Every effort should be made to deliver in an obstetrical center that is equipped with a neonatal intensive care unit to manage the neonate and to handle any complications that may arise.

Guidelines for managing labor are the same as for the nonaddicted patient. Once the patient's drug status has been ascertained, the physician is free to use whatever methods of anesthesia or analgesia which are deemed necessary to provide pain relief for labor and delivery. Addicted women often experience as much pain during labor as other women. It is unnecessary to withhold medications at that time under the misapprehension that they will contribute to the addictive process.

V. NEONATAL ABSTINENCE

The fact that drugs cross the placenta and reach the fetus creates potential problems for fetal development. These problems can be manifested as congenital abnormalities, fetal growth retardation, neonatal growth retardation, and neurobehavioral problems. In addition, one of the important effects of maternal drug use during pregnancy, especially use of drugs with a high potential for abuse, is that dependence develops in the fetus as well as in the mother. Thus, the fetus will experience withdrawal when the mother is withdrawn from her drug, or at term when the maternal drug use no longer provides the newborn with drugs.

Table 2 Laboratory Evaluation of the Pregnant Drug Addict

Blood work	Screening for infection	Urine tests	Cultures	Obstetric screening
Complete blood count with indices	Chest x-ray	Urinanalysis	Cervical culture for *Chlamydia trachomatis*	Ultrasound scan to confirm pregnancy after 6 weeks' gestation and serial scans for fetal measurement between 20 and 38 weeks' gestation
Fetoprotein (if between 16 and 18 weeks gestation)	Tuberculin skin test	Culture	Human immunodeficiency virus (HIV) antibody screen	
Rubella titer	Hepatitis B antigen and antibody	Toxicology	Cervical-rectal cultures for *Neisseria gonorrhoeae*	
Blood type	Serology			Cervical Pap smear
Rh determination	Venereal disease reaction level (VDRL)			
Coombs' test	Fluorescent treponemal antibody (lues) test (FTA)			
Sickle-cell prep, if indicated				

Symptoms of neonatal withdrawal from narcotics are usually present at birth, but may not reach a peak until 3–4 days of life, or as late as 10–14 days after birth [7]. Withdrawal from narcotics persists in a subacute form for 4–6 months after birth, with a peak in symptoms at around 6 weeks of age [8]. Abstinence symptoms in the neonate exposed to nonnarcotic drugs in utero have also been described for marijuana [9]. Although withdrawal from this drug does not appear to result in as severe a syndrome of abstinence as withdrawal from narcotics, the newborn does exhibit the irritability and restlessness, poor feeding, crying, and impaired neurobehavioral abilities that are characteristic of the neonatal abstinence syndrome.

The most common features of the neonatal abstinence syndrome [7], as outlined in Table 3, mimic aspects of an adult withdrawing from narcotics. Most significant for the neonate are the high-pitched cry, sweating, tremulousness, excoriation of the extremities, and gastrointestinal upset. In an effort to reduce the degree of withdrawal for the narcotic-exposed newborn, low-dose methadone maintenance programs for pregnant women have been developed, and it is now the general recommendation to maintain a pregnant woman on as low a dose of methadone as possible.

Treatment of the neonate for narcotic withdrawal should be supportive, since pharmacological therapy can prolong hospitalization and exposes the infant to additional agents which often are not necessary. Mothers should be taught to swaddle the withdrawing infant closely and tightly in a blanket. Use of a pacifier also soothes the infant's irritability and relieves the increased sucking urge experienced by the withdrawing infant. Frequent small feedings are best tolerated by the infant.

Pharmacological therapy with paregoric, diazepam, or phenobarbital (Table 4) should be based on evaluation of the infant through the use of one of the various abstinence scoring methods. Excessive weight loss or dehydration due to vomiting and diarrhea, inability of the infant to feed or sleep, fever unrelated to infection, or seizures are the most common clinical indications for drug treatment. Other causes for these symptoms, such as infection, metabolic abnormalities (hypoglycemia, hypocalcemia), hyperthyroidism, central nervous system hemorrhage, and birth anoxia should be considered before therapy is begun.

Infants treated with paregoric have improved and exhibit more efficient sucking behavior and better weight gain than infants treated with diazepam or phenobarbital [10,11]. A major concern, however, regarding the use of opiate preparations in neonates is the marked respiratory depressant effect, although infants manifesting narcotic withdrawal should be more tolerant of this drug than non–drug-exposed infants.

Diazepam rapidly suppresses narcotic withdrawal symptoms in the neonate. However, the newborn infant has a limited capacity to metabolize diazepam. Use of diazepam can be

Table 3 Signs and Symptoms of Neonatal Withdrawal

Tremors	Nasal stuffiness
Restlessness	Rapid respirations
Hyperactive reflexes	Frequent yawning
Vomiting, diarrhea	Sweating
Increased muscle tone	Excoriation of knees, elbows
High-pitched cry	Mottling of skin
Sneezing	Fever
Voracious sucking	Lacrimation
Sleeplessness	
Seizures	

Table 4 Pharmacological Therapy of Neonatal Narcotic Abstinence [10,11]

Medication	Dose	Note
Paregoric (anhydrous morphine 0.4 mg/ml)	0.2–0.5 ml/dose q 3–4 h	Taper off after symptoms for 4–5 days.
Diazepam icteric	1–2 mg q 8 h	Do not use in premature infant.
Phenobarbital	Loading dose: 16 mg/kg/24 h Maintenance dose: 2–8 mg/kg/24 h	Follow blood levels to maintain therapeutic levels. Decrease daily dose after symptoms stabilized to allow phenobarbital level to decrease by 10–20%/day.

associated with depression of the neonatal sucking reflex, and late-onset seizures have occurred in neonates after cessation of treatment with diazepam.

Phenobarbital will quiet the infant with neonatal withdrawal, but it does little for the gastrointestinal symptoms. Large doses of phenobarbital exert a marked sedative effect on the central nervous system of the infant and impair sucking. Blood levels of phenobarbital should be followed closely and adjusted according to the infant's symptoms and the abstinence score results. After the infant's symptoms have stabilized, the daily dose of phenobarbital should be decreased to allow the drug level to decrease by 10–20% per day.

Pharmacological therapy of infants with symptoms of abstinence due to exposure to nonopiate drugs is usually not necessary, since these infants rarely require any more than supportive therapy. If an infant in this situation should require pharmacological intervention, phenobarbital, given in the same manner as for opiate withdrawal described above, would be the medication of choice.

VI. OUTCOME: DRUGS OF ABUSE

A. Narcotics

Early studies of infants delivered to heroin-using mothers showed that these infants had a higher rate of perinatal morbidity and mortality than infants in the general population [7,12]. Common problems associated with heroin use during pregnancy were first-trimester spontaneous abortions, premature delivery, neonatal meconium aspiration syndrome, maternal/neonatal infections, including venereal diseases, and severe neonatal withdrawal [7,11,12]. Attempts to provide better control of these pregnancies were anchored in methadone maintenance programs in which pregnant women attended prenatal obstetrical clinics and received daily methadone to replace their use of street heroin. The initial methadone maintenance programs were successful in that the more consistent medical and nutritional care provided for these women resulted in improved pregnancy outcome. However, the high doses of methadone (80–120 mg/day) produced a more severe and prolonged period of abstinence for the newborn as compared to patterns of withdrawal for infants exposed to heroin.

These complications are avoided when the pregnant woman is placed on low-dose methadone maintenance, especially if the third-trimester dose of methadone is held at less than 20 mg.

Infants delivered to mothers who use narcotics (heroin, methadone, "T's and blues") have a significantly lower birth weight and length and a smaller head circumference than non–drug-exposed infants [13]. The inhibitory effects of narcotics on fetal growth, as well as the effects of inadequate maternal caloric and protein intake, can produce this fetal growth failure.

Infants exposed to narcotics in utero exhibit significant impairment in their interactive abilities, making them difficult to engage and to console. Narcotic-exposed infants are more tremulous and irritable than drug-free infants, demonstrating significant and unpredictable fluctuations in their emotional responses. These factors not only make these infants very difficult to cuddle and comfort, but also interrupt the normal processes of maternal/infant attachment that are so important to the early relationship between infant and mother [13,14].

Infants born to mothers maintained on methadone throughout pregnancy continue to be significantly smaller in weight and length compared to drug-free infants through 6–9 months of age [8], but usually catch up in weight and length by 12 months of age. This early stunting during a prolonged period of subacute withdrawal could be due to the direct effect of methadone on the hypothalamic-hypophyseal axis of the newborn. Following a period of slow excretion of the methadone, the plasma and tissue drug levels fall, the endocrinological effects of the drug subside, and neonatal growth recovers. The one exception is head circumference measurement for the opiate-exposed infants; it does not exhibit catch-up growth. The persistent reduction in head size in these infants is of concern, since small head size in young infants has been reported to be predictive of poor developmental outcome and may be an indicator of the prolonged high-risk status of these infants [14,15].

Two-year developmental follow-up of narcotic-exposed infants shows that their development, measured on the Bayley Scales of Infant Development, is within the normal range [14]. Of concern, however, is the fact that the infants demonstrate a downward trend in developmental scores by 2 years of age, a phenomenon not uncommon in infants from low socioeconomic groups. This observation suggests that the infants' environment with a lack of stimulation has a more direct influence on 2-year development than maternal drug use during pregnancy.

B. Cocaine

With the increasing use of cocaine in the general population, large numbers of women are using this drug during pregnancy [2–4]. Several reports have indicated that cocaine abuse during pregnancy is associated with a poor pregnancy and neonatal outcome.

Medical Complications of the Mother

In addition to the infectious complications associated with substance abuse, cocaine's powerful sympathomimetic effects can produce acute medical emergencies in the pregnant woman (Table 5).

Cardiac complications of cocaine intoxication include myocardial ischemia, arrhythmias, and cardiomyopathies. The initial cardiac effects are the result of catecholamine release and consist of tachycardia and hypertension. Low doses of cocaine usually cause stimulation of the myocardium and higher doses always produce myocardial depression with decreases in both the rate and force of contraction [16,17].

Cases of dilated cardiomyopathy following chronic cocaine use have been recently reported in nonpregnant addicts [18]. Two cases of cardiac myopathies have occurred in the postpartum period in pregnant women enrolled in our program at Northwestern Memorial Hospital. It is hypothesized that the stress of pregnancy places the women at increased risk of cocaine's cardiac effects.

There have been several reports of subarachnoid hemorrhage occurring shortly after cocaine use [19]. The etiology of the hemorrhages was felt to be due to the sudden increases

Table 5 Maternal Complications of Cocaine Use

Cardiovascular
  Myocardial ischemia
  Arrhythmias
  Cardiomyopathies
  Hypertension
Central nervous system
  Seizures
  Hperpyrexia
  Cerebrovascular accidents
Respiratory
  Pneumothorax
  Pulmonary dysfunction
  Perforation of the nasal septum
Gastrointestinal
  Ischemia of bowel with possible perforation
  Hepatotoxicity
Renal
  Rhabdomyolysis
  Renal failure

in blood pressure associated with acute cocaine intoxication. In addition to hemorrhage, cerebral infarction has also been reported.

Inhalation of cocaine can be associated with respiratory complications related to acute, direct effects from the drug. While many of the pulmonary complications are the result of chronic cocaine abuse, acute intoxication can result in respiratory failure or pulmonary edema [20,21].

Cocaine may damage the alveolar wall and therapy predispose patients to pneumothorax, pneumomediastinum, or pneumopericardium, especially when associated with a forced Valsalva maneuver used to intensify the euphoria that comes with cocaine smoking [22].

The oral ingestion of cocaine can produce gastrointestinal ischemia with possible death from gram-negative sepsis [23]. Hepatotoxicity with elevated hepatic enzymes in as many as 80% of cocaine and heroin users and jaundice have been reported associated with cocaine intoxication [24].

Cocaine Effects on the Fetus and Neonate

The increasing numbers of cocaine-exposed infants across the country are exhibiting their own unique set of problems. Recent data confirm that cocaine rapidly crosses the placenta, and hyperactivity of the fetus following maternal use of cocaine has been repeatedly demonstrated. There is a temporal association between cocaine use and the occurrence of abruptio placentae, as well as an association of cocaine use with the onset of uterine contractions and labor. Thus, there is an increased incidence of prematurity and its attendant complications among infants exposed in utero to cocaine [25,26].

Cocaine acts peripherally to inhibit nerve conduction and prevent dopamine and norepinephrine reuptake at presynaptic nerve terminals. This produces increased catecholamine levels with subsequent vasoconstriction, tachycardia, hypertension, and uterine contraction. The increased incidence of abruptio placentae and premature labor in cocaine-complicated pregnancies is thus consistent with these pharmacological actions of cocaine.

Intrauterine growth retardation also occurs in cocaine-exposed infants, a not surprising fact given the intermittent impairment of placental blood due to the vasoconstrictive action of cocaine [27,28]. Newborns who have been exposed to cocaine exhibit a high degree of irritability and tremulousness, with a deficiency in state control [26,27]. Case reports of perinatal cerebral infarctions occurring in infants whose mothers have used cocaine during the few days prior to delivery [29] are a severe example of the morbidity associated with intrauterine exposure to cocaine and are similar to intracerebral insults reported in adults who use cocaine.

The neurobehavioral changes for cocaine-exposed infants are in some areas more severe than changes noted for methadone-exposed infants. It is not yet fully understood whether the irritability and tremulousness found in cocaine-exposed infants is a syndrome due to withdrawal from the drug or a direct effect of cocaine on the central nervous system (CNS) of the infant. Differential outcomes of infants exposed to cocaine on only a few occasions during pregnancy as compared with infants exposed chronically throughout pregnancy show that early cessation of cocaine reduces the risk for premature delivery, fetal growth retardation, and neonatal morbidity [27].

C. Alcohol

The impact of alcohol on the health of the pregnant woman varies little from the nonpregnant adult. A high rate of hepatic dysfunction, anemia, and other complications of alcohol use occurs in the pregnant woman as well as the nonpregnant woman. However, studies have documented that alcohol use in pregnancy may have its greatest impact on the developing fetus [1,30,31], and that the fetal alcohol syndrome is one of the most common causes of mental retardation in the United States [30]. The notion that heavy maternal drinking is detrimental to offspring regained scientific status when Lemoine [32] and Jones and Smith [33] observed a common pattern of malformations in offspring of chronic alcoholic women. Jones and Smith coined the term fetal alcohol syndrome (FAS) to define a pattern of prenatal and postnatal growth deficiency, developmental delay, or mental retardation, microcephaly, fine motor dysfunction, and a characteristic facial dysmorphology. The initial publications describing FAS stimulated case reports from around the world, which have been followed by thousands of clinical, epidemiological, and experimental studies.

The body of findings has shown that ethanol and its metabolites have the potential to alter the growth and development of the embryo and fetus. These characteristics of alcohol toxicity in utero may occur in combination as the full spectrum of FAS, or any number of effects may be present (fetal alcohol effect, FAE). Fetal alcohol effects are considerably more common than the full-blown FAS.

Diagnosis of FAS

There are minimal criteria for the diagnosis of FAS:

1. Prenatal and or postnatal growth retardation (weight, length, and/or head circumference below the 10th percentile)
2. CNS involvement (signs of neurological abnormality, developmental delay, or intellectual impairment)
3. Characteristic facial dysmorphology with at least two of the following signs: (a) microcephaly; (b) microophthalmia, and/or short palpebral fissures; (c) poorly developed philtrum, thin upper lip, or flattening of the maxillary area.

In addition to the diagnostic signs, children with FAS have a higher frequency of nonspecific malformations than the general population (Table 6) [34,35].

Table 6 Fetal Alcohol Effects

Brain	Developmental delay or intellectual impairment (mental retardation)
Growth	Small head and body size and low birth weight
Eyes	Epicanthal folds, strabismus, ptosis, hypoplastic retinal vessels
Mouth	Poor suck, cleft lip, cleft palate
Ears	Deafness
Skeleton	Radioulnar synostosis, fusion of cervical vertebrae, retarded bone growth
Heart	Atrial and ventricular septal defects, tetralogy of Fallot, patent ductus arteriosus
Kidney	Renal hypoplasia, hydronephrosis, urogenital sinus
Liver	Extrahepatic biliary atresia, hepatic fibrosis
Immune	Increased infections—otitis media, upper
system	respiratory infections, immune deficiencies
Tumors	Nonspecific neoplasms
Skin	Abnormal palmar creases, irregular hair whorls

Alcohol's Actions

Clinical and experimental research findings point to multiple mechanisms which underlie alcohol's effects on fetal growth and development. Alcohol in high concentrations modifies cell functions throughout the body, affecting all organ systems. Direct and indirect actions have been observed on the maternal-placental-fetal system. Biochemical and pathophysiological effects of ethanol and its metabolite, acetaldehyde, can alter fetal development by disrupting cell differentiation and growth. Alcohol-induced alterations in maternal physiology and in the intermediate metabolism of carbohydrates, proteins, and fats can alter the environment in which the fetus develops. Chronic exposure to high doses of alcohol can interfere with the passage of amino acids across the placenta and with the incorporation of amino acids into proteins. The complete FAS results from the cumulative actions of high blood alcohol concentrations on the maternal-placental-fetal system throughout pregnancy [36].

Variability occurs in the nature and extent of the abnormalities seen in children exposed to alcohol in utero. It has been estimated that 2–10% of pregnancies complicated by alcohol produce children with FAS; another 30–40% have some of the adverse effects of FAE. The differences are related to several factors, including dose levels, chronicity of alcohol use, gestational stage and duration of exposure, and sensitivity of fetal tissue.

Reduction of heavy drinking has been associated with improved neonatal outcomes on growth parameters, somatic status, and/or CNS development in additional case reports and prospective studies [37]. In a program in Seattle, 80% of the women who drank alcohol heavily were able to modify their drinking pattern. Benefits among their children were described as "dramatic." The fetal alcohol effect occurred three times more often when mothers continued drinking than when mothers reduced drinking. Another program reported that 35% of at-risk women stopped drinking heavily. Increased neurobehavioral alterations were found in infants of women who continued to drink during pregnancy as compared with abstainers and with women who discontinued use by mid-pregnancy [38]. The observed benefits were attributed to cessation of drinking and not to maternal characteristics. The group of women who successfully abstained and the group who failed to respond to treatment were similar on demographic characteristics. No significant differences were found in patterns of alcohol consumption reported at the time of clinic registration. Among the women in the study, there were no differences in the prevalence of alcohol-related pathology, although the continued group had begun drinking at an earlier age and were more likely to meet criteria for the diagnosis of alcohol addiction.

Clinician's Role

Greater understanding of the mechanisms of alcohol's effects on fetal development has put new demands on prenatal care providers. Identification and treatment of problem-drinking women represents an important challenge for the prevention of alcohol- related birth defects. Since alcohol has the capacity to adversely affect each stage of fetal development, the earlier in pregnancy that heavy drinking ceases, the greater is the potential for improved outcome.

Recognition based on stereotypical ideas of the chronic alcoholic is ineffective. Pregnant women usually do not fit the stereotype of the alcoholic, since they are usually young and in the early stages of the disease. Although women who drink heavily differ statistically from other pregnant women on a series of behavioral and demographic traits, these traits have low predictive power and are not effective as specific clinical markers [39]. Blood and alcohol content in sweat and urine is not clinically useful. No direct measurements are currently available that will detect alcohol addiction before there is impairment of hepatic or hematopoietic function.

A brief Ten Question Drinking History (TQDH) has been developed which can be administered routinely as part of every intake examination (Table 7). The reliability of the questionnaire has been tested by Larsson, who reported good agreement between two occasions of history taking [40].

Separate, direct questions are asked about the frequency, quantity, and variability of the consumption of beer, wine, and liquor. Validity of self-reports has been shown to improve when specific questions are asked about each beverage. Inquiry about quantity, frequency, and variability of use further improves the accuracy of self-reports. The first nine questions ascertain present drinking patterns. Alcohol use is assumed, thereby diminishing moral projections. The tenth question explores changes in drinking habits during the past year. This allows for discussion of previous patterns, which often provides validation of reports of current use.

When the 10 questions are asked in a direct, nonjudgmental fashion, some patients will accept the clinician's concern and respond honestly. Simple introductory statements reassure the pregnant woman that the questions are being asked in an effort to improve pregnancy outcome. Patients who answer evasively should be calmly and firmly engaged in further discussion. Defensive reactions often indicate alcohol problems. Denial of alcohol and drug use remains high. Other chapters in this book outline approaches to diagnostic intervention of drug and alcohol addiction.

Administering the TQDH requires less than 5 min when women are not drinking at risk levels. For women who are addicted to alcohol, the questionnaire provides a basis for discussing

Table 7 Ten-Question Drinking History

Beer	How many times per week?
	How many cans each time?
	Ever drink more?
Wine	How many times per week?
	How many glasses each time?
	Ever drink more?
Liquor	How many times per week?
	How many drinks each time?
	Ever drink more?
Has your drinking changed during the past year?	

alcohol use and initiating supportive counseling, and referred for treatment of drug and alcohol addiction.

VII. SUMMARY

It is clear from current information that drug use and addiction by the pregnant woman has a major impact both on her health and that of her fetus. Thus, the physician's evaluation of every pregnant patient must be expanded to include an assessment of lifestyle. There is no indication that every pregnant woman should have a urine toxicology performed. However, every pregnant woman should have a complete substance abuse history taken by the health care professionals in a nonjudgmental, caring manner. In this way, women at risk can be identified and educational and therapeutic services initiated.

REFERENCES

1. Jones, K.L., et al. (1973). Pattern of malformation in offspring of alcoholic mothers. *Lancet 1*:1267–1271.
2. Chasnoff, I.J. (1989). Drug use and women: Establishing a standard of care. *Ann. N.Y. Acad. Sci. 562*:208–210.
3. NIDA Household Survey on Drug Abuse 1988 (1989). Population Estimates. National Institute of Drug Abuse, Rockville, Maryland.
4. Chasnoff, I.J., Landress, H., and Barrett, M. (1989). The Pinellas County Study. Presented before the Annual Meeting of the National Association for Perinatal Addiction Research and Education, Miami, Florida, September.
5. Chasnoff, I.J. (1988). Drug use in pregnancy: Parameter of risk. *Pediatr. Clin. North Am. 35*:1403–12.
6. Stark, M.J., and Nichols, H.G. (1977). Alcohol related admissions to a general hospital. *AIC Health Res. World Summer*: 11–14.
7. Finnegan, L.P., et al. (1975). Neonatal abstinence syndrome: Assessment and management, (R.D. Harbison, ed.), *Perinatal Addiction*. Spectrum Publications, pp. 141–158.
8. Chasnoff, I.J., Hatcher, R.P., and Burns, W.J. (1980). Early growth patterns of methadone-addicted infants. *Am. J. Dis. Child. 134*:1049–1051.
9. Fried, P.A. (1989). Marihuana use by pregnant women: Neurobehavioral effects in neonates. *Drugs Alcohol Depend. 6*:415–424.
10. Kron, R.E., et al. Neonatal narcotic abstinence: (1976). Effects of pharmo-therapeutic agents and maternal drug usage on nutritive sucking behavior. *J. Pediatr. 88*:637–641.
11. Finnetal, O.P. (1988). Neonatal abstinence syndrome: Assessment and pharmacotherapy, *Neonatal Therapy: An Update*, (F.F. Rubaltelli and B. Granati, eds.), Excerpta Medica, Amsterdam, pp. 122–146.
12. Kandall, S.R. (1977). Late complications in passively addicted infants. *Drug Abuse in Pregnancy and the Neonate*. (J.O. Rementeria, ed.), Mosby, St. Louis, p. 116.
13. Chasnoff, I.J., et al. (1982). Polydrug-and methadone-addicted newborns: A continuum of impairment? *Pediatrics 70*:210–213.
14. Chasnoff, I.J., et al. (1986). Prenatal drug exposure: Effects on neonatal and infant growth and development. *Neurobehav. Toxicol. Teratol.* 8357–8362.
15. Chasnoff, I.J., et al. (1984). Maternal nonnarcotic substance abuse during pregnancy: Effects on infant development. *Neurobehav. Toxicol. Teratol. 6*:277–280.
16. Karch, S.B., and Billingham, M.E. (1988). The pathophysiology and etiology of cocaine-induced heart disease. *Arch. Pathol. Lab. Med. 112*:225–230.
17. Cregler, L.L., and Mark, H. (1986). Cardiovascular dangers of cocaine abuse. *Am. J. Cardiol. 57*:1185–1186.
18. Weiner, R.S., Lockhart, J.T., and Schwartz, R.G. (1986). DIlated cardiomyopathy and cocaine abuse. *Am. J. Med. 81*:699–700.

19. Lichtenfeld, P.J., Rubin, D.B., and Feldman, R.S. (1984). Subarachnoid hemmorrhage precipitated by cocaine smoking. *Arch. Neurol. 41*:223–224.

20. Allred, R., and Ewer, S. (1981). Fatal pulmonary edema following intravenous freebase cocaine. *Ann. Emerg. Med. 10*:441–442.

21. Itkonen, J., Schnoll, S., and Glassworth, J. (1984). Pulmonary dysfunction in 'freebase' cocaine users. *Arch. Int. Med. 144*:2195–2197.

22. Luque, M.A., Cavallaro, D.L., Torres, M., et al. (1987). Pneumomediastinum, pneumothorax, and subcutaneous emphysema after alternate cocaine inhalation and marijuana smoking. *Pediatr. Emerg. Care 3*:107–109.

23. Nalbaudian, H., Sheth, N., Dietrich, R., and Georgion, J. (1985). Intestinal ischemia caused by cocaine ingestion. *Surgery 97*:374–376.

24. Marks, V., and Chapple, P.A.L. (1967). Hepatic dysfunction in heroin and cocaine users. *Br. J. Addict. 62*:189–195.

25. MacGregor, S., Keith, L., Chasnoff, I.J., et al. (1987). Cocaine use during pregnancy: adverse perinatal outcome. *Am. J. Obstet. Gynecol. 157*:686–690.

26. Chasnoff, I.J., Burns, W.J., Schnoll, S.H., and Burns, K. (1985). Cocaine use in pregnancy. *N. Engl. J. Med. 313*:666–669.

27. Chasnoff, I.J., Griffith, D.R., MacGregor, S.N., et al. (1989). Temporal drug affected infants. Patterns of cocaine use in pregnancy: Perinatal outcome. *J.A.M.A. 261*(12):1741–1744.

28. Bingol, N., Fuchs, M., Diaz, V., et al. (1987). Teratogenicity of cocaine in humans. *J. Pediatr. 110*:93–96.

29. Chasnoff, I.J., Bussey, M.E., Savich, R.E., and Stack, C.M. (1986). Perinatal cerebral infarction and maternal cocaine use. *J. Pediatr. 108*:456–459.

30. Abel, E.L., and Sokol, R.J. (1987). Incidence of fetal alcohol syndrome and economic impact of FAS-related anomalies. *Drug. Alcohol Depend. 19*:51–70.

31. Olegard, R., and Sabel, K.-G. and Aronsson, M. (1979). Effects on the child of alcohol abuse during pregnancy: Retrospective and prospective studies. *Acta Paediatr. S* (Suppl.) *275*:112–21.

32. Lemoine, P., Haorusseau, H., Borteyru, J.-P., and Menuet, J.-C. (1968). Les enfants de parents alcooliques: Anomalies observes. A propos de 127 cas (Children of alcoholic parents: Anomalies observed in 127 cases). *Quest Med. 21*:476–482.

33. Jones, K.L, and Smith, D.W. (1973). Recognition of the fetal alcohol syndrome in early infancy. *Lancet 2*:999–1001.

34. Rosett, H.L., and Weiner, L. (1984). *Alcohol and the Fetus: A Clinical Perspective*. New York, Oxford University Press.

35. Rosett, H.L. (1980). A clinical perspective of the fetal alcohol syndrome. *Alcohol. Clin. Exp. Res. 4*:119–122.

36. Fisher, S.E., Atkinson, M., Burnap, J.K., et al. (1982). Ethanol-associated selective fetal malnutrition: A contributing factor in the fetal alcohol syndrome. *Alcohol. Clin. Exp. Res. 6*:197–201.

37. Little, R.E., Young, A., Streissguth, A.P., and Uhl, C.N. (1984). Preventing fetal alcohol effects: Effectiveness of a demonstration project, in *CIBA Foundation Symposium 105, Mechanisms of Alcohol Damage in Utero*. Pitman Press, London, pp. 254–274.

38. Coles, C.D., Smith, I.E., Fernhoff, P.M., and Falek, A: Neonatal neurobehavioral characteristics as correlates of maternal alcohol use during gestation. *Alcohol. Clin. Exp. Res.*

39. Smith, I.E., Lancaster, J.S., and Moss-Wells, S: (1987). Identifying high-risk pregnant drinkers: Biological and behavioral correlates of continuous heavy drinking during pregnancy. *J. Studies Alcohol. 48*:304–309.

40. Larsson, G. (1983). Prevention of fetal alcohol effects: An antenatal program for early detection of pregnancies at risk. *Acta Obstet. Gynecol. Scand. 62*:171–178.

8

Women, Alcohol, and Drugs

Sheila B. Blume
South Oaks Hospital, Amityville, New York

I. INTRODUCTION: SOCIETAL ATTITUDES AND THE HIDDEN ADDICT

Human use of alcohol and other psychoactive drugs dates back to prehistory. Many of the early written records of mankind also document the existence of alcohol and drug problems, for which these societies developed a variety of legal controls [1]. The Old Testament makes many allusions to drinking and drunkenness. It is clear that intoxication among women was not unknown. The first Book of Samuel begins with the story of Hannah, the mother of Samuel, who is barren and prays for a child at the temple in Shiloh. She is observed silently moving her lips while "speaking inwardly" and is mistaken for a drunkard by the priest Eli. He advises her to stop drinking. Since the priests of the time were also the community's physicians, his advice was medical as well as spiritual.

Nearly all societies which have permitted alcohol use have developed separate and different standards of acceptable drinking for men and for women, dating back at least as far as the Law of Hammurabi [2]. These differences in drinking norms have evolved, in contemporary society, into a double-edged sword. On one hand, they protect women from the development of problematic drinking patterns (3-5), as will be further discussed below. On the other, they have been accompanied by intensely negative attitudes toward women who develop such problems, based on inaccurate stereotypes that are deeply ingrained in Western thought.

In the early days of ancient Rome the drinking of alcohol by women was strictly prohibited [6]. A law of Romulus provided the death penalty for women who drank. There are records of women having been put to death for the offense of having drunk wine or having been caught with the keys to the family wine cellar. It is interesting that the same law which prohibited women's drinking also forbade adultery by women. Writers of the time explained that alcohol was forbidden to women because it made them sexually promiscuous. The idea that women's drinking could be both abhorrent in itself and a cause of lascivious behavior was already well established in the ancient world. A very similar attitude was found among the early Israelites, as expressed in the following quotation from the Talmud, quoted by Gomberg [7]:

> One cup of wine is good for a woman;
> Two are degrading;
> Three induce her to act like an immoral woman;
> And four cause her to lose all self-respect and sense of shame.

In 1798, Immanuel Kant expressed an opinion about the sobriety of both Jews and women. He stated that both groups do not get drunk and avoid all appearance of drunkenness because their position in the community rests upon the belief of other in their piety and chastity:

> All separatists, that is, those who subject themselves not only to the general laws of the country but also to a special sectarian law, are exposed through their eccentricity and alleged chosenness to the attention and criticism of the community, and thus cannot relax in their self-control, for intoxication, which deprives one of the cautiousness, would be a scandal for them [8].

The idea that women are held to be a higher standard of behavior than men is often expressed as women being "put on a pedestal." The higher the pedestal, the greater the fall. Both female alcoholics and female addicts are considered "fallen women," and they are the victims of triple [or of a threefold] stigma. First, they are victims of the same stigma attached to all alcoholics and addicts. Pollsters have found that although the vast majority of Americans will agree that alcoholism is a disease, these same people also will agree that alcoholics are weak-willed and immoral. Acceptance of the disease concept of alcoholism remains only skin deep in our society, while the disease concept of other drug addiction is still a very new idea. The second part of the stigma is a result of the special standard of conduct expected of women. Behavior that is acceptable for men, as Kant pointed out, may be considereed scandalous for women. Consider the expression "drunk as a lord." Now consider its female counterpart, "drunk as a lady."

The third, and most injurious, is the pernicious sexual stigma attached to women who drink or use drugs. In our society, these women are automatically considered both promiscuous and acceptable targets for sexual aggression. The 1983 New Bedford, Massachusetts case, in which an intoxicated 22-year-old woman was gang-raped on a pool table in a bar, vividly illustrates society's perception. Many blamed the victim for her rape. During the trial of her attackers, demonstrators outside the courthouse carried signs protesting that she deserved what she got. The victim, an alcoholic woman, died 3 years later, in 1986, as a result of her disease [9]. The Neil Simon film *Only When I Laugh* contains a similar stereotype of the female alcoholic. It includes a scene in which the heroine, an alcoholic woman who has relapsed, is followed and beaten in an attempted rape by a man who had been sitting next to her in a bar. Later on, when asked what happened, she expresses the thought, "You get what you ask for."

Are these attitudes justified? Is it true that alcohol makes women promiscuous? Are women who drink the sexual aggressors rather than victims? Recent research sheds light on this important question. A series of studies by Sharon Wilsnack and her colleagues have explored the relationship between women's drinking and sexual behavior. Their work indicates that contrary to common belief, alcohol does not have this effect [10]. In an extensive survey of nearly 1000 women who used alcohol to some extent, only 8% said they had ever become less particular in their choice of sexual partner when they had been drinking. This proportion differed only slightly between lighter and heavier drinkers. On the other hand, 60% of the women surveyed said that someone else who was drinking had become sexually aggressive toward them. The percentage was constant for light drinkers, moderate drinkers, and heavier drinkers. Thus, the stereotype of women made promiscuous by alcohol is not merely inaccurate. It results in promoting the sexual victimization of drinking women.

This phenomenon is further explored by Fillmore [11]. In her general population study of social victimization caused by another person's drinking, Fillmore found that unlike men, women who drink in bars (that is, who are exposed to others while drinking) are far more likely to be victimized, even if they are not themselves heavy or problem drinkers.

Miller and her colleagues have studied the experiences of alcoholic women as victims [12,13]. Their studies compared 45 alcohol-dependent women recruited from Alcoholics Anonymous and a treatment program with 40 matched controls from a community sample. Thirty-eight percent of the alcoholic women reported that they had been victims of violent crime, as compared to only 18% of the controls. Sixteen percent of the alcoholic women had been raped as opposed to none of the controls [12]. These women were victimized not only by outsiders, but also by their own spouses. The alcoholic women had significantly more experience of spousal violence of every kind from verbal (insult, swearing) to serious assaults with fists or weapons [13].

The sexual stigma attached to women who drink alcohol has also been documented directly. George and his colleagues have studied the attitudes of college students toward men and women who drink, using videotapes and written descriptions of young adult dating scenes [14,15]. In one study, the scenes presented to the students were nearly identical. They varied only in the type of drink involved. Both male and female students rated the woman in the dating scene more sexually available and more likely to have intercourse if the scene showed her ordering an alcoholic beverage rather than a soft drink. Furthermore, she was rated even more likely to be sexually available if the male paid for the drinks than if they split the cost.

Finally, a study by Richardson and Campbell documents society's acceptance of the female drinker as a target of sexual aggression [16]. College students were given a written description of a rape scenario, based on an actual case. In it, the victim, cleaning up after a party in her apartment, was approached by a guest she hardly knew who offered to help. He then pulled her into a bedroom, struck her, and raped her. The story was presented in four versions: the male intoxicated, the female intoxicated, neither intoxicated and both intoxicated. In rating the participants in the scenario, both male and female students judged the rapist to be less responsible when he was drunk. The victim, on the other hand, was held more to blame when she was intoxicated. Furthermore, their ratings of the woman's character, but not the man's, showed significant differences when she was said to be drunk in the story. She was judged less moral and more aggressive if she had been intoxicated at the time of the rape. The ideas of the ancients seem to be alive and well in contemporary society.

The practical result of this intense social stigma applied to alcoholic- and drug-dependent women is to keep them in hiding [17]. Since the chemically dependent woman grows up in the same society as the rest of us, she applies these stereotypes to herself. She reacts to her problem with guilt and shame. She tends to drink and take drugs alone, often in the privacy of her kitchen or bedroom. For example, 84% of 116 alcoholic women studied in depth by Corrigan did their drinking at home [17]. Married women, employed women, and upper socioeconomic status women were most likely to drink alone. Partly for this reason, the nature and extent of the chemically dependent woman's drinking or other drug use is often not appreciated by her family and friends until she has reached an advanced state of her disease. In addition, although she may seek medical help repeatedly because of numerous physical problems, nervousness, and insomnia, the stereotype of the addicted female as the "fallen woman" makes health professionals unlikely to suspect these diagnoses in their well-dressed, socially competent female patients. A recent study from Johns Hopkins Medical School examined the prevalence of alcoholism among patients admitted to the university hospital. Although alcoholic patients were underrecognized on all but the psychiatric services, the study found that the alcoholic patients least likely to be correctly identified were those with private insurance, higher incomes and educations, and those who were female [18].

The chemically dependent woman seldom recognizes the basic nature of her own problem, since viewed from within, these substances are her attempt at solving the many other problems she perceives as her "real trouble." She thus brings many complaints to her medical visit, but seldom do these complaints include her dependence on alcohol or other drugs. More often than not she leaves the doctor's office with a prescription for an additional sedative drug rather than a referral for addiction treatment.

II. RECENT INTEREST IN WOMEN AND ADDICTION

In spite of the strong feelings of our society toward women and alcohol, relatively little research into the physiological, psychological, and sociological aspects of women's drinking was performed prior to the mid-1970s, when a nationwide movement encouraged by the National Council on Alcoholism (NCA) and the National Institute on Alcohol Abuse and Alcoholism (NIAAA) focused attention on this problem. Nearly all of the classic studies done on the physiology, biochemistry, and metabolism of alcohol had been done in males. The initial studies on the nature and course of the disease alcoholism were also done in men; for example, Jellinek's classic study of the course of the illness in 1000 members of Alcoholics Anonymous [19]. In 1976, the NCA established an office on women and a committee that coordinated the development of a nationwide network of task forces on women and alcohol. In 1980, the NCA adopted a policy position on women and alcoholism. The NIAAA has funded special studies on women and alcohol since 1972, and in 1978 sponsored a 4-day conference at Jekyll Island, Georgia, to review research on women and alcohol. The proceedings of that meeting were published as the NIAAA Research Monograph 1 [20]. A second conference and monograph were produced in 1986, updating the literature review and adding a section on public policy issues [21]. In addition, a further literature review was published by the NIAAA in 1988 [22].

The NIDA has also published a recent monograph on women's drug issues [23], although less research has been done in this area, and no parallel comprehensive literature review has been published.

III. PHYSIOLOGY AND PATHOPHYSIOLOGY

As has been mentioned, the early studies on the physiology and metabolism of ethanol were conducted on male subjects. Not until the 1970s did researchers realize that there are significant differences in the way men and women handle alcohol. Jones and Jones, in a series of studies, found that single doses of ethanol, under standard conditions, produced higher peak blood alcohol levels in women than in men given equal doses of ethanol per pound of body weight [24]. This may be explained, in part, by the higher average content of body water in men (65 $\pm$ 2%), than women (51 $\pm$ 2%) [25]. Since ethanol is distributed in total body water, a standard dose will be less diluted in a woman. The Joneses also found that their female subjects showed a great deal of day-to-day variability in peak blood alcohol levels, unlike the males. This was related in part to phases of the menstrual cycle, with highest peaks in the premenstrual phase [26]. However, this relationship between blood alcohol concentration (BAC) and the menstrual cycle has not been found by other investigators. Increased BAC variability [27], faster ethanol metabolism [28], and less marked acute alcohol tolerance have also been reported in women compared to men [27]. In practical terms, this means that a woman will both react more intensely to a given dose of alcohol and be less able than a man to predict the effects of any given amount of beverage alcohol she might consume.

Although much has been written about emotional and behavior changes related to the menstrual cycle, there have been few studies of women's drinking patterns in relationship to these changes. Sutker and colleagues studied the mood states and drinking patterns of 32 normally cycling nonalcoholic women. These women reported significantly more negative moods, more drinking to relieve tension or depression, and more solitary drinking during menstruation [29]. Since these drinking patterns are characteristic of alcohol dependence, this research suggests that the menstrual cycle may be a significant factor in the early development of pathological drinking patterns in women, and provides an important lead for future study.

Sex differences have also been found in the pharmacology of other psychoactive drugs. Since women have a greater proportion of body fat than men, lipid-soluble drugs such as diazepam and oxazepam have longer half-lives in women [30]. This may be true of some barbiturates and phenothiazines as well. As women age their proportion of body fat increases further, providing an increased reservoir for these fat-soluble drugs [31]. Little is known about the influence of the menstrual cycle on drug effects. In one study described by Mello, the effects of marijuana on mood and heart rate did not change during the menstrual cycle [32]. However, women with a history of regular marijuana smoking showed less intense intoxication, confusion, and heart rate increases than those who used the drug intermittently. Mello's review of research on the relationship between the menstrual cycle and the quantity and frequency of alcohol and marijuana use concludes that increased use in the premenstrual period correlates with premenstrual dysphoria rather than the cycle itself [32].

Several studies have examined the effects of drinking on the female reproductive system. Single doses of alcohol seem to have little effect on sex hormone levels [33,34]. However, inhibition of ovulation, decrease in gonadal mass, infertility and a wide variety of obstetrical, gynecological, and sexual dysfunctions have been reported in association with chronic heavy drinking [33–35]. Russell and Czarnecki studied the drinking patterns of 1500 patients in gynecological practices. They found a correlation between heavy drinking and self-reported menstrual distress [36]. This relationship was strongest in young women (under 30 years of age), in the less well educated, and in those who reported planning pregnancy in the next 2 years.

Wilsnack has recently reviewed research on drinking and sexuality in women [37]. Experimental paradigms studying the differential effects of expectation and pharmacology have found gender differences in the effects of single doses of alcohol on sexual arousal in normal adults [38]. In men, both self-reported feelings and physiological measurements of arousal increased in response to sexual stimuli when the subject believed he had consumed alcohol (whether or not he actually received it). In women, however, there was a dissociation between subjective feelings of arousal and physiological responses. Women who thought they had received an alcoholic beverage said they felt more aroused whether or not they actually consumed alcohol. This expectation effect was similar to that of men. However, their bodies reacted differently. Actual alcohol consumption had a negative linear relationship to physiological arousal in women. The same dissociation between subjective feelings of sexual arousal and actual physical arousal was found in a study on female orgasm [39]. Increasing blood alcohol levels (up to 0.075%) produced longer latency and decreased orgasmic intensity, although the women themselves reported feeling greater arousal and pleasure. Women suffering from alcoholism also report that they expect greater desire and enjoyment of sex after drinking, while at the same time they report a variety of sexual dysfunctions [40]. Recovering alcoholic women have been reported to avoid sex in early sobriety [41]. Physicians can be helpful to these patients by explaining the physiological depressant effect of alcohol on sexual functioning, and reassuring them that abstinence is likely to enhance their sexuality in the long run.

The reason for this curious tendency for women to believe they are sexually aroused by alcohol when in fact they are not, is most probably a result of culturally conditioned expectation. We have already examined traditional social attitudes dating from as far back as the early Romans and Israelites. Chaucer [42], in his *Canterbury Tales*, has his Wife of Bath say:

A woman in her cups has no defense
As lechers know from long experience

As Ogden Nash put it, "Candy is dandy but liquor is quicker" [43]. Yet a recent study of 69 sexually active young women, during which they kept daily diaries, did not show any effects of alcohol on sexual arousal. Furthermore, the women were less likely to initiate sexual activities when they had been drinking, yet they indicated on a retrospective questionnaire that they believed alcohol had enhanced their sexual enjoyment and activity [44]. The persistence of this belief is remarkable.

IV. ALCOHOL AND OTHER DRUGS IN PREGNANCY

A special problem for women is the influence of alcohol and other drugs on the development of the fetus during pregnancy. This subject is covered in depth in Chapter 6. The fetal alcohol syndrome (FAS) has a current estimated incidence of between one and three cases per 1000 live births [45], making it one of the three most frequent causes of birth defects associated with mental retardation, along with Down's syndrome and spina bifida. The FAS includes prenatal and postnatal growth retardation, central nervous system abnormalities, usually with mental retardation, a characteristic facial dysmorphism, and an array of other birth defects. Although full-blown FAS is seen almost exclusively in the offspring of alcoholic women, other fetal alcohol effects such as spontaneous abortion, reduced birth weight, and behavior changes have been associated with lesser levels of alcohol intake.

A variety of drugs of abuse have also been found to have adverse effects on pregnancy, causing spontaneous abortion, premature labor, and a variety of obstetric complications. Among these are cocaine [46], opiates [47], and polydrug or multiple substance abuse [48].

Offspring of mothers who are physically dependent on drugs at the time of delivery frequently suffer from the neonatal withdrawal syndrome, which has been described for alcohol and sedatives, but is most often seen in infants of opiate-dependent mothers, especially high-dose unsupervised methadone users. Infants undergoing withdrawal not only suffer agitation, irritability, difficulty in nursing, and disturbed sleep. They also experience interference in their ability to establish the mother-infant bonding thought to be critically important for later development [49].

Less information is available about specific birth defects caused by drugs of abuse other than alcohol. Lower birth weight has been associated with both tobacco and marijuana smoking [49]. Cocaine use has been linked to urinary tract malformations in one study, and also to abnormalities in newborn behavior [48].

Nursing mothers have traditionally been advised to drink beer or ale as a folk medicine. Since alcohol passes into breast milk in the same concentration as in the bloodstream, and since the newborn is totally dependent on breast milk for nourishment, this practice is unwise [50]. Likewise, cocaine enters breast milk, and cocaine intoxication via breast feeding has been reported in an infant [51]. The best advice to nursing mothers is abstinence.

V. OTHER HEALTH EFFECTS

Although the health effects of heavy drinking in women are uniformly negative, there is some evidence that low to moderate levels of alcohol use are associated with decreased risk of coronary disease and ischemic stroke. The same intake, however, is associted with elevated risk for subarachnoid hemorrhage [52]. The most likely mechanism for this protective effect would be increased high-density lipoprotein (HDL) levels which tend to be higher in consumers of alcohol. However, a recent large scale study of HDL in Finland has demonstrated a complex relationship between alcohol consumption, physical exercise, smoking, coffee consumption, and HDL levels [53]. More research will be needed to elucidate these relationships.

Increased risk for a number of cancers of the head, neck, and digestive system are known to be associated with alcohol consumption [45]. Of special interest to women is the relationship between alcohol and cancer of the breast. Several large studies have recently demonstrated a dose-response relationship between alcohol intake and risk in women (54–56], and another yielded evidence for a weak association at best [57]. At our present state of knowledge, the evidence seems to support a relationship between the two, but the mediating factors are not known. Speculations have ranged from changes in liver metabolism to stimulation of prolactin secretion [55].

Prolonged heavy drinking is also known to be an etiological factor in many diseases of the gastrointestinal, neuromuscular, cardiovascular, and other body systems [58]. There is growing evidence that women may be more vulnerable to some of these pathological effects of alcohol than men. Ashley and her colleagues compared the lifetime prevalence of various alcohol-related illnesses in 135 female and 736 male alcoholics treated as inpatients [59]. Although the women had been drinking to excess for a significantly shorter time (14.2 vs 20.2 years), their physical disease rates were comparable to the men's. The average duration of hazardous drinking before the first recorded occurrence of disease was shorter for almost all illnesses, including fatty liver, hypertension, obesity, anemia, malnutrition, gastrointestinal hemorrhage, and an ulcer requiring surgery.

Cirrhosis of the liver has been studied for sex differences by several researchers (60–62). These studies provide evidence that women develop liver damage at lower levels of alcohol intake (even accounting for differences in body weight) and for shorter periods of time when compared to men.

Neuropsychological impairment associated with prolonged heavy drinking has been extensively studied [63], but research has involved predominantly male subjects [64]. Jones and colleagues found evidence for cognitive deficits in 40 abstinent alcoholic women (mean abstinence: 21 weeks) compared to a matched group of normal women [65]. Likewise, Turner and Parsons found neuropsychological deficits in 54 alcoholic women. Comparing those who had an alcoholic parent or sibling with those who did not, women with familial alcoholism performed significantly worse [66]. In a comparison of the patterns of neuropsychological deficit in 25 alcoholic women to the characteristic impairments found in men, Silberstein and Parsons found evidence that deficits in women may be milder [64]. However, Acker found evidence of more severe impairment among women [67], and Jacobson found equally severe computed tomographic (CT) scan results in 119 male and 26 female alcoholics even though the women in the study had consumed markedly less alcohol over a shorter length of time [68].

VI. PATTERNS OF ALCOHOL AND OTHER DRUG USE AMONG WOMEN

The epidemiology of alcohol and other drug use and abuse is covered elsewhere in this volume. I will comment below on a few issues that are particularly important to women.

Surveys of drinking in the general population have uniformly found that women drink less than men. More women abstain at any age. The proportion of heavy drinkers, and the percentage of the population reporting drinking-related problems are uniformly lower for women [69]. The epidemiology of women's drinking has been reviewed by Wilsnack et al. [70] and by Fillmore [71]. There is little doubt that both drinking and alcohol problems in women have increased considerably since the end of World War II. Clinicians have reported an additional increase in the number of alcoholic women appearing for treatment during the past 10 years, particularly younger women. This perceived increase in the incidence of female alcoholism has been difficult to document in population studies but has been found in some areas of the country [72]. There is also evidence from a number of sources that younger cohorts of women may be showing higher rates of heavy-frequent drinking than the generations of women who preceded them. Engs and Hanson have shown an increase in both heavy drinking (from 4.4 to 11.5%), and in various alcohol-related problems in college women when comparing a 1982 survey with data obtained in 1974 [73]. Younger women may constitute an especially high-risk group.

Cloninger and his colleagues have shown a marked increase in prevalence of alcohol dependence in the male and female first-degree relatives of alcoholic patients when comparing studies using the same methodology performed in 1969 and 1983 [74]. In female relatives both male and female probands, alcoholism rose from 6.7% to nearly 21%. When the data were analyzed by age cohort, the authors found that the risk for development of alcoholism by age 25 rose dramatically for younger cohorts. Alcoholism was not only developing more frequently, but was also developing earlier. The authors conclude that the age of onset distribution of alcoholism in those women born in 1953 was similar to distribution in men born in 1938. Thus, the risk of alcoholism in the current generation of women in their study closely approximated that of men in their fathers' generation.

In the 1981 national survey of male and female drinking practices conducted by Wilsnack and her colleagues [70], those women who drank most heavily (the top 20% in intake) were over-sampled so that their behavior could be studied. The authors have reported on several aspects of their findings [10,70,75]. The researchers found the highest rates of alcohol-related problems in the youngest age group included in the study, age 21–34. This finding confirms that of Cloninger [74]. However, in the general population sample, the highest proportion of heavier drinkers was found in the 35–49 age group. Married women had the lowest overall problem rates, whereas those cohabiting in common law relationship had the highest. The demographic characteristics of women with the highest rates of alcohol-related problems among women who drink varied strongly with age [75]. In the 21- to 34-year-olds, those described as "role-less" (never married, not employed full time) were most likely to have problems. In the 35–49-year-olds, women characterized as "lost role" (separated or divorced, unemployed, their children not living at home) had the highest problem rates. In their oldest cohort, aged 50–64, the women characterized by "role entrapment" (married, children not living at home, not working outside the home) had most alcohol problems. This last group seems to resemble women with the so-called "empty nest" syndrome [76]. Wilsnack also noted a strong correlation between the drinking patterns of women and their "significant others," more so than for men. Thus, clinicians should carefully evaluate the drinking of the wives of their male alcoholic patients, rather than just make the assumption that she is the nondrinker of the pair.

Fillmore studied drinking patterns of both men and women longitudinally using general population samples surveyed at two points, 7 years apart [77]. She found that women's alcohol problems were more likely to remit than men's at all ages. Among the women, those who reported alcohol problems in their 30s were most likely to continue having problems. Men and women in their 30s had nearly equal rates of problem persistence.

In 1985, nearly 6 million adult American women were either alcohol abusers (nearly 2.5 million) or alcoholics (more than 3.3 million). This represents about 6% of the adult female population. By comparison, just over 12.1 million men, or about 14% of the male adult population, have serious alcohol problems. The proportion, then, is about two males to one female [78].

Patterns of other drug use and drug problems in women have also varied during recent American history. Women have been the primary abusers of therapeutic drugs (both prescribed and over-the-counter). In the late nineteenth and early twentieth centuries, before legal accessibility to many drugs was severely limited by law, drug dependence was common in American women [7]. Women of all social classes became dependent on a variety of "tonic wines" and medicinals containing opiates, which were purchased at the local pharmacy. One popular tonic, Vin Mariani, contained cocaine (as did Coca Cola) before the Harrison Narcotics Act of 1914. When such drugs became difficult to obtain, women did not shift in great numbers of illegal drugs. Instead, they became dependent on other prescribed drugs, such as the barbiturates and meprobamate of a few decades ago, and later the amphetamines and the so-called minor tranquilizers.

Today, American women remain more frequent users of prescribed drugs and less frequent users of cigarettes, as well as marijuana, cocaine, and other illegal drugs, compared to men. Although women begin alcohol and other drug use at a later age than men and use them less frequently, sex differences in use patterns are less marked in adolescents today than in previous generations. Researchers have referred to the "vanishing difference" between the sexes in the use of alcohol and other drugs. Roman, however, concluded that sex differences in alcohol intake seem to be persisting [22]. Among teens, cigarette smoking has become as common among girls as boys [79,80]. In addition, data from a 1985 national household survey indicate that among women of child-bearing age (18–34), 30% reported having used an illicit drug at least once during the previous year, and 18% had done so during the previous month [80].

VII. HEREDITY AND CHEMICAL DEPENDENCE IN WOMEN

Early studies seeking to separate the relative influences heredity and environment in alcoholism were either performed on all-male populations, contained too few women to reach conclusions, or failed to analyze males and females separately [81]. The Stockholm adoption study, as reported by Bohman and his colleagues [82–84] has yielded much information on inheritance patterns of alcohol problems in women as well as men. This group studied 1775 adults adopted by nonrelatives early in life. By comparing records of alcohol-related problems in the offspring of biological parents with and without records of alcohol abuse, they were able to distinguish two patterns of inheritance relevant to women. One pattern, which they called type 2, or male-limited, showed early-onset alcohol abuse associated with criminality in both biological father and son. Neither the biological mothers, nor the daughters of these fathers, had an increased incidence of alcohol problems, but the daughters had a high incidence of multiple somatic complaints. In contrast, the pattern they described as type 1, or millieu-limited, was characterized by alcohol abuse with adult onset, in both the male and female adopted-away offspring of biological parents who were alcohol abusers (both fathers and mothers). The rates of alcohol problems in these adoptees were influenced by characteristics of the adoptive home, unlike the male-limited type [83]. Thus, there is evidence that both heredity and environment play etiological roles in female alcohol problems, an important consideration for the design of prevention approaches.

Less is known about genetic influences on the origins of other drug dependencies, but there also may be an increased risk of such problems in those offspring of alcoholic parents who have been adopted and raised by nonrelatives. A recent study by Cadoret and his colleagues offers evidence for this hypothesis. Both hereditary and environmental factors proved to be important [84].

The search for specific markers that would identify individuals who carry a genetic predisposition for alcoholism has focused primarily on males [81]. However, researchers at McLean Hospital have compared a small number of nonalcoholic young women with and without first-degree relatives suffering from alcoholism [85]. They did not differ in blood alcohol levels attained after a measured dose of ethanol, nor were the rates of disappearance of alcohol from the blood different. However, the higher-risk women made fewer errors on a cognitive motor task and had less body sway under the influence of alcohol. These findings were comparable to those observed in male samples.

VIII. PSYCHOLOGICAL FACTORS

There is still a great deal of uncertainty about possible psychological factors which may predispose to alcoholism. Studies of clinical populations make it difficult to distinguish characteristics that might have been present before the onset of alcoholism from traits that are products or concomitants of the disease itself. Of the longitudinal studies of alcohol problems in which young people were given psychological tests and then followed into adulthood, few have included female subjects. The Oakland Growth Study identified general feelings of low self-esteem and impaired ability to cope at the junior high school and high school levels in girls who later become problem drinkers [86]. This was not true of the males [87]. In a 28-year follow-up of a study of drinking among American college students, Fillmore et al. found that factors predictive of problem drinking in later life differed considerably between males and females [88]. Different definitions were required for males and females to describe both "alcohol involvement" at the college level and "problem drinking" at follow-up. The best predictor of later drinking problems for college women was a high score on the "feeling adjustment" scale, which contained items such as drinking to relieve shyness, drinking to get high, drinking to be gay, and drinking to get along better on dates. Among men, those with "incipient problems" in college were most likely to show drinking problems at follow-up. In neither sex was the presence of overt alcohol problems in college the best predictor of drinking problems 27 years later, although college problem drinkers did have higher rates than the nonproblem college drinkers as a whole. These findings indicate that prevention efforts at the college level should not focus only on those women who have already developed alcohol problems, but also on those who drink to enhance their self-esteem and ability to function.

Various studies have demonstrated differences between men and women in the cognitive, emotional, and behavioral effects resulting from acute and chronic alcohol use. For example, Caudill and his colleagues found that either believing they had consumed moderate amounts of alcohol or actually doing so increased self-disclosure in male social drinkers. In women, actually drinking alcohol had no independent effect. If the women believed that they had consumed alcohol, however, they were less likely to talk about themselves [89]. Wilsnack [90,91] found that when nonalcoholic women drank they became more feminine in outlook as measured on the Thematic Apperception Test (TAT). This contrasted with nonalcoholic men, who tended to become more power oriented. Based on this finding as well as other evidence, a theory of sex-role conflict to explain alcoholism in women was developed. The theory postulated that the alcoholic woman has a strongly feminine identity at the conscious level (as noted, for example, on the M-F scale of the Minnesota Multiphasic Personality Inventory) but a masculine identification at an unconscious level. Alcohol, by enhancing feelings of femininity, relieves this conflict, thus increasing the risk of alcohol dependency. Beckman [92] reviewed this theory and presented her findings on a series of 120 alcoholic women (white, ages 20–59), matched with two control groups: 118 nonpsychotic women in psychiatric treatment for problems other than alcoholism, and 119 normal women. She found the predicted pattern of sex-role conflict in 23% of the alcoholic women, a higher percentage than in the treatment controls (16%) and normal controls (13%). When sex-role conflict was redefined to include both conscious femininity paired with unconscious masculinity, and also the reverse, there was no significant difference between the incidence of sex-role conflict in the alcoholic women (29%) and normal controls (27%). Sixty-six percent of the alcoholic women, 71% of the treatment controls, and 68% of the normal controls scored feminine on both conscious and unconscious measures. Those alcoholic women who manifested sex-role conflict differed from the remainder of alcoholic women in showing lower self-esteem and a more frequent history of having had an absent parent during childhood. Beckman also assessed "androgyny" (flexible utilization of traits considered stereotypically "masculine" and "feminine" by one's culture), and found the alcoholic women significantly less androgynous than the normal controls, but not different in this measurement from the women in treatment for other emotional disorders.

IX. SOCIAL AND CULTURAL FACTORS

Mention has already been made of the sex differences in norms for socially acceptable drinking behavior in most cultures. Cloninger has argued, from twin studies and studies of the families of alcoholic and sociopathic probands, that sex differences in the prevalence of these two disorders arise from different causes [93]. In the case of antisocial personality disorder, the higher prevalence of antisocial family members in female than in male probands indicates that a greater familial loading is needed to attain expression of the disorder in women than in men. No such difference was found in familial loading between male and female alcoholics. This argues for the predominance of environmental factors outside of the family in determining the lower prevalence of alcoholism in women. Sociocultural factors that protect women include, for example, the custom of drinking primarily in mixed groups (whereas men drink in both mixed and all-male groups), and the relatively limited range of occasions in women's lives in which drinking is expected.

Klee and Ames have used ethnographic and case study methods to analyze cultural factors that appeared to protect a group of 31 women married to heavy drinkers who had been employed at a large manufacturing plant that was closed [3]. Although many of the women had multiple risk factors for alcohol problems, such as family histories of heavy drinking or alcoholism, heavy drinking by husbands and by others in their social networks, and disruption in early family life, they themselves did not currently drink to excess. Some had earlier histories of heavy drinking. Protective factors identified included role modeling by these women's mothers, the belief that "partying" is acceptable for a woman only in teen and young adult years but not after she becomes a mother, the acceptance of drinking by men as part of male social networks, and the custom of women's drinking restricted to special occasions. Although these attitudes and values are not universally held in American society, similar factors were found to be associated with lower alcohol consumption in a general population sample of 1084 female residents of Baltimore, Maryland [4]. Women who believed more strongly in the equality of the sexes drank more than others, as did more educated women.

I earlier referred to sociocultural attitudes toward women's drinking as a double-edged sword. While stigma and stereotypes keep the chemically dependent woman from receiving help, and serve to promote the victimization of women, cultural expectations that encourage lower alcohol intake for women are protective. At present per capita consumption in American women is less than half as much as that of American men. Because of their lower body weight, greater sensitivity to alcohol, and special risk during pregnancy, if women were ever expected to match drink for drink with men, they would be likely to have more alcohol problems than men instead of less. Unfortunately, drinking norms in contemporary American society are changing. The advertising and marketing of alcoholic beverages sends messages that can, and do, change cultural norms. Manufacturers of these beverages see women today as a growth market. Because market research indicates that women drink much less than men but make a significant proportion of the purchases of beverage alcohol, women are being increasingly targeted by alcoholic beverage advertising [94]. Beverage manufacturers and retailers who used to cater primarily to a male market with advertisements emphasizing the masculinity of drinking, are now portraying the genteel refinement of feminine drinking [95]. They increasingly show women drinking with other women to encourage this custom. Advertisers are also trying to identify more and more times and places in which it can become appropriate to use alcohol, attempting to turn everyday occurrences into occasions that call for a drink. Thus, the cultural norms that have served as protection for women are in danger of vanishing.

To accomplish the goal of prevention of alcohol problems in women we must simultaneously work to combat stigmata and to preserve the custom of abstinence or moderation for women. Our best strategy would seem to be widespread education about the special sensitivity to alcohol in women, the teratogenicity of alcohol, the risk involved in using alcohol to medicate feelings of inadequacy or other emotional states, the risk of mixing alcohol and sedatives, and other relevant issues.

The frequent use by women of pscyhoactive medications, both prescription and over-the-counter, is socially approved in contemporary America. Education of health professionals about the risks of drug dependence and about appropriate prescribing practices must be accompanied by public education concerning the proper use of psychoactive drugs. Government regulations requiring special controls on drugs with a high abuse potential are additional strategies aimed at prevention of chemical dependency, especially in women. However, without changes in custom and cultural attitudes, these measures will not be fully effective.

The importance of sociocultural factors in causing and shaping women's problems with alcohol and other drugs also highlights the necessity to explore and utilize the ethnic or subcultural background of the addicted woman in treatment. For example, Carter points to the importance of the mother-daughter relationship in preserving the health and strength of the African-American family, and the role of this relationship in black women's recovery from chemical dependence [96]. Similarly, an understanding of the "corporate" culture for a female executive, and the values and expectations of the health professional's milieu, the military, and the campus can be helpful in treatment, just as an understanding of specific Native American and Hispanic American cultures is necessary in the treatment of their members. The better we understand these cultures, the more effective we can be at identifying strengths and challenges to our pateints' recovery.

X. CLINICAL CHARACTERISTICS OF CHEMICALLY DEPENDENT WOMEN

Many studies relating to women and alcohol in the medical literature have compared the characteristics of male and female alcoholics in clinical samples (e.g., see Refs. 17, 97, and 98). Common findings include the following.

1. Women start drinking and begin their pattern of alcohol abuse at later ages but appear for treatment at about the same age as male alcoholics. This points to a more rapid development or "telescoping" of the course of the illness in women [17]. Telescoping has been noted by Smith and Cloninger to be particularly characteristic of women who suffer from depressive illness before the onset of their alcohol dependence (the so-called affective alcoholic women, see below) [99].

2. Women in the general public drink less than men. So do alcoholic women. In one general population poll, for example, American women averaged 0.44 oz of absolute alcohol

daily compared to the male average of 0.91 [100]. In a study of 11,500 men and 2600 women accepted for treatment in NIAAA-sponsored alcoholism programs, women's intake averaged 4.5 oz of absolute alcohol per day (about 9 drinks) compared to the male average of 8.2 oz (about 16.5 drinks), although men and women had the same degree of impairment [100]. In addition to body weight and body water differences, differences in the use of other sedatives may also help explain this disparity. The equivalent of the male alcoholic's morning drink may be a morning Valium (diazepam) for an alcoholic woman. Her "nightcap" may contain less alcohol and more sedative drug. Thus, alcoholism should not be diagnosed as a function of quantity of intake alone [101]. Among the 150 women in treatment for alcoholism studied by Corrigan, while 25% sometimes drank as much as a fifth of hard liquor, 17% reported drinking less than five drinks a day when drinking [17]. As the alcoholic woman ages, her tolerance for both alcohol and other drugs falls and she will drink even less than before while still experiencing adverse health and social consequences from her drinking [30,31].

3. Alcoholic women are more likely to be divorced when they enter treatment, or to be married to or living with an alcoholic significant other [102].

4. Alcoholic women are more likely than alcoholic men to date the onset of pathological drinking to a particularly stressful event.

5. Both alcohol- and other drug-dependent women patients reaching treatment are more likely to report a wide variety of such symptoms of psychological distress as anxiety and depression, and to have a lower self-esteem than their male counterparts [17,103]. They are more likely to have a history of previous psychiatric treatment and, at least in nonclinical populations, to be classified as "dual diagnosis" (see below). A history of suicide attempts is also more frequently in female than male chemically dependent patients. Hesselbrock and her colleagues recorded such a history in 41% of 90 female alcoholic patients compared to 21% of 231 males treated in the same program [104]. Female suicide attempters showed more lifetime psychopathology and a higher rate of additional diagnoses of depression, other substance abuse, and obsessive-compulsive disorder, but not of antisocial personality disorder. They were also more likely to have had an alcoholic father (69 vs 38% for nonattempters).

6. Chemically dependent women are more likely to be motivated to enter treatment by health and family problems, whereas for the male, job and legal problems, particularly arrests for driving while intoxicated, are more prevalent.

7. Alcoholic women are more likely to present with histories of other substance abuse along with their alcoholism, particularly tranquilizers, sedatives, and amphetamines, although they are less likely to be abusers of illicit drugs. The drugs these women abuse have usually been prescribed by their physicians [105].

A series of studies from a combined alcoholism and drug-dependency treatment facility have compared women with alcohol dependence, other drug dependence, and various combinations of dependencies [106,107]. Looking at personality traits, self-concept, and psychopathology in 225 female patients, Carroll and his colleagues found greater similarities than differences between women when grouped by drug of choice. Differences between black and white patients were found to be more significant. Black women tested as more suspicious, guarded, self-protective, and likely to display anger [106]. The alcoholic women who did not abuse other drugs were noted to be significantly older than the others (average age 37 years compared to 26 years). Harrison and Belille analyzed data from 1776 adult women in rehabilitation treatment for chemical dependency according to age [108]. Those aged 18–30 years were more likely to have a family history of alcoholism, drug abuse, and familial violence; more frequently drank or used drugs with others; more often used marijuana, cocaine, other stimulants and hallucinogens; and complained more often of weight problems, sexual problems, restlessness, depression, and a lack of energy. Women over aged 30 were far more likely to drink daily (50 vs 35% of younger women), and to drink alone (36 vs 9%

of younger women), and more commonly used sedatives and tranquilizers. These differences were interpreted as a combined effect of age and cohort. They certainly document the changing nature of clinical case loads observed by treatment facilities that serve women.

Griffin and her colleagues compared 95 men and 34 women receiving hospital treatment for cocaine abuse [109]. Many of their findings were similar to those cited above for female alcoholics. The women in their study were likely to cite specific reasons for their drug abuse, live with a drug dependent partner, show more depression and guilt feelings, have a higher rate of major depression but less antisocial personality disorder, and to come to treatment with shorter histories of drug abuse. However, these women were somewhat younger at treatment than their male counterparts (average age 24.5 vs 29.0 years) and to have started drug use earlier (15.5 vs 18.5 years). This finding contrasts with female alcoholic patients and with opiate addicts treated in the same facility, who were older at admission and had begun drug use later than males. The significance of this finding is not clear at present, and it is not known whether this age difference is characteristic of female cocaine abusers in general.

XI. CASEFINDING FOR CHEMICALLY DEPENDENT WOMEN

Current surveys show that women are underrepresented in chemical dependence treatment. Data from the National Institute on Alcohol Abuse and Alcoholism indicate that the ratio of male to female problem drinkers is about 2 to 1 [78], whereas the ratio of males to females in treatment for alcohol problems, according to 1987 data, is 4 or 5 to 1 [110]. Thus, women are appropriately called the hidden alcoholics. As we have seen, women are more likely to drink alone. Their problems are more likely to be denied by their families than is the case with their male counterparts. This too is not astonishing, given the long history of stigma attached to women who drink. However, these are not the only reasons for the underrepresentation of women in treatment. The most common systematic casefinding methods in use today, including Employee Assistance Programs, Public Inebriate Programs, and especially Drinking Driver Programs, are very strongly male oriented [101]. A common male to female ratio in programs for persons convicted of driving while intoxicated or for public inebriates is about 9 to 1. Employee assistance programs, which use impaired job performance as a problem indicator and job jeopardy as a motivator, have also been more successful with men [111–113]. However, it is possible to improve this situation. Increased attention has recently been paid to devising more effective strategies to reach female employees [111,114]. One recent study of 378 female employees in 12 federal agencies found a high rate of alcohol problems (21.9%) among participants in an orientation program. Yet this figure turned out to reflect significant underreporting compared to estimates derived from a more anonymous method (the randomized response). This method yielded an estimate of 34.3% for the group [115].

Sensitivity to women's responses regarding their reasons for seeking alcohol treatment can also lead to the development of new and improved casefinding systems for women. Both alcoholic and drug-dependent women may be reached through systematic screening in the physician's office, in hospitals, and in medical clinics.

A number of recent studies provide excellent examples of such casefinding. Halliday and her colleagues studied two private gynecological practices, one in Boston and one in a Boston suburb. They used the simple, four-question CAGE test as an initial screening tool, followed by an interview employing the alcohol section of the Diagnostic Interview Schedule (DIS). They found that of 147 women visiting these offices for routine care, 12% satisfied the DSM-III (*Diagnostic and Statistical Manual of Mental Disorders*, 3rd Edition, American Psychiatric Association, Washington, D.C., 1980) diagnosis for alcohol abuse or dependence—more than twice the community rate. Of 95 women who had come for the treatment for premenstrual syndrome, 21% satisfied the diagnosis of alcohol abuse or dependence

[116]. Moore et al. screened consecutive admissions at The Johns Hopkins Hospital for alcoholism and found that 69 of 556 obstetrics patients (12.4%) and 30 of 242 gynecology patients (12.4%) were positive. Very few of these patients were diagnosed by their physicians [18].

Cyr and her colleagues at Brown University studied men and women coming to an ambulatory medical primary care unit in an urban teaching hospital for their first visit. This study used the Michigan Alcohol Screen Test (MAST), a 25-item questionnaire that focuses on drinking problems. Of the 147 women in the study, with an average of 37, 17% scored in the alcoholic range. Twenty-six percent of the 85 male patients screened were positive, a male to female ratio of 1.5:1.0 [117]. This ratio demonstrates the value of medical facilities as fertile ground for identification of alcoholic women. Another study of 347 primary care medical outpatients using the SMAST (Short Michigan Alcohol Screening Test) and DSM-III criteria, found that 11% of the women met criteria for alcohol abuse or dependence at some time in their lives [118].

Women's special problems with alcohol (including effects on pregnancy and the rapid progression of the late-stage physical complications of alcoholism in women), coupled with women's strong representation in medical facilities, reinforce the need for effective systematic screening, diagnosis, and referral of women with alcohol and drug problems in the health care system [119]. Such casefinding systems will not only serve to prevent the fetal alcohol syndrome and other fetal alcohol effects, they also have the potential to relieve much individual and family suffering.

XII. SCREENING FOR CHEMICAL DEPENDENCY IN WOMEN

There are a number of effective screening tools for alcoholism, both in the format of pencil-and-paper tests and structured interviews. The CAGE and MAST tests, cited above, are good examples. However, nearly all of these screens were developed and tested in predominately male populations [101]. One exception is the Health Questionnaire designed by Marcia Russell for the New York State Fetal Alcohol Syndrome prevention campaign in 1979 [120]. This simple self-test is meant to be filled out in the physician's waiting room, and can alert the clinician to emotional problems and drug dependence as well as alcohol dependence. It also provides information for estimating the patient's alcohol intake. The questionnaire has been slightly adjusted to include several drug-related questions [121].

Laboratory testing can also be helpful in screening. Hollstedt and Dahlgren [122] analyzed the records of 100 women undergoing their first episode of alcoholism treatment in the city of Stockholm. It was found that increased mean corpuscular volume (MCV) of the red blood cells was present in 48% of these women, and an increase in the enzyme gamma-glutamyl transferase (GGT) in 42%. If *either* an elevated MCV *or* an elevated GGT were considered the screening criterion, 67% of the alcoholic women were correctly identified.

Women who are primarily dependent on drugs other than alcohol may be less under-represented in treatment. Nationwide data collected in 1987 indicate that nearly one-third of all Americans in treatment for drug abuse were women [110]. However, may drug-dependent women remain in hiding. Urine screening for drugs of dependence remain an underutilized casefinding technique in medical settings. Social techniques of assessment and motivation can also be applied to reach drug-dependent women [123].

XIII. DIAGNOSIS AND DUAL DIAGNOSIS

Once the chemically dependent woman is identified through screening, a careful clinical assessment is extremely important. One major difference between the clinical presentation of alcoholism in women, as compared to men, is related to the presence of additional psychiatric diagnoses. Alcoholism or other drug dependence may be classified as primary when it develops in an individual with no preexisting psychiatric disorder, and secondary when another diagnosable illness is present before the pattern alcohol or drug abuse develops [124]. In a typical treatment population, primary alcoholism prevails. However, when alcoholism is secondary, there is a difference between men's and women's primary diagnoses. In men with secondary alcoholism, the most common primary diagnosis is antisocial personality disorder. Women's most prevalent primary diagnosis is major depression, a condition sometimes called affective alcoholism. This diagnosis must be based on a careful life history, since the presence of depressive symptoms at the time of treatment will not differentiate between primary and affective alcoholism.

Helzer and Pryzbeck [125] have added significantly to our knowledge in this area. Analyzing data from the Epidemiologic Catchment Area study of the prevalence of 44 "core" psychiatric diagnoses in nearly 20,000 American adults in a general community sample, they found that more than 13% of American adults satisfied a lifetime DSM-III diagnosis of alcohol abuse or dependence. Of those that satisfied an alcoholism diagnosis, 47% also met criteria for a second core psychiatric diagnosis. In contrast, of members of this community sample who had any core diagnosis, only 32% had a second psychiatric diagnosis. Thus, alcoholics in the general population were significantly more likely to have a "dual diagnosis" than persons with other psychiatric disorders. Their work also revealed significant differences between alcoholic men and women. First of all, women were more likely than men to have a dual diagnosis (65% of female alcoholics compared to 44% of males). Antisocial personality disorder, present in 15% of the alcoholic men and 10% of the women, was the only second diagnosis more common in males than females. A second diagnosis of drug abuse or dependence was found in 31% of women compared to 19% of men. Major depression was nearly four times as frequent in women (19 compared to 5%). Phobic disorder was diagnosed in 31% of the alcoholic women compared to 13% of men, and panic disorder in 7% of the women to 2% of the men. Even a diagnosis like mania, which was rare, occurred in 4% of the alcoholic women compared to 1% of alcoholic men. Some of the sex differences found may relate to the unusually high male to female ratio for alcohol abuse and dependence in the Epidemiological Catchment Area study (more than 5:1). This contrasts with previous studies using a variety of survey criteria. It may be that the women who satisfied the DSM-III diagnoses in this study were more severely affected than those in other studies. This might be related to the structure of the screening instrument used, the Diagnostic Interview Schedule (DIS).

The Helzer and Pryzbeck [125] study further clarifies the prevalence of dual diagnosis in female alcoholics by comparing the prevalence of the most frequent core diagnoses in alcoholic women to their prevalence among women in the total population. For example, 5% of the general population women satisfied a diagnosis of substance abuse or dependence, compared to 31% of the alcoholic women. Major depression was diagnosed in 7% of the women in the general community sample, but the rate nearly tripled in alcoholic women (19%). Similarly, the incidence of phobias in women with alcoholism was 31%, almost double the community rate (16%). Most telling was the finding that antisocial personality, which existed in only a fraction of a percentage of women in the community (0.31%), was diagnosed in 10% of the women alcoholics studied. In addition, Helzer and Pryzbeck [125] analyzed their data to separate primary from secondary alcoholism in those cases in which alcoholism and major depression were the two only diagnoses present. They found that in 78% of such men, the alcoholism was primary and the depression secondary (i.e., developed after the alcoholism). In the women, alcoholism was primary in only 34%. Two-thirds of the women had suffered from depression before developing alcoholism.

Treatment populations may be expected to have even higher rates of dual diagnoses than would be found in the general public. Helzer and Pryzbeck [125] reported that the number of additional diagnoses other than substance abuse, present along with the diagnosis of alcoholism in this community sample, was a very strong determinant of whether or not the individual had sought treatment, independent of the severity of the alcoholism itself. In their study, alcoholic women were more likely to have had some type of mental health treatment than men, although the nature and appropriateness of the treatment could not be judged by their data. However, their overall findings confirm the common sense expectation that more complicated, dual diagnosis cases are more likely to reach clinical attention.

Hesselbrock et al. [126] found, in a clinical sample of 90 women alcoholics, that 80% satisfied one or more additional lifetime psychiatric diagnoses. Another substance abuse was diagnosed in 38% of the sample, and 52% of the women were diagnosed as having major depression. Phobia was diagnosed in 44%, panic disorder in 14%, and obsessive-compulsive disorder in 13%. Twenty percent of the clinical sample of women satisfied diagnostic criteria for antisocial personality disorder. All other diagnoses were present in less than 10%. This profile differed significantly from the patterns shown by the 261 male alcoholics in the study. Among the males, 75% had one or more additional diagnoses, a difference from the female alcoholics which was not statistically significant. Forty-five percent had substance abuse, 32% had major depression, 20% had phobia, 8% had panic disorder, and 12% had obsessive-compulsive disorder. As in the community sample, antisocial personality was the only additional diagnosis in which males greatly outnumbered females. Forty-nine percent of the alcoholic men met these diagnostic criteria compared to 20% of the alcoholic women.

Both Helzer and Pryzbeck [125] and Hesselbrock et al. [126] identified major depression as the most common primary diagnosis in women with secondary alcoholism. Both studies indicate that depression was primary in approximately two-thirds of alcoholic women with depression. Depression was found to be primary in 41% of the alcoholic men who also had depression in the treatment sample compared to 22% in the general population sample.

Opiate addicts also show a high prevalence of both Axis I and Axis II dual diagnosis. Similar to the findings in alcoholics, Khantzian and Treece found Axis I disorders, particularly major depression, more frequent in opiate-addicted females and antisocial personality more prevalent in males [127]. Rounsaville and Kleber compared additional diagnoses in opiate addicts in treatment with an untreated community group of addicts [128]. Although their sample was largely male, the women differed in showing more amphetamine abuse and more affective disorder. Unlike the males, the community females had as much depression as the female treatment population.

In contrast to the above, Ross and her colleagues, studying 260 men and 241 women seeking treatment for alcohol and drug problems, found an equal prevalence of affective disorder in the two sexes [129]. This may have been influenced by the timing of their patient interviews, which was within the first few days of treatment. Women did show higher rates of anxiety disorders, sexual disorders, and bulimia, and lower rates of antisocial personality disorder. Other researchers have also found an association between eating disorders and psychoactive substance use disorders. In a study of 646 high school girls, 10.3% were bulimic and an additional 10.4% used purging at times to control weight [130]. These girls reported higher rates of cigarette and marijuana smoking and alcohol intoxication as well as more depression than their nonbulimic classmates. In a population of 35 bulimic women recruited through advertisements, 48.6% satisfied a DSM-III diagnosis of alcohol abuse, 22.9% alcohol dependence, 25.7% drug abuse, and 34.3% drug dependence [131]. The relatives of these women had high rates of alcoholism (60%) and drug abuse/dependence (22.9%). All of these rates were higher than controls. In our own eating disorder inpatient program at South Oaks Hospital, the staff found so many patients suffering from alcohol abuse and dependence that they started regular Alcoholics Anonymous (AA) meetings on the eating disorder unit and found them well-attended.

A study of gambling problems among inpatients admitted to South Oaks Hospital for alcohol and other drug dependence found the female patients far less likely than males to be compulsive or problem gamblers (6 vs 25%) [132].

A number of investigators have studied the relationship between psychoactive substance dependence and personality disorders. Several have studied borderline personality disorder (BPD). Nace and his colleagues surveyed a group of male and female alcoholic patients using a conservative definition of BPD and omitting substance-related criteria. They found that 12.8% satisfied a DSM-III diagnosis of BPD [133]. Although in the general population females are far more likely to suffer from this disorder than males, in this alcoholic population, males and females showed the same frequency. The borderline patients tended to be younger, and had more drug abuse, more suicide attempts, and more reports of craving for alcohol. One year after a 28-day inpatient program, followed by outpatient care and AA, the borderline patients did as well as the nonborderline patients as measured by decreased alcohol use [134]. Although the borderlines were a little bit worse in their drug use and interpersonal relations, they did respond well to treatment.

Vaglum and Vaglum, in a study from Norway [135], found a higher prevalence of BPD in 81 alcoholic women compared to 64 nonalcoholic psychiatric patient controls. Sixty-six percent of the alcoholic women but only 11% of the treatment control women satisfied a BPD diagnosis. Borderline personality disorder was six times as common as antisocial personality in the alcoholic sample. Loranger and colleagues studied 83 female inpatients with BPD [136]. In their sample, although 47% occasionally abused alcohol, only 3.6% met criteria for alcohol dependence. There was a very high incidence of parental alcoholism among the BPD patients. The authors interpreted their findings as supporting an independent but overlapping familial transmission of the two disorders.

Although far more research on BPD in relationship to addictive disorders is needed, the clinician should be alert to BPD in chemically dependent populations and to chemical dependence in patients with BPD. Specific treatment for chemical dependency, including 12-step programs, should be instituted for this dually diagnosed group.

There have been many studies on addiction in relation to antisocial personality disorder (ASP). Various patient groups have shown a prevalence for male alcoholics of between 10 and 55%, and for male opiate addicts from about 15% to over one-half. For alcoholic women, prevalence ranges more from 5 to 20%, depending on the patient group. For female addicts, higher rates are found, especially in criminal justice populations [137–139].

XIV. TREATMENT OF THE ALCOHOL OR OTHER DRUG DEPENDENT WOMAN

The sections on treatment in this volume deal in depth with the overall treatment of the psychoactive substance use disorders. Here I will touch upon a few gender-specific issues.

In detoxifying the chemical dependent woman, either on an inpatient or outpatient basis, special care must be given to the taking of a complete history of psychotropic drug use. Since women are more likely to be users and abusers of minor tranquilizers, sedatives, and stimulants, prolonged and/or unusual detoxification symptoms may be noted [140]. Substance abuse should always be considered in the differential diagnosis of delayed convulsions during alcohol withdrawal, along with head trauma and other causes of seizures.

During the rehabilitation phase, education on addiction for the patient and family are important for both sexes. In dealing with women, however, the effects of alcohol and other drugs on the fetus and the need for evaluation of the patient's children should be stressed.

Early in treatment the patient and her family should be introduced to the appropriate self-help groups. A female sponsor should be sought. There are all-female AA groups in some areas, and afternoon groups with associated babysitting for mothers of young children. An all-female self-help group, Women for Sobriety [141], is also available in many areas of the United States. Such groups help the chemically dependent woman identify with other women who have overcome their illness, instilling hope and allaying guilt and shame. This is particularly important in view of the social stigma discussed earlier in this chapter. As an additional aid in establishing a positive identity as a recovering woman, it is helpful to recommend that the patient read biographies and autobiographies of recovering chemically dependent women [141–146].

Psychotherapy during the initial treatment period may be performed individually or in groups. Mixed-sex groups, all-female groups, family groups, and couples' groups may all be used to good effect in treating the alcoholic woman. The treatment goals during this early phase include the establishment of abstinence and a beginning exploration of the previous role of alcohol and drugs in the life of the patient. With the relief of initial anxiety and depression, a great deal of buried anger may surface. This anger must be evaluated in terms of the patient's own psychological, interpersonal, and social reality, bearing in mind the effects of traditional sexism, the unequal societal roles assigned to women, and their special problems in self-esteem and identity. As treatment continues, a reevaluation of the patient's feelings about herself, her role, and the role of chemicals in her life becomes the major focus of treatment. Additional help may be needed through vocational rehabilitation, spiritual counseling, assertiveness training, or a wide variety of other services, depending on the needs of the individual.

In psychotherapy, special problems may arise when the chemically dependent woman is treated by a therapist accustomed to treating males. If the therapist measures success only in terms of adjustment to the societal stereotype of the female role, he or she may avoid helping the patient confront her feelings about individuality and independence, and thereby miss the best possible opportunity to enlarge her range of conscious choices about her life. This narrow "adjustment" goal may also fail to raise self-esteem and may reinforce dependent, childlike, or seductive behavior toward the therapist, rather than encouraging straightforward, aboveboard communication. Since the responsibility for her recovery must continue to rest squarely on the shoulders of the woman in treatment, dependence in the therapeutic interaction becomes a threat to that sobriety. Should the patient relapse during therapy, care must be taken not to reinforce this behavior by oversolicitousness or a level of interest not accorded her in the sober state. The therapist should always make sure that, while not rejecting the patient who relapses, he or she makes clear the expectation that the patient will return to the sober state and helps her make realistic plans to do so. The use of minor tranquilizers should be kept to a minimum because of the dangers of dependence.

A number of special treatment methods have been developed for the chemically dependent woman, but none has yet undergone statistical evaluation. Common themes in these methods are special sensitivity to the needs of women, provision for appropriate childcare, assertiveness training and preparation for more straightforward communication, special help for victims of physical and sexual abuse, therapy sensitive to cultural issues, and the provision of appropriate female role models. Particular attention should be paid to women who have been victims of abuse, either during childhood or in adulthood. In the study by Miller and her colleagues cited earlier, 67% of the alcoholic women reported that they had been the victims of sexual abuse by an older person during childhood. Only 28% of the matched community control group reported such abuse, a significant difference. The alcoholic women were not only more likely to have one such experience, but reported more frequent experiences over longer periods of time, especially if they were daughters of alcoholic parents. In these families, the father was not usually the aggressor. Rather, there was a lack of protection for the child, who was abused by others [147]. Routine admission history taking often fails to elicit information about these deeply shameful and sometimes repressed experiences. It is therefore imperative that gentle approaches to the subject of incest and abuse be made repeatedly throughout the treatment process.

In our hands at South Oaks Hospital, psychodrama has been a useful treatment modality for our female patients. Men and women participate together in this form of large-group psychotherapy [148]. The experience of playing the roles of other people and of switching roles with significant others helps the chemically dependent woman to develop insight and spontaneity, and to enlarge her repertory of behaviors.

Special populations of women needing specific attention include minority women [96,149], women in the military [150], women in the criminal justice system [151], and lesbian women [152–155].

XV. THE OUTCOME OF TREATMENT FOR WOMEN

Chemical dependency treatment may be a necessary, but not a sufficient condition to produce recovery in those chemical abusers who also suffer from a multitude of other problems. Treatment alone cannot be expected to succeed when needs for health care, housing, employment, job training, and social supports are unmet. However, treatment outcomes for those patients with established support systems in the community are very hopeful. The CATOR Studies tracked both adolescents [156] and adults [157] after inpatient rehabilitative treatment in a number of different facilities. For adolescents, girls had a slightly better recovery rate than boys. Seventy-four percent of the girls, compared to 66% of the boys completed inpatient treatment. Only 5% of the girls (vs 13% of the boys) were discharged due to behavior problems. Fifty percent of the 313 girls reinterviewed a year after treatment had remained abstinent compared to 40% of the 502 boys. Because of differences between former patients contacted for follow-up and those who could not be located, the overall recovery rate was not known. However, only one-third of the former patients contacted reported prolonged or multiple relapses.

Adult males and females from relatively stable socioeconomic environments had equal, high recovery rates. Approximately 53% of 1957 adult patients (55% married, 76% employed, homemakers or students) were followed for 2 years after discharge [157]. Of those interviewed, only 28% had relapsed to multiple or prolonged periods of substance use. Correcting for the influence of patients who were not contacted, the authors felt it was safe to conclude that about one-half of the men and women treated at the inpatient chemical dependency units studied maintained total abstinence for at least 2 years.

A number of reviews of alcoholism treatment outcome in women as compared to men have concluded that adult males and females treated together in the same programs do about equally well [158,159,101]. Less work has been done comparing the sexes in treatment for other drug dependence. Rounsaville et al. found that among opiate addicts, women had a higher treatment retention rate and experienced less legal problems at follow-up [160]. McLellan and his staff did not report sex differences in their study of three different populations of alcoholics and other drug abusers [161].

Several investigators have sought reliable prognostic factors predictive of treatment outcome. The McLellan study [161] found that the psychiatric severity scale of the Addiction Severity Index (ASI), a global measure of pretreatment psychiatric problems, was the best prediction of outcome for all groups [161]. Looking at specific psychopathology, Rounsaville et al. [162] tracked alcoholic men and women for 1 year after treatment. They found that those with the dual diagnosis of antisocial personality and alcoholism, whether male or female, had a poor outcome. However, women with the dual diagnoses of alcoholism and major depression did slightly better than average.

In a 2-year follow-up study of 127 patients suffering from major affective disorder, who also satisfied research diagnostic criteria for alcoholism, men and women had equal rates of remission from alcoholism [163]. Two-thirds had a remission of alcohol-related symptoms of at least 6 months and 45% did not relapse subsequently. Of the one-third who did not experience remission of their alcoholism, 17% died, mostly by suicide or violence. Patients with milder alcoholism of briefer duration remitted more quickly. Those with a diagnosis of schizoaffective disorder had a poorer prognosis, but the same did not apply to antisocial personality disorder.

Other researchers have focused on extra-treatment events and their influences on recovery. MacDonald followed 93 inpatient alcoholic women for 1 year after treatment [164]. He found that the number of life problems and the number of supportive relationships were the best predictors of favorable outcome. Being married was less important as a predictor than the supportive quality of the patient's marriage. Similar results were found by Havassy et al., who found a relationship between social support and time abstinent after detoxification from alcohol, methadone, and tobacco [165]. They also found that their female subjects experienced less social support than males.

Little is known about the stability of treatment outcome over many years. A sample of 103 alcoholic women treated in a public and private hospital in the late 1960s has been followed for 12 years by Smith and Cloninger [166]. The same factors that predicted a good outcome at 3 years (experienced by 41% of the women) predicted good outcome at 12 years (experienced by about one-half), 84% of women maintained the same outcome at 12 years as at 3. More shifted from poor to good outcome (24%) than from good to poor (9%). Predictors of poor outcome at both periods included early onset (under age 30), longer duration, loss of control, greater impairment, and antisocial personality disorder.

Wilsnack at al. looked at facotrs that predicted remission of problem drinking in their general population sample of women reinterviewed 5 years after their original survey. Women who experienced remission of their drinking problems were more likely to be under 35 or over 50 years old, divorced or separated, traditional in feminine traits and moral standards, free of sexual dysfunction, and not reporting heavy-drinking friends [167]. Thus, some of the same sociocultural factors seem to be associated with remission of alcohol problems in women in the general population and as have been implicated in protecting women from heavy and problem drinking.

Taking a broad look at the outcome literature, two major factors emerge: psychopathology on one hand and sociocultural factors on the other, particularly support by a social network that does not encourage alcohol and drug use by women. Both prevention and treatment efforts aimed at women will be more effective if they focus on these areas.

XVI. MORTALITY

Women suffering from alcoholism experience a high rate of mortality, both when compared to the general population of women and to rates of excess mortality in alcoholic men [168]. Mortality rates are especially high for alcoholic women who do not achieve recovery. The study by Smith and Cloninger discussed previously reported on the mortality rates of 103 alcoholic women [169]. Eleven years after discharge from treatment, 31% of the women were dead, at an average age of 51.5 years. Their mortality was 4.5 times the age-corrected general population rate, and they lost an average of 15 years from their expected lifespan. Those who attained abstinence, however, did not experience elevated mortality rates. A recent report from Sweden confirms these findings. Lindberg and Agren [170] followed nearly

4000 male and nearly 1000 female patients following hospital treatment for alcoholism over a period ranging from 2 to 22 years. The excess mortality was higher for the alcoholic women (5.2 times the expected rate) than for the men (3 times the expected rate). Causes of death in excess of expected rates for women were alcoholism, intoxication, cirrhosis, breast cancer, and a variety of types of violence. For males, the excess deaths were attributed to alcoholism, cirrhosis, pancreatitis, tuberculosis, pneumonia, intoxication, suicide, violence, heart disease, and cancer of the upper digestive tract, liver, and lung. The excess mortality rate was highest in the first year following treatment, but continued to be elevated throughout the follow-up period. Since the data were obtained from official death records, the alcoholism recovery status of the former patients was not known. However, from the causes of excess mortality it can be inferred that these deaths occurred predominantly in those who continued to drink.

XVII. PREVENTION AND THE REMOVAL OF TREATMENT BARRIERS: THE POLICY ISSUES

Prevention efforts aim either at avoiding alcohol and drug problem development (primary prevention) or early casefinding to prevent the damage of the full-blown disease (secondary prevention). Secondary prevention has been covered briefly in this chapter in Section XI. As for primary prevention, relatively little has been done to design educative prevention programs specifically for women or to evaluate women's programs [45,171]. Most education programs have concentrated on promoting abstinence during pregnancy, and thus preventing the fetal alcohol syndrome, fetal alcohol effects (FAE); and other problematic births. Additional prevention efforts have concentrated on physician education [172,173].

A recent paper has reviewed many of the public policy issues relevant to women and alohol, including availability and marketing of alcoholic beverages, highway safety, prevention of FAS/FAE, child abuse and neglect, custody and child care, and support for outreach, treatment, and research about women [174]. Research is sorely needed to evaluate the effects of beverage advertising aimed at women, since increases in heavier drinking in young women seem to be associated with an increase in alcohol problems, as noted above. A policy issue that has engendered much recent debate is that of health warnings, both in the form of alcoholic beverage labels [58] and as posters required to be displayed at the point of sale [175]. These measures specifically include messages on the dangers of drinking during pregnancy, and are therefore of special relevance to women. Warning labels will appear on alcoholic beverage containers by the end of 1989. Warning posters are now required in many states and local jurisdictions.

One of the important roles of government is the removal of barriers that keep chemically dependent people from obtaining the treatment they need. For women, a major barrier is the lack of child care. Many alcoholic and drug-dependent women are single parents, or, if married, lack the resources to provide adequate care for their children. In a multicity survey of services for alcoholic women conducted by the Woman to Woman program of the Association of Junior Leagues, the most frequently mentioned institutional barrier to treatment was the lack of child care services for women needing residential care [176]. A few model programs in several states have developed such services but the need is largely unmet [177,178].

Many women in need of chemical dependency treatment are single or divorced and unemployed or underemployed, leaving them without health insurance coverage. This is particularly true for black women [179]. The federal government attempted to improve this situation in 1984 by requiring that 5% of the funds granted to the states for alcohol, drug abuse, and mental health services be devoted to new or expanded services for women. This measure, which involved $63.5 million of these "block grant" funds was opposed by the states.

However, a study conducted by the National Council on Alcoholism concluded that the so-called women's set-aside had accomplished its purpose, by stimulating the initiation of a broad range of prevention, education, and treatment services, many of which were sorely needed [180]. The satisfaction of the Congress with this measure was demonstrated in that the set-aside was increased to 10% in the Omnibus Drug Bill of 1988.

An additional barrier to treatment may be found in the legal definitions of child abuse and neglect in force in the various states. In many states, the habitual or addictive use of alcohol or drugs by a parent makes the parent a child abuser/neglector by definition. This definition becomes a barrier, particularly for disadvantaged and single mothers who must rely on public social service agencies for child care in order to enter treatment. Asking for help in such a situation puts them in real jeopardy of losing custody of their children. Paradoxically, continuing their chemical dependency without seeking help does not, in general, have this effect. Child abuse laws can be altered in their language, not only to remove this barrier, but to provide an incentive for the alcoholic or addicted parent to accept treatment. The state of New York has revised its definitions so that an addicted parent who is participating in a program of recovery is no longer presumed to be guilty of abuse or neglect without additional evidence [174].

All of the public policy trends discussed above have been designed to improve the lot of women with alcohol and drug problems while preserving their individual rights and human dignity. However, there are other important and urgent policy issues currently under debate that pit the rights of the unborn fetus against those of the prospective mother who has chosen to bear the child [181,182]. Although the debate is most often framed in terms of compelling the mother to undergo cesarean section or other medical treatment against her will, for the sake of her fetus, the same principle (of prenatal child abuse) has been used to force pregnant women to abstain from alcohol and other drugs through threats of loss of custody or even incarceration. In 1986, a California woman whose premature infant died at age 5 days, allegedly because she took drugs while pregnant, was charged with criminal child neglect for not following medical advice during pregnancy [183]. Advances of knowledge in the field of teratology can put women at increasing risk for legal penalties if the principle of fetal rights becomes established in law.

Although public policy has come a long way since the early Roman death penalty for female drinkers, the relationship between women and mind-altering drugs still poses a difficult conundrum to human society. And it looks like the relationship will continue to be problematic for many years to come. We are in desperate need of more and better research. We have to know more about women's drinking patterns, risk factors, treatment needs, and differential effects of treatment by gender. However, if we apply even a portion of what we know right now, with vigor, we will be able to greatly improve the welfare of all American women.

REFERENCES

1. McCarthy, R.G. (ed. (1959). *Drinking and Intoxication*, New Brunswick, N.J. College and University Press and Rutgers Center of Alcoholic Studies.
2. Heath, D. (December 1986). Women and alcohol: Does gender make a difference? *Addict. Lett.*, pp. 5–7.
3. Klee, L., and Ames, G. (1987). Reevaluating risk factors for women's drinking: A study of blue collar wives, *Am. J. Prev. Med.*, 3:31–41.
4. Celentano, D.D., and McQueen, D.V. (1984). Alcohol consumption patterns among women in Baltimore, *J. Stud. Alcohol*, 45:355–358.

5. Samarasinghe, D.S., Dissanayake, S.A.W., and Wyesinghe, C.P., (1987). Alcoholism in Sri Lanka: An epidemiological study, *Br. J. Addict., 82*:1149–1154.

6. McKinlay, A.P. (1959). The Roman attitude toward women's drinking, *Drinking and Intoxication* (R.G. McCarthy, ed.), Free Press, Glencoe, Illinois, pp. 58–61.

7. Gomberg, E.S.L. (1986). Women: Alcohol and other drugs, *Perspectives on Drug Use in the United States*, (B. Segal, ed.), Haworth Press, New York.

8. Jellinek, E.M. (1941). Immanuel Kant on drinking, *Q. J. Stud. Alchol, 1*:777–778.

9. Rovner, S. (Nov. 1, 1988). Women, alcohol and sex: Troubled trio, *Washington Post*.

10. Klassen, A.D., and Wilsnack, S.C. (1986). Sexual experiences and drinking among women in a US national survey, *Arch. Sexual Behav., 15*:363–392.

11. Fillmore, K.M. (1985). The social victims of drinking, *Br. J. Addict., 80*:307–314.

12. Miller, B.A., and Downs, W.R. (1986). *Conflict and Violence Among Alcoholic Women as Compared to a Random Household Sample*, paper presented at the 38th Annual Meeting of the American Society of Criminology, Atlanta, Georgia.

13. Miller, B.A., Downs, W.R., and Gondoli, D.M. (1989). Spousal violence among alcoholic women as compared to a random household sample of women, *J. Stud. Alcohol, 50*:533–540.

14. George, W.H., Gournic, S.J., and McAfee, M.P. (1988). Perceptions of postdrinking female sexuality: Effects of gender, beverage choice and drink payment, *J. Appl. Soc. Psychol., 81*:1295–1317.

15. George, W.H., Skinner, J.B., and Marlatt, G.A. (April, 1986). *Male Perceptions of the Drinking Woman: Is Liquor Quicker?* Presented at the Eastern Psychological Association, New York.

16. Richardson, D., and Campbell, J. (1982). The effect of alcohol on attributions of blame for rape. *Pers. Soc. Psych. Bull., 8*:468–476.

17. Corrigan, E.M. (1980). Alcoholic women in treatment, *Oxford University Press*, New York.

18. Moore, R.D., Bone, L.R., Geller, G., Mamon, J.A., Stokes, E.J., and Levine, D.M. (1989). Prevalence, detection and treatment of alcoholism in hospitalized patients, *J.A.M.A., 261*:403–408.

19. Jellinek, E.M. (1952). Phases of alcohol addiction. *Q. J. Stud. Alcohol, 13*:673–684.

20. U.S. Dept. of Health, Education and Welfare (1980). *Research Monograph 1, Alcohol and Women*, DHEW Publication No. (ADM)80-835, Washington, D.C.

21. U.S. Dept. of Health and Human Services (1986). *Research Monograph 16, Women and Alcohol: Health-Related Issues*, DHHS Publication No. (ADM)86-1139, Washington, D.C.

22. Roman, P.M. (1988). *Women and Alcohol Use: A Review of the Research Literature*, U.S. Dept. of Health and Human Services, Washington, D.C.

23. Ray, B.A., and Braude, M.C. (1986). *Women and Drugs: A New Era for Research*. National Institute of Drug Abuse Research Monograph 65, U.S. Dept. of Health and Human Services, Washington, D.C.

24. Jones, B.M., and Jones, M.K. (1976). Women and alcohol: Intoxication, metabolism, and the menstrual cycle, *Alcohol Problems in Women and Children* (M. Greenblatt, and M.A. Schuckit, eds.), Grune & Stratton, New York, pp. 103–136.

25. VanThiel, D.H., Tarter, R.E., Rosenblum, E. et al. (1988). Ethanol, its metabolism and gonadal effects: Does sex make a difference? *Adv. Alcohol Subst. Abuse, 3–4*:131–169.

26. Hay, W.H., Nathan, P.E., Heermans, H.W., and Frankenstein, W. (1984). Menstrual cycle, tolerance and blood alcohol level discriminating ability, *Addict. Behav., 9*:67–77.

27. Wilson, J.R., and Nagoshi, C.T. (1987). One-month repeatability of alcohol metabolism, sensitivity and acute tolerance. *J. Stud. Alcohol, 48*:437–442.

28. Cole-Harding, S., and Wilson, J.R. (1987). Ethanol metabolism in men and women, *J. Stud. Alcohol, 48*:380–387.

29. Sutker, P.B., Libet, J.M., Allain, A.N., and Randall, C.L. (1983). Alcohol use, negative mood states, and menstrual cycle phases, *Alcoholism Clin. Exp. Res., 3*:327–331.

30. Barry, P.P. (1986). Gender as a factor in treating the elderly, *Women and Drugs: A New Era For Research* (B.A. Ray and M.C. Braude, eds.), National Institute of Drug Abuse Dept. of Health and Human Services, Washington, D.C., pp. 65–69.

31. Braude, M.C. (1986). Drugs and drug interaction in the elderly woman, *Women and Drugs: A*

New Era For Research (B.A. Ray and M.C. Braude, eds.), National Institute for Drug Abuse Research Monograph 65, U.S. Dept. of Health and Human Services, pp. 58–64.

32. Mello, N.K. (1986). Drug use and premenstrual dysphoria, *Women and Drugs: A New Era For Research* (B.A. Ray and M.C. Braude, eds.), National Institute of Drug Abuse Research Monograph 65, U.S. Dept. of Health and Human Services, pp. 31–48.

33. Van Thiel, D.H., and Gavaler, J.S. (1982). The adverse effects of ethanol upon hypothalamic-pituitary-gonadal function in males and females compared and contrasted, *Alcohol Clin. Exp. Res.*, *6*:179–185.

34. Mello, N.K. (1980). Some behavioral and biological aspects of alcohol problems in women, *Alcohol and Drug Problems in Women* (O.J. Kalant, ed.), Plenum Press, New York, pp. 263–298.

35. Gavaler, J.S. (1985). Effects of alcohol on endocine function in postmenopausal women: A review, *J. Stud. Alcohol, 46*:495–516.

36. Russell, M., and Czarnecki, D. (1986). Alcohol use and menstrual problems (abstract). *Alcoholism Clin. Exp. Res., 10*:99.

37. Wilsnack, S.C. (1984). Drinking, sexuality and sexual dysfunction in women, *Alcohol Problems in Women* (S.C. Wilsnack, and L.J. Beckman, eds.), Guilford Press New York, pp. 189–227.

38. Wilson, G.T., and Lawson, D.M. (1976). Effects of alcohol on sexual arousal in women, *J. Abnormal Psychol., 85*:489–497.

39. Malatesta, V.J., Pollack, R.H., Crotty, T.D., and Peacock, L.J. (1982). Acute alcohol intoxication and female orgasmic response, *J. Sex Res., 18*:1–17.

40. Beckman, L.J. (1979). Reported effects of alchol on the sexual feelings and behavior of women alcoholics and nonalcoholics, *J. Stud. Alcohol, 40*:272–282.

41. Apter-Marsh, M. (1982). *The Sexual Behavior of Alcoholic Women While Drinking and During Sobriety*, (Dissertation). Institute for Advanced Study of Human Sexuality, San Francisco.

42. Chaucer, G. (1951). *The Canterbury Tales*, translated by Nevill Coghill, Harmondsworth, England, Penguin Books, 1951.

43. Powell, D.J. (1980). Sexual dysfunction and alcoholism. *J. Sex Ed. Therapy, 6*:40–46.

44. Harvey, S.M., and Beckman, L.J. (1986). Alcohol consumption, female sexual behavior and contraceptive use. *J. Stud. Alcohol, 47*:327–332.

45. U.S. Dept. Health and Human Services (1983). *Fifth Special Report to the U.S. Congress on Alcohol and Health*, U.S. Dept. Health and Human Services, Washington, D.C.

46. Chasnoff, I.J., Burns, W.J., Schnoll, S.H., et al. (1985). Cocaine use in pregnancy, *N. Engl. J. Med., 313*:666–669.

47. Chasnoff, I.J., Burns, K.A., Burns, W.J., et al. (1986). Prenatal drug exposure: Effects on neonatal and infant growth and development, *Neurobehav. Toxicol. Teratol., 8*:357–362.

48. Chasnoff, I.J., Schnoll, S.H., and Burns, W.J. (1984). Maternal nonnarcotic substance abuse during pregnancy: effects on infant development, *Neurobehav. Toxicol. Teratol., 6*:277–280.

49. Deren, S. (1986). Children of substance abusers: A review of the literature, *J. Subst. Abuse Treat., 3*:77–94.

50. Blume, S.B. (1987). Beer and the breast-feeding mom, *J.A.M.A., 258*:2126.

51. Chasnoff, I.J., Lewis, D.E., and Squires, L. (1987). Cocaine intoxication in a breast-fed infant, *Pediatrics, 80*:836–838.

52. Stamper, M.J., Colditz, G.A., Willett, W.C., Speizer, F.E., and Hennekens, C.H. (1988). A prospective study of moderate alcohol consumption and the risk of coronary disease and stroke in women, *N. Engl. J. Med., 319*:267–273.

53. Salonen, J.T., Happonen, P., and Salonen, R. (1987). Interdependence of associations of physical activity, smoking and alcohol and coffee consumption with serum high-density lipoprotein cholesterol: a population study in eastern Finland, *Prevent. Med., 16*:647–658.

54. Longnecker, M.P., Berlin, J.A., Orza, M.J., and Chalners, T.C. (1988). A meta-analysis of alcohol consumption in relation to risk of breast cancer, *J.A.M.A., 260*:652–656.

55. Schatzkin, A., Jones, D.Y., Hoover, R.N., Taylor, P.R., Brinton, L.A., Ziegler, R.G., Harvey, E.B., Carter, C.L., Licitra, L.M., Dufour, M.C., and Larson, D.B. (1987). Alcohol consumption and breast cancer in the epidemiologic follow-up of the first national health and nutrition examination survey, *N. Engl. J. Med., 16*:1169–1173.

56. Willett, W.C., Stampfer, M.J., Colditz, Rosner, B.A., Hennekens, C.H., and Speizer, F.E. (1987). Moderate alcohol consumption and the risk of breast cancer, *N. Engl. J. Med., 316*:1174–1179.

57. Harris, R.E., and Wynder, E.L. (1988). Breast cancer and alcohol consumption: A study in weak associations, *J.A.M.A., 259*:2867–2871.

58. U.S. Dept. of the Treasury and U.S. Dept. of Health and Human Services (1980). *Report to the President and the Congress on Health Hazards Associated with Alcohol and Methods to Inform the General Public of these Hazards.* Washington D.C., U.S. Dept. of the Treasury.

59. Ashley, M.J., Olin, J.S., LeRiche, W.H., Kornaczewski, A., Schmidt, W., Jur, D., and Rankin, J.G. (1977). Morbidity in alcoholoics: Evidence for accelerated development of physical disease in women, *Arch. Intern. Med., 137*:883–887.

60. Wilkinson, P. (1980). Sex differences in morbidity of alcoholics, *Research Advances in Alcohol and Drug Problems in Women* (O.J. Kalant, ed.), Plenum Press, New York, pp. 331–364.

61. Gavaler, J.S. (1982). Sex-related differences in ethanol-induced liver disease: Artifactual or real? *Alcoholism Clin. Exp. Res.,* 186–196.

62. Hislop, W.S., Bouchier, I.A.D., Allan, J.G., Brunt, P.W., Eastwood, M., Finlayson, N.D.C., James, O., Russell, R.I., and Watkinson, G. (1983). Alcoholic liver disease in Scotland and North-eastern England: presenting features in 510 patients, *Q. J. Med. New Series, 52*:232–243.

63. Ryan, C., and Butters, N. (1983). Cognitive deficits in alcoholics, *The Pathogenesis of Alcoholism: The Biology of Alcoholism*, Vol. 7 (B. Kissin and H. Begleiter, eds.), Plenum Press, New York, pp. 485–538.

64. Silberstein, J.A., and Parson, O.A. (1980). Neuropsychological impairment in female alcoholics, *Currents in Alcoholism*, Vol. 7 (M. Galanter, ed.), Grune & Stratton, New York, pp. 481–496.

65. Jones, B.M., Jones, M.K., and Hatcher, E.M. (1980). Cognitive deficits in women alcoholics as a function of gynecological status, *J. Stud. Alcohol, 41*:140–146.

66. Turner, J., and Parsons, O.A. (1988). Verbal and nonverbal abstracting-problem-solving abilities and familial alcoholism in female alcoholics, *J. Stud. Alcohol, 49*:281–287.

67. Acker, C. (1986). Neuropsychological deficits in alcoholics: The relative contributions of gender and drinking history, *Br. J. Addict., 81*:395–403.

68. Jacobson, R. (1986). The contributions of sex and drinking history to the CT brain scan changes in alcoholics, *Psychol. Med., 16*:547–559.

69. Malin, H., Coakley, J., and Kaelber, C. (1982). An epidemiologic perspective on alcohol use and abuse in the United States, in National Institute on Alcohol Abuse and Alcoholism: *Alcohol and Health Monograph 1, Alcohol Consumption and Related Problems*, U.S. Dept. of Health and Human Services Publication No. (ADM)82-1190 99-153, Washington, D.C.

70. Wilsnack, S.C., Wilsnack, R.W., and Klassen, A.D. (1986). Epidemiological research on women's drinking, 1978–1984, in National Institute on Alcohol Abuse and Alcoholism: *Research Monograph 16, Women and Alcohol: Health-Related Issues*, U.S. Dept. of Health and Human Services Publication No. (ADM)86-1139 1–68, Washington, D.C.

71. Fillmore, K.M. (1984). When angels fall: Women's drinking as cultural preoccupation and as reality, *Alcohol Problems in Women* (S.C. Wilsnack and L.J. Beckman, eds.), Guilford, New York, pp. 7–36.

72. Hilton, M.E., and Clark, W.B. (1987). Changes in American drinking patterns and problems, 1967–1984, *J. Stud. Alcohol, 48*:515–522.

73. Engs, R.C., and Hanson, D.J. (1985). Drinking patterns and problems of college students, *J. Alcohol Drug Ed., 31*:65–83.

74. Cloninger, C.R., Reich, T., Sigvardsson, S., von Knorring, A.L., and Bohman, M. (in press). The effects of changes in alcohol use between generations on the inheritance of alcohol abuse, *Alcoholism: A Medical Disorder* (R. Rose, ed.), Raven Press, New York.

75. Wilsnack, R.W., and Cheloha, R. (1987). Women's roles and problem drinking across the lifespan, *Soc. Probl., 34*:231–248.

76. Curlee, J. (1969). Alcohol and the "empty nest," *Bull. Menninger Clin., 33*:165–171.

77. Fillmore, K.M. (1987). Women's drinking across the adult life course as compared to men's, *Br. J. Addict., 82*:801–811.

78. Williams, J.D., Stinson, F.S., and Parker, D.A. (1987). Demographic trends, alcohol abuse and alcoholism, 1985–1995. Epidemiology Bulletin #15, *Alcohol Health Res. World, 11*:80–83.

79. Clayton, R.C., Voss, H.L., Robbins, C., et al. (1986). Gender differences in drug use: An epidemiological perspective, *Women and Drugs: A New Era for Research* (B.A. Ray and M.C. Braude, eds.), National Institute of Drug Abuse Research Monograph 65, U.S. Dept. of Health and Human Services, Washington, D.C., pp. 80–99.

80. Gritz, E.R. (1986). Gender and the teenage smoker, *Women and Drugs: A New Era for Research* (B.A. Ray, M.C. Braude, eds.), National Institute of Drug Abuse Research Monograph 65, U.S. Dept. of Health and Human Services, Washington, D.C., pp. 70–79.

81. Russell, M., Henderson, C., and Blume, S.B. (1985). *Children of Alcoholics: A Review of the Literature*, Children of Alcoholics Foundation, New York.

82. Bohman, M., Sigvardsson, S., and Cloninger, C.R. (1981). Maternal inheritance of alcohol abuse; cross-fostering analysis of adopted women, *Arch. Gen. Psychiatry, 38*:965–969.

83. Cloninger, R.J., Sigvardsson, S., Gilligan, S.B., et al. (1988). Genetic heterogeneity and the classification of alcoholism, *Adv. Alcohol Subst. Abuse, 3–4*:3–16.

84. Cadoret, R.J., Troughton, E., O'Gorman, T.W., and Heywood, E. (1986). An adoption study of genetic and environmental factors in drug abuse, *Arch. Gen. Psychiatry, 43*:1131–1136.

85. Lex, B.W., Lukas, S.E., and Greenwald, N.E. (1988). Alcohol-induced changes in body sway in women at risk for alcoholism: a pilot study, *J. Stud. Alcohol, 49*:346–356.

86. Jones, M.C. (1971). Personality antecedents and correlates of drinking patterns in women, *J. Consult. Clin. Psychol., 36*:61–69.

87. Jones, M.C. (1968). Personality correlates and antecedents of drinking patterns in adult males, *J. Consult. Clin. Psychol., 32*:2–12.

88. Fillmore, K.M., Bacon, S.D., and Hyman, M. (1979). *The 27 Year Longitudinal Panel Study of Drinking by Students in College*, Report 1979 to National Institute of Alcohol Abuse and Alcoholism contract ADM 281-76-0015, Washington, D.C.

89. Caudill, B.D., Wilson, G.T., and Abrams, D.B. (1987). Alcohol and self-disclosure: Analyses of interpersonal behavior in male and female social drinkers, *J. Stud. Alcohol., 48*:401–409.

90. Wilsnack, S.C. (1976). The impact of sex roles on women's alcohol use and abuse, *Alcoholism Problems in Women and Children* (M. Greenblatt, and M.A. Schuckit, eds.), Grune & Stratton, New York.

91. Wilsnack, S.C. (1973). Sex role identity in female alcoholism, *J. Abnormal Psychol., 82*:652–664.

92. Beckman, L. (1978). Sex-role conflict in alcoholic women: myth or reality?, *J. Abnormal Psychol., 84*:408–417.

93. Cloninger, R.C., Christiansen, K.O., Reich, T., et al. (1978). Implications of sex differences in the prevalence of antisocial personality, alcoholism, and criminality for familial transmission, *Arch. Gen. Psychiatry, 35*:941–951.

94. Jacobson, M., Hacker, G., and Atkins, R. (1983). *The Booze Merchants*, CSPI Books, Washington, D.C.

95. Marsteller, P., and Karnchanopee (1980). The use of women in the advertising of distilled spirits, *J. Psychedelic Drugs, 12*:1–12.

96. Carter, C.S. (1987). Treatment of the chemically dependent black female: A cultural perspective, *Counselor, 5*:16–18.

97. Beckman, L.J. (1975). Women alcoholoics: A review of social and psychological studies, *J. Stud. Alcohol, 36*:797–824.

98. Gomberg, E.S. (1986). Women and alcoholism: Psychosocial issues, *Research Monograph 16, Women and Alcohol: Health-Related Issues*, U.S. Dept. of Health and Human Services, Publication No. (ADM)86-1139, Washington, D.C., pp. 78–120.

99. Smith, E.M., and Cloninger, C.R. (1981). Alcoholic females: Mortality at twelve-year follow-up, *Focus on Women, 2*:1–13.

100. Armor, D.J., Polich, J.M.,and Stambul, H.B. (1978). *Alcoholism and Treatment*, Wiley, New York.

101. Blume, S.B. (1980). Researchers on women and alcohol, *Research Monograph 1, Alcohol and*

Women, U.S. Dept. of Health, Education and Welfare, Publication No. (ADM)80-835, Washington, D.C., pp. 121-151.

102. Jacob, T., and Bremer, D.A. (1986). Assortative mating among men and women alcoholics, *J. Stud. Alcohol, 47*:219-222.

103. Beckman, L. (1978). Self-esteem of women alcoholics, *J. Stud. Alcohol, 39*:491-498.

104. Hesselbrock, M., Hesselbrock, V., Syzmanski, K., et al. (1988). Suicide attempts and alcoholism, *J. Stud. Alcohol, 49*:436-442.

105. Lyons, J., Welte, J., Hines, G., et al. (1979). *Outcome Study of Alcoholism Rehabilitation Units*, New York State Division of Alcoholism and Alcohol Abuse, Albany, New York.

106. Carroll, J.F.X., Malloy, T.E., Roscioli, D.L., and Godard, D.R. (1981). *Personality similarities and differences in four diagnosis groups of women alcoholics and drug addicts, J. Stud. Alcohol, 42*:432-440.

107. Carroll, J.F.X., Malloy, T.E., Roscioli, D.L., Pindjak, G.M., and Clifford, S.J. (1982). Similarities and differences in self-concepts of women alcoholics and drug addicts, *J. Stud. Alcohol, 43*:725-738.

108. Harrison, P.A., and Belille, C.A. (1987). Women in treatment: Beyond the stereotype, *J. Stud. Alcohol, 48*:574-578.

109. Griffin, M.L., Weiss, R.L., Mirin, S.M., and Lange, U. (1989). A comparison of male and female cocaine abusers, *Arch. Gen. Psychiatry, 46*:122-126.

110. National Institute on Alcohol Abuse and Alcoholism (1989). *Highlights from the 1987 Drug and Alcoholism Treatment Unit Survey*, Washington, D.C.

111. Trice, H.M., and Beyer, J.M. (1979). Women employees and job-based alcoholism programs, *J. Drug Issues, 9*:371-385.

112. Young, D.W., Reichman, W.R., and Levy, M.F. (1987). Differential referral of women and men to employee assistance programs: The role of supervisory attitudes, *J. Stud. Alcohol, 48*:22-28.

113. Brodzinski, J.D., and Goyer, K.A. (1987). Employee assistance program utilization and client gender, *Employee Assist. Q., 3*:1-13.

114. Cahill, M.H., Volicer, B.J., and Neuburger, E. (1982). Female referral to employees assistance programs: The impact of specialized intervention, *Drug Alcohol Depend., 10*:223-233.

115. Volicer, B.J., Cahill, M.H., Neuburger, E., and Arntz, G. (1983). Randomized response estimates of problem use of alcohol among employed females, *Alcoholism Clin. Exp. Res., 7*:321-326.

116. Halliday, A., Bush, B., Cleary, P., Aronson, M., and Delbanco, T.L. (1986). Alcohol abuse in women seeking gynecologic care, *Obstet. Gynecol., 68*:322-326.

117. Cyr, M.G., and Wartman, S.A. (1988). The effectiveness of routine screening questions in the detection of alcoholism, *J.A.M.A., 259*:51-54.

118. Cleary, P.D. Miller, M., Bush, B.T., Warburg, M.M., Delbanco, T.L., and Aronson, M.D. (1988). Prevalence and recognition of alcohol abuse in a primary care population, *Am. J. Med. 85*:466-471.

119. Blume, S.B. (1986). Women and alcohol: a review, *J.A.M.A., 256*:1467-1470.

120. Blume, S.B. (1981). Drinking and pregnancy, preventing fetal alcohol syndrome, *N.Y. State J. Med., 81*:95-98.

121. Blume, S.B. (1988). *Alcohol/Drug Dependent Women: New Insights into Their Special Problems, Treatment, Recovery*, Johnson Institute, Minneapolis, Minnesota.

122. Hollstedt, C., and Dahlgren, L. (1987). Peripheral markers in the female "hidden alcoholic," *Acta Psychiatr. Scand., 75*:591-596.

123. Leipman, M.R., Wolper, B., and Vasquez, J. (1982). Ecological approach for motivating women to accept treatment for drug dependency, *Treatment Services for Drug Dependence Women*, National Institute on Drug Abuse, Rockville, Maryland, pp. 1-61.

124. Schuckit, M., and Morrissey, E.R. (1976). Alcoholism in women: Some clinical and social perspectives with an emphasis on possible subtypes, *Alcoholism Problems in Women and Children* (M. Greenblatt and M.A. Schuckit, eds.), Grune & Stratton, New York, pp. 5-36.

125. Helzer, J.F., and Pryzbeck, T.R. (1988). The co-occurrence of alcoholism with other psychiatric disorders in the general population and its impact on treatment, *J. Stud. Alcohol, 49*:219-224.

126. Hesselbrock, M.N., Meyer, R.E., and Keener, J.J. (1985). Psychopathology in hospitalized alcoholics, *Arch. Gen. Psychiatry, 42*:1050–1055.

127. Khantzian, E.J., and Treece, C. (1985). DSM-III psychiatric diagnosis of narcotic addicts, *Arch. Gen. Psychiatry, 42*:1067–1071.

128. Rounsaville, B.J., and Kleber, H.D. (1985). Untreated opiate addicts: How do they differ from those seeking treatment? *Arch. Gen. Psychiatry, 42*:1072–1077.

129. Ross, H.E., Glaser, F.B., and Stiasny, S. (1988). Sex differences in the prevalence of psychiatric disorder in patients with alcohol and drug problems, *Br. J. Addict., 83*:1179–1192.

130. Killen, J.D., Taylor, C.B., Telch, M.J., Robinson, T.N., Maron, D.J., and Saylor, K.E. (1987). Depressive symptoms and substance use among adolescent binge eaters and purgers: A defined population study, *Am. J. Public Health, 77*:1539–1541.

131. Bulik, C.M. (1987). Drug and alcohol abuse by bulimic women and their families, *Am. J. Psychiatry, 144*:1604–1606.

132. Lesieur, H.R., Blume, S.B., and Zoppa, R.M. (1986). Alcoholism, drug abuse, and gambling, *Alcoholism Clin. Exp. Res., 10*:33–38.

133. Nace, E.P. Saxon, J.J., et al. (1983). A comparison of borderline and non-borderline alcoholic patients, *Arch. Gen. Psychiatry, 40*:54–56.

134. Nace, E.P., Saxon, J.J., et al. (1986). Borderline personality disorder and alcoholism treatment: A one-year follow-up study, *J. Stud. Alcohol, 47*:196–200.

135. Vaglum, S., and Vaglum, P. (1985). Borderline and other mental disorders in alcoholic female psychiatric patients: A case control study, *Psychopathology, 18*:50–60.

136. Loranger, A.W., and Tules, E.H. (1985). Family history in alcoholism and borderlione personality disorder, *Arch. Gen. Psychiatry, 42*:153–160.

137. Allen, M.H., and Frances, R.J. (1986). Varieties of psychopathology found in patients with addictive disorder, *Psychopathology and Addictive Disorder* (R.E. Meyer, ed.), Guilford Press, New York.

138. Hesselbrock, M.N., Hesselbrock, V.M., Babor, T.F., Stabenau, J.R., Meyer, R.E., and Weidenman, M. (1984). Antisocial behavior, psychopathology and problem drinking in the natural history of alcoholism, *Longitudinal Studies of Antisocial Behavior* (S.A. Mednick and K. VanDusen, eds.), Kleuver-Nijhoff, Boston, Massachusetts.

139. Schuckit, M., and Morrissey, M.A. (1979). Psychiatric problems in women admitted to an alcoholic detoxification center, *Am. J. Psychiatry., 136*:611–617.

140. Benzer, D., and Cushman, P. (1980). Alcohol and benzodiazepines: withdrawal syndromes, *Alcoholism Clin. Exp. Res., 4*:243–247.

141. Kirkpatrick, J. (1978). *Turnabout: Help For a New Life*, Doubleday, Garden City, New York.

142. Allen, C. (1978). *I'm Black and I'm Sober*, Comp Care, Minneapolis, Minnesota.

143. Meryman, R. (1984). *Broken Promises, Mended Dreams*, Little Brown, New York.

144. Robertson, N. (1988). *Getting Better Inside AA*, Morrow, New York.

145. Moran, M. (1985). *Lost Years: Confession of a Woman Alcoholic*, Doubleday, Garden City, New York.

146. Ford, B.B. (1987). *Betty: A Glad Awakening*, Doubleday, Garden City, New York.

147. Miller, B.A., Downs, W.R., Gondoli, D.M., and Keil, A. (1987). The role of childhood sexual abuse in the development of alcoholism in women, *Violence and Victims, 2*:157–172.

148. Blume, S.B. (1985). Psychodrama and the treatment of alcoholism, *Practical Approaches to Alcoholism Psychotherapy*, 2nd ed., (S. Zimberg, J. Wallace, and S.B. Blume, eds.), Plenum Press, New York.

149. Fernandez-Pal, B., Bluestone, H., Missouri, C., Morales, G., and Mizruchi, M.S. (1986). Drinking patterns of inner-city black Americans and Puerto Ricans, *J. Stud. Alcohol, 47*:156–160.

150. Jeffer, E.K., and Baranick, M. (1983). Drug abuse, the U.S. Army in Europe: Women and substance abuse, *Int. J. Addict., 18*:133–138.

151. Miller, B.A. (1981). Drugs and crime interrelationships among women in detention, *J. Psychoactive Drugs, 13*:289–295.

152. Scheafer, S., Evans, S. and Coleman, E. (1987). Sexual orientation concerns among chemically dependent individuals, *J. Chem. Depend. Treat., 1*:121–140.

153. Anderson, S.C., and Henderson, D.C. (1985). Working with lesbian alcoholics, *Social Work, 30*:518–525.

154. Diamond, D.L., and Wilsnack, S.C. (1978). Alcohol abuse among lesbians: A descriptive study. *J. Homosexuality, 4*:123–142.

155. Weathers, B. (1980). Alcoholism and the lesbian community, *Alcoholism in Women* (C.C. Eddy and J.L. Ford eds.), Kendall/Hunt, Dubuque, Iowa.

156. Harrison, P.A., and Hoffman, N.G. (1987). *CATOR Adolescent Residential Treatment, Intake and Follow-up Findings*: 1987 Report, Ramsey Clinic, St. Paul, Minnesota.

157. Hoffman, N.G., and Harrison, P.A. (1986). *CATOR 1986 Report, Findings Two Years After Treatment*, Ramsey Clinic, St. Paul, Minnesota.

158. Annis, H.M., and Leban, C.B. (1980). Alcoholism in women: Treatment modalities and outcomes, *Research Advances in Alcohol and Drug Problems*, Vol. 5 (O.J. Kalant, ed.), Plenum Press, New York, pp. 385–422.

159. Vannicelli, M. (1986). Treatment considerations, *Research Monograph 16, Women and Alcohol: Health-Related Issues*, U.S. Dept. of Health and Human Services, Publication No. (ADM)86-1139, Washington, D.C., pp. 130–153.

160. Rounsaville, B.J., Tierney, T., Crits-Christoph, K., Weissman, M.M., and Kleber, H.D. (1982). Predictors of outcome in treatment of opiate addicts, *Comprehen. Psychiatry, 23*:462–478.

161. McLellan, A.T., Luborsky, L., O'Brien, C.P., et al. (1986). Alcohol and drug abuse treatment in three different populations: Is there improvement and is it predictable? *Am. J. Drug Alcohol Abuse, 12*:101–120.

162. Rounsaville, B.J., Dolinsky, Z.S., Babor, T.F., and Meyer, R.E. (1987). Psychopathology as a predictor of treatment outcome in alcoholics, *Arch. Gen. Psychiatry, 44*:505–513.

163. Hasin, D.S., Endicott, J., and Keller, M.B. (1989). RDC alcoholism in patients with major affective syndromes: Two-year course, *Am. J. Psychiatry, 146*:318–323.

164. MacDonald, J.G. (1987). Predictors of treatment outcome for alcoholic women, *Int. J. Addict., 22*:235–248.

165. Havassy, B.E., Hall, S.M., and Tschann, J.M. (1987). Social support and relapse to tobacco, alcohol and opiates, *National Institute on Drug Abuse Problems of Drug Dependence*, Research Monograph No. 76, Rockville, Maryland.

166. Smith, E.M., Cloninger, R.C. (1989). *A Prospective 12-Year Follow-Up Study of Alcoholic Women II: Stability of Predictors of Outcome 3 Years and 12 Years After Treatment*. Unpublished.

167. Wilsnack, S.C., Wilsnack, R.W., and Klassen, A.D. (1989). *Women's drinking problems: A U.S. national longitudinal survey*. Paper presented at the American Public Health Association Annual Meeting, October.

168. Hill, S.Y. (1986). Physiological effects of alcohol in women, *Research Monograph 16, Women and Alcohol: Health-Related Issues*, U.S. Dept. of Health and Human Services, Publication No. (ADM)86-1139, Publication, Washington, D.C.

169. Smith, E.M., Cloninger, C.R., and Bradford, S. (1983). Predictors of mortality in alcoholic women: A prospective follow-up study, *Alcoholism Clin. Exp. Res., 7*:237–243.

170. Lindberg, S., and Agren, G. (1988). Mortality among male and female hospitalized alcoholics in Stockholm 1962–1983, *Br. J. Addict., 83*:1193–1200.

171. Wilsnack, S.C. (1980). Introduction: Prevention and education: Current status and research needs, *Research Monograph 1, Alcohol and Women*, U.S. Dept. of Health, Education and Welfare, Publication No. (ADM)80-835, Washington, D.C., pp. 163–190.

172. Little, R.E., Streissguth, A.P., Guzinski, G.M., Frathwohl, H.L., Blumhagan, J.M., and McIntyre, C.E. (1983). Change in obstetrician advice following a two-year community educational program on alcohol use and pregnancy, *Am. J. Obstet. Gynecol., 146*:23–28.

173. Weiner, L., Rosett, H.L., and Edelin, K.C. (1983). Behavioral evaluation of fetal alcohol education for physicians, *Alcoholism Clin. Exp. Res., 6*:230–233.

174. Blume, S.B. (1986). Women and alcohol: Public policy issues. *Research Monograph 16, Women and Alcohol: Health-Related Issues*, U.S. Dept. of Health and Human Services, Publication No. (ADM)86-1139, Washington, D.C., pp. 294–311.

175. Schechter, D.M. (1986). *Alcohol Warning Signs: How to Get Legislation Passed in Your City*, Center for Science in the Public Interest, Washington, D.C.

176. Association of Junior Leagues (1987). *Highlights of the Woman to Woman Survey Findings from 38 Communities in the U.S. and Mexico.*

177. Davis, T.S., and Hagood, L.A. (1979). In-home support for recovering alcoholic mothers and their families, *J. Stud. Alcohol, 40*:313–317.

178. Reckmon, L.W., Babcock, P., and O'Brien, T. (1984). Meeting the child care needs of the female alcoholic, *Child Welfare Leagues of America, 63*:541–546.

179. Amaro, H., Beckman, L.J., and Mays, V.M. (1987). A comparison of Black and White women entering alcoholism treatment, *J. Stud. Alcohol, 48*:220–228.

180. National Council on Alcoholism (1987). *A Federal Response to a Hidden Epidemic: Alcohol and Other Drug Problems Among Women.*

181. Nelson, L.J., and Milliken, N. (1988). Compelled medical treatment of pregnant women: Life, liberty and law in conflict, *J.A.M.A., 259*:1060–1066.

182. Rosner, F., Bennett, A.J., Cassell, E.J., Farnsworth, P.B., Landoldt, A.B., Loeb, L., Numann, P., Ona, Fu, Risemberg, H.M., Sechzer, P.H., and Sordillo, P.P. (1989). Fetal therapy and surgery: Fetal rights versus maternal obligations, *N.Y. State J. Med., 89*:80–84.

183. Lader, L. (1989). Regulating birth: Is the state going too far? *Newsday*, July 18, 1989, Melville, New York, p. 49.

9

Alcohol and Drug Addiction in the Elderly

Giovanni Caracci and Norman S. Miller
Cornell University Medical College, The New York Hospital-Cornell Medical Center, White Plains, New York

I. EPIDEMIOLOGY

The prevalence of alcohol dependence among the elderly has been determined in systematic epidemiological studies [1]. The prevalence of drug dependence in the geriatric age group is not as clearly documented as that for alcohol dependence, although there is considerable evidence that it is a significant problem, particularly, with prescription and over-the-counter medications. The use of illicit drugs by the geriatic population is generally not considered a common problem, although narcotic and other similar drugs are obtained by the elderly through prescriptions [2–4].

The rates of lifetime and recent prevalence of alcohol and drug dependence have been recently determined by the national cooperative study in five major cities in the United States—Baltimore, Los Angeles, New Haven, Durham, and St. Louis (Epidemiologic Catchment Area Program [ECA]) [1]. This study was unique because it determined the prevalence of actual diagnoses according to DSM-III-R (*Diagnostic and Statistical Manual of Mental Disorders*, 3rd Edition-Revised. American Psychiatric Association, Washington, D.C., 1987) criteria, whereas all preceding national studies had been based on estimates of consumption and of social, occupational and health consequences of alcohol and drug use.

II. ALCOHOL DEPENDENCE

The findings relevant to age were that the prevalence rates for alcohol dependence are higher for younger than for older ages and for men compared to women. For men, lifetime prevalence for alcohol dependence varied from 27% (ages 18–29) to 28% (ages 30–44), 21% (45–64 years), and *14% (65 years and over)*. Among women, the corresponding prevalence rates

Reprints Requests To: Norman S. Miller, M.D., 21 Bloomingdale Road, White Plains, New York 10605, (914) 997-5777 were 7.0, 6.0, 3.0, and 1.5%. The remission rates tended to rise consistently with increasing age. Although alcohol dependence is a disorder predominately of male predominance, there is substantial evidence that the prevalence for women is increasing dramatically, especially at the youngest ages (ages 18–29). Other studies of prevalence report wide variation in prevalence rates at all ages, mostly because of the inherent bias in the methods for ascertaining prevalence (i.e., estimates, not actual diagnostic criteria) [5–7]. (Table 1).

The age of onset of alcohol dependence for the age group 18–29 cohort was 17.8 years in men and 18.4 in women; for the age 30–59 cohort it was 24.2 years in men and 27.3 years in women; and for the *age 60+ cohort*, the age of onset was 31.0 years in men and 40.6 years in women [1] (Table 2).

III. EARLY AND LATE ONSET

There are two major explanations regarding the distribution of the prevalence and the age of onset of alcohol dependence in the geriatric population. One explanation is that alcohol dependence is a progressive disorder that has a peak prevalence in early to mid-adulthood [1]. The second explanation is that alcohol dependence can occur as a later onset phenomenon in the 60-year-old and older group engendered by factors in later life [8,9].

IV. DRUG DEPENDENCE

Among those of all ages who did not meet lifetime criteria for alcohol dependence, 3.5% had a diagnosis of illicit drug dependence, whereas in those with alcohol dependence, the rate of drug dependence was 18%. The lifetime prevalence rates for illicit drug dependence according to age were 17% for ages 18–29, 4% for ages 30–59, and *less than 1% for 60+ years old*. The prevalence rates for prescription medications are not available in the ECA study published thus far.

It has been well established that the elderly are the largest users of legal drugs in the national population, accounting for approximately 30% of all prescription [3,10–12]. The 1985 National Ambulatory Medical Care survey of office physicians revealed that for patients over 65 years of age, at least one drug was prescribed in more than 68% of office visits [12]. The most commonly prescribed drugs are cardiovascular medications, sedative/hypnotics, tranquilizers, and analgesics. It is estimated that 25% of all individuals of geriatric age (over 55) use psychoactive drugs and are at risk for development of drug abuse and dependence [11].

Table 1 Rates of Lifetime Alcohol Disorder by Age, Sex, and Race (All Sites)

Age	Men			Women		
	white	black	other	white	black	other[a]
18–29	29	13[b]	27	7	4[b]	5
30–59	24	32	29	4	7	5
60+	13	24	22	2	3	1
All ages	23	24	28	4	6	5

[a]This category is dominated by Los Angeles Hispanics, whose male rates exceed white, and whose female rates are below whites.
[b]The low rate in young blacks is found in all four sites with substantial black populations.
Source: From Ref. 1, used with permission.

Table 2 Onset, Remission, and Duration of Alcohol Disorders

Age at interview (years)	Mean age at onset (years)		Mean age at last symptom if none recent (years)		Mean duration (years)	
	men	women	men	women	men	women
18–29	17.8	18.4	21.3	20.8	3.5	2.4
30–59	24.2	27.3	32.6	33.5	8.4	6.2
60+	31.0	40.6	51.0	55.7	20.0	15.1

Source: From Ref. 1, used with permission.

The propensity of the elderly to use multiple drugs in addition to the high rate of use of at least one drug, and combined with their enhanced sensitivity to drug toxicity, accentuates the problem of psychoactive drug use in the elderly. It has been reported that as much as 20% of the patients admitted to a general hospital had a drug induced disorder. A study of nursing home residents (confirmed by other studies) revealed that 50% of them received psychotropic drugs, particularly, benzodiazepines, sedative/hypnotics, and antipsychotic drugs. Moreover, for the elderly living independently, analgesics, anxiolytics, and sedative/hypnotic drugs constitute the greatest source for the development of drug dependence and its consequences [10,13]. In a recent survey, as many as 33% of chronic daily benzodiazepine users were elderly (over 55) [14]. The use of benzodiazepines by the elderly is disproportionate to their numbers. In other survey data from the National Disease and Therapeutic Index indicate that 26% of benzodiazepine prescriptions for anxiety and 40% as hypnotics for sleep are given to patients 65 years of age and older [3].

V. THE PHYSICIAN AS THE SOURCE

In the vast majority of cases, the source of the drugs is the physician [11,12]. The general practitioner or primary care physician leads the list of physician types, followed by the psychiatrist. The physician's attitude toward drug abuse and dependence and in prescribing practices is a critical determinant in the frequency and prevalence of drug abuse and dependence in the geriatric population [11,12].

VI. ILLICIT DRUG USE

The use of illicit drugs such as cannabis, cocaine, and phencyclidine is not prevalent. The ECA study found illicit drug dependence to be less than 17% in the general population. Prevalence rates for patient populations for illicit drugs are much higher; as high as 60% among adult populations of alcoholics. Most information regarding illicit drug use among the elderly is obtained from small series or case reports. These suggest that the elderly may use cannabis, cocaine, or other drugs, although uncommonly [1,2,5]. However, one should always suspect illicit drug use in the presence of alcohol dependence and/or atypical psychiatric syndromes in the elderly.

VII. OVER-THE-COUNTER MEDICATIONS

Over-the-counter (OTC) medications are frequently a major source of drug toxicity and of abuse and dependence. Of the 69% of individuals over the age of 60 years old who use OTC drugs, 80% use alcohol. It is well known that OTC drug use increases with advancing age, especially in females, and approximately two-thirds of all persons over the age of 60 consume at least one nonprescription drug on a daily basis [4,16]. Over-the-counter drugs are defined as analgesics, antihistamines, anticholinergics, vitamins, laxatives, and others. Also, OTC drugs are less expensive to obtain without a prescription, and they may be taken mistakenly because of reduced cognition and judgment in some of the elderly [2].

VIII. SPECIAL POPULATIONS

The prevalence rates for alcohol and drug dependence are higher for special populations than in the general population of the elderly. The prevalence of alcohol and drug dependence is estimated to be 25–50% in general medical populations and 50–75% in general psychiatric populations [13,18]. The elderly comprise a majority of the general medical populations and a significant proportion of the general psychiatric populations. Furthermore, there is no significant age-related decrease in drinking problems associated with alcohol abuse and dependence in the elderly. The clinical diagnosis of alcohol and drug dependence in the geriatric population as determined by clinicians is considerably less than the actual prevalence rates as determined in the ECA studies [10,13,15].

IX. IDENTIFICATION AND DIAGNOSIS

A. Dependence Syndrome

The essential features of the dependence syndrome as defined by the DSM-III-R criteria include the behaviors of addiction and pharmacological tolerance and dependence. The behaviors of addiction are: (1) preoccupatoin with the acquisition of alcohol/drugs, (2) compulsive use, and (3) a pattern of relapse. Preoccupation is manifested by a persistent drive to acquire alcohol or a drug, and having alcohol or drug use a high priority. Compulsive use is continued use in spite of adverse consequences, and may or may not represent repetitive use. Relapse to the drug is manifested by an inability to reduce or abstain from the use of the drug in spite of recurrent, adverse consequences [6,17].

Tolerance is defined as either a loss of an effect at a particular dose, or the need to increase the dose to maintain the same effect. Dependence is defined as the onset of stereotypic and predictable signs and symptoms on cessation of a drug. Tolerance and dependence are not essential to the diagnosis of addiction, as the criteria for the dependence syndrome in DSM-III-R may be met without them. Furthermore, tolerance and dependence are not specific to addiction and may occur in the absence of addiction. Tolerance and dependence are particularly poor indicators of dependence on alcohol and drugs in the elderly because they do not develop dramatically. The ability to develop tolerance and dependence actually diminishes with increasing age. Clinically, tolerance and dependence for alcohol, anxiolytics, sedative/hypnotics, and other drugs develops only to a minimal or moderate extent in all ages, making them marginal clinical markers [6,17].

Denial is a common accompaniment of addiction. Making a diagnosis of drug or alcohol addiction is usually tenuous if only the patient's account is obtained. The patient's objective behavior regarding preoccupation with and compulsive use of alcohol/drugs and corroborative history from others are the key methods for making a proper diagnosis. Usually the patient will minimize or rationalize drug and alcohol use and their consequences. Direct confrontation is sometimes helpful in obtaining more information, but sometimes it may anger the patient. This reaction may be instructive in itself, as most nonaddicted people will not mind a sincere inquiry into possible harmful effects from alcohol and drugs [6,17].

The DSM-III-R criteria are difficult to apply in the case of the elderly when the diagnostic emphasis is on the consequences of the alcohol and drug use [15,17]. The consequences for drug use in the elderly are often considerably different than for younger individuals. The elderly do not have the same vulnerability for the development of consequences. For instance, the elderly are frequently not employed, live alone or apart from family, and do not experience significant legal problems as a result of their alcohol and drug dependence. Psychiatric and medical problems constitute the major consequences of drug and alcohol dependence.

X. COMMON PATTERNS OF USE OF ALCOHOL AND DRUGS

Many of the signs and symptoms produced by alcohol dependence are also produced by the benzodiazepines (BZDs) and sedative/hypnotic drugs. Anxiety, depression, and insomnia are frequent consequences of chronic alcohol intake of moderate to high doses in many, and in low doses in some. These are symptoms for which BZDs and sedative/hypnotics are frequently prescribed in alcoholics. Unfortunately, while the drugs may transiently relieve these symptoms, as did alcohol at one time, as long as the alcohol dependence continues, the need for the drugs will also continue as well as the consequences of the alcohol dependence. Drugs such as BZDs and sedative/hypnotics may be used as substitutes for alcohol when alcohol is not available [6,18].

Furthermore, as the BZDs and sedative/hypnotics are used repetitively, consequences from the dependence on them will develop. These consequences are sometimes indistinguishable from the original target symptoms for which the drugs were initially prescribed; namely, anxiety, depression, and insomnia. The development of pharmacological dependence and addiction causes anxiety, depression, and insomnia, which are often worse than the original symptoms. The adverse consequences from these drugs may occur whether the cause of the anxiety, depression, and insomnia is alcohol dependence, some other cause or is idiopathic [6,18].

XI. PSYCHIATRIC COMPLICATIONS

The psychiatric complications of alcohol and drug dependence are similar in the aged to those found in any population with some shift in emphasis. Anxiety and depression are common consequences of alcohol and drug dependence [13,16]. The expression of the central nervous system (CNS) in response to the effects of the alcohol and drugs is predictable. The depressant drugs such as alcohol, anxiolytics, and sedative/hypnotics produce depression during intoxication and anxiety during withdrawal. Mood sedation is a function of the intrinsic nature of the depressant drug, whereas symptoms of withdrawal are the discharge of catecholamines by the sympathetic nervous system. In contrast, stimulant drugs such as caffeine and ephedrine produce anxiety during intoxication and depression during withdrawal because withdrawal from CNS stimulants represents a depletion of catecholamines.

The depressants and stimulants in acute and chronic use during intoxication and withdrawal may produce frank psychotic symptomatology such as delusions and hallucinations. These are particularly troublesome for the elderly individuals who have diminished vision and hearing, and therefore are already vulnerable to misperception. Drug-induced delusions are frequently paranoid and terrifying, whereas the hallucinations are more often visual than auditory. The anticholinergic-, antihistaminic-, and stimulant-containing drugs may also induce delusions and hallucinations, particularly with chronic administration.

Psychotropic drugs are particularly liable to induce a dementia or delirium syndrome. A compromise of cognition is always a potential problem when alcohol, anxiolytic, sedative/hypnotic, anticholinergic, and antihistaminic drugs are used on a chronic basis individually or in combination. Impairments in cognition and memory from alcohol and drugs may be indistinguishable from other causes. Studies of alcohol-induced dementia cite age as the most important risk factor in the severity of the dementia, older alcoholics sustaining a more severe decline in intelligence [19]. This is supported by computed tomographic (CT) scans that reveal significant cerebral atrophy among alcoholics, particularly older alcoholics. Identification of an alcohol- or drug-induced dementia or delirium may prevent costly evaluations for other etiologies [6].

Some of the common psychiatric and medical consequences from alcohol and drug dependence do not fit precise diagnostic categories and pertain to intrapsychic and interpersonal disturbances which, nonetheless, can impair the individual significantly and severely.

Intrapsychic and interpersonal relationship difficulties which may arise in old age, such as dependency conflicts, isolation, and social withdrawal, are cardinal manifestations of alcohol and drug dependence. These are also common accompaniments of the aging process, and are often mistakenly confused with alcohol and drug dependence. A clinical caveat is to avoid attributing feelings of worthlessness, futility, and despair to old age and to suspect alcohol and drug dependence when these signs and symptoms are present.

Suicide is a particularly common problem associated with alcohol and drug dependence. Next to advancing age, alcohol and drug dependence are among the greatest risk factors for suicide. Men are more likely to commit suicide than women. The elderly are clearly weighted toward suicide as a complication from alcohol and drug use [5,12,13].

XII. MEDICAL COMPLICATIONS

The medical complications of alcohol and drugs are numerous, and are referable to the cardiovascular, gastrointestinal, metabolic, central nervous, and vascular systems. The psychotropic drugs and alcohol produce acute and chronic effects on these systems to result in substantial morbidity and mortality. Alcohol by itself leads to liver disease, hypertension, myocardial infarction, cardiac arrhythmias, stroke, peptic ulcer disease, immunosuppression, dehydration and electrolyte abnormalities, and accidents just to name some of the complications [6,20].

Delirium tremens (DT) as part of the abstinence withdrawal syndrome remains a significant source of morbidity and mortality. This condition is defined as confusion with hallucinations, tremors, and excessive autonomic discharge. The death rate from DT may be as high as 20–40% if appropriate treatment is not instituted in time [21]. The typical history is a chronic consumer of alcohol with a previous history of DT and significant elevation of vital signs in early withdrawal. Hypertension, tachycardia, and hyperthermia in the setting of coarse tremors of the extremities and body, anxiety, and agitation within hours of the last drink, represent an increased risk for the development of DT. Moreover, one-third of the cases of DT are preceded by an alcohol withdrawal seizure [20]. Delirium tremors must be differentiated from intoxication from stimulants.

Usually the withdrawal seizures occur within 12–24 h of cessation of drinking followed by the onset of the autonomic signs and the onset of terrifying hallucinations, extreme agitation, and delusions within 3–4 days. The total course is typically 1 week, followed by a period of prolonged prostration. The best alternative is to prevent DT if possible by adequate suppression of withdrawal with BZDs, hydration, and administration of thiamine and other B-complex vitamins.

The Wernicke-Korsakoff syndrome is a clinical syndrome seen in alcoholics, although not exclusively. The syndrome consists of a continuum of two disorders that are clinically distinct and related to a common pathogenesis; namely, a thiamine deficiency. The syndrome is a confusional state characterized by a clouded sensorium associated with one or more neurological abnormalities. Ataxia, ophthalmoplegia (commonly an unilateral or bilateral sixth nerve paresis), and peripheral neuropathy may occur in any combination with the delirium [20].

The total syndrome may last for weeks followed by a gradual clearing and a residual deficit for recent memory. The loss in recent memory is out of proportion to the relatively spared other cognitive functions. Confabulation or a tendency to rationalize the memory loss is a popular sign associated with the Wernicke-Korsakoff syndrome. Improvement usually occurs although a significant proportion of those affected will continue to suffer from the recent memory loss.

XIII. ETIOLOGY AND PATHOGENESIS

A. Biology of Inheritance to Alcoholism

The specific etiology of alcoholism and drug dependence is not known. What is known is that alcoholism is an inherited disorder [22]. Twin, adoption, familial and high-risk studies clearly demonstrate that the genetic background of an individual is an important determinant in the development of alcoholism [22]. Other factors are operative and pertain to the exposure to alcohol and drugs and the factors that control the exposure.

Those with a family history of alcoholism tend to have an earlier onset and a more rapid course of alcoholism. Familial alcoholics also appear to have a greater number and more serious consequences of alcoholism. Early-onset alcoholics may have a greater family history of alcoholism [8]. The later-onset alcoholics in mid-life and geriatric age groups appear to have less familial alcoholism [22]. Only a few studies have shown that a family history of alcohol dependence is present in drug dependents (cocaine and heroin) at similar rates for alcoholics [23].

B. Exposure

For the geriatric population, exposure to alcohol is determined by a number of conditions. The availability of alcohol and drugs is the rate-limiting step in exposure. While it may be under the ultimate control of the individual, availability of alcohol and drugs is influenced by many other less controllable factors. For instance, many retirement communities have cocktail hours, which by themselves are apparently harmless sources of congeniality and congregation to aide the social interaction. For those who have a genetic predisposition, repeated exposure to alcohol represents a risk of developing alcoholism.

Aging often brings freedom from children and rigors of a career, as well as an increasing independence in a marital relationship. The sense of fewer responsibilities may ease self-imposed controls, leading to greater use of alcohol and drugs.

XIV. DIFFERENTIAL DIAGNOSIS

Alcohol and drug dependence are primary disorders according to the dependence syndrome defined in DSM-III-R. The relationship to other disorders is better understood if the alcohol and drug dependence is recognized as producing virtually any psychiatric syndrome, particularly depression, anxiety, and cognitive difficulties in the elderly.

A. Relationship of Alcohol/Drug Dependence and Affective Disorder

Schuckit reviewed the relationship between alcoholism and affective disorders and delineated five possible types of interactions (may be modified for drug dependence as well): (1) alcohol (drugs) can cause depressive symptoms in anyone; (2) signs of transient serious depression can follow prolonged drinking (drug use); (3) drinking (drug use) can escalate during primary affective episodes in some patients, typically mania; (4) depressive symptoms from alcohol and drug use occur coincidentally in other psychiatric disorders; and (5) a small proportion of patients have independent alcoholism and affective disorder; i.e., 1% [24].

According to studies done under different conditions in all ages, the prevalence rates for depression among alcoholics were from 5 to 59% with the average around 15%. These rates are somewhat higher for females, as much as two- to three-fold in some studies. Exact rates for the elderly are not available, as most of the studies were performed on heterogeneous populations with respect to age.

Anxiety symptoms are very common among alcoholics and drug addicts. As with depression, most studies have examined the prevalence of anxiety disorders in the active or recent drinking/drug use state. Studies have reported rates for anxiety disorders in alcoholics as high as 63%. The patients had panic attacks, generalized anxiety, agoraphobia, social phobia, or in combinations when last drinking. The severity is found to be correlated with the most dependent on alcohol and drugs. The periods of heavy drinking and drug dependence upon alcohol were associated with an exacerbation of the anxiety disorder. Subsequent periods of abstinence were associated with substandard improvements in these anxiety states. These studies do not delineate age-related rates for the elderly [25].

B. Relationship of Alcohol/Drug Dependence and Dementia

The factor that is associated most with the decreased IQ in alcoholic is age. Older alcoholics show significantly greater deterioration in intelligence. It has also been reported that as many as 26% of the patients admitted to a general hospital had a drug-induced dementia because of adverse drug reactions as an explanation for the mental impairment. Given the high rate of drug use by alcoholics, the magnitude and frequency of reversible dementia related to alcohol and drugs are obvious.

C. Time Course for Alcohol/Drug–Induced Psychiatric Syndromes

The consequences of alcoholism and drug dependence are frequently confused with other psychiatric disorders. As discussed above, these consequences include anxiety, depression, insomnia, dementia, liver disease, hypertension, trauma, and peptic ulcer disease. A good way of distinguishing the consequences of alcohol and drug dependence from other psychiatric disorders is to identify and treat the former, and allow for a period of abstinence over time. If the psychiatric disturbances are caused by alcohol and drug dependence, eventually they will ameliorate and disappear despite initial worsening from the acute withdrawal. If the psychiatric disturbances persist or get worse, then they may be determined as independent and in need of the proper diagnosis and treatment.

Studies suggest that for depression, a period of 2–3 weeks will allow for the majority of the alcohol-induced depression to clear, although a longer period may be necessary for some cases. Anxiety symptoms typically improve within weeks of cessation of alcohol and drugs, although studies confirm that the withdrawal for BZDs may be prolonged; i.e., weeks or months. Alcohol- and drug-induced hallucinations and delusions typically resolve shortly after the period of intoxication, (i.e., in the case of stimulants), or may take weeks in the withdrawal from alcohol and sedative hypnotics. The dementia syndrome in alcoholics resolves with protracted abstinence over months and documented improvement occurs years after cessation of drinking.

XV. TREATMENT

Effective treatments for alcohol and drug dependence exist and are available to the elderly. As with every aspect of geriatric psychiatry, the attitude that the elderly are unable to benefit from treatment of alcoholism and drug dependence is to be avoided, although the treatment may be modified to take into considerations the physical and psychological differences associated with aging.

A. Reduced Tolerance to Drugs

Age-related changes in the distribution and metabolism of drugs may result in increased sensitivity to and prolonged effects from low levels of drugs, including alcohol. These age changes include a slowed metabolic breakdown of alcohol and drugs by hepatic enzymes, and a decreased lean body mass with a relative increase in body fat, reducing the intravascular volume. Serum proteins are also reduced, and in combination with the above factors, contribute to an increased free concentration of alcohol and drugs in the water compartment. Furthermore, the neuroreceptors are more sensitive to alcohol and drugs with advancing age [5,16].

Perhaps less well appreciated is the fact that some drugs accumulate by being taken up in the fat and muscle stores and persist for prolonged periods of time after the drug is discontinued. Because of slow release over time from the stores back into blood, the protracted effect of the drug on cognition, memory, and mood may be experienced for weeks to months even in the elderly who have reduced muscle mass and fat deposits [18].

As a result, the tolerance to alcohol and drugs is reduced in the elderly and the withdrawal syndrome from the dependence may be more severe and prolonged. Typically, the complete withdrawal from alcohol and drugs may take weeks to months in the aged compared to days or weeks in younger individuals. Clinically, this is important as detoxification may take considerably longer and require reduced doses of drugs used for detoxification. Correspondingly, the cognitive improvement, reduction in anxiety and depression, chronic pain, and insomnia originating from alcohol and drug dependence may resolve more gradually over an extended period of time. Patience is needed as rapid evaluations are frequently not possible in the population of elderly patients. Hospitalization may be indicated because of the associated medical risks of the elderly for outpatient detoxification from alcohol and drugs. Although the risks from inpatient hospitalization itself must be included in the decision to hospitalize, the added advantage of enhancing abstinence and compliance with detoxification within a structured environment is achieved. In the medically stable and motivated, outpatient detoxification is possible and may be desirable.

B. Treatment of Acute Withdrawal

The treatment of acute withdrawal should be modified for the elderly. Because of the enhanced sensitivity to drugs, including BZDs, doses required to suppress the signs and symptoms of withdrawal are usually one-half to one-third those required for middle-aged adults. Benzodiazepines are the drugs of choice, and short- to intermediate-acting forms may be used. Longer-acting preparations may result in an accumulation and undesired prolonged effects from the drugs.

There are many detoxification schemes available, employing various BZDs, including lorazepam, diazepan, and chlordiazepoxide. It suggested that the clinician become familiar with one type of BZD to maximize efficacy and minimize untoward effects. The author prefers chlordiazepoxide because it produces a smoother withdrawal without the cumulative sedation with its intermediate half-life. It also promotes less drug-seeking behavior than with many other BZDs.

The elderly patient should also receive daily 100 mg thiamine intramuscularly for 3 days if debilitated, and then orally as well as multivitamins daily. The thiamine should be administered before any intravenous dextrose is given to avoid precipitating Wernicke's encephalopathy by using up marginal stores of thiamine.

The patient may also need parenteral hydration with intravenous fluids if he or she is unable to take sufficient fluid by the oral route. It is important to assess daily the need for hydration in the acute withdrawal period when the water loss in an already dehydrated patient may be high. Also, the patient may be sedated from the medication used to treat the withdrawal and not take fluids as much as needed. Electrolytes should be checked as many elderly patients are on drugs that may promote electrolyte loss, as does vomiting and diarrhea from acute and chronic alcohol withdrawal.

The detoxification from BZD/barbiturate/sedative/hypnotic dependence in the elderly is adjusted to the duration of action of the drug that is being detoxified. Usually 2 weeks are sufficient to withdraw a patient from a shorter-acting preparation, such as aprazolam or secobarbital (Seconal), and 4 weeks from longer-acting preparations such as diazepam or meprobamate. The initial dose is determined from the estimated daily dose used by the patient. The dose equivalency is calculated according to conversion criteria in order to use a selected BZD, such as chlordiazepoxide (Table 3). The total calculated dose is reduced by 50%, given in three to four divided doses and tapered gradually over the desired time. Exact daily reductions in dose are not necessary, and may be accomplished every 2–3 days if a longer-acting benzodiazepine is used because of its tendency to be eliminated in a more gradual slope. It is suggested that the short-acting preparations not be tapered to withdrawal themselves because of the more intensive withdrawal effects from the stepper slope in the blood level of the drug during elimination. Longer-acting preparations will provide a more comfortable and safer withdrawal (Table 3).

C. Treatment of Coexisting Psychiatric Diseases

The treatment of coexisting psychiatric disorders may be necessary, particularly in the geriatric population in which affective and anxiety disorders and cognitive impairments are relatively common. After a sufficient period of abstinence from alcohol and drugs (discussed above), which should be individualized for each patient, the use of medications may be indicated. In general, medications should be instituted either when there is no improvement in affective or anxiety symptoms or a plateau has been reached after an initial period of improvement.

For depressive symptoms, antidepressants are indicated and may be administered using the same guidelines that apply to the treatment of affective disorders in general. Electroconvulsive therapy may be indicated. For anxiety symptoms, antidepressants again are indicated, and the use of BZDs should be avoided. For behavior control in dementia, neuroleptics may be used in doses and for indications in the treatment of dementia in general. For persistent insomnia, chronic pain, and obsessive disorders, the use of antidepressants and antipsychotics may be indicated.

However, it is important to bear in mind that the central nervous system changes that must occur for normal mood and sleep, such as a return of REM (rapid eye movement) sleep, restoration of neuroreceptor functions, and normal brain mass, may take weeks to months. Psychotropic medications may delay the return of these vital functions. Also, those who suffer from addiction (dependence) are prone to use the complaints of anxiety, depression, and chronic pain as justifications and represent drug-seeking behavior originating from the addiction. Medicating these symptoms is to be discouraged and avoided whenever possible.

Table 3 Dose Conversions[a] for Sedative/Hypnotic Drugs Equivalent to Secobarbital 500 mg and Diazepam 60 mg

Drug	Dose (mg)	Drug	Dose (mg)
Benzodiazepines		Glycerol	
alprazolam	6	meprobamate	2400
chlordiazepoxide	150	Piperidinedione	
clonazepam	24	glutethimide	1500
clorazepate	90	Quinazolines	
flurazepam	90	methaqualone	1800
halazepam	240		
lorazepam	12		
oxaxepam	60		
prazepam	60		
temazepam	90		
Barbiturates			
amobarbital	600		
butabarbital	600		
butalbital (in Fiorinal)	600		
pentobarbital	600		
secobarbital	600		
phenobarbital	180		

[a]For patients receiving multiple drugs (e.g., flurazepam 30 mg/day, diazepam 30 mg/day, phenobarbital 150 mg/day, each drug should be converted to its diazepam or secobarbital equivalent. In the preceding example the patient is receiving the equivalent dose of diazepam 100 mg/day or secobarbital 1000 mg/day [52].
Source: Adapted from Perry, P.J., and Alexander, B. (1986). Sedative/hypnotic dependence: Patient stabilization, tolerance, testing, and withdrawal. *Drug Bull. Clin. Pharmacol.*, 20:532–537.

D. Treatment of Addiction

An effective form of treatment currently being used for the treatment of alcohol and drug dependence is based on an abstinence approach and referred to as the AA model, which is named after the organization Alcoholics Anonymous. This form of treatment incorporates the practice of abstinence from alcohol and other psychoactive drugs. The aim of the treatment is to educate, confront the denial surrounding the alcohol and drug dependence, and provide alternative attitudes and lifestyle to those associated with alcohol and drug dependence. The patient is encouraged to accept his or her alcohol and/or drug dependence and to establish a commitment to recovery. The techniques used are group and individual therapies directed at the addiction and other aspects of the personality that are nonadaptive.

Family therapy is also provided to treat the codependency that exists in the family members and significant others. Codependency is a syndrome that shows many of the same characteristics of the dependence syndrome in the drug user; i.e., denial, minimization, and rationalization of the alcoholic and drug dependent. The codependent is the "enabler."

The so-called enabler is the person or system that allows the alcohol and drug dependence to continue. The enabler in a sense "allows" the alcoholic and drug dependent to continue to use alcohol and drugs. Without the enabler, many alcoholics and drug dependents would experience spontaneous remission or seek the necessary treatment. The enablers are many and frequently are apparently well-meaning family members, physicians, and friends. The enabling is often both conscious and unconscious and represents misguided efforts to help. Education and treatment for the enabler are available through education, group and individual therapy, and involvement in Alanon and Naranon [21].

The elderly may be placed in long-term treatment facilities that will provide the social and medical support that they need in addition to continued treatment of the alcohol and drug dependence. These facilities may be in the form of residential half-way houses or homes. The social supports and services may also be provided in the home setting if available through local government or private nurses.

Elderly people may do well in traditional forms of long-term treatment for alcoholism and drug dependence such as Alcoholics Anonymous and Narcotics Anonymous. It is important for them to select meetings which are made up of individuals in the same age group. Otherwise, the principles of these self-help groups are as applicable to the elderly as other ages.

Supportive and cognitive psychotherapies are often useful in guiding the elderly alcoholic toward a life without alcohol and as many other drugs as possible. The elderly will respond to confrontal and directive forms of psychotherapy for alcoholism and drug dependence as they do for other psychiatric illnesses. Studies have shown that cognitive group and individual therapies are effective in the treatment of major depression. These same therapies are also effective in the treatment of alcohol and drug dependence. Insight-oriented psychotherapy may be useful in those cases in which a desire to explore intrapsychic conflicts exists.

E. Prognosis and Outcome

The prognosis for untreated alcoholism and drug dependence in the elderly is poor. Alcoholism and drug dependence are chronic, progressive, relapsing disorders that require continuous treatment for permanent remission. Many alcoholics and drug dependents can and do stop using for periods of time, so that the ability to "quit" is not the measure of the overall prognosis. Rather, the ability to maintain abstinence is the best single predictor of prognosis.

Most well-designed studies in adults have demonstrated clearly that alcoholics cannot drink alcohol in a controlled fashion. To recommend moderation in alcohol or drug consumption in the elderly alcoholic is contraindicated. Moreover, after the detoxification period use of of BZDs and other sedative/hypnotic drugs is also contraindicated and will frequently induce a relapse to alcohol as welll as a dependence on the same drugs.

REFERENCES

1. Robins, L.N., Helzer, J.E., Przybeck, T.R., and Regier, D.A. (1988). Alcohol disorders in the community: A report from the epidemiologic catchment area, *Alcoholism: Origins and Outcomes*. Raven Press, New York.
2. Baum, C., Kennedy, D.L., and Forbes, M.B. (1985). Drug utilization in the geriatric age group. Geriatric Drug Use-Clinical and Social *Perspectives, 63–69.*
3. Schweizer, E., Case, W.G., and Rickles, K. (1989). Benzodiazepine dependence and withdrawal in elderly patients. *Am. J. Psychiatry, 146*:529–531.
4. Beers, M., Avorn, J.A., Sounerai, S.B., Everett, D.E., Sherman, D.S., and Salem, S. (1988). Psychoactive medication use in intermediate care facility residents. *J.A.M.A., 260*:3016–3024.
5. Atkinson, J.H., and Schuckit, M.A. (1983). Geriatric alcohol and drug misuse and abuse. *Adv. Subst. Abuse, 3*:195–237.
6. Hartford, J.T., and Samorajski, T. (1982). Alcoholism in the geriatric population. *J. Am. Geriatr. Soc., 30*:18.
7. Bienenfield, D. (1989). Substance abuse in the elderly. *Verwoerdt's Clinical Geropsychiatry*, 3rd ed. (D. Bienenfield, ed.), Williams & Wilkins, Baltimore.
8. Atkinson, R.M., Turner, J.A., Kofoed, L.L., and Tolson, R.L. (1985). Early versus late onset alcoholism in older persons. *Alcoholism Clin. Exp. Res., 9*:513–515.
9. Vaillant, G.E. (1983). *The Natural History of Alcoholism.* Harvard University Press, Boston.
10. Stephens, R.C., Haney, C.A., and Underwood, S. (1981). Psychoactive drug use and potential misuse among persons aged 55 years and older. *J. Psychoactive Drugs, 13*:185–193.

11. Beardsley, R.S., Gardocki, G.L., Larson, D.B., and Itidalgo, J. (1988). Prescribing of psychotropic medication by primary care physicians and psychiatrists. *Arch. Gen. Psychiatry, 45*:1117–1119.

12. Koch, H., and Knapp, D.E. (1987). Highlights of drug utilization in office practice, National Ambulatory Medical Survey, 1985. *Advance Data From Vital and Health Statistics, No. 134.* Dept. of Health and Human Services Publication No. (PHS) 87-1250 Maryland: Public Health Service, 1987.

13. Curtis, J.R., Geller, G., Stokes, E.G., Levine, D.M., and Moore, R.D. (1989). Characteristics, diagnosis and treatment of alcoholism in elderly patients. *J. Am. Geriatr. Soc., 37*:310–316.

14. Mellinger, G.G., Balter, M.B., and Uhlenhuth, E.H. (1984). Prevalence and correlates of the long-term regular use of anxiolytics. *J.A.M.A., 251*:375–379.

15. Whitcup, S.M., and Miller, F. (1987). Unrecognized drug dependence in psychiatrically hospitalized elderly patients. *J. Am. Geriatr. Soc., 35*:297–301.

16. Schuckit, M.A. (1983). A clinical review of alcohol, alcoholism, and the elderly patient. *J. Clin. Psychiatry, 43*:396–399.

17. Miller, N.S., and Gold, M.S. (1989). Suggestions for changes in DSM-III-R criteria for substance abuse disorders. *Am. J. Drug Alcohol Abuse, 2*:223–230.

18. Miller, N.S., and Gold, M.S. (1989). Identification and treatment of benzodiazepine abuse. *Am. Fam. Physician, 40*(4).

19. Parsons, O.A., and Leber, W.R. (1981). The relationships between cognitive dysfunction and brain damage in alcoholics: Causal, interactive or epiphenomenal. *Alcoholism Clin. Exp. Res., 5*:326–343.

20. Lieber, C.S. (1982). *Medical Disorders of Alcoholism: Pathogenesis and Treatment.* Saunders, Philadelphia.

21. Miller, N.S., Gold, M.S., Cocores, J.A., and Pottash, A.C. (1988). Alcohol dependence and its medical consequences. *N.Y. State J. Med. 88*:476–481.

22. Goodwin, D.W. (1985). Alcoholism and geriatrics: The sins of the father. *Arch. Gen. Psychiatry 42*:171–174.

23. Kosten, T.R., Rounsaville, B.T., and Kleher, H.D. (1987). Parental alcoholism in opioid addicts. *J. Nerv. Mental Dis. 8*:461–468.

24. Schuckit, M.A. (1986). Genetic and clinical implications of alcoholism and affective disorder. *Am. J. Psychiatry, 143*:140–147.

25. Small, P., Stockwell, T., Canter, S., and Hodgson, R. (1984). Alcohol dependence and phobic anxiety states. I. A prevalence study. *Br. J. Psychiatry, 144*:53–57.

10

Eating Disorders and Drug and Alcohol Addiction

James E. Mitchell, Richard L. Pyle, Elke D. Eckert, and Sheila Specker
University of Minnesota Hospital and Clinic, Minneapolis, Minnesota

I. INTRODUCTION

The risk for alcohol/drug addiction problems among patients with eating disorders appears to be increased compared to the risk for such problems in the general population, as does the risk for eating disorders among women with drug and alcohol problems. This chapter will discuss eating disorders, first offering an overview of these disorders and then focusing on the literature which addresses the interface between eating disorders and chemical dependency.

II. EPIDEMIOLOGY

The majority of the available research suggests that anorexia nervosa and bulimia nervosa are increasing in prevalence, although the exact magnitude of the increase is unclear. For example, Theander in 1970 examined the incidence of anorexia nervosa in Sweden over the period from 1930 to 1960 and noted a sharp increase [1]. A study from Monroe County, New York, also found a significant increase in the incidence from the periods 1960–1969 to 1970–1976 [2].

Epidemiological surveys of bulimia nervosa have focused primarily on college and high school populations, and an adequate population-based survey has yet to be done. However, the available epidemiological studies suggest that 1–4% of young women in late adolescence or early adulthood will meet rigid criteria for bulimia nervosa (3–6). Although very few cross-cultural studies has been reported, the available evidence also suggests that bulimia nervosa and anorexia nervosa are seen almost exclusively in industrialized societies where there is an abundance of food, and where a high value is placed on slimness as a model of attractiveness for young women. Many workers in the field believe quite strongly that the cultural pressure on girls and women to be thin leads many of them into unnecessary dieting, which predisposes to binge eating and subsequently to vomiting and the full bulimia syndrome.

In societies where models of attractiveness do not require women to be so thin, physicians report seeing these disorders very rarely. For example, in a study our group recently completed in Changsha, The People's Republic of China, we found practically no evidence of anorexia nervosa and bulimia nervosa (unpublished data). These disorders occur almost exclusively in women, with only 5–10% of the cases occurring in men [7].

Although it has been reported that anorexia nervosa predominates in upper socioeconomic groups, recent reports suggest a more equal distribution [8]. Both disorders are rare in blacks, but it has been suggested that the prevalence of eating disorders in blacks will increase as their socioeconomic status improves [9].

III. DIAGNOSIS

The DSM-III-R (*Diagnostic and Statistical Manual of Mental Disorders*, 3rd edition-Revised, American Psychiatric Association, Washington, D.C., 1987) diagnostic criteria for anorexia nervosa require an amount of weight loss which often results in physiological dysfunction as well as requiring body image distortion, fear of fatness, and amenorrhea. The bulimia nervosa criteria require binge-eating coupled with some behavior designed to promote weight loss or prevent weight gain. In reality, most patients who present for treatment with bulimia nervosa are self-inducing vomiting or abusing laxatives as weight-control techniques.

It is important to remember that there is considerable overlap between anorexia nervosa, bulimia nervosa, and some other eating problems. A subgroup of anorexia nervosa patients mainly restrict their caloric intake and lose weight. However, approximately half—the bulimic anorexia nervosa subgroup—also meet criteria for bulimia nervosa and receive both diagnoses. Members of this group primarily starve themselves, but periodically will overeat and then engage in vomiting and/or laxative abuse to prevent weight gain. This bulimic subgroup tends to have a worse prognosis and to have other associated problems such as depression and/or alcohol/drug addiction problems. Another group is the group of normal-weight bulimic women, some of whom will have a history of anorexia nervosa, but most of whom will be within 20% of ideal body weight. A subgroup of bulimia nervosa subjects, however, overlap with the overweight population. This group tends to be older and to have a later age of onset of their eating disorder. How they differ from obese binge eaters or "compulsive overeaters" is yet to be adequately studied.

IV. MEDICAL COMPLICATIONS

Anorexia nervosa and bulimia nervosa are similar to alcohol/drug addiction problems in that they can be associated with a variety of serious medical complications [10]. Anorexia nervosa in particular has a fairly high morbodity and mortality compared to other psychiatric disorders. Although bulimia nervosa is more benign overall, it still can be accompanied by serious complications. Because of the fact that many of the abnormalities encountered in anorexia nervosa result from starvation rather than eating behavior per se, we will discuss these two disorders independently.

A. Anorexia Nervosa

Signs and Symptoms

Most patients who present with anorexia nervosa have very few physical symptoms, despite the fact that they appear emaciated [10]. On questioning, most will report amenorrhea. Many will also report constipation, but most will state that they feel physically fine. Upon physical examination though the picture is often very different. Common findings include bradycardia, hypotension, and occasionally hypothermia, which can be severe. Some anorectics will develop lanugo. Rarely, peripheral edema or petechiae formation will be found.

Fluid and Electrolyte Abnormalities

Several fluid and electrolyte abnormalities have been described in anorexia nervosa [11]. Most commonly encountered is metabolic alkalosis. This is often seen in patients who are purging as well as fasting, and results from the contraction alkalosis secondary to dehydration. Many patients also will develop hypochloremia secondary to loss of chloride in the vomitus. Potassium deficits can be demonstrated in a minority of patients. The potassium loss is primarily through the kidney secondary to the hyperaldosteronism which results from the volume contraction. Hyponatremia is rare.

Neurological Complications

The relationship between eating disorders and central nervous system (CNS) dysfunction has been the source of considerable interest, both as a logical extension of the examination of various organ systems in these disorders, but also as a way of attempting to understand their pathophysiology, since many of the systems that control appetite and satiety are in the CNS. There have been isolated reports of individuals who have CNS lesions, including space-occupying lesions, presenting with anorectic symptoms. The possibility of such a presentation must always be considered, particularly in patients with unusual symptoms.

Available studies using computerized tomography or magnetic resonance imaging of the brain suggest evidence of ventricular dilatation and cortical atrophy in patients with anorexia nervosa when they are of low weight, with evidence of reversal after weight gain [12]. These changes are particularly interesting when we consider that many patients with anorexia nervosa have cognitive impairment when at low weight, which therefore may have a neuroanatomical basis.

Menstrual Dysfunction

Essentially all the neuroendocrine regulatory mechanisms become disrupted in patients who lose large amounts of weight [13]. This includes the development of amennorhea with hypofunctioning of the hypothalamo-pituitary-ovarian axis.

Low levels of triiodothyronine (T_3) are frequently demonstrated, since thyroid hormone is preferentially converted to reverse T_3, which is less metabolically active. A delayed or blunted thyroid-stimulating hormone (TSH) response to thyrotropin-releasing hormone (TRH) has also been described.

Fasting growth hormone levels are occasionally reported to be elevated, and several reports have documented a pathological growth hormone response to TRH stimulation or to glucose administration, although the results here are inconsistent. Fasting prolactin levels are usually normal, but elevated levels have been reported. Fasting hypoglycemia has been documented in a number of patients with anorexia nervosa.

Most patients with anorexia nervosa demonstrate a lack of suppression on the dexamethasone suppression test [13]. The elevated cortisol appears to reflect both an increase in secretion and a decrease in clearance.

Temperature Regulation

Some anorectics appear to have difficulty maintaining a stable core body temperature and have exaggerated fluctuations when exposed to extremes of temperature.

Cardiopulmonary Problems

A growing number of reports suggest that the cardiovascular system does not function properly in patients with anorexia nervosa when they are of low weight [14]. Electrocardiographic abnormalities have been described, most commonly bradycardia. Patients with anorexia nervosa also appear to be at increased risk for a variety of arrhythmias. Studies examining circulatory dynamics have shown a decrease in cardiac chamber dimensions, and some evidence of left ventricular functional impairment reflecting reduced cardiac contractility. A few cases of pneumomediastinum have also been reported.

Dental Problems

Problems in dentition result primarily from self-induced vomiting. Routine vomiting exposes the enamel of the teeth to the highly acidic gastric contents [15]. This results in decalcification of the lingual, palatal, and posterior occlusal surfaces of the teeth, which can be quite dramatic and is unfortunately irreversible.

Gastrointestinal Problems

Although the data in this area are conflicting, the most recent studies suggest that many patients with anorexia nervosa do have delayed gastric emptying which may contribute to their sense of bloating postprandially. A possible complication of anorexia nervosa, particularly during refeeding, is the development of gastric dilatation, which is serious and can be fatal [16].

Swelling of the salivary glands, particularly the parotid glands, has been seen in a subgroup of patients. However, the pathophysiology of this abnormality is not understood. Several case reports also suggest a relationship between anorexia nervosa and pancreatitis.

The loss of fat around the superior mesenteric neurovascular bundle can lead to compression of the duodenum and to obstruction. This is referred to as the superior mesenteric artery syndrome. This disorder can present with symptoms like anorexia nervosa, with intermittent vomiting after eating, but also can result from anorexia nervosa because of the weight loss. Therefore, this syndrome should always be considered in a differential diagnosis of anorexia nervosa.

Metabolic Problems

Elevated serum cholesterol is frequently reported, as well as elevated serum carotene. Trace mineral difficiencies, particularly of zinc, may contribute to the development and maintenance of anorexia nervosa. Liver function abnormalities are commonly reported and may worsen during the period of refeeding.

Bone

Many patients with anorexia nervosa will develop osteoporosis, which puts them at increased risk for fractures [17].

B. Bulimia Nervosa

Symptoms and Signs

Patients with bulimia nervosa frequently have many physical complaints when they seek treatment. Many complain of weakness, feeling "bloated," and dental problems [18].

On physical examination there are several signs that are of use diagnostically. The first is Russell's sign, which involves evidence of skin changes over the dorsum of the hand, generally pigmented callous formation or scarring resulting from using the hand to stimulate the gag reflex. Another diagnostic sign is hypertrophy of the salivary gland, particularly the parotid glands. A third diagnostic clue is the presence of dental enamel erosion, which is present in the majority of patients who have been vomiting at least three times a week for 4 years.

Fluid and Electrolytes

Females with bulimia nervosa are at risk for dehydration secondary to fluid losses from several sources, including vomiting, diuretic abuse, and laxative abuse [19]. The most common abnormalities are alkalosis, hypochloremia, and hypokalemia. Some patients who are abusing laxatives will be transiently acidotic secondary to the loss of bicarbonate-rich fluid in the stool with diarrhea.

Neurological Complications

Rau and colleagues in a series of reports discussed the possibility that abnormal electroencephalographic activity might be responsible for some cases of bulimialike symptoms [20,21]. However, these observations have not been validated by other groups.

Of interest are recent studies demonstrating that a significant minority of patients with bulimia nervosa will have brain cortical changes similar to those seen in anorexia nervosa, again suggesting that these patients are malnourished despite their apparently normal body weight.

Endocrine Problems

About half of patients with active bulimia nervosa will fail to suppress on a routine dexamethasone suppression test [13]. Many patients with bulimia nervosa have irregular menses, but few have the profound amennorhea seen among patients with anorexia nervosa [18].

A particularly interesting relationship concerns eating disorders and diabetes mellitus [22]. Several groups have reported cases or series of cases where these disorders coexist, and it appears that women with diabetes mellitus may be at increased risk for developing eating problems.

Pirke and colleagues have reported that patients with bulimia nervosa tend to have lower glucose levels, reduced T_3 levels, reduced plasma and norepinephrine levels, and elevated levels of free fatty acid and beta-hydroxybutryic acid [23]. This grouping of metabolic changes is indicative of dietary insufficiency and starvation, despite normal body weight.

V. COMORBIDITY BETWEEN EATING DISORDERS AND DRUG AND ALCOHOL ADDICTION

Early in the course of the description of bulimia and bulimia nervosa it became apparent that there was a high rate of alcohol and drug addiction among these individuals [24–29]. Several of these studies are summarized in Table 1. Several groups reported a high prevalence of current or past alcohol and drug addiction in this population. The data by Hudson et al. [31] are of particular importance given the fact that both groups used the Structured Diagnostic Interview Schedule (DIS) to make diagnoses of drug and alcohol addiction.

Table 1 Drug and Alcohol Abuse in Bulimics—Uncontrolled Studies

Ref.	Year	N	Age	Results
29	1981	34	24	High rate of drug/alcohol problems; 24% treated for CD
25	1983	49	17–49	31% lifetime prevalence of substance use disorder (DIS)
27	1985	275	24.8	34% history of drug/alcohol problems; 18% history of CD treatment
24	1986	112	24.9	Alcohol abuse and excess usage increased with age; to 50% by age 35
26	1987	70	18–45	49% lifetime prevalence of substance use disorder (DIS)
18	1987	22 22	<20 >25	More substance abuse and affective disorder in the latter age onset group (36 vs 5%)

In 1987, we reported that patients with a late onset of their eating disorder (beyond age 25) were significantly more likely to have associated drug and alcohol addiction and affective disorders compared to patients with a more common age of onset (less than 20) [28].

Several controlled studies have also been done in this population [30–33]. These are summarized in Table 2. In an epidemiological survey of freshman college students Pyle et al. [33], they found that there were more alcohol and drug problems among bulimic than nonbulimic students who had been identified through a questionnaire survey, and Bulik [30] found more alcohol and drug problems in bulimics compared to sex- and age-matched controls, as did Hudson et al. [31]. In another epidemiological survey, Killin et al. [32] found more problems with alcohol usage among females who also reported purging behavior compared to those who did not.

The data on anorexia nervosa are more limited and are summarized in Table 3 [34,35]. As can be seen, the figures here are somewhat lower than those among women with bulimia or bulimia nervosa. Of particular interest is the fact that when present, alcohol and drug addiction among anorectics seem to cluster in a bulimic subgroup rather than the restrictor subgroup.

VI. EATING DISORDERS IN DRUG AND ALCOHOL ADDICTION

A few studies examined the comorbidity for these two types of disorders by studying women who are already in treatment or who were presenting for treatment with drug and alcohol addiction. One such study (unpublished) by Eckert and Pyle compared the percentage of college students and drug and alcohol addicted women who met various criteria for abnormal eating behaviors. Significantly more males and females undergoing drug and alcohol addiction treatment met bulimia criteria and bulimia criteria coupled with weekly binge-eating. Using even more stringent research criteria, nearly seven times as many females in the chemically dependent population appeared to meet criteria for bulimia nervosa, while the rate in males was essentially identical. Hudson et al [36] also found a higher than expected rate of eating disorder problems in 143 women undergoing chemical dependency treatment.

Another interesting report by Jonas et al. in 1987 reported data using a structured clinical interview designed to diagnose eating disorders which was administered to 259 consecutive callers to the National Cocaine Hotline who met DSM-III-R criteria for cocaine abuse [37].

Table 2 Drug and Alcohol Abuse in Bulimics—Controlled Studies

Ref.	Year	N	Age	Results
33	1983	1355	College freshman	More alcohol and drug abuse in bulimics than nonbulimics (13.3 vs 3.6%)
30	1987	35 bulimics 35 healthy controls	30 31	More alcohol/drug abuse in bulimics (48%) than in age- and sex-matched healthy controls (8.6%)
31	1987	70 bulimics 28 bulimics	26 31	More total substance abuse disorders in bulimics (49%) vs controls (3%)
32	1987	1728	tenth graders	More drunkenness and drinking in female purgers (22%) than nonpurgers (6%)

Table 3 Drug and Alcohol Abuse in Anorectics

Ref.	Year	N	Age	Mean Results
34	1979	105	27.3	6.7% lifetime DSM-III diagnosis of alcohol abuse
25	1983	16	25	19% lifetime DSM-III diagnosis of substance abuse disorder (DIS)
35	1985	13	22.1	0% had diagnosis of alcohol or drug abuse (Feighner criteria)

Thirty-two percent of this sample met criteria for an eating disorder. Of these, 22% met DSM-III criteria for bulimia, 7% met the criteria for anorexia nervosa and bulimia, and 2% met the criteria for anorexia nervosa only. Interestingly, 44% of the callers who met the criteria for bulimia nervosa were males. Another interesting study was published by Lacey et al. in 1986, who studied 27 consecutively presenting alcoholic women between ages of 15 to 45. Eleven were bulimic and 16 were nonbulimic. The bulimics tended to be younger at presentation, to have had an earlier onset of problem drinking, and to weigh more, although they had a lower prevalence of alcoholism among their fathers. In a separate study, Lacey et al. [38] in 1983 reported the results of a treatment study of 30 severely bulimic outpatient women aged 17–45. A history of an alcohol abuse problem associated with bulimia was associated with a poor outcome.

VII. FAMILY STUDIES

Several studies have examined the prevalence of alcohol and drug addiction problems among relatives of patients with anorexia nervosa and bulimia nervosa. In 1970, Theander reported that 6.4% of the fathers and none of mothers of 94 women with anorexia nervosa had a drug or alcohol abuse problem [1].

Two controlled studies have reported data on the relatives of patients with bulimia nervosa. Bulik in 1987 compared the rate of alcohol and drug addiction problems in the first- and second-degree relatives of 35 bulimics and 35 healthy controls. Overall, 49% of the bulimics and 20% of the controls met the criteria for an associated alcohol or drug addiction problem. Hudson et al. in 1987 [25] reported a comparison of drug and alcohol addiction in the first-degree relatives of 69 bulimic women and 28 nonpsychiatric controls, and again found more drug and alcohol addiction in first-degree relatives than controls (19 vs 6.5% morbid risk). Therefore, the available studies suggest that the rate of alcohol and drug abuse problems is higher in the families of patients with bulimia nervosa than the families of controls.

VIII. OTHER STUDIES

Hatsukami et al. in 1986 reported a comparison of subjects with bulimia nervosa (N = 46) who did not have a history of alcohol or drug addiction and a group of patients with bulimia nervosa who had concurrent drug and alcohol addiction problems (N = 34) [39]. Those in the comorbidity group were more likely to be older at the time of evaluation, were significantly more likely to report abuse of diuretics as a weight control technique, and reported significantly more financial, social, and work problems compared to the other group. They were also more likely to report a history of suicide attempts, stealing behavior (both before and since the onset of the eating disorder), and prior inpatient and outpatient treatment. Specker et al.

(unpublished manuscript) found that among 70 female drug and alcohol addicts with a diagnosis of bulimia nervosa there was a high prevalence of the use of laxatives (66%), diuretics (26%), and diet pills (40%).

IX. WHY IS THERE AN INCREASED COMORBIDITY?

Although the literature in this area is convincing in that there is an exaggerated risk of alcohol and drug addiction problems among bulimic women, the reason for this comorbidity problem is unresolved [40,41]. Although some controlled trials have been done using patient populations and their relatives, the controls have been normals rather than other psychiatric controls. Therefore, it is unclear whether the increased comorbidity for these problems is unique to eating disorder patients or whether it reflects a more general risk factor for alcohol and drug problems among patients with emotional disorders.

Although several authors have commented that the eating disorder seems to frequently precede the development of the alcohol or drug addiction problem, this has not really been carefully studied and further work in this area is indicated. Another open question concerns the actual logistics of drug and alcohol addiction in this population. It would appear that some patients tend to binge eat when intoxicated, whereas others tend to substitute binge eating for alcohol and drug addiction. Therefore, we need to further study the actual patterns of these behaviors in this comorbidity group.

Several authors have pointed out that there are many similarities, both in cognitive and behavioral terms, between these two types of disorders. For example, both alcohol/drug addicts and patients with bulimia nervosa crave a certain substance, become dependent on its use, use it for mood-altering effects, and as a way of avoiding unpleasant effects and stress. Both types of disorders also can result in a variety of adverse psychosocial sequelae, including depression and social maladjustment as well as significant medical complications. These similarities and the comorbidity issue has led some to adopt the position that eating disorders are another form of addiction, to regard eating disorders as analogous to alcohol and drug addiction problems, and to treat eating disorders using traditional addiction treatment models. While a case can certainly be made for such an approach, at times such programs ignore a significant theoretical difference between these two types of disorders which has important implications for treatment. Patients with alcohol/drug addictions can be taught the necessity of avoiding the use of substances of abuse (abstinence), whereas patients with eating disorders need to learn to eat in a controlled fashion. They cannot avoid food; they need in a sense to master it. Therefore any approach which teaches them that they are powerless against the substance, and that they will be so indefinitely is, in our opinion, less than optimal.

X. TREATMENT IMPLICATIONS

How should these dual diagnoses patients be treated? There really are no empirical data in this regard. It would seem that the ideal situation would be to utilize a treatment program which incorporates treatment components for both alcohol/drug addiction and eating disorders into the same system. Some of these techniques would be quite similar, and others would be different, but presumably they could be integrated. This would avoid a common occurrence in the treatment of these disorders, in that one condition worsens while the other is improving during the treatment of the latter (e.g., the patient with bulimia who is admitted to the alcohol and drug treatment program and whose eating gets out of control).

The current state of affairs is that most of these patients end up first in treatment for alcohol/drug addiction. At minimum, the intervention for an eating disorder in this setting should include dietary management and support and limited access to food to preclude binge eating. Most alcohol and drug treatment programs see enough women with both diagnoses that it would seem feasible for them to have one therapist also trained to work with eating disorders, who could initiate therapy for this condition at least to the degree necessary to control their eating while they are in alcohol and drug treatment. Patients can then be referred to an appropriate eating disorders program. Ideally, both disorders could be treated concurrently, but few programs have the expertise and flexibility to accomplish such a task.

REFERENCES

1. Theander, S. (1970). Anorexia nervosa a psychiatric investigation of 94 female patients. *Acta Psychiatr. Scand.*, (Suppl.) *46*:1–194.
2. Jones, D.J., Fox, M.M., Babigian, H.M., and Hutton, H.E. (1980). Epidemiology of anorexia nervosa in Monroe County, New York: 1960–1976. *Psychosomatic Med.*, *42*:551–558.
3. Cooper, P.J., and Fairburn, C.G. (1983). Binge-eating and self-induced vomiting in the community—a preliminary study. *Br. J. Psychiatry*, *142*:139–144.
4. Halmi, K.A., Falk, J., and Schwartz, E. (1981). Binge-eating and vomiting: A survey of a college population. *Psychol. Med.*, *11*:697–706.
5. Pyle, R.L., Halvorson, P.A., Neuman, P.A., and Mitchell, J.E. (1986). The increasing prevalence of bulimia in freshman college students. *Int. J. Eating Disorders*, *5*:631–647.
6. Pyle, R.L., Mitchell, J.E., Eckert, E.D., Halvorson, P.A., Neuman, P.A., and Goff, G.M. (1983). The incidence of bulimia in freshman students. *Int. J. Eating Disorders*, *2*:75–85.
7. Mitchell, J.E., and Eckert, E.D. (1987). Scope and significance of eating disorders. *J. Consult. Clin. Psychol.*, *55*:628–634.
8. Garfinkel, P.E., and Garner, D.M. (1982). *Anorexia nervosa: A multidimensional Perspective*. Brunner/Mazel, New York.
9. Anderson, A.E., and Hay, A. (1985). Racial and socioeconomic influences in anorexia nervosa and bulimia. *Int. J. Eating Disorders*, *4*:479–487.
10. Mitchell, J.E. (1984). Medical complications of anorexia nervosa and bulimia. *Psychiatr. Med.*, *1*:229–255.
11. Warren, S.E., and Steinberg, S.M. (1979). Acid-base and electrolyte disturbances in anorexia nervosa. *Am. J. Psychiatry*, *136*:415–418.
12. Nussbaum, M., Shenker, I.R., and Marc, J., et al (1980). Cerebral atrophy in anorexia nervosa. *J. Pediatr.*, *96*:867–869.
13. Newman, M.M., and Halmi, K.A. (1988). The endocrinology of anorexia nervosa and bulimia nervosa. *Neurol. Clin. North Am.*, *6*:195–212.
14. Gottdiener, J.S., Gross, H.A., and Henry, W.L., et al. (1978). Effects of self-induced starvation on cardiac size and function in anorexia nervosa. *Circulation*, *58*:425–433.
15. Hellstrom, I. (1977). Oral complications in anorexia nervosa. *Scand. J. Dent. Res.*, *85*:71–86.
16. Saul, S.H., Dekker, A., and Watson, C.G. (1981). Acute gastric dilatation with infarction and perforation: Report of fatal outcome in patients with anorexia nervosa. *Gut*, *22*:978–983.
17. Treasure, J.L., Russell, G.F.M., Fogelman, I., and Murby, B. (1987). Reversible bone loss in anorexia nervosa. *Br. Med. J.*, *295*:474–475.
18. Mitchell, J.E., Seim, H.C., Colon, E., and Pomeroy, C. (1987). Medical complications and medical management of bulimia. *Am. Intern. Med.*, *107*:71–77.
19. Mitchell, J.E., Pyle, R.L., Eckert, E.D., Hatsukami, D., and Lentz, R. (1983). Electrolyte and other physiological abnormalities in patients with bulimia. *Psychol. Med.*, *13*:273–278.
20. Rau, J.H., and Green, R.S. (1978). Soft neurological correlates of compulsive eaters. *J. Nerv. Ment. Dis.*, *166*:435–437.
21. Rau, J.H., Struve, F.A., and Green, R.S. (1979). Electroencephalographic correlates of compulsive eating. *Clin. Electroencephalogr.*, *10*:180–189.
22. Hillard, J.R., Lobo, M.C., and Keeling, R.P. (1983). Bulimia and diabetes: A potentially life-threatening combination. *Psychosomatics*, *24*:292–295.

23. Pirke, K.M., Pahl, J., Schweiger, U., and Warnhoff, M. (1985). Metabolic and endocrine indices of starvation in bulimia: A comparison with anorexia nervosa. *Psychiatry Res.*, *14*:33–39.

24. Beary, M.D., Lacey, J.H., and Merry, J. (1986). Alcoholism and eating disorder in women of fertile age. *Br. J. Addict.*, *81*:685–689.

25. Hudson, J.I., Pope, H.G., Jonas, J.M., et al. (1983). Family history study of anorexia nervosa and bulimia. *Br. J. Psychiatry, 142*:133–138.

26. Hudson, J.I., Pope, H.G., Jonas, J.M., et al. (1987). A controlled family history study of bulimia. *Psychol. Med., 17*:883–890.

27. Mitchell, J.E., Hatsukami, D., Eckert, E.D., et al. (1985). Characteristics of 275 patients with bulimia. *Am. J. Psychiatry, 142*:482–485.

28. Mitchell, J.E., Hatsukami, D., Pyle, R.L., et al. (1987). Late onset bulimia. *Comp. Psychiatry, 28*:323–328.

29. Pyle, R.L., Mitchell, J.E., and Eckert, E.D. (1981). Bulimia: A report of 34 cases. *J. Clin. Psychiatry, 42*:60–64.

30. Bulik, C.M. (1987). Drug and alcohol abuse by bulimic women and their families. *Am. J. Psychiatry, 144*:1604–1606.

31. Hudson, J.I., Pope, H.G., Yurgelun-Todd, et al. (1987). Psychiatric disorders in bulimic outpatients. *Am. J. Psychiatry, 144*:1283–1287.

32. Killen, J.D., Taylor, C.B., Telch, M.J., et al. (1987). Evidence for an alcohol-stress link among normal weight adolescents reporting purging behavior. *Int. J. Eating Disorders, 6*:349–356.

33. Pyle, R.L., Mitchell, J.E., Eckert, E.D., et al. (1983). The incidence of bulimia in freshman college students. *Int. J. Eating Disorders, 2*:75–85.

34. Eckert, E.D., Goldberg, S.C., Halmi, K.A., et al. (1979). Alcoholism in anorexia nervosa. *Psychiatric Factors in Drug Abuse*, (R.W. Pickens, and L.L. Heston, eds.), Grune & Stratton, New York.

35. Viesselman, J.O., and Roig, M. (1985). Depression and suicidality in eating disorders. *J. Clin. Psychiatry, 46*:118–124.

36. Hudson, J.I., Weiss, R.D., Pope, H.G., et al. (in press). Eating disorders in hospital substance abusers. *J. Clin. Psychiatry*.

37. Jonas, J.M., Gold, M.S., Sweeney, D., et al. (1987). Eating disorders and cocaine abuse: A survey of 259 cocaine abusers. *J. Clin. Psychiatry, 48*:47–50.

38. Lacey, J.H., and Moureli, E. (1986). Bulimic alcholics: Some features of a clinical subgroup. *Br. J. Addict., 81*:389–393.

39. Hatsukami, D., Mitchell, J.E., Eckert, E.D., et al. (1986). Characteristics of patients with bulimia only, bulimia with affective disorder, and bulimia with substance abuse problems. *Addict. Behav., 11*:399–406.

40. Zweben, J.E. (1987). Eating disorders and substance abuse. *J. Psychoactive Drugs, 19*:181–192.

41. Scott, D.W. (1983). Alcohol and food abuse: Some comparisons. *Br. J. Addict., 78*:339–349.

III
Adolescents

11

Adolescent Alcohol and Drug Addiction and Its Consequences: An Overview

Dorynne Czechowicz
National Institute on Drug Abuse, Rockville, Maryland

I. INTRODUCTION

The use of tobacco, alcohol, and other drugs by our nation's youth has been recognized as a serious public health problem. The inappropriate use of chemicals involves both licit and illicit substances. Substances of abuse commonly include alcohol, tobacco, marijuana, cocaine and other stimulants, PCP and other hallucinogens, inhalants, sedative-hypnotics, opioids, and over-the-counter drugs. It has been estimated that the annual cost to our society of chemical dependency is approximately $205 billion, of which $140 billion is attributed to alcohol abuse and $65 billion to drug abuse [1]. In the United States, personal and social costs of alcohol and drug abuse resemble those of major physical illnesses such as cardiovascular disease and cancer.

Alcohol and other drug abuse has the most serious impact on developing children and youth. Initiating drug use at an early age can have far-reaching physical, psychosocial, and developmental consequences. Youthful users are more vulnerable to life-threatening accidents and injuries; impulsive and risk-taking behaviors; illegal activity; physical complications; sexually transmitted diseases, including acquired immune deficiency syndrome (AIDS); and impairment of memory, cognitive, and motor performance. In addition, the effects of psychoactive drugs on the emotional development of adolescents and young adults can interfere with their ability to address important developmental challenges at this stage, as well as subsequent stages of life.

The public, Congress, and the Administration have placed increased emphasis on the prevention and treatment of alcohol and drug abuse, especially among high-risk youth. With the passage of the Anti-Drug Abuse Act of 1986, the National Institute on Drug Abuse and the National Institute on Alcohol Abuse and Alcoholism have expanded epidemiological, prevention, and treatment research.

This chapter was adapted from Adolescent alcohol and drug abuse and its consequences, Dorynne Czechowicz, M.D., *Am. J. Drug Alcohol Abuse 14*(2), pp. 189–197 (1988).

II. PATTERNS OF SUBSTANCE ABUSE AMONG ADOLESCENTS

Substance abuse increased explosively among adolescents and young adults in the 1960s and 1970s and peaked in 1978. Recent data from two national surveys—the 1985 National Household Survey [2] and the 1986 National High School Senior Survey [3]—indicate that, among teenagers, the use of many illicit drugs has declined significantly from the peak levels attained during the 1970s. The one exception to this trend is cocaine abuse. However, alcohol and drug use remain prevalent in this population group. Of particular concern is the fact that youth are beginning their first drug experience at an early age. Specifically, these surveys found that:

Over half (58%) of all American youth have tried an illicit drug at least once before finishing high school.

Over one-third of adolescents have used an illicit drug other than marijuana by the 12th grade (age 12–17).

Approximately 5 million young people, age 12–17, have used marijuana at some time during their lives. Nearly 3 million of these young people are current users of marijuana.

At least 1 out of 25 high school seniors smokes marijuana on a daily basis. One in 5 smoke cigarettes daily. More females than males smoke cigarettes.

About one in 20 seniors (5%) drinks alcohol daily. Approximately 37% have consumed five or more drinks on a single occasion in the past 2 weeks.

About one in five adolescents aged 14–17 is a "problem drinker." The National Council on Alcoholism estimates that 3 million teenagers are problem drinkers.

Cocaine was tried by at least 17% of the seniors in the class of 1986.

While 82% of the seniors acknowledged the harmful effects of using cocaine regularly, *only* 34% saw much risk in experimenting with it.

One in 25 high school seniors has used "crack" cocaine at least once. Cocaine abuse is on the rise. The increased availability of the inexpensive, potent, smokable form of crack cocaine has contributed to the increased abuse of cocaine by younger age groups.

Cocaine use remains high among American college students, even though the use of most other drugs on campus has fallen substantially since 1980. Cocaine is readily available on college campuses, and many students perceive little risk in experimenting with this drug.

Alcohol is the licit drug abused most often by adolescents. Adolescents who drink are responsible for a significant number of highway accidents and fatalities, as well as for many cases of violent crime and suicide. Alcohol-related traffic accidents kill 8000 persons 15–24 years of age each year—the leading cause of death in this age group [4].

III. CONSEQUENCES OF ALCOHOL AND DRUG USE

Since the turn of the century, mortality rates in the general population have steadily declined and life expectancy has increased. However, for one age group, those aged 15–24 years, mortality rates have increased significantly since the early 1960s (5). All the leading causes of death and disability among young people are preventable. These include traffic accidents, other accidental trauma, suicide, and homicide, which account for approximately three-quarters of all mortality in this population. The contribution of alcohol and drug abuse to this tragedy is significant.

Alcohol and other drug abuse interferes with the developmental process in children and adolescents and can result in long-term physical, psychological, and social consequences. Youthful users are also more prone to developing accelerated onset of both tolerance and addiction.

IV. MARIJUANA ABUSE

Over the past decade there have been significant increases in the potency of marijuana; this, coupled with decreasing age of first use, has resulted in increasing concern about the long-term developmental effects in children and adolescents who are especially vulnerable to the physiological, behavioral, and psychological effects of marijuana. Recent studies have linked marijuana use to, e.g., chronic cough, emphysema, increased risk for lung cancer, endocrine problems such as decreased testosterone and gynecomastia, suppression of lutenizing hormone in women, immune system suppression, and alterations in blood pressure and tachycardia [6].

One of the major concerns about marijuana is the drug's effects on personality, cognitive capacities, and behavior. Δ-9-Tetrahydrocannabinal (THC), the principal psychoactive ingredient in marijuana, produces short-term memory loss, decreased attention span, and impaired perceptual motor coordination that can interfere with learning and school performance. Significant progress has been made recently in determining the effects of marijuana on the brain. There is evidence that chronic THC exposure damages and destroys nerve cells and causes other pathological changes in the hippocampus [6]. The neuronal loss appears to be identical to the loss seen with normal aging. This raises concerns that mild functional losses due to aging and chronic marijuana use could be additive, placing long-term marijuana users at risk for serious or premature memory disorders as they age.

V. COCAINE ABUSE

The population groups that seem more vulnerable to cocaine use include youth and young adults who have higher than average preexisting levels of tobacco, alcohol, and especially marijuana use. Because youth with *conduct problems* in early elementary school have higher risk of becoming heavy marijuana users, it is anticipated that these youth also may be more vulnerable to initiating cocaine use [7].

Parallel to the increasing use of freebase crack cocaine, there has been a three- to four-fold increase in reports of adverse medical consequences associated with cocaine use.

Cocaine is the most effective reinforcing drug known. It produces intense drug-taking behavior in all animal species studied, including man. There is evidence that chronic use of cocaine produces a disruption of attention and impairs performance over time. Chronic use can lead to severe depression and "cocaine psychosis." High doses can result in seizures. There is evidence that cardiovasculr effects, such as myocardial infarction, as well as myocarditis associated with cocaine use are being seen more frequently [7]. Since there is increasing use of the drug among young people, there is concern about the future mental and physical health of these individuals. Prospective epidemiological studies are needed to follow these young people into adulthood. There is emerging evidence that cocaine taken during pregnancy has adverse effects on the course of gestation and the fetus. Specifically, difficulties in carrying the baby to term and low birth weight are seen.

VI. RECOGNITION OF EARLY PATTERNS OF SUBSTANCE USE IN ADOLESCENTS AND YOUNG ADULTS

The earlier the diagnosis, the more successful the intervention is likely to be. The early stages of adolescent drug abuse may be missed because changes are often subtle and behavioral changes may be attributed to the normal maturation process that occurs during adolescence. There are some clues that are helpful to physicians and parents attempting to distinguish normal from pathological adolescent behavior.

Most often, the diagnosis of drug abuse is made on the basis of behavioral or physical changes that points to the need to investigate further—such as deterioration in school performance; impaired family relationships; personality changes, such as unpredictable mood swings; depression; withdrawn behavior and/or changes in friends and peer group; legal problems; and physical changes such as frequent cough, sore throat, and/or conjunctivitis [8].

VII. STAGES OF DRUG USE/ABUSE

In the nonmedical use of any drug, there are four basic stages of the drug dependence syndrome [9]. In each stage the pattern of use and the progression of signs and symptoms resulting from drug use are observable.

The first stage is experimentation, and initial use often occurs in social settings. Too many individuals still believe that experimentation with drugs is safe, and for certain drugs such as alcohol and tobacco, even normal.

The second stage is occasional or recreational use in which the adolescent actively seeks the euphoric effects of the psychoactive drug. The adolescent in this stage often develops expertise in the use of substances for mood regulation and does not perceive drug use as causing undesirable consequences.

In stage three, regular use occurs and there is intense preoccupation with and self-perceived need for the psychoactive drug. Adolescents in this stage have lost control over the use of drugs. These youngsters develop tolerance and frequently use multiple drugs. Their major concern is to attain a drug-induced euphoria. Psychosocial functioning deteriorates and may include antisocial behavior.

In the fourth stage, daily use of psychoactive drugs occurs. The adolescent now uses drugs to prevent negative feelings rather than seeking euphoria. Psychosocial functioning is significantly impaired, and the individual is no longer functioning productively in society.

The diagnosis of adolescent drug abuse in its early stages can often be made by asking the youngster, as well as the parent, about general health concerns, school performance, family and peer relationships, attitudes at home, and, of course, about drug use. In addition to a physical evaluation, proper use of the laboratory can assist in the diagnosis and management of drug use. Screening for drugs of abuse in the urine should be done as part of the physical examination. Results, of course, must be interpreted in light of the psychosocial history and physical findings.

VIII. RISK FACTORS FOR ADOLESCENT SUBSTANCE ABUSE: IMPLICATIONS FOR PREVENTIVE INTERVENTIONS FOR THE PSYCHIATRIST

In the past, drug use has often gone unrecognized by physicians trained to associate only the later stages of use with problems, but a high index of suspicion and increased awareness of the prevalence of substance abuse and the related health and social consequences will aid in the earlier recognition of substance abuse.

Physicians who are sensitive to biopsychosocial risk factors and to the symptoms that signal early drug involvement will be better able to detect drug use *before* the adolescent becomes dependent.

While some individuals discontinue the use of one or more abused substances after only brief experimentation, all too often initiating tobacco, alcohol, and other drug use leads to continuing patterns of use and dependence [10], especially when use of these substances begins at an early stage. Many young people who go on to serious involvement with illicit drugs have started with these substances. For girls, for example, tobacco use seems to be an especially important predictor of subsequent escalation of drug use.

Of course, this sequence of drug use is not absolute. In some communities, inhalants are the first drugs abused by children, particularly children in ethnic minority groups. In addition, some adolescents will try a drug, then stop using it.

There is increasing awareness and concern regarding the relationship between alcohol and drug abuse and associated behaviors. Robins and Przybeck noted that persons who initiated drug use very early (under age 15) or late (after age 24) were those who tended to develop the most dysfunctional drug use pattern [11]. Underlying psychiatric problems were associated with early and late onset of drug use. In contrast, most drug use initiated between ages 15 and 24, the period of greatest risk for initiation, appears to be related to peer and social influences rather than underlying psychiatric disorders.

Youngsters with low self-esteem, inadequate interpersonal skills, inadequate social skills, negative peer relationships, and impaired family relationships may be at increased risk. The evidence suggests that children of chemically dependent parents are probably the highest risk population because of genetic and/or environmental vulnerability. Children from disadvantaged and socially isolated families, including many minority children, are also at increased risk for substance abuse [12].

The presence of antisocial behavior; strong rebellious feelings; alienation from others; a lack of strong bonds to family, school, or church and other conventional social institutions; lack of sense of direction; and low self-esteem have been shown to increase susceptibility of drug use and abuse. The evidence of a positive relationship between childhood antisocial behavior and subsequent drug abuse is relatively consistent [12]. Early antisocial behavior has been found to predict adolescent substance abuse. In a sample of urban black first-grade male students, Kellam et al. [13] found a positive correlation between first-grade male aggressiveness—especially when accompanied by shyness—and frequency of substance use 10 years later.

Use of certain drugs by some adolescents may represent an attempt to cope with depression or anxiety. It is often difficult to differentiate drug-induced psychopathology from an underlying psychiatric disorder.

An interesting finding in an analysis of data on 18- to 30-year-olds from the National Institute on Mental Health's (NIMH) Epidemiological Catchment Area Program (ECA) suggests that a significant amount of drug abuse could possibly be prevented by prompt identification and effective treatment of preexisting and/or coexisting mental illness. Nineteen percent of male drug abusers were found to have had an earlier episode of depression or anxiety. Kandell and Davies also linked affective disturbance in adolescents with substance abuse [14].

IX. CONCLUSIONS

The psychiatrist can play an important role in the prevention and early intervention of substance abuse problems. Earlier recognition of youth and families who may be at increased risk is important. The assessment of every child should include a careful history regarding the possibility of substance abuse. Accurate diagnosis may be complicated by the problem of comorbidity. Diagnostic expertise is needed to assess which diagnosis is primary and how the use of substances may have precipitated, masked, or ameliorated psychiatric symptoms.

For children and youth believed to be in the initial stages of drug use, educating the patient and educating and counseling the parents is necessary. Failure to assess family functioning, problem behaviors in children and youth, parental alcohol and other drug use, parental attitudes toward drug use, etc., may lead to failure to recognize potential problems.

Psychiatrists involved in the treatment of children and youth presenting with behavioral and emotional problems should be alert to the possibility that drug use may be a contributing factor.

In order to intervene effectively with these patients, close cooperation between parents, educators, primary health care providers, and alcohol and drug abuse counselors is necessary.

REFERENCES

1. Harwood, H.J., Napolitano, D.M., Kristiansen, P.L., et al., *Economic Costs to Society of Alcohol and Drug Abuse and Mental Illness* (Report Prepared for the Alcohol, Drug Abuse, and Mental Health Administration, Research Triangle, North Carolina), Research Triangle Institute, Raleigh, North Carolina, 1984.

2. National Institute on Drug Abuse, *National Household Survey on Drug Abuse, 1985*, DHHS Publication No. (ADM-87-1539), Rockville, Maryland, National Institute on Drug Abuse, 1987.

3. Johnson, L.D., O'Malley, P.M., and Backman, J.H., *Drug Use among American High School Students, College Students and Other Young Adults* (National Institute on Drug Abuse—DHHS Publication No. (ADM-86-1450), U.S. Government Printing Office, Washington, D.C., 1986.

4. Bass, J., Gallegher, S., and Mehta, K., Unintentional injuries among adolescents and young adults, *Pediatr. Clin. North Am. 32*:31–39 (1985).

5. U.S. Department of Health and Human Services, *The Surgeon General's Report on Health Promotion and Disease Prevention*, U.S. Government Printing Office, Washington, D.C., 1980.

6. *Drug Abuse and Drug Abuse Research, the Second Triennial Report to Congress from the Secretary, Department of Health and Human Services* (DHHS Publication No. (ADM)87-1486), U.S. Government Printing Office, Washington, D.C., 1987.

7. Scientific perspectives on cocaine abuse. Report of a meeting sponsored by the National Institute on Drug Abuse, American Society for Pharmacology and Experimental Therapeutics and Committee on Problems of Drug Dependence, *Pharmacologist 29*:20–27 (1987).

8. Semlitz, L., and Gold, M., Adolescent drug abuse: Diagnosis, treatment and prevention, *Psychiatr. Clin. North Am.* 455–473 (1986).

9. Macdonald, D.I., Drugs, smoking, and adolescence, *Am. J. Dis. Child. 138*:117–125 (1984).

10. Kandel, D.B., and Logan, J.A., Patterns of drug use from adolescence to young adulthood: Periods of risk for initiation, continued use and discontinuation, *Am. J. Public Health 74*:660–666 (1984).

11. Robins, L.N., and Przybeck, T.R., Age of onset of drug use as a factor in drug abuse and other disorders, *Etiology of Drug Abuse: Implications for Prevention* (C.L. Jones and R.J. Battjes, eds.), (National Institute on Drug Abuse Research Monograph 56, DHHS Pub. No. (ADM)85-1335), U.S. Government Printing Office, Washington, D.C., 1985.

12. Hawkins, J.D., Lishner, D.M., Catalana, P.F., et al., Childhood predictors of adolescent substance abuse, *J. Child. Contemp. Soc. 18*(1 & 2):1–65 (1986).

13. Kellam, S.G., and Simon, M.C., Mental health in first grade and teenage drug, alcohol and cigarette use, *J. Drug Alcohol Depend. 5*:273–304 (1980).

14. Kandell, D.B., and Davies, M., Adult sequelae of adolescent depressive symptoms, *Arch. Gen. Psychiatry 23*:255–261 (1986).

12

Adolescent Drug and Alcohol Addiction: Diagnosis and Assessment

J. Calvin Chatlos
St. Mary Hospital, Hoboken, New Jersey

I. INTRODUCTION

The devastation of adolescent drug and alcohol addiction challenges modern medicine with an opportunity to develop and apply a holistic biopsychosocial approach to this cultural crisis. This chapter is designed to guide practitioners with a broad understanding of this rapidly developing field. It will begin with an elaboration of a biopsychosocial model [1,2] as it refers to adolescent chemical dependency (drug and alcohol addiction) and focus on diagnosis and assessment based on current research. The following chapter uses this biopsychosocial model and presents a treatment approach that can guide clinical efforts to meet this challenge.

Setting the stage for understanding the problem of adolescent and alcohol addiction requires essential data gathering. Data regarding the chemical use by the general population of adolescents has been released from the *1988 National Household Survey on Drug Abuse*. This survey, conducted every 2–3 years since 1971 by the Research Triangle Institute reports the nature and extent of drug use among the American household population aged 12 years and over. The most recent survey [3] revealed significant declines in the current use of all illicit drugs by youth. Among youth aged 12–17, current illicit drug use decreased from 18% in 1985 to 10% in 1988, led by the almost 50% decline in current marijuana use from 12 to 6.4% in 1988. The rate of cocaine use by youth in the past years decreased from 4.9% in 1985 to 3.4% in 1988, continuing the decrease begun since its peak use by 6.5% in 1982. This has been associated with an increase in the perceived great risk of use from 31% in 1985 to 53% in 1988. To place these figures in perspective, the 8% of youth that are current illicit drug users indicates over 2 million teenagers using illicit drugs last year!

Further information has been obtained from the University of Michigan research and reporting program entitled *Monitoring the Future: A Continuing Study of the Lifestyles and Values of Youth*. This survey provides an ongoing means of evaluating drug and alcohol use by a more select group of young people. This annual survey involving high school seniors and college students reports data on the use of 11 separate classes of drugs (including alcohol and nicotine), prevalence and recency of use, grade level and use, and attitudes and beliefs by peers, friends, and parents regarding drug use. Information in the most recent survey [4] reported annually by the National Institute of Drug Abuse (NIDA) revealed that a significant trend in drug use has been the decrease from peak lifetime prevalence of illicit drug use by 66% of high school seniors in 1981 and 1982 to 54% in 1988. During that time, marijuana use, the most widely used illicit drug, decreased from 59 to 47%, cocaine use decreased from 17 to 12%, alcohol use remained alarmingly steady at 93–92%, and cigarette use decreased from 71 to 66%. This period did not show a steady decline, but included a stall in the downward trend in 1985 with an increase in cocaine prevalence. Partly as a result of extensive media coverage about the widespread appearance of "crack" cocaine and the hazards of cocaine spurred by the cocaine-related deaths in 1986 of sports stars Len Bias and Don Rogers [5] the downward trend resumed.

Additionally noted in the survey is the increased drug use beyond adolescence and through the mid 20s with lifetime prevalence of any illicit drug use rising to 80%, marijuana use to 75%, and cocaine use to 40%. Elaborating further about more extensive use, 18% of high school seniors smoke cigarettes daily, 11% smoke half-a-pack or more a day; 2.7% smoke marijuana daily; and 4.2% drink alcohol daily, with 35% reporting having had five or more drinks in a row on at least one occasion during the 2 weeks just prior to the survey. Information in this survey also shows that the decrease in the use of marijuana and cocaine has mirrored an increase in perceived risk of harm in use in spite of continued or increased availability (Fig. 1).

These data provide an extensive background and continued tool for the understanding, diagnosis, and comprehensive treatment of adolescent drug and alcohol addiction.

How are we to understand this and respond?

II. HISTORY OF ADDICTION RESEARCH

The field of adolescent drug and alcohol addiction has developed and expanded dramatically in the past 5 years. Several excellent review articles [6,7] recently available, as well as a volume of *Pediatric Clinics of North America* [8] dedicated to chemical dependency, and the presence of a new *Journal of Adolescent Chemical Dependency* (1990) all highlight the progression of the field. The changes in understanding adolescent addiction are often reflected in the literature during the last 15 years and are often confusing to newcomers in the field. This section presents a model to place research and understanding about adolescent chemical dependency in a historical perspective that will allow more fruitful reading of the literature.

The historical progression of addiction research follows the developmental sequence leading to a biopsychosocial model as outlined by Schwartz [9], and parallels ideas regarding shifts in paradigm [10]:

Stage 1. Formistic. Clinical experience leads to comparing patients with the impression being formed of a category. This leads to questions regarding the (single) cause for these observations.

Stage 2. Mechanistic. Single-cause, single-effect research, often including control groups without the variable attempt to explain the observation. This progresses to reviewing the limits to the observation and the conditions under which it works and other effects in a situation.

Stage 3. Contextual. Competing "single" causes are found with moderating variables. A contextual awareness develops recognizing that what the mechanism is depends on how you look at it. The complexities increase to the point of requiring adaptation of an organistic-systems approach.

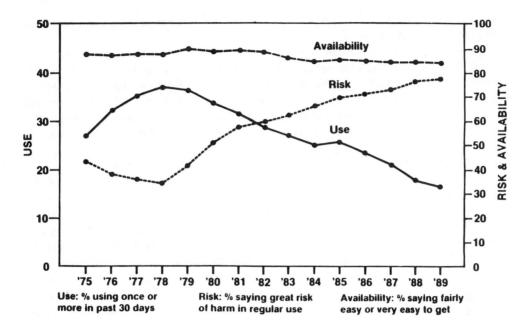

Figure 1 Trends in marijuana availability, perceived risk of regular use, and use in past 30 days high school seniors.

Stage 4. Organistic. A multicategory, multicase, multieffect interactive model is developed. Multivariant research designs uncover the importance of different variables and their relationship to the problem and to each other.

For years, research and ideas regarding addiction were based on alcoholism or heroin addiction in adults, since these drugs were often used exclusively as well as being more prevalent and accessible. This led to the definition of the category of alcoholism or opiate addiction and Stage 1 research.

Stage 2 research investigated single causes. During this stage there was a raging controversy over whether alcoholism was a disease or a moral problem. Researchers [11] concluded that alcoholism was variously:

A symptom of compulsion neurosis
A symptom of hysterical type neurosis
A symptom of social unrest
A symptom of underlying personality structure
Due to defective superego development and is therefore a moral question
A sign of a weak character and treatment . . . should be combined with punitive measures
No more a disease than thievery, or lynching

In 1960, Jellinek's *The Disease Concept of Alcoholism* [11] presented a contextual framework (Stage 3) for understanding alcoholism. He reviews historically the controversies regarding alcoholism, outlines the many competing "single causes," and progresses to develop an early organistic framework (Stage 4) and biopsychosocial model involving physiological, psychological, social, cultural, and economic factors. The disease concept of alcoholism was officially adopted by the American Medical Association in 1956. However, as late as 1968 the American Psychiatric Association in its *Diagnostic and Statistical Manual of Mental*

Disorders, 2nd Edition (DSM-II) classified alcoholism under personality disorders and other nonpsychotic mental disorders.

As other drug use became more prevalent in the 1960s and 1970s, added factors required inclusion in a biopsychosocial model. The focus shifted from alcoholism and single drug use to broader context of drug addiction. A paper by Sobell and Sobell [12] grouped substances together because of the presence of tolerance, physical dependence, and withdrawal symptoms.

In further understanding and elaborating an interactive model, Kandel [13,14] described stages of drug use, heralding a new focus on adolescents and a developmental approach. Four distinct developmental stages of progression were identified in longitudinal studies: (1) beer or wine, (2) hard liquor or cigarettes, (3) marijuana, and (4) other illicit drugs (Fig. 2). This concept of drug use being a developmental phenomena introduced new and critical factors to understanding addiction. Part of this impetus occurred as drug use became present at earlier ages [5], and clinicians working more with teenagers were investigating intervention efforts. A longitudinal study from 1969 to 1972 [15] of adolescent development demonstrated the association between onset of drinking and general increase in other socially deviant behaviors such as marijuana use, premarital intercourse, and problem drinking. Elaborating further on the developmental sequence and identifying problem drinking as a significant separate step, Donovan and Jessor [16] demonstrated a progressive scale of use with the following order: nonuse of drugs or alcohol, nonproblem use of alcohol, use of marijuana, involvement in problem drinking, use of one or more pills (amphetamines, barbiturates, or hallucinogens), and use of hard drugs (cocaine or heroin).

The interactive model was further elaborated in a longitudinal study from 1971 to 1972 [17] demonstrating that depressive mood was related to onset of marijuana use and predicted the use of other illicit drugs by marijuana users.

Interest also focused more specifically on the abuse of alcohol and drugs in the treatment population of adolescents. A study in 1981–1982 revealed specific characteristics of the adolescents in treatment compared to adults [18]. The adolescents used drugs at an earlier age, initiated use of multiple drugs more quickly, progressed to regular use of drugs more quickly, were more likely to come from violent homes and have been physically abused, had a higher incidence of suicide attempts, and had a first arrest at an earlier age.

Information similar to this was included as MacDonald [19] outlined stages of drug use in teenagers:

A. Stage 1. Experimentation/Learning the Mood Swing

This stage usually begins in junior high school with peer pressure to "try it," usually involving beer drinking, marijuana smoking, or some inhalant sniffing. This usually occurs at home, at a party, or "hanging out." There is often a desire to feel grown up. Small amounts of the drug are needed to get high and the person is usually quickly returned to a normal mood with no problems. The teenager has learned to use drugs to affect mood and affect the pleasure centers of the brain. To a young person, "What feels good must be good!"

B. Stage 2. Regular Use/Seeking the Mood Swing

More regular use begins with progressing to hard liquor or bouts of drinking to get drunk as use is more associated with dealing with stresses. Use begins to occur during the week and more drug is used, since the body develops tolerance. Problems occur such as missing school because of hangovers, missing time on a job, not performing as well on the sports team. Different drugs are tried and they may progress to using hallucinogens and pills. Socially, non–drug using friends may be dropped. More money may be needed, leading to stealing from family as well as lying to hide drug use. Moods may change rapidly and without

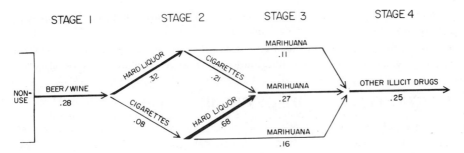

Figure 2 Major stages of adolescent involvement in drug use. Figures are probabilities of moving from one stage to another. (From Ref. 13, used with permission.)

explanation to being irritable, happy, angry, or even depressed. Interest in usual activities may change.

C. Stage 3. Daily Preoccupation/Preoccupation with the Mood Swing

More dangerous drugs are used more often with more problems developing in more areas of the adolescent's life. Drug use becomes a central focus of life as the teenager thinks about the last high, and where, when, and with whom the next high will occur. The preoccupation with drug use replaces thoughts and activities with family, school, and community. More serious problems develop that may involve stealing, breaking of other laws, and violence. Many mood changes occur as guilt, shame, loneliness, and depression, partially covered by denial are now mixed with withdrawal from or cravings for drugs. Attempts are made to cut down or quit, but are usually unsuccessful at this stage. Physical problems may develop.

D. Stage 4. Dependency/Using to Feel Normal

This final stage of addiction involves "hard" or more dangerous drugs in large amounts. Since the teenager has become surrounded by drug-using friends and situations, they no longer know what normal behavior is. Use has gotten out of control and life has become unmanageable in many areas—physical, psychological, social, family, school, and legally. There is also much guilt, shame, and self-hatred, which may lead to suicide thoughts and attempts. The teenager no longer gets as high and much more time and behavior is spent "trying to feel normal" and to avoid withdrawal symptoms.

The emphasis was now focused less on the drug itself and more on the addictive process [20,21]. Distinctions between previous terms of use, abuse and addiction were often limited. In 1980, DSM-III [22] distinctions were based on the presence or absence of tolerance. Distinctions also were made between psychological versus physical addiction. Research and progress in understanding cocaine, a drug once believed to be only psychologically addicting [23], led to a broader definition of addiction: An irresistible compulsion to use the drug at increasing doses and frequency even in the face of serious physical and/or psychological side effects and the extreme disruption of the user's personal relationships and system of values. The contextual shift supported the concept of adolescent chemical dependency (ACD) as a syndrome [6] that included aspects of extent of drug use, and consequences in physical, psychological and social areas of functioning. This is reflected in DSM-III-R (DSM-III-Revised) criteria [24]. Ralph and Barr [25] further identify characteristics of a specific adolescent behavioral chemical dependency–syndrome (ABCD-S) associated with depressive symptoms, hyperactivity, distractibility, restlessness, and other "problem behaviors."

With adults, it was also becoming more apparent that drug addiction or chemical dependency is frequently associated with other compulsive behaviors such as bulimia, gambling, compulsive sex, violence, and self-destructive behaviors. As reviewed in Donovan and Marlatt [21] for adults, the focus in research has led to a biopsychosocial model to comprehensively understand and assess the multidimensional aspects of addictive behaviors.

III. BIOPSYCHOSOCIAL MODEL OF CHEMICAL ADDICTION

An expression of a multidimensional biopsychosocial disease model for chemical dependency that has been useful at the Adolescent Center for Chemical Education, Prevention and Treatment (ACCEPT) program is diagrammed (Fig. 3).

This model is divided into parts that coordinate with research efforts that have approached chemical dependency (drug and alcohol addiction) investigating antecedent, concomitant, and maintenance factors.

Antecedents are those factors that occur before the onset of drug use. This predisposition is divided by Donovan [26] using alcoholism as an heuristic example, into four possible sources—genetic, constitutional, psychological, and sociocultural.

A. Genetic Basis for Addiction

Family, twin, and adoption studies [26–28] demonstrate evidence for a genetic basis that may predispose a person to alcoholism or produce a vulnerability. The 54% concordance rate for alcoholism in identical twins and a 38% rate in paternal twins support this genetic basis. Sons of alcoholic fathers have a four times greater chance of developing alcoholism than controls. Data regarding the genetics of drug abuse are not well defined and the strengths that this factor contributes in adolescent chemical dependency and in relation to specific drug addictions is yet to be determined.

B. Constitutional Basis for Addiction

Support for a constitutional basis comes from studies showing a high heritability of increased alcohol-elimination rates in male twins [29], higher levels of acetaldehyde in sons of alcoholics than in sons of nonalcoholics after an alcohol challenge [30], and lower activity of acetaldehyde

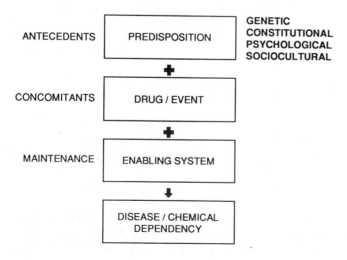

Figure 3   ACCEPT Biopsychosocial disease model.

dehydrogenase in sober alcoholics than in controls [31]. Evaluation of several other markers correctly distinguished 83% of controls and 70% of sons of alcoholics [32]. The role of tetrahydroisoquinoline (THIQ) in the brain as a result of alcohol administration may be related to its addictive potential [33]. As explained by Donovan [26], the constitutional factors may have a genetic basis or may be due to environmental influences.

C. Psychological Basis for Addiction

Psychological factors have been more thoroughly studied as predisposing factors to adolescent substance abuse. These have been reviewed in Isralowitz and Singer [34] and include: negative attitude toward school and low self-esteem, low sense of psychological well-being, low self-esteem regarding school, high rebelliousness, untrustworthiness, sociability and impulsive traits, tolerance of deviance, inconsistency between one's own and one's parents opinions about drug abuse, lower academic aspirations, low school achievement, dropping out of school, mental health problems, frequent cigarette smoking, disciplinary problems in school, and delinquent and deviant behavior. A longitudinal study of personality traits of adolescents assessed in 1969 was followed up on subsequent measures of substance abuse in 1980–1981 [35]. It demonstrated that high self-reported variables of obedience and law abiding, works hard and effectively, and feels valued and accepted correlated significantly with low drug and alcohol use. In addition, peer reports of low socialization were predictive of high drug and alcohol use. Variables in this factor associated negatively with drug use were orderliness, curious/interested, tender, determined/persistent, obedient, likes hard thinking, tries hard to achieve, feels in control, and works hard. Variables associated with high drug use were does not concentrate, immature interest, slow worker, cannot always be trusted, dependent, impulsive, not responsible, pessimistic, and not considerate.

D. Sociocultural Basis for Addiction

Sociocultural studies in adults [26,36] have demonstrated the effects of age, occupation, social class, and subcultural and religious affiliations on alcoholism. Sociocultural antecedents in adolescents have also been reviewed by Isralowitz and Singer [34] and include: parental use of hard liquor or drugs, parental divorce, parental arrest, lack of closeness between parents and children, high level of adolescent peer activity, drug use and problem behavior by close friends, broader society becoming a "drug culture," and portrayal of drugs as glamorous.

Drug use as well as problem drinking in adolescence [37] are associated with proneness to "problem behaviors" that also include behaviors such as delinquency and premarital sexual intercourse. The specific progression noted previously from nonuse, nonproblem use of alcohol, use of marijuana, problem drinking, use of pills, use of hard drugs was found to be correlated with increasing involvement in psychosocial proneness to problem behaviors. These included lower personal controls against problem behavior, less of an orientation toward parents than toward peers, higher social support for drinking, greater involvement in other problem behaviors, and lower involvement with conventional institutions of church and the schools.

E. Drug Factors

To all of these predisposing factors a *drug* is then introduced. Among teenagers, the major forces of introduction are peer pressure and availability of the drug [6]. Specific predictors of initiation into drug use in adolescence [38] include: peer group influence; prior participation in delinquent activities, low religiosity, academic performance, and interest in academic activities; personality factors such as depression, risk-taking, and low self-esteem; and parental factors, including poor quality of relationship with parents and parental role models for drug use such as drinking or taking medically prescribed psychoactive substances.

Certain factors are important for initiation into use of specific drugs—a developmental pattern of deviant or problem behaviors are predictive of first alcohol use [15], peer influences predict initiation into marijuana use, and depression and low parental closeness lead to initiation into use of illicit drugs other than marijuana [38]. Once introduced, the strong positive reinforcement of the drug euphoria, the negative reinforcement of the abstinence symptoms, and genetic and biochemical effects [6,39,40] interact with the personality to dominate the clinical picture. Newcomb and Harlow [41] have supported hypotheses that stressful life events lead to a perceived loss of control, development of meaninglessness, and use of drugs to cope with these stresses. This supports some of the learning factors that occur especially with progression into Stage 2 of chemical dependency as already described.

Various other concomitants to drug use as reviewed in Isralowitz and Singer [34] include genetic factors associated with acute toxic reactions to drugs, vulnerability to adverse effects of toxic substances on the brain during childhood and adolescence, dislike of school, less adequate problem-solving skills, lower expectation of getting one's needs met, lower religiosity, lower cognitive development, higher life stress, frequency of school absenteeism, early premarital intercourse, running away from home, sexual promiscuity, and perceived lack of parental support.

A cross-sectional study of substance abuse [42] demonstrated an increasing use of drugs associated with an increasing number of 12 risk factors—early alcohol intoxication, perceived adult drug use, perceived peer approval of drug use, perceived parental approval of drug use, school absences, poor academic achievement, distrust of teacher drug knowledge, distrust of parent drug knowledge, low educational aspirations, little religious commitment, emotional distress, and dissatisfaction with life.

F. Enabling System

The final factor is the enabling system. This is the system of all persons, places, and things surrounding the user that knowingly or unknowingly enable the progression of the chemical dependency [43]. This may include promoting use without knowledge of harmful effects, modeling drug use and dependence, denial of use, removal of consequences that would deter use, or economic incentives for continued use [44]. This system may include parents, teachers, friends, therapists, physicians, judges, lawyers, law enforcement personnel, and the broader aspects of a political and economic system. Singer and Anglin [45] demonstrated physicians' failure to identify alcohol and drug problems in adolescents.

Part of the understanding of the enabling system comes from data on factors that predict cessation of drug use. Some of the factors identified [38] are changes in social roles, especially assumption of new family roles such as marriage or childbirth; lower degree of involvement in drug use, and later age of initiation into use; less participation in delinquent activities prior and at present, including less recent arrests; more involvement in religious activities; and involvement in social contexts that are less supportive of drug use. There are also characteristics of families in which drug use is low [46]:

1. The offspring perceive more love from both parents, particularly their father.
2. There is less discrepancy between how the parents would ideally like their children to be versus how they actually perceive them, and their children are seen as more assertive.
3. Parents and their offspring's friends are compatible. Parents have more influence than peers and less approval of drug use is voiced (and displayed by parents and peers).
4. More spontaneous agreement is observed in problem solving, but if it does not occur, members are slower but more efficient in reaching solutions.

5. They function more democratically or quasidemocratically, with shared authority and better communication.
6. Low-risk families also manifest a "benevolent dictatorship" structure with diverisity of self-expression and adherence to traditional sex roles.
7. They also show religious involvement, more emphasis of childrearing, discipline, self-control, and less allowance of freedom for children.
8. There is an emphasis on family cohesion and togetherness and a greater ability to plan and have fun together.
9. Offspring are more enamored of control and obedience and also are generally reliable, honest, and sensible.
10. An important variable is their sense of family tradition—that the family had existed over generations—an ethos that engenders loyalty to family standards.

The interaction of the predisposition, drug effects and concomitant behaviors, and enabling system combine to produce the syndrome of chemical dependency. These factors lead chemical dependency to be understood as having several key features: primary, progressive, chronic, and multidimensional [47]. According to Gitlow and Peyser [48], *primary* means that:

> though the [alcoholic's] illness may begin from quite diverse psychological origins, once the disease of [alcoholism] has been grafted upon this personality structure, it dominates the clinical picture and eventually becomes the major determinant in both choice and efficacy of therapy.

Whatever the temporal process of predisposition, drug interaction, and enabling system, the person eventually acquires characteristics that are autonomous. Once alcohol or other drug addiction is grafted onto the personality, a new illness occurs that is inextricably intertwined. The intertwining develops as a result of specific effects of the drug and conditioning and learning effects of the body and behavior by the drugs [21,49].

This has important implications, since once the drug is removed physically, the patterned behaviors—drug urges or cravings, impulsiveness, paranoia, fearfulness, distrust—remain and are the focus of treatment. In addition, Morrison and Smith [6] have referred to a "biochemical-genetic" line that is crossed during addiction, after which the chemicals control the behavior. They deemed addiction to be an "urge" that precludes logical and rational thought processes. This has been elaborated specifically [50] in relation to neurotransmitter functioning. Another way of understanding this is associated with the paradox of control—as the person becomes stimulus responsive [51] based on interoceptive and exteroceptive stimuli that have been conditioned by drug use. Drug and alcohol use begins with the person controlling their experience of "learning the mood swing," but with these conditioning effects, eventually the environment of persons, places, and things controls the urges and drug-seeking behaviors. Thus progression is described as loss of control and is related to the person becoming more stimulus responsive.

Progressive means that due to conditioning and learned responses, physical adaptation of the body, and reinforcing effects of the enabling system the disease progresses. Data suggest that most adolescents that use drugs do not go on to develop dependency [52], and Wheeler and Malmquist [53] report that only 6–10% of adolescents meet the criteria for chemical dependency. Kandel, as noted previously, has described an association between depression and progression. It is important to remember that the progressive stage of the disease can be fatal. This is often not thought about with adolescents until we note the increased death rate of 15- to 24-year-olds, mostly due to accidents, homicides, and suicides, with about 50% believed to be drug- or alcohol-related [54–57].

This leads to an understanding of drug alcohol addiction as a *chronic* disease. This understanding is derived mainly from work with adults and is due to the predisposition of genetic and constitutional factors that persist, but also to possibly permanent effects of the drugs and conditioning. With adults, the present controversy regarding alcoholics returning to "controlled drinking" versus abstinence as the goal continues to test the limits of this understanding. With teenagers, the question of controlled use remains. As a result of experience with adult addiction and unknown information regarding the more specific nature of adolescent drug and alcohol addiction, treatment programs generally require abstinence as a goal.

IV. FAMILY FACTORS AND THE BIOPSYCHOSOCIAL MODEL

The biopsychosocial model as described emphasizes the role of family as a maintenance factor in the enabling system part of the equation. It is important to recognize that the family is an important aspect of all three factors—the antecedent (predisposition), concomitant (drug/event), and the maintenance. An interactive or reciprocal approach is required to understand how chemical dependency affects the entire family and how the entire family affects chemical dependency [58].

In addition to the family genetic factors mentioned previously, some of the antecedent factors involving the family that have been identified are birth order and sibling relationships [59], parental mental illness, divorce, separation and frequent geographic moves [60], and parental drug and alcohol addiction being a more important determinant of adolescent drug abuse than parental attitude toward substance abuse [61].

Problems often begin in early adolescence associated with new developmental issues [46]. The onset of puberty and sexuality heralds the developmental family issues of physical changes, identity formation, autonomy [62], and separation-individuation [63]. Dramatic physical and social changes during junior high school lead to an awareness of body function and self with experimentation in many areas as new behaviors are required to adapt to these changes. Drug and alcohol use readily becomes part of this experimentation physically and socially owing to strong peer pressures. As the adolescent progresses through stages of chemical dependency, the family is undergoing its own progression through stages of "coaddiction." Coaddiction refers to the emotional and behavioral dependency that the parents and family members develop with the addict that is similar to the dependency that the addict develops on drugs. Kaufman [58] describes the progression of codependency (coaddiction) that develops between adolescent and family:

> Drug-abusing adolescents generally refuse to follow parental rules for behavior at home. They associate with individuals whom their parents consider bad influences and bring them into the house. They come home just sufficiently later than curfews and without calling in a way that infuriates their parents. They drive the family car without permission and frequently get traffic citations which they can't afford to pay and which require parental court appearances. They are constantly in trouble at school, particularly through tardiness, absence, not paying attention, and unruly behavior, yet they develop a multiplicity of ways for intercepting messages from school to parents. Shoplifting as well as theft from and damage to friends' homes are also common and the adolescent may either conceal or flaunt these activities. Parents are lied to about needs for funds that are diverted to drugs and when these lies are discovered, parents are coerced into continuing to provide funds by threats of violence from debtors or of commission of crimes, and through promises of protection from incarceration. They continue to drink and to use drugs at home after they've been prohibited from doing so even with legal reinforcement. They lie about their substance abuse and destructive behavior and the lies themselves frequently become a major concern to parents. They also engage parents in frequent power struggles about whether they are high or have used drugs. This type of defiance leads many parents to feel they have totally lost control of their children.

Family members at this point have become preoccupied with the adolescent's behavior and their own inability to contain it, similar to the teenager's preoccupation with drugs and loss of control over use.

Some family factors that have been identified as concomitants of this progression are triangulation involving the marital dyad and the adolescent [64,63]; sibling relationships, including developing specific roles in the family [65]; patterns of intimacy and distance [63]; inconsistency in parental rule making and limit setting; use of denial; covert encouragement of behaviors; and impaired intergenerational mourning [66]. These factors contribute to ongoing interactions in which one person does or says something that is the stimulus for another's response, and that response in turn becomes the stimulus evoking further responses. These interactive patterns of developing coaddiction attempt to maintain a family homeostasis [46] that eventually becomes habitual and locks all family members into rigid, repetitive, and reactive patterns [63]. Blurred generational boundaries and intensely symbiotic or emotionally distant relationships are common [63]. A typical family pattern described in narcotics addicts [59] is that of an enmeshed mother and disengaged father. Of note, this may be more descriptive of white Protestant and black families with more enmeshment of fathers with sons in Jewish and Italian families, emphasizing the need to be aware of ethnic differences in families.

The family at this point has been described as dull and lifeless, only becoming alive when it is mobilized to deal with the crisis of drug abuse [66]. However, the joylessness may actually precede the drug use and reflect family predispositional patterns of behaviors. Maintenance factors in these systems are the use of guilt by teenagers and parents, physical symptoms of depression, anxiety or psychosomatic problems, and even parental suicide attempts blamed on the teenager [58]. Communication is most frequently negative and without praise for good behavior [67]. Levine [63] describes examples of unresolved mourning of family members maintaining substance abuse in "an ongoing death-like process with suicidal ramifications," highlighting the frequent fatal outcome in severely addicted teens and the importance of grief processes in family development.

All of these examples illustrate the use of the biopsychosocial model and the value of including the family in all factors of the process.

V. DUAL DIAGNOSIS AND THE BIOPSYCHOSOCIAL MODEL

Another factor that plays a significant role in the biopsychosocial model is that of psychiatric disorder. Dual diagnosis (chemical dependency and psychiatric disorder) has been recognized as a frequent aspect of adult alcoholism and addiction [68–70]. Only recently has dual diagnosis been recognized as associated with ACD. A review by Morrison and Smith [6] included depression [17,19,71], conduct disorder [72], attention deficit disorder [73], eating disorders [74], and borderline personality disorder [75]. A more recent review [7] includes associations between adolescent substance abuse and depression [76], bipolar disorder [71], antisocial behavior [77], attention deficit hyperactivity disorder [78], borderline personality disorder [79], and suicide [80,81]. Ralph and Barr [25] elaborates on the association of ADHD, learning disabilities, and chemical dependency. Bukstein [82] explores relationships of addiction in adolescents to affective disorders, conduct disorders and antisocial personality disorder, attention-deficit hyperactivity disorders, anxiety disorders, eating disorders, and schizophrenia.

A comparison of two studies done at Fair Oaks Hospital, a private psychiatric facility, is revealing of the situation. A retrospective study [83] of adolescents treated in 1980–1981 on an inpatient psychiatric unit assessed the presence of concomitant substance abuse using DSM-III [22] criteria. Of 41 patients in the study, 29 (71%) were abusing one or more drugs at admission. Of those 29, diagnosis was first made in 14 (48%) at admitting interview, 13 (45%) by admitting urine drug screen, and 2 (7%) at structured neuropsychiatric interview. The admitting urine drug screen was positive in 19 (65%) patients with a positive clinical history of addiction. A subsequent study was conducted by the same author [84] at the same hospital, but in 1987 after an adolescent substance abuse inpatient unit was established. A Structured Clinical Interview for DSM-III-R (SCID) of 60 consecutive adolescents admitted for substance abuse or dependence using DSM-III [24] criteria was conducted 4–6 weeks following admission. A SCID diagnosable Axis I illness was present in 53 (87%). The categories included conduct disorder 53 (88%), posttraumatic stress disorder 26 (42%), major depression eight (13%), simple phobia six (10%), social phobia five (7%), agoraphobia four (5.7%), bulimia three (5%), bipolar disorder two (3.3%), anorexia two (3%), and obsessive compulsive disorder one (1.5%). Considering the diagnosis of posttraumatic stress disorder, of note was that 11 (43%) had traumatic stressors precede the onset of addiction, and 15 (57%) had stressors follow and were related to addiction.

In reviewing studies of adolescents, a major impediment has been the lack of an adequate assessment tool for ACD. Using DSM-III [22] criteria is limited by the rarity in which physical signs of withdrawal occur in teenagers. Criteria for DSM-III-R [24] are more helpful and consistent with the use of a biopsychosocial model and syndrome concept for ACD. A recent study [85] using a new diagnostic tool based on DSM-III-R (24) criteria evaluated 73 drug clinic teenagers. They found affective disorder (unipolar or bipolar) to be most prevalent at 24.7%, ADHD with 20.5%, developmental disorder 15.1%, psychosis (delusions or hallucinations) 6.8%, eating disorder (anorexia or bulimia) 5.5%, and anxiety (separation, avoidant, or overanxious) disorder at 5.5%. As with adult studies, differential figures of ACD and psychiatric disorder appear to be related to the specific population (inpatients, outpatient, school, community), specific assessment criteria, stage of assessment or treatment at which evaluation was done, biases of historical recall, and possible specific referral network established.

A clinically useful approach to dual diagnosis uses the biopsychosocial model, and as elaborated by Kranzler and Liebowitz [86] acknowledges parallel biopsychosocial processes with a bidirectional interaction of two or more disorders that can occur at any level—antecedent, concomitant, or maintenance. For instance, depression has a predisposition that includes a strong genetic component. Concordance rates for depressive disorder in identical twins of 67% and in paternal twins of 15% as well as data from adoption studies support this [87]. The presence of constitutional factors in a predisposition are indicated by neuroendocrine studies that show abnormal biogenic amines and involvement of the hypothalamic-pituitary-adrenal axis [88]. Psychological and sociocultural factors, especially low socioeconomic status (SES) have been known to be relevant to depression [89]. In the psychiatric biopsychosocial model, rather than the drug being present, an event occurs. With depression, life events have been shown to be significantly related to the development of depression [90]. Because of the strong biological basis for depression, there may also be specific biological events that precipitate depression. The final factor of the enabling system and maintenance factors of depression have been poorly studied, though there has been a focus on the role of support systems or intimate relationships being protective of depression. As described in further detail [91], this model can be used in the understanding and treatment of affective disorders, eating disorders, posttraumatic stress disorder, conduct disorders and delinquency, attention deficit hyperactivity disorders, anxiety disorders, sexual dependence, and personality disorders such as narcissistic and borderline disorders commonly associated with chemical dependency. A review article [92] on eating disorders demonstrates the utility of this approach with anorexia and bulimia and supports the further development of this model.

Though the psychiatric disorder is often seen as more likely to be associated with antecedents or concomitants in our biopsychosocial model, it can be a part of the maintenance factors for ACD. The concerns regarding the relationship between ACD and psychiatric disorder are similar to those described with adults [93]:

1. Axes I and II psychopathology may serve as a risk factor for addictive disorders.
2. Psychopathology may modify the course of an addictive disorder in terms of rapidity of course, response to treatment, symptom picture, and long-term outcome.
3. Psychiatric symptoms may develop in the course of chronic intoxications.
4. Some psychiatric disorders emerge as a consequence of use and persist into the period of remission.
5. Substance-using behavior and psychopathological symptoms (whether antecedent or consequent) will become meaningfully linked over the course of time.
6. Some psychopathological conditions occur in addicted individuals with no greater frequency than in the general population, suggesting that the psychiatric disorder and the addictive disorder are not specifically related.

In reference to the biopsychosocial model, in relationship 1, the psychiatric disorder is part of the antecedents to ACD, relationships 2 and 3 are concomitant factors, relationships 4 and 5 are concomitant factors that progress into maintenance factors, and relationship 6 describes a parallel process. Much controversy and confusion in the literature focus on narrow perspectives regarding one or two of these relationships, often assuming they were mutually exclusive determinants. A study with adults [69] demonstrated specifics regarding these relationships and assessed temporal relationships of drug and alcohol abuse and onset of psychiatric disorder. A similar study with adolescents has not been done and would be extremely valuable. However, Bukstein [82] reviews the comorbidity of multiple psychiatric disorders and substance abuse in adolescents with a focus on the specific relationships described above by Meyer.

This suggests that an important distinction to make is that of primary/secondary [86] based on temporal onset. Schuckit [94] suggests the use of age at which the person first met criteria for a diagnosis rather than onset of individual symptoms. Heuristically this is useful, but it must be tempered by the likelihood of distortion in historical recall, especially after extensive drug and alcohol use. The utility of this primary/secondary distinction, first of all, clarifies the presence of two or more biopsychosocial syndromes. It furthermore focuses attention on the specific relationship at a single point in time (satisfaction of criteria) and then allows further investigation to understand the ongoing, interactive relationship of two coincident syndromes.

The utility of this model is demonstrated by a study with another focus in time [95] of events precipitating hospital admission for substance abuse. Even though psychiatric diagnoses were not stated, the symptom complex of resistance to authority, family dysfunction, and/or academic failure in conjunction with substance abuse suggest the presence of coincident conduct disorder as related to hospitalization. A helpful addition would have been to make a distinction between primary and secondary onset.

Further support of this use of the biopsychosocial model comes from a review by Schubert [96] demonstrating the concurrent presence of alcohol, drug, and antisocial personality. They suggest that an elaboration of Donovan's [26] etiological model, the basis for this model, should be applied to each of these three diagnoses and treatment should be designed to address them holistically. Longitudinal studies [15–17] already described have assisted in defining some of these interactive effects.

A frequent difficulty relates to the simultaneous presence in adolescents of conduct disorder, attention deficit hyperactivity disorder, learning disabilities, and addiction. Ralph and Barr [25] review these concerns and elaborate on factors to be considered in assessing and treating these disorders.

VI. ASSESSMENT

The complexity in understanding adolescent chemical dependency (ACD) (drug and alcohol addiction) has made assessment difficult and poorly standardized. Blum [97] notes that

> as one reviews the literature on drug abuse assessment one is left with a disquieting feeling of an "Alice in Wonderland" definition, namely, that "drug abuse" means exactly what you would like it to mean.

The role of extent of use for many years was the measure of addiction. DSM-III [24] emphasized frequency of use and impairment in social functioning with the presence of tolerance being the distinguishing factor between abuse and dependence. Studies previously described began to reveal specific characteristics of the adolescent population that required a broader approach. The multiple drug use and the association with stages of a syndrome, including other "problem behaviors," was described. Owen and Nyberg [98] noted that adolescent chemical dependency programs varied greatly in their assessment of ACD with most relying on subjective judgement, and nonstandardized or adult measures. DSM-III-R has incorporated the expanded biopsychosocial focus and makes a distinction between abuse and dependence on the extent of problem areas involved and the presence of tolerance and/or withdrawal symptoms. This lacks the developmental approach that would make this more useful with teenagers. Other issues regarding assessment and adolescent and adult differences have been reviewed by Blum [97].

With the increasing need for treatment, increasing number of treatment programs, and increasing costs of providing care, the demands for accurate diagnosis have escalated. In 1982, the Chemical Dependency Adolescent Assessment Project (CDAAP) was initiated in Minnesota. Its purpose was to develop a clinical standardized assessment battery to aid professionals in the identification, referral, and treatment of problems associated with adolescent alcohol and drug involvement. The project comprehensively reviewed efforts to date of ACD assessment [85]. This project, supported by a National Institute of Drug Abuse (NIDA) initiative [99] has been a major impetus in coordinating professional efforts at understanding and treating this problem comprehensively. It will be described in detail as part of a comprehensive evaluation of adolescents.

A. NIDA Adolescent Assessment—Referral System

The recognition of the need for a comprehensive biopsychosocial model in addressing adolescent issues and the importance and urgency related to the ACD syndrome has prompted a unique situation for adolescent medicine and psychiatry. The NIDA has developed a comprehensive Adolescent Assessment and Referral System program to coordinate efforts nationwide and across disciplines (Fig. 4).

The assessment package begins with the Problem Oriented Screening Instrument for Teenagers (POSIT), which includes 139 true or false questions that can be self-administered in 20–30 min. It is designed to identify youth in need of further assessment in 10 domains:

1. Substance Use/Abuse
2. Physical Health Status
3. Mental Health Status
4. Family Relationships

```
            Initial Identification
     of Adolescent as High Risk Youth
                    ↓

PROBLEM ORIENTED SCREENING INSTRUMENT FOR TEENAGERS (POSIT)
          Target functional areas that
   require more comprehensive diagnostic assessment
                    ↓

          COMPREHENSIVE ASSESSMENT BATTERY
          Selected BATTERY measures and POSIT
   scores yield individualized diagnostic assessment
                    ↓

          DIRECTORY OF ADOLESCENT SERVICES
     Matching of individualized assessment with
          characteristics of treatment programs
```

Figure 4 Schematic model for the NIDA adolescent assessment–referral system.

5. Peer Relationships
6. Educational Status
7. Vocational Status
8. Social Skills
9. Leisure and Recreation
10. Aggressive Behavior/Delinquency

To assist in further evaluation of problem domains, a comprehensive assessment battery of specific recommended instruments has been developed. The assessment of the substance use/abuse is done with the CDAAP tools to be described. The results of this extensive assessment are to be used to determine referrals to appropriate treatment centers using a Directory of Adolescent Services currently being developed. It is hoped that these assessment tools and organized referral use will lead to the development of guidelines for optimal client–treatment matching as described by Hester and Miller [100].

B. Interviewing and Drug and Alcohol Addiction Assessment

Evaluation of drug and alcohol use/addiction begins with a complete history. Excellent reviews on the interviewing process and guidelines for clinicians are provided by Anglin [101] and Farrow and Deisher [102]. It is recommended that information obtained by personal interview follow the domains identified in the POSIT and those measured in the CDAAP assessment questionnaires. The interviewing situation may reveal unnoted areas, elaborate identified problem areas, or identify sensitive issues that are withheld on a questionnaire. Information must also be obtained from other sources such as parents, teachers, referral sources, or other agencies involved.

The CDAAP battery was developed to provide standardized measures of the ACD syndrome. It consists of three separate instruments: the Personal Experience Screen Questionnaire (PESQ), a drug abuse screening questionnaire; the Personal Experience Inventory (PEI), a multidimensional questionnaire; and the Adolescent Diagnostic Interview (ADI), a DSM-III-R–based diagnostic interview [24].

The Personal Experience Screen Questionnaire (PESQ)* is a 38-item, self-administered 15-min questionnaire designed to screen for severity of chemical involvement. It is useful as an initial screening tool for preassessment to decide if a more complete assessment is warranted. School and chemical dependency clinic norms have been collected. The design includes assessment of "faking" tendencies and the problem severity scale is correlated highly with a similar scale on the more comprehensive Personal Experience Inventory.

The Adolescent Diagnostic Interview (ADI)** is a structured diagnostic interview requiring 45–60 min to determine whether the client meets DSM-III-R [24] diagnostic criteria for psychoactive substance use disorders. It begins by reviewing client and family background and also includes Axes 4 and 5, severity of psychosocial stressors, and global level of functioning. It also briefly screens for six other mental disorders (affective, attention deficit, developmental, psychosis, eating, and anxiety) using approximately five screening questions for each in a yes/no format. Data demonstrate a high degree of reliability and that DSM-III-R [24] criteria for substance use disorders appear valid for adolescents.

The Personal Experience Inventory (PEI)** is a 300-item, 45- to 60-min self-administered questionnaire designed to comprehensively evaluate the adolescent chemical dependency syndrome. The PEI consists of two parts: a Chemical Involvement Problem Severity Section (CIPSS) and a Psychosocial Section.

The CIPSS was developed clinically and empirically with identification of five basic dimensions of chemical use:

1. Personal Involvement with Chemicals. Measures global chemical use problem severity. Items focus on the specific reinforcing properties of chemicals in altering mood state, and assess dependency-related features including self-medication and restructuring activities for use.
2. Effects From Use. Items relate to chemical use associated with aversive psychological, physiological, and behavioral effects such as feeling out of control.
3. Personal Consequences. Items related to difficulties with friends, parents, school, and social institutions as a result of use of chemicals.
4. Social Benefits Use. Items reflect use associated with increased social confidence, peer acceptance, and interpersonal skills.
5. Polydrug Use. Items survey use of seven drug categories (marijuana, stimulants, tranquilizers, "downers," cocaine, hallucinogens, and opioids) other than alcohol.

Findings by CDAAP suggest that these five dimensions can adequately assess the chemical use severity. They are correlated with the symptoms in DSM-III-R [24] substance use disorders, and reflect the multidimensional aspect of adolescent chemical dependency described previously. Using statistical analyses, questions regarding specificity of the "syndrome" concept, and the ability to identify independent dimensions of ACD were evaluated. Factor analysis of the five scales demonstrated that a single factor could account for over 70% of the total variance and was unable to demonstrate independent dimensions, supporting the clinically described concept of an ACD "syndrome."

Research conducted in developing the Personal Involvement with Chemicals subscale also investigated the stagelike progression of ACD. Items included clinical signs, symptoms, and behaviors based on a psychological involvement with chemicals trait continuum. Testing using this scale demonstrated the presence of stages that were identified as (1) social/ recreational use, (2) mood-related use, (3) adjustment of activities to accommodate use,

---

*PESQ available at Adolescent Assessment Project, Publishing Division, 907 W. Arlington, St. Paul, MN 55117.
**ADI, PEI available at Western Psychological Services, 12031 Wilshire Blvd, Los Angeles, CA 90025.

(4) engaging in deceptive or deviant behavior to accommodate use, and (5) use indicative of physiological adaptation [85]. These data support the concept involving states of progression of ACD described clinically by MacDonald [19]. It also indicated that the quality of progression was similar to symptom progression often associated with adult alcoholism.

The Psychosocial Section measures aspects of psychological functioning that have been shown to be antecedent, concomitant, or maintenance factors in ACD. A Personal Risk Factor subsection includes scales of (1) negative self-image, (2) psychological disturbance, (3) social isolation, (4) uncontrolled behavior, (5) rejecting convention, (6) deviant behavior, (7) absence of goals, and (8) spiritual isolation. An Environmental Risk Factor subsection includes scales of (1) peer chemical environment, (2) sibling chemical use, (3) family pathology, and (4) family estrangement. In addition, a Specific Problem Screen questions for (1) need for psychiatric referral, (2) eating disorder signs/symptoms, (3) sexual abuse, (4) physical abuse (intrafamilial), (5) family chemical dependency history, and (6) suicide potential. These readily provide a screen for psychiatric problems often associated with ACD and would require further and more extensive evaluation.

C. Medical Evaluation

History

A complete medical history and physical and neurological examinations are required. These will assess antecedent medical problems that may predispose to the ACD syndrome or to problems that have resulted from its development. Specific symptoms that should alert pediatricians and other practitioners to substance abuse include fatigue, recurrent abdominal pain, chest pain, headaches, chronic coughing, and sore throat [101]. Also important to note are the inflamed acneiform skin problems and muscle wasting found in the severe hallucinogen abuser.

Specific aspects of the history should include prenatal risk exposure (i.e., medication, maternal drug use, cigarette smoking, or illness), perinatal injury (i.e., prematurity, respiratory distress, anoxia, jaundice), developmental disability, chronic disease, allergies, and accidents. The presence of chronic illness (asthma, diabetes, familial hypercholesterolemia) provides an opportunity for further education about the effects of specific chemicals and may provide added incentive for abstinence.

Information regarding sexual development, including Tanner Stage, age of onset of puberty and relationship to peer's development, sexual activity, and practices, including associated use of drugs and alcohol, provide insight into aspects of self-esteem often related to drug use.

Laboratory Studies

Laboratory evaluation should include CBC (complete blood cell count) and a comprehensive clinical profile (SMA) to assess any medical problems that may be the result of chemical use. Medical conditions in the differential diagnosis of substance-induced organic mental disorders includes temporal lobe disorder and other neurological diseases or lesions, head trauma, toxic or metabolic disorders, including hypoglycemia, diabetic ketoacidosis, hyper- and hypothyroidism, adrenocortical disease, vitamin deficiencies, and viral illnesses. Urine toxicology screens for chemicals of abuse should be obtained and guidelines [103,104] are helpful. Sexually active teenagers should be screened for pregnancy and sexually transmitted diseases, including HIV (human immunodeficiency virus). An electrocardiogram may reveal cardiac abnormalities that with continued drug use may be life threatening. A sleep-deprived electroencephalogram may indicate signs of temporal lobe dysfunction or other organic mental conditions often associated with delinquent and aggressive behaviors [105]. Neuroendocrine testing, using the DST (dexamethasone suppression test) [106] or the TRH (thyrotropin-releasing hormone) test [107], are helpful in assessing possible antidepressant-responsive depressions. However, to limit the effects of prior drug use on these tests, a 2- to 3-week period of abstinence is suggested.

Psychiatric Assessment

The assessment of psychiatric status begins with assessment of psychoactive substance–induced organic mental disorders [24] to include: drug and alcohol intoxication, withdrawal, withdrawal delirium, hallucinosis, delusional disorder, alcohol amnestic syndrome, posthallucinogen perception disorder, and organic mood syndrome. Often the "organic" nature is only determined by resolution after 2- to 4-weeks of chemical abstinence.

Psychiatric disorders in the differential diagnosis of organic mental syndrome should include [24] schizophrenia and other nonorganic psychotic disorders, manic episode, depression, panic disorder, generalized anxiety disorder, and factitious disorder and malingering. Morrison and Smith [6] also include mental retardation, specific developmental disorders, attention deficit hyperactivity disorder, conduct disorder, oppositional disorder, and personality disorders. Assessment strategies should include questions to determine whether the onset of symptoms or behavior of the psychiatric disorder are predisposing antecedents, concomitants that are independent, precipitated by or a result of substance abuse, and/or maintenance factors. The Adolescent Diagnostic Interview (ADI) described as part of the CDAAP can be instrumental in this assessment. Another evaluation tool is the Diagnostic Interview Schedule for Children (DISC) [108] that is currently being revised for DSM-III-R [24] criteria.

The psychiatric assessment ideally should occur after the resolution of the substance-induced organic syndromes. This would allow for accurate diagnosis and lessen the chance of beginning treatment with psychotropic medications and committing the patient to an extended period of medication use, such as with lithium or tricyclic antidepressants. However, the presence of emergency situations such as acute psychosis, severe psychomotor retarded depression with psychotic features, or dangerous manic behaviors require modification. An assessment must be made immediately and medication started for the emergency situation, based on a tentative diagnosis. Attempts should be made to stabilize the emergency situation and in a later controlled setting, decrease or discontinue medication and repeat the psychiatric evaluation both medication- and drug-free. This will allow a clearer diagnosis to be made free of drug effects. The acuteness of the emergency situation, the possibility and problems of long-term psychotropic medication maintenance, the possibility of loss of the patient for treatment due to delay and increase of psychotic or paranoid ideation, and the likelihood of substance-induced organic factors must all be considered in these decisions.

D. Family Assessment

The family as a significant influence on predisposition, concomitant, and maintenance factors has been elaborated. Family assessment is crucial both in understanding the syndrome in the specific family and in developing them as a major ally in treatment. Use of the bio-psychosocial model framework requires a systems theory approach to families [46]. Obtaining a family genogram with emphasis on chemical abuse and psychiatric disorders opens discussion and allows education about the Disease Concept. Assessment of current family chemical use may alert staff to family denial or possible drug and alcohol addiction of family members. Specific family issues to be aware of are outlined [46]. The systems approach to family emphasizes interactions and relationships which are best demonstrated in family interviews with the patient and all family members present. A focus on assessing the developmental level of the family [62] and identifying specific issues will allow a family developmental context for the understanding of the teen's addiction.

A standardized questionnaire, the Family Assessment Measure (FAM), [109] uses a process model of family functioning and can be completed by client and parents in 30 min. The Family Assessment General Scale measures the health of a family along dimensions of task accomplishment, role performance, communication, affective expression, involvement, control, and values and norms. A Dyadic Relationship Scale measures the relationships between specific family member pairs on the same dimensions noted above. A Self-Rating Scale measures each individual's perception of their own functioning in the family unit.

E. Psychosocial Assessment

The psychosocial assessment identifies predisposing risk factors, concomitants, and maintenance characteristics in understanding the indidvual's addiction. It is also valuable in identifying specific psychosocial strengths to support recovery and weaknesses and behaviors that may block recovery. Specific questions relevant to this extensive part of the assessment are elaborated by Anglin [101]. Detailed questions about peer relationships and involvement in risk-taking activities may reveal deviant behaviors that suggest more severe psychopathology than assessed by structured interview. Especially important in some regions of the country is involvement in cultlike activities that may include satanism and its cruelty to animals or people. Specific questions about aggressive behaviors, runaway behaviors, past physical and sexual abuse, promiscuity, and evidence of compulsive sexual activity may alert clinicians to problems that while initially controlled may appear later during the stress of treatment.

REFERENCES

1. Engel, G.L. (1977). The need for a new medical model: A challenge for biomedicine. *Science, 196*(Apr):129–136.
2. Engel, G.L. (1980). The clinical application of the biopsychosocial model. *Am. J. Psychiatry 137*(5):535–544.
3. *National Household Survey on Drug Abuse* (1989). National Institute of Drug Abuse, Rockville, Maryland.
4. Johnston, L.D., O'Malley, P.M., and Bachman, J.G. (1989). *Drug Use, Drinking, and Smoking: National Survey Results from High School, College and Young Adult Populations 1975–1988*. National Institute of Drug Abuse, Rockville, Maryland.
5. Johnston, L.D., O'Malley, P.M., and Bachman, J.G. (1988). *Illicit Drug Use, Smoking, and Drinking by America's High School Students, College Students, and Young Adults*, 1975–1987. National Institute of Drug Abuse, Rockville, Maryland.
6. Morrison, M.A., and Smith, Q.T. (1987). Psychiatric issues of adolescent chemical dependence. *Pediatr. Clin. North Am., 34*(2):461–480.
7. Bailey, G.W. (1989). Current perspectives on substance abuse in youth. *J. Am. Acad. Child Adolesc. Psychiatry 28*(2):151–162.
8. Rogers, P.D. (ed.) (1987). *Chemical dependency, Pediatr. Clin. North Am., 34*(2) (entire issue).
9. Schwartz, G.E. (1982). Testing the biopsychosocial model: The ultimate challenge facing behavioral medicine? *J. Consult. Clin. Psychol., 50*(6):1040–1053.
10. Kuhn, T.S. (1970). *The Structure of Scientific Revolutions*. University of Chicago Press, Chicago, Illinois.
11. Jellinek, E.M. (1960). *The Disease Concept of Alcoholism*. Hillhouse, New Haven, Connecticut.
12. Sobell, M.B., and Sobell, L.C. (1976). Assessment of addictive behavior, *Behavioral Assessment: A Practical Handbook* (M. Hersen and A.S. Bellack, eds.), Pergamon, New York. pp. 305–336.
13. Kandel, D.B. (1975). Stages in adolescent involvement in drug use. *Science 190*:912–914.
14. Kandel, D., and Faust, R. (1975). Sequence and stages in patterns of adolescent drug use. *Arch. Gen. Psychiatry 32*:923–932.

15. Jessor, R., and Jessor, S.L. (1975). Adolescent development and the onset of drinking: A longitudinal study. *J. Stud. Alcohol, 36*(1):27–51.

16. Donovan, J.E., and Jessor, R. (1983). Problem drinking and the dimension of involvement with drugs: A Guttman scalogram analysis of adolescent drug use. *Am. J. Public Health, 73*(5):543–552.

17. Paton, S., Kessler, R., and Kandel, D. (1977). Depressive mood and adolescent illicit drug use: A longitudinal analysis. *J. Genet. Psychol., 131*:267–289.

18. Holland, S., and Griffin, A. (1984). Adolescent and adult drug treatment clients: Patterns and consequences of use. *J. Psychoactive Drugs, 16*(1):79–89.

19. MacDonald, D.I. (1984). Drugs, drinking and adolscence. *Am. J. Dis. Child., 138*(2):117–125.

20. Peele, S. (ed.) (1985). *The Meaning of Addiction: A Compuslive Experience and Its Interpretation*. Lexington Books, Lexington, Massachusetts.

21. Donovan, D.M., and Marlatt, G.A. (1988). *Assessment of Addictive Behaviors*. Guilford, New York.

22. *Diagnostic and Statistical Manual of Psychiatric Disorders*, 3rd ed. (1980). American Psychiatric Association, Washington, D.C.

23. Dackis, C.A., and Gold, M.S. (1985). New concepts in cocaine addiction: The dopamine depletion hypothesis. *Neurosci. Biobehav. Rev. 9*:469–477.

24. *Diagnostic and Statistical Manual of Mental Disorders*, 3rd ed.-Revised (1987). American Psychiatric Association, Washington, D.C.

25. Ralph, N., and Barr, M.A. (1989). Diagnosing attention-deficit hyperactivity disorder and learning disabilities with chemically dependent adolescents. *J. Psychoactive Drugs, 21*(2): 203–215.

26. Donovan, J.M. (1986). An etiologic model of alcoholism. *Am. J. Psychiatry, 143*(1):1–11.

27. Goodwin, D.W. (1986). Heredity and alcoholism. *Ann. Behav. Med., 8*:3–6.

28. Mendelson, J., and Mello, N. (eds.) (1984). *Diagnosis and Treatment of Alcoholism*. McGraw-Hill, New York.

29. Vesell, E.S., Page, J.G., and Passananti, G.T. (1971). Genetic and environmental factors affecting ethanol metabolism in man. *Clin. Pharmacol. Therapeut., 12*:192.

30. Schuckit, M., and Rayses, V. (1979). Ethanol ingestion: Differences in acetaldehyde concentration in relatives of alcoholics and controls. *Science, 203*:54–55.

31. Thomas, M., Halsall, P., and Peters, T.J. (1982). Role of hepatic acetaldehyde dehydrogenase in alcoholism. *Lancet 8307*(2):1057–1059.

32. Schuckit, M.A., and Gold, E.O. (1988). A simultaneous evaluation of multiple markers of ethanol/placebo challenges in sons of alcoholics and controls. *Arch. Gen. Psychiatry, 45*(3):211–216.

33. Myers, R.D. (1978). Tetrahydroisoquinolines in the brain: The basis of an animal model of alcoholism. Alcoholism Clin. Exp. Res., 2:145–154.

34. Isralowitz, R., and Singer, M. (eds.) (1983). *Adolescent Substance Abuse: A Guide to Prevention and Treatment*. Haworth, New York.

35. Smith, G.M. (1986). Adolescent personality traits that predict young adult drug use. *Comprehen. Ther., 12*(2):44–50.

36. Vaillant, G.E. (1983). *The Natural History of Alcoholism*. Harvard University Press, Cambridge, Massachusetts.

37. Donovan, J.E., Jessor, R., and Jessor, L. (1983). Problem drinking in adolscence and young adulthood: A follow-up study. *J. Stud. Alcohol, 44*(1):109–137.

38. Kandel, D.B., and Raveis, V.H. (1989). Cessation of illicit drug use in young adulthood. *Arch. Gen. Psychiatry, 46*:109–116.

39. Carroll, J.F. (1986). Treating multiple substance abuse clients, *Recent Developments in Alcoholism*, Vol. 4. (M. Galanter, ed.), Plenum, New York, pp. 85–103.

40. Kauffman, J.F., Schaffer, H., and Burglass, M.E. (1985). The biological basics: Drugs and their effects, *Alcoholism and Substance Abuse: Strategies for Clinical Intervention*. (T.E. Bratter and G.G. Foerrest, eds.), Free Press, New York, pp. 107–136.

41. Newcomb, A.D., and Harlow, L.L. (1986). Life events and substance use among adolescents: Mediating effects of perceived loss of control and meaninglessness in life. *J. Personal. Soc. Psychol., 51*(3):564–577.

42. Newcomb, M.D., Maddahian, E., Skager, R., and Bentler, P.M. (1987). Substance abuse and psychosocial risk factors among teenagers: Association with sex, age, ethnicity and type of school. *Am. J. Drug Alcohol Abuse, 13*(4):413-433.
43. Wegscheider, S. (1981). *Another Choice: Hopes and Health for the Alcoholic Family.* Science and Behavior Books, Palo Alto, California.
44. Chatlos, J.C. (1987. *Crack: What You Should Know About the Cocaine Epidemic.* Putnam, New York.
45. Singer, M., and Anglin, T. (1986). The identification of adolescent substance abuse by health care professionals. *Int. J. Addict., 21*(2):247-254.
46. Huberty, D.J., Huberty, C.E., Hobday, K.F., and Blackmore, G. (1987). Family issues in working with chemically dependent adolescents, *Pediatr. Clin. North Am., 34*(2):507-521.
47. Winters, K. (1990). The need for improved assessment of adolscent substance involvement. *J. Drug Issues, 20*:487-502.
48. Gitlow, S.E., and Peyser, H.S. (eds.) (1980). *Alcoholism: A Practical Treatment Guide.* Grune & Stratton, New York.
49. Ray, B.A. (ed.) (1988). *Learning Factors in Substance Abuse.* National Institute of Drug Abuse, Research Monograph 84, Rockville, Maryland, pp. 122-140.
50. Talbott, G.D. (1984). Substance abuse and the professional provider: The need for new attitudes about addiction. *Ala. J. Med. Sci., 21*(2):150-155.
51. Bickel, W.K., and Kelly, T.H. (1988). The relationship of stimulus control to the treatment of substance abuse. *Learning Factors in Substance Abuse* (B.A. Ray, ed.), National Institute of Drug Abuse, Research Monograph 84. Rockville, Maryland, pp. 122-140.
52. Kandel, D.B., and Logan, J.A. (1984). Patterns of drug use from adolescence to young adulthood: I. Periods of risk for initiation, continued use and discontinuation. *Am. J. Public Health, 74*:660-666.
53. Wheeler, K., and Malmquist, J. (1987). Treatment approaches in adolescent chemical dependency. *Pediatr. Clin. North Am., 34*(2):437-447.
54. Garfinkel, B., Froese, A., and Hood J. (1982). Suicide attempts in children and adolescents. *Am. J. Psychiatry, 139*:1257-1261.
55. Douglass, R.L. (1983). Youth, alcohol and traffic accidents. *Recent Dev. Alcohol.* , Vol. 1:347-366, Plenum, New York.
56. Bass, J., Gallagher, S., and Mehta, K. (1985). Unintentional injuries among adolescents and young adults. *Pediatr. Clin. North Am., 23*:31-39.
57. Friedman, J. (1985). Alcohol and unnatural deaths in San Francisco youths. *Pediatrics, 76*:191-193.
58. Kaufman, E. (1985). Adolescent substance abusers and family therapy, *Handbook of Adolescents and Family Therapy.* Gardner Press, New York, pp. 245-254.
59. Kaufman, E. (1981). Family structures of narcotics addicts. *Int. J. Addict., 16*(2):273-282.
60. Gibbs, J.T. (1982). Psychosocial factors related to substance abuse among delinquent females: Implications for prevention and treatment. *Am. J. Orthopsychiatry, 52*(2):261-271.
61. Kandel, D.B. Kessler, R., and Margulies, R. (1978). Antecedents of adolescent initiation into stages of drug abuse. *J. Youth Adolesc., 7*:13-40.
62. Preto, N.G. (1988). Transformation of the family system in adolescence, *The Changing Family Life Cycle: A Framework for Family Therapy*, (B. Carter and M. McGoldrick, eds.), Gardner Press, New York, pp. 255-283.
63. Levine, B.L. (1985). Adolescent substance abuse: Toward an integration of family systems and individual adaptation theories. *Am. J. Fam. Ther., 13*(2):3-16.
64. Schwartzman, J. (1975). The addict, abstinence and the family. *Am. J. Psychiatry, 132*(2):154-157.
65. Cleveland, M. (1981). Families and adolescent drug use: Structural analysis of children's roles. *Fam. Proc., 20*:295-304.
66. Reilly, D.M. (1984). Family therapy with adolescent drug abusers and their families: Defying gravity and achieving escape velocity. *J. Drug Issues, 2*:381-391.
67. Reilly, D.M. (1976). Family factors in the etiology and treatment of youthful drug abuse. *Fam. Ther., 2*:149-171.

68. Mirin, S.M., Weiss, R.D., Michael, J., and Griffin, M.L. (1988). Psychopathology in substance abusers: Diagnosis and treatment. *Am. J. Drug Alcohol Abuse, 14*(2):139–157.
69. Ross, H.E., Glaser, F.B., and Germanson, T. (1988). The prevalence of psychiatric disorders in patients with alcohol and other drug problems. *Arch. Gen. Psychiatry, 45*(11):1023–1031.
70. Alterman, A.I. (ed.) (1985). *Substance Abuse and Psychopathology*. Plenum, New York.
71. Famularo, R., Stone, K., and Popper, C. (1985). Pre-adolescent alcohol abuse and dependence. *Am. J. Psychiatry., 142*(10):1187–1189.
72. Robins, L.N. (1978). Sturdy childhood predictors of adult antisocial behavior: Replications from longitudinal studies. *Psychol. Med., 8*:611–622.
73. Cantwell, D.P. (1978). Hyperactivity and antisocial behavior. *J. Am. Acad. Child Psychiatry, 17*:252–262.
74. Pyle, R.L., Mitchell, J.E., and Eckert, E.D. (1981). Bulimia: A report of 34 cases. *J. Clin. Psychiatry, 42*:60–64.
75. Masterson, J.F. (1972). *Treatment of the Borderline Adolescent: A Developmental Approach*. Wiley Interscience, New York.
76. Kashani, J.H., Keller, M.B., Solomon, N., Reid, J.C., and Mazzola, D. (1985). Double depression in adolescent substance abusers. *J. Affect. Disorders, 8*:153–157.
77. Clayton, R.R. (1986). Multiple drug use. *Recent Dev. Alcohol., 4*:7–38.
78. Gittelman, R., Mannuzza, S., Shenker, R., and Bonagura, N. (1985). Hyperactive boys almost grown up. I. Psychiatric status. *Arch. Gen. Psychiatry, 42*(10)937–947.
79. Loranger, A.W., and Tullis, E.H. (1985). Family history of alcoholism in borderline personality disorderes. *Arch. Gen. Psychiatry, 42*(2):153–157.
80. Fowler, R.C., Rich, C.L., and Young, D. (1986). San Diego suicide study II. Substance abuse in young cases. *Arch. Gen. Psychiatry, 43*(10):962–965.
81. Rich, C.L., Fowler, R.C., Fogarty, L.A., and Young, D. (1988). San Diego suicide study III. Relationships between diagnosis and stressor. *Arch. Gen. Psychiatry, 45*(6):589–592.
82. Bukstein, O.G., Brent, D.A., and Kaminer, Y. (1989). Comorbidity of substance abuse and other psychiatric disorders in adolescents. *Am. J. Psychiatry, 146*(9):1131–1141.
83. Roehrich, H., and Gold, M.S. (1986). Diagnosis of substance abuse in an adolescent psychiatric population. *Int. J. Psychiatry Med., 16*(2):137–143.
84. Roehrich, H.G., Jonas, J.M., and Gold, M.S. (1988). Phenomenology of adolescent drug addiction (personal communication).
85. Winters, K. (1990). Clinical considerations in the assessment of adolescent chemical dependency. *J. Adolesc. Chem. Depend., 1*:31–52.
86. Kranzler, H.R., and Liebowitz, N.R. (1988). Anxiety and depression in substance abuse: Clinical implications. *Med. Clin. North Am., 72*(4):867–883.
87. Gershon, E.S., Berrettini, W.H., and Goldin, L.R. (1989). Mood disorders: Genetics, *Comprehensive Textbook of Psychiatry V*. (H. Kaplan and B. Sadock, eds.), Williams & Wilkins, Baltimore, Vol. 1, pp. 879–888.
88. Schildkraut, J.J., Green, A.I., and Mooney, J.J. (1989). Mood disorders: Biochemical aspects. *Comprehensive Textbook of Psychiatry V*. (H. Kaplan and B. Sadock, eds.), Williams and Wilkins, Baltimore, Vol. 1, pp. 868–879.
89. Mollica, R.F. (1989). Mood disorders: Epidemiology. *Comprehensive Textbook of Psychiatry V*. H. Kaplan and B. Sadock, eds.), Williams & Wilkins, Baltimore, Vol. 1, pp. 859–868.
90. Hirschfeld, M.A., and Cross, C.K. (1982). Epidemiology of affective disorder: Psychosocial risk factors. *Arch. Gen. Psychiatry, 39*(1):35–46.
91. Chatlos, J.C. (1989). Adolescent dual diagnosis: A 12 step transformational model. *J. Psychoactive Drugs, 21*(2):189–201.
92. Yates, A. (1989). Current perspectives on the eating disorders: I. History, psychological and biological aspects. *J. Am. Acad. Child and Adolesc. Psychiatry, 28*(6):813–828.
93. Meyer, R.E. (1986). How to understand the relationship between psychopathology and addictive disorders: Another example of the chicken and the egg, *Psychopathology and Addictive Disorders*. (R.E. Meyer, ed.), Guilford, New York, pp. 3–16.

94. Schuckit, M. (1985). The clinical implications of primary diagnostic groups among alcoholics. *Arch. Gen. Psychiatry, 42*:1043–1049.

95. Williams, R.A., Feibelman, N.D., and Moulder, C. (1989). Events precipitating hospital treatment of adolescent drug abusers. *J. Am. Acad. Child Adolesc. Psychiatry, 28*(1):70–73.

96. Schubert, D.S., Wolf, A.W., Patterson, M.B., Grands, T.P., and Pendleton, L. (1988). A statistical evaluation of the literature regarding the associations among alcoholism, drug abuse, and antisocial personality disorder. *Int. J. Addict., 23*(8):797–808.

97. Blum, R.W. (1987). Adolescent substance abuse: Diagnostic and treatment issues. *Pediatr. Clin. North Am., 34*(2):523–537.

98. Owen, P.L., and Nyberg, L.R. (1983). Assessing alcohol and drug problems among adolescents: Current practices. *J. Drug Ed., 13*:249–254.

99. Rahdert, E.R., and Grabowski, J. (eds.) (1988). *Adolescent Drug Abuse: Analyses of Treatment Research*. National Institute of Drug Abuse Research Monograph 77. Rockville, Maryland.

100. Hester, R.K., and Miller, W.R. (1988). Empirical guidelines for optimal client-treatment matching, *Adolescent Drug Abuse: Analyses of Treatment Research* (E.R. Rahdert and J. Grabowski, eds.), National Institute of Drug Abuse, Research Monograph 77. Rockville, Maryland, pp. 27–39.

101. Anglin, T.A. (1987). Interviewing guidelines for the clinical evaluation of adolescent substance abuse. *Pediatr. Clin. North Am., 34*(2):381–398.

102. Farrow, J.A., and Deisher, R. (1988). A practical guide to the office assessment of adolescent substance abuse. *Pediatr. Ann., 15*:675–684.

103. Mackenzie, R.G., Cheng, M., and Haftel, A.J. (1987). The clinical utility and evaluation of drug screening techniques. *Pediatr. Clin. North Am., 34*(2):423–435.

104. Gold, M.S., and Dackis, C.A. (1986). Role of the laboratory in the evaluation of suspected drug use. *J. Clin. Psychiatry, 47*:17–23.

105. Lewis, D.O. (1983). Neuropsychiatric vulnerabilities and violent juvenile delinquency. *Psychiatr. Clin. North Am., 6*(4):707–714.

106. Carroll, B.J. (1986). Informed use of the dexamethasone suppression test. *J. Clin. Psychiatry, 47*(1):10–12.

107. Extein, I., and Gold, M.S. (1986). Psychiatric applications of thyroid tests. *J. Clin. Psychiatry, 47*(1):13–16.

108. Costello, A. (1987). Structured interviewing for the assessment of child psychopathology, *Basic Handbook of Child Psychiatry: Advances and New Directions* (J. Noshpitz, ed.), Basic Books, New York, pp. 143–152.

109. Skinner, H., Steinhauer, P., and Santa-Barbera, J. (1983). The Family Assessment Measure. *Canad. J. Commun. Ment. Health, 2*:91–105.

13

Adolescent Drug and Alcohol Addiction: Intervention and Treatment

J. Calvin Chatlos
St. Mary Hospital, Hoboken, New Jersey

I. INTRODUCTION

This chapter on intervention and treatment provides an extension of the ideas presented in Chapter 12 on Adolescent Drug and Alcohol Addiction: Diagnosis and Assessment. The treatment approach presented is based on the biopsychosocial disease model previously described and focuses on a comprehensive treatment for adolescents.

As the extent and severity of teenagers with drug use has increased during the past 10 years, the urgency and interest in treatment has followed. Treatment programs have proliferated even though research documenting the superiority of any single approach with adolescents has not been done. Adolescent chemical dependency (ACD) (drug and alcohol addiction) treatment has been mostly based on successful adult treatment programs developed by the Johnson Institute and Hazelden Foundation in Minnesota. This Minnesota Model [1,2] involves a short to intermediate inpatient program (28–60 days) with an intensive group therapy approach based on the Disease Concept and the 12 Steps of Alcoholics Anonymous (AA) [3] using chemical dependency counselors as primary therapists. Acute care is generally followed by extended aftercare for several months to over a year. Alternative care such as outpatient programs or day treatment programs have been developed using the concepts, approaches, and techniques already proven successful.

II. TREATMENT PROGRAMS

Treatment programs have generally been divided into outpatient, inpatient, residential, day care, and aftercare components. A review by Hoffman [1] of the various treatment approaches discusses some of the philosophic and practical dimensions regarding ACD treatment. In accord with most state mental health laws, treatment is to be accomplished in the "least restrictive setting." Currently, the determination of this has been poorly based on research and is usually determined by physical and economic availability [2]. The Cleveland Hospital in Cleveland, Ohio [4] has developed criteria for determining levels of care that are currently being tested for validity. Hoffman [1] reviews multiple issues regarding evaluation of ACD programs, assessment of outcome, and the information learned from CATOR [5]—a chemical abuse/addiction treatment outcome registry. The CATOR report includes symptom reports on about 2000 adolescents in treatment and outcome data on almost 1000. The broad range of demographic data provides information regarding treatment needs for these teenagers. A major impetus in research at this time is to provide guidelines to match specific client characteristics with specific treatment approaches [6]. Since few studies have been done on adolescents, potentially predictive variables have been derived from adult literature. These include: (1) problem severity, including problem duration, severity of dependence, or consequences; (2) concomitant psychopathology; (3) social stability, including measures of family functioning and dynamics; (4) neuropsychological functioning; (5) personality characteristics; (6) cognitive style; (7) locus of control; (8) perceived choice; (9) family history; and (10) stage of change.

III. ASSESSMENT

Clinically, many adolescent treatment programs determine treatment based on an assessment of the severity of the syndrome. Using descriptions of the stages [7] of progression of drug use from experimental to severe chemical dependency often guides the intervention and treatment placement.

A. Stage 1

An adolescent in Stage 1 of experimental use has usually had few consequences to motivate him or her for treatment. Even during later aspects of this stage, denial may limit patient and/or family motivation. If the teenager and family acknowledge a problem, intervention consists of education and counseling. These focus on the biopsychosocial disease model and ACD syndrome as described in Chapter 12, as well as specific medical consequences of drug use. The goal of this intervention (primary prevention) is to limit progression or to develop abstinence (Fig. 1). If the teen or family recognizes use but does not acknowledge a problem, an "abstinence contract" [8] is useful. An agreement is made with the clinician that the client will remain free of mood-altering drugs for a specified time, usually 4–6 weeks, which should involve urine screening. During that time, regular (at least weekly) contact should assess abstinence as well as refusal of opportunities to use, difficulty of refusal, necessity of changing lifestyle or social situations to avoid use, mood during abstinence, and extent, nature, and situation of drug urges if present. An inability to maintain this abstinence contract demonstrates severity of chemical dependency that is likely beyond Stage 1. This will also break through denial and open the family system to outpatient treatment.

B. Stage 2

A person at Stage 2, often referred to as regular use or abuse, may also have denial and difficulty acknowledging a problem. Occasionally at this stage, the teenager may recognize a problem and the family does not or vice versa. Abstinence contracting assists in demonstrating the extent of the problem and developing a family unity in seeking treatment as an outpatient (secondary prevention).

  Outpatient treatment is noted [9] to be fraught with denial of the problem by the client and/or family, basic adolescent mistrust of adult authority, continued association with addicts peer groups, unwillingness to abstain, and lack of motivation. These must be considered in the treatment choice. Other criteria outlined for outpatient treatment [10] include:

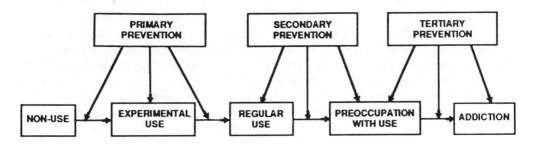

Figure 1 Types of intervention and stages of chemical dependency.

1. Absence of acute medical and/or psychiatric problems
2. Absence of chronic medical problems that would preclude outpatient treatment
3. Willingness to abstain from all mood-altering chemicals, and cooperation with random urine testing
4. No prior outpatient treatment failure
5. Extent to which the family is interested and able to become involved in treatment
6. Precipitant and motivation for treatment

Because Stage 2 use includes use of drugs to cope with stress and affective stages, more emphasis is required in assessing other areas of dysfunction and on psychotherapy and coping skills. Emphasis on group process and 12-Step self-help group support is useful. Outpatient treatment at this stage must be intensive and extended [11] to convey the seriousness of the problem and the commitment that is needed for successful treatment. Filstead and Anderson [11] describe a program of four times per week for 4 weeks, followed by twice a week for 4 weeks, and then once weekly for 12 weeks. During this course of treatment the family is expected to participate twice per week, once with the client as a total family unit and once as the parental couple. It is expected that parents will actively attend Alanon or Families Anonymous during this course of treatment while the teenager attends Alcoholics Anonymous (AA) and/or Narcotics Anonymous (NA).

Some rules have been described [11] that if violated during outpatient care lead to recommendations for a more restricted treatment setting, usually an inpatient setting. The rules are (1) no use of alcohol or other drugs for any reason, (2) no violent behavior, (3) regular attendance at therapy sessions, and (4) AA/NA meeting attendance. If any use of chemicals is suspected, urine screens are requested.

C. Stage 3

Stage 3, preoccupation with use demonstrates a significant drug and/or alcohol addiction. At this stage, many programs recommend inpatient treatment (tertiary prevention). This allows a structured environment to complete a comprehensive assessment and to maintain control and security to deal with any physical symptoms of withdrawal, or severe impulsiveness related to significant urges to use drugs or to act out (e.g., suicide, violence, sexual urges). The presence of any significant medical or psychiatric illness indicates the need for inpatient treatment.

During the initial evaluation, families may be resistant to the recommendation for inpatient care owing to a poor understanding of addiction, denial of the seriousness of the problem, poor understanding of the treatment process, or fears about inpatient settings. A trial at outpatient treatment often is used to educate families in chemical dependency. Similar to the contracting method noted above, it often demonstrates the teenager's inability to abstain and participate in an outpatient treatment program. This use of outpatient treatment assists families in benefitting more from the subsequent inpatient treatment referral. However, the person at Stage 3 is often engaged in more dangerous behaviors—socially and with more dangerous drugs. Failure at outpatient treatment may mean loss of the opportunity for inpatient treatment owing to stubborn refusal, runaway behaviors, or even worse—death due to accidents, overdose, homicide, or suicide, which is common in this stage [12–15]. Treatment in Stage 3 is often a psychiatric or medical emergency and may require immediate inpatient treatment or a very highly structured outpatient treatment (such as a partial day care program) with a motivated patient *and* family.

D. Stage 4

Stage 4 addiction constitutes an emergency crisis situation with teenagers and they should be treated as inpatients. The degree of structure and support needed to assess and treat associated medical and psychiatric problems, as well as to sustain treatment with severe cravings and urges to act impulsively requires inpatient support. This often requires not only the support of the family, but also that of the school, job, and often legal system.

IV. INPATIENT TREATMENT—A 12-STEP TRANSFORMATIONAL MODEL

Some practitioners believe that the only effective treatment for adolescent drug and alcohol addiction is inpatient treatment [2]. As described, a more usual approach is for adolescents that are in the later stages of daily preoccupation and severe addiction to be referred for inpatient treatment. As noted earlier, research efforts are aimed at screening ACD patients and matching them to a specific program or aspects of the program. Because of unresolved controversies regarding the length of time after abstinence that drug effects persist, the best time to evaluate for psychiatric psychopathology, the presence of extended denial in adolescents, and the need for a comprehensive approach to treatment in adolescents, these attempts may be limited. Therefore, ACD treatment must be approached as an extended evaluation concurrent with a comprehensive treatment.

The Transformational Model [16] developed at the Adolescent Center for Chemical Education Prevention and Treatment (ACCEPT) at Fair Oaks Hospital, Summit, N.J. provides a comprehensive treatment program. The structure provides an ongoing evaluation of disorders that leads to the clarification of specific needs for successful recovery. This program is designed to treat dual diagnosis patients, since the criteria for inpatient admission as described select a population that is predominantly dually diagnosed. This section will provide a detailed description of the ACCEPT inpatient treatment program to demonstrate many of the successful principles that can be modified in other settings. Often these modifications are determined by management factors such as staffing patterns, quality of staff, intensity and frequency of therapy, extensiveness of evaluation capabilities, and many economic factors. The principles of this model are adaptable to any inpatient or outpatient setting within the limitations noted.

This treatment design is based on the Minnesota Model with emphasis on group therapy, and has been described elsewhere [16] with a case study presentation. Concepts from short-term dynamic psychotherapy as developed by Davanloo [17,18] have been instrumental in the development of this model and the understanding of the biopsychosocial model presented earlier (see Chap. 12). Certain factors define this program:

1. Use of drug and alcohol addiction biopsychosocial disease model
2. Use of psychiatric biopsychosocial disease model

3. Treatment of the biological part of each disorder first
4. Emphasis on the "family disease" aspects of addiction and psychiatric disorders
5. Focus on a commitment to abstinence
6. Therapeutic progression using the 12 Steps of AA/NA
7. Structured program emphasizing "discipline" in recovery

For many inpatient programs where the focus is primarily on the psychiatric disorder, not using a 12-step approach, the use of this model must be modified. A structure must be arranged so that the issues of each Step as described are addressed. A specific program design incorporating these ideas within a psychiatric framework has not yet been described, partly owing to the lack of "spiritual" focus in psychiatric treatments.

The drug and alcohol addiction biopsychosocial model as presented fosters a systemic, holistic understanding of data gathered during the evaluation and guides understanding of further information obtained by the structured treatment process. The emphasis on chemical dependency as a disease assists families and patients in working through severe guilt feelings and the sense of being a failure, both prominent initially in treatment. Owing to its inclusion of "maintenance factors" and the enabling system, it fosters acceptance of responsibility in taking action to stop these behaviors and to stop the progression of the disease. This balance is often critical as some families use their "disease" to defensively continue to deny their responsibility in the process, and others victimizingly paralyze themselves by taking on full responsibility with resulting self-pity. An attempt to have each family member understand their role in the different factors in the equation is the initial focus in treatment.

As the addiction biopsychosocial model is presented, the use of this model in understanding the psychiatric disorders and dual or multiple diagnoses is also explained. Using this model with families fosters a holistic focus on the problem rather than splitting a focus on chemical dependency and/or a focus on psychiatric disorder. Clinical experience on dual diagnosis treatment units demonstrates how teenagers and family members can effectively use the focus on any single part of the problem (e.g., bulimia) to defensively block treatment progress. The position stated, "I'm only here for my bulimia, not my drug use!" assists continued denial.

Treatment requires a commitment to abstinence from drug and alcohol use. This is a long-term commitment that is renewed one day at a time. Most treatment programs believe this should be a life-long commitment to abstinence [1]. With information that adolescents grow out of substance abuse [19], further research about the need for abstinence is needed. However, the study by Kandel and Raveis [19] suggests that those young people that initiate drug and alcohol use at an early age and have extensive use are the ones that progress and are abusing chemicals years later. It is this group that is usually assessed at Stages 3 and 4, requiring inpatient treatment.

The requirement for abstinence is based on the understanding of chemical dependency as a primary illness, as described previously. This concept actually has two different parts that confuse clinicians owing to the terminology. First, the *primary* intervention must be removal of the drug from the person's system in order to stop progression of the illness. Second, since an autonomous primary disorder has developed, once the drug is removed physically, the person will continue with many of the patterned behaviors—drug urges and cravings, impulsiveness, paranoia, fearfulness, and distrust—that are now the focus of treatment. For this to occur, ACD must be treated as a major or primary focus with continued abstinence being a necessary part of treatment.

This is not to be confused with the distinction primary/secondary as noted in the chapter on assessment (see Chap. 12, Sect. III). This temporal distinction is helpful in understanding the development and interactions of the multiple syndromes. However, in the presence of drug and alcohol use and with the focus on treatment, this distinction has limitations. Primarily owing to historical recall being distorted by the use of drugs and alcohol, Kranzler and Liebowitz [20] suggest the treatment utility of distinctions based on persistence of symptoms. They describe characteristic symptoms of the transient states due to use of alcohol, stimulants, opiates, and sedative/hypnotics. As described in the chapter on assessment (See Chap. 12, Sect. VI.C), these drug-induced organic disorders must be resolved prior to an adequate psychiatric evaluation and treatment.

Following abstinence from alcohol or drugs, resolution of the organic disorders, and psychiatric evaluation, pharmacotherapy may be indicated for the persistent symptoms. Since there are no studies that have demonstrated the specific efficacy of medication in drug and addicted adolescents, intervention is guided by clinical and research experience with adults [21–23] or with non–drug addicted adolescents [24]. Clinical experience with ACD and dual diagnosis patients has shown similar responses of anxiety and depressive disorders, bulimia, posttraumatic stress, obsessive-compulsive, intermittent explosive, and personality disorders as has been demonstrated with adults.

In many cases, it is the expression and persistence of symptoms that is treated rather than a "disorder" satisfying full DSM-III-R (*Diagnostic and Statistical Manual of Mental Disorders*, 3rd Edition-Revised, American Psychiatric Association, Washington, D.C., 1987) criteria, especially those that are time related. For instance:

A 16-year-old girl with extensive cocaine and alcohol abuse was admitted for treatment. Initially she was mildly depressed and guarded but cooperative and engaged in treatment. During the subsequent 10 days, her affect became more depressed and tearful with psychomotor retardation, with paranoid ideation developing into delusions with ideas of reference, and a morbid preoccupation with death and past deaths of relatives. A dexamethasone suppression test done at 2 weeks abstinence failed to suppress. She was started on nortriptyline with increasing doses. Her mood responded within 4 days with decreased psychomotor retardation, but progressed to be euphoric with giggling, laughing inappropriately, and flight of ideas. She was diagnosed as having bipolar disorder, though there was no prior history of hypomanic or manic episodes and she did not satisfy time criteria for this disorder. She responded well and completed treatment maintained on lithium.

In addition to persistence of symptoms, in the structured program to be described, the failure to progress in an expected time, associated with significant intensity of symptoms, is often an indication for pharmacotherapy.

Thus, after resolution of the organic syndrome, in some patients in whom a psychiatric disorder is not diagnosable by history, progress through the structured treatment may precipitate symptoms that must then be treated pharmacologically. This is often seen with the development of panic attacks:

A 15-year-old female with a history of parental divorce at age 7 followed by multiple geographic moves was admitted with extensive cocaine, marijuana, and alcohol abuse. She was diagnosed as having conduct disorder with a history since junior high school of progressively increasing antisocial behaviors—poor school motivation, truancy, shoplifting, stealing, runaway episodes, and physical fights with involvement with knives. She also had a history of being raped at age 13, and since then had made a serious suicide attempt. She has also been involved for 2 years with satanism, including daily rituals and prior animal sacrifice.

She expressed motivation in treatment, but as she dealt with her involvement in satanism she developed extreme anxiety with sweating, restlessness, and palpitations.

During some group sessions this would occur and panic attacks would necessitate removal from groups. Since this appeared to have a separation anxiety component, she was started on imipramine, which was increased to 100 mg/day. During the next 5 days, her mood fluctuated with increasingly frightening dreams and thoughts about attacking a patient with a knife. As she was less overwhelmed by her panic while on medications, issues were worked through regarding rage at her father, the desire for power and revenge associated with satanism, and the guilt and fear of dying associated with betrayal of satan. Breakthroughs into feelings of loneliness and self-hatred were sufficient to continue treatment without further panic attacks.

The structured treatment program is designed to continually assess and explore the interface between psychobiological and psychodynamic aspects of disorders and treatment.

V. PSYCHOTHERAPEUTIC APPROACH

Traditionally, the psychotherapeutic approach to a chemically dependent person would be to attempt an understanding of their psychological development. By understanding specific issues and conflicts related to past life experiences, it was believed that the end result would be abstinence of drug use as diagrammed (Fig. 2). With addicts, knowledge and insight often did not lead to action regarding abstinence from chemical use. A more empowering approach is to begin with a commitment to abstinence. This has been known and utilized for years by the founders of Alcoholics Anonymous:

> But the actual or potential alcoholic, with hardly an exception, will be absolutely unable to stop drinking on the basis of self-knowledge [3].

The AA program *begins* with this commitment to abstinence.

As noted, once detoxification is complete and evidence of any significant drug-induced organic syndrome is absent, beginning with the commitment to abstinence leads to predictable effects. As teenagers meaningfully verbalize this commitment, certain emotional and behavioral reactions occur. These reactions display patterns of behavior that demonstrate their specific and individual psychobiological history. These patterns are referred to as "structures from the past" (Fig. 3), a neutral term that allows discussion by psychoanalytic therapists, self psychologists, developmental psychologists, behaviorists and learning theorists, cognitive and rational-emotive theorists, systems theorists, and others.

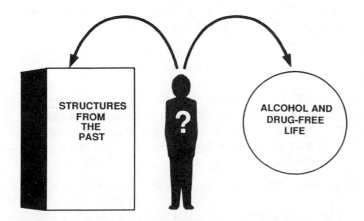

Figure 2 Traditional psychotherapeutic model.

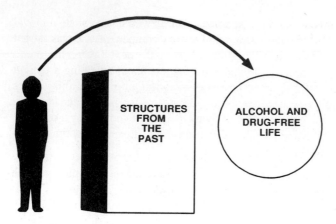

Figure 3 Commitment to recovery.

These patterns or structures from the past are the result of learned coping patterns, including ego defenses, perceptual and cognitive distortions that may or may not have occurred during drug use, and urges. Urges are vague poorly differentiated feelings that are strong motivators to specific actions, such as drug urges, sex urges, binge/purge urges, violence urges, or suicidal and self-mutilative urges. Understanding and working with urges is a key to successful transformation toward recovery. The focus on urges incorporates ideas presented in Chapter 12 regarding a possible biochemical-genetic barrier, and the concept of primary. The presence of urges demonstrates how the addiction is grafted onto the preexisting behavior and personality structure, creating a new and autonomous entity.

Using the biopsychosocial model with dual diagnosis patients requires that the commitment to abstinence be extended. As with addiction, other disorders such as depression, bulimia, posttraumatic stress disorder, sexual dependency, and attention deficit hyperactivity disorder become primary. Whatever the temporal process of predisposition to psychiatric disorder, events or drug interaction, and enabling or maintenance factors, the psychiatric disorder eventually acquires characteristics that are autonomous. Similar to addiction, the physiological aspects interact with emotional and behavioral learning and conditioning that are maintained by an enabling system. Therefore, as with chemical dependency, once the biological component of the psychiatric disorder is addressed, as with medications, a commitment to abstinence must still be the beginning. Because multiple disorders are being treated, this means a commitment to no drugs, no binging, purging, or compulsive dieting, and no sex, no depression, and no impulsive violent or suicidal behaviors.

VI. 12 STEPS

Because it is unrealistic to expect teenagers to be capable of making and keeping these commitments early in recovery, the 12 Steps of AA [3] are used as the foundation of the therapeutic process. In addition to using the 12 Steps as an educational tool and beginning attachment to the 12-Step fellowship in preparation for aftercare, the first five Steps are used as a powerful measure of progression and an impetus for change:

Step 1.   We admitted we were powerless over drugs and alcohol and that our lives had become unmanageable.
Step 2.   Came to believe that a power greater than ourselves could restore us to sanity.
Step 3.   Made a decision to turn our will and our lives over to the care of God—as we understood Him.

Step 4. Made a searching and fearless moral inventory of ourselves.
Step 5. Admitted to God, to ourselves, and to another human being the exact nature of our wrongs.

Patients are expected to make specific commitments to completion of each Step successively. Written work and behavioral assignments are provided that foster this progression. Completion occurs when a cognitive-behavioral-emotional shift is noted consistent with the foundation of the Step as outlined in AA [3]. This approach to treatment involves a powerful reframing [25] of the traditional psychotherapeutic approach. Its orientation to the results of abstinence has revealed a psychology regarding commitment to abstinence that is somewhat predictable within a structured setting using the 12 Steps. Within their commitment to each of the Steps, specific patterns of behavior occur which block progress in recovery. What is revealed is an association of memories of events with which this pattern developed, crystallized, or was significantly attached to this person's experience.

A 17-year-old male patient was motivated and progressed well to completion of his Step 1. Following this, his mood changed, he was not as active, was often confused, and appeared to be blocked in treatment. There was no clear explanation that could be seen until he developed complaints of pain in his leg. No physical signs of a problem were present. The patient soon after recalled an injury in which he broke a leg during a soccer game at a point in his life at which he and his father had many dreams of him becoming a professional athlete. He never did as well in athletics after this injury. The disappointment to his father and himself were not previously resolved and had resurfaced to block his progress in treatment. The disappointment and the victimizing self-pity associated with this event were blocks to his commitment to Step 2 and were part of his "insane" behaviors. Once this issue was examined, he was able to continue treatment successfully.

The therapeutic work involved identifying the structures from the past, recalling the events in detail, reexperiencing the thoughts, feelings, and behaviors associated with the event, and then acting in the present to produce a different result. Therapeutic techniques include processes and understandings from short-term dynamic psychotherapy [17], behavior and learning theory [26], and cognitive [27] or rational-emotive therapy [28].

An important insight into this process has come from Lane and Schwartz [29]. They approached the treatment of psychiatric disorders from a cognitive-developmental viewpoint. Five developmental levels of emotional experience were described: (1) bodily sensations, (2) body in action, (3) individual feelings, (4) blends of feelings, and (5) blends of blends of feelings. Transformations occur as one breaks through into an experience of a new level of awareness. Clinically, as teenagers progress through treatment, this process occurs. Typically teenagers enter treatment with only impulsive actions and awareness of no feelings. They will progress into an awareness of single feelings, usually only anger. Further breakthroughs occur as awareness of guilt and shame appear, and they progress into further distinctions to include a full range of emotional experiences.

As mentioned previously, specific blocks to progress may be biologically related as depression, panic attacks, or other anxiety symptoms develop. Their appearance clinically may indicate specific information about the teenager's psychobiological history. The significance of the timing of these symptoms in this structure remains to be explored.

An important determinant of the progress is the focus on urges. Often, part of the structure from the past includes urges and associated behaviors—drug seeking, or acting out sexually, violently or self-destructively, or with runaway behaviors. Important therapeutic contributions and dynamic understandings of urges have come from the self psychological theorists [30] and the role of addictive trigger mechanisms (ATMs) in compulsive behaviors. Using their psychodynamic framework, ATMs are described as any substance (alcohol, drugs, or food), behavior (compulsive eating, purging), or attachment with which a person becomes obsessively involved and which functions as an archaic self-object. Addictive trigger mechanisms produce a dissociative alteration of self-experience and are related to archaic self-object fantasies and moods of euphoric bliss. Archaic self-object fantasies are described as powerful affect-laden images related to intense experiences of admiration and exhibition, or security and merger. The accompanying moods of bliss produce powerful antianxiety and antidepressant effects that protect the addict from painful states of depressive emptiness, deple-tion, and deadness, or from anxious feelings of self-fragmentation or falling apart and going to pieces. In psychotherapeutic work with these teenagers, their abstinence from the ATMs creates urges that when explored further reveal the presence of specific emotional states, often related to these archaic self-object fantasies. Therapeutic work leads to resolution of these deficit states and simultaneously an expansion of emotional awareness as described by Lane and Schwartz [29]. Thus, urges provide an opportunity for further investigation of the link between psychodynamic and psychobiological processes:

> A 16-year-old male with a history of parental separation at age 2, with mother's remar-riage and stepfather's leaving at age 7, was admitted for marijuana and mixed substance dependence. His medical history included several years of left-sided headaches that were associated with flashing lights and nausea and were diagnosed at age 13 as migraine headaches with a normal EEG and CT scan. Initially in treatment he was generally guarded and presented a "macho" image of bravado. Work initially in treatment revealed many issues with authority, and he developed mood lability with intermittent angry episodes and eventually migraine attacks. He acknowledged severe drug urges and the desire to run away at this time. During one of these attacks he stated that the therapist talking to him at that moment was like beating something into his head. He recalled how his stepfather had hit him in the head and repeatedly criticized him, calling him a wimp. He recalled wishes to hit his stepfather but with fears of destructive annihilation. His headache worsened as anger was directed toward the therapist. A breakthrough occurred as he identified the disappointment in not having a father emotionally available and cried for the first time in treatment. He tearfully related how he wanted his father and step-father to be proud and to admire him as being a strong son. This occurred in the presence of a smile and the relief of the migraine attack, which did not return throughout treatment.

These understandings have created a different framework regarding time in the therapeutic process. The transformation process allowing progression to more complex levels of emo-tional awareness is limited primarily by the patient's openness and willingness to become self-aware and self-expressive, or the therapist's limitation in identifying feeling states rather than by time factors. Clinically, in the structured program as described, character transfor-mation has occurred in time frames significantly shorter than previously described:

> A 17-year-old male with a history of parental divorce at age 7 and classification by the Child Study Team as emotionally disturbed was admitted with a history of mixed substance abuse with extensive marijuana and hallucinogen use. His history included attention deficit hyperactivity disorder and conduct disorder progressing since age 11 with lying, steal-ing, property destruction, fire setting, cruelty to animals, truancy, and driving without a license. His drug use began at age 14. He also developed self-destructive behaviors with self-inflicted knife wounds and cigarette burns to his arms and legs, jumping off a two-story building and fracturing his ankle in a suicide attempt, and two other suicide attempts. He was diagnosed as having borderline personality disorder with many of the behaviors beginning prior to drug use, but exacerbated significantly by it.

Initial treatment included mood lability, irritability, and aggressive outbursts, including hitting a staff member. As structure was present and he reviewed consequences of his drug use, he expressed much guilt and shame and developed a depressive mood with suicidal ideation. Staff interventions assisted him in continued tearful expression of loneliness and sadness for what he had done to himself. Working through many issues related to resentments toward a physically abusive stepfather, absence of his father, and anger at women led to resolving of the depression. As this occurred his irritability, restlessness, and poor attention decreased and allowed further engagement in therapy. Many issues regarding codependency on his alcohol-using mother were focused on. He also expressed apologies for past behaviors with family members. During the termination phase he was very sensitive to separations and worked through many issues regarding separations and rejections as he prepared himself for placement in a Halfway House and later independent living to get away from a chaotic home situation. Two-year follow-up showed that he was sober and maintaining a job and independent living situation. Inpatient treatment was 9 weeks.

A. Relapse Education

Another advantage of this model is the manner in which education to prepare and deal with relapse is an integral part of the treatment process. As previously mentioned, when making a meaningful commitment to successively taking each of the Steps, patients react with behaviors that block progress. This may range from aggressive assaults, overwhelming guilt or shame, depression with hopelessness and suicide attempts, feelings of failure and withdrawal, sexual urges and acting out, binging and purging behaviors, and multiple urges that may be acted on or verbalized. These behaviors are viewed as *patterns of relapse* and a sign that their commitment is strong rather than that they are failing. This reframing allows patients to identify specific events in their lives that are associated with these behaviors. It also assists patients in the recognition that the often perceived crisis of urges presents an opportunity for further self-discovery. By remaining abstinent from ATMs, a feeling state with associated memories and fantasies (archaic self-object) can be identified. This identification can be used to lead to further self-fulfillment and self-expression. This fosters a powerful shift from a focus on illness to empowering recovery.

B. Therapeutic Progression

Step 1

Use of this treatment model has demonstrated a predictable progression through each of the Steps highlighting specific issues often associated with dual diagnoses [16]. After breaking through initial denial, guilt, and shame are experienced as patients review the consequences of their drug use. The ability to accomplish this appears partly related to the locus of control and the ability for introspection. Some persons with severe conduct disorders and "sociopathic" personality traits have a limited ability to experience guilt and shame and may be identified early in treatment. Issues of authority and discipline highlight the cognitive distortions and paranoid defenses as complaints of "brainwashing" occur. Staff are perceived as punishing parents or law enforcement persons with whom they have previously had bad experiences. Severe distortions and paranoia may indicate an underlying schizophrenia or schizophreniform disorder. The confrontation method is designed to highlights this and to distinguish it from the cognitive distortions and mistrust of the patient with borderline personality disorder. Schizophrenia or schizophrenialike disorders begin to display primary process thinking. These patients are not appropriate for this type of treatment, and must be placed in a more supportive therapeutic environment. The patients with borderline personality disorder develop more organized thought processes with confrontation. However, they also develop overwhelming urges with acting out behaviors—to use drugs, to have sex, to binge or purge, to commit suicide or self-mutilate, to be violent, or to run away. With structure, the "abandonment depression" [31] breaks through. This loneliness and depression is common as teenagers begin to perceive their life without drugs, without drug-using friends, and without behaviors used to previously cope with feelings of loneliness and alienation. The presence of persistent depressive symptoms must be evaluated for an underlying major depressive disorder often evident with psychomotor retardation or psychotic processes. These teenagers have responded well to antidepressant medications. For some patients, the development of intense paranoid feelings may be indicative of secrets regarding unexposed criminal behavior (i.e., murder or abuse) and issues of confidentiality must be addressed before treatment can continue.

Adolescents with learning disabilities and prior social and school failure experience overwhelming feelings of failure with behaviors of giving up. They frequently equate treatment with school, and staff as teachers or critical parents. When addressed properly with remedial support and development of alternative coping strategies, treatment becomes one of their successes in recovery [32].

Step 2

Step 2 begins with the reading of a comprehensive drug chart to parents, breaking through family denial, and opening a family system to building new relationships. Step 2 is referred to as one of the spiritual steps of AA. The word *spiritual* often has religious associations that may block understanding by both patients and professionals. Understanding spirituality as the "quality of our relationships to whatever or whomever is most important in our life" [33] allows concepts of object relations theory to be applicable and fosters better understanding of this Step by professionals.

Spiritual can also be referred to as those feelings that touch the heart and soul of a human being. This is similar to what Bettelheim [34] described in *Freud and Man's Soul*. This Step requires looking at past religious experiences, including those that have emotional attachments and cognitive distortions, often fostering magical thinking and the "Santa Claus concept" of a Higher Power.

Step 2 often deals with the deepest levels of mistrust and alienation as addicted teenagers feel betrayed by their family, by the world, and by God. There is a reexperiencing of the losses of relationships, such as by divorce or separation, as well as disappointments in the ideal models of family and parents, or the loss of goals. Some of the most painful disappointments are related to the loss of trust or self-worth of the physically or sexually abused adolescent, who feels victimized by the world. Therapeutic work on unresolved grief issues and hopelessness are necessary owing to the recurrence of severe self-destructive behaviors including increased purging, depression, violence and self-mutilation.

The focus on spirituality also assists identification of adolescents involved in satanism and other cultlike activities. The spiritual focus fosters experience of intense rage, hatred, and sadistic revenge that is often associated with issues of power and humiliation as well as covering feelings of inadequacy and mortifying shame. Often these teenagers have an underlying schizotypal or schizoid personality disorder requiring treatment. Owing to the intense countertransference issues that arise in dealing with teenagers at this stage, emphasis on reality testing, projection, and projective identification is critical for success.

Emphasis during this Step is on group process and support. For most teenagers this is against their sense of "individualism," and appears to be antithetical to the developmental task of separation-individuation. As described by Ehrlich [35], the paradox of these Steps requires interpretation of the language and experience to teenagers.

The focus of Step 2 on relationships leads to clarification of family issues in detail. If patients are the children of alcoholics or other drug-abusing parents, issues of their codependence become prominent as they noticeably focus on other's behaviors rather than on themselves. It is necessary for these children of alcoholics that these issues be dealt with currently rather than waiting further in recovery, since if they are left unresolved this will often lead to an early relapse or withdrawal from treatment if not addressed.

Step 3

Step 3 is designed to consolidate treatment gains. It emphasizes making choices and taking responsibility as it relates to "surrendering" defensive patterns of the structures from the past [36]. This step is instrumental in facilitating character transformation. Its focus on overcoming past defensive patterns, identity changes, and adopting new behaviors is often difficult for persons with a narcissistic personality disorder. Some "images" or identity changes that are related to the narcissistic self and are mostly defensive are those of the drug or street image, macho image, rebellious/anarchist image (often seen in followers of the skinhead movement), victim image of the abused, and recently the drug dealer image. Surrendering of these images brings up issues of "not being remembered" and "not feeling significant," reflective of past life experience patterns. For many kids, especially the sexually dependent, the identity is so pervasive that it is experienced as if they were dying, with precipitation of acute panic attacks often related to a separation anxiety disorder or posttraumatic stress disorder with traumatic experiences at an early age.

Sexual feelings are often the last defense and the strongest attachment against feelings of abandonment, loneliness, isolation, and alienation. Helpful distinctions are made between sexuality and intimacy. Adopted teenagers often regress as "adoption" into a recovering community is experienced through past emotional experiences of loss and abandonment related to being adopted by their family. This is consistent with previous recognition of the resistance to treatment that occurs among adopted patients [37].

The role of this Step in the separation-individuation process of adolescence is recognized by scheduling Family Week (see Sect. VIII) treatment at this stage. Many teenagers are unable to complete this Step without concrete experiences with family members and a direct resolution of major family conflicts.

Step 4

Step 4 is designed to foster personal responsibility and growth for continued self-motivated recovery. This Step aims at self-acceptance and acceptance by others to "form a true partnership with another human being" [3]. The openness at this point in successful treatment allows teenagers to deal with issues of intimacy and sexuality with an emotional maturity consistent with their age.

Patients are asked to choose a specific character trait that has been present in themselves throughout treatment. For instance, the arrogance of the perfectionist, the self-pity of the victim, the fear of living of the suicide attempter, or the fear of loneliness of the sexually dependent. They choose another patient who reactivates this character structure, and in front of the peer group demonstrate how to use Steps 1 through 3 to overcome this. When done successfully, a breakthrough and transformation occurs during the Step 4 presentation that is nearly overwhelming in its expression of the courage in the human spirit and emotionally moves all in attendance.

Step 5

Step 5 is best described by a quote from *Twelve Steps and Twelve Traditions* [38]: "It amounts to a clear recognition of what and who we really are, followed by a sincere attempt to become what we could be." This Step is done privately with the hospital chaplain, who is involved as a member of the treatment team. He leads a regular grief group and spirituality group as well as being available to discuss any concerns about the concept of a Higher Power.

He describes the experience of patients completing Step 5 as one of overwhelming honesty and sharing of gratitude by the patient for what he or she has gained during treatment.

At this point, the person has demonstrated choice, responsibility, willingness, and openness that will form a working partnership with the family, friends, and sponsors to continue recovery.

VII. FAMILY TREATMENT

Family treatment is designed as a conjoint treatment with family members expected to be engaged in their own treatment for codependency. It is based on information reviewed by Stanton [39] and a family systems theory [8,40–42] with elements of behavioral [43] treatments applied. The two major goals of family therapy with ACD are to:

1.   Restructure the maladaptive aspects of the family system
2.   Establish an ongoing method for abstinence and recovery [8]

The confused, angry, and beleagured families that have been part of the codependency process described in Chapter 12 need structure and guidance [8]. Details of the treatment program expectations are outlined below:

1.   All family and household members and significant others are expected to participate.
2.   A "family intervention" will occur within 72 h of admission onto the treatment unit.
3.   Family attendance at 2 week-night evenings in a multifamily group.
4.   Attendance at a Family Week (Monday through Friday) midway in treatment.
5.   Attendance at Alanon/Families Anonymous meetings weekly.
6.   Optional attendance of siblings in a siblings group once a week.
7.   Abstinence from all mood-altering chemicals during the course of treatment.
8.   Commitment to the 12 Steps of Alanon as a process for recovery.
9.   Attendance in an aftercare program following treatment that may be 6–12 months in duration.

The expectation of abstinence by family members can be extremely valuable. It serves several purposes [41,8]:

1.   Allows therapeutic work to be done without the active influence of chemical use
2.   Assists family members in empathically recognizing the difficulties that the adolescent's commitment to abstinence entails
3.   Screens for family member chemical dependence

As with the adolescent, families are expected to make commitments to full participation in the treatment program through the first three Steps of Alanon. In a structured program like this, deviations assist in identifying family blocks to recovery or conflicts with other priorities. These blocks, similar to the adolescent treatment, are often associated with structures from the past, or unresolved family developmental issues. Identification of these may require additional individual family sessions to foster working through and continued engagement in treatment.

A. Siblings Group

A siblings group is for brothers and sisters of all ages. It offers an opportunity for siblings to acknowledge and express their feelings and receive support and attention. Often this group is the only place they can go to talk freely about the crisis that the family is experiencing. Siblings often develop specific roles in the family that foster inflexibility and maintenance of the family dysfunction [44,45]. Some roles may be (1) the "hero" and doing academically well or superior in school, (2) "lost" or ignored by the parents, (3) victimized or scapegoated (criticized by parents or siblings), or (4) also using drugs or alcohol. The group setting without parents allows a compassionate setting for their concerns to be expressed.

B. Family Intervention

The family intervention occurs initially in treatment when the parents are generally over-whelmed and frightened. Parents have usually felt out of control as the child controls the family with manipulative behaviors as described in Chapter 12. This technique was developed by the Johnson Institute, Minneapolis Minnesota and has been adapted for use with teenagers. It assists in overcoming the denial of the harmful effects of their drug use as well as denial that the parents may still have regarding the severity of the problem. Often teenagers will become poorly engaged in treatment if they believe that a parent is not fully supportive of their treatment. This is an opportunity to dispel these illusions of "rescue" regarding the parents' commitment to treatment.

Parents are given specific instructions for the intervention. They are individually asked to list harmful situations or incidents with their teenager and the effect that it had on them personally and on relationships. The intervention is then conducted by the therapist as parents individually present this to the teenager who is expected to make no response or comments. It is often the first opportunity for the addicted teenager to hear family members when he or she is drug free. A successful intervention assists both teenager and family members to break through the denial and begin awareness of the guilt, shame, and sense of failure that have been avoided by chemical dependence and codependent behaviors.

C. Multifamily Groups

The multifamily groups [39] are a critical element in treatment. One of these groups weekly is a "beginners" group for parents whose children have recently entered treatment. The emphasis is largely educational, preparing them for involvement in the remainder of the program. Preparation includes:

1. Introduction to the Disease Concept and the biopsychosocial model of drug and alcohol addiction and dual diagnosis
2. Introduction to group process
3. Identification of feelings and use of "I" statements
4. Introduction to the 12 Steps of Alanon
5. Introduction to concepts of enabling, codependency, detachment, defenses, spirituality, commitment

The educational preparation and the compassionate support of other parents during this crisis, and relief as they detach from their codependent reactivity to their child provides hope and an openness to further therapeutic work. The advanced multifamily group continues with educational lectures and is more therapeutic in design. It assists parents in understanding themselves, their role in the addictive process, and its relationship to their family of origin. They learn to understand the predisposing and maintenance factors as well as the interactive effect that the chemical use of their teenager has had on them. This group is both supportive and confrontational. It also prepares families for Family Week as well as supports their involvement with Alanon and/or Families Anonymous.

VIII. FAMILY WEEK

Family Week is an intensive educational-psychotherapeutic experience whose goal is to restructure family patterns to support recovery. Ideally, it occurs when the adolescent has integrated

Step 2 and family members have acknowledged Step 1 for co-addicts. It takes place Monday through Thursday for 6 h daily, and Friday morning is a final summary and recommendations are given. Three to four families participate simultaneously with two co-therapists. Specific areas that are addressed by lecture or group process include:

1. Review of the Disease Concept and the biopsychosocial model
2. Review of personal commitment to abstinence from mood-altering drugs
3. Setting of personal goals for the week
4. Focus on commitments and structures from the past
5. Group rules and the role of group process in recovery
6. Barriers to communication/defenses
7. Issues, resentments, and secrets withheld and/or unresolved
8. Family roles and family interactions, including family of origin

Family Week begins with the foundation of the program—the biopsychosocial model of the Disease Concept and the commitment to abstinence. These are established firmly as goals for the week are expressed. The goal setting establishes a structure for the week as well as alerts the therapist to participants' self-awareness, openness and manner of communication, and problem solving. As with the adolescent, the structure provided by the 12 Steps of Alanon is a major focus.

As the group works to understand this model, and in an attempt to dislodge the inflexible behavior patterns that maintain the enabling system, each individual's role in the family is explored. Emphasis is on an interactive understanding between teenager, parents, and siblings and an identification of feelings beyond anger and fear. This process is facilitated as the family of origin portion of structures from the past is demonstrated in family interactions.

Most family interactions are done in a "fishbowl" arrangement in which one family circles together to deal with specific issues while other participants observe. Often, therapy involves a delicate balancing between individual family work and group process. By the middle of the week, tracking of group themes becomes a powerful tool in reinforcing group process and setting the stage for future group involvements. An interesting phenomenon that remains to be explored is the stages of group development that occur during a Family Week. Clinical experience has demonstrated the progression of the group through developmental stages related to each of the first three Steps of AA, with issues similar to those described with the adolescents as they progress through treatment. The possibility of developing a group therapy model integrating distinctions of the 12 Steps is evident.

The concept of triangulation [46,44] is presented and demonstrated within family interactions to foster each member in extricating themselves from the inflexible system. Emphasis and demonstration of triangulation is extremely useful in assisting parents in removal from coaddiction patterns. This often leads to discussions on triangulation in the family of origin and values and behaviors that have been continued through the generations. This provides an opportunity for families to change the several generations of maintenance factors for chemical dependence.

As triangulation issues in interactions are effectively worked through, by mid-week the emphasis is on parents/couples and often requires couples-focused therapy to be done in the group. This is a critical time in the process as the level of group intimacy is tested and strengthened depending on the degree of honesty and openness present. This is often determined by the degrees to which families are shame-bound systems. In a very successful group, parents and children discuss secrets and resentments never before expressed as they develop a strong desire for further closeness. Issues regarding sexual behavior, including unknown pregnancies, abortions, rape, or extra-relationship affairs are discussed. Issues of family violence and abuse often associated with other chemically dependent family members are openly worked through. Many issues related to the adult child of alcoholics syndrome occur at this point and require identification with chemical use. An emphasis on experiences of full expression and forgiveness provide further impetus for continued recovery.

The final day allows family members to evaluate themselves in terms of their original goals and personal learning experiences. Requirements for aftercare and continued recovery are reviewed as emphasis is given to the ongoing nature of recovery. Family system recommendations are also made by the therapists. This may involve recommending couples or family therapy, or extended service placement for the adolescent such as a halfway house, or residential care placement.

Family Week can be powerfully effective in not only restructuring maladaptive aspects of the family system, but it also establishes an experience of behaviors and group process required for continued abstinence and fulfilling recovery.

IX. DISCHARGE PLANNING

The final stage of treatment focuses on discharge planning. This involves establishing a structure for the continuation of recovery. This includes a detailed home contract specifying curfew hours, friends that will support recovery, places and situations to be avoided, and after-school activities, including aftercare and attendance at AA/NA meetings. Life goals for 6 months to a year are identified, such as obtaining a GED or completing school, attendance at college or vocational school, specific jobs for career development, and specific leisure activities. Aspects of AA/NA support group attendance, developing of relationships, and choosing of "sponsors" are important in the transition from the hospital.

X. CONCLUSIONS

Chapters 12 and 13 have attempted to provide clinicians with both a historical and clinical orientation to adolescent chemical dependency in a rapidly growing field. A biopsychosocial disease model was described to emphasize the multidimensional approach needed in assessing and treating adolescents. The dynamic model is designed to facilitate further research on antecedents, concomitants, and maintenance factors and to assist social systems in developing interventions. A Transformational Model for treatment utilizing the 12 Steps of AA describes a combined extended evaluation and treatment approach to include dual and multiply diagnosed adolescents. The combination of the biopsychosocial understanding and the Transformational Model of treatment allows professionals from multiple disciplines to work using various paradigms. These models have been extremely empowering to patients, staff, educators, parents, and the general public in assisting adolescents to transform the crisis of addiction into the opportunity of living with integrity, vitality, and excellence.

REFERENCES

1. Hoffman, N.G., Sonis, W.A., and Halikas, J.A. (1987). Issues in the evaluation of chemical dependency treatment programs for adolescents. *Pediatr. Clin. North Am., 34*(2):449–459.
2. Wheeler, K., and Malmquist, J. (1987). Treatment approaches in adolescent chemical dependency. *Pediatr. Clin. North Am., 34*(2):437–447.
3. *Alcoholics Anonymous* (1984). 3rd ed. Alcoholics Anonymous World Services, New York.
4. *Cleveland Criteria* (1989). Greater Cleveland Hospital Association, Cleveland, Ohio.
5. Harrison, P.A., and Hoffman, N.G. (1987). *CATOR 1987 Report: Adolescent Residential Treatment Intake and Follow-up findings*. CATOR, St. Paul, Minnesota.
6. Hester, R.K., and Miller, W.R. (1988). Empirical guidelines for optimal client-treatment matching, *Adolescent Drug Abuse: Analysis of Treatment Research* (E.R. Rahdert and J Grabowski, eds.), National Institute of Drug Abuse Research Monograph 77, pp. 27–39.

7. MacDonald, D.I. (1984). Drugs, drinking and adolescence. *Am. J. Dis. Child.*, *138*(2):117–125.

8. Kaufman, E. (1985). Adolescent substance abusers and family therapy, *Handbook of Adolescents and Family therapy* (M. Mirkin and S. Koman, eds.), Gardner Press, New York, pp. 245–254.

9. Bailey, G.W. (1989). Current perspectives on substance abuse in youth. *J. Am. Acad. Child. Adolesc. Psychiatry, 28*(2):151–162.

10. Semlitz, L., and Gold, M.S. (1986). Adolescent drug abuse: Diagnosis, prevention and treatment. *Psychiatr. Clin. North Am., 9*(3):455–473.

11. Filstead, W.J., and Anderson, C.L. (1983). Conceptual and clinical issues in the treatment of adolescent alcohol and substance misuers, *Adolescent Substance Abuse: A Guide to Prevention and Treatment* (R. Isralowitz and M. Singer, eds.), pp. 103–116. Haworth, N.Y.

12. Douglass, R.L. (1983). Youth, alcohol and traffic accidents. *Recent Dev. Alcohol.,* Vol. 1: 347–366, Plenum, New York.

13. Bass, J., Gallagher, S., and Mehta, K. (1985). Unintentional injuries among adolescents and young adults. *Pediatr. Clin. North Am., 23*:31–39.

14. Friedman, J. (1985). Alcohol and unnatural deaths in San Francisco youths. *Pediatrics, 76*:191–193.

15. Garfinkel, B., Froese, A., and Hood, J. (1982). Suicide attempts in children and adolescents. *Am. J. Psychiatry, 139*:1257–1261.

16. Chatlos, J.C. (1989). Adolescent dual diagnosis: A 12 step transformational model. *J. Psychoactive Drugs, 21*(2):189–201.

17. Davanloo, H. (1980). *Short-Term Dynamic Psychotherapy.* Jason Aronson, New York.

18. Davis, D.M. (1989). Intensive short-term dynamic psychotherapy in the treatment of chemical dependency, part I. *Int. J. Short-Term Dynam. Psychother., 4*(1):61–88.

19. Kandel, D.B., and Raveis, V.H. (1989). Cessation of illicit drug use in young adulthood. *Arch. Gen. Psychiatry, 46*:109–116.

20. Kranzler, H.R., and Liebowitz, N.R. (1988). Anxiety and depression in substance abuse: Clinical implications. *Med. Clin. North Am., 72*(4):867–883.

21. Mirin, S.M., Weiss, R.D., Michael, J., and Griffin, M.L. (1988). Psychopathology in substance abusers: Diagnosis and treatment. *Am. J. Drug Alcohol Abuse, 14*(2):139–157.

22. Galanter, M., Castaneda, R., and Ferman, J. (1988). Substance abuse among general psychiatric patients: Place of presentation, diagnosis, and treatment. *Am. J. Drug Alcohol Abuse, 14*(2):211–235.

23. Spitz, H.I., and Rosecan, J.S. (1987). *Cocaine Abuse: New Directions in Treatment and Research.* Brunner/Mazel, New York.

24. Geller, B. (1988). Pharmacotherapy of concomitant psychiatric disorders in adolescent substance abusers, *Adolescent Drug Abuse: Analyses of Treatment Research*, (E.R. Rahdert and J. Grabowski, eds.), National Institute of Drug Abuse Research Monograph 77. Rockville, Maryland, pp. 94–112.

25. Bandler, R., and Grinder, J. (1982). *Reframing: Neurolinguistic Programming and the Transformation of Meaning.* Real People Press, Moab, Utah.

26. Ross, A.O. (1981). *Child Behavior Therapy.* Wiley, New York.

27. Beck, A.T. (1978). *Cognitive Therapy of Depression.* Guilford Press, New York.

28. Ellis, A., and Bernard, M.E. (eds.) (1985). *Clinical Applications of Rational-Emotive Therapy.* Plenum, New York.

29. Lane, R.D., and Schwartz, G.E. (1987). Levels of emotional awareness: A cognitive developmental theory and its application to psychopathology. *Am. J. of Psychiatry, 144*(1):133–143.

30. Ulman, R.B., and Paul, H. (1990). The addictive personality disorder and "Addictive Trigger Mechanisms" (ATMs): The self psychology of addiction and its treatments, *Progress in Self Psychology*, Vol. 6, pp. 129–156 (A. Goldberg, ed.), Analytic Press, Hillsdale, New Jersey.

31. Masterson, J.F. (1972). *Treatment of the Borderline Adolescent: A Developmental Approach.* Wiley Interscience, New York.

32. Ralph, N., and Barr, M.A. (1989). Diagnosing attention-deficit hyperactivity disorder and learning disabilities with chemically dependent adolescents. *J. Psychoactive Drugs, 21*(2):203–215.

33. Bjorklund, P.E. (1983). *What is Spirituality?* Hazelden, Center city, Minnesota.

34. Bettelheim, B. (1983). *Freud and Man's Soul.* Knopf, New York.

35. Ehrlich, P. (1987). 12 Step principles and adolescent chemical dependence treatment. *J. Psychoactive Drugs, 19*(3):311–317.

36. Tiebout, H.M. (1949). The act of surrender in the therapeutic process. *Q. J. Stud. Alcohol.*, *10*:48–59.
37. Fullerton, C.S., Goodrich, W., and Berman, L.B. (1986). Adoption predicts psychiatric treatment resistances in hospitalized adolescents. *J. Am. Acad. Child. Psychiatry, 25*(4):542–551.
38. Alcoholics Anonymous (1985). *Twelve Steps and Twelve Traditions.* Alcoholics Anonymous World Services, New York.
39. Stanton, M.D. (1979). Family treatment approaches to drug abuse problems: A review. *Fam. Proc., 18*(3):251–280.
40. Graham, L.C. (1985). A developmental model for family systems. *Fam. Proc., 24*(2):139–150.
41. Huberty, D.J., Huberty, C.E., Hobday, K.F., and Blackmore, G. (1987). Family issues in working with chemically dependent adolescents. *Pediatr. Clin. North Am., 34*(2):507–521.
42. Quinn, W.H., Kuehl, B.P., Thomas, F.N., and Joanning, H. Families of adolescent drug abusers: Systemic interventions to attain drug-free behavior. *Am. J. Drug Alcohol Abuse, 14*(1):65–87.
43. Bry, B.H. (1988). Family-based approaches to reducing adolescent substance use: Theories, techniques, and findings, *Adolescent Drug Abuse: Analyses of Treatment Research* (E.R. Rahdert and J. Grabowski, eds.), National Institute on Drug Abuse Research Monograph 77. Rockville, Maryland.
44. Levine, B.L. (1985). Adolescent substance abuse: Toward an integration of family systems and individual adaptation theories. *Am. J. Fam. Ther., 13*(2):3–16.
45. Cleveland, M. (1981). Families and adolescent drug use: Structural analysis of children's roles. *Fam. Proc., 20*:295–304.
46. Schwartzman, J. (1975). The addict, abstinence, and the family. *Am. J. Psychiatry, 132*(2):154–157.

IV
Diagnosis

14

Nosology of Drug and Alcohol Addiction

Norman S. Miller
Cornell University Medical College, The New York Hospital–Cornell Medical Center, White Plains, New York

I. INTRODUCTION

The DSM-III-R (*Diagnostic and Statistical Manual of Mental Disorders*, 3rd Edition-Revised, American Psychiatric Association, Washington, D.C., 1987) criteria are significant steps in defining an operational approach to diagnosing alcohol and drug addiction [1,2]. However, these criteria do not yet reflect, fully, state of the art concepts of addiction, abuse, tolerance, and dependence for diagnosis and treatment. Further revisions are offered as suggestions to make the criteria more relevant and useful.

II. NOSOLOGY

A. Class Name

The term *substance* is overly inclusive and not denotative to represent the chemicals, alcohol and drugs. Substances include food and other nondrug stuffs. The term *drug* defines a pharmacologically active substance that has distinctive chemical effects on the brain. Alcohol is a drug [3].

The class name of Drug Use Disorders is an exact designation of the major agents in this group of disorders; namely, drugs. Other important considerations such as emotional and attitudinal connotations pertaining to "drugs" are retained.

B. Abuse and Addiction

The difference between the terms *abuse and addiction* is distinct and commonly confused, as they are used interchangeably incorrectly. Both mean abnormal use of a drug. However,

---

This chapter was adapted from Suggestions for changes in DSM-III-R criteria for substance abuse disorders, Norman S. Miller, M.D. Mark S. Gold, M.D., *Am. J. Drug Alcohol Abuse 15* (2), pp. 223–230 (1989).

abuse is a relative term that depends on the standard of use for a particular society. Addiction is a universal term that is independent of societal norms for use and can be identified as a distinct pattern of loss of control of drug use in any setting [4–6].

The term abuse is improperly used in the DSM-III-R, where it is defined as (1) continued use despite knowledge of having a persistent or recurrent social, occupational, psychological, or physical problem that is caused or exacerbated by use of the psychoactive substance, (2) recurrent use in situations in which use is physically hazardous. These criteria more accurately fit the definition of addiction [7].

Addiction is a behavioral pattern of drug use that is defined as a preoccupaton with the acquisition of a drug, compulsive use of a drug, and a propensity to relapse to the use of drugs [4,6].

Preoccupation with the acquisition is illustrated in DSM-III-R by criteria (3) a great deal of time spent in activities necessary to get the substance (e.g., theft), taking the substance (e.g., chain smoking), or recovering from its effects, and (5) important social, occupational, or recreational activities given up or reduced because of substance use. The drug-seeking behavior is evident in these criteria. The high priority and time assigned to acquiring the drug supercedes other responsibilities, pleasures, and important interpersonal relationships [7].

Compulsive use is continued use of a drug in spite of adverse consequences. Compulsiveness often is associated with regular use but not necessarily as binge use may be compulsive. The criteria in DSM-III-R that illustrates compulsive use are (1) substance often taken in larger amounts or over a longer period than the person intended, (4) frequent intoxication or withdrawal symptoms when expected to fulfill major role obligations at work, school, or home (e.g., does not go to work because hung over, goes to school or work "high," intoxicated while taking care of his or her children), or when substance use is physically hazardous (e.g., drives while intoxicated), and (6) continued substance use despite knowledge of having a persistent or recurrent social, psychological, or physical problem that is caused or exacerbated by the use of the substance (e.g., keeps usingheroin despite family arguments about it, cocaine-induced depression, or having a ulcer made worse by drinking). The frequent intoxication and continued use despite recurrent problems or adverse consequences is compulsive use of the drug. Correct identification of the consequences of the compulsive drug use is critical. A caution is urged at this juncture to not reverse the antecedent drug use and the consequences. Disturbances or difficulties in interpersonal relationships, psychological (mood), and physical states are likely to follow compulsive drug use than cause it [7,8].

Relapse is the *sine qua non* of addictive behavior. The criterion that illustrates relapse is (2) persistent desire or one or more unsuccessful efforts to cut down or control substance use. Abnormal use of a drug may lead to adverse consequences in a given individual in a particular setting at sometime. However, if a "recurrent" pattern of loss of control that leads to adverse consequences is identified, then preoccupation and compulsiveness with drug use are confirmed. Unsuccessful attempts to reduce or eliminate drug use with adverse consequences are indicative of relapse in addiction.

A simplification of the first six criteria to the three components of addictive behavior allows for an easier conceptualization and ultimately an accurate operationalization for the diagnosis of addiction to drugs and alcohol. Some of the present criteria in DSM-III-R actually represent examples of addictive behavior. However, as the criteria now stand, a diagnosis of "dependence" can be made without any of the criteria of addictive behavior. All that is needed is the identification of tolerance and dependence as illustrated in criteria (7), (8), and (9) as any three criteria of the nine are required to make the diagnosis of dependence. The major difficulty with using only criteria (7), (8), and (9) is that tolerance and dependence can occur in the absence of addiction.

C. Tolerance and Dependence

Tolerance and *dependence* are pharmacological terms that describe adaptations of the body to the presence of alcohol and drugs. Tolerance is defined as the need to increase the dose of a drug to maintain the same effect or the diminution of an effect at a particular dose. Dependence is the onset of a predictable and sterotypic set of signs and symptoms on the cessation of the use of the drug [9–11].

The criterion that illustrates tolerance is (7) marked tolerance: need for markedly increased amounts of the substance (i.e., at least a 50% increase) in order to achieve intoxication or desired effect, or markedly diminished effect with continued use of the same amount. The criteria that illustrate dependence are (8) characteristic withdrawal symptoms (see specific withdrawal syndromes under Psychoactive Substance-induced Organic Mental Disorders), and (9) substance often taken to relieve or avoid withdrawal symptoms (7).

Tolerance and dependence develop in response to the regular use of alcohol and a variety of drugs. Tolerance and dependence represent the body's attempt to achieve a new set point to maintain homeostasis or normal function in the presence of the drug. Tolerance may be viewed as an adaptation to the presence of the drug and dependence as the deadaptation to the absence of the drug. Addiction or addictive use of a alcohol and drugs may or may not be present. The identification of tolerance and dependence do not necessarily imply addiction or the loss of control of the use of alcohol and drugs. Tolerance and dependence are often associated with addiction, however, because of the frequent use of alcohol and drugs [11,12].

An example of the development of tolerance and dependence without addiction is the use of potent analgesics in the management of pain. Tolerance and dependence often occur, but addictive pursuit of the narcotic drug does not necessarily develop. Tolerance and dependence may develop with the chronic use of alcohol without the presence of an addiction. Furthermore, the presence of tolerance and dependence may be difficult to establish with addictive use of some drugs such as cannabis, cocaine, and even alcohol [13]. The criteria used for tolerance and dependence determine whether they will be identified. The requirement for at least a 50% increase to establish the presence of tolerance will sometimes make it difficult to identify tolerance to some drugs. The choice of the figure of 50% is unclear. If strict physiological criteria are required for dependence, then withdrawal from cannabis will not be seen. However, if anxiety, depression, and appetite and sleep disturbances are used as criteria for describing physiological withdrawal, then dependence to cannabis and cocaine are identifiable.

If the diagnosis of substance dependence is to describe a spectrum of behaviors that indicate an addiction to drugs, then to fulfill criteria (7), (8), and (9) will not satisfy for the diagnosis as they do not describe an addiction. As emphasized, tolerance and dependence occur in the absence of addiction to alcohol and drugs. The inclusion of tolerance and dependence in the criteria may be useful as indicators of regular use but not as specific definitions of the syndrome of alcoholism and drug addiction.

D. Dependence Syndrome

Finally, the use of the term *dependence* should be dropped from the diagnostic nomenclature as a primary term. Again, dependence is a pharmacological term that does not define addiction. Its continued use promotes confusion because of the misrepresentation of dependence to denote addiction. The two may coincide in alcohol and drug use but are different in definitions and implications. The term *dependence* may be retained to describe the physiological adaptation that occurs in the development of pharmacological dependence.

E. Denial

The phenomenon of denial is important to emphasize in the diagnosis of substance dependence. Denial in alcoholics and drug addicts is commonly present and makes the identification of any criteria difficult. The denial concerns drug use as well as the consequences of the drug use. The behaviors of addiction and the development of tolerance and dependence are not readily identifiable because of the denial. Corroborative historical sources are often needed to obtain the information to include or exclude the diagnosis. The denial originates from the addiction and toxic effects of the drug use, and itself is a reliable indicator of the presence of addiction [14,15].

F. Polydrug Diagnosis

The use of multiple drugs and alcohol is the rule in young alcoholics and drug addicts; as many as 80% of alcoholics under the age of 30 are addicted to at least one other drug [16]. Over 80% of cocaine addicts are addicted to alcohol and 50% are addicted to cannabis [17,18]. The need to use the class diagnosis of "drug" addict rather than single out individual drugs has important practical implications. The treatment of only one drug addiction in a multiple drug addict or monodrug addict reduces the probability of success. Most drug addicts and alcoholics need to abstain from all drugs with a potential for developing addiction [8].

G. Other Psychiatric Diagnosis

Because alcohol and drugs can produce virtually any psychiatric symptom or syndrome, the diagnosis of an additional psychiatric syndrome or disorder is difficult in the presence of an alcohol and drug addiction. The need to observe and follow the clinical state of the drug addict for a period of time during acute, subacute, and protracted withdrawal in the abstinent state is frequently necessary to establish another psychiatric diagnosis. Alcoholic hallucinosis, alcohol- and cocaine-induced anxiety and depression, and hallucinogen-induced psychosis are examples of "psychiatric symptoms" that may persist for weeks to months following cessation of use. Premature intervention with unnecessary treatment modalities may interfere with establishing the correct diagnosis and the institution of effective treatment modalities.

III. SUMMARY

Specific suggestions for further revisions are listed for convenience.

1. Redefine confusing terminologies of *abuse* and *dependence*. Retain them as descriptive terms for drug use but not as diagnostic categories.
2. Adopt the term *addiction* as the major diagnostic category in lieu of *dependence syndrome*.
3. Use the class name *drug* instead of substance to denote pharmacological importance in addiction to drugs and alcohol.
4. Clarify *tolerance* and *dependence* as pharmacological criteria for drug use and eliminate them as criteria for drug and alcohol addiction.
5. Emphasize essential characteristics that are keys to understanding addiction to alcohol and drugs such as loss of control, denial, preoccupation, compulsivity, and relapse.
6. Acknowledge the primary nature of addiction as the origin of psychiatric symptoms.
7. Emphasize the commonalities of the vulnerability to alcohol and drugs; that the similarities between drugs (alcohol) of addiction may be greater than the differences.
8. Acknowledge the influence of alcohol/drug addiction on mood, cognition, and personality.

REFERENCES

1. Rounsaville, B.J., Spitzer, R.L., and Williams, J.B.W. Proposed changes in DSM-III substance abuse disorders: Description and rationale, *Am. J. Psychiatry, 143*:463–468 (1986).
2. Rounsaville, B.J., Kosten, T.R., Williams, J.B.W., and Spitzer, R.I. A field trial of DSM-III-R psychoactive substance dependence disorders, *Am. J. Psychiatry, 144*:3 (1987).
3. Benet, L.Z., and Sheiner, L.B., Introduction, *The Pharmacological Basis of Therapeutics*, 7th ed. (A.G. Gilman, L.S. Goodman, T.W. Rall, and F. Murad, eds.), Collier Macmillan, New York, (1985), pp. 1–2.
4. Jaffe, J.H. Drug addiction an drug abuse, *The Pharmacological Basis of Therapeutics*, 6th ed. (L.S. Goodman, and A.G. Gilman, eds.), Macmillan, New York (1983).
5. Robins, L.D. The diagnosis of alcoholism after DSM-III, *Psychiatry Update: The American Psychiatric Association Annual Review, Vol. III* (L. Grinspoon, ed.), American Psychiatric Press, Washington, D.C. (1984).
6. Edwards, G., Arif, A., and Hodgson, R. Nomenclature and classification of drug and alcohol related problems, *Bull. W.H.O. 59*:225–242 (1981).
7. *Diagnostic and Statistical Manual. American Psychiatric Association Psychoactive Substance Use Disorders*, pp. 165–185, American Psychiatric Association Press (1987), pp. 165–185.
8. Miller, N.S. A primer of the treatment process for alcoholism and drug addiction, *Psychiatry Lett., 5*(7):30–37 (1987).
9. Hoffman, F.G. *A Handbook on Drug and Alcohol Abuse*, 2nd ed., Oxford University Press (1983).
10. Ritchie, J.M. The aliphatic alcohols, *The Pharmacological Basis of Therapeutics*, 7th ed. (A.G. Gilman, L.S. Goodman, T.W. Rall, and F. Murad, eds.), Collier Macmillan, New York (1985).
11. Hill, M.A., and Bangham, A.D. General depressant drug dependency: A biophysical hypothesis, *Adv. Exp. Med. Biol., 59*:1–9 (1975).
12. Miller, N.S., Dackis, C.A., and Gold, M.S. The neurochemistry of addiction, tolerance and dependence, *J. Subst. Abuse Treat. Vol. 4*, pp. 197–207 (1987).
13. Gold, M.S., and Verebey, K. The psychopharmacology of cocaine, *Psychiatr. Ann. 14*(10):714–723 (1984).
14. Jellinek, E.M. *The Disease Concept of Alcoholism*, Hillhouse Press, New Brunswick, New Jersey (1981), pp. 139–148.
15. Milam, J.R., and Ketchum, K. *Under the Influence*, Madrona Publishers (1981).
16. Galizio, M., and Maish, S.A. *Determinants of Substance Abuse*, Plenum Press, New York (1985). pp. 383–424.
17. Miller, N.S., and Gold, M.S. Alcohol Use in Cocaine Addicts, *Subst. Abuse, 9*(4):216–221 (1988).
18. Miller, N.S., and Gold, M.S. The diagnosis of cannabis dependence in cocaine addicts, *J. Subst. Abuse, 2*(1):107–111 (1990).

15

Criteria for Diagnosis

Therese A. Kosten and Thomas R. Kosten
Yale University School of Medicine, New Haven, Connecticut

I. INTRODUCTION

Classification of psychiatric disorders, such as drug dependence, is an important issue for clinicians and researchers. Successful treatment as well as research on the etiology of these disorders is contingent on having a valid and reliable method for assessing diagnoses. While errors in making psychiatric diagnoses may not seem as critical as making errors in other medical specialties, misclassification of patients can still lead to poor treatment or false conclusions of the etiology of the disorder. Thus, it is crucial that the best criteria for diagnosing drug dependence (addiction) be established. This is done by gathering as much information about the disorder as possible from clinical and research sources. The first purpose of this chapter is to discuss the importance of creating and using accurate diagnostic criteria for drug dependence; the second purpose is to present the current diagnostic systems for classifying drug dependence along with the support for their use.

The structure of the chapter covers five general topics. First, we will discuss why classifications systems are useful in psychiatry, and how they are developed and tested. Second, we will review different approaches to developing classification systems for drug dependence. Third, past drug dependence classification systems will be presented. Fourth, we will review the development of and empirical support for the "dependence syndrome," which is the basis of many current classification systems. Fifth, we will present some of the current instruments that are used to diagnose drug dependence.

II. CLASSIFICATION SYSTEMS IN PSYCHIATRY

A. Developing Classification Systems

Psychiatric phenomena, like all behavioral constructs, are complex. This complexity not only creates difficulties in treatment, prevention, and research in psychiatry, but also hinders communication [1]. It is laborious to describe to colleagues all the features of an individual's behavior, some of which may not be relevant for the purposes of your discussion. For example, describing a person's characteristics of auditory hallucinations, paranoid delusions, loose associations, chronic deterioration in social adjustment, and other interpersonal deficits is more tedious than labeling the symptoms as schizophrenia and then discussing the course of treatment or current research for this disorder. Thus, classification systems allow us to reduce these complexities into a short-hand categorical term.

While ease of communication is increased, we may lose some of the subtleties of the individual's behavior by classifying them into a discrete category. This loss is particularly problematic when it goes unrecognized. For example, two clinicians who are discussing schizophrenia may have very different conceptualizations of the role of affective symptoms in this disorder, since these symptoms are not explicitly considered except as exclusions leading to other diagnosis. Disagreements may be due to these different conceptualizations, not to the differences in treatment or research conceptualizations. Thus, classification systems must have a great deal of face validity in psychiatry [1]. That is, the experts must have a high level of consensus about what cluster of symptoms constitutes a case of schizophrenia.

Before establishing these consensus criteria, there should be an awareness of what assumptions are necessary and what assumptions are not necessary to make when developing a classification system. Because current classification systems in psychiatry are based on description not on explanation, one does not need to assume that there is a specific psychological etiology nor a biological dysfunction underlying the disorder. While a psychiatric classification system based on description appears atheoretical and purposely devoid of an etiological bias, it has been argued that description is not devoid of explanation [2]. Descriptions involve choosing which salient symptoms will be used for the definition of the syndrome and which symptoms will not be used. This inclusion/exclusion process implies that some symptoms are more important in accounting for the history or treatment response of the disorder. Thus, etiology and theory are present in this descriptive process. Nonetheless, a descriptive approach to classification allows greater proximity to the data, so that it is easier to reassess the classification system, if necessary.

A second assumption is that while classification systems categorize a relatively distinct set of symptoms or signs as a particular syndrome, the category does not need to be totally discrete, nor must its members be homogeneous. Syndromes become syndromes because a cluster of symptoms appear together in individuals in a somewhat systematic, or at least nonrandom manner. Yet, not all symptoms are necessary to classify an individual as a case. Nor is it necessary to assume that the categories are so discrete that there is no continuity with other disorders or with normality.

A final assumption of these psychiatric classifications is that these syndromes are undesirable. That is, they interfere with the functioning of the individual and are a cause of distress. Thus, when we classify particular behavioral syndromes, we have eased communication among clinicians and researchers, which in turn, should help our treatment and research strategies.

B. Usefulness of Classification Systems

In our discussion about developing classification systems in psychiatry, we mentioned many uses for this approach. First, we stated that classification allows ease of communication. Second, we stressed that the behavioral features of the categories should be fairly unique. This is important in order to be able to differentiate members of the category from nonmembers; this is often referred to as descriptive validity. Third, classification of individuals by their cluster of symptoms and signs should help us to predict their treatment outcome. In other words, classification systems should have predictive validity. Finally, although not always inherent in classification systems, the ability to scale severity of cases is useful. Clearly, this aspect would help our predictive power, as more severe cases of drug dependence have poorer outcome [3].

Predictive validity is also based on the second use of the category. Errors in assignment are problematic. False-positives (assigning noncases to the category) and false-negatives (not assigning cases to the category) decrease the validity of our system. Moreover, these mistakes lead to poor or no treatment strategies and misinterpretation of research results. Spitzer and Williams [1] suggest that false-negative diagnoses are less costly than false-positive diagnoses. A false-positive diagnosis could lead to expensive and even toxic treatment; whereas false-negative diagnoses probably lead to a delay in treatment, which in psychiatry, is not usually fatal. However, there are the obvious exceptions of suicide and psychosis that often lead to difficult clinical decisions in emergency settings.

C. Testing Classification Systems

The next step in developing a classification system is to test whether the categories are reliable and valid. Reliability in classification systems is the extent to which there is agreement about classification of individuals by different diagnosticians [1]. Reliability can exist in the absence of validity when two raters accurately and consistently agree upon classifications, but these classifications have little meaning. In drug dependence, this situation can exist with urine toxicology results. The urine results can have excellent reliability as biochemical tests, but the results have little meaning when there is no psychiatric context. For example, a positive opiate urine test in an overdosed patient with needle track marks is a meaningful context for diagnosing drug dependence, whereas a positive opiate urine in a cancer patient being treated for pain relief with increasing doses of opiates is not a meaningful context for a drug dependence diagnosis. Yet, both patients have reliable laboratory diagnoses of opiate use. The specific context gives meaning to these cases and suggests different treatment approaches.

Validity can exist with little reliability, if the category is meaningful, but there is no good method for accurately and consistently classifying cases. An example of this situation has been repeatedly demonstrated with alcoholism diagnoses in medical patients. Routine clinical diagnoses by clinicians not specializing in drug dependence rarely diagnosis alcoholism in these patients [4].

There are several ways of designing and executing reliability studies [5]. Reliability studies use multiple diagnosticians who rate the same cases through (1) written case vignettes, (2) videotaped interviews, (3) live interviews done by one interviewer and observed by another, or (4) live interviews done at different times. There are advantages and disadvantages to each method. The case vignette design is the least expensive, but is less stringent because there are minimal sources of variability in rating. This is because the vignettes are fixed and there is no interviewing style variance. These same limitations exist in the second design of videotaped interviews, except viewing the interview leads to less homogeneous responses than reading case studies. Similarly, having observers watch an interviewer leads to high agreement because one person determines the interview style. In addition, during the live interview, the observers can be influenced by watching the interviewer's cues and gestures.

Finally, the test-retest is the most stringent of the reliability designs. In this design, a subject is interviewed at two different times, usually by two different raters. The number of sources of variation are greater in this design and include (1) subject variance, (2) occasion variance, and (3) observation or interpretation variance. Separating the different sources of variation is often difficult. The subject may vary in their recollection of events, especially when the time interval between occasions is large. And different interviewers may elicit different information or interpret the data differently. Presumably, if the same method of interview is used, then there should be no contribution of variance from the method.

Classification systems are based on criteria that have face validity. Face validity involves drug dependence experts agreeing on a relatively comprehensive list of descriptive elements inherent in drug dependence. Several of these criteria must be met simultaneously in order to maximize specificity of the diagnosis. For example, using an illicit drug once should not be the only qualification for meeting a drug dependence criterion, as many nondrug addicts would fit this criterion. Moreover, more criteria, in which only a few in any combination are required for a diagnosis, usually allows greater sensitivity. This will enhance the probability of finding drug dependence cases within a heterogeneous population. Thus, good face validity with a reasonable number of criteria should provide a classification system that has good sensitivity and specificity.

There are a variety of study designs to test other types of validity in classification systems. Descriptive validity assesses how unique the characteristics of the category are among cases already in a drug dependence treatment setting compared to patients in an unrelated setting, such as a general outpatient psychiatry group, or a health care clinic. Those who meet criteria for drug dependence should include almost all patients in the drug treatment program, whereas patients meeting these criteria should be relatively uncommon in the other groups.

There are other types of validity that reflect the methodological aspects of making diagnoses. New diagnostic approaches should classify cases and noncases similar to an established method or criterion source. And classification of individuals by these different methods should measure the same thing. The former aspect is termed procedural validity by Spitzer and Williams [1], and the latter is known as concurrent validity. In a sense, these aspects of validity are like reliability, except that we are measuring the reliability of two methods, not of two diagnosticians. Moreover, one diagnostic method has to be considered the "standard" by which the other diagnostic method is judged.

The criteria developed for a category should reflect future events. The course of the disorder, the complications, recovery, and response to treatments should show some specificity, if the category is unique. This aspect of classification systems is predictive validity [1]. Predictive validity is assessed through follow-up studies that chart the course of the disorder. There are several things to assess. First, if many cases show recovery, whereas many others show deterioration, then the group was probably composed of at least two different categories, not one. Second, if follow-up studies reveal that certain treatments are more effective for one category than another, then we have further evidence for predictive validity. Note that we may assess this aspect of validity in the relative absence of a theoretical basis for the disorder even if the treatments are theory driven. Finally, specific problems can be associated with certain disorders. For example, suicide is more common in depressed opiate addicts than in antisocial opiate addicts [6].

Finally, the ultimate goal of classification is to have construct validity [1]. This type of validity goes beyond our descriptive ability and tests the extent to which our classification system can be used as evidence to support an etiological theory. Thus, construct validity is explanatory. For example, successful categorizing of alcohol or drug dependence allows us to study familial patterns of alcoholism or its relationship to biological and environmental determinants. The relative genetic contribution to schizophrenia, diagnosed by different criteria, was studied by Gottesman [7]. These studies gave evidence for construct validity of this diagnostic category.

III. ASSESSMENTS OF DRUG DEPENDENCE WITH DIFFERENT APPROACHES

A. Description vs Explanation

As we discussed earlier, currently established criteria for the classification of drug dependence are based on description rather than explanatory or etiological models. Describing phenomena generally precedes explaining it and, because research on drug dependence is relatively new, description is the current phase of inquiry [8]. Describing which people are affected under which circumstances and its consequences, can be done using different perspectives, including psychological (personality or behavioral), social, and biological perspectives. Thus, we will discuss next how drug dependence has been assessed by these different etiological approaches.

B. Is There an Addictive Personality?

Many early studies of drug dependence were predicated on the notion that there is an "addictive" personality [9–13]. This idea is based on a number of assumptions. First, it assumes that drug dependence is a trait. Since traits are aspects of the individual that are fairly permanent and stable, then this assumes that drug dependence behaviors will be persistent. The second assumption is that there is a premorbid tendency to abuse drugs. Although a few longitudinal studies have been done recently in order to determine which individuals are at high risk for drug dependence [14], the addictive personality hypothesis predates these studies. Also, these studies are often based on retrospective data from relatively few patients. Moreover, although certain personality traits may be more common in drug addicts, such as sensation seeking [15], it is not clear if these traits would predict future drug dependence in a longitudinal study.

Finally, the notion of an addictive personality as a category of diagnosis carries with it all the assumptions we discussed earlier about the validity of making diagnoses. One such assumption is that the category be fairly homogenous; members would show similar characteristics and treatment outcome. This assumption has not held up. Recent studies in drug dependence have found that drug dependence diagnoses can coexist with a wide range of personality disorders [16–19]. The coexistent disorders have predictive validity on specific outcomes. For example, antisocial personality disorder predicts more legal problems at follow-up than those without this personality diagnosis [18]. This and other coexistent personality disorders tend to show predictive validity on specific outcomes, which does not support the notion of a single, addictive personality type [20].

One potential problem in the available studies of personality disorders in drug addicts is that even the most recent studies are based on the DSM-III [44] or earlier diagnostic systems, and many of these criteria for personality disorder overlap with criteria for drug dependence. Studies using the DSM-III-R (revised DSM-III, published in 1987) criteria for drug dependence, which have less overlap with criteria for personality disorders, are not yet available. This overlap problem is evident for the most common personality disorder among drug addicts; i.e., antisocial personality disorder [21–22]. Some of the criteria for antisocial personality include an inability to sustain work behavior or parenting behavior, and no respect for the law. The older, DSM-III [44] drug dependence criteria reflected these behaviors as well. The second most common personality disorder we found among opioid addicts was borderline personality [23]. Two diagnostic criteria for borderline personality are self-damaging acts and impulsiveness, which may be expressed as drug taking. This is another possible overlap in the diagnoses of drug dependence and a personality disorder. These overlaps in criteria may reflect a true propensity for personality traits in drug addicts. Studies using the new DSM-III-R criteria, which do not overlap as much with the criteria for these two personality disorders, may provide more homogeneous subgroups within drug addicts. However, it is unlikely that these studies will support a unitary "addictive personality" hypothesis. Even the most common personality disorder in drug addicts—antisocial personality—accounts for only a minority of patients.

C. Is Drug Dependence a Social Phenomena?

A second etiological approach to understanding drug dependence is as a social phenomenon. It would be hard to argue that drug dependence does not have a social component in its etiology, as it is necessary to be exposed to drugs in order to potentially abuse drugs. Indeed, a sociological perspective holds that the social context in which drugs are used gives the meaning to drug use [24]. Research has shown that drug sampling in adolescents is influenced by both parental and peer factors [25]. Later in the course of drug dependence, coping strategies, which are argued to have a social learning basis [26], may be an important factor in the individual's ability to abstain from drugs. There are also differences in perception of and rationalization for drug use, and the control over its use across drug addicts [24].

Social consequences of drug dependence have been a critical component of most classification systems used to define drug dependence. Certainly, one underlying assumption in the classification of psychiatric disorders is that the disorder is associated with social impairment. Indeed, if this holds for most psychiatric disorders, then how can we show specificity in diagnoses? A case in point, which was alluded to earlier, is how do we make the criteria for antisocial personality and drug dependence distinct when trouble with the law is often common to both disorders?

In fact, the committee that suggested the revisions for drug dependence disorders for DSM-III-R argued strongly and convincingly against the continued practice of using social consequences as criteria for drug dependence diagnoses [27]. Because the criteria for diagnoses determine the base rates of disorders, any change in society over time or across different cultures would lead to varying rates of diagnoses. For example, recent changes in society have lead to tougher drunk driving laws. If alcohol dependence is based on arrests owing to drinking, then the rates of alcoholism should increase with this change in the laws. In addition, there are certain social situations that make it easier to hide a drug habit, such as being a physician where access to drugs is easier, or being independently wealthy and not working, so that job functioning would not be affected by a drug habit. Moreover, social consequences of alcohol use have been shown to be dependent on cultural variations, not on level of consumption [28].

D. Possible Behavioral Etiology of Drug Dependence

Drug use begins with intermittent exposure or experimentation before escalation to more regular use and the usual concepts of abuse or dependence. Clearly, this represents a change in behavior. However, the mechanisms underlying the altered behavior are unknown. Similarly, relapse to dependence after abstinence is a behavioral change with unknown mechanisms.

Some researchers have speculated that drug-abusing behavior changes owing to learning or conditioning [29,30]. Wikler [29] theorized that cues that have been associated with drug taking come to elicit physiological withdrawal responses. These conditioned withdrawal responses then lead to continued drug taking to relieve withdrawal symptoms or to relapse after abstinence. The cues that become conditioned can include environmental stimuli associated with drug taking (e.g., drug paraphernalia, drug-using friends), or emotional states, such as anger or anxiety. These conditioned cues are similar to those described in Siegel's learning theory of drug dependence [30]; however, the unconditioned responses differ. Siegel theorized that cues come to elicit conditioned physiological responses that are opposite to those included by the drug itself. These compensatory responses are hypothesized to prepare the addict for the anticipated onslaught of the drug [30]. For example, an opiate addict sees an opiate-using friend in a familiar area where drugs have been taken. The addict begins to experience hypothermia, increased heart rate, and other opiate withdrawal symptoms. These responses are either compensatory responses that were conditioned through past opiate use [30], or are themselves the responses that were conditioned [29]. In either case, drug use becomes highly probable in this situation.

Another behavioral explanation for the etiology of drug dependence comes from motivation theory. Solomon and Corbit [31] propose that the motivation to use drugs is acquired through an opponent-process theory. The first uses of a drug elicit two processes: the first set of drug responses is due to the immediate physiological effects of the drug, whereas the second set of responses, which are slower to occur, are opposite in direction to the first set. In becoming drug addiction, the first process is considered pleasurable, whereas the second, opponent process is aversive. It is the later set of responses that is hypothesized to lead to drug addiction as the responses become stronger with conditioning and the first set of responses become weaker with conditioning [31].

There are many other theories of motivation, and we have suggested that they be applied to drug dependence behavior in order to better understand its etiology [32]. One reason that motivation theory would be useful in the study of drug dependence is methodological. For example, Miller [33] proposed that the proper measurement of motivation is not consumption, rather it is the effort involved in obtaining the goal; in this case drugs. This aspect of drug use has not been studied as a criterion for drug dependence, but it promises to be a useful one for consideration.

At present, there are some criteria for diagnosing drug dependence that reflect motivation, but they are ambigious in their origin, so that tests of Solomon and Corbit's [31] theory are difficult to do. For example, the criterion of replacing former enjoyable activities with drug-using activities can reflect either or both of two processes. First, this may reflect that drug use is more pleasurable than the other activities. Second, the negative opponent process may lead to the acquired motivation to use drugs, as Solomon and Corbit suggest.

E. Biological Assessment of Drug Dependence

Although the premise of establishing criteria for drug dependence diagnosis was to use a descriptive, atheoretical approach, any clinician or researcher would have to acknowledge that biological factors influence the etiology of this disorder. Moreover, biological tests of drug dependence appear to be more objective than, for example, self-reports or behavioral tests. There are three obvious biological factors associated with the diagnosis of drug dependence. First, the drug in question can be present in biological fluids (e.g., blood, urine, or breath). Second, chronic use of some drugs, notably alcohol, can cause physiological damage (e.g., cirrhosis of the liver, or breakdown of myelin sheaths in the nervous sytem). Third, many drugs of dependence are associated with stereotypical withdrawal syndromes [34–35]. The questions are whether these biological factors can be used as criteria for diagnosing drug dependence and will they apply to all drugs or only certain drugs?

One problem with using biological criteria for diagnosing drug dependence is in the validity and reliability of testing the presence of drug in the biological fluids. Reliability is compromised because some drugs are difficult to detect if use occured over 24 h earlier. Thus, the timing of sample collection is crucial. The validity of using the presence of drug in biological fluids as a criterion for drug dependence is questionable. Does the presence of drug signify dependence or occasional, recreational use? Clearly, biological tests need to be used in combination with psychological or behavioral assessments.

The second problem in assessing drug dependence through biological methods can be illustrated by the use of biological markers in alcoholism. There are several physiological changes that occur with long-term, chronic alcohol intake, such as liver damage. Alterations in liver enzyme levels, such as heightened gamma-glutamyl transpeptidase (GGT) levels, have been used to detect chronic alcohol use [36]. This test has not been shown to be very sensitive or specific. Sensitivity was found to be low when screening alcoholism in a health survey; only one-third of alcoholics were detected with the GGT test [37], probably because alcohol dependence can begin before serious physiological damage occurs. Specificity is compromised with the GGT test because high GGT levels can be due to chronic barbiturate or other drug use, or even non–drug-related liver disease [38]. Although this is only one example, it exemplifies that there can be high rates of false-positives and false-negatives that compromise the validity and reliability of biological tests.

The third biological factor associated with drug dependence is the presence of withdrawal symptomatology. Withdrawal symptoms can occur with chronic use of a drug even before long-term physical damage can be detected. Moreover, examining withdrawal symptoms is more indicative of dependence than detecting the presence of drug in biological fluids. Thus, this type of biological test may be the most sensitive and specific assessment of drug dependence. Unfortunately, withdrawal symptoms have been described in only a few drugs, such as opiates [34] or alcohol [39], and may not be a useful tool for all drugs of dependence.

Severity of opiate withdrawal, as assessed by a naloxone challenge test, has a high specificity for physical dependence on opiates [40], but it has to be considered in a behavioral or psychological context, such as street heroin use or prescribed opiate use for chronic pain relief. Opiate withdrawal in street heroin addicts has a limited, although significant correlation with degree of opiate dependence, as defined by the DSM-III-R criteria [41]. Thus, opiate dependence may be reliably assessed with the biological test of withdrawal symptomatology, but a valid diagnosis will depend on additional behavioral factors. Further research in this area of drug dependence for other drugs is warranted.

IV. PAST DRUG CLASSIFICATION SYSTEMS

A. Early Diagnostic and Statistical Manuals

The first edition of the *Diagnostic and Statistical Manual of Mental Disorder* (DSM) of the American Psychiatric Association (APA) was published in 1952, at about the same time that international nosology classified drug addiction [42]. This International Classification of Diseases (ICD) system was developed and revised under the aegis of the World Health Organization (WHO).

Drug addiction and alcoholism were classified as types of Sociopathic Personality Disturbances in the original DSM [42] and in DSM-II [43]. There was no differentiation by type of drug of dependence in DSM; however, DSM-II did distinguish alcohol and other types of drugs. The other additional feature of DSM-II was the capability to classify severity of addiction. However, the terminology used in DSM-II and in other classification systems had semantic ambiguity. Terms like *dependence, abuse, addiction*, and *habitual* use are not readily distinguished in our language. Thus, these terms needed definitions that were clear and precise. However, these terms and the corresponding diagnostic criteria were not clear, so that making diagnoses of drug addiction and alcoholism was fairly subjective and could only be done by well-trained professionals.

B. Diagnostic and Statistical Manual III

The development of DSM-III [44] was influenced by the nosological research of that time [45,46]. These groups developed the Feighner criteria that were later refined into the Research Diagnostic Criteria (RDC). Their approach was to develop diagnostic tools that used unambiguous decision rules, were atheoretical, and were based on empirical findings.

The criteria for drug addiction and alcoholism were very different in DSM-III compared to its predecessors. Diagnoses of drug addiction and alcoholism were determined by the presence of two things: signs of tolerance or withdrawal and impaired behavioral and social functioning. Terms and categories for drug addiction and alcoholism were clearly defined, including *abuse* and *dependence*. These terms had precise definitions and unambiguous criteria. Dependence was distinguished from abuse by the presence of tolerance or withdrawal, for those drugs associated with these phenomena. Both categories included additional criteria based on duration of use, pathological pattern of use, and impaired functioning. Finally, a specific number of criteria were necessary to diagnose these disorders.

There were several advantages and disadvantages to the DSM-III criteria for drug and alcohol dependence. The advantages included clarity and reliability of diagnoses [44]. The disadvantages included the lack of the capability to scale severity. Moreover, its reliance on consequences of drug or alcohol dependence failed to identify many patients who were either early in their development of dependence or who could avoid these consequences [47].

V. DEVELOPMENT OF THE DEPENDENCE SYNDROME

A. Original Concept Used for Alcohol

The dependence syndrome was proposed to describe the clinical features of problem drinkers [48]. Although this was certainly not the first attempt to classify alcoholism (e.g., see Ref. 49), Edwards and Gross attempted to relate clinical features to emergent psychobiological ideas of dependence, such as those of Wikler [29], which we discussed earlier. Another aspect of the dependence syndrome was that its elements were conceived to be independent, conceptually and statistically, from the social consequences of alcohol use. Thus, this concept was quite different from the American DSM-III concept.

The essential elements of the dependence syndrome, as designed by Edwards and Gross [48], are listed in Table 1. The first element is narrowing of the drinking behavior repertoire. This can be seen when drinking occurs with the same ritual as every morning or every midday as a substitute for lunch. It will also occur regardless of what day it is (i.e., work or weekend day). The second element is salience of drink-seeking behavior. That is, the person continues to drink despite adverse consequences. These adverse consequences could be negative remarks from family and friends, or drinking behavior has taken priority over other activities, such as sports or spending time with the family. Tolerance is the third element of the dependence syndrome. This can be determined by either behavioral or biological indicators. Behaviorally, the person will probably report needing more alcohol to reach intoxication. Biologically, this person could function normally at blood alcohol levels that would be associated with intoxication and dysfunction in a nontolerant person. The fourth element of persistent withdrawal symptoms is related to amount and duration of alcohol use, with increasing severity of withdrawal symptoms when drinking is stopped or blood alcohol levels fall [39,50]. Withdrawal symptoms can include tremor, nausea, sweating, mood disturbance, and many others. The fifth element is related to the previous one, where the dependent person drinks to alleviate these withdrawal symptoms. The sixth element, compulsion to drink, is difficult to characterize precisely. It may be described as loss of control over drinking behavior, craving to drink, or persistent thoughts about alcohol. The final element is the

Table 1 Dependence Syndrome Elements and DSM-III-R Criteria

Dependence Syndrome Elements	DSM-III-R Criteria
1. Narrowing of repertoire	Not represented in DSM-III-R
2. Salience	Frequent intoxication or withdrawal symptoms when expected to fulfill major role obligations at work, school, or home, or when substance use is physically hazardous.
	Important social, occupations, or recreational activities given up or reduced because of substance abuse.
	Continued substance use despite knowledge of having a persistent or recurrent social, psychological, or physical problem that is caused or exacerbated by the use of the substance.
3. Tolerance	The need for markedly increased amounts of the substance in order to achieve intoxification or desired effect, or markedly diminished effect with continued use of the same amount.
4. Withdrawal	Characteristic withdrawal symptoms.
5. Withdrawal avoidance	Substance often taken to relieve or avoid withdrawal symptoms.
	Substance often taken in larger amounts or over a longer period than the person intended.
	A great deal of time spent in activities necessary for obtaining the substance, taking the substance, or recovering from its effects.
7. Reinstatement liability	Persistent desire or one or more unsuccessful efforts to cut down or control substance use.

rapid, reinstatement of the syndrome after abstinence. If a dependent person stops drinking for a period of time and then resumes drinking, the length of time it takes to return to the original level or amount of drinking is short. It is considerably shorter than the original amount of time to reach that level of alcohol consumption.

These cognitive, behavioral, and physiological symptoms are thought to be related to a common psychobiological process that occurs when a person abuses alcohol. Moreover, these elements are postulated to exist on a continuum; thus, severity of cases can be assessed.

Edwards and Gross [48] and Edwards [51] were modest in their presentation of the dependence syndrome. It was not represented as a theory or even a hypothesis, but simply as "a provisional description of a clinical syndrome" [48], or as "a concept as stimulus to enquiry" [51]. Nonetheless, their work has served as a hypothesis in that it has stimulated much research and much criticism. Because the concept of the dependence syndrome was developed with an atheoretical, clinical descriptive approach, researchers and clinicians of many orientations have criticized it. Behaviorists claim the concept is too subjective or not empirically driven: Terms such as craving or compulsion are too ill defined for them. While these terms would not be objectionable to phenomenologists, they dislike the heavy reliance on behavioral or biological explanations. Biologists find the biological aspects too nondescript or not testable. Socially oriented researchers dislike the fundamental principle of the dependence syndrome's independence from social consequences. However, these criticisms have helped to enhance this concept and refine its elements.

B. The ICD System Is Based on the Dependence Syndrome

The alcohol dependence syndrome became the basis for the revision of the ICD by the WHO expert committee in 1981 [52]. Moreover, the concept, which was originally developed for alcohol, was now extended for all drugs of dependence. The reason for this extension was that these psychoactive drugs (defined below) share many properties, such as their use can lead to tolerance, drug-seeking behavior, or neuroadaption. These and other terms are described below.

Edwards et al. [52] proposed some terminology to be used in this revised ICD. First, the term *drug* was considered too broad, because it implies any chemical entity used for therapeutic or nontherapeutic purposes. It is the psychoactive drugs that are of interest because they alter mood and behavior. Specifically, it targets those psychoactive drugs that are likely to be self-administered owing to their reinforcing properties and used nontherapeutically.

A second term defined by Edwards et al. [52] was *neuroadaptation*. This term was offered to replace the older notion of physical dependence. Neuroadaptation occurs when a drug that had been used chronically is stopped or is displaced from its site of action. A constellation of withdrawal signs and symptoms can occur that are specific to the biological mechanisms inherent to the drug. Neuroadaptation is usually accompanied by tolerance, a third term included by Edwards et al. [52] in their formulation of the dependence syndrome. Tolerance has many facets, including pharmacodynamic and metabolic tolerance. Because it is possible for a person to show signs of neuroadaptation, but not signs of dependence (see below), this term was proposed.

Another term that has been proposed is *drug dependence*, or the *dependence syndrome*. This term is meant to avoid the dualism of physical dependence, defined earlier, and psychological dependence. Indeed, drug dependence is conceived as a sociopsychobiological construct, a holistic approach. The term *abuse* was recommended to be replaced by more specific terms like *unsanctioned use* or *hazardous use*.

C. The Dependence Syndrome Is the Basis of DSM-III-R

The changes in classification for the DSM-III-R were also based on the dependence syndrome as described by Rounsaville et al. [27]. First, they proposed replacing the class term *substance use disorders*, which was used in DSM-III, with *psychoactive substance use disorders*. This distinction was thought necessary to avoid misinterpretation of substances as meaning food or water.

The second proposal was changing the distinction between abuse and dependence. As we discussed earlier, abuse was distinguished from dependence, in DSM-III, by the presence of withdrawal or tolerance. However, Rounsaville and colleagues [27] argued that there were several problems with this distinction. Both the use of social consequences and tolerance or withdrawal as criteria were considered weak. In addition, these criteria for abuse and dependence can be inconsistent across drugs and across individuals.

The crux of the distinction between these terms are the revised criteria, which are presented in Table 1. First, the use of social and occupational consequences as criteria for dependence was considered problematic. As we discussed earlier (Sect. III.B), evaluating social consequences can be difficult because of changing social mores or differences across cultures. This would lead to changes in base rates of drug and alcohol cases between these classification systems. The older system is not sensitive to those who are developing abuse or to those who have the financial or occupational capacity to avoid social consequences.

Second, the use of tolerance or withdrawal to establish a diagnosis of dependence was criticized for several reasons. One criticism is that tolerance, or increasing the amount used, is variable among individuals owing to the ability of tolerance to develop through different mechanisms. Another problem with tolerance as a criterion is that its development differs among drugs. And specific effects of drug can develop tolerance at different rates [53]. In addition, some individuals develop cross tolerance to other drugs or reverse tolerance, where decreased amounts are needed to reach the desired effect. Finally, this criterion, because of these properties, lacks sensitivity and specificity. It may not be sensitive enough to identify early cases of drug dependence, or it may not exclude those patients in whom use is not excessive, but tolerance developed easily. Similar arguments to these can be made for the use of withdrawal as a criterion. The main objection is not whether to use either tolerance or withdrawal, but it was the heavy emphasis that was placed on them in DSM-III.

The criteria for DSM-III-R had several advantages over the old system. Removing social consequences from the criteria for diagnoses of drug dependence should lead to greater sensitivity and specificity for the reasons discussed earlier. Retaining tolerance and withdrawal was useful, as was decreasing the reliance on these criteria for diagnoses of dependence. Finally, by making the criteria similar across different drug use categories, DSM-III-R is easier to use. These criteria reflect the research and theories of drug and alcohol dependence developed in the last 2 decades as well as the clinical features.

One disadvantage to the revised criteria in DSM-III-R is that they were such a radical departure from their predecessor that it may be difficult for clinicians and researchers to switch gears. Another disadvantage was that the criteria were adopted with very little fieldwork. Thus, at the time, the dependence syndrome had reasonable face validity for nonalcoholic drugs of dependence, but little evidence for descriptive, procedural, or concurrent validity. The reliability and validity of the dependence syndrome among drugs will be discussed next.

VI. EMPIRICAL SUPPORT FOR THE DEPENDENCE SYNDROME

A. Reliability and Validity Studies

The internal consistency and reliability of the dependence syndrome in alcohol was studied by Skinner and Allen [54]. Using a 29-item scale based on the dependence syndrome elements, they found that the majority of the items correlated well with the scale. Moreover, the internal consistency reliability estimate [55] was high. Thus, the dependence syndrome was found to be consistent and reliable for alcohol.

One of the postulates of the dependence syndrome was that its elements constitute a unidimensional scale. The results described above support the unidimensionality of the scale. In addition, the results of the factor analysis on these alcohol items showed that one factor accounted for about one-third of the variance; the second and third factors accounted for less than 8% of the variance each [54]. Thus, further evidence for the postulate that dependence constitutes a unidimensional scale was given.

We conducted a study testing, first, the generalizability of the dependence syndrome among different drugs, and second, two of the postulates of the dependence syndrome, on which these criteria were based. These postulates are unidimensionality and independence from social consequences [56]. The dependence elements were examined among a cross section of drug addicts and non–drug-abusing psychiatric patients using item-scale correlations, Guttman scaling, and factor analysis. The drugs studied include opiates, alcohol, cocaine, stimulants, sedatives, cannibis, and hallucinogens.

We found excellent internal consistency for the items, based on Cronbach's alpha [55] and on the item-scale correlations. The best internal consistency was seen for opiates, then cocaine, and then alcohol, stimulants, and hallucinogens. Sedatives and cannabis were the least internally consistent of the drugs. Opiate items were also the most tightly clustered and highly correlated with the overall dependence scale. These results suggested that the elements formed cumulative, unidimensional scales.

Further support for this postulate was provided by the excellent reproducibility coefficients obtained when we performed Guttman scaling techniques. High reproducibility coefficients indicate that the items approximate a unidimensional scale [57]. Finally, additional support for the unidimensionality concept was provided by the results of the factor analysis done separately by drug. Single factors accounted for a substantial amount of the variance for opiates, alcohol, and cocaine. The other drugs had two or three factors with eigenvalues above 1.

We then correlated the dependence items with the scores on the Addiction Severity Index (ASI) [58], which scales problem severity in several psychosocial areas. This tested the postulate that the dependence items are independent of psychosocial consequences. Although there were a larger number of significant correlations than expected by chance alone; most of the ASI scales were relatively independent of the dependence syndrome scale. In particular, none of the ASI scores correlated with the dependence scale for opiates, stimulants, sedatives, or cannabis. Thus, our study showed modest support for the postulate of independence from psychosocial consequences, very good support for the postulate of unidimensionality, and strong support for the use of the dependence syndrome across different classes of drugs.

Further support for the postulate that drug dependence is independent of social consequences of drug use was provided by Skinner and Goldberg [59] in a sample of opiate addicts. Factor analysis of the 20-item drug scale showed support for this notion. The first factor was described as a "dependence" factor, and included items reflecting withdrawal symptoms and the inability to stop drug use. The second factor was characterized as a "social problems" factor. Items included neglecting family, job loss, and family complaints of drug use. Thus, the distinction of dependence from social problems appears particularly robust in opiate addicts based on these two studies [56,59]. Although the reliability and validity of the dependence syndrome concept may be weak for some drugs; thus far, the concept appears to fit dependence on opiates quite well.

B. How Well Does Dependence Relate to Other Variables?

A number of studies have assessed the concurrent validity of the dependence syndrome by studying how well it is related to other, more established measures of drug and alcohol use. The first and most basic assumption of concurrent validity is to test how well dependence is associated with measures of drug use (e.g., length of use, amount of use). Support of this has been mixed. For alcoholics, dependence correlated well with daily quantity of alcohol and with lifetime alcohol consumption measures [54]. Among opiate addicts, recent use measures have correlated with dependence, including use in the past 2 months [59], number of doses [60], and severity of naloxone-precipitated opiate withdrawal [41]. However, years of opiate use have not correlated with dependence [41,60].

Measurements of use may be problematic and unreliable, since they are based on recall. Furthermore, consumption measures should not be expected to be good indicators of dependence [32]; rather, measures of effort to obtain the drug, or "motivation" would be more indicative of dependence based on Miller's results in feeding behavior [33]. Motivation to obtain drugs may be a more appropriate measure, particularly for illicit drugs, since more barriers must be overcome to get these illicit drugs. These illicit drug barriers may explain the moderate discrepancy between the predictive utility of use measures in alcohol dependence (licit drug) compared to use measures for opiate dependence (illicit drug).

The relationship of dependence to biological tests has supported the dependence syndrome. Severity of dependence was related to the "priming effect" of a drink in alcoholic patients [61]. Severity of dependence was also correlated with the severity of naloxone-precipitated withdrawal in opiate addicts [41]. Moreover, we found that the correlation was heightened when we removed the tolerance and withdrawal symptoms from the dependence scale, indicating that a more purely "behavioral" assessment of dependence associated well with the biological indicator of withdrawal severity. The identification of these biological variables that are associated with severity of dependence is a needed area of investigation.

The procedural validity of the DSM-III-R criteria for measuring alcohol and drug dependence was assessed in a small-scale field trial [47]. The study assessed the agreement in categorizing cases of alcohol and drug dependence using DSM-III vs DSM-III-R in two settings: an inpatient, psychiatric unit and in an outpatient drug dependence unit. The results showed that the best agreement was obtained when the number of criteria met in DSM-III-R was three (compared to two or four). Reliability was moderate for cannabis and poor for hallucinogens. However, reliability was excellent for alcohol, stimulants, opiates, and cocaine. The rates of diagnoses were greater in the DSM-III-R diagnostic system. The authors argue that this is due to the removal of the requirement for social consequences, suggesting that this new system will better identify early cases of alcohol and drug dependence.

C. Predictive Validity of the Dependence Syndrome

The predictive validity of the dependence syndrome, or how well this measure is associated with treatment outcome, has been studied more for alcohol than for other drugs of dependence. Babor, Rounsaville, and colleagues [62,63] found that severity of alcohol dependence, based on a 15-item self-report, correlated with some measures of treatment outcome at 1 year. The number of these outcome measures that correlated with dependence was somewhat greater in male alcoholics than in female alcoholics. For male alcoholics, severity of dependence predicted craving, number of drinking days, and alcohol consumption per day, but not the length of time they stayed in treatment. The results were similar for female alcoholics except that number of drinking days, the significant variable with the least predictive power in males, did not correlate with dependence.

Another gender difference was seen when severity of dependence at intake, based on this self-report, was compared to derived severity measures in four areas based on DSM-III criteria assessed at outcome, 1 year later. The DSM-III is based on a categorical approach, not a dimensional one, as in DSM-III-R. However, these authors devised dimensional measures of DSM-III alcohol dependence/abuse by summing all positive responses to items in four areas. These areas included (1) pathological pattern of use, (2) impaired social functioning, (3) alcohol-related physical conditioning, and (4) withdrawal symptoms. Severity of dependence/abuse based on all four DSM-III scales was predicted by dependence based on DSM-III-R for male alcoholics only. Interpretation of these results for male alcoholics is somewhat difficult because of the long-time period between assessments (1 year). The data either suggest that DSM-III-R assesses severity of alcoholism similarly as DSM-III in males, if one considers this a test-retest study design of relability, or the data suggest that dependence, based on DSM-III-R, can predict degree of alcoholism 1 year later even though a different instrument was used. Since DSM-III assessment was based on lifetime report, the interpretation of good reliability is warranted. However, both interpretations of the results from the Rounsaville and Babor studies [62–64] suggest that DSM-III-R criteria may only be appropriate for certain demographic groups.

The severity of alcohol dependence has had only modest capability of predicting actual success in treatment. In one study, alcohol dependence was assessed at intake using a 29-item scale and patients were then randomly assigned to one of three treatment modalities (inpatient, outpatient, or brief, primary care). Showing up for treatment, after a 1- to 2-week waiting period, could be predicted by severity of alcohol dependence in the outpatient sample and in the total pooled sample, but not in the other two samples. Other studies have found that alcohol dependence was not related to success in various types of treatments [62,63,65].

Unfortunately, many of these studies have used different scales and instruments to measure dependence. Although these instruments are all based on the principles of the dependence syndrome, it is hard to determine whether conflicting results are due to subtle differences in methodology. Babor [62] argues further that the differences in statistical methods may also lead to different results. Several demographic factors, such as gender, may need to be controlled in these studies, either statistically (i.e., with partial correlations or logistic regressions) or methodologically.

Very few studies have been done on the predictive validity of the dependence syndrome for other drugs of dependence. Babor [62] reanalyzed data collected from two follow-up (1.0- or 2.5-year) studies of opiate addicts to assess the predictive utility of dependence in this drug-abusing population. Using the drug severity scores from the ASI, which were found to correlate well with dependence scores in another study, these authors found that drug severity at intake correlated with drug severity at outcome in one of the two samples. However, this instrument was not designed specifically to test the dependence syndrome principles. Moreover, this sample was comprised of male opiate addicts only, and a separate analysis by gender in the second sample did not show a relationship between the two drug severity measures.

We assessed the predictive utility of the dependence syndrome in a 1-year follow-up of methadone-maintained opiate addicts [66]. When we controlled for race, gender, and age, using stepwise regression procedure, we found that greater opiate dependence predicted shorter treatment length. Further analyses showed that this relationship between dependence and treatment success was very good for white addicts, but poor for nonwhite addicts. Thus, race is another factor that influences the results of these studies. Overall, it appears that the dependence syndrome may be predictive of outcome for white male drug addicts, but this predictive validity has not been shown for nonwhites or for women.

VII. INSTRUMENTS USED FOR MAKING DIAGNOSES

A. Types of Diagnostic Instruments

Drug dependence diagnoses are determined by eliciting information from the patient through careful questioning procedures. These procedures can have different formats, such as a self-report questionnaire or an interview, each of which have different advantages and disadvantages. The factors that are weighed in choosing a format include efficiency, reliability, richness of data, level of training of the personnel, and whether there are cognitive limitations in the patients (i.e., illiteracy or severe brain damage).

There are a number of instruments available to diagnose drug dependence which have been tested for validity and reliability. These will be presented shortly. If, however, you want to develop your own interview or modify one that already exists, there are several factors you should consider. First, do the questions truly reflect the criteria you purport to assess? Second, how many questions are necessary to provide an accurate diagnosis without being redundant or time consuming? Third, do the questions have clarity so that reliable and meaningful answers can be obtained? Finally, the reliability and validity issues discussed in Section II must be addressed. All these issues need to be considered in the context of parsimony. If a new instrument is to be developed, will it have any advantage over the existing ones to merit its development?

B. Self-Reports as Diagnostic Instruments

The self-report is a very efficient method of data collection; it requires little staff time to administer. Reliability can be quite good if the self-report is brief and simple enough so that the patients understand it. The patients must be literate and be able to follow simple written directions. The Drug Abuse Screening Test [67] is an example of a self-report that assesses the severity of drug dependence and is based on the principles of the dependence syndrome. It has been shown to be a sensitive instrument for detecting drug dependence diagnoses in an alcohol population [67].

C. Using Interviews to Assess Drug Dependence

Interviews are less efficient than self-reports to administer, but the data that can be obtained from them are much richer. A full diagnostic interview can take from 1 to 2 h; however, if your interest is only in alcohol and drug dependence, the interview will be much shorter (about 0.5 h).

Interviews can be unstructured where an experienced clinician questions the patient and can explore spontaneously specific aspects of the patient's problems. The richness of data obtained with unstructured interviews is usually greater than those data obtained with structured interviews. Structured interviews lead the diagnostician through a series of questions, which may also have probes suggested to gather further information or skip-out sections to save time. Efficiency and reliability are two advantages of the structured interview over the unstructured interview. In addition, the structured interviews that were designed for research [45,46] can be administered by personnel with less extensive training than a psychiatrist (i.e., social workers or others with clinical training), or even by lay interviewers.

D. Structured Interviews to Assess Drug Dependence

The Schedule for Affective Disorders and Schizophrenia (SADS) is a structured interview devised by Spitzer and his colleagues [68] to reduce variance in diagnoses due to interview style. This interview is designed to elicit symptoms, signs, and history in a systematic manner in order to provide an adequate data base for determining psychiatric diagnoses. The criteria on which this interview is based were also developed by Spitzer and colleagues [69] and are known as the *Research Diagnostic Criteria* (RDC). The RDC are a set of operational definitions for several psychiatric disorders with specific rules for making diagnosis.

The comparative utility of the SADS/RDC interview, which can be administered by paraprofessional, clinical interviewers, was assessed in an opiate-abusing population [70]. The diagnoses made using the SADS/RDC structured interview was compared to diagnoses made by psychiatrists using open-ended interviews and DSM-III criteria. The two diagnostic methods were very similar in their ability to diagnose opiate dependence, which is not surprising, since this was the population being studied. The ability of the SADS/RDC to detect diagnoses of other drug dependence, including alcohol, was considerably better than that of the unstructured, psychiatric interview. The authors conclude that the discrepancy in classifying other drug dependence disorders was due to information variance. That is, the SADS/RDC raters systematically asked about each type of drug used. Although psychiatrists attempted to be thorough by keeping a mental checklist of drugs used, they could only be reliable in their diagnoses of current and recent drug use. This is likely due to the tendency of psychiatrists to accept the patient's evaluation of his or her drug use problem.

Another structured interview that was developed is the Diagnostic Interview Schedule (DIS) [71]. This instrument was devised to make diagnoses based on criteria for three systems: (1) DSM-III, (2) RDC, and (3) Feighner criteria [45]. Moreover, these diagnoses can be determined using a computer program. The DIS has some advantages over the SADS/RDC. The DIS provides greater detail in its questions and probes. It also provides flexibility in defining "current" in order to comply with the three different criterion systems.

The DIS was found to be highly reliable in classifying alcohol and drug dependence diagnoses by all three systems when compared to diagnoses made by psychiatrists [71]. Moreover, it was highly specific and very sensitive for these disorders.

The Composite International Diagnostic Interview (CIDI) was written at the request of the World Health Organization (WHO) and the United States Alcohol, Drug Abuse, and Mental Health Administration (ADAMHA) Task Force on Psychiatric Assessment Instruments [72]. This structured interview was developed with questions based on the Present State Examination items (PSE) [73], the ICD-10, and the American Psychiatric Association's DSM-III. It is modeled on the DIS interview with added questions to elicit the PSE items that were not already covered by DIS items. The PSE has been used extensively in clinical research (see Ref. 74), and the DIS, as described earlier, has been used in large-scale epidemiological studies (see Ref. 75).

The CIDI, like the DIS, is fully structured and can be administered by lay clinicians. There is a special Substance Abuse Module (CIDI-SAM) that covers most drugs of dependence in detail and is designed to assess severity and course of dependence. The module has been based on the dependence syndrome principles [52]. In addition to these principles and those of the DIS, the CIDI-SAM assesses specific withdrawal symptoms, route of administration, periods of abstinence, and length of dependence. The module can be used as a separate interview apart from the rest of the CIDI. The CIDI is in the process of being field tested [72].

The Structured Clinical Interview for DSM-III-R (SCID) has a structured, yet flexible format so that it can be administered by trained clinicians, who are free to make unstructured probes to clarify diagnoses. There is a drug dependence section that covers the DSM-III-R criteria in detail and is designed to assess severity and course of dependence. The clinician input is also critical in determining final diagnoses, a feature distinguishing it from the DIS and from the CIDI-SAM.

VIII. FUTURE DIRECTIONS

Future directions in the classification of drug addicts will depend on the reliability and validity of the dependence syndrome for a full range of abused drugs beyond alcohol. The current classification systems used in the United States (DSM-III-R) and internationally (ICD-10) are both based on the dependence syndrome concept [48]. The usefulness and limitations of this system have been discussed. The dependence syndrome is based on clinical wisdom and current psychological and biological research ideas. This gives it the advantage of having a framework in which to be tested. Other advantages include the ability to scale severity of the drug dependence and its dependence from social consequences of drug use. The latter is useful for making comparisons across cultures. The greatest disadvantage of the current diagnostic system is that little research has been done on it with drugs of dependence other than alcohol, but this will be the challenge for future research.

Clearly, there is a great need for future research on the usefulness of the dependence syndrome concept as criteria for drug dependence. First, we should assess whether the classification systems are reliable using a test/retest design. Second, more studies need to address whether these criteria have predictive utility. Third, more research is needed on whether this concept will be appropriate for all drugs of dependence or for only those that are associated with withdrawal syndromes. Fourth, the diagnoses of drug dependence need to be assessed for overlap with other Axes I and II diagnoses. This will help determine the extent of heterogeneity of the drug-abusing population. Finally, the development of biological tests that correlate with diagnoses of dependence will help facilitate the reliability of making drug dependence diagnoses [76].

Another important issue in refining the criteria for diagnosing drug dependence is whether these criteria are appropriate for all demographic groups. Previous research has shown that there are gender and race differences with the criteria being more relevant for white, male drug addicts. Whether these demographic differences are taken into account when diagnosing and scaling drug dependence is another issue that needs to be addressed when more research has been conducted. This will likely be met with controversy, as it has been for intelligence tests and scholastic aptitude tests [77].

ACKNOWLEDGMENTS

Support was provided by the National Institute on Drug Abuse Center Grant P50-04050 and Research Scientist Development Award K02-DA00112 to TRK.

REFERENCES

1. Spitzer, R.L., and Williams, J.B.W. (1980). Classification of mental disorders and DSM-III, *Comprehensive Textbook of Psychiatry* (H. Kaplan, A. Freedman, B. Sadock, eds.), 3rd ed., Vol. 1, Williams & Wilkins, Baltimore, pp. 1035–1072.
2. Kaplan, A. (1963). *The Conduct of Inquiry: Methodology for Behavioral Science*, Harper & Row, New York.
3. Rounsaville, B.J., Kosten, T.R., Weissman, M.M., and Kleber, H.D. (1986). Prognostic significance of psychopathology in treated opiate addicts, *Arch. Gen. Psychiatry, 43*:739–745.
4. Chang, G., and Astrachan B.M. (1988). The emergency department surveillance of alcohol intoxication after motor vehicle accidents, *J.A.M.A., 260*:2533–2536.
5. Grove, W.M., Andreasen, N.C., McDonald-Scott, P., Keller, M.B., and Shapiro, R.W. (1981). Reliability studies of psychiatric diagnosis, *Arch. Gen. Psychiatry, 38*:408–413.
6. Kosten, T.R., and Rounsaville, B.J. (1988). Suicidality among opioid addicts: 2.5 year follow-up, *Am. J. Drug Alcohol Abuse, 14*:357–369.
7. Gottesman, I.I., and Shields, J. (1972). *Schizophrenia and Genetics: A Twin Study Vantage Point*, Academic Press, New York.
8. Bentler, P.M. (1978). The interdependence of theory, methodology, and empirical data: Causal modeling as an approach to construct validation, *Longitudinal Research on Drug Use: Empirical Findings and Methodological Issues* (D.B. Kandel, ed.), Hemisphere, Washington, D.C. pp. 226–302.
9. Dahlstrom, W.G., Welsh, G.S., and Dahlstrom, L. (1975). *An MMPI Handbook: Research Applications*, Vol. 2, rev. ed., University of Minnesota Press, Minneapolis.
10. English, G.E., and Tori, C.A. (1973). Psychological characteristics of drug abuse clients seen in a community mental health center, *J. Commun. Psychol., 1*:403–407.
11. Overall, J.E. (1973). MMPI personality patterns of alcoholics and narcotic addicts, *Q. J. Stud. Alcohol, 34*:104–111.
12. Penk, W.E., Fudge, J.W., Robinowitz, R., and Neman, R.S. (1979). Personality characteristics of compulsive heroin, amphetamine, and barbiturate users, *J. Consult. Clin. Psychol., 47*:583–585.
13. Zuckerman, M., Sola, S., Masterman, J., and Angelone, J.V. (1975). MMPI patterns in drug abusers before and after treatment in therapeutic communities, *J. Consult. Clin. Psychol., 43*:286–296.
14. Kandel, D.B. (1978). *Longitudinal Research on Drug Use: Empirical Findings and Methodological Issues*, Hemisphere, Washington, D.C.
15. Kosten, T.A., and Rounsaville, B.J. Opiate addicts exhibit sensation-seeking trait, American Psychiatric Association Meeting, 1990.
15. Alkane, H., Lieberman, L., and Brill, L.A. (1967). A conceptual model of the life cycle of addiction, *Int. J. Addict., 2*:221–240.

17. Hawks, D.V. (1970). The epidemiology of drug dependence in the United Kingdom, *Bull. Narcotics, 2*:21–22.
18. Rounsaville, B.J., Weissman, M.M., Kleber, H.D., and Wilber, C. (1982). Heterogeneity of psychiatric diagnosis in treated opiate addicts, *Arch. Gen. Psychiatry, 39*:161–166.
19. Salmon, R., and Salmon, S. (1977). The causes of heroin addiction—a review of the literature, *Int. J. Addict., 12*:679–696.
20. Kosten, T.A., Kosten, T.R., and Rounsaville, B.J. (1989). Personality disorders in opiate addicts show prognostic specificity, *J. Subst. Abuse Treat., 6*:163–168.
21. Khantzian, E.J., and Treece, C.J. (1980). Heroin addiction: The diagnostic dilemma for psychiatry, *Psychiatric Factors in Drug Abuse* (R.W. Pickens and L.L. Heston, eds.), Grune & Stratton, New York, pp. 21–45.
22. Rounsaville, B.J., Eyre, S.L., Weissman, M.M., and Kleber, H.D. (1983). The antisocial opiate addict, *Adv. Alcohol Substance Abuse, 2*:29–42.
23. Kosten, T.R., Rounsaville, B.J., and Kleber, H.D. (1983). Concurrent validity of the addiction severity index, *Comp. Psychiatry, 23*:572–581.
24. Alksne, H. (1981). The social bases of substance abuse, *Substance Abuse: Clinical Problems and Perspectives* (J.H. Lowinson and P. Ruiz, eds.), Williams & Wilkins, Baltimore, pp. 78–90.
25. Dishion, T.J., Patterson, G.R., and Reid, J.R. (1988). Parent and peer factors associated with drug sampling in early adolescence: Implications for treatment, *Adolescent Drug Abuse: Analyses of Treatment Research* (E.R. Radhert, and J. Grabowski, eds.), National Institute of Drug Abuse Research Monograph 77, U.S. Dept. Health Human Services, Bethesda, Maryland, pp. 69–93.
26. Bandura, A. (1977). Self-efficacy: Toward a unifying theory of behavioral change, *Psychol. Rev., 84*:191–215.
27. Rounsaville, B.J., Spitzer, R.L., and Williams, J.B.W. (1986). Proposed changes in DSM-III substance use disorders: Description and rationale, *Am. J. Psychiatry, 143*:463–468.
28. Makela, K. (1978). Level of consumption and social consequences of drinking, *Research Advances in Alcohol and Drug Problems* (Y. Israel, H. Kalant, R.E. Popham, W. Schmidt, and R.G. Smart, eds.), Plenum Press, New York, Vol. 7, pp. 207–246.
29. Wikler, A. (1973). Dynamics of drug dependence, *Arch. Gen. Psychiatry, 28*:611–616.
30. Siegel, S. (1979). The role of conditioning in drug tolerance and addiction, *Psychopathology in Animals: Research and Treatment Implications*, Academic Press, New York, 143–168.
31. Solomon, R.L., and Corbit, J.D. (1974). An opponent-process theory of motivation: I. Temporal dynamics of affects, *Psychol. Rev., 81*:119–145.
32. Kosten, T.A., and Kosten, T.R. (1989). The dependence syndrome concept as applied to alcohol and other substances of abuse, *Recent Developments in Alcoholism*, Vol. 8, (M. Galanter, ed.), Plenum Press, New York, pp. 47–68.
33. Miller, N.E. (1967). Behavioral and physiological techniques: Rationale and Experimental designs for combining their use, *The Handbook of Physiology*, Vol. VI. The Alimentary Canal, American Physiological Society, Rockville, Maryland, pp. 51–61.
34. Kleber, H.D. (1981). Detoxification from narcotics *Substance Abuse: Clinical Problems and Perspectives* (J.H. Lowinson and P. Ruiz, eds.), Williams & Wilkins, Baltimore, pp. 317–338.
35. Gawin, F.H., and Kleber, H.D. (1986). Abstinence symptomatology and psychiatric diagnosis in cocaine abusers, *Arch. Gen. Psychiatry, 43*:107–113.
36. Rosalki, S.G., and Rau, D. (1972). Serum-glutamyl transpeptidase activity in alcoholism, *Clin. Chimica Acta, 39*:41–47.
37. Kristenson, H., and Trell, E. (1982). Indicators of alcohol consumption: Comparisons between a questionnaire (Mm-MAST), interviews and serum gamma-glutamyl transferase (GGT) in a health survey of middle-aged males, *Br. J. Addict., 77*:297–304.
38. Babor, T.F., Ritson, E.B., and Hodgson, R.J. (1986). Alcohol-related problems in the primary health care setting: a review of early intervention strategies, *Br. J. Addict., 81*:23–46.
39. Mello, N.K., and Mendelson, J.H. (1970). *J. Pharmacol. Exp. Ther., 175*:94.
40. Wang, R.I.H., Wiesen, R.L., Lamid, S., et al. (1974). Rating the presence and severity of opiate dependence, *Clin. Pharmacol. Ther., 16*:653–658.

41. Kosten, T.A., Jacobsen, L.K. and Kosten, T.R. (1989). Severity of precipitated opiate withdrawal predicts drug dependence by DSM-III-R criteria, *Am. J. Drug Alcohol Abuse, 15*:237–250.
42. *Diagnostic and Statistical Manual of Mental Disorders* (1952). American Psychiatric Association, Washington, D.C.
43. *Diagnostic and Statistical Manual of Mental Disorders* (1968). American Psychiatric Association, Washington, DC.
44. *Diagnostic and Statistical Manual of Mental Disorders*, 3rd edition (1980). American Psychiatric Asociation, Washington, D.C.
45. Feighner, J.P., Robins, E., Guze, S.G., et al. (1972). Diagnostic criteria for use in psychiatric research, *Arch. Gen. Psychiatry, 26*:57–63.
46. Spitzer, R.L., Endicott, J., and Robins, E. (1973). Research diagnostic criteria: Rationale and reliability, *Arch. Gen. Psychiatry, 35*:773–782.
47. Rounsaville, B.J., Kosten, T.R., Williams, J.B.W., and Spitzer, R.L. (1987). A field trial of DSM-III-R psychoactive substance dependence disorders, *Am. J. Psychiatry, 144*:351–355.
48. Edwards, G., and Gross, M.M. (1976). Alcohol dependence: Provisional description of a clinical syndrome, *BR. Med. J., 1*:1058–1061.
49. Jellinek, E.M. (1960). *The Disease Concept of Alcoholism*, Hillhouse, New Brunswick, Connecticut.
50. Mendelson, J.H. (1964). Experimentally induced chronic intoxication and withdrawal in alcoholics, *Q. J. Stud. Alcohol.*
51. Edwards, G. (1986). The alcohol dependence syndrome: A concept as stimulus to enquiry, *Br. J. Addict., 81*:171–183.
52. Edwards, G., Arif, A., and Hodgson, R. (1981). Nomenclature and classification of drug- and alcohol-related problems: A WHO memorandum, *Bull. WHO, 59*:225–242.
53. Jaffe, J.H. (1985). Drug addiction and drug abuse, *The Pharmacological Basis of Therapeutics*, 5th ed. (L.S. Goodman, and A. Gilman, eds.), Macmillan, New York, pp. 532–584.
54. Skinner, H.A. and Allen, B.A. (1982). Alcohol dependence syndrome: Measurement and validation, *J. Abnorm. Psychol., 91*:199–209.
55. Cronbach, L.J., and Furby, L. (1970). How should we measure "change"—or should we? *Psychol. Bull., 74*:16–21.
56. Kosten, T.R., Rounsaville, B.J., Babor, T.F., Spitzer, R.L., and Williams, J.B.W. (1987). Substance-use disorders in DSM-III-R: Evidence for the dependence syndrome across different psychoactive substances, *Br. J. Psychiatry, 151*:834–843.
57. Guttman, L.A. (1944). A basis for scaling quantitative data, *Am. Sociol. Rev., 9*:139–150.
58. McLellan, A.T., Luborsky, L. Woody, G.E., and O'Brien, C.P. (1980). An improved diagnostic evaluation instrument for substance abuse patients, *J. Nerv. Mental Dis., 168*:26–33.
59. Skinner, H.A., and Goldberg, A.E. (1986). Evidence for a drug dependence syndrome among narcotic users, *Br. J. Addict., 81*:479–484.
60. Sutherland, G., Edwards, G., Taylor, C., Phillips, G., Gossop, M., and Brady, R. (1986). The measurement of opiate dependence, *Br. J. Addict., 82*:485–494.
61. Hodgson, R., Rankin, H., and Stockwell, T. (1979). Alcohol dependence and the priming effect, *Behav. Res. Ther., 17*:379–387.
62. Babor, T.F., Cooney, N.L., and Lauerman, R.J. (1987). The dependence syndrome concept as a psychological theory of relapse behavior: An empirical evaluation of alcoholic and opiate addicts, *BR. J. Addict., 82*:393–405.
63. Rounsaville, B.J. Dolinsky, Z.S., Babor, T.F., and Meyer, R.E. (1987). Psychopathology as a predictor of treatment outcome in alcoholics, *Arch. Gen. Psychiatry, 44*:505–513.
64. Hesselbrock, M., Babor, T.F., and Hesselbrock, V. (1983). Never believe an alcoholic? On the validity of self report measures of alcohol dependence and related constructs, *Int. J. Addict., 18*:593–609.
65. Orford, J., and Keddie, A. (1986). Abstinence or controlled drinking in clinical practice: A test of the dependence and persuasion hypotheses, *Br. J. Addict., 81*:495–504.
66. Kosten, T.A., Bianchi, M.S., and Kosten, T.R. Use predicts treatment outcome, not opiate dependence or withdrawal, *Proc. Committee Probl. Drug Dependence.* NIDA Research Monograph No. 95, U.S. Department of Health & Human Services, pp. 459–460.

67. Skinner, H.A. (1981). The primary syndromes of alcohol abuse: Their measurement and correlates, *Br. J. Addict., 76*:63–76.
68. Spitzer, R.L., and Endicott, J. (1979). *Schedule for Affective Disorders and Schizophrenia*, Biometrics Research Division, New York State Dept. of Mental Hygiene, Albany.
69. Spitzer, R.L., Endicott, J., and Robins, E. (1979). *Research Diagnostic Criteria*, Biometrics Research Division, New York State Dept. of Mental Hygiene, Albany.
70. Rounsaville, B.J., Rosenberger, P. Wilber, C., Weissman, M.M., and Kleber, H.D. (1980). A comparison of the SADS/RDC and the DSM-III: Diagnosing drug abusers, *J. Nerv. Mental Dis., 168*:90–97.
71. Robins, L.N., Helzer, J.E., Croughan, J., and Ratcliff, K.S. (1981). National institute of mental health diagnostic interview schedule, *Arch. Gen. Psychiatry, 38*:381–389.
72. Robins, L.N., Wing, J., Wittchen, H.U., Helzer, J.E., Babor, T.F., Burke, J., Farmer, A., Jablenski, A., Pickens, R., Regier, D.A., Sartorius, N., and Towle, L.H. (1988). The composite international diagnostic interview, *Arch. Gen. Psychiatry, 45*:1069–1077.
73. Wing, J.K., Cooper, J.E., and Sartorius, N. (1974). *The Description and Classification of Psychiatric Symptoms: An instructional manual for the PSE and CATEGO System*, Cambridge University Press, London.
74. Sartorius, N., Jablensky, A., Korten, A., Ernberg, G., Anker, M., Cooper, J.E., and Day, R. (1986). Early manifestations and first-contact incidence of schizophrenia in different cultures: A preliminary report on the initial evaluation phase of the WHO collaborative study of determinants of outcome of severe mental disorders, *Psychol. Med., 16*:909–928.
75. Myers, J.K., Weissman, M.M., Tischler, G., Holzer, C., Leaf, P., Orvaschel, H., Anthony, J., Boyd, J., Burke, J., Kramer, M., and Stoltzman, R. (1984). Six-month prevalence of psychiatric disorders in three communities, *Arch. Gen. Psychiatry, 41*:959–967.
76. Meyer, R.E., and Kranzler, H.R. (1988). Alcoholism: clinical implications of recent research, *J. Clin. Psychiatry, 49*:8–12.
77. Benbow, C.P., and Stanley, J.C. (1983). Sex differences in mathematical reasoning ability: More facts, *Science, 222*:1029–1031.

16

Alcoholism as a Medical Disorder

Samuel B. Guze, C. Robert Cloninger, Ronald Martin, and Paula J. Clayton
Washington University School of Medicine, St. Louis, Missouri

I. INTRODUCTION

Physicians have been forced to confront the clinical significance of alcoholism for hundreds, if not thousands, of years, but, until quite recently, such interest was focused primarily on the many medical complications of heavy drinking. These included, especially, a variety of disorders of the nervous system and gastrointestinal tract, some cardiovascular conditions, including hypertension, and a striking vulnerability to infections, particularly pneumonia and tuberculosis. During these many years, however, few physicians considered the *causes* of alcoholism as properly within the province of medicine. Moral defect or weakness was the usual explanation, and physicians left such matters to others.

The acceptance, more recently, of alcoholism as a medical disorder has meant primarily that physicians are expected to be interested in and concerned about the causes of alcohol abuse as well as in the many adverse consequences of such abuse. Approaching alcoholism using the "medical model" has meant that characteristic strategies applied in the rest of medicine to understand etiology, pathogenesis, clinical course, outcome, response to treatment, and epidemiology are appropriate for alcoholism as well. Thus, efforts have been launched to learn more about the course of alcohol abuse, its "natural history," and its epidemiological characteristics. At the same time, biological variation as a hypothesis to explain why some individuals become alcoholics, whereas others do not (despite apparently similar environments) shapes much research, and, together with growing evidence of some hereditary predisposition, suggests that some molecular or cellular variation, at least partially under genetic control, may prove very important in etiology.

This chapter was adapted from *Alcoholism as a Medical Disorder* by Samuel B. Guze, C. Robert Cloninger, Ronald Martin and Paula J. Clayton. In *Comprehensive Psychiatry*, Vol. 27 No. 6 November–December 1986, pp. 501–510, copyright 1986. Reprinted by permission of the W.B. Saunders Company.

Work from Washington University over the past 15 years has contributed significantly to a renewed and widespread interest in the genetics and epidemiology of alcoholism. This report will extend certain observations and provide new data bearing on the diagnosis and course of alcoholism as well as on its associated psychopathology and its concentration in families.

The Washington University Psychiatry Clinic 500 Study was begun in 1967 to develop a new sample of patients in whom to verify previous findings in a variety of disorders, and thus verify the validity of these findings. The patients were selected over a period of 28 months in such a way as to represent a true cross section of the clinic's population in terms of age, sex, race, other demographic variables, psychiatric disorders, extent of prior psychiatric treatment, etc. The patients were evaluated initially using a structured, psychiatric interview and systematic diagnostic criteria. After the index phase of the study, 1249 first-degree relatives were exained over a 4-year period by a separate team of investigators, blind to the data obtained at index concerning any individual patient, and using the same structured interview and diagnostic criteria. The third phase of the study consisted of a 6- to 12-year follow-up of the index patients, carried out by yet another team, also blind to information obtained at index and to that from the relatives, again using the same interview and diagnostic criteria. After the follow-up interviews, additional record information was obtained from physicians, clinics, and hospitals, and a second diagnosis was made based on all available information, except for that obtained at index and from the family members. In this report, the follow-up diagnoses are those made on the basis of the interview *and* records.

II. METHODS

Further details concerning selection of patients, relatives, interview protocol, diagnostic criteria, interviewers, follow-up records, and findings concerning a number of psychiatric disorders at index and at follow-up, and correlations between index patients and relatives are to be found in previous reports [1–30]. This chapter will present data concerning the consistency of the diagnosis of alcoholism over the period of the follow-up, the pattern of psychiatric disorders associated with alcoholism, and the distribution of psychiatric disorders among the first-degree relatives of the probands.

The criteria for the diagnosis of alcoholism are presented in Table 1. Symptoms in at least three groups were required for a diagnosis of definite alcoholism; symptoms in only two groups led to the diagnosis of probable alcoholism. These criteria reflect a definition of alcoholism based on recurrent drinking in the face of *repeated*, social, legal, or medical complications of alcohol use. The diagnosis of *primary* alcoholism was used for patients in whom alcoholism was the only psychiatric disorder present or in whom the alcoholism began *before* other psychiatric disorders. The diagnosis of *secondary* alcoholism was used for cases of alcoholism beginning *after* the onset of other psychiatric disorders.

III. RESULTS

A. Consistency of Alcoholism Diagnoses

Table 2 presents data concerning the distribution of alcoholism diagnoses at index and at follow-up. Seventy patients received an alcoholism diagnosis at index: 51 definites and 19 probables. Twenty-eight of these were considered to be primary alcoholics and 42 were considered to be secondary alcoholics. At follow-up, 111 patients received an alcoholism diagnosis: 94 definite and 22 probable. Of these, 40 were considered primary and 76 secondary.

Table 1 Criteria for Diagnosis of Alcoholism

Group 1
1. Any manifestation of alcohol withdrawal such as tremulousness, convulsions, hallucinations, or delirium
2. History of medical complications, e.g., cirrhosis, gastritis, pancreatitis, myopathy, polyneuropathy, Wernicke-Korsakoff syndrome
3. Alcoholic blackouts, i.e., amnesic episodes during drinking not accounted for by head trauma
4. Alcoholic binges or benders (48 h or more of drinking associated with default of usual obligations: must have occurred more than once to be scored as positive)

Group 2
1. Patient has not been able to stop drinking when he wanted to do so
2. Patient has tried to control drinking by allowing himself to drink only under certain circumstances, such as only after 5 PM, only on weekends, or only with other people
3. Drinking before breakfast
4. Drinking nonbeverage forms of alcohol, e.g., hair oil, mouthwash, Sterno, etc.

Group 3
1. Arrests for drinking
2. Traffic difficulties associated with drinking
3. Trouble at work because of drinking
4. Fighting associated with drinking

Group 4
1. Patient thinks he drinks too much
2. Family objects to his drinking
3. Loss of friends because of drinking
4. Other people object to his drinking
5. Feels guilty about his drinking

Definition alcoholism, symptoms in at least three groups; probable alcoholism, symptoms in two groups.

Of the 24 cases at index with a diagnosis of definite primary alcoholism, 23 received an alcoholism diagnosis at follow-up (96%), though three were considered probable primary cases and 11 received diagnoses of definite secondary alcoholism. Of the four cases of probable primary alcoholism at index, all received definite alcoholism diagnoses at follow-up (100%), though one case was considered secondary.

Of the 27 cases at index with definite secondary alcoholism, 24 received an alcoholism diagnosis at follow-up (89%), though nine were now diagnosed as primary alcoholism (eight definite and one probable). Of the 15 cases at index with probable secondary alcoholism, eight received alcoholism diagnoses at follow-up (53%), though one of these was considered a definite primary alcoholic, six were definite secondary cases, and only one remained a probable secondary case.

Thus, a total of 59 (84.3%) of the 70 index cases with alcoholism received an alcoholism diagnosis at follow-up, though there was some shifting with regard to the primary/secondary classification and with regard to the definite/probable division. The consistency was higher for primary cases (96.4%) than for secondary ones (76.2%). The lowest consistency was seen in the probable secondary cases, in whom only 53.3% received an alcoholism diagnosis at follow-up.

At the same time, 57 patients (13.3%) who received no alcoholism diagnosis at index received such a diagnosis at follow-up. Of these, 40 were definite cases and 17 probable, whereas 15 were considered primary and 42 secondary cases.

Table 2 Consistency in the Diagnosis of Alcoholism

Alcoholism diagnoses at index	Alcoholism diagnoses at follow-up					
	definite primary no. (%)	probable primary no. (%)	definite secondary no. (%)	probable secondary no. (%)	none no. (%)	total no. (%)
Definite primary	9 (37.5)	3 (12.5)	11 (45.8)	0 (0)	1 (4.2)	24 (100)
Probable primary	3 (75)	0 (0)	1 (25)	0 (0)	0 (0)	4 (100)
Definite secondary	8 (29.6)	1 (3.7)	15 (55.6)	0 (0)	3 (11.1)	27 (100)
Probable secondary	1 (6.7)	0 (0)	6 (40)	1 (6.7)	7 (46.7)	15 (100)
None	10 (2.3)	5 (1.2)	30 (7)	12 (2.8)	373 (86.7)	430 (100)
Total	31 (6.2)	9 (1.8)	63 (12.6)	13 (2.6)	384 (76.8)	500 (100)

Obviously, there were two major forms of inconsistency: those who received no alcoholism diagnosis at index, but were considered to have such a problem at follow-up and those who had received an alcoholism diagnosis at index but none at follow-up. Characteristics at index of such inconsistent subjects were analyzed in an effort to account for the inconsistency.

When the index records of the first group of patients were reviewed, it was decided, in order to maximize any differences, to compare only those who had received a definite diagnosis at follow-up to those who had not received any alcoholism diagnosis at either time. The data indicate that the subjects whose alcoholism was recognized only at follow-up were younger at index than those who never developed recognizable alcoholism (32.1 years of age vs 37.6) and yet had reported more alcoholism symptoms at index (0.95 mean symptoms vs 0.18) and more frequently had reported a history of drinking (93 vs 61%) as well as many of the individual alcoholism symptoms, such as family objecting (25 vs 5%), self-evaluation of drinking excessively (25 vs 4%), feeling guilty about drinking (7.5 vs <1%), fighting associated with drinking (7.5 vs <1%), and blackouts (12.5 vs 1%). All of these differences were statistically significant at the 0.05 level or better. Thus, it appears that individuals whose alcoholism was only diagnosable at follow-up had reported more symptoms of alcoholism at index, despite being younger, but had needed more time for the full disorder to become evident.

A comparison between those whose inconsistency was based on an alcoholism diagnosis at index but not at follow-up, and those who received alcoholism diagnoses at both index and follow-up revealed that the inconsistent subjects (at index) had reported fewer total alcoholism symptoms (a mean of 4.4 vs 7.8), and lower frequencies of many individual symptoms, such as benders (18 vs 51%), loss of control (9 vs 41%), blackouts (27 vs 73%), and manifestations of withdrawal (9 vs 46%). All of these differences were statistically significant at the 0.05 level or better. Thus, these inconsistent subjects at index had reported fewer and less severe features of alcoholism. However, not all of this inconsistency was explained in this way: of the 34 patients at index who reported six or more symptoms, at follow-up, two (6%) received no alcoholism diagnosis, suggesting strongly that denial accounted for some of inconsistency.

Overall, the concordance for *any alcoholism diagnosis at the two interviews* was moderately high (Cohen's Kappa = 0.56; Yule's Y = 0.71; X^2 = 170.46, $P < 10^{-6}$) even though alcoholism was more frequent at follow-up (23 vs 14%, McNemar's X_2 = 31.12, $P < 10^{-6}$). *Among those who were ever alcoholic*, concordance was substantial for primary cases (Kappa = 0.25; X^I = 8.11, $P < 0.01$) but not for secondary cases (Kappa =

-0.09; $\blacktriangledown^2 = 1.45$, *P* not significant), and for definite cases (Kappa $= 0.15$; $\blacktriangledown^2 = 4.70$, *P* $= 0.03$) but not probable cases (Kappa $= -0.13$, $\blacktriangledown^2 = 2.27$, *P* not significant). That is, while primary alcoholism and definite alcoholism were frequently diagnosed *in the same patient* at both examinations, secondary alcoholism and probable alcoholism were not. Any shift between primary and secondary or between definite and probable diagnoses, as well as any new cases developing during the period of follow-up, lowered the concordance value in these analyses.

B. Association with Other Psychiatric Disorders

Table 3 lists other psychiatric diagnoses at follow-up that were found to be significantly associated with alcoholism. A comparison between alcoholic female probands and nonalcoholic female probands indicated that the alcoholism was significantly associated with secondary depression (60 vs 24.7%), Briquet's syndrome (37.8 vs 18.3%), antisocial personality (17.8 vs 4.3%), and drug dependence (17.8 vs 2.5%). All of these differences were highly significant as noted in the table. There was no significant association between alcoholism and anxiety neurosis, phobic neurosis, obsessional neurosis, schizophrenia, organic brain syndrome, or primary affective disorder. Similarly, alcoholism in the male probands was significantly associated with secondary depression (52.1 vs 20%), secondary mania (4.2 vs 0.0%), and antisocial personality (25.4 vs 12.4%). There was no significant association with anxiety neurosis, phobic neurosis, obsessional neurosis, schizophrenia, organic brain syndrome, primary affective disorder (unipolar or bipolar), or drug dependence.

C. Patterns of Illness in First-Degree Relatives

Table 4 presents the findings concerning alcoholism in first-degree relatives. The results are presented by sex of probands and by sex of relatives. In all combinations, the prevalence of alcoholism was higher among the relatives of alcoholic probands compared to other probands, though not all of the differences were statistically significant, at least partially because of small Ns in some comparisons. The data indicate that the proband's sex did not influence the rate of alcoholism in the relatives, while the sex of the relatives was obviously important. For example, regardless of the proband's sex, the rate of alcoholism in relatives, divided by sex, was essentially the same: 6.3% in female relatives of male probands and 5.9% in female relatives of female probands, 27.1% in male relatives of male probands and 27.3% of male relatives of female probands. On the other hand, the rate of alcoholism was 15.2 and 15.5% in male relatives of male and female probands, respectively, whereas the rate was 6.1 and 9.7 in female relatives of male and female probands, respectively.

Table 3 Other Psychiatric Disorders Associated With Alcoholism at Follow-up

	Male Probands			Female Probands		
	Alcoholic (N = 71) (%)		Others (N = 105) (%)	Alcoholic (N = 45) (%)		Others (N = 279) (%)
Secondary depression	52.1	(*P* = 0.0001)	20.0	60.0	(*P* = 0.0001)	24.7
Secondary mania	4.2	(*P* = 0.0336)	0.0	0.0		0.0
Antisocial personality	25.4	(*P* = 0.0267)	12.4	17.8	(*P* = 0.0005)	4.3
Briquet's syndrome	1.4	(*P* = 0.8029)	1.9	37.8	(*P* = 0.0029)	18.3
Drug dependence	15.5	(*P* = 0.0987)	7.6	17.8	(*P* = 0.0001)	2.5

Table 4 Alcoholism in First-Degree Relatives

	Proband alcoholic (%)		Proband nonalcoholic (%)
Alcoholism in all relatives of all probands	15.3	$(P = 0.001)$	8.7
Alcoholism in all relatives of male probands	15.2	$(P = 0.002)$	6.1
Alcoholism in all relatives of female probands	15.5	$(P = 0.054)$	9.7
Alcoholism in male relatives of all probands	27.2	$(P = 0.010)$	16.8
Alcoholism in female relatives of all probands	6.1	$(P = 0.013)$	2.3
Alcoholism in female relatives of male probands	6.3	$(P = 0.0145)$	0.73
Alcoholism in female relatives of female probands	5.9	$(P = 0.1812)$	2.8
Alcoholism in male relatives of male probands	27.1	$(P = 0.0137)$	12.6
Alcoholism in male relatives of female probands	27.3	$(P = 0.1218)$	18.3

No statistically significant correlation was found between alcoholism in the probands and any other disorder in the relatives besides alcoholism. Specifically, no significant association was found with antisocial personality, Briquet's syndrome, drug dependence, or primary affective disorder (unipolar or bipolar). This was also true when the probands and relatives were divided by sex. It should be noted, however, that when such sex-based comparisons were carried out, some of the cells were quite small, thus raising the possibility of type II errors.

The high frequency of secondary depression in both male and female alcoholic probands and the absence of any significantly increased frequency of primary affective disorder in the first-degree relatives of these probands suggested a comparison of the rates of primary affective disorder in the relatives when the alcoholic probands were divided into those with and those without an associated secondary depression. The findings were clear-cut: the percentage of relatives with primary unipolar affective disorder when the probands received diagnoses of secondary depression was 9.6%; the figure was 9.4% when no secondary depression was present. The comparable figures for primary bipolar affective disorder were 0.0 and 0.05%. These results indicate that the high frequency of secondary depression in the alcoholic probands was not the result of a familial affective disorder.

IV. DISCUSSION

Several features of the data are especially noteworthy: first, the high prevalence of alcoholism. At index, 14% of the probands received an alcoholism diagnosis; at follow-up, the figure was 22%. Further, 8% of the female probands received an alcoholism diagnosis at index, with the number increasing to 14% at follow-up; the comparable figures for male probands being 24 and 40%. Thus, alcoholism represented a major component of the disorders seen in our psychiatry clinic. This reflects recent findings from the National Epidemiological Catchment Area study that the prevalence of alcoholism in the general population is quite high and may be rising [31]. For example, the prevalence of alcoholism in three participating centers ranged between 19.1 and 28.9% for males and between 4.2 and 4.8% for females. The figures from St. Louis were 28.9% for males and 4.3% for females.

The rates of alcoholism at follow-up (which was close in time to the epidemiology study) were higher in our patients than in the St. Louis general population, especially among the women, but the high rates in the general population suggest strongly that the findings in the patients are valid. Alcoholism is clearly a major clinical problem as well as a major public health problem. All physicians, including psychiatrists, must be alert to its presence and carefully consider it in the differential diagnosis of a wide variety of clinical conditions.

The consistency of the diagnosis of alcoholism, while not perfect, is reassuring. It suggests that the great majority of patients with alcoholism cooperate with the physicians if the physicians seriously explore the history of drinking and its consequences. Obviously, some patients will deny symptoms on one occasion that they have reported on another [32], but there is little evidence that this occurs much more frequently in alcoholism than in other clinical conditions. The data indicating that an important part of the inconsistency results from early or mild cases have been reported before [33]. The finding suggests that physicians and others continue to be alert for the possibility of alcoholism in individuals who are young, report only a few symptoms, and who may be in an early phase of the illness.

The association of alcoholism with depression, mania, antisocial personality Briquet's syndrome, and drug dependency has been recognized repeatedly, especially in psychiatric facilities [34,35]. It may be that these associated conditions increase the likelihood that an individual with alcoholism will seek or be referred for psychiatric help. This could partially account for the increased frequency of the associated disorders in alcoholics seen by psychiatrists.

It is significant that these clinical associations in the probands were not accompanied by any statistically significant increases in the prevalences of the same conditions among first-degree relatives. In fact, when the probands were divided into those with and without associated depression, with and without associated antisocial personality, etc., the frequency of the associated disorder among the first-degree relatives was not increased to a statistically significant degree among the relatives of probands with the associated condition compared to those without the associated condition. For example, the prevalence of antisocial personality was not significantly higher in the relatives of alcoholic probands with associated antisocial personality than in the relatives of alcoholic probands without associated antisocial personality. For antisocial personality, Briquet's syndrome, drug dependence, and mania, the relatively small number of cases with the particular association may not have permitted valid statistical tests, but this is less likely to be the case in the association with depression, which occurred in over half of the cases of alcoholism. It is, therefore, important to note that the frequency of primary depression in the relatives of probands with alcoholism and secondary depression and in the relatives of probands with alcoholism without depression was almost identical. This indicates that, for investigational purposes at least, the secondary depressions so often associated with alcoholism should be distinguished from primary depressions that are so often familial. The data suggest that it is highly unlikely that most alcoholism is a manifestation of an underlying primary depressive disorder. On the other hand, the association between alcoholism and mania warrants further study, and it will require large samples of patients with both alcoholism and mania.

Furthermore, over the period of follow-up, in a significant number of patients, the diagnosis changed between primary and secondary alcoholism, or vice versa. This resulted from different reporting by the patient or different interpretation by the physician about the presence of associated psychiatric disorders and the chronology of such associations. The ultimate significance of the primary/secondary distinction must await additional research, but the data, thus far suggest that the clinical picture and course of the alcoholism and the familial prevalence of alcoholism are the same in the two forms.

The concepts and strategies of the medical model have proven to be appropriate and useful in the study of alcoholism. Many investigators are now pursuing the lead of genetic variability in the vulnerability to alcoholism by trying to identify clinical and experimental "markers," and using these in "high-risk" studies. The addition of molecular biological principles and tools to these efforts offer great promise. It cannot be a coincidence that, as these research efforts have gathered momentum, an increasing number of physicians, including psychiatrists, have been approaching patients therapeutically with renewed interest and enthusiasm.

REFERENCES

1. Woodruff, R.A., Jr., Clayton, P.J., and Guze, S.B. Hysteria: An evaluation of specific diagnostic criteria by the study of randomly selected psychiatric clinic patients. *Br. J. Psychiatry, 115*:1243–1248 (1969).
2. Guze, S.B., Woodruff, R.A., Jr., and Clayton, P.J. Hysteria and antisocial behavior: Further evidence of an association. *Am. J. Psychiatry, 127*:957–960 (1971).
3. Woodruff, R.A., Clayton, P.J., and Guze, S.B. Hysteria: Studies of diagnosis, outcome, and prevalence. *JAMA, 215*:425–428 (1971).
4. Woodruff, R.A., Guze, S.B., and Clayton, P.J. Unipolar and bipolar primary affective disorders. *Br. J. Psychiatry, 119*:33–38 (1971).
5. Woodruff, R.A., Guze, S.B., and Clayton, P.J. The medical and psychiatric implications of anti-social personality (sociopathy). *Dis Nerv Syst., 32*:712–714 (1971?.
6. Guze, S.B., Woodruff, R.A., and Clayton, P.J. A study of conversion symptoms in psychiatric outpatients. *Am. J. Psychiatry, 128*:643–646 (1971).
7. Guze, S.B., Woodruff, R.A., Clayton, P.J. Secondary affective disorders: A study of 95 cases. *Psychol. Med., 1*:426–428 (1971).
8. Woodruff, R.A., Guze, S.B., and Clayton, P.J. Anxiety neurosis among psychiatric outpatients. *Compr. Psychiatry, 13*:165–170 (1972).
9. Woodruff, R.A., Guze, S.B., and Clayton, P.J. Divorce among psychiatric outpatients. *Br. J. Psychiatry, 121*:289–292 (1972).
10. Woodruff, R.A., Clayton, P.J., and Guze, S.B. Suicide attempts and psychiatric diagnosis. *Dis. Nerv. Syst., 33*:617–621 (1972).
11. Guze, S.B., Woodruff, R.A., and Clayton, P.J. Sex, age, and the diagnosis of hysteria (Briquet's syndrome). *Am. J. Psychiatry, 129*:745–748 (1972).
12. Woodruff, R.A., Guze, S.B., Clayton, P.J., et al. Alcoholism and depression. *Arch. Gen. Psychiatry 28*:97–100 (1973).
13. Woodruff, R.A., Jr., Guze, S.B., and Clayton, P.J. Alcoholics who see a psychiatrist compared with those who do not. *Q. J. Stud. Alcohol., 34*:1162–1171 (1973).
14. Guze, S.B., Woodruff, R.A., Jr., and Clayton, P.J. Psychiatric disorders and criminality. *JAMA, 227*:641–642 (1974).
15. Woodruff, R.A., Jr., Guze, S.B., and Clayton, P.J. Psychiatric illness and season of birth. *Am. J. Psychiatry, 131*:925–926 (1974).
16. Woodruff, R.A., Jr., Clayton, P.J., and Guze, S.B. Is everyone depressed? *Am. J. Psychiatry, 132*:627–628 (1975).
17. Guze, S.B., Clayton, P.J., and Woodruff, R.A., Jr. The significance of psychotic affective disorders. *Arch. Gen. Psychiatry, 32*:1147–1150 (1975).
18. Woodruff, R.A., Jr., Clayton, P.J., and Guze, S.B. Psychiatric diagnoses within a group of adolescent outpatients, *Life History Research in Psychopathology*, Vol. 4, University of Minnesota Press, Minneapolis, 1975.
19. Woodruff, R.A., Jr., Clayton, P.J., Cloninger, C.R., et al. A brief method of screening for alcholism. *Dis. Nerv. Syst., 37*:434–435 (1976).
20. Liskow, B.I., Clayton, P.J., Woodruff, R.A., et al. Briquet's syndrome, hysterical personality, and the MMPI. *Am. J. Psychiatry, 134*:1137–1139 (1977).
21. Cloninger, C.R., Martin, R.L., Clayton, P., et al. A blind follow-up an family study of anxiety neurosis: Preliminary analysis of the St. Louis 500, (D.F. Klein, and J. Rabkin, eds.), *Anxiety: New Research and Changing Concepts*. Raven, New York, 1981.
22. Guze, S.B., Cloninger, C.R., Martin, R.L. et al. A follow-up and family study of schizophrenia. *Arch. Gen. Psychiatry, 40*:1273–1276 (1983).
23. Martin, R.L., Cloninger, C.R., Guze, S.B., et al. Mortality in a follow-up of 500 psychiatric outpatients. I. Total mortality. *Arch. Gen. Psychiatry, 42*:47–54 (1985).

24. Martin, R.L., Cloninger, C.R., Guze, S.B., et al. Mortality in a follow-up 500 psychiatric outpatients. II. Cause-specific mortality. *Arch. Gen. Psychiatry, 42*:58–66, 1985.

25. Cloninger, C.R., Martin, R.L., Guze, S.B., et al. Diangosis and prognosis in schizophrenia. *Arch. Gen. Psychiatry, 42*:15–25 (1985).

26. Cloninger, C.R., Martin, R.L., Guze, S.B., et al. Current status of schizophrenia as a disease concept, (M. Alpert ed.), *Controversies in Schizophrenia*. Guilford, New York, 1985, pp. 12–24.

27. Martin, R.L., Cloninger, C.R., Guze, S.B., et al. Frequency and differential diagnosis of depressive syndromes in schizophrenia. *J. Clin. Psychiatry, 46*:9–13 (1985).

28. Guze, S.B. Cloninger, C.R., Martin, R.L., et al. A follow-up and family study of Briquet's syndrome. *Br. J. Psychiatry* (in press).

29. Martin, R.L., Cloninger, C.R., Guze, S.B., et al. Excess among psychiatric patients: The importance of unnatural death, substance abuse disorders, antisocial personality, and homosexuality. *Acta. Psychiatr. Belg.* (submitted).

30. Cloninger, C.R., Martin, R.L., Guze, S.B., et al. Somatization disorder in men and women: A prospective follow-up and family study. *Am. J. Psychiatry* (submitted).

31. Robins, L.N., Helzer, J.E., Weissman, M.M., et al. Lifetime prevalence of specific psychiatric disorders in three sites. *Arch. Gen. Psychiatry, 41*:949–958 (1984).

32. Martin, R.L., Cloninger, C.R., and Guze, S.B. The evaluation of diagnostic concordance in follow-up studies. II. A blind, prospective follow-up of female criminals. *J. Psychiatr. Res., 15*:107–125 (1979).

33. Goodwin, D.W., Crane, J.B., and Guze, S.B. Felons who drink: An 8-year follow-up. *Q. J. Stud. Alcohol, 32*:136–147 (1971).

34. Hesselbrock, M.N., Meyer, R.E., and Keener, J.J. Psychopathology in hospitalized alcoholics. *Arch. Gen. Psychiatry, 42*:1050–1055 (1985).

35. Schuckit, M.A. The clinical implications of primary diagnostic groups among alcoholics. *Arch. Gen. Psychiatry, 42*:1043–1049 (1985).

17

Drug and Alcohol Addiction as a Disease

Norman S. Miller
Cornell University Medical College, The New York Hospital–Cornell Medical Center, White Plains, New York

I. DISEASE CONCEPT

A. Definitions of Disease

Most definitions of disease easily accommodate alcoholism as a disease. The basic question is often not whether or not alcoholism may qualify as a disease, as that issue has been confirmed by clinical experience and scientific documentation. Certainly, the classification of alcoholism as a disease is beyond the stage of a concept for those who must diagnose and treat alcoholism as well as those who suffer from the disease of alcoholism [1,2].

When studies have been performed inquiring about the nature of the disease alcoholism and whether or not it is a disease, some interesting results have been obtained. In 1979, a study revealed that 85% of general practitioners agree that alcoholism is a disease—the same percentage that regarded coronary artery disease, hypertension, and epilepsy as a disease. A 1988 Gallop poll found that when the public was asked if alcoholism were a disease, 78% agreed strongly, 10% agreed somewhat, 6% disagreed somewhat, 5% disagreed strongly, and 1% had no opinion. But the poll indicated that the exact meaning of "disease" remains unclear in the public mind. Asked which of a number of options describe their feelings about alcoholism, 60% said it is a disease or illness, 31% a mental or psychological problem, 23% a lack of will power, 16% a moral weakness, and 6% were unsure. (The total is greater than 100% due to multiple responses.)

Unfortunately, the classification of alcoholism as a disease remains only partially accepted by many who are responsible for decisions that affect vast numbers of those who suffer from alcoholism. The reasons are complex and require an understanding more of metaphysical and ethical theory, and the emotional impact that alcoholism has on individuals and society than an appreciation of the scientific evidence. At the heart of the debate over the classification of alcoholism as a disease is the persistent notion that it is a moral degeneration, over which the individual must exercise will power to solve the moral dilemma and an emotional conflict that alcohol is used to self-medicate. Underlying the moral concept of alcoholism is that the ability to exercise free will is unimpaired, and the individual chooses to drink excessively and has complete control over that decision. Alcoholism then is a willful expenditure of one's immoral character as other sins of gluttony and self-destruction. And that the twisted and distorted emotional state compels someone to seek relief in alcohol [3].

For many, alcoholism is not regarded as a primary disorder and does not stand on its own as a self-sufficient disease. That is why terms associated with other psychiatric disorders, such as anxiety and depression, are employed to define alcoholism. Because the stigma of alcoholism is greater than that of mental illness, it is preferable to have anxiety and depression as diseases rather than is alcoholism (drug addiction).

Webster's Ninth New Collegiate Dictionary [4] defines disease as an impairment of the normal state of the living animal or plant body that affects the performance of the vital functions; a sickness is listed as a synonym. An obsolete definition is "trouble." This is a relatively inclusive definition that would allow many conditions to qualify as a disease. *Dorland's Illustrated Medical Dictionary, Twenty-Seventh Edition*, 1988, contains a definition of disease as "any deviation from or interruption of the normal structure or function of any part, organ, or system (or combination) of the body that is manifested by a characteristic set of symptoms and signs, and whose etiology, pathology, and prognosis may be known or unknown" [5]. Most dictionaries define disease as an illness, a sickness. Alcoholism (drug addiction) fits exactly into this definition because an addiction to alcohol and drugs is a definite morbid process that produces characteristic and identifiable signs and symptoms affecting many organ systems in the body.

A very stringent definition of disease is provided by Koch's Postulates that require several criteria be fulfilled before an entity can be called the cause of disease. The essential features are to identify the agent that is causing a sickness, isolate it from the host, and then give it to another host to see if it causes the same disease, and once again isolate the agent as the source of the disease to identify it as the cause [6].

Alcoholism fulfills these criteria by observing the characteristic behaviors in the setting of drinking, remove the alcohol, and give it to another vulnerable individual. The ingestion of alcohol will initiate the disease, alcoholism, in the second alcoholic as in the first. Koch originated these criteria to demonstrate that bacteria caused certain diseases; however, it can be seen that just a bacterium may be identified as a cause of pneumonia, alcohol may be identified as a cause of alcoholism. Other questions remain, of course, and that is why some people develop pneumonia, and others alcoholism. Although some liberty has been taken by applying Koch's Postulates to alcoholism, the analogous conditions exist between the introduction of alcohol into a genetically vulnerable individual and the infection by a bacterium in a susceptible host [6].

B. History of the Disease Concept

The history of the disease concept dates back to early Greek times when Hippocrates, the father of medicine, set down explanations of observations of disease he made in the fifth century B.C. He postulated that diseases were caused by an imbalance in the elements of earth, air, fire, and water and other ingredients of nature. Psychiatric disorders were caused by being possessed by evil spirits which overtook the body and mind. Medicine progressed rather slowly as even as late as the nineteenth century, certain medical diseases, such as syphilis, and most psychiatric disorders, including schizophrenia, manic-depressive illness, and alcoholism, were considered defects of character and moral degeneracies [7].

It was not until the early nineteenth century that mental illness acquired the legitimacy of a disease. Physicians in the United States first recognized alcoholism as a disease through the writings of Benjamin Rush, who among other contributions was the founder of the American

Psychiatric Association. Rush identified alcoholism as a disease in which alcohol serves as the causal agent, loss of control over drinking behavior as the characteristic symptom, and total abstinence as the only effective cure. Curiously, the field of alcoholism has not yet surpassed this simple but brilliant clinical observation made by a discerning psychiatrist [8].

Alcoholism fully arrived as a disease in the mid-twentieth century when physicians for the first time acknowledged as an official body that alcoholism was a disease [9]. The American Medical Association had published an official declaration in a journal article entitled "Hospitalization of Patients with Alcoholism," [3] in which The Council on Mental Health, its Committee on Alcoholism, and the profession in general recognized the syndrome of alcoholism as an illness which justifiably should have the attention of physicians. Although this statement constitutes the formal acceptance of the disease concept of alcoholism by the American medical profession as a whole, it does not mean that acceptance among physicians is unanimous or even a majority [3].

The disease concept of alcoholism, however, has never in reality been adopted and forwarded in any systematic way by physicians on any large scale. Throughout medical history there have been only a few physicians who have supported and formulated the disease concept of alcoholism. Dr. William Silkworth while working with alcoholics in Towns Hospital in New City arrived at a simple formula to explain his clinical observations of alcoholism. He ascertained that alcoholism is a physical allergy to alcohol, which exits in only those who are destined to become alcoholics, and not in those who are temperate drinkers [10].

Dr. Harry Tiebolt, a psychiatrist, worked closely with members of Alcoholics Anonymous to forward some formalization of the disease concept espoused by the recovered alcoholics. He published in leading medical journals about psychodynamic concepts which could be used to describe the intrapsychic phenomena in the disease of alcoholism. He emphasized the importance of the psychological defense mechanisms of denial, rationalization, and minimization in the propagation of alcoholism [11].

However, the popularization of the disease concept of alcoholism originates from the nonphysician E.M. Jellinek who wrote a lengthy, scholarly book entitled, *The Disease Concept of Alcoholism* [3]. In the book, he analyzed data and opinion from a variety of sources and arrived at the conclusion that a majority of the evidence favors that alcoholism is a disease. He basically views alcoholism as an addiction similar to other drug addictions. He also pointed out that the term *alcohol addiction* would not gain favor because of the stigma attached to the term addiction.

The growth of Alcoholics Anonymous and the development of effective treatment of alcoholism (drug addiction) has contributed greatly to the credibility of the disease concept. However, a parallel accumulation of scientific evidence has provided the long-awaited documentation of the disease concept of alcoholism. The genetic studies of alcoholism have clearly established that alcoholism has similar characteristics to other diseases because the genetic basis of alcoholism is transmitted through genetic material. Important investigations have revealed that genetic messages are encoded in the genes. These genes are composed of biochemical components, called deoxyribonucleic acid (DNA), which can be isolated. The gene for alcoholism has not been identified as yet [12].

II. ALCOHOLISM (DRUG ADDICTION) AS A DISEASE

A. Addiction to Alcohol and Drugs

Because of the enormous overlap between alcoholism and drug addiction in the contemporary alcoholic, it is almost useless to discuss alcoholism as a disease without also including drug addiction as a disease. Although there are differences, particularly in the consequences between the use of alcohol and drugs, the essential characteristics of the diseases are identical. Therefore, the consideration of alcoholism as a disease must include drug addiction also as a disease [13].

Addiction is defined by behaviors of addiction which are the preoccupation with the acquisition of alcohol (drugs), compulsive use of alcohol (use in spite of adverse consequences), and a pattern of relapse to alcohol and drugs in spite of adverse consequences. Pervasive to the three criteria for addiction is a loss of control underlying the preoccupation, compulsive use, and relapse. The addictive use of alcohol inevitably leads to the development of adverse consequences because of the persistent loss of control. This loss of control, once established, is to exist for a lifetime. In other words, the alcoholic and drug addict will not be able to use alcohol or drugs without experiencing a consistent loss of control, at some point following a resumption of use after a period of abstinence [14,15].

The primary foundation of alcoholism as a disease rests on the acceptance of the loss of control over alcohol by the alcoholic. The loss of control is the cardinal manifestation of the disease [16]. The loss of control is the essential feature that leads to the multitude of adverse consequences. The loss of control is manifested in many aspects of the alcoholics life, including disturbances in interpersonal relationships, and medical, psychiatric, and spiritual consequences. The key point that is difficult for dissenters of the disease concept to accept is that the alcoholic has lost this control over the use of alcohol because of a disease of the body, mind, and spirit. The dissenter to the disease concept contends that the alcoholic has chosen to drink because of an exercise of the will although often to relieve some intolerable condition. The fallacy in the free will concept of alcoholism is clear but difficult to refute if the loss of control explanation of alcoholism is not accepted.

Several studies have been performed to examine the loss of control over alcohol use in alcoholics. Several studies have demonstrated that alcoholics cannot use alcohol normally or nonaddictively over their lifetime once the diagnosis of alcoholism is made. One longitudinal study confirmed that less than 1% of the alcoholics drank without serious consequences, and there was significant doubt that even that 1% drank normally. However, other studies present findings that alcoholics can be taught to drink normally over time. Some studies bring alcoholics into the laboratory and ask questions and observe the drinking behaviors of the alcoholics. The findings are that some alcoholics do not show a loss of control with the use of alcohol [15].

There are several methodological problems with studying alcoholics in the cross-sectional state as well as over time, particularly in the active state of drinking or alcoholism. The central problem is the denial that is part of the disease of alcoholism. This denial may lead to difficulties in establishing the criteria for the diagnosis as well as identifying the adverse consequences. Any underestimation of the denial will lead to problems in confirming the loss of control in the alcoholics. Corroborative history from outside sources who know the alcoholic is often necessary to penetrate or circumvent the denial. Not all studies take these precautions in their methods [14].

According to the first step in Alcoholics Anonymous, the alcoholic must accept his or her loss of control over alcohol (drugs), although not explicitly stated, that extends over a lifetime. "We admitted we were powerless over alcohol—that our lives had become unmanageable" [30]. The word *powerless* is equivalent to the loss of control, and the word *unmanageable* represents the adverse consequences of the powerlessness. In order for the alcoholic to begin recovery from the alcoholism, responsibility for the loss of control must be assumed. A common reason for relapse to alcoholic drinking is an inability or unwillingness to accept this fundamental aspect of the disease. Relapse because of the lack of acceptance of the loss of control may occur after a brief or prolonged period of abstinence such as years.

It is much easier for the alcoholic to comprehend the first step and recognize the loss of control over alcohol if it is attributed to a disease. Because will power over the loss of control of alcohol use is ultimately ineffective, insistence on correcting a weak character or treating an underlying psychiatric or emotional disorder will not prevent relapse to alcohol (drugs). The alcoholic is already filled with self-condemnation and a further exaggeration of the guilt by making the alcoholic at "fault" for his or her abnormal drinking will impede the alcoholic's accepting responsibility for the alcoholism and its consequences [17].

B. Genetics of Alcoholism

The most important breakthrough in confirming that alcoholism is a disease since Jellinek published his book [11] is the finding that alcoholism is an inherited disorder. Many scientific studies have clearly documented that alcoholism has a genetic component to it, as do many other medical and psychiatric disorders. Plutarch noted in biblical times that "Drunkard begot drunkards" [12].

The genetic studies have used four major methods for studying alcoholism as a primary disease. The first method was utilized by Jellinek himself, who termed *familial alcoholism* as a diagnostic category. Jellinek and many others found that alcoholism ran in families, such that an alcoholic had a much greater chance of having a family member who is alcoholic than a nonalcoholic. In fact, the studies on families of alcoholics have found that over 50% of the alcoholics have a family history positive for alcoholism. Furthermore, if an alcoholic had at least one family member who was alcoholic, they were likely to have additional family members who were alcoholics [12].

The family studies led to attempts to control for environmental influences to determine that genetic disposition was responsible for the transmission of the alcoholism. Adoption studies performed abroad and in the United States have shown dramatically that biological background plays a determining role in the development of alcoholism. In the adoption studies, alcoholic and nonalcoholic adoptees were separated from their biological parents before 6 months of age and raised apart without contact or knowledge of their parents. The alcoholic adoptees were found to have biological parents who were alcoholics much more often than the nonalcoholic adoptees. Furthermore, whether or not the foster parents living with adoptees were alcoholics did not determine the development of alcoholism in the adoptees. In other words, the biological parents and not foster parents determined alcoholism in the adoptees, and who the adoptees lived with did not influence whether or not they became alcoholic. The genetic makeup of the adoptees determined the development of alcoholism, and not the environment [12].

The twin studies are also revealing in confirming a genetic predisposition to alcoholism. Identical twins are more likely to be concordant for alcoholism than fraternal twins according to many studies performed in the United States and abroad. Concordance for alcoholism means that the twin pairs both had the alcoholism, whereas discordance means that only one was alcoholic. Furthermore, identical twins have the exact same genes or genetic makeup, whereas fraternal twins are like brothers and sisters who share half of the same genes. The greater rate of alcoholism among identical twins is confirmation that the genetic predisposition is important in the development of alcoholism [12].

The high-risk studies have shown those who are at risk to develop alcoholism share characteristics with alcoholics and have characteristics that are different than nonalcoholic. A high-risk individual is not alcoholic but has a blood relative who is an alcoholic. The importance of high-risk studies is that there may be markers that we can identify which are specific for alcoholism, and that are present before the onset of alcoholism. Some of these markers are abnormal neurophysiological findings, such as seen on the electroencephalograph and evoked potentials and biochemical and behavioral measurements. These findings confirm that alcoholism has genetic features that can be identified by scientific methods, as can other medical and psychiatric disorders [12].

III. HEAVY DRINKING

A. Epidemiological Catchment Area Study

Heavy drinking does occur in the absence of alcoholism, and as such may not be considered a disease. Heavy drinking does not include addictive drinking, so that by definition, loss of control over alcohol is not present. What distinguishes heavy drinking from alcoholism is that the heavy drinker can and often will quit or abstain when the consequences from the drinking are serious enough to warrant it. The ability to control drinking to ward off adverse consequences is the hallmark of the heavy drinker, whereas the alcoholic continues in spite of the adverse consequences.

According to a large national study in which 20,000 people were interviewed in five cities, the Epidemiological Catchment Area Study (ECA) found that heavy drinking occurred in about the same number of the population as did alcoholism. The overall prevalence rate of alcoholism is 15% as is the category of heavy drinking [18].

Many heavy drinkers go on to develop alcoholism, but many may also quit drinking. Heavy drinkers may be considered at high risk to develop alcoholism as drinking, particularly, in high consumption rates, is a risk factor for the development of alcoholism.

B. Heavy Drinking as a Counter to Alcoholism as a Disease

Some opponents to alcoholism as a disease offer heavy drinking as a explanation of alcoholism. Fingarette argued in a book entitled *Heavy Drinking: The Myth of Alcoholism as a Disease* [19] that alcoholism is not a disease, and in fact does not exist. He concludes that alcoholics do not experience a loss of control over alcohol use, and presents several studies to support his contention. He ignores many studies that do show loss of control in alcoholics as well as the self-report of thousands to millions of alcoholics in recovery who attest to their powerlessness over the use of alcohol.

Fingarette unfortunately categorically discounts the vast amount of genetic evidence for alcoholism as a disease by denying the findings of the studies. He does not provide a critical analysis of the scientific methods employed in the large number of genetic studies. He does not account for the large number of alcoholics who have a family history of alcoholism i.e. 50% of alcoholics.

Curiously, Fingarette's definition of heavy drinking would qualify for many clinicians' definition of alcoholism. He affirms that heavy drinking becomes a central activity with consequences affecting the drinkers life. This definition of heavy drinking is essentially one of addictive drinking in which a preoccupation and compulsive use of alcohol is characteristic. He falls short of calling heavy drinking alcoholism.

Importantly, Fingarette asserts that alcoholics are not helpless; that they can take control of their lives. "In the last analysis, alcoholics must want to change and choose to change." He concludes that alcoholism is not a disease; the assumption of personal responsibility, however, is a sign of health, while needless submission to spurious medical authority is a pathology. Proponents of the disease concept would not disagree with Fingarette on any of those points. The cornerstone of recovery according to the disease concept of alcoholism is personal responsibility. The alcoholic must assume responsibility for his or her alcoholism (drug addiction) before recovery can begin and certainly be maintained. This is true of many diseases, particularly chronic ones that are not curable.

The alcoholic is helpless alone against the disease of alcoholism, just as a victim of hypertension is helpless without proper treatment. However, with an acceptance of alcoholism as a medical disease and the indicated treatment, the alcoholic becomes mater of his or her destiny. Finally, the alcoholic must ultimately want and choose to change as the essential treatment of alcoholism is a fundamental change in attitude and personality over time that results from active and voluntary involvement in a treatment program for alcoholism as a disease.

Although Fingarette uses the concept of alcoholism in his description of heavy drinking, he does not want to consider alcoholism a disease [19]. His effort to refute alcoholism as a disease is a rejection of basic definitions such as addiction, and is not based on scientific, empirical evidence. His resistance to the disease concept is not new and not rare as the stigma associated with alcoholism is age old. Fingarette, as many others, does not accept the classification of alcoholism as a disease. Moreover, if alcoholism is not a disease, then treatment is not necessary, and the need to stop drinking is not urgent. Unfortunately, Fingarette offers little alternative to his rejection of alcoholism as a disease.

IV. ALTERNATIVE THEORIES TO ALCOHOLISM AS A DISEASE: SELF-MEDICATION HYPOTHESIS

A. Psychoanalysis

Psychodynamic theory has provided a useful conceptualization and terminology for the description of some of the intradynamic processes involved in alcoholism (drug addiction). The terms of *conscious* and *unconscious* and *defense mechanisms* are particularly helpful is describing the character of the addictive process and the intrapsychic consequences of the addictive mode. Conscious and unconscious denial, minimization, rationalization, and other psychodynamic processes are psychological mechanisms by which alcoholism is perpetuated and sustained intrapsychically [20].

However, psychoanalytic theory neither explains addictive behavior nor provides a framework for the treatment of addiction. The existence of unconscious conflicts does not lead to addictive use, and the uncovering and resolution of these unconscious conflicts do not lead to a cure or an arrest of the addiction. In fact, the continued expression of an addiction can lead to serious and significant psychodynamic conflicts that will require treatment of the addiction.

Nonetheless, psychoanalytic theory has reflected a popular view of alcoholism that has existed for centuries. This historical view is that alcoholism is caused by some other disorder or disease than alcoholism; i.e., alcoholism is not a primary disease. In other words, alcoholism may exist but is not a disease as such, rather it is secondary to or a manifestation of an underlying, causative disorder. The psychoanalytic model has attempted to explain alcoholic drinking by a number of psychodynamic theories.

The ego is the mediator between the powerful forces of the impulsive id and the punitive superego, which operate in the unconscious mind according to psychoanalytic thinking. Whenever there is a conflict between these primitive drives, guilt may result, and the ego is in a dissonant state. The disharmony in the ego by its failed attempts to mediate conflict motivates the ego to seek relief in escape, such as through drinking to forget and to relieve tension [21].

Although this explanation may be valid for alcohol and drug "use," it does not account for addictive use, nor is it indicative of a disease. Psychoanalytic theory only provides a rationale for motivated use of alcohol and drugs but does not explain why alcoholics continue to use alcohol and drugs long after the benefits outweigh the adverse consequences. The conflicts created by addictive drinking often exceed those that may have motivated the drinking in the first place. The original distress to the ego is lost in the overwhelming disruption from diseased drinking.

Furthermore, according to psychodynamic principles, once the conflicts are resolved through psychotherapy, which may be extensive and prolonged, the alcoholic will no longer need to drink to self-medicate the underlying distress to the ego. The major drawback to this approach is that it often fails to work unless the drinking behavior is terminated. The alcoholic is either unable or unwilling to abstain from alcoholic by solving underlying conflicts. According to the disease model, the drinking must cease and other behaviors conducive to continued abstention must be instituted before the conflicts can be assessed and resolved by the alcoholic.

Studies have also been performed which have shown that no particular personality type predisposes one to the development of alcoholism. Vaillant [22] showed that all personality types were represented among alcoholics from a large group of individuals he followed for a prolonged period of time to deterine if a particular type of personality was more likely to become alcoholic. Several other studies have found similar results.

However, there does seem to be a core personality that is acquired from having the disease of alcoholism active over time. The core personality is characterized by narcissistic, antisocial, immature, and dependent traits. These traits may or may not have been predominant in the alcoholic before the development of alcoholism. Of course, these are traits that are present to some extent in most individuals and become exaggerated in the alcoholic.

B. Biological Psychiatry

The self-medication hypothesis is used in the biological psychiatry approach in that alcoholism (drug addiction) is due to some other illness. In this case, the major psychiatric illnesses are anxiety, depression, and personality disorders. The emphasis is on the need to self-medicate with alcohol and drugs the distress that originates from the underlying psychiatric disease.

A common example is the diagnoses of anxiety and depression and the use of alcohol and drugs. The theory is that because depression produces psychological pain, the sufferer of depression will use alcohol and drugs to obtain relief as in the psychoanalytic model. Once again, this is a model that is based on the popular and old conception of motivated use of alcohol and drugs. It not only fails to justify addictive or disease use, but it also does not fit the clinical picture of what actually happens in alcoholics and those who are depressed [23].

Studies have clearly shown that alcohol and drug use produces depression but do not substantiate that depression leads to alcohol and drug use. In one study, three groups were given alcohol and their mood and affect were measured. The three groups were depressed alcoholics, depressed nonalcoholics, and nondepressed nonalcoholics (normals). Surprisingly, the depressed alcoholics showed the least benefit in euphoria and improved affect from the drinking of alcohol. The depressed nonalcoholic received the greatest followed by the normals. These observations confirm that alcoholics do not drink to feel better because drinking makes them feel worse. It appears that alcoholics drink in spite of the depression and not because of it. Moreover, the assumption that alcoholics drink because of the depression is derived from effects produced by alcohol in depressed nonalcoholic and not those produced in alcoholics [24].

Furthermore, when the drinking behavior of manic-depressives who are not alcoholics was examined, similar conclusions were found. Manic-depressives showed that they reduced their drinking during their depressive episodes and increased their drinking during their manic episodes. The reason for increased drinking during mania is that many behaviors of excess are greater with the hyperactivity and poor judgment of the manic. The reason for reduced drinking during depression may be related to the overall effects of alcohol, which is to depress the mind and mood. Alcohol is categorized as a depressant by its pharmacological actions on the brain.

No studies have demonstrated that anxiety leads to addictive drinking and drug use. Once again, there are many anecdotal reports whereby that interpretation is forwarded but is not substantiated. It is generally accepted that anxiety leads to alcohol and drug use, but only assumed that addictive use is a manifestation of an underlying anxiety disorder.

However, studies have clearly shown that alcohol and drugs produce anxiety in either the intoxicated state or during withdrawal. For instance, chronic alcohol intake produces repetitive withdrawal states during which anxiety is produced as a function of the discharging sympathetic nervous system. Similarly, cocaine induces the sympathetic nervous system to produce rather severe states of anxiety, including panic disorders, as with alcohol.

The biological models of addiction are important to consider because they stress a underlying biochemical mechanism for behavior, mental life, and psychiatric disorders. Because alcoholism represents in part a physical "allergy" to alcohol, the basis is some change in the brain chemistry that is responsible for the expression of the disease of alcoholism when alcohol interacts with the brain cells. Further studies into the neurochemical origins of psychiatric disease will help our understanding of the origins of alcoholism and drug addiction because both classes of disorders are rooted in abnormalities in brain function.

V. ADAPTIVE VS DISEASE MODEL FOR ALCOHOLISM (DRUG ADDICTION)

A. Origins

The adaptive model is a popular framework that is reflective of an ancient conception that is used to understand alcoholism and drug addiction, and has evolved into psychosocial theories. These psychosocial theories originate from notions of causality in religion and morality, and late nineteenth and early twentieth century psychology. The religious concept of free will and will power in disease has continued throughout centuries. People became ill because of a lack of moral character and "true grit." Many of the psychosocial theories remain cemented in moral causality [25].

The disease model evolved for not only alcoholism and drug addiction, but for other medical, surgical, and psychiatric conditions. The principle reasons for the adoption and application of the disease model is that it fits the observations and provides a pragmatic approach that works for diagnosis and treatment.

The adaptive model is intuitively appealing to the mind but does not withstand scientific validation. The mind can just as intuitively arrive at the conclusion that the earth is flat and is at the center of the universe, as ancient philosophers did, or to the contrary that the earth is round and is part of a solar system around which it revolves. Scientific validation needs to demonstrate the fallacies of the intuitive mind. The disease model is as deterministic, probabilistic, and mechanical as science itself. The scientific model has been an effective way for medicine to advance. To revert back to the adaptive model with emotional suppositions and religious intonation is to impede medical progress, and unfortunately remain with a model that does not work.

B. Causality

According to the disease model, the interaction between alcohol or a drug and the brain is responsible for the initiation of the disease. The disease model states that a genetic vulnerability is expressed as a predisposition to develop an addiction when exposed to alcohol and drugs. Alcohol and drugs are thought to affect neurotransmitters in key areas of the brain to sustain addictive behavior [27]. The drive states such as hunger, thirst, sex, and others are associated with a reward system in the limbic system in an ancient portion of the brain. An effect of alcohol and drugs is to stimulate both the drive states and the reward center, and may produce a link between all of them through memory in the hippocampus of the limbic system [28].

In this way alcoholism and drug addiction are "biochemical diseases," just as are manic-depressive illness and schizophrenia. The biochemical theories for these psychiatric disorders are no further advanced than those for alcoholism and drug addiction. The biochemical cause of manic-depressive disease and schizophrenia is based on hypotheses about neurotransmitter affects in the brain that have much promise but are yet to be proven. There are several biochemical theories of alcoholism and drug addiction involving the same neurotransmitter systems, such as dopamine, serotonin, gamma-aminobutyric acid (GABA), and others, which are though to be operative in the expression of the other psychiatric disorders [27].

Environmental stress, availability, attitudes, and morality regarding alcohol and drugs are important factors that determine exposure to alcohol or drugs but do not cause addiction as claimed by the adaptive model. The disease model further states that economic, family, individual, psychological, psychiatric, physical, social, and moral consequences ensue from addictive drug use. The important link in the disease model is that the consequences result from and do not cause addiction.

The adaptive model states the reverse; i.e., the economic, family, individual and social problems, stresses, evils, and depravities lead to addictive use. The alcoholic prior to the onset of alcoholism has failed to achieve maturity in economic independence, self-reliance, and responsibility toward others. Because of these failures, the individual seeks and chooses to use alcohol and drugs to further self-destruction. The important ingredients to the equation in the adaptive model is that the addiction results from a lack of adult maturity through environmental problems.

Although this may be an appealing theory, it does not explain why some individuals choose alcohol and drugs, whereas others do not. It also does not account for the vast numbers of individuals who do not come from deprived backgrounds yet develop alcoholism. The majority of alcoholics have jobs, families, and a reasonable integration into society. It is the minority of alcoholics who are disadvantaged and deprived.

C. Pragmatism and Empiricism

Because the recovery from the disease alcoholism relies heavily on personal responsibility, the alcoholic is an active participant in the recovery process. In the adaptive model, the alcoholic is consumed by outside forces that conspire to undermine his maturity. Accordingly, the alcoholic is a victim within a network of forces which undermine maturity and will power. However, all diseases begin with the concept that the individual is responsible for possessing but not causing the disease. The diabetic has inherited the genes for diabetes but did not determine the physical or genetic predisposition for the disease with which he or she was born.

The disease model has gained whatever popularity it has today because it fits scientific inquiry, promotes medical progress, and works for the alcoholic. The adaptive model still has appeal where knowledge is lacking or not accepted. In this way the adaptive model is useful as a framework to form an hypothesis. Hopefully with continued research and accumulated knowledge, the true nature of the disease of alcoholism and drug addiction will further emerge.

VI. LEGAL DECISIONS REGARDING ALCOHOLISM AS A DISEASE

A previous case that reached the Supreme Court of the United States resulted in the ruling

> that the drinking of intoxicating liquor might develop from a harmless indulgence into a baneful disease of chronic disease alcoholism. It is common knowledge and the warning is evident that indulgence in intoxicating liquors, unless restrained . . . , leads to excessive indulgence and one need not be warned that if continued, the craving for alcoholic liquor may lead to habitual drunkenness and the unfortunate self-imposed consequences [3].

In this decision, the court acknowledges not only that alcoholism is a disease, but that this is common knowledge. It also believes that the individual is responsible for the taking the risks of drinking alcohol in the first place in face of a multitude of evidence that the consumption of alcohol can lead to chronic alcoholism. The self-imposed consequences originate from the decision to drink and not the disease of alcoholism according to this interpretation [3].

A Pennsylvania court decided [11]

> A caveat must be entered. We do not hold that chronic alcoholism is as a matter of law a self-inflicted injury. Our decision is that the evidence which the trial judge found credible justifies the conclusion that the disability suffered by this insured was self-inflicted.

A Maryland court rules [3]

> There is no evidence on the record legally sufficient for the jury to find that the chronic alcoholism of the insured is the result of his conscious purpose or design . . . . On the contrary the testimony tends to show that he had vainly exercised his will to restrain and control his desire. The result of his disease is a weakness of will and of character which caused him to yield to liquors. The drinking in the first stages was voluntary but there was not testimony that the drinker was then aware of the latent danger in his habit; and so while his consumption of liquor was a voluntary act, yet his ignorance of its insidious effect does not make the act a voluntary exposure of himself to the unexpected danger of the disease of chronic alcoholism. The result of the indulgence of an appetite does not necessarily determine that the result was self-inflicted because if the actor does not apprehend or is ignorant of the danger of his act, he may not be held to have voluntarily inflicted upon himself the consequences.

This decision covers the aspect of the insidious nature of alcoholism, and because of denial the alcoholic is often not aware of the severity of the drinking as well as the consequences from the drinking. Inherent but not explicitly stated is the loss of control over the alcohol use and the subsequent adverse consequences of the alcoholism.

The United States Supreme Court recently ruled that two alcoholics were not entitled to benefits from the Veterans Administration because they suffered from chronic alcoholism. The court was clear that it decided not to rule on whether or not alcoholism is a disease. It restricted its decision as to whether or not the alcoholics were guilty of willful misconduct. The court did not deny that the source of the willful misconduct was the disease of alcoholism. The court was careful to avoid a legal debate over a condition which rests on scientific and medical evidence [29].

Finally, the courts on many levels—municipal, county, state, and federal—regularly take into consideration the disease of alcoholism in rendering its decisions regarding the individual and the consequences of alcoholism. The courts do not excuse the alcoholic of the consequences of the alcoholism, which would only enable the alcoholic to continue drinking. What the courts do is to provide the alcoholic with a choice: Face the full punishment for the offense related to the alcoholism or accept a plan for retribution.

The legal system allows for remorse and restitution for many crimes, and frequently adjusts the sentence accordingly. It is a consistent practice for the judge to allow the alcoholic to accept responsibility for the treatment of his or her disease, express regret for the consequences, and demonstrate restitution by voluntarily choosing to undergo a formal treatment program for the alcoholism. In this way, alcoholism has no special place, and holds the alcoholic accountable for his or her alcoholism, and most importantly provides society with a corrective approach to a widespread disease. Thousands of alcoholics have initiated recovery with this particular legal intervention.

VII. TREATMENT OF THE DISEASE OF ALCOHOLISM

A. Comparisons to Other Diseases

The treatment of the disease alcoholism illustrates the paradoxical nature of many aspects of a disease with a strong physical component which also has so many behavioral and mental effects. Of interest is that alcoholism compares favorably to other well-accepted "medical" diseases.

Modern physicians are more uncertain about the diagnosis of coronary heart disease as a disease because the "root" etiologies are attributable to lifestyles under the individual's control and not an invasion of some external forces rendering the individual a victim. The diagnosis of coronary artery disease has become increasingly complex. Many different factors which are subject to error are integrate into a diagnosis of coronary artery disease, including personal reports from the patient and electrocardiographic findings.

Interestingly, effective treatment of early coronary heart disease depends much more on changing lifestyles than receiving medical treatments. Coronary artery disease has been associated with certain diets high in fats, obesity, type A, or hard driving, stress-oriented personalities, smoking, and high blood pressure. All of these conditions are believed to be under control of the will of the individual, and for this reason alone, coronary artery disease may be becoming less of "disease" in the sense that is readily accepted by the public [22].

It may be that any condition that involves some volition on the part of the individual to initiate or maintain will never fully qualify as a disease. A paradox is that in order to recover from alcoholism, an individual must exercise some commitment of will toward abstinence from alcohol consumption according to the disease concept. However, the term *disease* explicitly means that the individual has lost the capacity to consistently control how much and how often he or she drinks and the ability to accurately predict the consequences of the drinking. From where does the control arise to offset the autonomous state of addiction?

Alcoholism is also like essential hypertension in that neither has a known specific etiology but both conditions cause physical disease. Hypertension is heavily affected by social factors and may even have chronic alcohol consumption such as in alcoholism as a cause. Alcohol withdrawal is characterized by a discharging of the sympathetic nervous system which results in an elevation of blood pressure and pulse rate. The physical and psychological adverse complications from hypertension are as diverse as those caused by alcoholism [22].

The preferred treatment of hypertension is frequently a change in diet, loss of weight, reduction in stress, and changes in those aspects of the lifestyle that come under the power of the will. The treatment of alcoholism requires a change in lifestyle and attitudes in some ways similar to hypertension. Furthermore, the adverse consequences of alcoholism accrue in both conditions if left untreated, generally, the greater the number, the longer the course of the diseases.

Diabetes mellitus is another disease that has a physical basis in the expression of elevated blood sugar (hyperglycemia) and a medication, insulin, treatment. However, the diabetic must take responsibility for the disease in order to self-inject the insulin. If the diabetic is unwilling or unable to self-administer the treatment, serious consequences may follow, just as in the case of the alcoholic who must accept responsibility for the disease alcoholism and its treatment to avoid adverse consequences.

B. Obstacles to the Treatment of Alcoholism

Referring back to the ideal concept of disease, the individual who has a disease is a victim who has no control over its onset and progression. This notion may have originated in ancient biblical and mythological times when the gods intervened in the helpless victim's life to produce some unfortunate change. The god may have been angry and decided to punish someone because of a reason unrelated to that person, or the individual was responsible for a wrong but not in line with the severity of the punishment. At any rate, the god produced a victim, and the victim was not responsible for the malady possessing them.

A patient with cancer or a genetic disease is an example of a victim. A cancer victim is someone who has developed a malignancy, which is an uncontrolled growth of a tissue in the body. The tissue growth overtakes the normal functions of the organs, and eventually the ability of the body to sustain life is lost. We do not ordinarily hold the individual responsible for the cancer. Yet how else will the individual seek and accept any treatment that is available? The individual who continues to deny he or she either has or can have cancer will not seek early diagnosis and treatment. Are not these choices conscious decisions over which the individual has control and the freedom to exercise that control? How many victims of cancer see themselves as invincible and unrealistically avoid believing they may develop cancer, thereby avoiding the responsibility of seeking treatment.

Moreover, studies have shown that individuals may have more control over the onset and development of cancer than we had previously thought. For many types of cancer, prevention is becoming a reality. In some cases, lung cancer may be caused by cigarette smoking, cervical cancer may be a result of certain sexual practices and whether or not one has been pregnant, stomach cancer may be associated with particular types of diets, and breast cancer may be associated with taking birth control pills.

Many of the modern day diseases have been traced to environmental conditions that initiate and sustain diseases, and in which volition and responsibility play an active role.

Perhaps a difference is that other mental and physical diseases do not affect the "spirit" of the victim as does alcoholism. It is important to note that the spiritual disease develops as a result of the alcoholism and does not cause the alcoholism. Therein lies the basic difficulty for some in accepting alcoholism as a disease. Alcoholics act against their values and standards (id impulses and faulty ego integration with poor judgment) and as a consequence appear immoral and feel guilty (excessive superego). Because denial is such a large part of the disease, the alcoholic must deny the spiritual malady in order to continue the drinking in the same way denial is used in other aspects of the alcoholic's drinking practices and consequences.

At some point in order for the alcoholic to recover, he or she must resolve the conflicts between the twisted conscience and the distorted perceptions of reality. The source of the conflicts is the uncontrolled drinking that must cease and abstinence maintained before any meaningful resolution can take place. Alcoholism is a three-part disease, beginning with the physical allergy or predisposition to drink in an uncontrolled pattern. It is a mental illness that is the obsession that either the alcoholic has or will have control of the drinking at sometime either in the present or future despite repeated evidence to the contrary. And it is a spiritual disease that results from the compulsive use of alcohol, in which the alcoholic drinks and lives in conflict with himself or herself and others.

Another misconception that prevents alcoholism from being accepted as a disease is that those who judge the alcoholic and alcoholic drinking view drinking through their own experiences with alcohol. By definition, normal drinkers control the amount they drink and have no consistent pattern of adverse consequences from their drinking. Unfortunately, because of this introspective position, they apply their experience with alcohol to the alcoholic who cannot control his or her drinking. The two realities do not match and alcoholism is considered a lack of will power over alcohol that the normal drinker appears to possess. In actuality, because of genetic predisposition to alcoholism, the ability to drink consistently with control may be under genetic control and not under the will of the individual as much as previously considered.

The obstacle that may produce the greatest difficulty is the religious dogma that drinking is a sin or at least excessive drinking is a sin or morally wrong. This is a view that is responsible for moral judgments that condemn alcoholics, and only serve to prevent diagnosis and treatment. How many people would come forth to complain about a health problem if the it were judged to be a moral problem.

A prevalent view that obstructs treatment is that alcoholism is caused by another, underlying condition. This practice risks further injury to the alcoholic, promotes unnecessary and sometimes harmful treatment, and delays the alcoholic from receiving the proper treatment. Alcoholism is a primary disorder that is caused by an interaction between alcohol and a physical (genetic) predisposition, and is influenced by environmental (psychological) factors. Alcoholism frequently leads to or causes other conditions.

C. Pharmacological Treatment

A major factor determining whether or not a clinical state is accepted as a disease is the use of pharmacological agents. The use of medications is consistent with the passive, victim state so important to the disease concept. A drug requires limited volitional action on the part of the victim to treat the disease other than taking the medications and tolerating any side effects.

There are no known medications that specifically treat alcoholism or drug addiction. The lack of a pharmacological agents makes it less appealing to the scientifically-oriented physician who seeks a drug solution to diseases. However, alcoholism (drug addiction) is similar to other diseases such as hypertension, coronary artery disease, and cancer for which there are no pharmacological agents to treat their root causes.

REFERENCES

1. Guze, S.B., Cloninger, C.R., Martin, R., and Clayton, P.J. (1988). Alcoholism as a medical disorder, *Alcoholism: Origins and Outcome*, (R.M. Rose and J. Barret, eds.), Raven Press, New York, pp. 83–94.
2. Gordis, E. (1989). Guest editorial: The disease concept of alcoholism. *Psychiatr. Hosp.*, *20*(4):151–152.
3. Jellinek, E.M. (1960). *The Disease Concept of Alcoholism*. College and University Press, New Haven, Connecticut. In association Hillhouse Press, New Brunswick, New Jersey.
4. *Webster's Ninth New Collegiate Dictionary* (1986). Merriam-Webster, Springfield, Massachusetts.
5. *Dorland's Illustrated Medical Dictionary* (1988). 27th ed., Saunders, Philadelphia.
6. Koch's Postulates (1882). Die Aetiologie der Tuberculose. *Berlklin. Wschr.*, *19*:221–230.

7. Adler, M.J., McGill, V.J. (1963). *Biology, Psychology and Medicine*. Encyclopedia Britannica, Chicago.
8. Rush, B. (1970). *An Inquiry into the Effects of Spirituous Liquors in the Human Body*. Thomas and Andrews, Boston.
9. Meyer, R.E. (1988). Overview of the concept of alcoholism, *Alcoholism: Origins and Outcome*, (R.M. Rose and J. Barrett, eds.), Raven Press, New York.
10. *The Doctor's Opinion* (1976). Alcoholics Anonymous World Services, Inc., New York City.
11. Tiebout, H.M. (1953). Surrender versus compliance in therapy. *Q. J. Stud. Alcohol., 14*:58–68.
12. Goodwin, D.W. (1985). Alcoholism and genetics. *Arch. Gen. Psychiatry, 42*:171–174.
13. Bowman, K.M., and Jellinek, E.M. (1941). Alcohol addiction and its treatment. *Q. J. Stud. Alcohol., 2*:98–176.
14. Miller, N.S., and Gold, M.S. (1989). Suggestions for changes in DSM-III-R criteria for substance use disorders. *Am. J. Drug. Alcohol Abuse, 15*(2):223–230.
15. Helzer, J.E., Robins, L.N., Taylor, J.R., et al. (1985). The extent of long-term moderate drinking among alcoholics discharged from medical and psychiatric treatment facilities. *N. Engl. J. Med., 312*(26):27.
16. Edwards, G., and Gross, M.M. (1976). Alcohol dependence provisional description of a clinical syndrome. *BR. Med. J., 1*:1058–1061.
17. Milam, J.R., and Ketchum, K. (1981). *Under the Influence*. Madrona Publishers.
18. Robins, L.N., Helzer, J.E., Przybeck, T.R., and Regier, D.A. (1988). Alcohol disorders in the community: A report from the epidemiologic catchment area, *Alcoholism: Origins and Outcome* (R.M. Rose and J. Barrett, eds.), Raven Press, New York, pp. 15–28.
19. Fingarette, H. (1988). *Heavy Drinking: The Myth of Alcoholism as a Disease*. University of California Press, Los Angeles, California.
20. Brenner, C. (1974). *An Elementary Textbook of Psychoanalysis*. Doubleday, New York.
21. Khantzian, E.J. (1985). The self medication hypothesis of addictive disorders: Focus on heroin and cocaine dependence. *Am. J. Psychiatry, 142*(11):1259–1264.
22. Vaillant, G.E. (1983). *The Natural History of Alcoholism: Causes, Patterns and Paths to Recovery*. Harvard University Press, Cambridge, Massachusetts.
23. Schuckit, M.A., (1983). The history of psychiatric disorders. *Hosp. Commun. Psychiatry, 34*(11):1022–1027.
24. Mayfield, D. (1979). Alcohol and affect: Experimental studies, *Alcoholism and Affective Disorders* (D.W. Goodwin and C.K. Erickson, eds.), SP Medical and Scientific Books, New York.
25. Alexander, B.K. (1987). The disease and adaptive model of addiction: A framework evaluation. *J. Drug Issues*.
26. Miller, N.S., and Gold, M.S. (1990). The disease and adaptive models of addiction: A reevaluation. *J. Drug Issues, 20*(1):129–135.
27. Tabakoff, B., and Hoffman, P.L. (1980). Alcohol and neurotransmitters, *Alcohol Tolerance and Dependence* (Rigter, H. and Crabbe, J.C., eds.), Elsevier, New York.
28. Miller, N.S., Dackis, C.A., and Gold, M.S. (1987). The relationship of addiction, tolerance and dependence: A neurochemical approach. *J. Subst. Abuse Treat., 4*:197–207.
29. Seessel, T.V. (1988). Beyond the Supreme Court ruling on Alcoholism as willful misconduct: It is up to Congress to act. *J.A.M.A., 259*(2):248.
30. Alcoholics Anonymous. Alcoholics Anonymous World Services, Inc., New York.

18

Biochemical Markers for Alcoholism

Arthur W. K. Chan
Research Institute on Alcoholism, Buffalo, New York

I. INTRODUCTION

The progression from excessive alcohol consumption to alcoholism is often accompanied by manifestations of social and medical problems. Therefore, physicians and health care personnel have a sizable opportunity to encounter people with health problems associated with alcohol abuse or alcoholism. In fact, it has been estimated that at least 20% of the patients visiting physicians will qualify for an alcoholic diagnosis (Schuckit, 1984b, 1985, 1987b). Unfortunately, alcoholism or early stages of excessive drinking often remain unrecognized in general medical practice and in hospitals (Brown, Carter, and Gordon, 1987; Coulehan et al., 1987; Moore & Malitz, 1986; Reid et al., 1986; Schuckit, 1987b, Skinner et al., 1986). Schuckit (1987b) has suggested several factors that could contribute to the underdiagnosis of alcoholism. These include inadequate training in diagnosing alcoholism, lack of understanding of the usual course of alcoholism, and erroneous stereotyping of the alcoholic by physicians. Many clinicians do not think that self-reported data can be used as reliable tools in the detection of early alcohol abuse (Eckardt, Rawlings, and Martin, 1986). This may be because few physicians have received formal instruction on how to integrate historical information, laboratory data, and results of physical examinations specifically to arrive at a diagnosis of alcoholism (Schuckit, 1987b). Moreover, clinicians may be reluctant to spend time administering structured interviews and questionnaires. Some examples of simple screening tests are the CAGE (Ewing, 1984; Mayfield, McLeod, and Hall, 1974), the Michigan Alcoholism Screening Test (MAST) (Selzer, 1971), the Reich interview (Reich et al., 1975), and the self-administered alcoholism screening test (SAAT; Davis et al., 1987). Several reviews have dealt with the detection of alcoholism by questionnaires or structured interviews (Babor & Kadden, 1985; Hays & Spickard, 1987; Jacobson, 1976; Miller, 1976; Skinner, Holt,

This chapter was adapted from *Children of Alcoholics: Critical Perspectives*, edited by Michael Windle and John S. Searles. Copyright 1990, reprinted by permission from The Guilford Press, New York, NY.

and Israel, 1981; Wilkins, 1974). Since the usefulness of questionnaires for alcoholism screening in a medical setting may be limited because of vulnerability to deliberate falsification or unconscious denial (Babor and Kadden, 1985), objective methods such as biochemical indicators are generally preferred by clinicians.

Several reviews have summarized the pros and cons of old and new biological markers for alcoholism and heavy drinking (Cushman et al., 1984; Eckardt et al., 1986; Holt, Skinner and Israel, 1981; Lumeng, 1986; Salaspuro, 1986; Schuckit, 1986, 1987b; Skinner and Holt, 1987; Watson et al., 1986). The primary objective of this chapter is to review and evaluate research on biochemical markers for alcoholism, with emphasis on work involving children of alcoholics (COAs).

II. TYPES OF MARKERS

As Hill, Steinhauer, and Zubin (1987) have pointed out, the term *marker*, as commonly used by alcohol researchers, carries the same meaning as *indicator*, not the more restrictive meaning of marker used in genetic studies. In the latter studies, marker generally denotes an enduring heritable trait that usually has a known pattern of inheritance. For convenience of referring to published works, marker will be used synonymously with indicator in this chapter. However, it should be emphasized that at the present state of alcoholism research, a true genetic marker of alcoholism has not been detected.

Two major types of markers can be categorized: vulnerability (trait) markers and state markers. As the term implies, vulnerability markers identify people who may be vulnerable to developing alcoholism, even before they have consumed alcohol. State markers reflect the physiological, pathological, and biochemical changes in the body elicited by chronic and excessive alcohol intake. Ideally, both types of markers should be highly specific (few false-positives) and sensitive (few false-negatives). The predictive accuracy of these markers should not be affected by non–alcoholism-related factors such as age and sex differences, smoking, other drug use, and concomitant diseases. An ideal state marker would be capable of detecting regular drinkers as well as binge drinkers and would be sufficiently sensitive to distinguish light drinkers from heavy drinkers.

Since COAs, especially sons of alcoholic fathers, are known to have an increased risk of developing alcoholism (Goodwin, 1979), a logical and frequently used approach to identify putative vulnerability markers is to compare people having a positive history of familial alcoholism (FHP) with those having a negative history of familial alcoholism (FHN). A vulnerability marker should be present in a significantly larger proportion of FHP subject than in FHN subjects. Also, the same marker should be detectable in a sizable proportion of alcoholics. However, an indicator that appears to differentiate alcoholics from nonalcoholic controls may be either a state marker or a persistent characteristic of a vulnerability marker. It should be emphasized that persons who test positive for a vulnerability marker may not develop alcoholism throughout their lifetimes. Likewise, persons who test normal for a vulnerability marker are not immune to developing alcoholism. Not all (less than half) alcoholics have a positive history of familial alcoholism and most COAs will not develop alcoholism. A vulnerability marker should be detectable before a person is exposed to alcohol, and it should persist during the development of alcoholism as well as during abstinence. Hill, Steinhauer, and Zubin (1987) have speculated that it is theoretically possible to have a vulnerability marker that is detectable before a person is exposed to alcohol but not during the onset of alcoholism, and that reappears after recovery from alcoholism. They have also speculated that a marker might be detectable before and during the onset of alcoholism, but that it might be normalized after the cessation of alcohol abuse. However, these different types of vulnerability markers have yet to be found. The use of prepubertal boys who have not yet been exposed to alcohol to identify putative vulnerability markers presents the risk of missing postpubertal markers and those markers that appear only after exposure to alcohol intake (Begleiter et al., 1984; Behar et al., 1983).

State markers may or may not be reversible after long durations of abstinence from alcohol, and those that persist may be categorized erroneously as vulnerability markers. Residual state markers may or may not be detectable in persons undergoing the alcoholism phase of their lives (Hill, Steinhauer and Zubin, 1987). Reversible state markers can be used to monitor treatment outcome and to detect relapses. Investigators have not determined whether those who are vulnerable to developing alcoholism are more susceptible to the damaging effects of alcohol. If this were the case, it would probably lead to an earlier appearance of state markers in vulnerable than in nonvulnerable persons having the same duration and quantity of alcohol intake. This is an empirical question not yet answered.

III. STATE MARKERS

Most investigations of proposed markers for excessive alcohol consumption involve comparisons between a group of known alcoholics, usually in a treatment center, and a group of nonalcoholics or abstainers matched on a number of relevant variables. This approach does not distinguish persistent state markers from vulnerability markers. Nevertheless, the knowledge gained from these studies can be applied by clinicians to improve their diagnostic accuracy. It also provides a basis to investigate whether persistent differences between alcoholics and controls are potential trait markers. Less often investigated is the use of single or multiple putative markers for the early identification of alcohol abuse in the general population or in special population groups such as young adults, pregnant women, drunk-driving offenders, and those needing medical attention. Similarly, not many putative markers have been tested for their correlations with self-reported alcohol intake within groups of individuals over a given period.

A. Conventional Markers

Table 1 summarizes the diagnostic values of the more conventional or older markers of excessive alcohol consumption. Part A of the table lists tests currently in general use; part B lists tests that have proved less sensitive and specific or too cumbersome for routine clinical use. Given the large numbers of publications dealing with these tests, the references cited are not meant to be comprehensive, but are representative of either review articles or papers dealing directly with the particular test.

The only true indicator of alcohol intake is the detection of ethanol or one of its metabolites, namely, acetaldehyde and acetate, in a subject's body fluids. However, the relatively rapid elimination of these compounds renders them less useful as markers of alcohol abuse. Nevertheless, determinations of the level of alcohol in blood, urine, or breath have been found very effective in emergency hospital admissions, drunk-driving offenses, and in the follow-up of alcoholism treatment programs. Although the presence of alcohol does not distinguish acute from chronic alcohol intake, under certain circumstances it can be highly suggestive of abusive alcohol consumption. Thus, a blood alcohol level higher than 300 mg/dl recorded at any time, or a level higher than 100 mg/dl recorded during a routine medical examination, can be regarded as a strong indicator of alcoholism (National Council on Alcoholism, 1972). Likewise, a blood alcohol level exceeding 150 mg/dl in a patient without gross evidence of intoxication strongly suggests alcohol abuse and tolerance to alcohol. Using a sensitive method of detection involving gas chromatography–mass spectrometry, Tang (1987) found that ethanol concentrations in urine of 11 alcoholics after 14 days of abstention were at least seven times

Table 1 Older, Conventional Markers for Excessive Alcohol Intake

Marker[a]	Diagnostic capability
	Part A
Ethanol (National Council on Alcoholism, 1972; Tang, 1987)	Low sensitivity because of rapid elimination; useful in cases of intoxication; urinary ethanol levels may be more sensitive.
Aspartate aminotransferase (ASAT) (Matloff, Seligran, and Kaplan, 1980; Nishimura and Teschke, 1983; Salaspuro, 1986)	Increased activity in 30–75% of alcoholics; primarily an indicator of liver disease, but nonspecific for alcoholism; useful as an adjunct in diagnosis when combined with other tests.
Alanine aminotransferase (ALAT) (Cohen and Kaplan, 1979; Skude and Wadstein, 1977)	Same limitations as ASAT. A ratio of ASAT to ALAT greater than 2 is highly indicative of alcoholic etiology of liver disease.
Gamma-Glutamyltransferase (GGT) (Holt, Skinner and Israel, 1981; Salaspuro, 1986)	Most commonly used test. Activity elevated in 35–85% of alcoholics or heavy drinkers; nonspecific for alcoholism because it is also increased in liver diseases, other drug intake, and concomitant disease states. Useful as an adjunct in diagnosis when combined with other tests. Particularly useful in monitoring treatment results or in motivation of patients.
Mean corpuscular volume (MCV) (Holt et al., 1981; Salaspuro, 1986; Watson et al., 1986)	Elevated values in 31–96% of alcoholics; low specificity because other diseases and drug intake can increase MCV values. Less sensitive but more specific than GGT. Very useful as an adjunctive test.
	Part B
α-Amino-n-butyric acid to leucine ratio (Chick et al., 1982; Herrington et al., 1981)	Increased in alcoholics but also in patients with either alcoholic or nonalcoholic liver disease; values dependent on nutritional status; low sensitivity and specificity.
Glutamate dehydrogenase (GDH) (Jenkins et al., 1982; Mills et al., 1981; Van Waes and Lieber, 1977)	Nonspecific for alcoholism; increased levels in patients with recent alcohol excess and in those with fatty liver or alcoholic hepatitis. Not very reliable as marker of liver cell necrosis in alcoholics.
Lactate dehydrogenase (LDH) (Konttinen, Hartel, and Louhija, 1970; Nygren and Sundblad, 1971; Watson et al., 1986)	Tendency to increase in some isoenzyme levels in intoxicated chronic alcohol abusers. Nonspecific.
Erythrocyte δ-aminolevulinic acid dehydrase (Flegar-Mestric, Tadej, and Subic-Albert, 1987; Hamlyn, Hopper, and Skillen, 1979)	Level reduced in more than 90% of recently drinking alcoholics; also reduced transiently following acute alcohol intake in non-alcoholic normal subjects. Low sensitivity.
High-density lipoprotein (HDL) cholesterol (Barboriak et al., 1980; Devenyi et al., 1981; Hartung et al., 1983)	Values increased in 50–80% of alcoholics, and also in nonalcoholics drinking 75 gm of ethanol daily for 5 weeks; alcoholics with liver diseases may show decreased levels. Low sensitivity and specificity. Most changes are within normal limits.

(continued)

Table 1   *(Continued)*

Marker[a]	Diagnostic capability
Uric acid (Drum, Goldman and Jankowski, 1981; Holt et al., 1981; Watson et al., 1986)	Hyperuricemia is frequently associated with alcoholism and heavy alcohol intake. Low sensitivity and specificity.
Ferritin (Kristenson, Fex, and Trell, 1981; Valimaki, Harkonen, and Ylikahri, 1983)	Elevated levels in alcoholics and heavy drinkers; levels revert to normal with 2 weeks' abstinence. Primarily an indicator of hepatic dysfunction; nonspecific for alcoholism.

[a]Unless otherwise specified, tests are for serum or plasma samples.

higher than those of social drinkers (excluding heavy drinkers) and 10 times higher than those of control subjects who had not consumed alcohol during the 7 days before the test. In the morning following the day of admission, alcoholics had an average urine ethanol level nearly 160 times that found in light drinkers. The ability to detect ethanol in the urine even after 2 weeks abstinence greatly improves the reliability of the test as an indicator of heavy alcoholic consumption. Tang speculated that the source of ethanol in the urine might have been from ethanol conjugates. Because the number of heavy drinkers studied was very small, further investigations are needed to determine whether the measurement of ethanol in urine may be a specific marker for excessive alcohol intake. One possible limitation is the confounding effect of acute alcohol intake several hours before urine samples are taken.

None of the tests in Table 1, when used alone, has sufficient sensitivity and specificity to be a reliable marker of alcoholism or to be used as a screening test for heavy alcohol consumption. Nevertheless, clinicians can use an abnormal result as a reason for questioning a patient's drinking more closely. This applies especially to tests such as those for gamma-glutamyltransferase (GGT) and mean corpuscular volume (MCV). These two tests, and especially the one for GGT, have been widely used with varying degrees of success as adjunctive instruments in the diagnosis of alcoholism and as screening tests for those arrested for drinking and driving (Dunbar et al., 1985; Gjerde, Sakshaug, and Morland, 1986), adolescent alcohol use (Westwood, Cohen and McNamara, 1978) drinking in middle-aged men (Chick, Pikkarainen, and Plant, 1987; Peterson et al., 1983), and maternal alcohol abuse and fetal alcohol effects (Hollstedt and Dahlgren, 1987; Ylikorkala, Stenman, and Halmesmaki, 1987), as welll as epidemiological indicators of alcohol consumption (Gjerde et al., 1987). However, neither test is an adequate substitute for a careful medical history and full clinical examination in the diagnosis of alcoholism or alcohol abuse (Barrison, Ruzek, and Murray-Lyon, 1987). Bernadt et al., (1982) have advocated the use of short questionnaires such as the brief MAST, the CAGE, and the Reich interview in favor of eight laboratory tests (including those for GGT and MCV) for the routine screening of alcoholism in hospital patients. These investigators tested only the efficacy of single laboratory tests and did not use combinations of tests and sophisticated statistical methods such as discriminant function analyses. Other investigators have reported less successful results with the short questionnaires (Babor and Kadden, 1985).

Not listed in Table 1 are a large number of laboratory tests that are routinely requested by physicians to aid them in general diagnoses. These include tests for glucose, urea nitrogen, creatinine, calcium, phosphorus, total protein, albumin, globulin, iron, sodium, potassium, magnesium, zinc, chloride, carbon dioxide, total bilirubin, alkaline phosphatase, creatine kinase, isocitrate dehydrogenase, ornithine carbamyl transferase, and hematological variables such as red and white cell counts, hematocrit, and hemoglobin levels. Each of these tests, used separately, is a poor marker of alcoholism or alcohol abuse. By using various combinations of these tests, however, or by combining them with those listed in Table 1, diagnostic efficiency can be greatly improved (Eckardt et al., 1986; Watson et al., 1986).

B. Combined Tests

In general, combinations of large numbers of tests have yielded better results than combinations of a few tests (e.g., Clark et al., 1983; Cushman et al., 1984; Korri, Nuutinen, and Salaspuro, 1985; Morgan, Colman, and Sherlock, 1981; Sanchez-Craig and Annis, 1981). The best results have been obtained by using statistical forms of pattern recognition, called discriminant function analyses, on laboratory test batteries. For example, using a quadratic discriminant function analysis (QDA) of 24 laboratory tests, Ryback, Eckardt, and Pautler (1980) and Ryback et al., (1982) correctly identified 100% of medical ward alcoholics, 100% of nonalcoholic patients, and 94% of treatment program alcoholics. The alcoholic subjects in these studies had many years of heavy drinking and most of them had severe symptoms of alcoholism. Therefore, it is not surprising that other studies involving different samples of alcoholics or heavy drinkers reported slightly less impressive results, yet still with high specificity and sensitivity. For example, Ryback and Rawlings (1985) used the same technique to study a much younger, less impaired group of alcoholics who had an average of less than 5 years of heavy drinking; most of the laboratory tests were within the normal range. They achieved correct identification of 75.5 and 73.8% of alcoholics, and 90.3 and 95.9% of nonalcoholics with rank QDA and rank linear discriminant analysis (LDA), respectively. Discriminant function and analysis of a small number of tests in young adults did not achieve sufficient sensitivity in discriminatory power (Bliding et al., 1982). In contrast, using a large number of tests, Stamm, Hansert, and Feuerlein (1984) reported a sensitivity of 86% and a specificity of 87% by optimizing decision limits for the discrimination of male alcoholics from other nonalcoholic patients. Using a stepwise LDA of 31 laboratory tests, Chan, Welte, and Whitney (1987) correctly classified 89% of young adult (age 18–28 years) alcoholics and 92% of nonalcoholics. Beresford et al. (1982) reported a correct classification of 79% of alcoholic patients and 80% of nonalcoholic patients, using an LDA of 28 tests. However, the lower sensitivity and specificity might have resulted because their patient population had a wide age range (18–83 years), their definition of alcoholism was based solely on the CAGE interview, and the data were for a mixed population of men and women.

Other investigators have used discriminant function analysis of a panel of blood tests to identify heavy drinkers in selected population groups. Cowan, Massey, and Greenfield (1985) reported 96–99% correct classification of young (18–23 years) male heavy drinkers based on a measure of binge consumption for quantity/frequency of heavy drinking, and 90–92% correct classification based on maximum number of drinks per occasion as an index of heavy drinking. Similarly, Hillers, Alldredge, and Massey (1986) correctly classified 91% of persons who reported consumption of less than or more than four drinks (48 gm of ethanol) per day, using QDA of 15 blood tests. When the number of blood tests used was increased to 24 or 33, the correct classifications were 98 and 100%, respectively. The investigators cautioned that the percentage correctly classified may be inflated owing to an excessive number of blood tests for the number of subjects. They recommended a minimum subject to variable ratio of 10:1. Other researchers have suggested smaller ratios; namely, 3:1 (Solberg, 1978) and 5:1 (Schnitt and Dove, 1986). Less successful results have been reported in two studies of health screening subjects in which correct classifications of heavy drinkers were less than 50% in one (Shaper et al., 1985) and 92% in another (Whitfield et al., 1981). These may be due to the use of one set of discriminant functions for a diverse group of populations.

As Ryback and Rawlings (1985) have pointed out, it is unlikely that one set of discriminant functions will correctly define all types of drinkers.

It should be stressed that the use of discriminant function analysis to develop a screening instrument for alcoholism is still in its infancy (Schnitt and Dove, 1986). There is a need for further research to be undertaken to optimize and refine this method before it can be effectively applied to early detection of heavy drinking. Perhaps different sets of discriminant functions are needed to correctly define heavy drinkers with different characteristics, such as history of other drug intake, health status, age range, sex, number of years of heavy drinking, frequency and quantity of alcohol consumption, and familial history of alcoholism. The sensitivity and specificity of discriminant analyses can possibly be improved by combining laboratory tests with data from rapid interviews such as CAGE or the brief MAST, as well as with one or more of the newer biochemical markers such as those discussed in the next section (Persson and Magnusson, 1988). Bernadt, Mumford, and Murray (1984) performed discriminant analysis of three rapid interviews (CAGE, brief MAST, and Reich) and nine laboratory tests. They found that a combination of Reich interview and GDH level achieved 100% sensitivity and about 80% of specificity for excessive drinking and alcoholism.

The advantages of using discriminant function analysis of a large panel of laboratory tests are: (1) Nearly all the tests are those commonly ordered by physicians during regular physical examinations or hospital admissions. Most of them can be performed using automated procedures. The test results can complement the physician's diagnosis based on clinical symptoms and personal interview. (2) Abnormal test results can be used to advantage by the physician in counseling patients to overcome any denial response. (3) Classification accuracy is not changed by long abstinence (Eckardt et al., 1984; Ryback et al., 1985). (4) Good discrimination can be achieved even though values for the laboratory tests are within the normal range. (5) The automated test batteries are economically reasonable, being equivalent in cost to only two or three separate laboratory tests (Ryback et al., 1980). Limitations of the method are: (1) It cannot be used effectively in persons over 65 years of age because 50% would be classified as alcoholics even though they are not (Ryback et al., 1980; Ryback et al., 1983). Fortunately, persons older than 65 constitute a relatively small proportion of chronic alcoholics. (2) Accuracy of classification is dependent on a precise separation of the groups under study; that is, precisely clear definitions are needed for alcoholics versus nonalcoholics and heavy drinkers versus light drinkers.

Another method that is potentially valuable for the early identification of heavy drinking involves a combination of clinical signs, medical history, laboratory tests, and alcohol questionnaires collectively called the Alcohol Clinical Index (Skinner et al., 1986; Skinner and Holt, 1987; Skinner et al., 1984). Widespread use of this relatively simple method by properly trained physicians or health care professionals is very likely to result in a substantial improvement in the ability of physicians to diagnose alcohol abuse or alcoholism. Whether the method is sufficiently sensitive to detect those who drink heavily but are without clinical signs of alcohol-related complications needs to be tested.

C. Newer Markers

Table 2 summarizes the more recent biochemical markers for alcoholism or alcohol abuse. These tests are not part of the automated blood test batteries. The two urine tests, for dolichol and alcohol-specific product, have the advantage of being noninvasive in sample collection, compared with blood tests. The disadvantages of the dolichol test are that moderate alcohol intake for 10 days does not cause an increase in urinary dolichol levels and that the half-life decay for increased urinary dolichol is about 3 days (Roine, 1988). Another disadvantage is its low specificity (see Table 2) (Roine et al., 1988). Measurements of serum acetate and

Table 2 Newer Markers of Excessive Alcohol Intake

Marker[a]	Diagnostic capability
Acetate (Korri, Nuutinen, and Salaspuro, 1985; Nuutinen et al., 1985; Salaspuro et al., 1987; Roine et al., 1988)	Elevated level during ethanol oxidation is indicative of metabolic tolerance to alcohol. Specificity of increased acetate level is 92% and sensitivity is 65% for both alcoholism and heavy drinking. Requires presence of ethanol for analysis; therefore is useful only in intoxicated cases.
Urinary dolichol (Pullarkat and Raguthu, 1985; Roine, 1988; Roine et al. 1987; Roine et al., 1989b; Salaspuro et al., 1987)	Increased excretion in alcoholics and in other disease states. Values normalize within 1 week of abstinence. Low specificity because elevated levels are frequently seen in infections, malignancies, and during pregnancy.
Urinary alcohol-specific product (Tang et al., 1986)	Presumably breakdown product of acetaldehyde-protein adduct. Levels very low in controls but increased 17 times in chronic alcoholics; values return to normal after 2 weeks' abstinence. In one study specificity was 100% and sensitivity was 79%.
Ratio of mitochondrial ASAT (m-ASAT) to total ASAT (Nalpas et al., 1984; Nalpas et al., 1986; Okuno et al., 1988)	Increased ratio in alcoholics with or without liver disease; 93–100% sensitivity. After abstinence of 1 week, m-ASAT decreases by more than 50%.
Transferrin variant (Chapman, Sorrentino, and Morgan, 1985; Gjerde et al., 1988; Stibler, Borg, and Allgulander, 1980; Stibler, Borg, and Joustra, 1986; Storey et al., 1987; Vesterberg, Petran, and Schmidt, 1984)	Variant with isoelectric point 5.7 was elevated in alcoholics and heavy drinkers (consumption of more than 60 gm alcohol per day for 10 days). Levels decreased 50% after 14 days' abstinence. High sensitivity and specificity, but less successful results also have been reported.
Red cell morphology (Homaidan et al., 1986)	Elevated number of triangulocytes in alcoholics (range 2.6–18%) compared with healthy controls (0–0.5%). Slow and laborious test.
Acetaldehyde-hemoglobin adduct (Hoberman and Chiodo, 1982; Homaidan et al., 1983; Lucas et al., 1988; Peterson et al., 1985)	Tends to be elevated in alcoholics compared with normal volunteers, but unreliable as marker of alcohol abuse. Sensitivity and specificity as marker of heavy drinking not studied in large samples.
Antibodies against acetaldehyde adults (Hoerner et al., 1988; Israel et al., 1986; Niemela et al., 1987)	Elevated antibody titers found in 73% of alcoholics; 39% of patients with non-alcoholic liver diseases also had elevated levels.
Erythrocyte aldehyde dehydrogenase (Agarwal et al., 1987; Fantozzi et al., 1987; Lin, Potter, and Mezey, 1984; Palmer and Jenkins, 1985; Towell et al., 1986)	Activity generally decreased in chronic alcoholics, but increased activity has been reported. Low sensitivity and specificity. No correlation between daily alcohol intake or degree of liver injury and level of enzyme activity.

(continued)

Table 2 *(Continued)*

Marker[a]	Diagnostic capability
Apolipoprotein A-I and A-II (Malmendier and Delcroix, 1985; Puchois et al., 1984; Puddey et al., 1986)	Both increased in intemperate drinkers. Only A-II levels correlate significantly with self-reported alcohol intake. A-II may be more sensitive indicator of excessive alcohol intake than HDL cholesterol. Combination of GGT and A-II detected 72.9% of heavy drinkers; GGT alone detected only 59%.
2.3-Butanediol (Rutstein et al., 1983; Wolf et al., 1983)	Levels greater than $5\mu M$ in severely alcoholic men after drinking distilled spirits, with sensitivity to 79%. Only 1 of 22 controls had level above 5 μM.
Platelet adenylate cyclase (Tabakoff et al., 1988; Tsuchiya et al., 1987)	Enzyme activity after stimulation with agents such as cesium fluoride significantly lower in alcoholics; long-lasting changes detectable in alcoholics abstinent for one to four years. Combined with another test, has sensitivity and specificity of approximately 75%.

[a]Unless otherwise specified, tests are for serum or plasma samples.

2,3-butanediol have little value as screening instruments for early identification of alcoholism because their detection, especially that of acetate, is dependent on the presence of ethanol. Nevertheless, increased serum acetate could be used for the screening of problem drinking among drunken drivers (Roine et al., 1988). Tests in which abnormal values revert toward normal values within 1 or 2 weeks of abstinence may not be sufficiently sensitive and specific to identify binge drinkers or alcoholics in recent remission. Thus, nearly all of the tests in Table 2 fall into this category, except platelet adenylate cyclase, which may be a vulnerability marker. On the other hand, these tests may be good markers for monitoring abstinence in alcoholics under treatment. Because these tests are relatively new, investigations have been primarily confined to comparisons between known alcoholics and nonalcoholics. It is to be expected that the sensitivity and specificity of each test will decrease when it is applied as a screening test in populations with drinkers having different intake levels. For example, Stibler, Borg, and Joustra (1986) reported that 89% of their alcoholic subjects had elevated serum levels of abnormal transferrin ($Tf_{5.7}$); but in another study (Gjerde et al., 1988) only 68% of those who reported alcohol consumption above 40 gm/day had elevated $Tf_{5.7}$ values. The two tests, for m-ASAT and $Tf_{5.7}$, that were reported to have relatively high sensitivity and specificity in identifying alcoholics with a mean age of over 35, did not have sufficiently high sensitivity to identify young adult (mean age under 25) alcoholics (Chan et al., 1989). Although both tests showed significantly elevated levels compared with controls, there were many overlapping values between the alcoholics and controls. Depending on the cutoff limits, the sensitivity range for either test was only 15–50%, while specificty ranged from 82–96%. These authors speculated that the lower sensitivity and specificity could be due to a shorter duration of heavy drinking or to a greater resilience in young adults with regard to the damaging effects of alcohol. Another important factor is the number of days elapsed since a subject's last drink because elevated levels might revert to normal values faster in young adults.

There have been no investigations using discriminant function analysis of combinations of these newer markers in conjunction with the more conventional markers, as well as with questionnaire data. This approach is very likely to improve the sensitivity and specificity of these tests as screening instruments for excessive alcohol intake.

D. Miscellaneous Tests

The following biochemical variables need to be further investigated for their potential usefulness as markers of alcoholism or heavy drinking.

Lysosomal Glycosidases

Increased β-hexosaminidase levels have been reported in 94.4% of chronic alcoholics with acute ethanol intoxication (Hultberg, Isaksson, and Tiderstrom, 1980). After 7–10 days of abstinence, about half of the alcoholic patients had normalized values of the enzyme (Isaksson et al., 1985). The same investigators reported that consumption of 60 gm of alcohol daily for 10 days also significantly increased serum β-hexosaminidase activity.

Immunoglobulins (Ig)

Elevated serum IgA and IgE levels are often seen in chronic alcoholics (Hallgren and Lundin, 1983; Iturriaga et al., 1977). Although IgA may also be increased in nonalcoholic liver diseases, the IgA/IgG ratio can be used to separate alcoholic from nonalcoholic origin of the liver damage (Iturriaga et al., 1977).

Serotonin Uptake

Platelet affinity for serotonin was significantly increased in alcoholics on admission for treatment and in alcoholics with short and long (up to 11 years) durations of abstinence (Boismare et al., 1987). Neiman, Beving, and Malmgren (1987) also reported an increased affinity for serotonin in recently admitted alcoholics, but found that this effect was transient and that normal affinity was restored during detoxification. Further investigations are needed to establish whether this test could be a marker for alcohol dependence.

Response to Thyrotropin-Releasing Hormone (TRH)

Alcoholics who had been abstinent for more than 20 days showed a blunted thyroid-stimulating hormone (TSH) response to TRH, compared with healthy controls (Casacchia, Rossi and Stratta, 1985). A persistently blunted response was also reported in 31% of male alcoholics who were abstinent for 2–29 years (Loosen et al., 1983). The blunted response was postulated to be a trait marker for alcoholism. This possibility is discussed further in the section on vulnerability markers below.

Neurophysins

The polypeptide neurophysin II was elevated in the sera of alcoholics who also showed elevated levels of common blood markers for alcoholism such as GGT (Legros et al., 1983). These patients admitted to greater alcohol and less anxiolytic drug intake immediately before admission.

Alkaloid Condensation Products

The condensation of acetaldehyde with endogenous biogenic amines of the indolamine or catecholamine classes results in the formation of tetrahydroisoquinolines or tetrahydro-β-carbolines. These products have been postulated to play a role in the development of alcoholism (Collins, 1985; Myers, 1985). Although some of these products, in particular salsolinol, have been detected in the urine of alcoholic subjects, the results might have been confounded by the presence of these alkaloids in foods and beverages, by methodological inconsistencies, or by possible artifactual condensations (Adachi et al., 1986; Collins, 1985; Hirst, Evans, and Gowdey, 1987; Matsubara et al., 1986; Rommelspacher and Schmidt, 1985).

Methanol

One of the congeners in alcoholic beverages is methanol. Because its metabolism by liver alcohol dehydrogenase can be inhibited by ethanol, high blood methanol levels could be present after prolonged drinking, especially in alcoholics whose liver function is compromised. Since methanol is oxidized rapidly after the disappearance of ethanol from blood, its clinical usefulness is limited to situations in which blood alcohol levels of 0.2 gm/L or more are present (Roine et al., 1989a). It has been reported that some alcoholics have supplemented their regular intake with cleansing solutions containing up to 80% methanol (Martensson, Olofsson, and Heath, 1988), resulting in high blood methanol levels. Increased blood methanol levels are often detected in drunken drivers, and it has been suggested that a level exceeding 5 to 10 mg/L is indicative of alcohol-related problems (Bonte, Kuhnholz, and Ditt, 1985).

E. Age, Sex, and Race Differences

Ryback and Rawlings (1985) suggested that subpopulations of women, including those who are menstruating, menopausal, and those taking estrogen supplements, can create problems for diagnostic instruments if men and women are grouped together. Sex differences in some blood variables have been documented (Vital and Health Statistics, 1982); for instance, men have significantly higher serum iron levels, hemoglobin, and hematocrit but lower MCV than women. It has been suggested that MCV is a better indicator of excessive alcohol consumption in women than in men, and that women are more susceptible to the hematological toxicity of ethanol (Chalmers et al., 1980). Discriminant analysis of several blood chemistry items yielded better sensitivity and specificity for detecting female as opposed to male heavy drinkers (Chalmers et al., 1981). These findings are consistent with reports that women are more susceptible to the damaging effects of alcohol (e.g., Gavaler, 1982). Age and sex differences in the responses of alcoholic inpatients to a self-administered alcoholism screening test have been reported (Davis and Morse, 1987). Depending on the diagnostic instrument used, it may be necessary to have different criteria for the definition of alcoholism for subjects of different age groups and sex. This is an important issue because investigations of putative biochemical markers of excessive alcohol intake rely heavily on the accurate classification of comparison groups by an independent method.

Some blood variables change with age; for instance, mean corpuscular hemoglobin levels and MCV increase with age regardless of sex and race (Vital and Health Statistics, 1982). Older heavy drinkers will generally have more years of exposure to alcohol than younger heavy drinkers, and such a difference may affect the discriminatory power of biochemical tests for alcoholism or heavy drinking. For example, the inappropriateness of several biochemical tests to screen young heavy drinkers has been reported (Bliding et al., 1982). Another related issue is, again, the possibility that young drinkers may be more resilient to the damaging effects of ethanol than older drinkers. During periods of abstinence, biochemical variables may revert to normal values much more quickly in young drinkers than in older drinkers. Therefore, it is important to elicit information from research subjects about the number of days that elapsed since they last drank alcohol. These issues have not been adequately examined.

No studies have systematically examined whether racial differences (e.g., between whites and blacks) exist in terms of the various biochemical markers for alcoholism or heavy drinking. Only one marker, cupro-zinc superoxide dismutase of erythrocyte lysates, has been reported to be increased in black alcoholics, compared with black or white controls (Del Villano et al., 1979). There was too much overlap in enzyme activity between alcoholics and healthy controls to render the test a good marker for alcoholism in black patients. Nevertheless, it is possible that blacks and whites may show different blood chemistry profiles after chronic heavy alcohol intake, especially since blacks and whites show differences in some blood variables—for instance, whites of both sexes had consistently higher mean hematocrit and hemoglobin levels, higher MCV, and higher white blood cell counts. The mean serum iron levels of black females were lower than those of white females for all age groups (Vital and Health Statistics, 1982). Daily and dietary intake of thiamine and other vitamins was lower in blacks than in whites (Koplan et al., 1986; Vital and Health Statistics, 1982). Racial differences in alcohol dehydrogenase (ADH) and aldehyde dehydrogenase (ALDH) are discussed in the following section on vulnerability (trait) markers.

IV. VULNERABILITY MARKERS

A. Methodological Issues

Several reviews have summarized the genetic aspects of alcoholism and research involving those presumed to be at high risk for the future development of alcoholism; namely, COAs (e.g., Braude and Chao, 1986; Corder, McRee, and Rohrer, 1984; Deren, 1986; el-Guebaly, 1986; Goodwin, 1987; National Institute on Alcohol Abuse and Alcoholism [NIAAA], 1985; Russell, Henderson, and Blume, 1984; Schuckit, 1986). It should be emphasized that this high-risk group may not be homogeneous in terms of risk for development of alcoholism because only about one-third of the group will become alcoholics (Schuckit et al., 1982). Within the COA group there are those who are truly at risk and those who are not truly at risk because some FHP subjects may not have inherited a trait, or their relatives may have been misdiagnosed as alcoholics. Environmental factors also play important roles in the development of alcoholism. Likewise, the so-called low-risk group can loosely be considered as consisting of the same two subcategories because not all these people are immune to becoming alcoholics. Given these possible sources of error in comparing high-risk and low-risk groups (i.e., FHP vs FHN subjects), it is imperative that sample sizes be sufficiently large to enable adequate testing of the null hypothesis (Sher, 1983).

Other approaches to investigations of high-risk populations include studies involving COAs who were adopted and reared by nonalcoholics parents and studies of multiple generations of single families to search for markers that are unique in alcoholic relatives, but are absent in nonalcoholic relatives (Schuckit, 1986, 1987a). Both methods are expensive and difficult to carry out. The former method is largely dependent on availability of adoption records (which may be hard to obtain), whereas the latter method requires controlling for many factors such as age, lifestyle, and drinking history. Investigations involving comparisons between cohorts of FHP and FHN subjects, however, remain more popular, practical, and economically feasible. Further, it should be stressed that the biochemical variables that are different in FHP and FHN subjects may not necessarily be genetically influenced. Thus, the term *genetic marker* has been inappropriately used for some of the putative trait markers, even though no evidence in support of genetic transmission of the marker is available. It is also essential to conduct follow-up studies of the same populations of FHP and FHN subjects. Reports of this kind of study have yet to appear because this research approach is so new.

Several approaches can be used in the search for putative trait markers in FHP subjects: (1) Individual and natural variations in the biochemical factor need to be ascertained. (2) The responses of the marker to acute ethanol administration can be studied, and these should be compared with data on the same variable in alcoholics. One main drawback of this approach is that it is difficult to differentiate primary drug effects from secondary effects caused by stress, anxiety, or other responses to drug intake. (3) When alcoholics are used in the investigation, confounding effects of alcohol withdrawal or acute intoxication need to be accounted for. Tests involving the administration of ethanol to abstinent alcoholics may be hindered by ethical concerns.

B. Markers in COAs and Alcoholics

Table 3 summarizes research on biochemical markers in which investigators compared alcoholics with nonalcoholics and FHP subjects with FHN subjects. Where the results on both cohorts are similar, they suggest that the biochemical variable involved may be a vulnerability marker. However, where the results are dissimilar, interpretation of the data becomes more difficult. It may mean either that the biochemical variable is not a vulnerability marker or that the putative trait marker might have been altered by chronic alcohol intake.

Acetaldehyde

Several studies (reviewed by Di Padova, Worner, and Lieber, 1987) have shown that alcoholics have higher levels of blood acetaldehyde than normal controls after the ingestion of alcohol. However, this is not a consistent finding; some findings were confounded by problems with the analytical method (Eriksson and Peachey, 1980; Nuutinen, Lindros, and Salaspuro, 1983; Nuutinen et al., 1984). Di Padova et al. (1987) evaluated the blood levels of acetaldehyde after alcohol ingestion in abstinent and nonabstinent alcoholics. They found that the elevated acetaldehyde levels seen in nonabstinent alcoholics returned to normal values after 2 weeks of abstinence, suggesting that altered acetaldehyde metabolism in alcoholics is not a primary preexisting effect. Schuckit and Rayses (1979) reported that FHP subjects had higher acetaldehyde concentrations after alcohol ingestion than FHN subjects. However, this finding might have been confounded by artifactual acetaldehyde formation in the blood samples. The results of Schuckit and Rayses (1979) were not confirmed in two other studies (Behar et al., 1983; Eriksson, 1980). Therefore, there is not sufficient evidence to indicate that acetaldehyde is a vulnerability marker. However, there is strong evidence to suggest that increased acetaldehyde levels in Oriental subjects who show the flushing reaction after drinking alcohol may deter them from becoming heavy drinkers (reviewed by Chan, 1986); that is, acetaldehyde may be a negative vulnerability marker, or a protective marker. The higher levels of acetaldehyde in flushing subjects are caused by an unusually less active liver aldehyde dehydrogenase isozyme (ALDHI). Although not very likely, the possible contribution of an atypical alcohol dehydrogenase cannot be ruled out (Chan, 1986). Schuckit and Duby (1982) reported that FPH subjects showed higher levels of facial flushing in response to ethanol than did FHN subjects (10 vs 3%). The higher incidence of flushing in FHP subjects is still much less than that seen in Oriental populations (47–85%). It is doubtful whether the increased flushing in FHP subjects is a vulnerability marker. As Chan (1986) has pointed out, the flushing phenomenon cannot be the sole explanation for differences in incidence of alcoholism among different racial groups.

Prolactin

Acute ethanol ingestion generally causes an increase in the anterior pituitary hormone prolactin within 30 min, with a return toward baseline by 90 min in normal volunteers and nonabstinent chronic alcoholics. This finding is not universally consistent (Cicero, 1983). In two studies of COAs, one with and the other without placebo controls, FHP subjects had lower prolactin levels at 150 min after a low (0.75 ml/kg) or high (1.1 ml/kg) dose of ethanol (Schuckit, Parker, and Rossman, 1983; Schuckit, Gold and Risch, 1987b). These results seem to provide some basis for the previous findings that FHP subjects reported significantly less intense feelings of intoxication than FHN subjects, even though there were no differences

Table 3 Biochemical Variables in Alcoholics and COAs

Blood marker	Alcoholics[a]	COAs[b]
Acetaldehyde	Increased in nonabstinent subjects after alcohol intake. No difference after 2 weeks' abstinence.	Elevated levels after alcohol ingestion in one study, but no difference found in two other studies.
Prolactin	Resting level normal or slightly reduced in abstinent subjects. Increased after acute ethanol use in normal subjects and in drinking chronic alcoholics.	No difference in basal level. Initial (30 minutes) increase after acute ethanol intake, followed by decline; significantly lower levels 150 minutes after ethanol use.
Cortisol	Basal level increased in non-abstinent alcoholics but appears normal during abstinence. Acute ethanol intake causes increase in normal subjects and in drinking alcoholics.	No difference in basal level. Transient (30 minute) increase after a high dose of ethanol followed by decline past basal level yielding significantly lower levels.
Transketolase	Decreased affinity (lower K_m) for thiamine pyrophosphatase in cultured fibroblasts of male subjects.	Decreased affinity (lower K_m) for thiamine pyrophosphate in males.
Response to TRH	Blunted response in abstinent alcoholics.	Higher basal and peak thyrotropin levels in males.
Monoamine oxidase (MAO)	Generally reduced activity even after long abstinence, but conflicting results have been reported.	Lower activity; also lower V_{max}.

[a]Compared with nonalcoholics.
[b]FHP vs FHN subjects.

in peak blood ethanol levels (Hill et al., 1987; Schuckit, 1980, 1981, 1984c, 1985; O'Malley and Maisto, 1985; Pollock et al., 1986). The use of a placebo control is essential especially since Newlin (1985) clearly demonstrated that FHP subjects show a significantly enhanced antagonistic placebo response compared with FHN subjects; the former had a larger heart rate decrease than the latter after consuming what was believed to be malt liquor but was actually dealcoholized beer. The relationship between the group difference in postethanol prolactin levels and ethanol dose is not fully understood (Schuckit et al., 1987b).

Cortisol

Most human studies indicate that the cortisol level increases in normal human volunteers and in nonabstinent alcoholics after drinking ethanol if the dose is high enough (Cicero, 1983; Schuckit, Gold, and Risch, 1987a). In abstinent alcoholics during acute withdrawal, cortisol levels after an ethanol challenge may be decreased or increased. The inconsistent findings are probably due to confounding effects of withdrawal reactions (Cicero, 1983). In two studies, one with and the other without placebo controls, FHP subjects demonstrated lower cortisol levels after alcohol ingestion (0.75 or 1.1 ml/kg) than FHN subjects (Schuckit, 1984a; Schuckit et al., 1987a). These data are consistent with previous reports showing family group differences in ethanol-induced decrements in performance and self-reported feelings of intoxication (O'Malley and Maisto, 1985; Pollock et al., 1986; Schuckit, 1980, 1984c, 1985).

However, like the results for prolactin, these interesting and important findings do not provide any clue as to whether the group differences in ethanol response are genetically controlled or directly tied to an alcoholic predisposition (Schuckit et al., 1987a, 1987b). Follow-up studies of the same subjects will probably shed some light on the matter.

Schuckit reported at the 1988 annual meeting of the Research Society on Alcoholism that the adrenocorticotropic hormone (ACTH) response to a challenge dose of ethanol was significantly less in FHP than in FHN subjects. This hormone stimulates the human adrenal cortex to secrete cortisol and other steroids. Schuckit also found that the continuation of cortisol and ACTH provided a better classification (83%) of FHP subjects than did cortisol alone (67%).

Transketolase

One of the neurological complications of severe alcoholism is the Wernicke-Korsakoff syndrome (Greenberg and Diamond, 1985). Both thiamine deficiency and neurotoxic effects of ethanol per se can contribute to the disorder. There may be a genetically determined abnormality in the thiamine-requiring enzyme, transketolase, which predisposes individuals to developing Wernicke-Korsakoff syndrome (Blass and Gibson, 1977, 1979). Thus, transketolase from skin fibroblasts of patients with alcoholism-related Wernicke-Korsakoff syndrome had a 10-fold decrease in affinity (high K_m) for thiamine pyrophosphate compared with enzyme from the cells of normal subjects. Reproductibility of these results has been questioned (Greenberg and Diamond, 1985). Nevertheless, Mukherjee et al. (1987) confirmed the same K_m abnormality in cultured fibroblasts of patients with alcoholism-associated Wernicke-Korsakoff syndrome, familial chronic alcoholic males, and more importantly, male offspring of alcoholics without any history of alcoholism. The finding in the last group suggests a genetic predisposition to thiamine deficiency, but does not necessarily allow the inference that such abnormality predisposes FHP subjects to developing alcoholism. Longitudinal studies are needed before further conclusions can be reached. Also, the results of Mukherjee et al. (1987) need to be replicated with a larger sample size.

Response to TRH

Moss, Guthrie, and Linnoila (1986) studied the responses of thyrotropin to TRH. They found that sons of familial alcoholics had significantly higher basal thyrotropin levels, peak thyrotropin levels, and thyrotropin areas under the curve than did male controls. No differences were found between daughters of familial alcoholics and female controls. The findings are in contrast to the persistent blunting of the thyrotropin response seen in some abstinent alcoholics. The neurochemical basis for the differential response has yet to be investigated.

Monoamine Oxidase

Monoamine oxidase (MAO) is a mitochondrial enzyme known to be under genetic control (Lykouras, Moussas, and Markianos, 1987). It catalyzes the oxidative deamination of biogenic amines and has an important role in regulating mood and behavior. Several studies have reported reduced platelet MAO activity in alcoholics (e.g., Alexopoulous, Lieberman, and Frances, 1983; Brown, 1977; Faraj et al., 1987; Fowler et al., 1981; Major and Murphy, 1978; Sullivan et al., 1979), with some reporting that individuals with the lowest MAO activity also had the highest incidence of familial alcoholism (Alexopoulous et al., 1983; Lykouras et al., 1987; Major and Murphy, 1978; Sullivan et al., 1979). Because there was a great deal of overlap in activity of the enzyme in alcoholics and controls, some studies did not report lower MAO activity in alcoholics, but there was a trend toward lower activity in subgroups of individuals (Lykouras et al., 1987; von Knorring et al., 1985; von Knorring, Oreland, and von Knorring, 1987). For example, A.L. von Knorring et al. (1985) and L. von Knorring et al. (1987) found that MAO activity was normal in type 1 alcoholics (characterized by late-onset alcoholism and few social complications) but was clearly low in type 2 alcoholics (characterized by early onset, use and abuse of other drugs, and several social complications). The latter finding was confirmed by Pandey et al. (1988). Likewise, Lykouras et al. (1987) reported that only those alcoholics with at least one alcoholic first-degree relative showed a trend toward lower MAO activity. If lower MAO activity is a vulnerability marker rather than a state marker of alcohol abuse, the enzyme activity should remain low after periods of abstinence. Data on recovering alcoholics appear to support the vulnerability concept, but the possibility of long-lasting effects of chronic alcohol intake cannot be ruled out (Faraj et al., 1987; Giller and Hall, 1983; Giller et al., 1984; Sullivan et al., 1978). Transient increases in MAO activity during the initial period of abstinence have also been reported (Agarwal, et al., 1983; Wiberg, 1979). Faraj et al. (1987) suggested that measurements of MAO function, including the kinetic parameter V_{max}, constitute a more reliable biochemical marker for alcoholism. This approach has not been used in studies of COAs, but lower MAO activity has been demonstrated in FHP subjects compared with FHN subjects (Alexopoulos et al., 1983; Schuckit, et al., 1982). Because abnormalities in platelet MAO activity are also common in patients with various psychiatric disorders (Major et al., 1985), the use of this enzyme alone may not definitely identify vulnerability to alcoholism. It needs to be combined with other trait markers if better separation of those genuinely at risk from those not at risk is desired.

Combination of Markers

Only one report has appeared in which several trait markers were used simultaneously to classify high-risk and low-risk subjects (Schuckit and Gold, 1988). The investigators compared a sample of 30 male FHP and 30 matched FHN subjects on the following measures: postethanol changes in subjective feelings, static ataxia, and plasma levels of prolactin and cortisol. Using a stepwise discriminant function analysis of these measures, they found that four items (subjective feelings after high ethanol dose, cortisol values at two time points after high dose, and prolactin results after low dose) combined to correctly classify 83% of FHN subjects and 70% of FHP subjects. It is hoped that future investigations will explore the potential usefulness of including additional variables, such as those discussed above, in the discriminant analysis of FHP-FHN pairs. Schuckit and Gold (1988) suggested that resting eye blink rate may be a good candidate. Other potentially useful variables that have been demonstrated to differ between FHP and FHN subjects are behavioral, cognitive, and neurophysiological parameters such as verbal IQs, auditory word span performance, reading comprehension, the P300 wave component of event-related potentials, and electroencephalographic patterns.

Miscellaneous Markers

A major metabolite of the neurotransmitter serotonin, 5-hydroxyindoleacetic acid (5-HIAA), has been reported to be low in the cerebrospinal fluid of alcoholics (Ballenger, et al., 1979) and depressed relatives of alcoholics who themselves are not alcoholics (Rosenthal et al., 1980). Low levels of 5-HIAA have also been associated with several kinds of violent behavior (Virkkunen et al., 1987). Most of the subjects have alcoholism problems. Thus, 5-HIAA may be a potential vulnerability marker, at least for a subgroup of FHP subjects; namely, those with type 2 alcoholic personalities. Prospective studies with young FHP and FHN subjects who have not been exposed to alcohol need to be conducted to confirm this hypothesis. Since low levels of another monoamine metabolite, 3-methoxy-4-hydroxyphenylglycol, and a blood glucose nadir during glucose tolerance testing are found to coexist with low 5-HIAA levels in most arsonists (Virkkunen et al., 1987), these two may also be potential vulnerability markers that warrant further investigation.

Ledig et al. (1986) investigated eight enzymes, all known to be genetically determined, in alcoholics and controls with the aim of locating differences in phenotype distributions. Only one enzyme, glyoxalase-I in erythrocytes, showed a significant increase in frequency in phenotype 1 and a significant decrease in phenotype 2 in male alcoholics compared with controls. No differences were found between alcoholic and normal women. The investigators stated that the male-limited difference in glyoxalase phenotype 1 remain after alcohol withdrawal, but the duration of abstinence was not specified. Further studies of this enzyme in COAs and in families over several generations are needed to support the hypothesis that males with phenotype 1 of glyoxalase may be predisposed to alcoholism.

Hulyalkar, Nora, and Manowitz (1984) found a relatively high occurrence of the electrophoretic variant of arylsulfatase-A in mentally ill patients with alcoholism. Arylsulfatase-A is a lysosomal enzyme that catalyzes the conversion of sulfatides to cerebroside and sulfate. The abnormal enzyme is not primarily associated with mental illness. These investigators hypothesized that persons in whom the abnormal enzyme is expressed may be at risk for the neuropathological effects of alcohol. More research is needed to test this hypothesis.

A number of clinical reports have suggested the possibility that the development of alcoholic liver diseases might have a genetic basis. For example, HL-A antigens have been implicated as immunogenic markers of alcoholism and alcoholic liver disease (e.g., Saunders et al., 1982; Saunders and Williams, 1983; Shigeta et al., 1980), However, the findings are primarily confined to demonstrating a higher frequency of certain HL-A antigens in patients with alcoholic cirrhosis compared with healthy controls. Only the report by Hrubec and Omenn (1981) provides empirical support for the genetic basis of alcoholic cirrhosis. These investigators found a twin concordance rate for alcoholic cirrhosis of 14.6% for monozygotic twins and 5.4% for dizygotic twins from a study of more than 15,000 male twin pairs.

V. ANIMAL STUDIES

Although there are no complete models of human alcoholism (Deitrich and Spuhler, 1984), the use of animal models to assess genetic influences on various aspects of alcoholism serves to provide guidance for human investigations by indicating promising leads out of the myriad possibilities. Animal studies on molecular and neurochemical mechanisms of actions of alcohol are indispensable because analogous studies in humans would be either impractical or unethical. These studies can lead to the design of better pharmacological interventions to prevent or treat alcoholism. Furthermore, the availability of genetically pure strains of mice and rats that differ in their responses to alcohol will greatly facilitate the search for vulnerability markers of alcoholism. These animal models will also enhance our understanding of the molecular and biochemical mechanisms underlying the development of tolerance to and physical dependence on alcohol, preference for alcohol, and differences in sensitivity to alcohol. The reader is referred to reviews summarizing the development of and research on the many animal models of alcoholism (e.g., Collins, 1986; Crabbe et al., 1985; Deitrich and Spuhler, 1984; Kosobud and Crabbe, 1986; Li et al., 1986; McClearn and Erwin, 1982).

VI. CONCLUSIONS

There is compelling evidence to indicate that for some individuals genetic predisposition plays an important role in the development of alcoholism. However, environmental influences are equally important. Irrespective of whether individuals have the inherited risk of developing alcoholism, the early identification of those who drink heavily, preferably before any medical, economic, and social complications have set in, should remain a priority in our society. It follows that appropriate primary and secondary prevention strategies need to be developed to target the at-risk populations (Miller, Nirenberg, and McClure, 1983). Perhaps different intervention and prevention strategies are required for those who might develop milieu-limited alcoholism and those at risk for the male-limited form of hereditary alcoholism. In addition, prospective and retrospective investigations are needed to help identify the relevant environmental factors that also play important roles in the development of alcoholism. Some recommendations for future research pertaining to biochemical markers for alcoholism are listed below:

1. There is a need for further population studies to identify subcategories of genetic predisposition to alcoholism.

2. Studies of at-risk populations need to be continued to identify new trait markers. These should also include alcoholics and nonalcoholics with or without a family history of alcoholism. One unique approach is to compare those who have a multigenerational history of alcoholism with those who have a unigenerational history of alcoholism (Begleiter, presented at the 1988 meeting of the Research Society on Alcoholism). Follow-up investigations of young COAs previously tested for the presence of trait markers may reveal important information regarding the development of alcoholism, other drug abuse, or psychiatric problems. They should also provide useful data concerning environmental influence.

3. Multivariate analysis, such as discriminant analysis of several trait markers (Schuckit and Gold, 1988), is a very promising tool in the early identification of those who are genuinely at risk. The same battery of tests needs to be applied to alcoholics to determine whether they can be classified accurately and to test the hypothesis that chronic alcohol intake does not alter trait markers.

4. Currently available biochemical markers do not possess 100% sensitivity and specificity as screening devices in apparently healthy populations. Nevertheless, several promising methods, reviewed in this chapter, can be refined for routine clinical use to complement information on medical and drinking history and physical symptoms gathered by clinicians. Because of the inherent advantages of routine laboratory tests and the relatively high sensitivity and specificity that can be attained by using discriminant analyses of a battery of these tests, further investigations are needed to refine and optimize discriminant functions for various groups. As Ryback and Rawlings (1985) have suggested, it is unlikely that one set of discriminant functions will correctly define the universe of alcoholic versus nonalcoholic drinking patterns. It is necessary to define populations more precisely based on data such as quantity and frequency of alcohol intake, number of years of heavy drinking, whether ambulatory or nonambulatory, inpatient or outpatient, other drug intake, age, sex, smoking, and health status. Besides the standard laboratory tests, newer markers and responses to short diagnostic questionnaires such as the CAGE, MAST-10, or Reich interview, can also be included to improve overall diagnostic efficiency.

5. Although much emphasis has been placed on the identification of vulnerability markers, it may be equally fruitful to investigate the existence of negative vulnerability markers, which protect individuals from developing alcoholism. The use of longitudinal research designs to study FHP subjects who do not develop alcoholism represents one possible approach that may reveal important biological as well as environmental factors relevant to this issue.

6. There is an urgent need for physicians to be better educated about how to diagnose alcoholism (Barnes and O'Neill, 1984; Schuckit, 1987b).

7. Continued investigation with various animal models will sharpen foci in the search for specific behavioral, physiological, and biochemical traits associated with inherited risk for alcoholism. These include factors underlying preference for alcohol, development of tolerance and dependence, neurochemical actions of acute and chronic alcohol intake, and initial sensitivity to ethanol.

ACKNOWLEDGMENTS

The expert review and comments of Dr. Mikko Salaspuro are gratefully acknowledged. I thank Carol Tixier for her skillful typing and Donna L. Schanley for proofreading.

REFERENCES

Adachi, J., Mizoi, Y., Fukunaga, T., Ueno, Y., Imamichi, H., Ninomiya, I., and Naito, T. (1986). Individual difference in urinary excretion of salsolinol in alcoholic patients. *Alcohol, 3*:371–375.

Agarwal, D.P., Philippu, G., Milech, U., Ziemsen, B., Schrappe, O., and Goedde, H.W. (1983). Platelet monoamine oxidase and erythrocyte catechol-*o*-methyltransferase activity in alcoholism and controlled abstinence. *Drug Alcohol Depend., 12*:85–91.

Agarwal, D.P., Volkens, T., Hafer, G., and Goedde, H.W. (1987). Erythrocyte aldehyde dehydrogenase: Studies of properties and changes in acute and chronic alcohol intoxication. In H. Weiner and T.G. Flynn (eds.), *Enzymology and Molecular Biology of Carbonyl Metabolism*. New York: Alan R. Liss, pp. 85–101.

Alexopoulos, G.S., Lieberman, K.W., and Frances, R.J. (1983). Platelet MAO activity in alcoholic patients and their first-degree relatives. *Am. J. Psychiatry, 140*:1501–1504.

Babor, T.F., and Kadden, R. (1985). Screening for alcohol problems: Conceptual issues and practical considerations. In N.C. Chang and H.M. Chao (eds.), *Early Identification of Alcohol Abuse*, NIAAA Research Monograph No. 17, U.S. Government Printing Office, Washington, D.C., pp. 1–30.

Ballenger, J.C., Goodwin, F.K., Major, J.F., and Brown, G.L. (1979). Alcohol and central serotonin metabolism in man. *Arch. Gen. Psychiatry, 36*:224–227.

Barboriak, J.J., Jacobson, G.R., Cushman, P., Herrington, R.E., Lipo, R.F., Daley, M.E., and Anderson, A.J. (1980). Chronic alcohol abuse and high density lipoprotein cholesterol, *Alcoholism, 4*:346–349.

Barnes, H.N., and O'Neill, S.F. (1984). Early detection and outpatient management of alcoholism: A curriculum for medical residents. *J. Med. Ed., 59*:904–906.

Barrison, I.G., Ruzek, J., and Murray-Lyon, I.M. (1987). Drinkwatchers—Description of subjects and evaluation of laboratory markers of heavy drinking. *Alcohol Alcohol., 22*:147–154.

Begleiter, H., Porjesz, B., Bihari, B., and Kissin, B. (1984). Event-related brain potentials in boys at risk for alcoholism. *Science, 225*:1493–1496.

Behar, D., Berg, C.J., Rapoport, J.L., Nelson, W., Linnoila, M., Cohen, M., Bozevich, C., and Marshall, T. (1983). Behavioral and physiological effects of ethanol in high-risk and control children: A pilot study. *Alcoholism, 7*:404–410.

Beresford, T., Low, D., Hall, R.C.W., Adduci, R., and Goggans, F. (1982). A computerized biochemical profile for detection of alcoholism. *Psychosomatics, 23*:713–720.

Bernadt, M.W., Mumford, J., and Murray, R.M. (1984). A discriminant-function analysis of screening tests for excessive drinking and alcoholism. *J. Stud. Alcohol, 45*:81–86.

Bernadt, M.W., Mumford, J., Taylor, C., Smith, B., and Murray, R.M. (1982). Comparison of questionnaire and laboratory tests in the detection of excessive drinking and alcoholism. *Lancet, 1*:325–328.

Blass, J.P., and Gibson, G.E. (1977). Abnormality of a thiamine-requiring enzyme in patients with Wernicke-Korsakoff syndrome. *N. Engl. J. M., 297*:1367–1370.

Blass, J.P., and Gibson, G.E. (1979). Genetic factors in Wernicke-Korsakoff syndrome. *Alcoholism, 3*:126–134.

Bliding, G., Bliding, A., Fex, G., and Tornqvist, C. (1982). The appropriateness of laboratory tests in tracing young heavy drinkers. *Drug Alcohol Depend., 10*:153–158.

Boismare, F., Lhuintre, J.P., Daoust, M., Moore, N., Saligaut, C., and Hillemand, B. (1987). Platelet affinity for serotonin is increased in alcoholics and former alcoholics: A biological marker for dependence? *Alcohol Alcohol., 22*:155–159.

Bonte, W., Kuhnholz, B., and Ditt, J. (1985). Blood methanol levels and alcoholism. In M. Valverius (ed.), *Punishment and/or Treatment for Driving Under the Influence of Alcohol and Other Drugs*, Stockholm, International Committee on Alcohol, Drugs and Traffic Safety, pp. 255–259.

Braude, M.C., and Chao, H.M. (eds.), (1986). *Genetic and Biological Markers in Drug Abuse and Alcoholism*, NIDA Research Monograph No. 66, U.S. Government Printing Office, Washington, D.C.

Brown, S.A. (1977). Platelet MAO and alcoholism. *Am. J. Psychiatry, 134*:206–207.

Brown, R.L., Carter, W.B., and Gordon, M.J. (1987). Diagnosis of alcoholism in a simulated patient encounter by primary care physicians. *J. Fam. Pract., 25*:259–264.

Casacchia, M. Rossi, A., and Stratta, P. (1985). Thyrotropin-releasing hormone test in recently abstinent alcoholics. *Psychiatry Res., 16*:249–251.

Chalmers, D.M., Chanarin, I., MacDermott, S., and Levi, A.J. (1980). Sex-related differences in the haematological effects of excessive alcohol consumption. *J. Clin. Pathol., 33*:3–7.

Chalmers, D.M., Rinsler, M.G., MacDermott, S., Spicer, C.C., and Levi, A.J. (1981). Biochemical and haematological indicators of excessive alcohol consumption. *Gut, 22*:992–996.

Chan, A.W.K. (1966). Racial differences in alcohol sensitivity. *Alcohol Alcohol., 21*:93–104.

Chan, A.W.K., Welte, J.W., and Whitney, R.B. (1987). Identification of alcoholism in young adults by blood chemistries. *Alcohol, 4*:175–179.

Chan, A.W.K., Leong, F.W., Schanley, D.L., Welte, J.W., Wieczorek, W., Rej, R.O., and Whitney, R.B. (1989). Transferrin and mitochondrial aspartate aminotransferase in young adult alcoholics. *Drug Alcohol Depend., 23*:13–18.

Chapman, R.W., Sorrentino, D., and Morgan, M.Y. (1985). Abnormal heterogeneity of serum transferrin in relation to alcohol consumption: A reappraisal. In N.C. Chang and H.M. Chao (eds.), *Early Identification of Alcohol Abuse*, NIAA Research Monograph No. 17, U.S. Government Printing Office, Washington, D.C., pp. 108–114.

Chick, J., Pikkarainen, J., and Plant, M. (1987). Serum ferritin as a marker of alcohol consumption in working men. *Alcohol Alcohol., 22*:75–77.

Chick, J., Longstaff, M., Kreitman, M.P., Thatcher, D., and White, J. (1982). Plasma μ-amino-n-butyric acid leucine ratio and alcohol consumption in working men and in alcoholics. *J. Stud. Alcohol, 43*:583–587.

Cicero, T.J. (1983). Endocrine mechanisms in tolerance to and dependence on alcohol. In B. Kissin and H. Begleiter (eds.), *The Biology of Alcoholism*, Vol. 7, Plenum Press, New York, pp. 285–357.

Clark, P.M., Holder, R., Mullet, M., and Whitehead, T.P. (1983). Sensitivity and specificity of laboratory tests for alcohol abuse. *Alcohol Alcohol., 18*:261–269.

Cohen, J.A., and Kaplan, M.M. (1979). The SGOT/SGPT ratio—An indicator of alcoholic liver disease. *Digest. Dis. Sci., 24*:835–838.

Collins, A.C. (1986). Genetics as a tool for identifying biological markers of drug abuse. In M.C. Braude and H.M. Chao (eds.), *Genetic and Biological Markers in Drug Abuse and Alcoholism*, NIDA Research Monograph No. 66, U.S. Government Printing Office, Washington, D.C., pp. 57–70.

Collins, M.A. (1985). Alkaloid condensation products as biochemical indicators in alcoholism. In N.C. Chang and H.M. Chao (eds.), *Early Identification of Alcohol Abuse*, NIAAA Research Monograph No. 17, U.S. Government Printing Office, Washington, D.C., pp. 255–257.

Corder, B.F., McRee, C., and Rohrer, H. (1984). A brief review of literature on daughters of alcoholic fathers. *N.C. J. Ment. Health, 10*:37–43.

Coulehan, J.L., Zettler-Segal, M., Block, M., McClelland, M., and Schulberg, H.C. (1987). Recognition of alcoholism and substance abuse in primary care patients. *Arch. Intern. Med., 147*:349–352.

Cowan, R., Massey, L.K., and Greenfield, T.K. (1985). Average, binge and maximum alcohol intake in healthy young men: Discriminant function analysis. *J. Stud. Alcohol, 46*:467–472.

Crabbe, J.C., Kosobud, A., Young, E.R., Tam, B.R., and McSwigan, J.D. (1985). Bidirectional selection for susceptibility to ethanol withdrawal seizures in *Mus musculus. Behav. Genet., 15*:521–536.

Cushman, P., Jacobson, G., Barboriak, J.J., and Anderson, A.J. (1984). Biochemical markers for alcoholism: Sensitivity problems. *Alcoholism, 8*:253–257.

Davis, L.J., and Morse, R.M. (1987). Age and sex differences in the responses of alcoholics to the self-administered alcoholism screening test. *J. Clin. Psychol., 43*:423–430.

Davis, L.J., Hurt, R.D., Morse, R.M., and O'Brien, P.C. (1987). Discriminant analysis of the self-administered alcoholism screening test. *Alcoholism, 11*:269–273.

Deitrich, R.A., and Spuhler, K. (1984). Genetics of alcoholism and alcohol actions. In R.G. Smart, H.D. Cappell, F.B. Glaser, Y. Israel, H. Kalant, R.E. Popham, W. Schmidt, and E.M. Sellers (eds.), *Research Advances in Alcohol and Drug Problems*, Vol. 8, Plenum Press, New York, pp. 47–98.

Del Villano, B.C. Tischfield, J.A., Schacter, L.P., Stilwil, D., and Miller, S.I. (1979). Cupro-zinc superoxide dismutase: A possible biologic marker for alcoholism (studies in black patients). *Alcoholism, 3*:291–296.

Deren, S. (1986). Children of substance abusers: A review of the literature. *J. Subst. Abuse Treat., 3*:77–94.

Devenyi, P., Robinson, G.M., Kapur, B.M., and Roncari, D.A.K. (1981). High-density lipoprotein cholesterol in male alcoholics with and without severe liver disease. *Am. J. Med., 71*: 589–594.

Di Padova, C., Worner, T.M., and Lieber, C.S. (1987). Effect of abstinence on the blood acetaldehyde response to a test dose of alcohol in alcoholics. *Alcoholism, 11*:559–561.

Drum, D.E., Goldman, P.A., and Jankowski, C.B. (1981). Elevation of serum uric acid as a clue to alcohol abuse. *Arch. Intern. Med., 141*:477–479.

Dunbar, J.G., Ogston, S.A., Ritchie, A., Devgun, M.S., Hagart, J., and Martin, B.T. (1985). Are problem drinkers dangerous drivers? An investigation of arrest for drinking and driving, serum γ-glutamyltranspeptidase activities, blood alcohol concentrations, and road traffic accidents: The Tayside safe driving project. *Br. Med. J., 290*:827–830.

Eckardt, M.J., Rawlings, R.R., and Martin, P.R. (1986). Biological correlates and detection of alcohol abuse and alcoholism. *Prog. Neuro-Psychopharmacol. Biol. Psychiatry, 10*:135–144.

Eckardt, M.J., Rawlings, R.R., Ryback, R.S., Martin, P.R., and Gottschalk, L.A. (1984). Effects of abstinence on the ability of clinical laboratory tests to identify male alcoholics. *Am. J. Clin. Pathol., 82*:305–310.

el-Guebaly, N. (1986). Risk research in affective disorders and alcoholism: Epidemiological surveys and trait markers. *Canad. J. Psychiatry, 31*:352–361.

Eriksson, C.J.P. (1980). Elevated blood acetaldehyde levels in alcoholics and their relatives: A reevaluation. *Science, 207*:1383–1384.

Eriksson, C.J.P., and Peachey, J.E. (1980). Lack of difference in blood acetaldehyde of alcoholics and controls after ethanol ingestion. *Pharmacol. Biochem. Behav., 13*:101–105.

Ewing, J.A. (1984). Detecting alcoholism. The CAGE questionnaire. *J.A.M.A., 252*:1905–1907.

Fantozzi, R., Caramelli, L., Ledda, F., Moroni, F., Masini, E., Blandina, P., Botti, P., Peruzzi, S., Zorn, A.M., and Mannaioni P.F. (1987). Biological markers and therapeutic outcome in alcoholic disease: A twelve-year survey. *Klin. Wochenschr., 65*:27–33.

Farej, B.A., Lenton, J.D., Kutner, M., Camp, V.M., Stammers, T.W., Lee, S.R., Lolies, P.A., and Chandora, D. (1987). Prevalence of low monoamine oxidase function in alcoholism. *Alcoholism, 11*:464–467.

Flegar-Mestric, Z., Tadej, D., and Subic-Albert, N. (1987). Validity of 5-aminolevulinate dehydratase activity (5-ALAD) for the discrimination of alcoholics and nonalcoholics with chronic liver disease. *Clin. Biochem., 20*:81–84.

Fowler, C.J., Wiberg, A., Oreland, L., Danielsson, A., Palm, U., and Winblad, B. (1981). Monoamine oxidase activity and kinetic properties in platelet-rich plasma from controls, chronic alcoholics, and patients with nonalcoholic liver disease. *Biochem. Med., 25*:356–365.

Gavaler, J.S. (1982). Sex-related differences in ethanol-induced liver disease. Artifactual or real? *Alcoholism, 6*:186–196.

Giller, E., Jr., and Hall, H. (1983). Platelet MAO activity in recovered alcoholics after long-term abstinence. *Am. J. Psychiatry, 140*:114–115.

Giller, E., Jr., Nocks, J., Hall, H., Stewart, C., Schmitt, J., and Sherman, B. (1984). Platelet and fibroblast monamine oxidase in alcoholism. *Psychiatry Res., 12*:339–347.

Gjerde, H., Sakshaug, J., and Morland, J. (1986). Heavy drinking among Norwegian male drunken drivers: A study of γ-glutamyltransferase. *Alcoholism, 10*:209–212.

Gjerde, H., Amundsen, A., Skog, O.J., Morland, J., and Aasland, O.G. (1987). Serum gamma-glutamyltransferase: An epidemiological indicator of alcohol consumption? *Br. J. Addict.*, 82:1027–1031.

Gjerde, H., Johnsen, J., Bjorneboe, A., Bjorneboe, G.-E.A.A., and Morland, J. (1988). A comparison of serum carbohydrate-deficient transferrin with other biological markers of excessive drinking. *Scand. J. Clin. Lab. Invest.*, 48:1–6.

Goodwin, D.W. (1979). Alcoholism and heredity: A review and hypothesis. *Arch. Gen. Psychiatry*, 36:57–61.

Goodwin, D.W. (1987). Genetic influence in alcoholism. *Adv. Intern. Med.*, 32:283–298.

Greenberg, D.A., and Diamond, I. (1985). Wernicke-Korsakoff syndrome. In R.E. Tarter and D.H. Van Thiel (eds.), *Alcohol and the Brain, Chronic Effects*, Plenum Press, New York, pp. 295–314.

Hallgren, R., and Lundin, L. (1983). Increased total serum IgE in alcoholics. *Acta Med. Scand.*, 213:99–103.

Hamlyn, A.N., Hopper, J.C., and Skillen, A.W. (1979). Assessment of δ-aminolevulinate dehydrase for outpatient detection of alcoholic liver disease: Comparison with γ-glutamyltransferase and causal blood ethanol. *Clin. Chim. Acta*, 95:453–459.

Hartung, G.H., Foreyt, J.P., Mitchell, R.E., Mitchell, J.G.M., Reeves, R.S., and Gotto, A.M. (1983). Effect of alcohol intane on high-density cholesterol levels in runners and in inactive men. *J.A.M.A.*, 249:747–750.

Hays, J.T., and Spickard, W.A. (1987). Alcoholism: Early diagnosis and intervention. *J. Gen. Intern. Med.*, 2:420–427.

Herrington, R.E., Jacobsen, G.R., Daley, M.E., Lipo, R.F., Biller, H.B., and Weissgerber, C. (1981). Use of the plasma α-amino-n-butyric acid: leucine ratio to identify alcoholics. *J. Stud. Alcohol*, 42:492–499.

Hill, S.Y., Steinhauer, S.R., Zubin, J. (1987). Biological markers for alcoholism: A vulnerability model conceptualization. In P.C. Rivers (eds.), *Alcohol and Addictive Behavior: Nebraska Symposium on Motivation, 1986*, University of Nebraska Press, Lincoln, pp. 207–256.

Hill, S., Armstrong, J., Steinhauer, S.R., Baughman, T., and Zubin, J. (1987). Static ataxis as a psychobiological marker for alcoholism. *Alcoholism*, 11:345–348.

Hillers, V.N., Alldredge, J.R., and Massey, L.K. (1986). Determination of habitual alcohol intake from a panel of blood chemistries. *Alcohol Alcohol.*, 21:199–205.

Hirst, M., Evans, D.R., and Gowdey, C.W. (1987). Salsolinol in urine following chocolate consumption by social drinkers. *Alcohol Drug Res.*, 7:493–501.

Hoberman, H.D., and Chiodo, S.M. (1982). Elevation of the hemoglobin Al fraction in alcoholism. *Alcoholism*, 6:260–266.

Hoerner, M., Behrens, U.J., Worner, T.M., Blacksberg, I., Braley, L.F., Schaffner, F., and Lieber, C.S. (1988). The role of alcoholism and liver disease in the appearance of serum antibodies against acetaldehyde adducts. *Hepatology*, 8:569–574.

Hollstedt, C., and Dahlgren, L. (1987). Peripheral markers in the female "hidden alcoholic," *Acta Psychiatr. Scand.*, 75:591–596.

Holt, S., Skinner, H.A., and Israel, Y. (1981). Early identification of alcohol abuse: 2. Clinical and laboratory indicators. *Canad. Med. Assoc. J.*, 124:1279–1295.

Homaidan, F.R., Kricka, L.J., Clark, P.M.S., Jones, S.R., and Whitehead, T.P. (1983). Acetaldehyde–hemoglobin adducts: An unreliable marker of alcohol abuse. *Clin. Chem.*, 30:480–482.

Homaidan, F.R., Kricka, L.J., Bailey, A.R., and Whitehead, T.P. (1986). Red cell morphology in alcoholics: A new test for alcohol abuse. *Blood Cells*, 11:375–385.

Hrubec, Z., and Omenn, G.S. (1981). Evidence of genetic predisposition to alcoholic cirrhosis and psychosis: Twin concordances for alcoholism and its biological end points by zygosity among male veterans. *Alcoholism*, 5:207–215.

Hultberg, B., Isaksson, A., and Tiderstrom, G. (1980). β-Hexosaminidase, leucine aminopeptidase, cystidylaminopeptidase, hepatic enzymes and bilirubin in serum of chronic alcoholics with acute ethanol intoxication. *Clin. Chim. Acta*, 105:317–323.

Hulyalkar, A.R., Nora, R., and Manowitz, P. (1984). Arylsulfatase A variants in patients with alcoholism. *Alcoholism*, 8:337–341.

Isaksson, A., Blanche, C., Hultberg, B., and Joelsson, B. (1985). Influence of ethanol on the human serum level of β-hexosaminidase. *Enzyme, 33*:162–166.

Israel, Y., Hurwitz, E., Niemela, O., and Arnon, R. (1986). Monoclonal and polyclonal antibodies against acetaldehyde-containing epitopes in acetaldehyde-protein adducts. *Proceedings of the Natl. Acad. of Sci., 83*:7923–7927.

Iturriaga, H., Pereda, T., Etevez, A., and Ugarte, G. (1977). Serum immunoglobulin A changes in alcoholic patients. *Ann. Clin. Res., 9*:39–43.

Jacobson, G. (1976). *The Alcoholism: Detection, Diagnosis and Assessment*. Human Sciences Press, New York.

Jenkins, W.J., Rosalki, S.B., Foo, Y., Scheuer, P.J., Nemesanszky, E., and Sherlock, S. (1982). Serum glutamate dehydrogenase is not a reliable marker of liver cell necrosis in alcoholics. *J. Clin. Pathol., 35*:207–210.

Konttinen, A., Hartel, G., and Louhija, A. (1970). Multiple serum enzyme analysis in chronic alcoholics. *Acta Med. Scand., 188*:257–264.

Koplan, J.P., Annest, J.L., Layde, P.M., and Rubin, G.L. (1986). Nutrient intake and supplementation in the United States (NHANES II), *Am. J. Public Health, 76*:287–289.

Korri, U.-M., Nuutinen, H., and Salaspuro, M. (1985). Increased blood acetate: A new laboratory marker of alcoholism and heavy drinking. *Alcoholism, 9*:468–471.

Kosobud, A. and Crabbe, J.C. (1986). Ethanol withdrawal in mice bred to be genetically prone or resistant to ethanol withdrawal seizures. *J. Pharmacol. Exp. Ther., 238*:170–177.

Kristenson, H., Fex, G., and Trell, E. (1981). Serum ferritin, gammaglutamyltransferase and alcohol consumption in healthy middle-aged man. *Drug Alcohol Depend., 8*:43–50.

Ledig, M. Doffoel, M., Ziessel, M., Kopp, P., Charrault, A., Tongio, M.M., Mayer, S., Bockel, R., and Mandel, P. (1986). Frequencies of glyoxalase I phenotypes as biological markers in chronic alcoholism. *Alcohol, 3*:11–14.

Legros, J.J., Deconinck, I., Willems, D., Roth, B., Pelc, I., Brauman, J., and Verbanck, M. (1983). Increase of neurophysin II serum levels in chronic alcoholic patients: Relationship with alcohol consumption and alcoholism blood markers during therapy. *J. Clin. Endocrinol. Metab., 56*:871–875.

Li, T.K., Lumeng, L., McBride, W.J., Waller, M.B., and Murphy, J.M. (1986). Studies on an animal model of alcoholism. In M.C. Braude and H.M. Chao (eds.). *Genetic and Biological Markers in Drug Abuse and Alcoholism*, NIDA Research Monograph No. 66, U.S. Government Printing Office, Washington, D.C., pp. 41–49.

Lin, C.C., Potter, J.J., and Mezey, E. (1984). Erythrocyte aldehyde dehydrogenase activity in alcoholism. *Alcoholism, 8*:539–541.

Loosen, P.T., Wilson, I.C., Dew, B.W., and Tipermas, A. (1983). Thyrotropin-releasing hormone (TRH) in abstinent alcoholic men. *Am. J. Psychiatry, 140*:1145–1149.

Lucas, D., Menez, J.F. Bodenez, P., Baccino, E., Bardou, L.G., and Floch, H.H. (1988). Acetaldehyde adducts with haemoglobin: Determinations of acetaldehyde released from haemoglobin by acid hydrolysis. *Alcohol Alcohol., 23*:23–31.

Lumeng, L. (1986). New diagnostic markers of alcohol abuse. *Hepatology, 6*:742–745.

Lykouras, E., Moussas, G., and Markianos, M. (1987). Platelet monoamine oxidase and plasma dopamine-β-hydroxylase activities in non-abstinent chronic alcoholics. Relation to clinical parameters. *Drug Alcohol Depend., 19*:363–368.

Major, L.F., and Murphy, D.L. (1978). Platelet and plasma amine oxidase activity in alcoholic individuals. *Br. J. Psychiatry, 132*:548–554.

Major, L.F., Hawley, R.J., Saini, N., Garrick, N.A., and Murphy, D.L. (1985). Brain and liver monoamine oxidase type A and type B activity in alcoholics and controls. *Alcoholism, 9*:6–9.

Malmendier, C.L., and Delcroix, C. (1985). Effect of alcohol intake on high and low density lipoprotein metabolism in healthy volunteers. *Clin. Chim. Acta, 152*:281–288.

Martensson, E., Olofsson, U., and Heath, A. (1988). Clinical and metabolic features of ethanol-methanol poisoning in chronic alcoholics. *Lancet, 1*:327–328.

Matloff, D.S., Seligran, M.J., and Kaplan, M.M. (1980). Hepatic transaminase activity in alcoholic liver disease. *Gastroenterology, 78*:1389–1392.

Matsubara, K., Fukushima, S., Akane, A., Hama, K., and Fukui, Y. (1986). Tetrahydro-β-carbolines in human urine and rat brain—No evidence of formation by alcohol drinking. *Alcohol Alcohol.*, *21*:339–345.

Mayfield, D.G., McLeod, G., and Hall, P. (1974). The CAGE questionnaire: Validation of a new alcoholism screening instrument. *Am. J. Psychiatry, 131*:1121–1123.

McClearn, G.E., and Erwin, V.G. (1982). Genetic influence in biological mechanisms in alcohol-related behaviors: Animal models. In *Alcohol Consumption and Related Problems,* Alcohol and Health Monograph No. 1, U.S. Department of Health and Human Services, Library of Congress, Washington, D.C., pp. 271–285.

Miller, W.R. (1976). Alcoholism scales and objective assessment methods: A review. *Psychol. Bull. 83*:649–674.

Miller, P.M., Nirenberg, T.D., and McClure, G. (1983). Prevention of alcohol abuse. In B. Tabakoff, P.B. Sutker, and C.L. Randall (eds.), *Medical and Social Aspects of Alcohol Abuse,* Plenum Press, New York, pp. 375–397.

Mills, P.R., Spooner, R.J., Russell, R.I., Boyle, P., and MacSween, R.N.M. (1981). Serum glutamate dehydrogenase as a marker of hepatocyte necrosis in alcoholic liver disease. *Br. Med. J., 283*:754–755.

Moore, R.D., and Malitz, F.E. (1986). Underdiagnosis of alcoholism by residents in an ambulatory medical practice. *J. Med. Ed., 61*:46–52.

Morgan, M.Y., Colman, J.C., and Sherlock, S. (1981). The use of a combination of peripheral markers for diagnosing alcoholism and monitoring for continued abuse. *Br. J. Alcohol Alcohol., 16*:167–177.

Moss, H.B., Guthrie, S., and Linnoila, M. (1986). Enhanced thyrotropin response to thyrotropin releasing hormone in boys at risk for development of alcoholism. *Arch. Gen. Psychiatry, 43*:1137–1142.

Mukherjee, A.B., Svoronos, S., Ghazanfari, A., Martin, P.R., Fisher, A., Roecklein, B., Rodbard, D., Staton, R., Behar, D., Berg, C.J., and Manjunath, R. (1987). Transketolase abnormality in cultured fibroblasts from familial chronic alcoholic men and their male offspring. *J. Clin. Invest., 79*:1039–1043.

Myers, R.D. (1985). Alkaloid metabolites and addictive drinking of alcohol. In N.C. Chang and H.M. Chao (eds.), *Early Identification of Alcohol Abuse,* NIAAA Research Monograph No. 17, U.S. Government Printing Office, Washington, D.C., pp. 268–284.

Nalpas, B., Vassault, A., LeGuillou, A., Lesgourgues, B., Ferry, N., Lacour, B., and Berthelot, P. (1984). Serum activity of mitochondrial aspartate aminotransferase: A sensitive marker of alcoholism with or without alcoholic hepatitis. *Hepatology, 4*:893–896.

Nalpas, B., Vassault, A., Charpin, S., Lacour, B., and Berthelot, P. (1986). Serum mitochondrial aspartate aminotransferase as a marker of chronic alcoholism: Diagnostic value and interpretation in a liver unit. *Hepatology, 6*:608–614.

National Council on Alcoholism, Criteria Committee (1972). Criteria for the diagnosis of alcoholism. *Am. J. Psychiatry, 129*:127–135.

National Institute on Alcohol Abuse and Alcoholism (NIAAA). (1985). *Alcoholism: An Inherited Disease,* U.S. Department of Health and Human Services, Rockville, Maryland.

Neiman, J., Beving, H., and Malmgren, R. (1987). Platelet uptake of serotonin (5-HT) during ethanol withdrawal in male alcoholics. *Thrombosis Res., 46*:803–809.

Newlin, D.B. (1985). Offspring of alcoholics have enhanced antagonistic placebo response. *J. Stud. Alcohol, 46*:490–494.

Niemela, O., Klajner, F., Orrego, H., Vidins, E., Blendis, L., and Israel, Y. (1987). Antibodies against acetaldehyde-modified protein epitopes in human alcoholics. *Hepatology, 7*:1210–1214.

Nishimura, M., and Teschke, R. (1983). Alcohol and gamma-glutamyltransferase. *Klin. Wochenschr., 61*:265–275.

Nuutinen, H., Lindros, K.O., and Salaspuro, M. (1983). Determinants of blood acetaldehyde level during ethanol oxidation chronic alcoholics. *Alcoholism, 7*:163–168.

Nuutinen, H.U., Salaspuro, M.P., Valle, M., and Lindros, K.O. (1984). Blood acetaldehyde concentration gradient between hepatic and antecubital venous blood in ethanol-intoxicated alcoholics and controls. *Eur. J. Clin. Invest., 14*:306–311.

Nuutinenm, H., Lindros, K., Hekali, P., and Salaspuro, M. (1985). Elevated blood acetate as an indicator of fast ethanol elimination in chronic alcoholics. *Alcohol, 2*:623–626.

Nygren, A., and Sundblad, L. (1971). Lactate dehydrogenase isoenzyme patterns in serum and skeletal muscle in intoxicated alcoholics. *Acta Med. Scand. 189*:303–307.

Okuno, F., Ishii, H., Kashiwazaki, K., Takagi, S., Shigeta, Y., Arai, M., Takagi, T., Ebihara, Y., and Tsuchiya, M. (1988). Increase in mitochondrial GOT (m-GOT) activity after chronic alcohol consumption: Clinical and experimental observations. *Alcohol, 5*:49–53.

O'Malley, S.S., and Maisto, S.A. (1985). The effects of family drinking history on responses to alcohol: Expectations and reactions to intoxication. *J. Stud. Alcohol, 46*:289–297.

Palmer, K.R., and Jenkins, W.J. (1985). Aldehyde dehydrogenase in alcoholic subjects. *Hepatology, 5*:260–263.

Pandey, G.N., Fawcett, J., Gibbons, R., Clark, D.C., and Davis, J.M. (1988). Platelet monoamine oxidase in alcoholism. *Biol. Psychiatry, 24*:15–24.

Persson, J., and Magnusson, P.H. (1988). Comparison between different methods of detecting patients with excessive consumption of alcohol. *Acta Med. Scand., 223*:101–109.

Peterson, B., Trell, E., Kristensson, H., Fex, G., Yettra, M., and Hood, B. (1983). Comparison of gamma-glutamyltransferase and other health screening tests in average middle-aged males, heavy drinkers and alcohol nonusers. *Scand. J. Clin. Lab. Invest., 43*:141–149.

Peterson, C.M., Nguyen, L., Fantl, W., Stevens, V., Hawthorne, G., and Blackburn, P. (1985). Acetaldehyde adducts with hemoglobin. In N.C. Chang and H.M. Chao (eds.), *Early Identification of Alcohol Abuse*, NIAAA Research Monograph No. 17, U.S. Government Printing Office, Washington, D.C., pp. 68–77.

Pollock, V.E., Teasdale, T.W., Gabrielli, W.F., and Knop, J. (1986). Subjective and objective measures of response to alcohol among men at risk for alcoholism. *J. Stud. Alcohol, 47*:297–304.

Puchois, P., Fontan, M., Gentilini, J.L., Gelez, P., and Fruchart, J.C. (1984). Serum apolipoprotein A-II, A biochemical indicator of alcohol abuse. *Clin. Chim. Acta, 185*:185–189.

Puddey, I.B., Masarei, J.R.L., Vandongen, R., and Beilin, L.J. (1986). Serum apolipoprotein A-II as a marker of change in alcohol intake in male drinkers. *Alcohol Alcohol., 21*:375–383.

Pullarkat, R.K., and Raguthu, S. (1985). Elevated urinary dolichol levels in chronic alcoholics. *Alcoholism, 9*:28–30.

Reich, T., Robins, L.N., Woodruff, R.A., Taibleson, M., Rich, C., and Cunningham, L. (1975). Computer-assisted derivation of a screening interview for alcoholism. *Arch. Gen. Psychiatry, 32*:847–852.

Reid, A.L.A., Webb, G.R., Hennrikus, D., Fahey, P.P., and Sanson-Fisher, R.W. (1986). General practitioners' detection of patients with high alcohol intake. *Br. Med. J. 293*:735–737.

Roine, R.P. (1988). Effects of moderate drinking and alcohol abstinence on urinary dolichol levels. *Alcohol, 5*:229–231.

Roine, R.P., Turpeinen, U., Ylikahri, R., and Salaspuro, M. (1987). Urinary dolichol—a new marker of alcoholism. *Alcoholism, 11*:525–527.

Roine, R.P., Korri, U.M., Ylikahri, R., Penttila, A., Pikkarainen, J., and Salaspuro, M. (1988). Increased serum acetate as a marker of problem drinking among drunken drivers. *Alcohol Alcohol., 23*:123–126.

Roine, R.P., Eriksson, C.J.P., Ylikahri, R., Penttila, A., and Salaspuro, M. (1989a). Methanol as a marker of alcohol abuse. *Alcoholism, 13*:172–175.

Roine, R.P., Humaloja, K., Hamalainen, J., Nykanen, I., Ylikahri, R., and Salaspuro, M. (1989b). Significant increases in urinary dolichol levels in bacterial infections, malignancies and pregnancy but not in other clinical conditions. *Ann. Med., 21*:13–16.

Rommelspacher, H., and Schmidt, L. (1985). Increased formation of β-carbolines in alcoholic patients following ingestion of ethanol. *Pharmacopsychiatry, 18*:153–154.

Rosenthal, N.E., Davenport, Y. Cowdry, R.W., Webster, M.H., and Goodwin, F.K. (1980). Monoamine metabolites in cerebrospinal fluid of depressive subgroups. *Psychiatry Res., 2*:113–119.

Russell, M., Henderson, C., and Blume, S. (1984). *Children of Alcoholics: A Review of the Literature*, New York State Division of Alcoholism and Alcohol Abuse, Buffalo.

Rutstein, D.D., Veech, R.L., Nickerson, R.J., Felyer, M.E., Vernon, A.A., Needham, L.L., Kishsore, P., and Thacker, S.B. (1983). 2,3-Butanediol: An unusual metabolite in the serum of severely alcoholic men during acute intoxication. *Lancet, 2*:534–537.

Ryback, R.S., and Rawlings, R.R. (1985). Biochemical correlates of alcohol consumption. In N.C. Chang and H.M. Chao (eds.), *Early Identification of Alcohol Abuse*, NIAAA Research Monograph No. 17, U.S. Government Printing Office, Washington, D.C., pp. 31–48.

Ryback, R.S., Eckardt, M.J., and Pautler, C.P. (1980). Biochemical and hematological correlates of alcoholism. *Res. Commun. Chem. Pathol. Pharamcol., 27*:533–550.

Ryback, R.S., Eckardt, M.J., Rawlings, R.R., and Rosenthal, R.S. (1982). Quadratic discriminant analysis as an aid to interpretive reporting of clinical laboratory tests. *J.A.M.A., 248*:2342–2345.

Ryback, R.S., Eckardt, M.J., Negron, G.L., and Rawlings, R.R. (1983). The search for a biochemical marker in alcoholism. *Subst. Alcohol Actions/Misuse, 4*:217–224.

Ryback, R.S., Rawlings, R.R., Faden, V., and Negron, G.L. (1985). Laboratory test changes in young abstinent male alcoholics. *Am. J. Clin. Pathol., 83*:474–479.

Salaspuro, M. (1986). Conventional and coming laboratory markers of alcoholism and heavy drinking. *Alcoholism, 10*:5S–12S.

Salaspuro, M.P., Korri, U.-M., Nuutinen, H., and Roine, R. (1987). Blood acetate and urinary dolichols—new markers of heavy drinking and alcoholism. *Prog. Clin. Biol. Res., 241*:231–240.

Sanchez-Craig, M., and Annis, H.M. (1981). γ-Glutamyltranspeptidase and high density lipoprotein cholesterol in male problem drinkers: Advantages of a composite index for predicting alcohol consumption. *Alcoholism, 5*:540–544.

Saunders, J.B., and Williams, R. (1983). The genetics of alcoholism: Is there an inherited susceptibility to alcohol-related problems? *Alcohol Alcohol., 18*:189–217.

Saunders, J.B., Haines, A., Portmann, B., Wodak, A.D., Powell-Jackson, P.R., Davis, M., and Williams, R. (1982). Accelerated development of alcoholic cirrhosis in patients with HLA-B8. *Lancet, 1*:1381–1384.

Schnitt, J.M., and Dove, H.G. (1986). Issues in the development of alcoholism screening models using discriminant function analysis of blood profiles. *Subst. Abuse, 7*:38–51.

Schuckit, M.A. (1980). Self-rating of alcohol intoxication by young men with and without family histories of alcoholism. *J. Stud. Alcohol, 41*:242–249.

Schuckit, M.A. (1981). Peak blood alcohol levels in men at high risk for the future development of alcoholism. *Alcoholism, 5*:64–66.

Schuckit, M.A. (1984a). Differences in plasma cortisol after ingestion of ethanol in relatives of alcoholics and controls: Preliminary results. *J. Clin. Psychiatry, 45*:374–376.

Schuckit, M.A. (1984b). *Drug and Alcohol Abuse: A Clinical Guide to Diagnosis and Treatment*. Plenum Press, New York.

Schuckit, M.A. (1984c). Subjective responses to alcohol in sons of alcoholics and controls. *Arch. Gen. Psychiatry, 41*:879–884.

Schuckit, M.A. (1985). Ethanol-induced changes in body sway in men at high alcoholism risk. *Arch. Gen. Psychiatry, 42*:375–379.

Schuckit, M.A. (1986). Biological markers in alcoholism. *Prog. Neuro-Psychopharmacol. Biol. Psychiatry, 10*:191–199.

Schuckit, M.A. (1987a). Biological vulnerability to alcoholism. *J. Consult. Clin. Psychol., 55*:301–309.

Schuckit, M.A. (1987b). Why don't we diagnose alcoholism in our patients. *J. Fam. Pract., 25*:225–226.

Schuckit, M.A., and Duby, J. (1982). Alcohol-related flushing and the risk for alcoholism in sons of alcoholics. *J. Clin. Psychiatry, 43*:415–418.

Schuckit, M.A., and Gold, E.O. (1988). A simultaneous evaluation of multiple markers of ethanol/placebo challenges in sons of alcoholics and controls. *Arch. Gen. Psychiatry, 45*:211–216.

Schuckit, M.A., and Rayses, V. (1979). Ethanol ingestion: Differences in blood acetaldehyde concentrations in relatives of alcoholics and controls. *Science, 203*:54–55.

Schuckit, M.A., Parker, D.C., and Rossman, L.R. (1983). Ethanol-related prolactin responses and risk for alcoholism. *Biol. Psychiatry, 18*:1153–1159.

Schuckit, M.A., Gold, E., and Risch, C. (1987a). Plasma cortisol levels following ethanol in sons of alcoholics and controls. *Arch. Gen. Psychiatry, 44*:942–945.

Schuckit, M.A., Gold, E., Risch, C. (1987b). Serum prolactin levels in sons of alcoholics and control subjects. *Am. J. Psychiatry, 144*:854–859.

Schuckit, M.A., Shaskan, E., Duby, J., Vega, R., and Moss, M. (1982). Platelet monoamine oxidase activity in relatives of alcoholics. Preliminary study with matched control subjects. *Arch. Gen. Psychiatry, 39*:137–140.

Selzer, M. (1971). The Michigan Alcoholism Screening Test: The quest for a new diagnostic instrument. *Am. J. Psychiatry, 127*:1653–1658.

Shaper, A.G., Pocock, S.J., Ashby, D., Walker, M., and Whitehead, T.P. (1985). Biochemical and haematological response to alcohol intake. *Ann. Clin. Biochem., 22*:50–61.

Sher, K.J. (1983). Platelet monoamine oxidase activity in relatives of alcoholics. *Arch. Gen. Psychiatry, 40*:466.

Shigeta, Y., Ishi, H., Takagi, S., Yoshitake, Y., Hirano, T., Takata, H., Kohno, H., and Tsuchiya, M. (1980). HLA antigens as immungenetic markers of alcoholism and alcoholic liver disease. *Pharmacol. Biochem. Behav., 13*(Suppl. 1):89–94.

Skinner, H.A., and Holt, S. (1987). *The Alcohol Clinical Index: Strategies for Identifying Patients with Alcohol Problems*, Alcoholism and Drug Addiction Research Foundation, Toronto.

Skinner, H.A., Holt, S., and Israel, Y. (1981). Early identification of alcohol abuse: 1. Critical issues and psychosocial indicators for a composite index. *Canad. Med. Assoc. J., 124*:1141–1152.

Skinner, H.A., Holt, S., Schuller, R., Roy, J., and Israel, Y. (1984). Identification of alcohol abuse using laboratory tests and a history of trauma. *Ann. Intern. Med., 101*:847–851.

Skinner, H.A., Holt, S., Sheu, W.J., and Israel, Y. (1986). Clinical versus laboratory detection of alcohol abuse: The alcohol clinical index. *Br. Med. J., 292*:1703–1708.

Skude, G., and Wadstein, J. (1977). Amylase, hepatic enzymes and bilirubin in serum of chronic alcoholics. *Acta Med. Scand., 201*:53–58.

Solberg, H.E. (1978). Discriminant analysis. *CRC Crit. Rev. Clin. Lab. Sci., 9*:209–242.

Stamm, D., Hansert, E., and Feuerlein, W. (1984). Detection and exclusion of alcoholism in men on the basis of clinical laboratory findings. *J. Clin. Chem. Clin. Biochem., 22*:79–96.

Stibler, H., Borg, S., and Allgulander, C. (1980). Abnormal microheterogeneity of transferrin—a new marker of alcoholism? *Subst. Alcohol Actions/Misuse, 1*:247–252.

Stibler, H., Borg, S., and Joustra, M. (1986). Micro anion exchange chromatography of carbohydrate-deficient transferrin in serum in relation to alcohol consumption (Swedish Patent 8400587-5). *Alcoholism, 10*:535–544.

Storey, E.L., Anderson, G.J., Mack, U., Powell, L.W., and Halliday, J.E. (1987). Desialylated transferrin as a serological marker of chronic excessive alcohol ingestion. *Lancet, 1*:1292–1294.

Sullivan, J.L., Stanfield, C.N., Maltbie, A.A., Hammett, E., and Cavenar, J.O. (1978). Stability of low blood platelet monoamine oxidase activity in human alcoholics. *Biol. Psychiatry, 13*:391–397.

Sullivan, J.L., Cavenar, J.O., Maltbie, A.A., Lister, P., and Zung, W.W.K. (1979). Familial biochemical and clinical correlates of alcoholics with low platelet monoamine oxidase activity. *Biol. Psychiatry, 14*:385–394.

Tabakoff, B., Hoffman, P.L., Lee, J.M., Saito, T., Willard, B., and De Leon-Jones, F. (1988). Differences in platelet enzyme activity between alcoholics and nonalcoholics. *N. Engl. J. Med., 318*:134–139.

Tang, B.K. (1987). Detection of ethanol in urine of abstaining alcoholics. *Canad. J. Physiol. Pharmacol., 65*:1225–1227.

Tang, B.K., Devenyi, P., Teller, D., and Israel, Y. (1986). Detection of an alcohol specific product in urine of alcoholics. *Biochem. Biophys. Res. Commun., 140*:924–927.

Towell, J.F., Barboriak, J.J., Townsend, W.F., Kalbfleisch, J.H., and Wang, R.I.H. (1986). Erythrocyte aldehyde dehydrogenase: Assay of a potential biochemical marker of alcohol abuse. *Clin. Chem., 32*:734–738.

Tsuchiya, F., Sirasaka, T., Ikeda, H., Hatta, Y., Watanabe, J., and Saito, T. (1987). Platelet adenylate cyclase activity in alcoholics. *Jpn. J. Alcohol Drug Depend., 22*:366–372.

Valimaki, M., Harkonen, M., and Ylikahri, R. (1983). Serum ferritin and iron levels in chronic male alcoholics before and after ethanol withdrawal. *Alcohol Alcohol., 18*:255–260.

Van Waes, L., and Lieber, C.S. (1977). Glutamate dehydrogenase: A reliable marker of liver cell necrosis in the alcoholic. *Br. Med. J., 2*:1508–1510.

Vesterberg, O., Petren, S., and Schmidt, D. (1984). Increased concentrations of a transferrin variant after alcohol abuse. *Clin. Chim. Acta, 141*:33–39.

Virkkunen, M., Nuutila, A., Goodwin, F.K., and Linnoila, M. (1987). Cerebrospinal fluid monoamine metabolite levels in male arsonists. *Arch. Gen. Psychiatry, 44*:241–247.

Vital and Health Statistics (1982). Series II #232. U.S. Department of Health and Human Services, Washington, D.C.

von Knorring, L., Oreland, L., and von Knorring, A.L. (1987). Personality traits and platelet MAO activity in alcohol and drug abusing teenage boys. *Acta Psychiatr. Scand., 75*:307–314.

von Knorring, A.L., Bohman, M., von Knorring, L., and Oreland, L. (1985). Platelet MAO activity as a biological marker in subgroups of alcoholism. *Acta Psychiatr. Scand., 72*:51–58.

Watson, R.R., Mohs, M.E., Eskelson, C., Sampliner, R.E., and Hartmann, B. (1986). Identification of alcohol abuse and alcoholism with biological parameters. *Alcoholism, 10*:364–385.

V

Pharmacology of Drugs/Alcohol

19

Cocaine

James Cocores
Fair Oaks Hospital, Summit, New Jersey

A. Carter Pottash and Mark S. Gold
Fair Oaks Hospital, Summit, New Jersey, and Delray Beach, Florida

I. INTRODUCTION

The current cocaine epidemic shares many similarities with other illnesses which have plagued the world. Unlike other rapidly disseminating diseases, the cocaine epidemic does not involve transfer of a microorganism from individual to individual. Instead, the development of cocaine addiction relies on an interaction among various psychological, biological, and social factors. The current status is grim. An estimated 50 tons of cocaine, worth about 50 billion dollars, enters the United States each year. Twenty-five million Americans have experimented with cocaine and about 1.2 million are addicted users. There are 3000 neophytes trying cocaine each day [1]. Clinicians should recognize the signs early so that treatment can begin as soon as possible.

Primary prevention of cocaine addiction is also important. The development of cocaine addiction involves three basic phases, which include experimentation, casual or social use, and dependence [2]. Educational awareness should be tailored to each phase. Emphasis on the medical and psychiatric consequences of cocaine addiction are probably most effective in the very young, who presumably have not yet experimented. In addiction, educators should extend the topic of cocaine addiction to include the broader heading of chemical addiction. The place that "gateway" drugs such as marijuana, alcohol, and even volatile substances [3] take in the development of cocaine addiction needs to be emphasized. But individuals who have experimented with cocaine and have evolved into the casual-use stage have already started to develop a denial system which renders them partially immune to the above-mentioned education strategies. Casual users, therefore, need to dissect and learn about the seductive and cunning transition from innocent casual use to the bondage of cocaine addiction. Individuals who are already cocaine addicted need to learn about treatment and recovery [4]. Increased awareness of the treatment options that are available serve to decrease fear and serves to muster the courage needed to seek and comply with treatment. A comprehensive educational approach is useful when addressing family members and friends of cocaine addicts. Family education helps foster the clinical–family member alliance often required to engage the cocaine addict into treatment [5].

The 1988 National Household Survey on Drug Abuse, which showed significant declines in the "current use" of illicit drugs by Americans nationwide, but also indicated continued severe problems with heavy drug users, especially frequent users of cocaine. The survey conducted in the fall of 1988 showed a decrease of 37% in current use of illicit drugs compared with results of the most recent previous Household Survey, conducted in 1985. In other words, based on survey responses, persons who used marijuana, cocaine, or any other illicit drug within the last 30 days dropped from 23.0 million in 1985 to 14.5 million in 1988. In addition, users of any illicit drug within the last year decreased almost 25%, from 37 to 28 million.

The number of current cocaine users also dropped, by 50%, from 5.8 million in 1985 to 2.9 million in 1988, and those who used cocaine in the past year fell from 12 to 8 million.

However, the 1988 survey found continued intense use of cocaine within the cocaine-user population. Some 862,000 individuals used cocaine once a week or more, compared with 647,000 in 1985; and some 292,000 individuals used the drug daily or almost daily, compared with 246,000 in 1985.

Cocaine use was highest among the unemployed (4.6%) and those aged 18–25 (4.5%). The survey also found there were almost half a million current "crack" users among the 2.9 million current cocaine users.

II. HISTORY

For centuries coca leaves, from which cocaine is obtained, have been used by natives of South America to increase endurance. It has been estimated that cocaine's anesthetic and central nervous system stimulant properties were recognized by inhabitants of South America as long ago as 1500 B.C. The Incas incorporated the coca plant in many of their religious rituals. The leaves have been chewed by natives of Bolivia and Peru for thousands of years. It was not until the mid-1800s that cocaine was popularized in Europe. Cocaine was considered safe by the 1890s. Over 50 cocaine-containing drinks and elixirs were available to the public by the turn of the twentieth century. Cocaine was the only local anesthetic available for medical use prior to the introduction of procaine in 1905 [5]. Cocaine was an ingredient found in wine (Vin Mariani) and other beverages (Coca-Cola) regularly consumed in the United States before 1914 [6]. Despite the Harrison Narcotic Act, which limited the use and distribution of cocaine, drug use continued at epidemic proportions in the late 1920s [7]. Cheaper, "safer," and longer-acting central nervous system stimulant alternatives, the amphetamines, began their popularity in the 1930s. This set the stage for the amphetamine epidemic which extended through the early 1970s. But by then even amphetamine abusers recognized the dangers of amphetamines in expressed slogans such as "speed kills." Awareness of the dangers of amphetamine use among the medical community and society contributed to the progressive restriction of the amphetamines to schedule II. In 1973, two national commissions on drug abuse did consider the dangers of amphetamines but did not link cocaine with substantial morbidity [8,9]. One of the precipitants to the cocaine explosion of the 1980s was the commonly held popular belief that cocaine was safe. Some researchers viewed cocaine as a relatively safe, nonaddicting euphroic agent as recently as 1980 [10]. Between 1976 and 1986, there was an increase of more than 15-fold in cocaine-related emergency room visits, deaths, and admissions to cocaine treatment programs [11]. By 1986, it was estimated that 3 million people abused cocaine regularly and almost 15% of the U.S. population had tried cocaine [12]. Cocaine dependence was not listed as a separate diagnostic category until 1987 [13]. The medical, social, and psychological consequences of cocaine abuse became clearly evident by the turn of 1990. The news was spread by the scientific community [1], politicians, educators, and the media. Their efforts may have contributed to recent reports of declining first-time cocaine users. But reports of increasing amphetamine abuse, "ice," in Hawaii and on the West Coast serve to underscore the need for continued education around the general topic of addiction rather than specific drug epidemics as they arise.

III. BACKGROUND

Cocaine is extracted from the leaves of *Erythroxylon coca* and other species of *Erythroxylon* trees indigenous to the eastern Andes of South America. South America clearly generates and harvests the largest coca leaf crop even though the plant is cultivated in Southeast Asia, the United States, and Europe. Bolivia and Peru are clearly the largest producers of the crop. Only two of the 250 varieties of coca possess enough cocaine to give farmers incentive enough to grow the crop. Cocaine is probably the highest yielding cash crop in the world. It is only one of 14 alkaloids found in coca leaves. *Theobroma cacao* (chocolate) and *Cocos nucifera* (coconut palm) are not related to coca despite similar-sounding names. Coca leaves are processed into a light brown paste, which is further refined into a white sugarlike powder.

IV. ROUTES OF ADMINISTRATION

The addiction liability of oral cocaine use is far less than that of the intranasal route because of the time lag in the onset of pharmacological effects after oral use. The low brain delivery of cocaine after oral administration is due to first-pass hepatic biotransformation, which prevents 70–80% of the dose from reaching the systemic circulation. Cocaine hydrochloride is rarely used orally in the United States today, but was common when cocaine could be purchased in over-the-counter beverages. Coca leaf chewing on the other hand is a common practice in South America. The leaves are toasted and then chewed with an alkaline material. The combined alkaline wad enhances buccal absorption.

Cocaine hydrochloride is a water-soluble salt, which is usually sniffed. The white powder is commonly sold in 1-gm quantities, which is about the size of a sugar packet. Cocaine hydrochloride does not vaporize and is not smoked. A portion of the packet contents is usually spilled onto a smooth clean surface such as a small mirror. The powder is broken up finely with a razor blade then separated into thin uniform lines. A straw, rolled up dollar bill, or piece of paper is then inserted into a nostril while the other nostril is obstructed with a finger. Each line of cocaine is sniffed into the sinuses in this manner. Cocaine is absorbed across the sinus membranes and into the blood stream. Local vasoconstriction limits absorption of the alkaloid. This is a major reason why sniffers usually develop addiction at a slower rate when compared to smokers. Up to 50% of cocaine addicts seeking treatment are intranasal users [14]. Nasal vasoconstriction leads to necrosis with subsequent nose bleeds and septal perforations.

Cocaine hydrochloride decomposes if smoked. Only after it has been chemically altered to form "free base" can cocaine be smoked. Free-base cocaine is prepared by mixing cocaine hydrochloride with a solvent such as ether. Once dissolved the mixture is dried. The resulting free base is smokable and extremely addicting. The addiction potential is analogous to the decreased addiction potential of oral nicotine compared to that of cigarette smoking [15]. The lungs provide a large surface area for diffusion of cocaine directly into the blood stream. Cocaine base is extremely addicting because of the almost immediate and complete transfer of cocaine to the brain. Cocaine blood levels reached by smoking approach those levels resulting from intravenous (IV) use. Free-base and crack cocaine smoking have toxic effects on the lungs [16]. Crack is ready-to-use, low-priced cocaine free base. No chemical preparation is needed. Traffickers have increased their drug volume sales by making the most addictive form of cocaine less expensive, purer, and more convenient. It is similar to marketing methods employed by fast-food chains. Three or four small rocks of crack are typically sold in a vial which generally costs between 10 and 20 dollars. The term *crack* was derived from the crackling sound heard when the small creamy colored rocks are ignited.

Intravenous cocaine use is a less widespread method of drug administration when compared to crack or sniffing. One of the reasons for this is probably related to the fear of using a needle and the related health risks. Intravenous cocaine is frequently used in conjunction with heroin. Heroin reduces the uncomfortable side effects of tension and irritability that are associated with intravenous cocaine abuse. Lack of sterile IV techniques contribute to a wide spectrum of medical complications [17]. Systemic infections such as septic pulmonary embolus, brain abscesses, bacteremia, and bacterial endocarditis result. Intravenous cocaine users often share needles and increases the chance of transmitting hepatitis A, B, non-A, non-B, and acquired immunodeficiency syndrome (AIDS) [18].

The route of administration chosen is the primary factor determining the onset of drug effect, the concentration of cocaine in the brain, and the rate of progression from abuse to dependence (Table 1) [19]. Other important factors which contribute to the rate at which addiction evolves include frequency of use, technique employed with the particular route of administration chosen, the purity of the drug sample, and how predisposed the user is to cocaine addiction. The latter predisposition may be genetic or the result of an experience as a chronic substance user.

V. PSYCHOLOGICAL AND SOCIAL CONTRIBUTING FACTORS

It is believed that the cocaine addict originally uses the drug for a number of reasons, including peer pressure, boredom, curiosity, and recreation. The majority of cocaine addicts once believed that their occasionl cocaine use was benign and they could stop if the frequency increased to more dangerous proportions. Cocaine delivers a predominantly euphoric reward and repeated use occurs as a means of again achieving pleasure. The euphoric state is not forgotten and haunting recollections often flood consciousness. A dysphoric state rapidly follows the cocaine-induced euphoria. The dysphoria is a negative reinforcer that also contributes to continued cocaine use. Although cocaine withdrawal lacks the severe physical discomfort seen in other drug addictions, such as opiate addiction, it is characterized by equal if not more severe psychological discomfort in the form of cocaine craving. Cocaine's powerful action on the reward system in the brain possesses a greater positive reinforcement property. The etiology of cocaine addiction involves an interplay between positive and negative reinforcers.

Some cocaine addicts start using the drug in an effort to medicate an underlying psychological problem such as depression. The self-medication hypothesis of cocaine addiction [20] applies to a subpopulation but clearly does not explain or apply to the majority of cocaine addiction cases. Even when the self-medication hypothesis does apply to a cocaine addict, the clinician must still emphasize the need for drug treatment or rehabilitation.

Environmental factors contribute to the development of cocaine dependence. For example, the increased availability and low cost of crack in metropolitan areas of the continental United States fuels the progression of cocaine addiction in these areas, whereas amphetamine addiction is much more common in Hawaii. Even the gateway drugs leading to cocaine addiction vary from one place to the next. For example, alcohol or marijuana are common gateway drugs in metropolitan areas, whereas gasoline sniffing among adolescent native

Table 1 Differential Effects Dependent on Routes of Cocaine Administration

Administration		Initial onset of action (s)	Duration of "high" (min)	Average acute dose (mg)	Peak plasma levels (ng/ml)	Purity (%)	Bioavailability (% absorbed)
Route	Mode						
Oral	Cocoa leaf chewing	300–600	45–90	20–50	150	0.5–1.0	
Oral	Cocaine HCl	600–1800		100–200	150–200	20–80	20–30
Intranasal	"Snorting" Cocaine HCl	120–180	30–45	5 × 30	150	20–80	20–30
Intravenous	Cocaine HCl	30–45	10–20	25–50 >200	300–400 1000–1500	7–100 × 58	100
Smoking Intrapulmonary	Coca paste Freebase Crack	8–10	5–10	60–250 250–1000	300–800 800–900 ?	40–85 90–100 50–95	6–32

Americans of the Southwest is not uncommon [3]. Gateway drugs are commonly involved in drug addiction, but not always. Also, social norms regarding drug addiction vary among countries, states, towns, and families. These differences help determine drug of choice and can alter the rate at which drug addiction progresses.

The interplay of social, psychological, and biological factors forms the foundation of cocaine addiction. Cocaine addiction is similar to other diseases in this regard. For example, the risk of developing coronary heart disease increases with the identification of a genetic predisposition. But the status of a person's environment and personality serve to further express or suppress a familial predisposition.

VI. NEUROCHEMICAL FACTORS

Cocaine produces euphoria by activating reward pathways in the brain. Reward or pleasure is mediated by activating dopamine in mesolimbic and mesocortical pathways. Several neurotransmitter systems in the brain may contribute to the many effects of cocaine. Indirect evidence for the involvement of various neurotransmitters in the brain has been found in animal studies and by extrapolation of subjective and objective cocaine effects in humans.

Many of the effects may be attributed to the dopamine system. Specifically, cocaine rapidly blocks the reuptake of the dopamine neurotransmitter into its presynaptic nerve terminal for storage by the vesicles. The reuptake mechanism is the principal means of termination of action of the neurotransmitter. Blockade of the reuptake mechanism results in a greater concentration and a longer duration of action of dopamine [21]. The acute effect of cocaine on the dopamine neurons in vitro is to stimulate enhanced dopamine activity by dopamine reuptake blockade and by increased dopamine synthesis.

Dopamine appears to be intimately involved in the "reward" center located in the limbic system. Dopamine neurons in the central nervous system (CNS) originate in the ventral tegmental area and project to the limbic structures, which include the nucleus accumbens (meoslimbic pathways) and the frontal cortex (mesoortical pathways). The mesolimbic and mesocortical pathways are linked to the reward system, the neurons of which originate in the lateral hypothalamus. These neurons descend as part of the median forebrain bundle and terminate in the ventral tegmental area, where they synapse on dopamine neurons.

The subjective and objective effects of cocaine can be correlated with the demonstrated actions of cocaine on neurons in the various locations in the brain. The limbic system is the substrate for mood, drive states such as hunger and sex, memory, and reward behavior. The basal ganglia are the substrate for motor behavior. The substantial nigra neurons that contain dopamine project to the caudate nucleus and putamen. The amygdala and septal areas control mood and contain dopamine neurons [22].

Animals avidly press a layer for electrical stimulation when electrodes are placed in these dopamine pathways, whereas dopamine-receptor blockers or lesions of these pathways eliminate self-administration of stimulants [23]. Central nervous system addiction to cocaine is best conceptualized in terms of neurotransmitter-induced physiological reinforcement rather than the presence of physical abstinence symptoms [24].

VII. COCAINE ADDICTION

The diagnostic category of cocaine dependence has only recently been added to the list of mental disorders [13]. Cocaine withdrawal differs from opiate or alcohol withdrawal. The predictable withdrawal syndrome associated with cocaine abuse has been less convincing when compared to the delirium tremens or severe bone pain associated with other drug addictions. Nevertheless, tolerance to cocaine develops very rapidly and varies with dose, duration, and the route of administration selected.

Addiction to cocaine is defined as the preoccupation with the acquisition and compulsive use of cocaine, with relapse. Loss of control is pervasive and is the *sine qua non* of addictive behavior. The cocaine addict continues to seek and use cocaine in spite of sometimes overwhelming psychiatric, medical, legal, and financial consequences.

Tolerance and dependence regularly occur, but may be difficult to ascertain in the clinical interview because of the denial of the extent and the amount of use of cocaine by the addict. Cocaine addicts frequently increase the amount of use dramatically in an attempt to maintain certain cocaine effects. The dependence syndrome is characterized by the withdrawal, or "crash," that occurs in the abstinent state [22,25]. Tolerance to and dependence on opiates readily occur, although they are greater and more clearly definable in the case of narcotics. The addiction to either cocaine or opiates is similar in the strength and type of preoccupation with acquisition, compulsive use, and relapse to either drug.

The strength of the addiction is illustrated by experiments performed on *Rhesus* monkeys. These monkeys were allowed to self-administer cocaine by pressing a bar. The cocaine was available in unlimited amounts over indefinite periods of time. All the monkeys pressed the bar to receive cocaine until inanition and death. The loss of control for self-administration of the cocaine was sufficiently potent to produce disregard for the instincts of self-preservation. The behavior in the *Rhesus* monkeys is readily seen in humans who pursue without regard for health and welfare, as manifested by loss of large sums of money, liberty, and life [23,24].

Cocaine addicts describe tolerance in terms of "chasing the high." For example, free basers achieve a level of euphoria which is not surpassed on a given day despite continued smoking throughout the day. Cocaine addiction is characterized by increased frequency of use, increased amounts of cocaine used, and the inability to stop despite consequences. Cocaine-addicted persons have been using other drugs for the characteristic dysphoria and irritability of cocaine withdrawal, the crash, with a variety of drugs which include heroin and the benzodiazepines. Beer, marijuana, and other alcoholic beverages are the most commonly employed drugs used to reduce the discomfort of cocaine withdrawal. This is why most cocaine addicted persons are polydrug abusers. This often leads to dual addiction and the need for extended inpatient detoxification.

Alcoholism and other drug abuse diagnoses are highly prevalent among cocaine addicts. Ninety-eight percent of cocaine addicts have used marijuana before initiating cocaine use. More than 80% have used alcohol before using cocaine. Furthermore, alcohol is used before marijuana in the sequence of drug use in the natural history of the progression to cocaine addiction [26].

In a study of 263 inpatients who were given a structured psychiatric interview, 83% qualified for DSM-III-R [13] diagnoses of cocaine and alcohol dependence. Alcohol was the first drug used, at an average age of 14 years, followed by marijuana at an average age of 15 years, and eventually cocaine at 22 years. These findings also correlate with others that confirm 80% of alcoholics below the age of 30 use at least one other drug addictively, often marijuana and then cocaine [27].

Acute detoxification, or "crashing," from cocaine frequently does not require more than supervised supportive psychological treatment by professionally trained nurses and physicians. The depression, somnolence, hyperphagia, anxiety, paranoia, and craving subside gradually over days. No significant alterations in vital signs, withdrawal seizures, or delirium usually occur. Relapse to cocaine usually results, however, unless some outside, experienced intervention is provided.

Acute hospitalization may be indicated for special consequences of chronic cocaine use that include suicide risk, inability to abstain from cocaine, and other associated drug use such as alcohol, which may require supervised detoxification. Acute detoxification is not sufficient to prevent relapse. Professional treatment and rehabilitation aimed at the addictive process are required in order for the addict to achieve and maintain the desired goal of abstinence. Abstinence is necessary, as the cocaine addict, by virtue of the addiction, is unable to moderate the amount and frequency of cocaine intake so as to avoid adverse consequences.

The most problematic cocaine withdrawal symptom is craving, or the desire to use cocaine. Despite the dysphoria, depression, financial problems, associated crimes, family dysfunction, health problems, and other consequences that develop with cocaine addiction, the drug addict's priority is obtaining more cocaine. The intensity and severity of cocaine craving surpasses most other drugs of abuse. Both psychosocial and neurochemically based cocaine cravings predominate during the early phases of cocaine abstinence. The cocaine crash and craving is believed to be a function of dopamine depletion, though the neurotransmitter does not function unilaterally. For example, acetylcholine turnover usually increases when dopamine is depleted [28]. Therefore, cocaine-induced catecholamine depletion may activate acetylcholine, which also contributes to increased prolactin and anergy [29]. The more cocaine the abuser uses the more likely he or she is to experience overwhelming drug craving. The cocaine-induced neurotransmitter imbalance is believed to reverse during the early phase of cocaine abstinence back to the premorbid state. Cocaine cravings that are believed to originate from neurotransmitter imbalances decrease in magnitude and frequency during the first few months of abstinence. Psychosocial factors such as people, places, and things associated with cocaine addiction may continue to trigger cocaine craving or thoughts of cocaine for years or even for life. Certain environmental cues can trigger cocaine reminiscing. The reminder may graduate to preoccupation with cocaine or can be converted into physical symptoms. For example, one drug counselor employed by our clinic has abstained from cocaine for over 7 years and still experiences perspiration and numbness of the upper lip when watching a cocaine documentary on television.

Comprehensive cocaine addiction treatment must therefore address both medical and psychological aspects of the disease. Pharmacological interventions may include benzodiazepines (chlordiazepoxide), desipramine, or bromocriptine. The theory is that the dopamine is overcome by the dopamine agonist effect of bromocriptine. The usual doses are listed in Table 2. Beta blockers, such as propranolol, may be effective in neutralizing

Table 2 Bromocriptine Regimen for Cocaine Withdrawal

Day	Bromocriptine dose[a] (mg)	Frequency
1–2	1.25	Twice a day
3–4	1.25	Three times/day
5–6	2.5	Twice a day
7–11	2.5	Three times/day
12–14	5	Twice a day
15–20	b	b

[a]Titration of the dose is necessary with anticraving and antiwithdrawal effects weighted against possible side effects. Lower doses than those listed above are often sufficient. Maintenance bromocriptine may be necessary if symptoms recur after discontinuation.
[b]Decrease by approximately 50% every 2 days.

the peripheral effects of the catecholamine by blocking the sympathetic effects at the target organs.

The tricyclic antidepressants, bromocriptine, and propranolol alone will not significantly promote abstinence from cocaine. These agents may help reduce the relapse to cocaine in the ensuing weeks only if combined with other group and individual therapies, and self-help groups such as Alcoholics Anonymous, Narcotics Anonymous, and Cocaine Anonymous. Effective inpatient and outpatient treatment exists. Abstinence-based programs for other drugs, such as alcohol, also work for the cocaine addict. The long-term management rests with the group and individual therapies and the self-help groups.

Effective treatment is available for cocaine addiction. The morbidity and mortality can be significantly reduced by prevention. Prevention is initiated by education and a willingness to eliminate cocaine as an alternative. An awareness of the catastrophic power of cocaine hopefully will lead to its return to a chapter in history in which it will only be remembered. Treatment will be discussed elsewhere in this volume.

VIII. GENETICS OF COCAINE ADDICTION

The genetic predisposition to alcoholism may extend to cocaine addiction. When the same 263 patients were studied by the family history and study methods, approximately 50% of the cocaine addicts had at least a first- or second-degree relative with a diagnosis of alcohol dependence [27]. These findings of a positive family history of alcoholism in cocaine addicts, combined with the high prevalence of cocaine and other drug use among alcoholics under the age of 30, suggest a common vulnerability to cocaine addiction and alcoholism. More studies are needed to confirm this hypothesis of a universal vulnerability to cocaine and alcohol addictions [30,31].

IX. MEDICAL CONSEQUENCES

It is clear that cocaine is not and never was a benign drug. There is no amount of cocaine and no route of use that is medically safe. The most serious side effect is death. Death has been reported after oral, intranasal, free-base, and intravenous use. Death by cocaine may be ushered in by symptoms of confusion or convulsions. Often no warning signs appear. The victim collapses suddenly and dies. Death usually occurs because of status epilepticus, stroke, myocardial infarctions, respiratory paralysis, arrhythmia, and hyperthermia. The latter can be striking because of cocaine's direct effect on the temperature-regulating centers and peripheral vasoconstriction. Hyperthermia can lead to seizures and possibly cardiac arrhythmias. Cocaine is arrhythmogenic and has been associated with sinus tachycardia, ventricular premature contractions, ventricular tachycardia, and fibrillation. The arrhythmias presumably occur because of relative hypoxia and elevated catecholamine levels associated with cocaine intoxication. Cerebrovascular accidents have also been reported with cocaine abuse. Fatalities also result from crimes committed by cocaine addicts. Dangerous situations often arise during drug transactions, which include assault and murder. Also, judgment and timing are impaired by cocaine, which contribute to job-related injuries and motor vehicle accidents. A common cause of death involves the use of cocaine by alcohol-intoxicated individuals prior to operating a motor vehicle. The short-lived cocaine-induced alert mental status is rapidly replaced by the somnolence of alcohol intoxication while driving.

A commonly held myth among cocaine addicts is that only people with preexisting medical disorders experience fatalities from cocaine. The fact is that cocaine does not discriminate. Rather, cocaine abusers with preexisting medical disorders substantially increase their risk of worsening medical complications further. An individual with a preexisting seizure disorder is more likely to precipitate a cocaine-induced seizure. But most people who report a history of cocaine-induced seizures have no prior seizure history. In fact, repeated doses of cocaine may have a cumulative or kindling effect. That is, repeated small doses produce the same symptoms that one large dose may have produced previously, leading to seizures or other neurological problems [32]. Likewise, individuals with coronary artery disease or arrhythmias increase their risk of developing fatal cardiac complications. Arteriovenous malformations and aneurysms can rupture and result in stroke because of cocaine-induced hypertension.

A common medical complication of cocaine addiction is dental problems. This is due in part to decreased salivary secretion in the oral cavity plus the anesthetic effect and pain-relieving effect of cocaine. Dentists are in the position of not only recognizing cocaine abuse, but also nicotine addiction and bulimia. As with bulimia, generalized malnutrition and vitamin B_b, vitamin C, and thiamine deficiencies are common with chronic cocaine abuse. Decreased sexual interest and sexual dysfunction are common in cocaine addiction [33]. Other complications include nasal septum necrosis and perforation, loss of smell, sinusitis, aspiration pneumonia, reduced carbon monoxide diffusing capacity in the lungs, abnormal blood glucose levels, and a diminished immune response.

Cocaine causes vasoconstriction in the placenta, which may result in decreased blood flow to the fetus and uterine contraction. The rate of spontaneous abortion among cocaine addicts is higher than that among women who use heroin [34]. In addition to abruptio placentae, cocaine has been associated with stillbirths and skull and heart defects in the fetus. Infants exposed to cocaine are at a higher risk of developing congenital malformations, perinatal mortality, neurobehavioral impairments, learning disabilities, and sudden infant death syndrome.

X. PSYCHIATRIC COMPLICATIONS

Acute cocaine intoxication can produce euphoria, impulsivity, sexual preoccupation, rapid thoughts, impaired judgment, grandiosity, increased psychomotor activity, decreased inhibition, depression, and hypervigilant and compulsive repetitive behavior. These signs and symptoms may be confused with mania or a manic episode and depression as in affective disorders. Such effects in over 80% of cocaine users [35]. The central nervous system stimulation and euphoria become a prominent desirable memory and force behind continued cocaine use. The brief pleasurable experience which last only minutes is followed by uncomfortable symptoms characterized by dysphoria. The crash is ushered in by severe depression, agitation, and anxiety [25]. In addition to cocaine craving, craving for sleep ensues. The desire to sleep and reverse the negative side effects of crashing often leads to additional substance abuse with sedatives such as alcohol, marijuana, or benzodiazepines. Cocaine withdrawal symptoms mimicking dysthymic disorder or major depression [13] often persists for days, weeks, and sometimes months. Despite uncomfortable withdrawal symptoms, thoughts about the pleasures of cocaine can persist for months. The extent of cocaine addiction and the method of administration used often allows the clinician to predict the severity of withdrawal symptoms and the length of time they may persist. Ths information is important when differentiating drug-induced symptoms from those resulting from underlying mental disorders.

Symptoms of paranoia and paranoid psychosis regularly result from cocaine abuse and may be confused with schizophrenia. The rapid cocaine-induced fluctuation of symptoms from elation to depression can be indistinguishable from bipolar disorder [36]. The fatigue, low self-esteem, decreased interest in pleasurable activities, poor concentration, low energy level, and social isolation that constitute cocaine withdrawal is often difficult to differentiate from dysthymic disorder or major depression. Cocaine-induced states of severe panic attacks with doom and a belief in impending death are common among cocaine users [37]. Cocaine abuse has been misdiagnosed as attention deficit disorder [38], and often leads to a variety of sexual dysfunctions [39]. These are some of the more common mental disorders which are confused with cocaine addiction. Cocaine-induced or exacerbated mental illness also contributes to crimes. Cocaine addiction has also been linked to armed robbery, domestic violence (spouse and child), rape, and murder [40]. Because cocaine abuse can mimic or coexist with any mental problem, psychiatric diagnoses should not be generated before a drug-free evaluation period [41]. A minimum of biweekly supervised random comprehensive urine drug screens is essential when a drug-free evaluation period is attempted on an outpatient basis. Atypical mood should alert the primary care physician to cocaine as a possible cause in all but the very young and the very old.

The cocaine epidemic has drawn considerable attention to the field of drug and alcohol addiction. It seems as though a day does not pass without at least one citation of cocaine on television, in a newspaper, or in a medical journal. Reminders of the drug are found on many street corners and even in the names of beverages we drink. There is much fuss in the wake of cocaine's devastation. Even though other drugs have been and continue to be just as devastating, cocaine demands the most attention because of the speed with which it progresses. The road to alcohol addiction can be traveled for a half century before it is recognized. Individuals addicted to opiates can continue their lives relatively intact for decades before they or anyone else notices the addiction. Often it takes a diangosis of AIDS or endocarditis for an opiate addict to consider entering treatment. In fact, we have admitted numerous opiate addicts with over 10 years of daily opiate use who were brought to treatment following a mere 6-month involvement with cocaine. Most cocaine addicts advance from casual use to dependent status in less than 5 years. Some addicts go from neophyte status to addict in less than 6 months. Cocaine has surpassed other drugs by reducing the usual 40-year evolution span of addiction down to a few years. When used as an example and placed in the context of other drug addictions, cocaine addiction strongly facilitates the understanding of drug and alcohol addiction. The cocaine epidemic has also motivated much new research which has furnished many missing pieces to the incomplete puzzle of drug and alcohol addiction.

REFERENCES

1. Gold, M.S. (1984). *800-COCAINE*, Bantam Books, New York, p. 27.
2. Cocores, J.A., and Gold, M.S. (1989). Recognition and crisis intervention treatment with cocaine

abusers, *Crisis Intervention Handbook* (A.R. Roberts, ed.), Wadsworth, Pacific Grove, California, p. 216.

3. Cocores, J.A. (1989). Volatile Substance Abuse, *Drugs of Abuse* (A.J. Giannini and A.E. Slaby, eds.), Medical Economics, Oradel, New Jersey, p. 265.

4. Cocores, J.A. (1990). *800-COCAINE Guide to Alcohol and Drug Recovery*, Villard Books, New York, p. 218.

5. Cocores, J.A. (1987). Co-addiction: A silent epidemic, *Fair Oaks Psychiatry Lett.*, *5*:5.

6. Lee, D. (1981). *Cocaine Handbook: An Essential Reference*, And/Or Press, Berkeley, Califoria, p. 85.

7. Gawin, F.H., and Ellinwood, E.H. (1988). Cocaine and other stimulants, *N. Engl. J. Med.*, *318*:1173.

8. Strategy Council on Drug Abuse. (1973). *Federal Strategy for Drug Abuse and Traffic Prevention*, Government Printing Office, Washington, D.C.

9. National Commission on Marijuana and Drug Abuse (1973). *Drug Use in America, Problem in Perspective: Second Report of the National Commission on Marijuana and Drug Abuse*, National Institute on Drug Abuse, Washington, D.C., March.

10. Grinspoon, L., and Bakalar, B.J. (1980). Drug dependence: Non narcotic agents, *Comprehensive Textbook of Psychiatry* (H.I. Kaplan, A.M. Freedman, and B.J. Sadock, eds.), 3rd ed., Williams & Wilkins, Baltimore, p. 889.

11. National Institute on Drug Abuse, Division of Epidemiological and Statistical Publication. Cocaine Client Admissions (1987). DHHS publication no. (ADM), p. 87.

12. Adams, E.H. Gfroerer, J.C., and Rouse, B.A. (1986). Trends in prevalence and consequences of cocaine use, *Adv. Alcohol Subst. Abuse*, *6*:49.

13. American Psychiatric Association (1987). *Diagnostic and Statistical Manual of Mental Disorders*, 3rd ed., revised, Washington, D.C.

14. Gawin, F.W., and Kleber, H.D. (1985). Cocaine use in a treatment population: Patterns and diagnostic distinctions, *NIDA Res. Monogr. Ser.*, *61*:182.

15. Cocores, J.A., Sinaikin, P., and Gold, M.S. (1989). Scopolamine as treatment for nicotine polacrilex dependence, *Ann. Clin. Psychiatry*, *1*:51.

16. Weiss, R.D., Goldenheim, P.D., and Mirin, S.M. (1981). Pulmonary dysfunction in cocaine smokers, *Am. J. Psychiatry*, *138*:1110.

17. Gold, M.S., and Estroff, T.W. (1985). The comprehensive evaluation of cocaine and opiate abusers, *Handbook of Psychiatric Diagnostic Procedures* (R.C.W. Hall and T. Beresford eds.), Spectrum, New York, p. 213.

18. Estroff, T.W., and Gold, M.S. (1986). Medical and psychiatric complications of cocaine abuse with possible points of pharmacological treatment, *Controversies in Alcoholism and Substance Abuse*, Haworth, New York, p. 61.

19. Verebey, K., and Gold, M.S. (1988). From cocaine leaves to crack: The effects of dose and routes of administration in abuse liability, *Psychiatr. Ann.*, *18*(9):513–520.

20. Khantzian, E.J. (1985). The self-medication hypothesis of addictive disorders: Focus on heroin and cocaine dependence, *Am. J. Psychiatry*, *142*:1259.

21. Miller, N.S., and Gold, M.S. (1988). The human sexual response and alcohol and drugs, *J. Subst. Abuse Treat.*, *5*:171–177.

22. Miller, N.S., Dackis, C.A., and Gold, M.S. (1987). The relationship of addiction, tolerance and dependence to alcohol and drugs: A neurochemical approach, *J. Subst. Abuse Treat.*, *4*: 197–207.

23. Wise, R.A. (1984). Neural mechanisms of the reinforcing actions of cocaine, *NIDA Res. Monogr. Ser.*, *50*:15.

24. Dackis, C.A., and Gold, M.S. (1985). New concepts in cocaine addiction: The dopamine depeletion hypothesis. *Neurosci. Biobehav. Rev.*, *9*:469.

25. Gawin, F.H., and Kleber, H.D. (1986). Abstinence symptomatology and psychiatric diagnosis in cocaine abusers, *Arch. Gen. Psychiatry*, *43*:107.

26. Miller, N.S. (1987). A primer of the treatment process for alcoholism and drug addiction, *Psychiatry Lett*, *5*(7):30–37.

27. Miller, N.S., Gold, M.S., Belkin, B.M., et al. (in press). Family history and diagnosis of alcohol dependence in cocaine dependence. *Subst. Abuse.*

28. Risch, S.C., Janowsky, D.S., and Siever, L.J. (1982). Cholinomimetic induced co-release of prolactin and beta-endorphin in man, *Psychopharmacol. Bull., 18*:26.

29. Janowsky, D.S., and Risch, S.C. (1984). Cholinomimetic and anticholinergic drugs used to investigate an acetylcholine hypothesis of affective disorders and stress, *Drug Dev. Res. 4*:125.

30. Galizio, M. (1985). *Determinants of Substance Abuse*, Plenum Press, New York.

31. Goodwin, D.W. (1983). Familial alcoholism: A separate entity, *Subst. Alcohol Actions/Misuse, 4*:129-136.

32. Post, R.M., and Kopanda, R.T. (1976). Cocaine, kindling and psychosis, *Am. J. Psychiatry, 133*:627.

33. Cocores, J.A., Dackis, C.A., and Gold, M.S. (1986). Sexual dysfunction secondary to cocaine abuse in two patients, *J. Clin. Psychiatry, 47*:384.

34. Chasnoff, I.J., Burns, W.J., Schnoll, S.H., and Burns, K.A. (1985). Cocaine in pregnancy, *N. Engl. J. Med., 313*:666.

35. Gold, M.S., Washton, A.M., and Dackis, C.A. (1985). Cocaine abuse. Neurochemistry, phenomenology and treatment. *NIDA Res. Monogr. Ser., 61*:130.

36. Cocores, J.A., Patel, M.D., Gold, M.S., Pottash, A.C. (1987). Cocaine abuse, attention deficit disorder, and bipolar disorder, *J. Nerv. Ment. Dis., 175*:431.

37. Jeri, F.R., Sanchez, C.C., Del Pozo, T. (1980). Further experience with the syndromes produced by coca paste smoking, *Cocaine 1980* (F.R. Jeri, ed.), Pacific Press, Lima, Peru, p. 9.

38. Cocores, J.A., Davies, R.K., Mueller, P.S., and Gold, M.S. (1987). Cocaine abuse and adult attention deficit disorder, *J. Clin. Psychiatry, 48*:376.

39. Cocores, J.A., Miller, N.S., Gold, M.S., and Pottash, A.C. (1988). Sexual dysfunction in abusers of alcohol and cocaine, *Am. J. Drug Alcohol Abuse, 14*:169.

40. Miller, N.S., Gold, M.S., and Herridge, P. (1989). *Violent Behavior and Cocaine*, Society for Neuroscience, 19th Annual Meeting, Phoenix, Arizona.

41. Cocores, J.A. (1990). Treatment of the dually diagnosed adult drug user, *Dual Diagnosis Patients* (A.E. Slaby and M.S. Gold, eds.), Marcel Dekker, New York, p. 344.

20

Marijuana

Mark S. Gold

Fair Oaks Hospital, Summit, New Jersey, and Delray Beach, Florida

I. INTRODUCTION

The risks and consequences of marijuana* use have been intensively debated in the United States for more than 50 years. Unfortunately, the discussion has often relied more on rhetoric and hysteria than on objective scientific evidence. More than simply a medical issue, the controversy over marijuana has been defined in terms of beliefs, values, and political persuasion.

However valid these various perspectives may be, they have created a troubling climate for physicians. In an effort to lend scientific support for their positions, proponents and opponents alike have selectively cited or dismissed the scientific research that has been conducted, and have drawn conclusions that go far beyond the limits justified by the underlying evidence. Anecdotal evidence has been presented as conclusive and poorly controlled or even discredited studies continue to be referenced. Perhaps most disturbing is the practice of citing the *lack* of evidence as evidence itself—that is, of citing inconclusive studies as evidence of marijuana's safety.

Although much of this confusion has been generated by advocates who lack rigorous scientific training, it has muddied the waters for physicians who require a clear and objective understanding of the risks of marijuana abuse. In addition, it has clouded the physician's role. The physician's concern with marijuana use is very straightforward: Does it cause health problems? If so, how can these problems be prevented or treated?

The answer to the first is an unequivocal yes. Marijuana use has been shown to cause a variety of physical and psychological problems. Although some of these disorders are still

This chapter was adapted from *Marijuana* by Mark S. Gold copyright 1989, Plenum Publishing Corporation, reprinted with permission.
*Except where specifically noted, the term *marijuana* in this chapter refers to marijuana and its derivatives, including haskish, haskish oil, and delta-9-tetrahydrocannabinol (delta-9-THC).

the subject of scientific debate, many of them are well established. Moreover, they are progressive rather than self-limiting, and are responsive to medical treatment. Thus, the justification for medical intervention is clear.

II. AN OVERVIEW OF CANNABINOIDS*

Cannabis sativa is an annual plant that grows both wild and under cultivation throughout the tropical and temperate zones. It may grow as high as 20 feet. (Formerly the Indian variety of marijuana was classified as a separate species, *C. indica*, but it has since been reclassified as a subspecies of *C. sativa*.]

Closely related to the hops plant (although very different in appearance), cannabis is dioecious; that is, it grows as separate male and female plants. The male plant is taller and usually dies after the flowering cycle. The female, by contrast, is smaller and bushier. It secretes a resin that covers the flowering tops and nearby leaves. The resin is more abundant when the plant is grown in tropical areas, leading to speculation that its function is to retard moisture loss.

Traditionally, the flowering tops and adjacent leaves of the female have been cultivated for their psychoactive properties. Hashish consists primarily of the resin. It was long believed that male plants were not psychoactive; however, recent studies reveal that the males and females have similar potencies [2].

The most common psychoactive compound in marijuana is delta-9-tetrahydrocannabinol (delta-9-THC), but the plant contains more than 60 related compounds known as cannabinoids [1,3]. Most of them have no known psychoactive properties and unknown physiological effects. Marijuana's psychoactive effects are predominantly caused by delta-9-THC.

The potency of marijuana varies greatly. When marijuana is grown by traditional methods, the highest concentration of cannabinoids is found in the flowers of the female plant. However, *C. sinsemilla*, a seedless variety, has been widely cultivated by domestic growers in recent years, and concentrations of THC are much higher throughout the plant.

This increased potency has drastically changed the picture of marijuana use. For example, a typical marijuana cigarette in the early 1970s might contain 1% THC by weight and perhaps 10 mg of THC [4]. Today a high-quality marijuana cigarette might contain as much as 150 mg of THC—or twice as much if it is laced with hashish oil [4]. Thus, the user today can easily be exposed to doses as high as 300 mg from a single joint. Studies have shown that a daily dose of 180 mg of THC a day for 11–21 days produces a defined withdrawal syndrome [5].

III. FORMS AND TYPES OF MARIJUANA

Marijuana and its derivatives are used in a variety of forms (Table 1), and go by a variety of names throughout the world, including "pot," "grass," "herb," "tea," "reefer," "Mary Jane," "ganja," "bhang," "charas," "kif," and "dagga." Marijuana is most often dried and smoked. It may be rolled into a cigarette (known as a "joint," "reefer," or, less commonly, "spliff"), or smoked in a pipe. Water pipes (sometimes called "bongs" or "hookahs") are often used to humidify the smoke and permit deeper inhalation.

---

*Two different numbering schemes exist for cannabinoids. The more common dibenzopyran system is used here. In addition, it must be kept in mind that a number of cannabinoid isomers exist. The (−)-*tarns* isomer of delta-8-THC and delta-9-THC, which are the most pharmacologically active as well as the ones that occur naturally in the marijuana plant, are the ones referred to in this discussion.

Table 1 Forms and Types of Marijuana

Marijuana
  Prepared from dried leaves and flowers of the *Cannabis sativa* plant. Potency: 1% THC and up
  (early 1970s); 6–14% THC (current strains of domestic sinsemilla)
Hashish
  Prepared by collecting the resin secretedby cannabis leaves or by boiling the plant. It is pressed
  into bricks or cakes. Potency: 10–20% THC.
Hashish oil
  Prepared by distilling the plant in organic solvents. Potency: 15–30% THC.

Sources: Nahas, G.G. *Marijuana in Science and Medicine.* Raven, New York, 1984. Cohen, S. Marijuana, in *American Psychiatric Association: Annual Review.* Washington, D.C., American Psychiatric Press, Vol. 5, 1986. Mann, P. *Marijuana Alert.* McGraw-Hill, New York, 1985. Gold, MS. *The Facts About Drugs and Alcohol.* Bantam, New York, 1986.

Marijuana may be refined into hashish or the more potent hashish oil, which is then smoked. Any of these substances may also be ingested orally—typically baked into brownies or cookies—causing less potent but more long-lasting effects. THC is very insoluble in water, making it difficult to prepare injectable solutions. Indeed, virtually the only known cases of intravenous administration of cannabinoids occur in research studies; the practice is virtually unknown among regular users.

IV. THE HISTORY OF MARIJUANA USE

Cannabis sativa grows wild throughout most of the tropical parts of the world. Historically its seeds have been used for animal feed, its fiber for hemp rope, and its oil as a vehicle for paint. But its widest use throughout history has been for its intoxicating properties.

With alcohol and opium, marijuana is one of the oldest known intoxicants. The reason is simplicity itself: It requires only minimal cultivation and preparation before use.

The oldest known written record of marijuana (The term *marijuana* (i.e., "Mary Jane") apparently comes from Mexico, where it was originally a slang term for cheap tobacco [6].) use comes from the records of the Chinese Emperor Shen Nung in 2727 B.C. [7]. It is believed to have first been cultivated in Asia and was used in India as early as 2000 B.C. in religious ceremonies [8,9]. Written evidence of its use in the Middle East dates from about 500 A.D., though some have suggested that it is referred to in the Old Testament [10,11]. The ancient Greeks and Romans were familiar with cannabis; the Greek physicians Dioscordes and Galen mention it in connection with the treatment of otitis media, and Herodotus describes its being thrown upon hot stones to release its vapor [12,13].

From the Middle East, the use of cannabis spread throughout the Islamic Empire throughout North Africa. Its use was not without its detractors. The Emir Soudouni Schekhounia of Arabia outlawed it in 1378, and the Arab historian Al Magrii blamed the decline of Egyptian society on it [14,15].

Cannabis spread to the western hemisphere in 1545, when Spaniards imported it to Chile for the use of its fiber [16]. It may have come by way of African slaves even earlier [16]. By the eighteenth century it was known in Europe. Carolus Linnaeus assigned it the name *Cannabis sativa* in 1735 [17].

Hemp was grown in the American settlements of Jamestown, Virginia, in 1611 and in New England by 1629. Though it was primarily grown during the colonial period for the manufacture of rope, there is evidence that its psychoactive properties were known to the colonists. George Washington, for example, is known to have grown hemp at Mount Vernon, and careful study of his diaries have led some to conclude that he separated the potent female plants for his personal "medicinal" use.

Though the drug had been touted as a natural herbal cure and used by physicians in India, England, and Egypt, it was not used widely in the United States until the 1840s, when it became popularized within and outside of medical circles by the writings of Dr. W.B. Oshavghwessy, Jacques Joseph Moreau, and Fitz Hugh Ludlow [8,18]. From 1850 to 1942, cannabis was listed in the *U.S. Pharmacopeia*, and pharmaceutical firms such as Parke-Davis, Lilly, Squibb, and Burroughs-Wellcome marketed preparations containing cannabis [7]. "Hashish houses" emerged in large American cities during the last half of the nineteenth century, but use of the drug was limited to a small, fashionable group [7]. Marijuana use proliferated in the United States during the 1920s, perhaps partially as a result of soldiers' exposure to it in Central America and the Caribbean or due to Prohibition.

In 1937, marijuana was effectively outlawed by the federal Marijuana Tax Act. Its passage was due in large part of a campaign of hysteria and misinformation orchestrated by Harry J. Anslinger, the Commissioner of the Federal Bureau of Narcotics. Anslinger's portrayal of marijuana as a drug that immediately and irrevocably led to homicidal insanity did much to set the tone for very harsh criminal sanctions against the drug, including, in Georgia, the penalties of life imprisonment or death for selling marijuana to a minor [7].

Marijuana use became widely popular within the youthful counterculture in the 1960s. Its use increased steadily through the 1960s and 1970s, peaking in 1979. Since then its use has declined dramatically.

V. CURRENT-USE PATTERNS

When the use of marijuana first became widespread, most of the supplies came from foreign sources. Marijuana came primarily from South and Central America (bearing such names as Colombian Gold, Panama Red, and Acapulco Gold), or from the Orient (e.g., Thai sticks). Hashish and hash oil usually came from the Middle East or Mediterranean, often by way of Europe. Most of it entered the country through Florida and California, as well as major ports such as New York.

Although these foreign sources still exist, the marijuana scene has changed drastically in the past decade as a result of illicit domestic production. Faced with the need to grow marijuana clandestinely in relatively small areas, domestic producers have used sophisticated breeding and cultivation techniques to vastly increase the potency of their crop, and thus its market value. Indeed, marijuana is available on the street today that is hundreds of times more potent than the typical street pot of the late 1960s and early 1970s. This single fact has made obsolete much of what we once knew about the risks and consequences of marijuana use.

A. Who Uses Marijuana?

Two national surveys provide the best evidence available about who uses marijuana. The first, the National Household Survey, has been conducted regularly since 1971. It is based on a random sample of persons 12 years of age and older living in households in the coterminous United States. The Second, *Student Drug Use in America*, has sampled high school students since 1975; survey respondents include each year's high school students as well as a portion of the previous year's respondents. The surveys do not include certain groups: The first fails to reach those who do not have regular addresses or who live in institutional settings, such as military barracks or student dormitories; the second omits those who do not reach their sensor year in high school. In light of evidence that both of these groups may be more likely to use marijuana, these studies probably understate marijuana use to some extent. Also, of course, they rely on self-reporting of illicit behavior, further suggesting that they understate actual use.

Even so, the results of these studies are illuminating (Table 2). Petersen [19] summarizes them as follows:

1. Both marijuana experimentation and current use (within the month preceding the survey) have increased markedly since the 1960s. Between 1971 and 1982 (the latest year for which data was complete at the time of Petersen's report), the percentage of youth (ages 12–17) who had ever used (marijuana) nearly doubled—from 14% to 27.3%. Among those aged 18 to 25, an increase of over 50% occurred in the same period—from 39.3 to 64.3%. The percentage of those currently using (i.e., those reporting use in the 30 days prior to the survey) is roughly half that of those who have ever used. This has been a consistent pattern over time for young adults and adolescents.
2. Among high school seniors, nearly half (47.3%) of the class of 1975 had experimented with marijuana, compared with about 60% of the classes of 1978 to 1982 and 50% in the class of 1987. As with other adolescent and young adult groups, the percentage of current users is approximately half that of those who have ever tried the drug.
3. Daily use has not been surveyed in the National Household Survey, but among high school seniors, it rose from 6 to nearly 11% between 1975 and 1978 and has since fallen to 3.3% in the class of 1987.

Petersen [19] noted other significant findings from the National Household Survey and other studies. Briefly, these studies showed that:

1. The lower the age of initial use of alcohol and cigarettes, the more likely the individual is to use marijuana.
2. The age of first use of marijuana has decreased steadily.
3. Daily use of marijuana (i.e., 20 or more days per month) is positively correlated with absenteeism and poor academic performance and negatively correlated with religious involvement and plans to attend college.
4. Daily use is more common among seniors who are socially active and who spend little time at home.
5. Use of other drugs is much more common among seniors who use marijuana on a daily basis than among less frequent users, nearly half of daily marijuana users currently use amphetamines and almost a third of them use cocaine.

The National Household Surveys show that marijuana is the most popular illicit drug used in the United States [20]. A recent national survey indicated that some 15 million Americans smoke marijuana at least monthly; 9 million smoke it at least once a week; and 6 million smoke it daily [21]. In 1987, one high school senior in 25 smoked marijuana every day; nearly one in four are current users [22,23]. Half of high school seniors report that they have tried the drug (Table 2). More than half of all marijuana users report that they first tried the drug between the sixth and ninth grades [24]. Males are more likely to be users than females [19].

Marijuana is often used in conjunction with other drugs. The 1984 senior survey showed that 5% of daily marijuana users also reported daily alcohol use; 7% reported current (i.e., in the preceding 30 days) use of amphetamine or cocaine, and 2% current use of other illicit drugs [25]. Recent reports indicate a new form of marijuana known as AMP that is soaked in formaldehyde [26]. Other adulterants that have been reported include insect spray, LSD, amphetamines, strychnine, stramonium leaves, rat poison, and catnip [27,28]. The herbicide

Table 2 High School Senior Drug Use: 1975–1986

| | Class of | | | | | | | | | | | |
	'75	'76	'77	'78	'79	'80	'81	'82	'83	'84	'85	'86
	Ever used (%)											
Marijuana/hashish	47	53	56	59	60	60	60	59	75	55	54	51
Inhalants[a]	NA	NA	NA	NA	18	17	17	18	18	18	18	20
amyl and butyl nitrites	NA	NA	NA	NA	11	11	10	10	8	8	8	9
Hallucinogens[b]	NA	NA	NA	NA	18	16	15	14	14	12	12	12
LSD	11	11	10	10	10	9	10	10	9	8	8	7
PCP	NA	NA	NA	NA	13	10	8	6	6	6	5	5
Cocaine	9	10	11	13	15	16	17	16	16	16	17	17
Heroin	2	2	2	2	1	1	1	1	1	1	1	1
Other opiates	9	10	10	10	10	10	10	10	9	10	10	9
Stimulants[c]	NA	NA	NA	NA	NA	NA	NA	28	27	26	26	23
Sedatives	18	18	17	16	15	15	16	15	14	13	12	10
barbiturates	17	16	16	14	12	11	11	10	10	10	9	8
methaqualone	8	8	9	8	8	10	11	11	10	8	7	5
Tranquilizers	17	17	18	17	16	15	15	14	13	12	12	11
Alcohol	90	92	93	93	93	93	93	93	93	93	92	91
Cigarettes	74	75	76	75	74	71	71	70	71	70	69	68

Marijuana
359

Used in last year (%)

	40	45	48	50	51	49	46	44	42	40	41	39
Marijuana/hashish	40	45	48	50	51	49	46	44	42	40	41	39
Inhalants[a]	NA	NA	NA	NA	9	8	6	7	6	7	8	9
amyl and butyl nitrites	NA	NA	NA	NA	7	6	4	4	4	4	4	5
Hallucinogens[b]	NA	NA	NA	NA	12	11	10	9	8	7	8	8
LSD	7	6	6	6	7	7	7	6	5	5	4	5
PCP	NA	NA	NA	NA	7	4	3	2	3	2	3	2
Cocaine	6	6	7	9	12	12	12	12	11	12	13	13
Heroin	1	1	1	1	1	1	1	1	1	1	1	1
Other opiates	6	6	6	6	6	6	6	5	5	5	6	5
Stimulants[c]	NA	NA	NA	NA	NA	NA	NA	20	18	18	16	13
Sedatives	12	11	11	10	10	10	11	9	8	7	6	5
barbiturates	11	10	9	8	8	7	7	6	5	5	5	4
methaqualone	5	5	5	5	6	7	8	7	5	4	3	2
Tranquilizers	11	10	11	10	10	9	8	7	7	6	6	6
Alcohol	85	86	87	88	88	88	87	87	87	86	86	85
Cigarettes	NA	NA	NA	NA	NA	NA	NA	NA	NA	NA	NA	NA

(continued)

Table 2 *Continued*

								Class of					
	'75	'76	'77	'78	'79	'80	'81	'82	'83	'84	'85	'86	
						Used in past month (%)							
Marijuana/hashish	27	32	36	37	37	34	32	29	27	26	26	23
Inhalants[a]	NA	NA	NA	NA	3	3	3	3	3	3	3	3
amyl and butyl nitrites	NA	NA	NA	NA	2	2	1	1	1	1	2	1
Hallucinogens[b]	NA	NA	NA	NA	5	4	5	4	4	3	4	4
LSD	2	2	2	2	2	2	3	2	2	2	2	2
PCP	NA	NA	NA	NA	2	1	1	1	1	1	2	1
Cocaine	2	2	3	4	6	5	6	5	5	6	7	6
Heroin	*	*	*	*	*	*	*	*	*	*	*	*
Other opiates	2	2	3	2	2	2	2	2	2	2	2	2
Stimulants[c]	NA	NA	NA	NA	NA	NA	NA	11	9	8	7	6
Sedatives	5	5	5	4	4	5	5	3	3	2	2	2
barbiturates	5	4	4	3	3	3	3	2	2	2	2	2
methaqualone	2	2	2	2	2	3	3	2	2	1	1	1
Tranquilizers	4	4	5	3	4	3	3	2	3	2	2	2
Alcohol	68	68	71	72	72	72	71	70	69	67	66	65
Cigarettes	37	39	38	37	34	31	29	30	30	29	30	30

Daily users (%)

Marijuana/hashish	6.0	8.0	9.1	10.7	10.3	9.1	7.0	6.3	5.5	5.0	4.9	4.0
Inhalants[a]	NA	NA	NA	NA	0.1	0.2	0.2	0.2	0.2	0.2	0.4	0.4
amyl and butyl nitrites	NA	NA	NA	NA	0.0	0.1	0.1	0.0	0.2	0.1	0.3	0.5
Hallucinogens[b]	NA	NA	NA	NA	0.2	0.2	0.1	0.2	0.2	0.2	0.3	0.3
LSD	0.0	0.0	0.0	0.0	0.0	0.0	0.1	0.0	0.1	0.1	0.1	0.0
PCP	NA	NA	NA	NA	0.1	0.1	0.1	0.1	0.1	0.1	0.3	0.2
Cocaine	0.1	0.1	0.1	0.1	0.2	0.2	0.3	0.2	0.2	0.2	0.4	0.4
Heroin	0.1	0.0	0.0	0.0	0.0	0.0	0.0	0.0	0.1	0.0	0.0	0.0
Other opiates[c]	0.1	0.1	0.2	0.1	0.0	0.1	0.1	0.1	0.1	0.1	0.1	0.1
Stimulants[c]	NA	NA	NA	NA	NA	NA	NA	0.7	0.8	0.6	0.4	0.3
Sedatives	0.3	0.2	0.2	0.2	0.1	0.2	0.2	0.2	0.2	0.1	0.1	0.1
barbiturates	0.1	0.1	0.2	0.1	0.0	0.1	0.1	0.1	0.1	0.0	0.1	0.1
methaqualone	0.0	0.0	0.0	0.0	0.0	0.1	0.1	0.1	0.0	0.0	0.0	0.0
Tranquilizers	0.1	0.2	0.3	0.1	0.1	0.1	0.1	0.1	0.1	0.1	0.0	0.0
Alcohol	5.7	5.6	6.1	5.7	6.9	6.0	6.0	5.7	5.5	4.8	5.0	4.8
Cigarettes	26.9	28.8	28.8	27.5	25.4	21.3	20.3	21.1	21.2	18.7	19.5	18.7

[a]Inhalants—adjusted for underreporting of amyl and butyl nitrites.
[b]Hallucinogens—adjusted for underreporting of PCP.
[c]Stimulants—adjusted for overreporting of nonprescription stimulants.
NA indicates data not available
*Indicates less than 0.5%

Terms

Ever used: Used at least one time.
Used in last year: Used at least once in the 12 months prior to survey.
Used in past month: Used at least once in the 30 days prior to survey.
Daily users: Used 20 or more times in the month before survey.
Source: National Institute on Drug Abuse, Monitoring the Future Study, 1986

paraquat has been found on marijuana samples in the past as a result of government eradication programs in Mexico, but the practice has been discontinued. Adulterants may cause acute psychosis and physical toxicity.

Marijuana use is not only widespread but evenly distributed. In the early 1960s, its use was largely confined to urban coastal areas, but currently its use is fairly uniform across regions and in both urban and rural communities.

Surveys show that marijuana use by high school seniors increased steadily from the late 1960s to 1979, at which time it began to drop [29]. Many rationales have been offered to explain the recent decline, including the development of effective prevention and educational programs and a generalized swing to more conservative values among students.

Although the figures showing a decline in use are encouraging, two new trends are not so reassuring. First, the initiation into marijuana use is beginning at earlier and earlier ages. The second trend is the vastly increased potency mentioned previously. Little is known about the developmental effects of marijuana when its use begins in childhood or very early adolescence; in addition, the long-term effects of high-potency strains of marijuana have never been studied because these strains never existed until just a few years ago. Each of these trends alone is alarming enough; together they present some very troubling, and still unanswered, questions.

Indeed, they even cast some doubt on the validity of the trend seen in the survey data referred to above. As pointed out in *Marijuana and Health*, the 1982 Institute of Medicine study, the decline could simply be an artifact, with heavy users of marijuana becoming increasingly underrepresented in the survey sample (i.e., high school seniors) owing to absenteeism and dropouts associated with earlier and more intensive involvement with the drug [29].

B. Affected Ages

The 1985 National Household Survey revealed that 62 million Americans—roughly a third of the population older than 12—have tried marijuana at least once. Among persons aged 18–25, some 5 million (about 60%) have done so [30]. The same source showed that 19.9% of youths (ages 12 to 17), 36.8% of young adults (ages 18 to 25) and 9.5% of older adults (26 years of age and older) used marijuana in the preceding year. Current users (i.e., use within the preceding 30 days) among these same groups were, respectively 12.2, 22, and 6.5%, respectively [21]. With the exception of the aged 26 + group, these figures have shown a considerable decline from their peaks in 1979. For example, current use among these groups in 1979 versus 1985 was 16.7 versus 12.2%; 35 versus 22%; and 6 versus 6.5%, respectively. The figures for lifetime use and use within the preceding 30 days show similar trends.

Use during the 18–25 age span seems to be mostly due to social factors rather than to underlying psychological problems and in many cases, cessation of use occurs spontaneously once the user reaches early adulthood. In fact, those cases where onset of use occurs before age 13 or after age 24 are far more likely to involve psychiatric disorders, and these persons are at very high risk of progressing to addiction [21].

VI. CANNABINOID PHARMACOLOGY

Marijuana is a unique psychoactive agent; its chemistry and pharmacology do not fit well within any other class of mind-altering drugs. In low doses, it has paradoxical effects, acting both as a stimulant and depressant. In higher doses depressant effects predominate [31]. In addition to its action on the central nervous system (CNS), marijuana also affects the immune system, reproductive system, and cardiovascular system [31].

Though marijuana is widely used, its pharmacology is poorly understood. It is often difficult to draw firm conclusions from the research that has been conducted, for a number of reasons. First, marijuana is not a single drug, but a complex mix: More than 60 cannabinoid compounds have been isolated from marijuana smoke. Further, measurements of active levels of cannabinoids in body tissues is difficult because of their high potency; doses as low as 10 μg of delta-9-THC/kg of body weight are sufficient to cause a "high" [32]. In addition, marijuana's effects vary widely across species, and long-term effects are difficult to extrapolate from short-term human studies.

These and other methodological complexities help explain why uncertain and often contradictory results that have been obtained in marijuana research since the 1960s. For example, some researchers have conducted studies using "standard" marijuana cigarettes supplied by the federal government; others have used preparations of marijuana extracts, primarily delta-9-THC. Dosages have varied widely in different studies, as have the mode of ingestion (oral, intravenous, inhalation) and vehicles (ethanol, Tween 80, dimethylsulfoxide [DMSO], and others). In addition, the subjects in these studies are not easily comparable; for obvious reasons, many studies have been conducted in vitro or using animal subjects. Human subjects have at times included nonusers, "moderate" users, and "heavy" users, categories that are often inconsistent from one study to another.

The studies are also complicated by the increasing potency of illicit marijuana over the past two decades. With today's marijuana being, on the average, about five times as powerful as that of the 1960s, the current "moderate" user would be ingesting much larger doses of cannabinoids than the average "heavy" user of, for example, 1977. And, finally virtually all of the experimental studies involving humans have looked at *short-term* effects; practical considerations make long-term or longitudinal studies all but impossible to conduct.

For all these reasons, current research offers only a very sketchy outline of the pharmacology and effects of marijuana. Despite the fact that it is one of the most widely abused psychoactive drugs in the world, we know far less about it than, for example, narcotics (whose effects and chemistry are relatively straightforward), or such synthetic compounds as amphetamines and benzodiazepines, which because of their therapeutic value have been studied under controlled conditions and in well-defined populations. These caveats must be kept in mind when considering the conclusions presented in this chapter.

Of the 60-odd cannabinoids found in marijuana smoke, only 14 have been studied in depth: delta-9-THC—the most common and most psychoactive one; delta-8-THC; cannabidiol (CBD); and cannabionol (CBN). Behavioral studies in animals also show that various constituents found in marijuana have additive or antagonistic effects, a fact that helps explain the varying potencies found in different marijuana preparations, and the often inconsistent results of experimental studies.

Some debate has existed over whether marijuana's main constituent, delta-9-THC, acts directly on the CNS, or whether it first must be metabolized to 11-OH-delta-9-THC, which studies have shown to be more potent than the parent compound. However, recent studies, for example, one in which delta-9-THC was injected into the cerebroventricle of squirrel monkeys, support the idea that delta-9-THC is directly psychoactive, and need not be converted metabolically to produce its effects [33].

VII. PHARMACOKINETICS

A key factor in the pharmacokinetics of cannabinoids, and one that distinguishes them from the majority of drugs, is that they are highly soluble in lipids, although showing only very slight solubility in water. This fact seems to play an important role in the way they are metabolized and in their psychoactive effects, although the mechanism of these actions is far from clear. In addition, cannabinoids' lipid solubility helps explain the extremely long half-life of these compounds, because they are retained by lipids within the body.

A. Route of Administration

Smoking

The most common route of administration of cannabinoids, at least when they are used illicitly, is by smoking. Marijuana smoke contains approximately 0.3 to >3% delta-9-THC (about 10% in hashish) [34]. It also contains numerous other substances, including other cannabinoids (which may exert unknown synergistic or antagonistic effects) as well as tars, carbon monoxide, and most other substances found in tobacco smoke (with the exception of nicotine).

The actual amount of THC ingested by smoking depends on a number of factors: (1) the speed at which it is smoked, (2) puff duration, (3) volume inhaled, and (4) the amount of time the user withholds expiration after inhalation [32,34]. The use of a pipe does significantly increase cannabinoid transfer: About 20% of delta-9-THC present in marijuana is transferred when a mariguana cigarette is smoked in its usual fashion, versus about 45% with a pipe [35,36]. Two factors that users widely believe to affect potency—humidification (by use of a water pipe) and the type of cigarette paper—do not influence the percentage of transfer of delta-9-THC [37].

In addition to active smoking, persons may be passively exposed to marijuana smoke in social situations. Some controversy exists over whether such passive smoking can produce intoxication (a "contact high"). One study found that some subjects showed subjective and physiological effects after passive exposure to extremely heavy exposure (16 marijuana cigarettes). Subjective effects were mild after passive exposure to the smoke of four marijuana cigarettes (and were not significantly different from placebo responses), but were more pronounced after exposure to the smoke of 16 marijuana cigarettes. *Physiological* effects, by contrast, were mild and highly variable; in most cases, the difference in physiological response between marijuana and placebo failed to reach significant levels, even after exposure to the smoke of 16 marijuana cigarettes [38]. Curiously, however, this same exposure resulted in urine cannabinoid levels similar to those seen after active smoking of one marijuana cigarette.

Ingestion

Orally ingested delta-9-THC is converted by intestinal acids into 11-hydroxy-delta-9-THC, a compound with a pharmacological profile virtually identical to delta-9-THC. Ingestion produces effects similar to those seen with smoking; however, they are less intense and of longer duration.

Intravenous Administration

Generally, intravenous administration of cannabinoids has been limited to research studies, because of the limited availability of purified delta-9-THC and the difficulty of preparing intravenous solutions. In general, plasma profiles with intravenous administration are the same as for smoking [39]. However, some difficulties occur because of the insolubility of cannabinoids in water. Various vehicles have been used, such as Tween 80 and ethanol, but their use may affect study results, especially ethanol, whose psychoactive effects are similar in many respects to those of the cannabinoids.

B. Mechanisms of Action

Surprisingly little is known about cannabinoids' mechanism of action. One study raises the possibility that cannabinoids may act on benzodiazepine receptors. In addition, cross tolerance of cannabinoids with ethanol and other depressants raises the possibility that some of their effects are due to general CNS depression. Some researchers have suggested that they act on specific cannabis receptors. No such receptors have been identified, but as alterations to the THC structure erase the psychoactive effects, it seems plausible that a specific receptor is matched to psychoactive THCs [40].

At least some of the differences among psychoactive THCs may be caused by differences in penetration, distribution, or elimination from the CNS [41]. This seems to be the case with delta-9-THC and 11-OH-delta-9-THC [42–44]. Although some drugs have been shown to reverse or block cannabis effects, Martin suggests that these phenomena are more likely due to drug interactions (i.e., indirect action) than to specific antagonism [45].

C. The Compartment Model

The time relationship between cannabinoid administration and serum levels is complex; moreover, subjective psychological effects do not correlate well with serum levels. This fact suggests a complex mechanism of action, possibly involving a one- or two-compartment model. Chiang et al. describe an empirical two-compartment model to describe the lag, and note that 1–4 h after smoking a marijuana cigarette, effects are directly proportional to mean THC levels [46].

VIII. EFFECTS OF CANNABINOIDS

A. Effects of Chronic Use

One of the most unusual findings regarding delta-9-THC is that of Lemberger et al., who concluded that it disappears more quickly from the plasma of chronic users than that of nonusers [47]; however, this finding has been challenged by others [48]. What is clear is that persons with a history of heavy use achieve higher plasma levels of delta-9-THC than naive users who smoke the same amount of marijuana; presumably the difference is due to more efficient smoking techniques [49,50].

B. Behavioral Effects

The reported subjective psychological effects of cannabinoids, which include excitement and dissociation of ideas, enhancement of the senses, distortions of time and space, delusional thinking, impulsiveness, illusions, and hallucinations, are accompanied by objective behavioral changes, including a deterioration of psychomotor performance, diminished attention span and memory, and reduced physical strength [31].

Animal studies of cannabinoids reveal widely varying behavioral effects, but several appear consistently. One is a hyperreflexive response to specific stimuli accompanying the overall sedative effects. This sedative-hyperreflexive effect results in unusual behavioral responses. For example, groups of white mice exhibit a so-called "popcorn" response: when one mouse lands on another mouse, it in turn jumps, causing a chain reaction that eventually subsides as all the mice become sedated once again [51].

This sedative-hyperreflexive combination is unique among CNS depressants. Although some other depressants and stimulants may show paradoxical effects under certain circumstances, none of them do so with the consistency of cannabinoids, and only the cannabinoids cause hyperreflexia throughout the period of CNS depression [51].

Animals receiving delta-9-THC sleep a great deal in the 24 h following administration [52], when aroused, they exhibit hyperreflexive behavior. These and other effects show that cannabinoids have a very long duration of action—24 h or more, and an even longer half-life (see Sect. VIII.C).

C. Effects on Motor Skills

Marijuana clearly causes a deterioration of motor skills. For example, 94% of those whose plasma concentrations of delta-9-THC exceeded 25–30 ng/ml failed a standard roadside sobriety test administered 90 min after smoking despite the fact that by plasma levels of THC had dropped drastically by the time the test was administered. Some 60% of them failed the test 150 min after smoking [53].

The effects on motor skills has particular relevance to the role of marijuana in traffic accidents and other types of accidents. Although epidemiological studies are hampered by methodological difficulties, in particular, the poor correlation between blood levels of cannabinoids and their effects, experimental studies show that marijuana impairs many of the fundamental skills needed for safe driving, including coordination, tracking, perception, and vigilance. Similarly, performance in driving simulators and on the road is demonstrably poorer after marijuana use [54]. Studies further demonstrate that the importance of marijuana and alcohol on driving skills are addictive [54].

These results are generally consistent with findings that the marijuana "high" persists long after plasma THC levels have dropped. Thus, unlike alcohol, delta-9-THC plasma levels alone are a poor indicator of marijuana-related motor skill impairment. In general, motor skills are impaired for hours or even days after use.

One study of pilots who were exposed to marijuana found significant impairment in flying skills as long as 24 h after impairment. Especially disturbing is the fact that the pilots themselves were unaware of their impairment [55].

These effects on motor skills have significant implications regarding the consequences of marijuana use. Especially the fact that these effects persist for relatively long periods of time after use, and that this carry-over effect is not perceived by the user nor accurately reflected in blood-THC levels, suggests that the role of marijuana in traffic accidents and other types of accidents is vastly underestimated. Indeed, marijuana arguably poses a greater risk to drivers even than alcohol, whose effects are relatively short-lived and accompanied by a subjective sense of intoxication.

Assessment of the risks of drugs tends to focus on *direct* effects, but these and similar studies demonstrate that the *indirect* effects may be even more profound. Although it is difficult to estimate these effects with accuracy, they must be considered as part of the overall cost, to the individual and to society, of drug abuse.

D. Effects on Cognitive Functioning

The effect of marijuana on attention has been studied using a variety of cognitive tests [56]. These studies show that subjects consistently do more poorly after receiving even moderate amounts of marijuana. Some of the specific impairments found have included confusion, loss of directedness, and the ability to simultaneously remember information (e.g., numbers) and manipulate it to achieve a goal.

Other studies show that marijuana's effects on attention are marked but complex [56]. Short-term memory appears to be affected more strongly than does retrieval of information that is already present in memory. In word-recognition tests, in which subjects are asked to identify words that were previously read aloud to them, subjects receiving marijuana tended to accept more incorrect words from a list that was supplied to them, and when asked to write as many words as they could recall, were able to remember fewer words than subjects receiving placebo. In tests of free recall, in which subjects are given a book to read and later asked to recall the contents, those receiving marijuana recalled less and included fewer content words. Experimental evidence has not confirmed the perceived enhanced sensory awareness (e.g., visual or auditory acuity) reported by users [56].

IX. AMOTIVATION AND AGGRESSION

An often-cited, but anecdotal, consequence of marijuana use is the amotivational syndrome, a loosely defined concept involving disinterest, apathy, and antisocial behavior. Some of these effects are characteristic of CNS depressants in general. Whether a distinct amotivational syndrome can be ascribed to marijuana use is open to question. The term is imprecise, though it is clear from clinical observation that some adolescents who use marijuana appear flat in affect and devoid of the drive and energy normally seen in adolescents.

As a CNS depressant, marijuana would be expected to *decrease* aggression. However, animal studies generally show that delta-9-THC *increases* aggressive behavior, especially in animals who are deprived of food or sleep or otherwise stressed. [57,58]. For example, administration of marijuana extract or delta-9-THC causes aggression in rats that have been deprived of food for 20 h [59–61], and increases deaths among rats.

Other studies, however, cloud this picture. Low doses (0.5 and 1.0 mg/kg) of delta-9-THC *reduced* schedule-induced aggression in pigeons [62], whereas delta-8- and delta-9-THC reduced isolation-induced aggressiveness in mice and Chinese hamsters [63]. One group of researchers studying the effects of cannabinoids on sleep-deprived rats concluded that their effects depend on the animals' state, producing CNS depression in normal rats but increasing aggressiveness and irritability when administered to stressed rats.

We have no clear understanding of how cannabinoids affect the neurotransmitter system to cause or potentiate aggression in laboratory animals. Large doses of atropine block cannabis-induced aggression in sleep-deprived rats, suggesting that the cholinergic nervous system is involved [61]. Other studies point to a role for dopamine and serotonin in cannabinoid-induced aggression [58,64].

For the most part, cannabinoids' effects on aggression are inconsistent across species, and Dewey's review of the literature concludes that these and other studies are *not* predictive of cannabinoids' effects on aggression in human beings.

X. TOLERANCE

The development of tolerance to the effects of cannabinoids is difficult to characterize. For example, one study failed to find significant tolerance to the effects of delta-9-THC, as measured both by pulse rate and subjective reports, unless subjects repeatedly self-administered large doses of the drug [65]. In another study, regular marijuana users reported increased elation after smoking marijuana, but their pulse rates showed no significant increase [66]. In the same study, intermittent and occasional smokers exhibited the opposite effects, with *no* significant marijuana-induced elation, but *did* show significant increases in pulse rate. In other words, regular use of marijuana seems to intensity (and thus presumably reinforce) the subjective "high." When these subjects were given oral nabilone (a synthetic cannabinoid) and oral delta-9-THC, they experienced a significant increase in pulse rate but no elation. These results are confusing and to some extent counterintuitive. However, one unequivocal finding from the study was that among these three compounds, marijuana proved to be the most powerful reinforcer by far.

Some researchers have suggested that marijuana tolerance is *dispositional*; that is, caused by changes in the way the drug is stored or metabolized [67]. Others, including Agurell et al., believe that tolerance is primarily functional, a conclusion supported by studies showing similar patterns of drug distribution and metabolism in heavy users and light users.

XI. CORRELATION BETWEEN PLASMA LEVELS AND SUBJECTIVE EFFECTS

Taken alone, plasma levels of psychoactive cannabinoids and subjective reports of the high are not closely correlated. However, when these two values are charted against time on a graph (Fig. 1), a revealing pattern emerges. After intravenous administration of delta-9-THC, plasma levels drop quickly at first, and then more slowly. The subjective high, however, rises to a sharp peak over the first 30 min, and then drops off gradually and uniformly.

As noted previously, this pattern has led some to speculate that delta-9-THC must first be metabolized to 11-hydroxy-delta-9-THC before it becomes psychoactive [68]. According to this theory, the initial drop in delta-9-THC levels represents conversion to 11-hydroxy-delta-9-THC, which in turn accounts for the rise in the subjective high. However, if this theory were correct, intravenous administration of 11-hydroxy-delta-9-THC would be

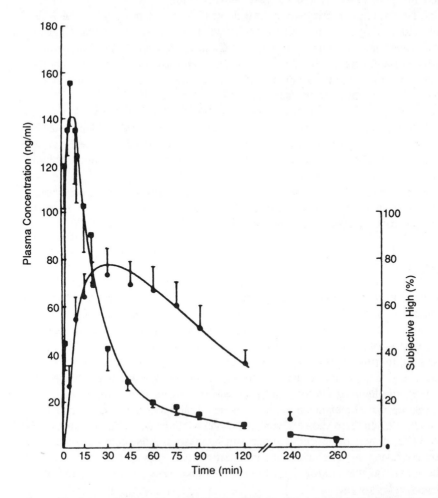

Figure 1 Plasma THC concentration-time (■) and subjective high-time (●) after smoking one 2.5% THC cigarette ($\overline{X} \pm$ SE; $n =$). *Solid curves* are computer fits to the data.

expected to create an instantaneous high. It does not; in fact, it shows a pattern virtually identical to that of delta-9-THC [69,70].

Another possible explanation, though not well supported by experimental studies, is that the lag observed on the graph is caused by slow penetration of psychoactive cannabinoids into the brain [71]. Agurell et al. [67] suggest that the reasons could involve "the time required to start the biochemical effects or, speculatively, to penetrate to the receptor, or displace a possible endogenous ligand"; however, they caution that these explanations are only speculation, and that causes of the lag remain unknown [63].

XII. FORMATION AND EXCRETION OF METABOLITES

Some 80 metabolites of delta-9-THC are known [72]. Of these, 7-hydroxy-delta-9-THC and 6[beta]-hydroxy-delta-9-THC are capable of producing marijuanalike symptoms and increased pulse rate. The others are believed to be essentially nonpsychoactive. About two-thirds of these metabolites are excreted in feces and about one-third in the urine. As noted previously, the metabolites are excreted slowly, with only about half the dose eliminated after 2–3 days [72]. In fact, traces of cannabinoid metabolites may be found as long as several weeks after marijuana [48]. Neither delta-9-THC nor CBD are excreted unchanged in the urine, although traces of CBN may be found. Delta-9-THC is excreted in feces [72].

XIII. ANTICONVULSANT EFFECTS OF CANNABINOIDS

At least one cannabinoid, cannabidol (CBD), shows some anticonvulsant action, and researchers have investigated its potential as a anticonvulsant medication. Because it is chemically unrelated to other anticonvulsants, it could offer an alternative for those in whom other drug therapies fail to control seizures. Studies of CBD's anticonvulsant properties have been rare, in large part because of the difficulty of preparing CBD, and thus far inconclusive [73,74].

XIV. SUMMARY

As the preceding discussion shows, some facets of cannabinoid pharmacology are understood with a fair degree of certainty, whereas for others the evidence is inconclusive and contradictory. In general, the psychoactive components of marijuana exert an overall depressive effect on the central nervous system, with some paradoxical stimulatory components. They are very potent, with active plasma levels in the nanogram range, but even in relatively high doses they do not possess the immediately life-threatening potential of such other psychoactive drugs as opiates, cocaine, barbiturates, or alcohol.

Cannabinoids are soluble in lipids, but almost entirely insoluble in water. It is likely that they are bound up in fatty tissues, and slowly excreted from these tissues over the course of several days, accounting for their long half-life.

The psychoactive mechanism(s) of these drugs is unknown, although the bulk of current evidence suggests that they act on some type of receptors. Though chemically unrelated to other psychoactive compounds, the evidence suggests that may act to some degree on similar sites within the CNS. For example, they show some cross tolerance with ethanol, and appear to exert antianxiety and anticonvulsant effects via benzodiazepine receptors. A few cannabinoids show antiemetic activity.

Beyond this handful of relative certainties, however, many controversies continue to surround the pharmacology of cannabinoids. For example, their long-term effects (over the course of years, versus the days or weeks that typical studies examine) are controversial but largely unexplored for our culture. The reasons for these gaps are numerous. Certainly the drugs' illicit nature as well as the almost total lack of a therapeutic role for them make long-term studies difficult. Another less obvious, but still important, factor is marijuana's low acute toxicity; unlike the case with heroin or cocaine, acute marijuana use, in and of itself, rarely comes to the attention of emergency physicians. But though marijuana's effects are far less dramatic than those of "killer drugs" such as heroin or cocaine, it does not follow that it is harmless. As discussed in the chapters that follow, marijuana is definitely contraindicated for those in whom the developmental process is not yet complete; that is, children and adolescents. Unfortunately, this is the very group that uses it most heavily.

Because patients will often deny the consequences of long-term marijuana use—for obvious reasons—it is exceedingly difficult to establish links between illness and long-term use through population studies. For example, adolescents commonly enter emergency rooms with problems that they attribute to cocaine overdose or problems, even though they have been using marijuana before or simultaneously with the cocaine. Similarly, auto accidents are often attributed to alcohol use despite the fact of concurrent marijuana use. For all these reasons, the true incidence of marijuana-induced effects are unknown, and almost certainly understated.

XV. MEDICAL PROBLEMS

Marijuana causes a number of medical problems, including respiratory ailments, impaired immunity, and reproductive disturbances. Often the symptoms are subtle and nonspecific, and the link with marijuana use not immediately apparent; thus, a careful history is important. Although acute respiratory discomfort can be eased with symptomatic treatment, abstinence is the only effective long-term treatment for all of these conditions. The limited evidence from long-term studies suggests that most of the medical effects are reversible with cessation of marijuana use. However, the psychological and developmental effects of marijuana on adolescents, as with other developmental injuries, may not be reversible.

A special concern is marijuana use during pregnancy. Numerous studies show that maternal marijuana use has direct deleterious effects on the developing fetus. A link between marijuana use and low birth weight is well established; similarly, marijuana has been shown to increase the risk of complications during pregnancy. In addition, case reports and animal research strongly suggests that marijuana is a teratogen, a finding that is consistent with its known mutagenic and carcinogenic properties, and that it can cause fetal hypoxia resulting in impaired growth, prematurity, and fetal brain damage.

XVI. RESPIRATORY EFFECTS

Inhaled smoke from any source harms lung tissue and epithelial cells lining the airways, as well as the immune cells found in the lungs. All of these effects can make the lungs more vulnerable to infection, and can complicate or trigger respiratory disorders [75].

Marijuana and tobacco smoke are chemically similar (except that marijuana smoke contains cannabinoids and tobacco smoke contains nicotine), and the effects of marijuana smoking parallel those seen in tobacco smokers. Smoking habits of the two groups are not identical; marijuana users tend to smoke less, but they inhale more deeply, do not use filters, and smoke the cigarette down to the butt. Thus, it seems reasonable to conclude that marijuana smoking carries similar risks of lung cancer, emphysema, chronic bronchitis, and other respiratory ailments as does cigarette smoking.

The cardiovascular effects of tobacco, however, are related to nicotine. Although cannabinoids are known to cause short-term cardiovascular changes, these effects are very different from those caused by nicotine. The long-term consequences on the cardiovasular system are essentially unknown, and cannot be extrapolated from evidence related to cigarette smoking.

A. Acute Effects

The acute effects of marijuana smoking on ventilation are dose dependent [26]. Smaller doses (one cigarette or less) stimulate ventilation, in conjunction with an increased metabolic rate and heightened response to CO_2 as a regulatory stimulant. Larger doses, by contrast, may have the opposite effect. Curiously, intravenous administration of delta-9-THC has relatively little effect on ventilation rates or respiratory response to CO_2.

Marijuana smoke is a powerful bronchodilator, persisting as long as 60 min after smoking. Again, delta-9-THC administered intravenously has much less potent bronchodilatory action though its pulmonary effects may persist as long as 6 h. The mechanism of action for bronchodilation is not clear, but involves neither beta-adrenergic stimulation nor blockade of receptors in smooth muscle [77].

In addition to bronchodilation, heavy marijuana smoking (at least 4 days per week for 6–8 weeks) results in mild airway obstruction [78]. One study found that these effects were incompletely reversed 1 week after cessation of smoking, suggesting that long-term heavy marijuana smoking "could lead to clinically significant and less readily reversible impairment of pulmonary function [79].

Contaminated marijuana may result in respiratory infections or other disease. The use of paraquat herbicide on illegal marijuana crops is well publicized. Marijuana harvested after it has been sprayed with paraquat can result in severe lung damage. Currently, the spraying of marijuana crops with paraquat has been discontinued by law enforcement authorities; however, its use in the future has not been precluded [80].

In addition to chemical contamination, marijuana may also be contaminated by infectious agents, especially aspergillus organisms. One researcher found aspergilli in 11 of 12 marijuana samples tested [81]. Aspergilli can cause severe respiratory infections as well as subacute infections that may easily be overlooked [82].

B. Chronic Effects

Studies of hashish-smoking American soldiers stationed in West Germany have revealed a number of respiratory ailments associated with heavy hashish use. One study involved 31 soldiers who smoked 100 gm or more of hashish a month for 6–15 months. The study found that the primary ailments in this group were respiratory (bronchitis, sinusitis, asthma, and rhinopharyngitis) [83]. A third of the soldiers had sputum-producing coughs, difficulty in breathing, and wheezing after 3–4 months of hashish use. Chest radiographs and sputum cultures were normal, and antibiotics failed to resolve the symptoms.

The condition, which was so severe that all of the affected soldiers were unable to work and four required hospitalization, resolved after they decreased their hashish consumption. Pulmonary tests administered 3 days after they reduced their intake of hashish showed mild airway obstruction. The patients responded to isoproterenol, leading the researchers to surmise that reversible bronchospasm, accumulation of fluid in the bronchi, or both, were responsible for the symptoms.

Another study of 200 soldiers who sought medical attention for problems related to hashish smoking found that inflammation of the mouth and back of the throat and persistent rhinitis were common [84]. Symptoms were relieved by antibiotics, decongestants, and phenylephrine, but returned with continued smoking.

Additional evidence of chronic respiratory effects comes from Jamaica, where both heavy marijuana usage and bronchitis are common [85]. However, many Jamaican marijuana users are also heavy tobacco smokers, which clouds the relationship between marijuana and bronchitis. Other studies in Jamaica [86] and Costa Rica [87] found no difference in the incidence of respiratory illness among marijuana smokers and nonsmokers.

A well-controlled study of 74 persons who had smoked marijuana for 2–5 years found a mild but significant increase in air flow resistance in the large airways, with no effect on conventional pulmonary tests [88].

Auerbach [89] found evidence of chronic bronchitis among heavy hashish users. Physical examinations revealed abnormal respiratory sounds (rhonchi, wheezes, and rales), though chest x-rays were normal. Lung capacity was 15–40% below normal, and in six of the 20 patients studied, biopsies showed abnormal bronchial tissue resembling that of older heavy tobacco smokers as well as atypical cells not found in tobacco smokers.

C. Pulmonary Immune Effects

The effect of marijuana smoke on alveolar macrophages is not clear. In vivo studies using macrophages from rat lungs show a decrease in bactericidal activity [85–93], but another report [94] showed no significant effect of marijuana smoke (or tobacco smoke) on macrophage activity.

D. Neoplastic Changes in the Lung

Correlation of marijuana smoking with lung cancer presents difficult methodological problems because of lung cancer's long latency period, the tendency not to report a history of marijuana use, and the concurrent use of tobacco by many marijuana smokers. Laboratory studies, however, show that elements of marijuana smoke are mutagenic and, therefore, likely to be carcinogenic [95–97]. In addition, chemical analysis of marijuana smoke reveals many known carcinogens. Delta-9-THC, however, does *not* appear to be mutagenic [98–99].

Tennant's [100] and Henderson's [84] studies of American service personnel showed numerous cellular abnormalities associated with heavy hashish smoking. These effects were worse among patients who smoked both hashish and tobacco than among those who smoked only tobacco. Thus, the cellular effects of the two substances seem to be additive.

XVII. CARDIOVASCULAR EFFECTS

Marijuana smoking results in an almost immediate increase in heart rate and blood pressure, which can aggravate existing cardiac insufficiency or hypertension. In healthy young adults, smoking 10 mg of marijuana increases the heart rate by as much as 90 beats/min; the effect lasts about one hour [101]. This tachycardia seems to result from both parasympathetic and sympathetic stimulation of the cardiac pacemaker [102–108]. However, studies with propranolol have yielded contradictory answers to the question of whether beta-adrenergic stimulation is involved [102,105–108].

Although cardiac output may increase by as much as 30% after smoking marijuana, blood pressure rises only modestly (if at all), indicating decreased peripheral resistance [109]. Large doses of delta-9-THC have resulted in opposite effects, causing a *drop* in systolic and diastolic blood pressure [110] and in heart rate [111–115]. Some degree of tolerance to these hemodynamic effects occurs among chronic users of marijuana. The changes in cardiac function are not permanent; even in long-term users, they can be reversed by cessation of smoking [112–115].

A. Coronary Artery Disease

The long-term cardiovascular risks of marijuana are unknown. It is clear, however, that marijuana can aggravate existing heart conditions. It is known to cause changes in the electrocardiogram [102,116]. It increases the work of the heart in ways that are characteristic of stress [117], and in all probability can trigger arrhythmias or even myocardial infarction in patients suffering from preexisting coronary artery disease. In addition, by dulling the pain of angina, it can cause the patient to delay taking antianginal medications, which can further contribute to cardiac damage [117]. Increased catecholamine levels as a result of marijuana smoking can stimulate myocardial tissue and trigger arrhythmias [118].

Marijuana also causes postural hypotension, thereby aggravating coronary artery disease or cerebrovascular insufficiency. And marijuana smoke, like tobacco smoke, can cause the formation of carboxyhemoglobin in the bloodstream, thus compromising the blood's oxygen-carrying capacity [117].

B. Other Cardiovascular Effects

Chronic administration of large doses of delta-9-THC promotes sodium retention, and leads to increases in body weight and plasma volume [112–114]. The increased plasma volume seems to be caused by the decrease in orthostatic hypertension that occurs with chronic use [119], but the mechanisms by which delta-9-THC promotes sodium retention are not clear.

XVIII. NEUROLOGICAL EFFECTS

The long-term neurological consequences of marijuana intoxication are unknown. Early studies using pneumoencephalography suggested that long-term marijuana users had cerebral atrophy, but this research suffered from serious methodological and technological limitations and has not been supported by later studies employing better patient selection and computed tomography (CT) [120,121].

One study, in which rhesus monkeys received delta-9-THC over a 5-year period, revealed atrophy of the caudate nucleus and frontal portion of the brain, as measured by CT scanning. The authors caution, however, that the implications of these results are uncertain, especially as regards the effects of long-term marijuana use on humans [122].

Despite anecdotal reports that marijuana induces seizures in patients with preexisting seizure disorders, the bulk of the evidence suggests that this is not the case [121]. In fact, some cannabinoids have been shown to have antiepileptic properties.

XIX. REPRODUCTIVE EFFECTS

A. Male Reproductive System

Marijuana is antiandrogenic, and a number of its constituents, including delta-9-THC, bind to androgen receptors. In addition, marijuana may act on estrogenic receptors [123]. In males, marijuana diminishes testosterone production and inhibits reproductive function [124]. The magnitude and duration of these effects are not well established. One study of 20 men who used marijuana at least 4 days a week for 6 months found lowered testosterone levels [124]. The testosterone levels, though lower than those of controls, were still within normal range in all but two subjects. Levels of follicle-stimulating hormone (FSH) and sperm counts were also lower in marijuana smokers. The results of this study suggested that all of these effects were dose dependent.

However, the study did not control for the use of other drugs concurrently with marijuana. Another study involving men in a research ward who smoked government-supplied marijuana found no suppression of plasma testosterone levels [125]. Follicle-stimulating hormone counts were not reported.

Further research has yielded equally inconsistent results. Hembree et al., found a decrease in sperm motility, increased numbers of abnormal sperm, and eventually a decline in sperm counts among subjects who received high doses of marijuana for 5–6 weeks [126]. They concluded, based on this and other evidence, that marijuana interfered with sperm production by acting directly on the seminiferous tubular epithelium, and not by suppressing gonadotropins. A Costa Rican study, by contrast, found no evidence of suppressed testosterone levels among subjects who had regularly smoked marijuana for at least 10 years [87]. Rats exposed to marijuana from a smoke machine for 30 days exhibited lowered sperm counts, but so did rats exposed to smoke that was free of cannabinoids [127]. However, the rats receiving marijuana smoke had an increased number of abnormal sperm forms.

The conclusions that can be drawn from these conflicting studies are at best tentative. Marijuana is antiandrogenic, but it is not known whether the effects translate into decreased libido or impaired fertility. Also unknown is the persistence of these effects—whether they resolve spontaneously after discontinuation of marijuana use, and whether tolerance develops with continued use. Although the effects on developing sexual organisms, that is, adolescents, are not known, it is reasonable to assume that they would be more significant, and perhaps long lasting, than among adults.

B. Female Reproductive System

Marijuana causes hormonal disruption of the female reproductive cycle. Women who use marijuana four times a week or more have shorter luteal phases, resulting in shorter menstrual cycles. In addition, plasma prolactin levels are elevated and testosterone levels are depressed. Galactorrhea has been reported in as many as 20% of these cases [128]. One study has found impaired fertility among women who use marijuana [129]; however, it suffers from severe methodological flaws and its findings have been challenged [130]. Animal studies, however, show a suppression of ovarian function and interference with gonadotropin and estrogenic activity in females [131–138] as well as amenorrhea [139].

C. Teratogenicity and Effects on Pregnancy

Animal studies as well as anecdotal evidence suggests other disturbing effects among chronic users of relatively low doses of marijuana [140–147]. Female monkeys given oral doses of 2.4 mg/kg of delta-9-THC for 1–4 years showed a subsequent pattern characteristic of high-risk pregnancies, including a higher than normal rate of miscarriage and death of offspring in the early postnatal period [148,149]. Fetal anomalies and neonatal deaths are increased by prenatal marijuana use [155]. Moreover, animal studies consistently show that exposure to marijuana during pregnancy causes growth retardation of the fetus. The underlying mechanism seems to include both direct effects on the fetus and suppression of maternal appetite and weight gain [150–152]. In addition, marijuana may reduce the fetal blood supply [156]. Also, symptoms consistent with the fetal alcohol syndrome have been observed [153,154]. Indeed, the fetal alcohol syndrome is five times more likely when the mother is a user of marijuana [155].

There is some evidence that the use of marijuana close to the delivery date may prolong and complicate labor. Precipitate labor and meconium passage are more frequent in marijuana users than in control groups. However, other studies of women who smoked marijuana but were otherwise in good health and had good living conditions showed no significant effects from prenatal marijuana use [151–153,155]. It seems reasonable to conclude from these studies that marijuana may exacerbate other risk factors in pregnancy.

Delta-9-THC crosses the placental barrier [151,152,154] and accumulates in mother's milk. Some studies suggest that marijuana use may interfere with lactation and/or diminish the milk supply by inhibiting prolactin secretion [151,152,154]. Rodent studies show significant levels of THC in nursing infants as a result of maternal exposure to THC, and infant monkeys whose mothers are given THC prove to be lethargic and slow to gain weight. One study [147] found a variety of abnormal responses in newborns whose mothers used large amounts of marijuana during pregnancy. These responses included increased startle reflex, tremors, poor self-quieting, and failure to habituate to light. At 1 month after birth, the visual effects remained in half the infants, and tremors were present in a fourth of them.

XX. IMMUNE IMPAIRMENT

Animal studies provide evidence that marijuana impairs the immune system [157]. Human studies are more contradictory, but several do demonstrate mild immunological impairment as a result of marijuana use. The impairment appears to be reversible with cessation of use [148]. In otherwise healthy subjects, this impairment of the immune system is not accompanied by increased susceptibility to infectious disease; a sufficient reservoir of immunity remains to resist infection [148]. However, the impairment may well come into play in patients who are immunocompromised or otherwise at risk of infection. For example, the use of marijuana as an antiemetic for cancer patients is ill advised in light of the immunosuppressive effects of antineoplastic agents.

In addition, the immunosuppressive effects take on added importance in light of the total picture of marijuana abuse if, for example, marijuana use is part of a pattern of multiple drug use. It would be reasonable to assume that patients who use intravenous drugs along with marijuana might be at increased risk of developing blood-borne infections, including hepatitis. Similarly, the smoking of contaminated marijuana combined with immune system impairment would seem to place users at heightened risk of respiratory infection. Further, long-term immune system impairment is likely to increase the risk of cancer. All of these effects are speculative, but they should be kept in mind by the practitioner who may be seeing chronic marijuana users in clinical practice.

XXI. SUMMARY

Marijuana causes a variety of medical problems. The most pronounced effects are on the respiratory system, and for the most part appear to result from the direct action of marijuana smoke on lung tissues. These acute respiratory effects are dose dependent and reversible with cessation of use. In addition, marijuana smoke is almost certainly carcinogenic, and although the long-term risk of lung cancer from marijuana smoking has not been established, it is probably similar to the risk from cigarette smoking. If a patient smokes both cigarettes and marijuana, we would expect the effects to be additive at least.

Marijuana use, especially chronic use or use by adolescents, also results in systemic effects on the male and female reproductive systems, and in all likelihood on the immune system as well. It is difficult to estimate the ultimate course or severity of these systemic effects; although most seem to resolve spontaneously with cessation of marijuana use, the data are very sparse.

When considered in light of the long-term psychological effects of marijuana use, these medical problems raise some disturbing issues. Because their signs and symptoms are subtle and often nonspecific (for instance, the low-normal hormonal levels and marginally impaired immune responses) they are likely to be overlooked or attributed to other sources. But the clinical picture of these somatic disturbances may parallel and reinforce the nonspecific psychological disturbances that accompany long-term marijuana use. For example, a patient may present a host of vague complaints, such as decreased libido, frequent respiratory infections, mild depression, and sleep disturbances, all of which may be mutually reinforcing and yet difficult to diagnose. In fact, the patient may present an entirely unrelated complaint without realizing the effect that marijuana use is having on his or her general well-being. In all these cases, a diagnosis of marijuana dependency may easily be overlooked, especially because the clinician has no baseline to compare against the patient's current condition.

For patients presenting with these sorts of nonspecific symptoms, marijuana use should always be considered as an element in the differential diagnosis. Even when other etiological factors are identified, marijuana use may be a contributing factor. Because the initial symptoms are nonspecific, it may be difficult to show clear improvement resulting from abstention. Even so, abstinence in these cases is more than simply prudent; it is well justified by the evidence from animal and human studies.

REFERENCES

1. Turner, C.E. Cannabis: The plant, its drugs, and their effects. *Aviation Space Environ. Med.* *54*:363–368 (1983).
2. Pillard, R.C. Marihuana. *N. Engl. J. Med. 283*:294 (1970).
3. Turner, C.E. *The Marijuana Controversy: Definition of Research Perspectives and Therapeutic Claims*. American Council for Drug Education, 1981.
4. Mann,, P. *Marijuana Alert*. McGraw-Hill, New York, 1985.
5. Jones, R.T., Benowitz, W., and Bachman, I. Clinical studies of cannabis tolerance and dependencies. *Ann. N.Y. Acad. Sci. 282*:21–239 (1976).
6. Snyder, B.H. *Uses of Marijuana*. Oxford University Press, New York, 1971.
7. Brecher, E.M., et al. *Licit and Illicit Drugs: The Consumers Union Report on Narcotics, Stimulants, Depressants, Inhalants, Hallucinogens, and Marijuana—Including Caffeine, Nicotine and Alcohol*. Boston, Little Brown, 1972.
8. Nahas, G.G. *Keep Off the Grass*. Pergamon, New York, 1979.
9. Nahas, G.G. *Marijuana in Science and Medicine*. Raven, New York, 1984.
10. Creighton, C. On indications of the hashish—vice in the Old Testament. *Janus 1902*:8.
11. Clay, M. *The Song of Solomon in the Book of Grass*. Grove, New York, 1967.
12. Walton, R.P. *Marijuana: America's New Drug Problem*. Lippincott, Philadelphia, 1938.
13. Giannini, A.J., Slaby, A.E., and Giannini, J.D. *Handbook of Overdoses and Detoxification Emergencies*, 3rd ed. Medical Examination, New York, 1985.
14. Rosenthal, F. *The Herb Hashish versus Moslem Medieval Society*. Leiden, Brill, Netherlands, 1972.
15. Lewin, L. *Phantastica: Narcotic and Stimulating Drugs—Their Use and Abuse*. [Reprint of 1924 edition.] Dutton, New York, 1964.
16. Hoffman, F. *A Handbook on Drug and Alcohol Abuse*, 2nd ed. Oxford University Press, 1983.
17. Winek, C.L. Some historical aspects of marijuana. *Clin. Toxicol. 10*:243–253 (1977).
18. Grinspoon, L., and Bakalar, J.B. Marihuana, J.H. Lowinson and P. Ruiz (eds). *Substance Abuse: Clinical Problems and Perspectives*. New York, Williams and Wilkins, 1981.
19. Petersen, R.D. Marijuana overview, M. Glantz (ed.). *Correlates and Consequences of Marijuana Use*. National Institute on Drug Abuse, Rockville, Maryland, 1984.
20. Fishburne, P.M., Abelson, H.I., and Cisin, I. *National Survey on Drug Abuse: Main Findings: 1979*. U.S. Government Printing Office, 1980 [DHHS publication no. (ADM) 80–976], Washington, D.C.
21. National Institute of Drug Abuse: *NIDA Capsules: Highlights of the 1985 National Household Survey on Drug Abuse*. Rockville, Maryland, 1986.
22. National Institute of Drug Abuse: *NIDA Capsules: High School Senior Drug Use 1975–1986*. Rockville, Maryland, 1987.
23. Schwartz, R.H. Marijuana: An overview. *Pediatr. Clin. North Am. 34*(2):305–317 (1987).
24. Anonymous: Alcohol and other drug abuse among adolescents. *Metropolitan Insurance Company Statistical Bulletin 65*(7):4–73 (1984).
25. Kandel, D. Adolescent drug abuse. *J. Am. Acad. Child Psychiatry 20*:573–577 (1982).
26. Millman, R.B., and Sbriglio, R. Patterns of use and psychopathology in chronic marijuana users. *Psychiatr. Clin. North Am. 9*(3):533–545 (1986).

27. Yamaguchi, K., and Kandel, D.B. Patterns of drug use from adolescence to young adulthood. II. Sequence of progression. *Am. J. Public Health 74*:668–672 (1984).

28. Jessor, R., Jessor, S.L. *Problem Behavior and Psychosocial Development: A Longitudinal Study of Youth.* Academic, New York, 1977.

29. Institute of Medicine: *Marijuana and Health.* National Academy, Washington, D.C., 1982.

30. Miller, J.A., and Cisin, I.H. Highlights from the National Survey on Drug Abuse 1979. U.S. Government Printing Office, 1980 [DHHS publication no. (ADM) 80-1302], Washington, D.C.

31. Dewey, W.L. Cannabinoid pharmacology. *Pharmacol. Rev. 38*(2):151–178 (1986).

32. Agurell, S., Halldin, M., Lindgren, J.E., et al. Pharmacokinetics and metabolism of delta-1-tetrahydrocannabinol and other cannabinoids with emphasis on man. *Pharmacol. Rev. 38*(1):23 (1986).

33. Lemberger, L., McMahon, R., and Archer, R. The role of metabolic conversion on the mechanisms of actions of cannabinoids, M.C. Braude and S. Szara (eds.). *Pharmacology of Marihuana*, Vol. I, Raven, New York, 1976, pp. 125–133.

34. Agurell, S., Halldin, M., Lindgren, J.E., et al. Pharmacokinetics and metabolism of delta-1-tetrahydrocannabinol and other cannabinoids with emphasis on man. *Pharmacol. Rev. 38*(1):22 (1986).

35. Agurell, S., and Leander, K. Stability, transfer, and absorption of cannabinoid constituents of cannabis (hashish) during smoking. *Acta. Pharm. Suec. 8*:391–402 (1971).

36. Davis, K.H., Jr., McDaniel, I.A., Jr., Cadwell, L.W., and Moody, P.L. Some smoking characteristics of marijuana cigarettes, S. Agurell, W.L. Dewey, and R.E. Willette (eds). *The Cannabinoids: Chemical, Pharmacologic, and Therapeutic Aspects.* Academic, New York, 1984, pp. 97–109.

37. Perez-Reyes, M., Diguiseppi, S., Davis, K.H., Schindler, V.H., and Cook, C.E. Comparison of effects of marijuana cigarettes of three different potencies. *Clin. Pharmacol. Ther. 31*:617–624 (1982).

38. Cone, E.J., and Johnson, R.E. Contact highs and urinary cannabinoid excretion after passive exposure to marijuana smoke. *Clin. Pharmacol. Ther. 40*:247–256 (1986).

39. Agurell, S., Halldin, M., Lindgren, J.E., et al. Pharmacokinetics and metabolism of delta-1-tetrahydrocannabinol and other cannabinoids with emphasis on man. *Pharmacol. Rev. 38*(1):40 (1986).

40. Harvey, D.J. Pharmacology, metabolism, pharmacokinetics, and analysis of the cannabinoids, *ISI Atlas of Science: Pharmacology 1987.* ISI, Philadelphia, 1987, pp. 209–210.

41. Martin, B.R. Cellular effects of cannabinoids. *Pharmacol. Rev. 38*(1):54 (1986).

42. Schou, J., Prockop, L.D., Dahlstrom, G., and Rohde, C. Penetration of delta-9-tetrahydrocannabinol and 11-OH-delta-9-tetrahydrocannabinol through the blood-brain barrier. *Acta. Pharmacol. Toxicol. 41*:33–38 (1977).

43. Perez-Reyes, M., Simmons, J., Brine, D., Kimmel, G.L., Davis, K.H., and Wall, M.E. Rate of penetration of delta-9-tetrahydrocannabinol and 11-hydroxy-delta-9-tetrahydrocannabinol to the brain of mice, G. Nahas (ed.). *Marihuana: Chemistry, Biochemistry, and Cellular Effects.* Springer-Verlag, New York, 1976, pp. 179–185.

44. Gough, A.L, and Olley, J.E. Catalepsy induced by intrastriatal injections of delta-9-THC and 11-OH-delta-9-THC in the rat. *Neuropharmacology 17*:137–144 (1978).

45. Martin, B.R. Cellular effects of cannabinoids. *Pharmacol. Rev. 38*(1):56 (1986).

46. Chiang, C.W.N., Barnett, G., and Brine, D. Systemic absorption of delta-9-tetrahydrocannabinol after ophthalmic administration in the rabbit. *J. Pharm. Sci. 72*:136–138 (1983).

47. Lemberger, L., Silberstein, S.D., Axelrod, J., and Kopin, I.J. Marihuana: Studies on the disposition and metabolism of delta-9-tetrahydrocannabinol in man. *Science 170*:1320–1322 (1970).

48. Dackis, C.A., Pottash, A.L.C., Annitto, W., and Gold, M.S. Persistence of urinary marijuana levels after supervised abstinence. *Am. J. Psychiatry 139*:1196–1198 (1982).

49. Ohlsson, A., Lindgren, J.E., Wahlen, A., Agurell, S., Hollister, L.E., and Gillespie, H.K. Plasma delta-9-tetrahydrocannabinol concentrations and clinical effects after oral and intravenous administration and smoking. *Clin. Pharmacol. Ther. 28*:409–416 (1980).

50. Ohlsson, A., Lindgren, J.E., Wahlen, A., Agurell, S., Hollister, L.E., and Gillespie, H.K. Single dose kinetics of deuterium labelled delta-1-tetrahydrocannabinol in heavy and light cannabis users. *Biomed. Mass. Spectrom.* 9:6–10 (1982).

51. Dewey, W.L. Cannabinoid pharmacology. *Pharmacol. Rev.* 38(2):153 (1986).

52. Dewey, W.L. Cannabinoid pharmacology. *Pharmacol. Rev.* 38(2):154 (1986).

53. Reeve, V.C., Grant, J.D., Robertson, W., Gillespie, H.K., and Hollister, L.E. Plasma concentrations of delta-9-tetrahydrocannabinol and impaired motor function. *Drug Alcohol Depend.* 11:167–175 (1983).

54. Moskowitz, H. Marihuana and driving. *Accid. Anal. Prev.* 17:323–345 (1985).

55. Yesavage, J., Leirer, V.O., Ditman, J., and Hollister, L.E. "Hangover" effects of marijuana intoxication on aircraft pilot performance. *Am. J. Psychiatry* 142:1325–1329 (1985).

56. Murray, J.B. Marijuana's effects on human cognitive functions, psychomotor functions and personality. *J. Gen. Psychol.* 113(1):23–55 (1986).

57. Fujiwara, M., Ibii, N., Kataoka, Y., and Ueki, S. Effects of psychotropic drugs on delta-9-tetrahydrocannabinol-induced long-lasting muricide. *Psychopharmacology* 68:7–13 (1980).

58. Carlini, E.A., and Lindsey, C.J. Effect on serotonergic drugs on the aggressiveness induced by delta-9-tetrahydrocannibinol in REM-sleep-derived rats. *Braz. J. Med. Biol. Res.* 15:281–283 (1982).

59. Fujiwara, M., and Ueki, S. The course of aggressive behavior induced by a single injection of delta-9-tetrahydrocannabinol and its characteristics. *Physiol. Behav.* 22:535–539 (1979).

60. Carlini, E.A., Hamaoui, A., and Martz, R.M.W. Factors influencing the aggressiveness induced by delta-9-tetrahydrocannabinol in food-deprived rats. *Br. J. Pharmacol.* 44:794–804 (1972).

61. Musty, R.E., Lindsey, C.J., and Carlini, E.A. 6-Hydroxydopamine and the aggressive behavior induced by marihuana in REM sleep-deprived rats. *Psychopharmacology* 48:175–179 (1976).

62. Cherek, D.R., Thompson, T., and Kelly, T. Chronic delta-9-tetrahydrocannabinol administration and schedule-induced aggression. *Pharmacol. Biochem. Behav.* 12:305–309 (1980).

63. Ten Ham, M., and Van Noordwijk, J. Lack of tolerance to the effects of two tetrahydrocannabinols on aggressiveness. *Psychopharmacology* 29:171–176 (1973).

64. DeSouza, and Neto, J.P. Effects of anti-acetylcholine drugs on aggressive behavior induced by cannabis sativa in REM sleep-deprived rats. *J. Pharm. Pharmacol.* 30:591–592 (1978).

65. Babor, T.F., Mendelson, J.H., Greenberg, I., and Kuehnle, J.C. Marihuana consumption and tolerance to physiological and subjective effects. *Arch. Gen. Psychiatry* 32:1548–1552 (1975).

66. Mendelson, J.H., and Mello, N.K. Reinforcing properties of oral delta-9-tetrahydrocannabinol, smoked marijuana, and nabilone: Influence of previous marijuana use. *Psychopharmacology* 83:351–356 (1984).

67. Agurell, S., Halldin, M., Lindgren, J.E., et al. Pharmacokinetics and metabolism of delta-1-tetrahydrocannabinol and other cannabinoids with emphasis on man. *Pharmacol. Rev.* 38(1):28 (1986).

68. Lemberger, L., Weiss, J.L, Watanabe, A.M., Galanter, I.M., Wyatt, R.J., and Cardon, P.V. Delta-9-tetrahydrocannabinol: Temporal correlation of the psychological effects and blood levels after various routes of administration. *N. Engl. J. Med.* 276:685–688 (1972).

69. Lemberger, L., Crabtree, R.E., and Rowe, H.M. 11-Hydroxy-delta-9-tetrahydrocannabinol: Pharmacology, disposition, and metabolism of a major metabolite of marihuana in man. *Science* 170:1320–1322 (1972).

70. Perez-Reyes, M., Timmons, M.C., Lipton, M., Davis, K.H., and Wall, M.E. Intravenous injection in man of delta-9-tetrahydrocannabinol and 11-hydroxy-delta-9-tetrahydrocannabinol. *Science* 177:633–635 (1972).

71. Agurell, S., Halldin, M., Lindgren, J.E., et al. Pharmacokinetics and metabolism of delta-1-tetrahydrocannabinol and other cannabinoids with emphasis on man. *Pharmacol. Rev.* 38(1):31 (1986).

72. Agurell, S., Halldin, M., Lindgren, J.E., et al. Pharmacokinetics and metabolism of delta-1-tetrahydrocannabinol and other cannabinoids with emphasis on man. *Pharmacol. Rev.* 38(1):34 (1986).

73. Ames, F.R., and Cridland, S. Anticonvulsant effect of cannabidiol, letter. *S. Afr. Med. J. 69*:14 (1986).
74. Cunha, J.M., Carlini, E.A., Pereira, A.E., et al. Chronic administration of cannabidiol to healthy volunteers and epileptic patients. *Pharmacology 21*:175–185 (1980).
75. Anonymous: Effects of marijuana on the respiratory and cardiovascular systems, in Institute of Medicine. *Marijuana and Health*. National Academy Press, Washington, D.C., 1982, p. 57.
76. Vachon, K., FitzGerald, M.X., Solliday, N.H., et al. Single-dose effect of marijuana smoke: Bronchial dynamics and respiratory-center sensitivity in normal subjects. *N. Engl. J. Med. 288*:985–989 (1973).
77. Zwillich, C.W., Doekel, R., Hammill, S., and Weil, J.V. The effects of smoked marijuana on metabolism and respiratory control. *Am. Rev. Respir. Dis 118*:885–891 (1978).
78. Shapiro, B.J., Tashkin, D.P. and Frank, I.M. Effects of beta-adrenergic blockade and muscarinic stimulation upon cannabis bronchodilation, M.C. Braude, S. Szara (eds.). *Pharmacology of Marijuana*. Raven, New York, 1976.
79. Tashkin, D.P., Shapiro, B.J., Lee, E.Y., and Harper, C.E. Subacute effects of heavy marijuana smoking pulmonary function in healthy young males. *N. Engl. J. Med. 294*:125–129 (1976).
80. Hollister, L.E. Health aspects of cannabis. *Pharmacol. Rev. 38*(1):11 (1986).
81. Kagan, S.L. Aspergillus: An inhalable contaminant of marijuana. *N. Engl. J. Med. 304*:483–484 (1981).
82. Schwartz, I.S. Marijuana and Fungal infection. *Am. J. Clin. Pathol. 84*:256 (1985).
83. Tennant, F.S., Preble, M., Prendergast, T.J., and Ventry, P. Medical manifestations associated with hashish. *J.A.M.A. 216*:1965–1969 (1971).
84. Henderson, R.L., Tennant, F.S., and Guerry, R. Respiratory manifestations of hashish smoking. *Arch. Otolaryngol 95*:248–251 (1972).
85. Hall, J.A.S. *Testimony in marihuana—hashish epidemic hearing of the Committee of the Judiciary U.S. Senate*. U.S. Government Printing Office, Washington, D.C., 1975.
86. Rubin, V., and Comitas, L. *Ganja in Jamaica: A Medical Anthropological Study of Chronic Marijuana Use*. Mouton, The Hague, 1975.
87. Hernandez-Bolanos, J., Swenson, E.W., and Coggins, W.J. Preservation of pulmonary function in regular heavy, long-term marijuana smokers. *Am. Rev. Resp. Dis. 113*(Suppl.):100 (1976).
88. Tashkin, D.P., Calvarese, B.M., Simmons, M.S., and Shapiro, B.J. Respiratory status of seventy-four habitual marijuana smokers. *Chest 78*:699–706 (1980).
89. Auerbach, O., Stout, A.P., Hammond, E.C., and Garfinkel, L. Changes in bronchial epithelium relation to cigarette smoking and in relation to lung cancer. *N. Engl. J. Med. 265*:253–267 (1961).
90. Huber, G.L., Simmons, G.A., McCarthy, C.R., et al. Depressants effect of marijuana smoke on antibacterial activity of pulmonary alveolar macrophages. *Chest 68*:769–773 (1975).
91. Huber, G.L., Pochay, V.E., Shea, J.W., et al. An experimental animal model for quantifying the biologic effects of marijuana on the defense system of the lung, G.G. Nahas, and W.D.M. Paton (eds.). *Marihuana: Biological Effects. Analysis, Metabolism, Cellular Responses, Reproduction, and Brain*. Pergamon, Oxford, England, 1979, pp. 301–328.
92. Huber, G.L., Shea, J.W., Hinds, W.E., et al. The gas phase of marijuana smoke and intrapulmonary antibacterial defenses. *Bull. Eur. Physiopath Resp. 15*:491–503 (1979).
93. Huber, G.L., Pochay, V.E., Pereira, W., et al. Marijuana, tetrahydrocannabinol, and pulmonary antibacterial defenses. *Chest 77*:403–410 (1980).
94. Drath, D.B., Shorey, J.M., Price, L., and Huber, G.L. Metabolic and functional characteristics of alveolar macrophages recovered from rats exposed to marijuana smoke. *Infect. Immun. 25*:268–272 (1979).
95. Busch, F.W., Seid, D.A., and Wei, E.T. Mutagenic activity of marihuana smoke condensates. *Cancer Lett. 6*:319–324 (1979).
96. Seid, D.A., and Wei, E.T. Mutagenic activity of marihuana smoke condensates. *Pharmacologist 21*:204 (1979).
97. Wehner, F.C., Van Rensburg, S.J., and Thiel, P.G. Mutagenicity of marijuana and transkei tobacco smoke condensates in the salmonella/microsome assay. *Mutat. Res. 77*:135–142 (1980).

98. Glatt, H., Ohlsson, A., Agurell, S., and Oesch, F. Delta-1-tetrahydrocannabinol and 1-alpha, 2-alpha-epoxyhexahydrocannabinol: Mutagenicity investigation in the Ames test. *Mutat. Res.* 66:329–335 (1979).

99. Van Went, G.F. Mutagencity testing of three hallucinogens: LSD, psilocybin and delta-9-THC, using the micronucleus test. *Experientia 34*:324–325 (1978).

100. Tennant, F.S., Guerry, R.L, and Henderson, R.L. Histopathologic and clinical abnormalities of the respiratory system in chronic hashish smokers. *Subst. Alcohol Misuse 1*:93–100 (1980).

101. Anonymous: Effects of marijuana on the respiratory and cardiovascular systems, in Institute of Medicine. *Marijuana and Health*. National Academy Press, Washington, D.C., 1982, p. 66.

102. Beaconsfield, P., Ginsburg, J., and Rainsbury, R. Marihuana smoking: cardiovasclar effects in man and possible mechanisms. *N. Engl. J. Med. 287*:209–212 (1972).

103. Martz, R., Brown, D.J., Forney, R.B., et al. Propranolol antagonism of marihuana-induced tachycardia. *Life Sci. 11*:999–1005 (1972).

104. Sulkowski, A., Vachon, L., and Rich, E.S. Propranolol effects on acute marihuana intoxication in man. *Psychopharmacology 52*:47–53 (1977).

105. Bright, T.P., Kiplinger, G.F. Brown, D., et al. Effects of beta-adrenergic blockade on marijuana-induced tachycardia, *National Academy of Sciences: Report of the 33rd Annual Scientific Meeting of the Committee on Problems of Drug Dependence*, Vol. 2. Washington, D.C., 1971.

106. Perez-Reyes, M., Lipton, M.A., Timmons, M.C., et al. Pharmacology of orally administered delta-9-tetrahydrocannabinol. *Clin. Pharmacol. Ther. 14*:48–55 (1973).

107. Kanakis, C.J., Pouget, J.M., and Rosen, K.M. The effects of delta-9-tetrahydrocannabinol (cannabis) on cardiac performance with and without beta blockage. *Circulation 53*:703–707 (1976).

108. Tashkin, D.P., Soares, J.R., Hepler, R.S., Shapiro, B.J., and Rachelefsky, G.S. Cannabis 1977. *Ann. Intern. Med. 89*:539–549 (1978).

109. Anonymous: Effects of marijuana on the respiratory and cardiovascular systems, Institute of Medicine. *Marijuana and Health*. National Academy Press, Washington, D.C., 1982, p. 67.

110. Kochar, M.S., and Hosko, M.J. Electrocardiographic effects of marihuana. *J.A.M.A. 225*:25–27 (1973).

111. Bernstein, J.G., Becker, D., Babor, T.F., and Mendelson, J.H. Physiological assessments: Cardiopulmonary function, J.H. Mendelson, A.M. Rossi, and R.E. Meyers, (eds.). *The Use of Marijuana: A Psychological and Physiological Inquiry*. Plenum Press, New York, 1974.

112. Benowitz, N.L, and Jones, R.T. Cardiovascular effects of prolonged delta-9-tetrahydrocannabinol ingestion. *Clin. Pharmacol. Ther. 18*:287–297 (1975).

113. Benowitz, N.L., and Jones, R.T. Effects of delta-9-tetrahydrocannabinol on drug distribution and metabolism. *Clin. Pharmacol. Ther. 22*:259–268 (1977).

114. Benowitz, N.L., and Jones, R.T. Prolonged delta-9-tetrahydrocannabinol ingestion: Effects of sympathomimetic amines and autonomic blockades. *Clin. Pharmacol. Ther. 21*:336–342 (1977).

115. Nowlan, R., and Cohen, S. Tolerance to marijuana: Heart rate and subjective "high." *Clin. Pharmacol. Ther. 22*:550–556 (1977).

116. Johnson, S., and Domino, E.F. Some cardiovascular effects of marihuana smoking in normal volunteers. *Clin. Pharmacol. Ther. 12*:762–768 (1971).

117. Anonymous: Effects of marijuana on the respiratory and cardiovascular systems, Institute of Medicine: *Marijuana and Health*. National Academy Press, Washington, D.C., 1982, p. 72.

118. Anonymous: Effects of marijuana on the respiratory and cardiovascular systems, Institute of Medicine. *Marijuana and Health*. National Academy Press, Washington, D.C., 1982, p. 70.

119. Anonymous: Effects of marijuana on the respiratory and cardiovascular systems, Institute of Medicine: *Marijuana and Health*. National Academy Press, Washington, D.C., 1982, p. 69.

120. Campbell, A.M.G., Evans, M., Thomson, J.L.G., Williams, M.J. Cerebral atrophy in young cannabis smokers. *Lancet* :1219–1225 (1975).

121. Anonymous: Effects of marijuana on the brain, Institute of Medicine: *Marijuana and Health*. National Academy Press, Washington, D.C., 1982, p. 87.

122. McGahan, J., Dublin, A., and Sassenrath, E. Long-term delta-9-tetrahydrocannabinol treatment. *Am. J. Dis. Child. 138*:1109–1112 (1984).

123. Purohit, V., Ahluwahlia, B.S., and Vigersky, R.A. Marijuana inhibits dihydrotestoserone binding to the androgen receptor. *Endocrinology 107*:848–850 (1980).

124. Kolodny, R.C., Masters, W.H., Kolodner, R.M., and Toro, G. Depression of plasma testosterone levels after chronic intensive marijuana use. *N. Engl. J. Med. 290*:872–874 (1974).

125. Mendelson, J.H., Kuehnle, J., Ellingboe, J., and Babor, T.F. Plasma testosterone levels before, during, and after chronic marihuana smoking. *N. Engl. J. Med. 291*:1051–1055 (1974).

126. Hembree, W.C., Nahas, G.G., Zeidenberg, P., and Huang, H.F.S. Changes in human spermatozoa associated with high-dose marihuana smoking, G.G. Nahas, and W.D.M. Paton (eds.). *Marihuana: Biological Effects. Analysis, Metabolism, Cellular Responses, Reproduction, and Brain*. Pergamon, Oxford, England, 1979, pp. 429–439.

127. Huang, H.F.S., Nahas, G.G., and Hembree, W.C. Effects of marihuana inhalation on spermatogenesis of the rat, G.G. Nahas and W.D.M. Paton (eds.). *Marihuana: Biological Effects. Analysis, Metabolism, Cellular Responses, Reproduction, and Brain*. Pergamon, Oxford, England, 1979, pp. 419–427.

128. Cohen, S. Marijuana and reproductive functions. *Drug Abuse and Alcohol. Newslett. 13*:1 (1985).

129. Bauman, J.E., Kolodny, R.C., Dornbusch, R.L., and Webster, S.K. Efectos endocrinos del use cronico de la mariguana en mujeres, *Simposio Internacional Sobre Actualizacion en Mariguana*. Tlalpan, Mexico, July 1979, vol. 10, pp. 85–97. [Cited in Institute of Medicine: *Marijuana and Health*. National Academy Press, Washington, D.C., 1982, p. 97.

130. Anonymous: Effects of marijuana on the brain, Institute of Medicine. *Marijuana and Health*. National Academy Press, Washington, D.C., 1982, p. 98.

131. Chakravarty, I., Sengupta, D., Bhattacharyya, P., and Ghosh, J.J. Effect of treatment with cannabis extract on the water and glycogen contents of the uterus in normal and estradiol-treated prepubertal rats. *Toxicol. Appl. Pharmacol. 34*:513–516 (1975).

132. Dixit, V.P., Arya, M., and Lohiya, N.K. The effect of chronically administered cannabis extract on the female genital tract of mice and rats. *Endokrinologie 66*:365–368 (1975).

133. Nir, I., Ayalon, D., Tsafiri, A., et al. Suppression of the cyclic surge of luteinizing hormone secretion and of ovulation in the rat by delta-1-tetrahydrocannabinol. *Nature 243*:470–471 (1973).

134. Ayalon, D., Nir, I., Cordova, T., et al. Acute effect of delta-1-tetrahydrocannibinol on the hypothalamo-pituitary-ovarian axis in the rat. *Neuroendocrinology 23*:31–42 (1977).

135. Marks, B.H. Delta-1-tetrahydrocannabinol and luteinizing hormone secretion. *Prog. Brain Res. 39*:331–338 (1973).

136. Tyrey, L. Delta-9-tetrahydrocannabinol suppression of episodic luteinizing hormone secretion in the ovariectomized rat. *Endocrinology 102*:1808–1814 (1978).

137. Besch, N.F., Smith, C.G., Besch, P.K., and Kaufman, R.H. The effect of marihuana (delta-9-tetrahydrocannabinol) on the secretion of luteinizing hormone in the ovariectomized Rhesus monkey. *Am. J. Obstet. Gynecol. 128*:635–642 (1977).

138. Asch, R.H., Fernandez, E.O., Smith, C.G., and Pauerstein, C.J. Precoital single doses of delta-9-tetrahydrocannabinol block ovulation in the rabbit. *Fertil Steril 31*:331–334 (1979).

139. Asch, R.H., Smith, C.G., Siler-Khodr, T.M., and Pauerstein, C.J. Effects of delta-9-tetrahydrocannabinol during the follicular phase of the Rhesus monkey (*Macaca mulatta*). *J. Clin. Endocrin. Metab. 52*:50–55 (1981).

140. Braude, M.C., and Ludford, J.P. *Marijuana Effects on the Endocrine and Reproductive Systems*. U.S. Government Printing Office, Washington, D.C., 1984, pp. 115–123.

141. Anonymous: Effects of marijuana on other biological systems, Institute of Medicine: *Marijuana and Health*. National Academy Press, Washington, D.C., 1982, p. 99.

142. Gerber, W.F., and Schramm, L.C. Effects of marihuana extract on fetal hamsters and rabbits. *Toxicol. Appl. Pharmacol. 14*:276–282 (1969).

143. Linn, S., and Schoenbaum, S.C. The association of marijuana use with outcome of pregnancy. *Am. J. Public Health 73*:1161 (1983).

144. Hingston, R., et al. Effects of maternal drinking and marijuana use on fetal growth and development. *Pediatrics 70*:539–546 (1982).

145. Abel, E.L. Prenatal exposure to cannabis: A critical review of effects on growth, development, and behavior. *Behav. Neurol. Biol. 29*:137 (1980).

146. Qazi, Q.H., Mariano, E., Milman, D.H., and Beller, E.,and Crombleholme, W. Abnormalities in offspring associated with prenatal marihuana exposure. *Dev. Pharmacol. Ther.* 8:141–148 (1985).

147. Jones, K.L., and Chernoff, G.F. Effects of chemical and environmental agents, R.K. Creasy, and R. Resnik (eds.). *Maternal Fetal Medicine*. Saunders, Philadelphia, 1984.

148. Anonymous: Effects of marijuana on other biological systems, Institute of Medicine: *Marijuana and Health*. National Academy Press, Washington, D.C., 1982, p. 100.

149. Sassenrath, E.N., Banovitz, C.A., and Chapman, L.F. Tolerance and reproductive deficit in primates chronically drugged with delta-9-THC. *Pharmacologist* 21:201 (1979).

150. Fried, P.A., Buckingham, M., and Von Kulmiz, P., Marijuana use during pregnancy and prenatal risk factors. *Am. J. Obstet. Gynecol. 146*:992–994 (1983).

151. Institute of Medicine: *Marijuana and Health*. National Academy Press, Washington, D.C., 1982.

152. Pinkert, T.M. (ed.). *Current Research on the Consequences of Maternal Drug Abuse*. NIDA Researrch Monograph 59. Department of Health and Human Services, Rockville, Maryland, 1985.

153. Braude, M.C., Ludford, J.P. (eds.). *Marijuana Effects on the Endocrine and Reproductive Systems: A RAUS Review Report*. NIDA Research Monograph 44. Department of Health and Human Services, Rockville, Maryland, 1984.

154. Fehr, K.O., and Kalant, H. (eds.). *Addiction Research Foundation/World Health Organization Meeting on Adverse Health and Behavioral Consequences of Cannabis Use*. Addiction Research Foundation, Toronto, 1983.

155. Marijuana and reproductive functions. *Psych. News* (Sep. 19): 13 (1986).

156. Murthy, et al. Long-term effects of marihuana smoke on uterine contractility and tumour development in rats. *West Indian J. Med. 34*:244 (1985).

157. Anonymous: Effects of marijuana on other biological systems, Institute of Medicine: *Marijuana and Health*. National Academy Press, Washington, D.C., 1982, p. 105.

21

Phencyclidine

A. James Giannini
Ohio State University, Columbus, Ohio

I. INTRODUCTION

Phencyclidine (PCP) is the prototypical member of a group of arylcyclohexylamines known as the "dissociatives." The name phencyclidine itself is the generic name of 1-(1-phenyl-cyclohexyl)piperidinehydrochloride. It was first released by Parke-Davis Laboratories in 1958 as a sedating anesthetic which produced an inconsistent amnesia. A particular benefit of this drug was that it caused no respiratory depression. Unfortunately, phencyclidine also produced postanesthetic depression, agitation, delirium, paranoia, psychosis, and occasional violence. As a result, it was removed from the pharmacopeia in 1965, two years later, it was reintroduced as a veterinary tranquilizer [1].

It was as a veterinary medication that phencyclidine entered the drug culture. It was first reported as a drug of abuse in the Haight Ashbury district of San Francisco in the late 1960s, where it received the name of the peace pill. Within 6 months, the abuse of phencyclidine had spread nationwide. Nationally, phencylidine became known as angel dust or PCP. It was an inexpensive, highly popular street drug, producing a unique combination of effects, including paradoxical excitation and sedation, hallucinations, anesthesia, dissociations, and euphoria. Phencyclidine was relatively easy to make and could be taken by a number of routes. These modalities of intake included smoking, insufflation ("snoring"), inhalation of fumes, ingestion, intravenous and intramuscular injection, enema, and douching [2].

Because of the above reasons, the abuse of phencyclidine burgeoned. By the early 1970s, it accounted for 25% of all mind-altering drugs then in use. During this time, approximately 6% of all Americans in the age group 12–17 had knowingly abused phencyclidine at least one time, whereas nearly another 15% those persons aged 18–25 had knowingly abused the drug. Because phencyclidine can be taken by a variety of routes and its effects mimic those of nearly all major neurotransmitters systems, it was used to adulterate such drugs as cocaine, amphetamine, lysergic acid, heroin, methaqualone, barbiturates, marijuana, ethychlorvinyl, methamphetamine, and dioxymethyalineamphetamine. As a result, nearly two-thirds of all phencyclidine is sold surreptitiously as an adulterant for another street drug. With both knowing and unknowing purchases of phencyclidine accounted for, it has been recently demonstrated that nearly 25% of all adults in the United States in 1988 have abused phencyclidine at least one time [3,4].

Phencyclidine was a legal drug until 1970 when it was removed from legal production by the Comprehensive Drug Abuse Prevention and Control Act. This drove phencyclidine production underground, where it was easily manufactured from piperidine precursors. Phencyclidine was easily prepared using piperidine, ether, other easily obtained amino acids, and a platinum catalyst (readily obtained from any automobile catalytic converter) or nickel catalyst (approximately $3.00 in American nickel coins). In response to this, U.S. Congress passed the Psychotropic Substances Act in 1978, which restricted the sale and manufacture of these piperidine precursors. This Act did not, however, in any way reduce the production or supply of phencyclidine or its analogues [5].

Phencyclidine is seen as a drug of downward demographic mobility. It is knowingly abused in the predominantly industrial areas in the United States. Key areas of addiction include the Chicago-Pittsburgh megalopolis, southern New York state, northern New Jersey, the greater Detroit area, metropolitan St. Louis, and southern California. The typical addict's profile is that of a 20-year-old white blue-collar male with a high school education employed in an unskilled or semiskilled occupation. Thirty-five percent of all knowing abusers become addicted to this drug. Phencyclidine is abused in the slums of the United States, where it is most often combined with cocaine. When combined with free-base cocaine, this form is known as space-base super-base, or majo [6].

In addition to those mentioned previously, common street names for phencyclidine include angel mist, animal crackers, cadillac, crystal, hog, shermies, surfers, and zombie dust. When dusted over marijuana, it is known as crystal joint or stepped on grass. When combined with cocaine hydrochloride, it is called snuff. It is occasionally mixed with heroin and called speed ball [1,2,7,8].

Phencyclidine presents a legal nightmare. It has been associated with multiple assaultive acts, including suicide, rape, and particularly brutal homicides. Self-inflicted burn injury, enucleation and disemboweling are representative examples of these suicidal and homocidal acts. Because of the usual unknowing nature of phencyclidine ingestion, and the amnestic effects produced, many individuals have committed brutal acts while under its influence and remembered none of their actions. Since phencyclidine is an anesthetic, various defensive techniques by the victim, including clubbing, biting, stabbing, and even gun shot wounds have little effect on the PCP-powered aggressor. The view of criminal culpability under phencyclidine is still under an evolutionary process. Verdicts in various cases in different legal jurisdictions in the United States have produced equally varied results. In some cases, phencyclidine has reduced the sentence, not affected the sentence in other cases, and in some cases in which the ingestion was involuntary, not guilty verdicts have been handed down. Generally, legal defenses have centered about two conditions: (1) inability to refrain from the criminal action and (2) inability to distinguish right from wrong [9].

II. CHEMICAL STRUCTURE

Phencyclidine belongs to the arylcyclohexylamines, a group of psychoactive drugs which are both pharmacologically and behaviorally distinct from all other classes of street drugs. It is composed of a phenyl group, a piperidine group, and a cyclohexyl ring. Crystallography studies have indicated that a electron-dense region in the area of the aromatic ring and the cyclohexyl ring are both required to produce specific psychoactive effects. Because of its cyclohexyl spine, phencyclidine when dissolved exists in equilibrium between two comformations with a phenyl grouping on both the axial and equatorial planes. The receptor activity of phencyclidine occurs when the phenyl group is in the axial plane. Phencyclidine's potency as a dissociative is thought to be a function of its three-ring structure and its unsaturated bond. Aliphatic analogues and bicyclic analogues have much less activity [10,11].

Replacement of the phenyl group with a thienyl group produces TCP, 1-(1-2-thienylcyclohexyl)piperidine, the most potent of all dissociatives. Substititing a pyrrolidine group for the piperindine group, results in the synthesis of PHP, 1-(1-phenylcyclohexyl)pyrrolidine, which is a frequent byproduct in the production of illicit PCP. It is only slightly less effective then PCP itself. It has particular abusive desirability that it is not detected in the thin-layer chromotographic analysis used by forensic laboratories [5,10–12].

The only legal analogue of phencyclidine is ketamine hydrochloride, which is sold under the trade name Ketalar for limited use in anesthesia. Ketamine has a 2-O-chloralphenyl-1-2-methylaminecyclohexanone configuration. Ketamine is a bicyclic, and it is markedly less potent than phencyclidine. The chloride side chain off the phenyl group further decreases its potency. Ketamine can be further modified to form PCE (cyclohexamine), N-ethyl-1-phenylcyclohexylamine, which is a byproduct of phencyclidine manufacture, and is also an active metabolite of phencyclidine [11].

III. METABOLISM AND EXCRETION

Response time to phencyclidine is a function of the delivery system. When phencyclidine is injected intravenously, there is a near-instantaneous response time of approximately 1–2 s. Inhalation of phencyclidine fumes brings a response within 30–60 s. Smoking phencyclidine causes effects to appear within 1–5 min, whereas ingestion delays an appearances of response time to about 20 min. The half-life of PCP ranges from 10 to 90 h, but some physicians have reported prolonged effects lasting up to 5 days [13].

Phencyclidine is a weakly basic compound with a pKa estimated between 8.5 and 9.5. It is readily lipid soluble and fairly soluble in chloroform, rather insoluble in alcohol, but absolutely insoluble in ether. Preparing PCP as a hydrochloric salt increases its solubility to 1:6 in water and in alcohol and 1:2 in chloroform. It does not, however, affect its ether solubility. In chloride form, PCP is a white, odorless, poorly crystalline powder with a melting point of about 230 °C and a molecular weight of 279.9 AWU. Owing to its mid-range pKa, PCP is very liquid soluble and is rapidly absorbed from the gastrointestinal tract. Initially, the acidic content of the stomach causes ionization of phencyclidine. Phencyclidine is temporarily trapped in the stomach, since the ionized form does not usually cross membrane barriers. However, in passing from the stomach into the relatively alkaline contents of the intestines, PCP is transformed into a nonionized lipophilic form. At the intestinal level, phencyclidine is reabsorbed and recirculated throughout the enteroheptic route. It is the enterohepatic circulation which accounts for the many frequent exacerbations and remissions seen during PCP intoxication. Ionization also occurs in the relatively acidic environment of the urinary bladder. Once phencyclidine and its active metabolites pass into the urinary tract, it is removed, from further reabsorption and recirculation by the body [14].

When phencyclidine is smoked, it is absorbed at about approximately a 40% rate. In addition, pyrrolysis of phencyclidine produces PC, 1-phenylcyclohexene, which is about 50% as active as PCP. Inhaled PCP and PC are trapped within the buccal mucosa, the bronchial tissue, and the lungs. From there, it is released to the systemic circulation. Both PCP and PC are excreted by the renal route [13,15].

Regardless of the mode of intake, PCP and all of its metabolites are excreted predominantly through the renal route. Ninety-five percent of phencyclidine is excreted renally, about 4.5% is excreted through the biliary-fecal route, and trace amounts are lost through the skin and tears. Two to ten percent of PCP can also be removed from the body via breast milk in nursing mothers. Fifty percent of all PCP is excreted in unchanged form. Renal clearance varies according to the pH of the urine. It averages approximately 0.38 L/min; nonrenal clearance averages 3.5 L/min [16].

Metabolism of PCP is hepatic; inactive forms of metabolites are formed by glucoronidation and hydroxylation. Approximately half of all PCP is excreted in unmetabolized form. The most common active metabolite is PHP, N-4-hydroxypiperidinephencyclidine and 4-hydroxycyclophencyclidine. The most common inactive metabolite is 4-dyhydroxy-cyclopiperidine [6].

It is estimated that about 35% of phencyclidine is free in the plasma, and it is therefore capable of crossing the blood-brain barrier. Binding occurs predominantly with albumin and 1-α-acid glycoprotein. High-density lipoproteins seem not to to be important in phencyclidine binding. Since a relatively large amount of phencyclidine circulates in unbound form, the effects of phencyclidine are not responsive to changes in binding capacity [17].

IV. NEUROTRANSMITTER ACTION

Central effects of phencyclidine are most often associated with increased glucose utilization in the areas of the limbic cortex, cingulate gyrus, the motor strip, the thalamus, and nucleus accumbens. Paradoxically, decreased activity is found in the auditory system. (Perhaps, this is the reason auditory hallucinations seldom occur in phencyclidine psychosis.) There is both stimulation and inhibition in various areas of the hypothalamus. Glucose utilization is also increased in certain discrete areas in the hippocampus such as the hippocampal body and the cingulate and antroventral thalamic projections. Phencyclidine also acts at multiple neurotransmitter systems and receptor sites [18,19].

A. PCP Receptor

Two PCP-specific receptor sites have been located. The first is a high-affinity binding site within the NDMA (N-methyl-D-aspartate) receptor channel [20]. This site is stimulated by glutamate, but it is irreversibly antagonized by metaphit, which acylates the receptor. It is noninteractive with either haloperidol, chlorpromazine, pimozide, naloxone, or the experimental drug SKF 10,047. While there is no known endogenous ligand for this site, another experimental drug, MK-801, which does act at this site, is being used as an investigatory tool [21,22].

When phencyclidine is given to the laboratory rat, 99.6% binds to the high-affinity PCP receptor with the remainder bound to all other receptor sites. The number of high-affinity PCP receptors in the rat is eight times greater than opiate receptors and four times greater than muscarinic receptors. Phencyclidine high-affinity receptors are located throughout the brain. Major sites of action include the hippocampus and its projections as well as the cingula. Minor areas of activity are found in the corpus callosum, inferior colliculi, locus ceruleus, medulla oblongata, and anterior pons. Interestingly, there have been no identified sites of activity in the cerebellum or spinal cord. This receptor type may act to prevent neuronal death through anoxia or hypoglycemia. In this way, abusers may be protected during periods of high-dose intoxication [20,22].

A second, low-affinity, PCP receptor site has also been isolated. It is insensitive to the effects of naloxone, haloperidol, chlorpromazine, and MK-801. Metaphit seems also not to interact with this site. In contradistinction, N-allylnormetazocine agonizes this site. No known endogenous ligand exists. The distribution of receptors sites has not yet been mapped [23].

B. Sigma Receptor

The sigma receptor was formerly considered to be an opioid receptor because it binds the opiate drug SKF-10,047. Unlike all opioid receptors, it is, however, insensitive to naloxone. The function of this receptor site and the hypothetical associated endogenous ligand are both unknown. Haloperidol antagonizes this receptor, but chlorpromazine and other phenothiazines are generally ineffective here [24].

C. Acetylcholine

Phencyclidine exerts an inhibitory action at cholinergic receptors in the central and peripheral nervous systems and the muscular system [25]. This action is due to its possession of the typical structure of anticholinergic drugs: It has a cationic head, a large hydroxy group, and a phenyl group. This arrangement is a characteristic of all dissociative compounds. Peripherally, PCP exerts an antinicotinic action in striate muscle. It also blocks potassium conduction and delays release of the neurotransmitter. While blocking neuromuscular transmission PCP depresses the rate of amplitude [20], causing a decrease in the rise of the action potential and actually prolongs it. As a result, PCP decreases voltage and concentration-dependent peak current and plate current [26]. A similar blockade of the potassium channel by PCP also depresses acetylcholine-induced secretion of catecholamines in the adrenals [27]. This depression was reversed with physostigmine and ingested calcium [28]. The role of calcium was not receptor direct but due to coupling of phencyclidine to nicotinic receptors [29]. This coupling has been hypothesized to be secondary to configurational changes of the receptor sites than of the PCP molecule itself. It is competitive with acetylcholine at muscarinic sites. There is also good evidence that PCP and other dissociatives act directly to block the cholinergic ionophore. It then decouples the linkage between this potassium ionaphore and nicotinic receptors. There is also a complex blockage of cholinergic-linked ion channels. Collaterally, phencyclidine seems to block both pseudocholinesterase and butylcholinesterase activity [30].

This anticholinergic activity produces specific behavioral effects, including catalepsy. The dissociatives produce hypersynchronous slow-wave activity on the electrocephlogram. These EEG changes have been reversed by physostigmine salicylate, a reversible inhibitor of cholinesterase [31]. When phencyclidine decreased an accuracy spatial alternation performance in rats, accuracy was improved by use of three separate muscarinic agents: pilocarpine, aracoline, and oxytremorine [32]. Clinically, physostigmine salicylate has been used to treat some of the symptoms of low-dose phencyclidine intoxication [33]. When physostigmine salicylate, 2 mg, was given intramuscularly, it decreased the frequency of resting tremor as well as horizontal and vertical nystagmus. It was also noted to reduce anxiety, conceptual disorganization, excitement, disorientation, and suspiciousness [25,33].

D. Dopamine

Several lines of evidence point to a role for dopamine in contributing to phencyclidine intoxication. Chronic phencyclidine use is associated with decreased levels of prolactin. Accordingly, there is a diminished response of thyroid-stimulating hormone when stimulated by thyroid-releasing hormone [34]. Phencyclidine has also been shown to enhance the effect of amphetamine-induced stereotypy [33]. The dopamine DA-2 blocker, haloperidol, has been shown to reverse both stereotypy and the prolactin suppression [35]. In the rat, at least, PCP also downregulates spiroperidol binding sites and increases their density in the striatum [36]. In clinical studies comparing such mixed DA-1 and DA-2 neuroleptics as chlorpromazine and fluphenazine with specific DA-2 neuroleptics such as pimozide and heloperidol there was a significantly greater response to the latter group of dopamine blockers [37–39].

Phencyclidine seems to act as a nonamphetamine stimulant at the storage vesicles in contradistinction to amphetamine which stimulates the release of newly synthesized dopamine [40]. In addition to causing release, PCP blocks reuptake, thus prolonging the action of dopamine in the presynatic cleft, but also reducing the recycling of the dopamine metabolite homovanillic acid. Thus, the overall supply of dopamine is decreased and may contribute to the global depression associated with phencyclidine addiction and abuse [41]. The increased release of dopamine seems to be due to a phencyclidine-induced prolonged action potential, which in turn is dependent upon phencyclidine's interaction with the presynaptic potassium channels [42]. Phencyclidine also seems to inhibit dopamine accumulation in the presynaptic vesicles and in synaptosomes.

While phencyclidine has strong hypertensive effects, this does not seem to be due to increased levels of peripheral dopamine. Rather, effects are due to increased stimulation of noradrenergic and adrenergic release in the adrenal medulla [43]. In fact, phencyclidine seems to have a minimal pheripheral dopaminergic role.

The addictive potential of phencyclidine resides in its effects on the teleomesencephalic system. Its dopamine agonism stimulates this primary "reward" system. Phencyclidine's dopaminergic effects seem to be mediated by opioids, since naloxone will block both low-dose "highs" as well as high-dose dysphoric episodes.

E. Opioid Systems

Anesthetic effects of phencyclidine and the other dissociatives especially ketamine, are due to their opiatelike properties [44]. Behaviorally, phencyclidine has been shown to affect both μ- and σ-opioid receptors. The μ-agonist, morphine, increases metenkephlin-induced phencyclidine ataxia, which is in turn blocked by naloxone [44]. In addition, patients have reported cross tolerance between phencyclidine and morphine. Methadone can suppress phencyclidine-induced behavior in rats, and meperidine can cause a similar effect in humans [45]. Acute phencyclidine intoxication causes decreased levels of metenkephlin in the striate bodies, medulla oblongata, mid brain and pons [46]. Acutely, phencyclidine increases metenkephlin. This points to a stimulatory-depletion role on the opioid system similar to phencyclidine's action on dopamine. In comparing the dissociatives with morphine, both phencyclidine and ketamine produce anesthetic effects equal to that of morphine. However, the duration of action of phencyclidine is at least one and one-half as long as that of either morphine or ketamine [45].

F. Gamma–Aminobutyric Acid

The role of the dissociatives on the GABA-ergic system is confusing and somewht controversial. Since phencyclidine seems to work at numerous receptor sites, an intellectual incision with Occam's razor suggests that it may in fact have GABA-antagonistic properties. It is well known that most initial effects of acute phencyclidine intoxication can be attenuated by administration of benzodiazepines (BZDs). Again, it is an open question as to whether this effect of benzodiazepine agonism of BZD receptors and GABA receptors might be an actual or pseudoeffect. Alternatively, BZD may indirectly attentuate the actions of PCP at multiple receptor sites and systems throughout the brain by inducing a relative shutdown. Certainly, more direct-acting GABA-ergic agonists such as both barbiturates and methaqualone are not particularly effective in treating phencyclidine intoxication [6].

G. Serotonin

The least evidence for phencyclidine action occurs at serotonergic receptor sites [5]. Phenomenologically, many of the phencyclidine-induced states are similar to those induced by lysergic acid diethylamide (LSD) and mescaline. There have been reports of geometricization of figures, vivid visual hallucinations, catelepsy, depersonalization, derealization, astral projections, and bodily misperceptions. Studies of REM-phase sleep produce similar tracings in both phencyclidine- and LSD-treated patients [6]. There also appears to be cross tolerance to mescaline, psilocybin, and lysergic acid. Rats' performance in two-level drug discrimination tests can often not distinguish LSD and mescaline from phencyclidine. However, in contradistinction to the above evidence, post-LSD depression has been reported to respond only to fluoxetine, a pure serotonergic antidepressant, whereas phencyclidine withdrawal depression responds best to desipramine, a predominantly noradrenergic antidepressant [6].

V. GENERAL PRESENTATION OF INTOXICATION

The presentation signs of phencyclidine intoxication varies according to the dosage. These tend to occur at all levels of intoxication and are useful when making quick diagnostic assumptions in the office or the emergency room. Eight signs, the majority of which are usually always present, have been arranged in useful mnemonic form to aid learning. They are [47]:

Rage
Enlarged pupils
Delusions

Dissociatives
Amnesia
Nystagmus
Excitation
Skin dry and red

Other common, but not consistent, features include ataxia, dysarthria, hyperacusis, hypertension, rigidity, and seizures. While the severity of many of these signs are dose dependent, the actual signs tend to present across the full range of dosages. The effects of the PCP receptor tends to modulate effects of other sites during acute intoxication [48].

VI. TREATMENT OF INTOXICATION: THE ANTIDOTAL STRATEGY

As has been demonstrated above, phencyclidine works at a number of receptor sites. Consequently, there is no one specific antidote for acute intoxication as there is, for example, in cocaine or opiate abuse. Specific antidotal strategies have evolved to treat the presentation of specific symptom complexes. The antidotal model is based on the hypothesis that specific symptom clusters are caused by a predominance of activity of one specific neurotransmitter system [19]. This dose-dependent receptor specificity is thought to be due to the function of the particular dosage. Clinically, the major symptoms are due to the actions at cholinergic, dopaminergic, and opioid receptors [49,50]. Accompanying this specific antidotal strategy is a generalized "ion trapping" approach.

At low levels of abuse, with a dosage range of 1–10 mg, PCP acts predominantly as an anticholinergic compound. In addition to the signature horizontal nystagmus and red dry skin, there is photodermititis and mydriasis. The EKG often shows ST depression, T-wave flattening or inversion, arrythmias, widening of the QRS interval, and occasionally progression of U waves. Occasionally, circus rhythms and Q waves are seen. Treatment with this presentation is the same as for all anticholinergic presentations. Give physostigmine salicylate, 2 mg, intramuscularly every 20 min until psychosis remits or the QRS interval contracts to less then 10 mm [33,51]. It should be noted that in using physostigmine, occasionally an emergency arises which results in bronchial secretion plugging the respiratory system. Because of this problem, it is recommended that a trachial suction pump be available. Other peripheral complications caused by anticholinergic effects respond to physostigmine treatment. To assess this, the physician should auscultate the abdomen and palpate the area of the bladder. Obtain a flat plate x-ray of the abdomen should it be available to help further assist in the diagnosis. Foley catheters can be used to assist urination. A careful assessment of fluid intake and urinary output can be used to follow the course of phencyclidine intoxication much as the anticholinergic effects as can an EKG monitor [41].

Hypertensive crises often occur in phencyclidine intoxication and are due to atropinic actions upon the adrenal medulla. By blocking cholinergic receptors, large amounts of norepinephrine are released. To block these catecholiminergic effects, administer propranolol, 1 mg, intravenously by the titration method. If the patient is an asthmatic, propranolol should not be used. In the latter case, give diaoxide, 2.5 mg/kg, intravenously in a 10- to 30-s infusion [6].

At levels of moderate intoxication (from 5 to 15 mg) there seems to be a predominant dopaminergic effect [14]. Presentations include seizures, myoclonus, stereotypy, violence, paranoia, delusions, excitement, agitation, fever, hypersalivation, mutism and hyperreflexia. The clinical manifestations seem to be a result of dopaminergic actions at DA-2 receptors in the striatal and mesolimbic areas [52]. Since phencyclidine's dopaminergic actions occur at predominantly DA-2 receptors, it is recommended that DA-2 antagonists be prescribed. Haloperidol, 5 mg q 20 min, generally will block all the above symptoms by the second to fifth dose [53]. Usually anticholinergics such as diphenhydramine or benztropine maleate are not necessary because of phencyclidine's anticholinergic properties. If haloperidol is ineffective, give pimozide, another DA-2 antagonist, 2–5 mg, every 20–30 min [39]. In comparison with other neuroleptics, the butyrophenones, haloperidol and pimozide, where found to be superior to all phenothiazines, molidones, and loxapine. This is probably because much of phenothiazine's action is diffused between DA-1 and DA-2 receptors, whereas the butyropohenones are much more specifically acting agents. It cannot be stressed enough that the aliphatic and the piperidine phenothiazines are to be avoided because of their strong anticholinergic effects. When used as antidotal medications, the combined anticholinergic effects of aliphatics or piperidines with phencyclidine may precipitate cardiac arrythmias and occasionally produce a fatality [39].

Some clinical researchers have used GABA-ergic drugs to treat the medium-dosage range of phencyclidine intoxication. They have hypothesized that PCP is mutually antagonistic to GABA receptors in the mesolimbic and striatal systems. It may also hypothesized that PCP can cause a reduction in GABA concentration at these areas. Benzodiazepines as well as the experimental compound, baclofen, have been shown useful to treat agitation caused by phencyclidine, ketaine, PCP, PHP, and PCE [6]. Convulsions which occur when dopaminergic systems are stimulated can respond to diazepam, 2–5 mg, by slow intravenous push [53]. While benzodiazepines are undoubtedly useful, it should be stressed that they also inhibit hepatic metabolism. As a result, the half-life of PCP can be prolonged sometimes by as much as 100–200%.

At very high dosage ranges of PCP intoxication of more then 15 mg the opioid systems seem to predominate [57]. Fever can reach as high as 103 °F. Arrythmias are more frequent and the patient complains of encopresis. Tactile as well as visual hallucinations occur. The patient is hypertensive and hyporeflexic. Opisthotonus occurs and the rate of convulsions are much more frequent. Patients may become catatonic. This latter symptom is a very poor prodromal sign, since it leads to coma and possible death [53].

There is some indication that this dosage range produces a dopaminelike presentation which is under control of the opioid systems. Haloperidol should again be tried. If this is not successful by the third dosage, then give the synthetic opiate meperidine, 50 mg, intravenously every 20 min. While meperidine is not significantly more effective then haloperidol, in controlled studies it did seem to improved those cases which are haloperidol resistent [45]. Although there have been some reports of the success of naloxone administration in the treatment of PCP intoxication, it should be noted tht this medication can cause hyperthermia in low-dose phencyclidine intoxication and hypothermia in high-dose phencyclidine intoxication [7]. It should, therefore, be used only with great caution and limited to cases in which haloperidol, pimozide, and meperidine have all failed. If hyperthermia goes beyond 103 °F, cooling blankets and bathes should be given immediately.

Since the patient is anesthetic and paranoid, he or she is capable of great violence. There are numerous reports of medical and nursing personnel being seriously injured and even killed by phencyclidine-intoxicated patients who were later amnestic for the entire episode [14]. Because of the agitation and anethesia, patients can tear their own muscle tissue without awareness. Myoglobinuria can be a more than an occasional and can have a potentially lethal result. Urine should be checked and if positive, the patient should be treated by renal dialysis as soon as possible. Again, anticholinergic medications are to be avoided if meperidine is used at this dosage range [54]. Not only may they enhance the anticholinergic action of phencyclidine, but some evidence suggests that anticholinergics may also enhance opiate action in much the same manner as tripelenamine enhances the effects of pentazocine.

Ion trapping is a concept which utilizes the relative insolubility of the ionized form of phencyclidine to isolate it from the systemic circulation. To accomplish this isolation, the environments of the gastrointestinal tract and bladder are acidified and the phencyclidine isolated and sequestered. To isolate recently ingested phencyclidine, administer magnesium sulfate into the stomach via nasogastric tube at a dosage of 0.3 gm/kg. This will maintain the inactive ionized state and also stimulate fecal elimination. When phencyclidine is used in any form, inject 1000 mg of ascorbic acid every 6 h for the first day and then give 1000 mg/day orally thereafter. It is the key player in the ion trapping protocol. Ascorbic acid acidifies the urine and, therefore, renders ionized phencyclidine incapable of reentering the systemic circulation. To speed the elimination of this ionized form, give furosemide, 40 mg intramuscularly in combination with a 0.9 N sodium chloride an intravenous drip at maximum amount of centimeters tolerated per minute.

Some clinicians have recommended that phencyclidine patients be pushed to drink cranberry juice to further acidify the urine. Cranberries are a source of hippuric acid, a urinary acidifying agent. It is questionable, however, that this acid has much addictive clinical effect. It is imperative that a urinary pH of 5.5 or lower be maintained. With ascorbic acid, renal clearance can be boosted from 0.3 L½min to 3.0 L/min. Also, without ascorbic acid, the urinary route accounts for only 9% of total secretion. Urinary acidification can increase this rate so that the proper pH elimination of the urinary tract is boosted to approximately 70%.

Ascorbic acid also plays a direct role on the central nervous system. It has been shown to significantly increase haloperidol's activity in treating phencyclidine as well as amphetamine psychosis [55]. It has also been noted that ascorbic acid has direct antipsychotic effects in phencyclidine intoxication independent of those of haloperidol's effects [55,56]. While mandelamine is also a useful acidifying agent, it lacks ascorbic acid's direct effect in psychosis and interactive effects with haloperidol.

Long-term phencyclidine addiction predisposes the patient to the postwithdrawal state. Patients seem to be lethargic, depressed, and without ambition. There are disturbances in appetite and sleep. Diurnal mood variations have been noted. Libido is much decreased and this is seen as a component of the overall anhedonic state [49]. Desipramine, 200–300 mg q day, maintained over a 3- to 8-month period has proven quite effective in treating this [57]. Desipramine should never be started in cases of high levels of intoxication owing to exacerbation of anticholinergic effects. Rather it should be prescribed 2–3 days after initial antipsychotic treatment.

Special problems occur in treating the pregnant or nursing mother who abuses phencyclidine. Since phencyclidine as lipid soluble, it passes through the placental barrier. Indeed, it has been reported to pass into the amniotic fluid and umbilical cord blood [58]. Affected children are born with persistent hypertonicity, tremor, increased startle reflex, elevated serum bilirubin, coarse tremors, and, occasionally, generalized spasticity. There have also been single case reports of mongoloid features [59]. In the neonate, acidification has usually resulted in a significant metabolic acidosis. Neurological symptoms can be partially treated with maintenance phenobarbitol, 5 mg/kg/day for 7–10 days. Phencyclidine also passes into the breast milk and affects nursing infants [60]. The presentation is again dependent upon the relative dosage. Except in cases of high levels of intoxication, the best treatment is withdrawal. Pharmacological treatment should be approached with extreme caution in this age group.

REFERENCES

1. Giannini, A.J. PCP-Detecting the abuser. *Med. Aspects Hum. Sexual. 21*(1):100 (1987).
2. Giannini, A.J., and Slaby, A.E. *Handbook of Overdose and Detoxification Emergencies*, Medical Examination, New Hyde Park, New York, 1983.
3. DiPalma, J.R. Phencyclidine: Angel dust. *Am. Fam. Physician 20*:120–122 (1979).
4. Sioris, L., and Krenselok, E. Phencyclidine intoxication. *Am. J. Hosp. Pharm. 35*:1362–1366 (1978).
5. Giannini, A.J., Loiselle, R.H., and Giannini, M.C. Phencyclidine and the dissociatives. *Med. Psychiatry 3*(3):197 (1987).
6. Giannini, A.J., and Slaby, A.E. *Drugs of Abuse*, Medical Economics, Oradell, New Jersey, 1989.
7. Giannini, A.J., and Price, W.A. PCP: Management of acute intoxication. *Med. Times 113*(9):43 (1985).
8. Peterson, R.C., and Stillman, R.C. Phencyclidine—An overview. *N.I.D.A. Res. Monogr. Serv. 21*:1–17 (1978).
9. Ohio *vs* Burke, 1983.
10. Snyder, S.H. Phencyclidine. *Nature 285*:355 (1980).
11. Kalii, A. Structure-activity relationship of phencyclidine derivatives. *Psychopharmacol. Bull. 16*:54 (1980).
12. Budd. R.D. PHP, a new drug of abuse. *N. Engl. J. Med.* 303–588 (1980).
13. Cook, C.E., Brine, D.R., and Jeffcoat, A.R. Phencyclidine disposition after intravenous and oral doses. *Clin. Pharmacol. Ther. 31*:625 (1982).
14. Giannini, A.J. *Biological Foundation of Clinical Psychiatry*. Elsevier/Medical Examination, New York, 1986.
15. Freeman, A.S., and Martin, B.R. Quantification of PCP and identification of PCE as a pyrolysis product. *J. Pharmacol. Sci. 70*:1002 (1981).
16. Domino, E.F. *Phencyclidine: Historical and current perspectives*. NPP Books, Ann Arbor, 1981.
17. Giles, H.G., Corrigall, W.A., and Khouw, W.A. Plasma binding of phencyclidine. *Clin. Pharmacol. Ther. 3*:77 (1982).
18. Davis, B.M., and Beech, H.R. The effects of 1-arylcyclohexylamine on twelve normal volunteers. *J. Ment. Sci. 106*:912 (1960).
19. Giannini, A.J., and Giannini, M.C. Antidotal strategies in phencyclidine intoxication. *Int. J. Psychiatry Med. 14*:315 (1984).

20. Computon, R.P., Contreras, P.C., and O'Donohue, T.L. The NDMA antagonists, 2-amino-7-phosphoheptarate, produces PCP-like behavioral effects in rats. *Eur. J. Pharmacol.* (in press).

21. Vincent, J.P., Kartulouski, D., and Geneste, P. Interaction of phencyclidine with a specific receptor in rat membranes. *Proc. Natl. Acad. Sci. U.S.A.* 76:4678 (1979).

22. Maragos, W.F., Chu, D.C.M., and Grenamyre, J.T. High correlation between localization of TCP binding and NDMA receptor. *Eur. J. Pharmcol.* 123:173 (1986).

23. Rafferty, M.F., Mattson, M.V., and Giannini, A.E. A specific acetylating agent for the [3H] phencyclidine receptors in rat brain. *F.E.B.S.* 181:318 (1985).

24. Martin, W.R., and Eades, C.G. Effects of morphine and malorpine-like drugs in chronic spinal dogs. *J. Pharmacol. Exp. Ther.* 197:516 (1976).

25. Castellani, S., Adams, P.M., and Giannini, A.J. Physostigmine treatment of acute phencyclidine intoxication. *J. Clin. Psychiatry* 43:10 (1982).

26. Vincent, J.P., Bidards, J.N., and M. Lazdowski. Identification and properties of phencyclidine binding sites in nervous tissue. *Fed. Proc.* 42:2570 (1983).

27. Malave, A., Borowitz, J.L., and Yim, G.K.W. Block by phencyclidine of acetycholine barium induced adrenal catecholamine secretion. *Life Sci.* 33:516 (1983).

28. Oswald, R.E. Effects of calcium on the binding of phencyclidine to acetycholine receptor-rich membrane fragments from Torpedo California electroplague. *J. Neurochem.* 41:1077 (1983).

29. Gabrielevitz, A., Kloog, Y., and Kalin, A. Interaction of phencyclidine and adamuntyl derivatives with muscarinic receptors. *Life Sci.* 26:89 (1980).

30. Kloog, Y., Rehavi, M., and Maayani, S. Anticholinesterase and antiacetylcholinesterase activity of phenylclclohexylamine derivatives. *Eur. J. Pharmacol.* 45:221 (1977).

31. Winters, W.D., and Kott, K.J. Nonpharmacological interaction ketamine and physostigmine, diazepam and propranolol. *Proc. West. Pharmacol. Soc.* 19:230 (1976).

32. Glick, S.D., Cox, R.D., and Maayani, S. Anticholinergic behavioral effects of phencyclidine. *Eur. J. Pharmacol.* 59:103 (1979).

33. Castellani, S., Giannini, A.J., and Adams, P.M. Physostigmine and haloperidol treatment of acute phencyclidine intoxication. *Am. J. Psychiatry* 139:508 (1982).

34. Giannini, A.J., Malone, D.A., and Loiselle, R.H. Blunting of TSH response to TRH in chronic cocaine and phencyclidine abusers. *J. Clin. Psychiatry* 48:25 (1987).

35. Lasarsky, D., Saller, C.F., and Bayard, M.A. Effects of phencyclidine on rat prolactin dopamine receptor and locomotor activity. *Life Sci.* 32:2725 (1983).

36. Robertson, H.A. Chronic phencyclidine-like binding produces a decrease in 3H-spiroperidol binding in rat straitum. *Eur. J. Pharmacol.* 78:363, 1982.

37. Castellani, S., Giannini, A.J., and Boeringa, J.A. Phencyclidine intoxication: Assessment of possible antidotes. *J. Toxicol. Clin. Toxicol.* 19(3):313 (1982).

38. Giannini, A.J. Eighan, M.J., and Giannini, M.C. Comparison of haloperidol and chlorpromazine in the treatment of phencyclidine psychosis: Role of the DA-2 receptor. *J. Clin. Pharmacol.* 61:401, 1980.

39. Giannini, A.J., Nageotte, C., and Loiselle, R.H. Comparison of chlorpromazine, perphenazine, haloperidol and pimozide in the treatment of phencyclidine psychosis. *J. Toxicol. Clin. Toxicol.* 22:573 (1985).

40. Vickroy, T.M., and Johnson, K.M. Effects of phencyclidine on the release and synthesis of newly formed dopamine. *Neurophamacology* 22:839 (1983).

41. Giannini, A.J., and Gold, M.S. Cocaine abuse: Demons within. *Primary Care/Emerg. Decision* 4(9):34 (1988).

42. Blaustein, M.P., and Ickowicz, R.K. Phencyclidine in nanomolar concentrations binds to synaptosomes and blocks potassium channels. *Proc. Natl. Acad. Sci. U.S.A.* 80:3855 (1983).

43. Robertson, H.A. Chronic d-amphetamine and phencyclidine: Effects on dopamine agonist and antagonist binding sites in the central and peripheral nervous systems. *Brain Res.* 267–279 (1983).

44. Castellani, S., Giannini, A.J., and Adams, P.M. Effects of naloxone, metenkephlin and morephine on phencyclidine-induced behavior in the rat. *Psychopharmacology* 78:76 (1982).

45. Giannini, A.J., Loiselle, R.H., and Giannini, M.C. Comparison of chlorpromazine and meperidine in the treatment of phencyclidine psychosis. *J. Clin. Psychiatry 46*:52 (1985).

46. Nabeshima, T., Hiramatsu, M., and Amano, M. Chronic phencyclidine increase methionine enkephlin in mouse striatum. *Neurosci. Lett. 37*:69–74 (1983).

47. Giannini, A.J. Red Danes. *Primary Care 3*(11):53 (1987).

48. Giannini, A.J. Catecholamine depletion suggested as biological tie between cocaine withdrawal and depression. *Natl. Inst. Drug Abuse Notes 2*(2):5 (1987).

49. Giannini, A.J. Drug abuse and depression. *Neurobiol. Aging 9*(1):26 (1988).

50. Giannini, A.J., Armbrechet, C.A., and King, M.S. Anxiolytic response to buspirone in chronic cocaine and phencyclidine dine abusers. *J. Clin. Pharmacol. 27*:705 (1987).

51. Giannini, A.J., and Castellani, S. A case of PHP intoxication treated with pysostigmine. *J. Toxicol. Clin. Toxicol. 19*:505 (1982).

52. Giannini, A.J., Kalavsky, S., and Loiselle, R.H. Possible role of the DA-2 receptor in phencyclidine psychosis. *Soc. Neurosci. Abst. 9*:33 (1983).

53. Giannini, A.J., and Price, W.A. PCP intoxification. A step-by-step approach. *Emerg. Decisions 3*:57 (1982).

54. Giannini, A.J., Giannini, M.C., and Lazarus, H.D. Absence of response to histamine-1 blockage in phencyclidine toxicity. *J. Clin. Pharmacol. 26*:716 (1986).

55. Giannini, A.J., Loiselle, R.H., and Giannini, M.C. Augmentation of haloperidol by ascorbic acid in phencyclidine intoxication. *Am. J. Psychiatry 144*:1207 (1987).

56. Giannini, A.J. Ascorbic acid and dopamine activity. *Am. J. Psychiatry 145*:905 (1988).

57. Giannini, A.J., Malone, D.A., and Giannini, M.C. Treatment of chronic cocaine and phencyclidine abuse with desipramine. J. Clin. Pharmacol. 26:211 (1986).

58. Kaufman, K.R., Petruska, R.A., and Pitts, F.N. PCP in amniotic fluid and breast milk. *J. Clin. Psychiatry 44*:296 (1983).

59. Strauss, A.A., Houchang, P., and Madanlou, H.D. Neonatal manifestations of maternal PCP abuse. *Pediatrics 68*:550 (1981).

60. Nicholas, J.M., Lipschitz, J., and Schreiber, F.C. Phencyclidine—Its transfer across the placenta as well as into breast milk. *Am. J. Obstet. Gynecol. 143*:143 (1982).

22

The Volatile Agents

A. James Giannini
Ohio State University, Columbus, Ohio

I. INTRODUCTION

Inhalation of volatile agents, although commonly thought of as a phenomenon of the post–World War II period, dates back at least 2500 years. It has been reported by contemporaries that the ancient oracles of Delphi utilized natural carbon dioxide vents to induce a trancelike state. Other oracles of that time created trance-inducing fumes by burning laurel leaves in a copper calyx [1]. A carbon dioxide–induced hypoxia was reportedly generated by the berserkers and dervishes of the Arab Ascendancy. It was the Arab chemists of the medieval era who discovered the distillation process and made volatiles available [2]. However, they were not used as drugs of abuse until the advent of the twentieth century.

Nitrous oxide and other anesthetics were the first mass produced and popularly abused inhalants. In addition to its use in the operating theater, nitrous oxide was widely abused in the parlors of middle-class Victorian America. An avant-garde host or hostess would see to it that the guests were supplied with nitrous oxide. This "laughing gas" was passed about from person to person so that the euphoriant effects could be shared by all of the party goers. Nitrous oxide abuse was also supplemented by abuse of chloroform and ether, which produced similar results in similar circumstances. These effects were quickly soon sought after by many Americans and the various forms of laughing gases became available for use by adolescents and adults and later children in America's amusement parks. It has also been reported by Frank Harris that laughing gas was also a popular aid in the bordellos of the United States, France, and the United Kingdom [3,4].

Petroleum distillates became a source of abuse after mass production of the automobile. The needs of the automotive engine as well as the privacy afforded by the automobiles's interior soon made gasoline-sniffing afficionadoes out of members of the rumble-seat set. In England, G.T. racing enthusiasts would inhale the fumes generated by pouring camphor on red-hot iron ingots. Abuse of petroleum distillates declined during the 1920s. This was probably in response to the more enticing charms of bathtub gin and other forms of illegal alcohol during Prohibition [5].

In the 1930s, gasoline sniffing again became a minor rage. Also, other forms of inhalant abuse became popular in small subcultures. The advent of the seltzer bottle, popularized by Fred Astaire movies and other similar movies, provided a form of easily obtainable compressed carbon dioxide in the form of "charges." These were gas cartridges which helped put sparkle in the mixers and spritzers of the art deco era. Also abused for similar purposes was the acetone found in nail polish remover and nail polish as well as the numerous solvents found in some French perfumes. By the 1950s, adolescent hobbiests were able to choose from a large menu of volatile agents. Rubber cement was a widely used adhesive which contained large amounts of isopropanol, toluene, acetone, styrene, xylene, and hexane. Model paint spray was also a source of isopropanol and toluene. Plastic glues were rich sources for acetone and toluene. Toluene, naphtha, and acetone as well as methylene, chloride, methanol, and benzene were used to produce paint lacquers. Nitrogenated inert compound gases also became popularily abused as they propelled the whipped cream of the war babies' palates as well as the delirium of their parents so inclined to abuse [6].

In the late 1960s and early 1970s, marijuana- and tobacco-containing cigarettes were soaked in formaldehyde to produce intense hallucinatory effects. Spray paint also became not only a source of graffiti but one of brain abuse. Toluene or chlorinated aliphatic paint was sprayed into plastic bags and inhaled by the abusers. By the 1980s, trichlorethylene-containing typewriter fluid became such an abused product that many Fortune 500 companies had to store their supply of this commodity under lock and key.

Today, with one exception, solvent abuse is limited to the young. That single exception are the nitrites, which are used as sexual aids by middle-aged and elderly men [7]. Except for this specific group, most substance abusers are white and black males under the age of 14. Abuse of inhalants has continued at a steady level from 1975 to the present. Even when initial abuse starts, the likelihood of solvent addiction continuing past the high school years is quite minimal. Twenty percent of all American high school students have reported experimenting with inhalants at least once during their high school career. Another 10% have abused the nitrites, although not for sexual purposes. Addiction, however, is limited to less than one high school senior per thousand. Highest abuse has been reported on North American Indian reservations. In the Coulehan study, over 11% of Navajo high school students were reported to have tried sniffing gasoline, whereas 7.5% were addicted [8].

It was also further reported in other studies that nearly all children on a number of American Indian reservations have experimented with gasoline. As a high abuse-potential group, nearly one in five Native Americans abuse solvents more than once, and 5–10% are addicted to them. Another high-abuse group are American Hispanics. While only about 20% of all teenage Americans abuse inhalants, it has been reported that a 25–30% occasional abuse rate is seen and 0.5% addiction rate is seen in Hispanics [9].

The most commonly abused volatiles are those which contain chlorinated aliphatic compounds or toluene. Also in widespread abuse are the aromatic hydrocarbons, carbon dioxide and other propellents, glue, and spray paint. Nitrates are seen only in specific population groups. Since the halogenated hydrocarbons are the most dangerous of all the inhalants, they are seen most often in emergency room reports and on police blotters [10].

The volatiles remain popular for four reasons: their availability, the absence of legal sanction against their purchase, their low-cost, and the rapid onset of mind-altering effects. The inhaling of solvents usually produces effects within seconds or minutes. The "high" usually is associated with euphoria, loss of inhibitions, and increased aggressiveness or sexual performance.

Unfortunately, the high associated with solvents is associated with a syndrome of sudden death. Most of these deaths are derived from, but not limited to, the aerosol sprays. The major cause of death is cardiac arrythmia. This arrythmia arises from a variety of functions, including hypercapnea, increased psychosomotor activity, and stress. It is felt that these three factors then potentiate the effects of an epinephrine rush upon the heart. Other sources of death include laryngospasm. The halogenated hydrocarbons, especially Freon, are the compounds most associated with the laryngospasms. Progressive central nervous system depression with failing respiratory responses are another major source of death. A minor source of death is caused by gastroesophageal reflux into the respiratory tract owing to central suppression of the gag reflex. Indirectly, death may result from inhalation of volatiles through plastic bags. The combination of sedation, central nervous system depression, and suffocation produce death by asphyxiation.

An addiction syndrome occurs with the use of volatiles. It is estimated that 5% of those who experiment with the various volatiles become addicted. The sites of addiction are the dopaminergic "reward" centers of the teleomesencephalic system. While the ultimate mechanism appears to be dopaminergic, there may be GABA-ergic or enkephalinergic mediation. There is also some preliminary research which indicates cross tolerance exists between various volatile agents. The typical withdrawal symptoms which follow cessation of volatile abuse usually occur within 6–24 h after the last dose. The withdrawal complex includes anxiety, insomnia, irritability, cramping, parathesias, fine resting tremors, and, occasionally, seizures. Delirium tremens has also been reported with toluene and naphthalene abuse [11].

Teratogenic effects vary from solvent to solvent. Some studies report congential deformities in the children of volatile-abusing mothers, whereas other studies report no such abnormalities. While the data are not conclusive, it would behoove those physicians treating volatile abusers to warn them of possible adverse effects on their unborn child [12]. The general intoxication with volatiles involves several stages. It progresses from euphoria through an excitatory phase, which is followed by a phase of confusion, concluding with a final phase of central nervous depression. In the first phase, there is a feeling of grandiosity, euphoria, and excitement. These sensations are accompanied by visual, auditory hallucinations; lightheadedness; nausea and vomiting; sensations that one's head is expanding and body is floating; and a frontal headache. If volatile use persists, there is a period of confusion, the patient exhibits a lost of inhibitions, and there are delusions of vulnerability, impulsivity, and feelings that one's head or body is floating. There are also associated frontal headaches, tinitis, blurred vision, double vision, photosensitivity, photophobia, conjunctivitis with rhinitis, and protracted coughing. At the end of the phase, there is persistent vomiting, diarrhea, myalgia, arthralgia, and anginalike chest pain. In the final and most dangerous phase, the patient loses all control of coordination as well as urine and anal sphincter tone. There is dysarthria, hyporeflexia, and seizures. Persistent use of volatiles at this point usually results in a terminal cardiac arrest or respiratory arrest. Addiction may result after 3–6 months of frequent abuse [13–15].

II. TOXICITY OF VARIOUS VOLATILES

A. Alcohols

The most commonly abused alcoholic solvents are ethanol, methanol, and isopropanol [16–17]. Methanol, or wood alcohol, is the most dangerous member of this group. It is used in solvents, paints, and resin. Initial symptoms include abdominal cramping, severe pancephalic headache, emesis which may be projectile, nausea with vertigo, and generalized weakness. A delayed effect of methanol is caused by hepatic metabolism of methanol to form formaldehyde. Formaldehyde then causes edema of the retina. The effects of an edematous retina include blurred vision, photophobia, arreflexia, and persistent mydriasis. Continued high levels of formaldehyde abuse cause eventual blindness. It is also associated with sterility in the male.

Formaldehyde is in turn metabolized to formic acid, which is associated with destruction of the ganglionic cells, the caudate, and the putamen [16].

Isopropanol is also found in paints as well as perfumes. Its most common source of abuse is rubbing alcohol. High levels of ingested or inhaled isopropanol can cause severe central nervous depression and it is associated by a depression period. Death by isopropanol narcosis is not an uncommon result. Isopropanol is metabolized to acetone in the liver and then secreted through the lungs. Treatment for acute intoxication is hemodialysis. There is no known treatment for the effects of chronic abuse. Ethanol inhalation or addiction is generally not the severe health problem that ethanol ingestion is.

B. Nitrites

The nitrites involve a rather unique group in that they are abused primarily by middle-age and elderly men [18–21]. Nitrites tend to produce arterial dilation and have thus been used in the treatment of angina pectoris and cyanide and sulfate poisoning. As such, they are able to produce sustained penile erection and delay ejaculation by the vasodilation of the penile artery. Amyl nitrite perles are available from pharmacies for the treatment of angina, and in factory dispensaries in the chemical industry where potentially poisonous compounds such as cyanide and sulfites are produced. They are commonly sold as a black market drug to heterosexual males, although they have gained increased popularity with homosexual men.

In addition to the enhancement of orgasm, there are acute effects of giddiness, dizziness, and syncope, which are believed to be associated with hypotension and cerebral ischemia secondary to the vasodilation. Other effects have included confusion, methemoglobinemia, tachycardia, and convulsions. A sudden death syndrome results from cardiac and central effects.

Addiction is associated with a distinct set of symptoms which include abdominal cramping, cyanosis, diarrhea, emesis, giddiness, persistent hypertension, changes in libido, nausea, and tachypnea. If in response to these symptoms or owing to a lack of supply, the nitrite abuser discontinues the use of the nitrite, he usually experiences postural hyportension, postural weakness, severe headaches, and dizziness. Withdrawal symptoms usually disappear after several days. Analgesics, such as aspirin or even morphine, do not generally help the cramping or pain. Cyanosis is due to methemoglobinemia. If methemoglobinemia is greater than 30%, it is imperative to give oxygen as soon as possible, usually via a Venturi mask. Methyline blue 1% solution is usually administered at 0.1–0.2 ml/kg. After improvement is seen, some authors advise a treatment with ascorbic acid, 500 mg, intravenously q 2 h for the next 24 h.

Another source of nitrites are the isobutyl nitrites, which have recently been made illegal. Commonly, isobutyl nitrites are sold in sex shops as room deodorizers. This is quite strange because the usual nickname of isobutyl is "locker room" or "sweat sock." The odor is quite foul, but it does produce the same sexual response as does amyl nitrite. A further problem with isobutyl nitrite is that it is of industrial-level purity rather than USP purity. Problems may therefore result from contaminants. Addiction potential is equivalent to that of any nitrate.

C. Gasoline

Gasoline is a mixture of numerous aliphatic hydrocarbons and aromatic hydrocarbons, olefins, paraffins, and naphthenes [22–24]. The butane, hexane, pentane, heptane, and octane all tend to have sedating properties. The paraffins produce a drunken state. Usually, inhalation causes ataxia and dizziness with a intense visual hallucination, narcosis, syncope, respiratory paralysis, and death. These symptoms are progressive as the duration and intensity of the gasoline sniffing continues. Addiction to gasoline is associated with persistent ataxia, choreiform movements, confusion clonus, and moderately strong, resting, intention, and physiological tremors. Most long-term changes are, however, associated with lead poisoning owing to the treatment of gasoline with tetraethyl lead.

D. Aromatics

The major aromatics include benzene and toluene [25–30]. Other important aromatics are naphthalene, styrene, and xylene. Benzene itself is used as a vehicle for pigments. As such, it is found in nearly all plastics, paints, lacquers, resins, thinners, stains, and varnishes. Benzene is metabolized in the liver by sulfation. This produces other equally toxic compounds, including phenols, catechols, quinols, and mercapopuric acid.

Initial exposure produces euphoria, dizziness, and fatigue. Continued inhalation of benzene causes the symptoms to progress to dizziness, fatigue, severe headache, vertigo, dyspnea, and finally cardiac or respiratory arrest. The mechanisms progress as per other volatiles.

Addiction abuse produces many pathologies of the hemtopoietic system. These include anemia, dyscrasias, glucopenia, and thrombocytopenia. It appears that the metabolites of benzene inhibits both ribonucleic acid (RNA) and deoxyribonucleic acid (DNA) synthesis, and in turn may also cause chromosome damage.

Toluene is very closely related to benzene and is also used as a pigment vehicle. Interestingly enough, while it has had great abuse potential, toluene was introduced primarily to replace benzene owing to the latter compound's toxic effects on the hematopoietic system. Toluene's effects are essentially sedating. Effects range from extreme fatigue to acute renal damage, which can occur even after only one-time use, blood dyscrasia, cardiac arrest, liver damage, convulsions, lose of cerebellar dysfunction, encephalopathy and respiratory arrest.

Addiction to toluene may produce rhabdomyolysis and hypophosphatemia. There have been some gastrointestinal complaints, including hematemesis, projectile diarrhea, and projectile vomiting. Neurological effects include peripheral neuropathy, encephalopathy, optic neuropathy, and persistent ataxia. Objective changes include a direct optic neuropathy as well as formation of cataracts, retinal tearing, retinal hemorrhaging, and opacities. In patients with glucose-6-phosphate dehydrogenase (G-6-PD) deficiencies, sudden death is a possibility. Those groups at risk for G-6-PD deficiency include those of Mediterranean and Jewish ancestry and blacks.

Styrene is an industrial solvent used in the manufacture of plastic and synthetic rubber. Acute inhalation produces irritation of the eyes, nose, and throat as well as depressogenic effects. It is excreted primarily by the kidneys, and high doses can result in renal shutdown.

Naphthalene is a common volatile which is found in mothballs and toilet bowl deodorants. It can be used directly when mothballs are crushed inside of a plastic bag and the fumes inhaled. Naphthalene is also used to produce "scrap iron." Scrap iron is a concoction in which mothballs are dissolved in denatured ethanol to render it potable. This cocktail is then filtered through crushed charcoal briquets and then drunk.

Naphthalene abuse does not produce much of a "rush" or the high of most of the other volatiles. Acute inhalation is associated with profuse diaphoresis, nausea, emesis, and headaches. However, some abusers use it to attenuate symptoms of delirium tremens. This is probably why its greatest source of abuse is among derelict alcoholics. Addiction may lead to hemolytic anemia, hypocalemia, secondary to distal renal tubular acidosis and cataracts. Renal shutdown is always a possibility in the abuse of naphthalene.

The last of the benzene derivatives is xylene. Xylene's industrial use is varied. It is found in many types of varnishes, dyes, lacquers, cements, resins, cleaning fluids, and paints. It is also used in the commercial production of gasoline, and natural and synthetic rubbers. Its acute affects are consistent with all the other benzene derivatives except for naphthaline;

i.e., acute depression, feelings of extreme relaxation, and narcosis. Addiction has been reported to produce corneal damage and hemorrhagic pulmonary edema.

E. Halogenated Hydrocarbons

Halogenated hydrocarbons are basically limited to those hydrocarbons which have been chlorinated or fluorinated [31–32]. Brominated hydrocarbons are scarcely available in the United States. The chlorinated hydrocarbons tend to be cardiotoxic and can damage the kidneys and liver, whereas fluorinated hydrocarbons tend to reduce the contractility of the heart, producng ventricular arrythmias and occasionally death. Some of the halogenated hydrocarbons have specific effects. Carbon tetrachloride, for example, is a highly toxic compound which can produce changes in the heart, kidneys, lungs, spleen, and liver. Chloroform in addition to producing edema of the above organs, can produce hemorrhage of the brain and spinal cord. Trichloroflouromethane, a hydrocarbon with three chlorine and one flourine atom per molecule, is among the most toxic of the chlorinated hydrocarbons. It is associated with cerebral edema, cardiac arrythmia, cardiac arrest, hepatic necrosis, and renal necrosis.

Methachloroform is used as a solvent in the cosmetic industry and also as a industrial solvent for cleaning large machinery. Its use, both intentional and accidental, has been associated with epinephrine-sensitive arrythmias, peripheral vasodilatation, and decreased cardiac contractility. Because of its lethality, addiction potential is low.

F. Ketones

The most commonly abused ketone is acetone [33–34]. Other commonly abused ketones include methyethyl ketone and methyl and butyl ketone. Acetone is found primarily in lacquers, nail polish remover, and various oils and is used as a pigment vehicle. Acute abuse of acetone can produce dizziness, lightheadedness, feeling that one's head is floating, giddiness, and an overall feeling of well-being. This is associated with all the mucouse membranes. Addiction is associated with hepatic necrosis followed by hepatic failure.

Both methylethyl ketone and methyl and butyl ketone are used as solvents in the plastic industry as well as in the production of pigment vehicles. The rushes associated witth their abuse are essentially the same as that produced by acetone except they are more intense. Other chronic effects include dermatitis, peripheral numbness, congestion, and necrosis of the liver and kidneys, and emphysema.

G. Nitrous Oxide

Nitrous oxide (laughing gas) was the first of the volatiles available in the United States [35–36]. It is also used as a propellant for whipping cream and as an additive in automobile gases. Nitrous oxide still is used as an anesthetic. It is little used in hospital surgery and commonly found in the dentist's office for use in most outpatient dental work and oral surgery. The hallmark of nitrous oxide is extreme giddiness and euphoria associated with laughing. Analgesia and visual, auditory and tactile hallucinations are present, and sensations that the body is floating and astral projections occur. Unsupervised use of nitrous oxide has also been reported to produce severe respiratory depression, followed by respiratory arrest, coma, and hypoxic brain damage. Chronic abuse of nitrous oxide has produced a syndrome which includes ataxia, weakness in the lower extremities, impotence, loss of sphincter control, and tingling or shooting pains traveling down the spine after the head is flexed or extended. Some case studies have reported that these signs can mimic poliomyelitis, Guillain-Barré syndrome, and multiple sclerosis. There is no antidotal treatment for either acute or chronic nitrous oxide poisoning. Addiction potential is nonexistent.

H. Treatment

The treatment of the intentional volatile abuser is frustrating for psychiatrist and clinical toxicologists alike [37–41]. Unlike many other drugs of abuse, the volatile agents can produce irreversible damage to the major organs of the body. In spite of the damage which is obvious to the abuser, there tends to be little motivation to quit. In addition, there is much cross abuse from one volatile agent to another. The high availability of volatile agents plus the lack of criminal sanction of their purchase and use renders therapy difficult.

Nevertheless, some authors have reported limited success in treating this class of abusers. Some therapists have used behavior modification, whereas others have relied upon traditional psychotherapy. In the case of adolescents, one must always be ready to confront the denial of the patient and his or her parents. The confrontation and admission of abuse is a small but very necessary first step of treatment. Peer group therapy and counseling are also useful. However, in many cases, the volatile abuser tends to have a somewhat superior attitude to other "illegal" abusers, and therefore tends not to identify with them. It has been found by this author as well as others that therapy groups limited to solvent abusers produce much more fruitful results. In many drug units, a separate submodule can be formed for the abusers of volatile agents. Once this step is taken, the initial therapy can work on the abuser's motivation(s) for initiation of volatile inhalation. These usually involve themes of alienation, despair, rejection, and hopelessness. However, it is up to the therapist to not dwell too heavily on these themes because these tend only to reinforce the patients' rationalization for volatile abuse. Rather, one should admit the adversity of the circumstance and the environment, but then shift the group process to deal with themes of personal responsibility. Fears of helplessness can be enlarged to demythologize the "good rush" of the volatile agents. Loss of motoric and sphincter control or sensory decrements tend to emphasize current or projective loses and punctuate the group process. It is important that the physical and neurological damage sustained by the abuser be used as a warning rather than a justification of continued volatile abuse.

Occupational therapy, physical therapy, and vocational rehabilitation have all been seen as useful adjuncts in the treatment of volatile abusers. Tricyclic, bicyclic, and tetracyclic antidepressants have not been particularly useful in the treatment of the anomie and angst seen in this class of substance abusers. Outpatient therapy should be split, utilizing the services of the psychotherapist as well as the traditional "anonymous" programs. In treatment, office therapy should involve several weekly sessions of intermediate length rather then one lengthy psychotherapy session. This is because of the impulsivity profile of the abuser as well as the short attention span which may be the result of volatile abuse. Narcotics Anonymous (NA) provides good adjunctive therapy as does family therapy. The family therapy should be used not so much to educate the parents or spouse into becoming auxilliary police experts in detecting volatile abuse, but rather as ancillary friends who can detect those situations which proceed and precipitate episodes of volatile abuse. To encourage the production of a family unit which will support the abuser and not be destroyed by him, it is strongly encouraged that family members attend the NA meetings.

REFERENCES

1. Ramsay, W. *Asianic Elements in Greek Civilization*. Yale, New Haven, Connecticut, 1928.
2. Al-Makkari, A. *History of the Moslem Dynasties in Spain*. (Tr. M. Gayangos). Macmillan, London, 1840.
3. Smith, G. *When the Cheering Stopped*. MacLeod, Toronto, 1974.
4. Lewis, S. *Arrowsmith*. Harcourt, Brace, New York, 1925.

5. Purdy, K. *Encyclopedia of Automobile Racing*. Morrow, Philadelphia, 1962.

6. Mauries, P. *Vies oublies*. Promeneur, Paris, 1989.

7. Giannini, A.J., Slaby, A.E., and Giannini, M.C. *Handbook of Overdose and Detoxification Emergencies*. Medical Examination/Excerpta Medica, New Hyde Park, New York, 1983.

8. Inhalant use. *N.I.D.A. Notes 2*:20–21 (1988/1989).

9. Inhalant Data in D.A.W.N. Rockville, Maryland, *N.I.D.A. Div. Epidemiol.*, (June 1988).

10. Giannini, A.J., and Slaby, A.E. *Drugs of Abuse*. Medical Economics, Oradell, New Jersey, 1989.

11. Faucett, R.L., and Jensen, R.A. Addiction to the inhalation of gasoline fumes in a child. *J. Pediatr. 41*:364 (1952).

12. Goodwin, J.M., Geil, C., Groden, B., et al. Inhalant abuse, pregnancy, and neglected children. *Am. J. Psychiatry 138*(8):1126 (1981).

13. Aviado, D.M. Preclinical pharmacology and toxicology of halogenated solvents and propellants, *Review of Inhalants: Euphoria to Dysfunction* (C.W. Sharp and M.L. Brehm, eds.), US Government Printing Office, Washington, D.C., 1977.

14. Bass, M. Sudden sniffing death. *J.A.M.A. 212*:2075,2079 (1970).

15. Baerg, R., and Kimberg, D. Centrilobular hepatic necrosis and acute renal failure in solvent sniffers. *Ann. Intern. Med. 73'*713–720 (1970).

16. White, J., and Carlson, G. Epinephrine-induced cardiac arrythmias in rabbits exposed to trichloroethylene: Potentiation by ethanol. *Toxicol. Appl. Pharmacol. 60*:466–471 (1981).

17. Couri, D., and Nachtman, J.P. Toxicology of alcohols, ketones, and esters—Inhalation, *Review of Inhalants: Euphoria to Dysfunction* (C.W. Sharp, and M.L. Brehm, eds.), U.S. Government Printing Office, Washington, D.C. 1977.

18. Cohen, S. The volatile nitrites. *J.A.M.A. 241*:2077–2078 (1979).

19. Mason, D.T., and Braunwald, E. The effects of amyl nitrite on arteriolar and venous tone. *Circulation 32*:755–766 (1965).

20. Lange, W.R., Haertzer, C.A., Hickey, J.V., Snyder, F.R., Dax, E.M., and Jaffee, J.H. Nitrite inhalants: Patterns of abuse in Baltimore and Washington, D.C. *Am. J. Drug Alcohol Abuse 14*:24–39 (1988).

21. Bruckner, J.V., and Peterson, R.G. Review of the aliphatic and aromatic hydrocarbons, *Review of Inhalants: Euphoria to Dysfunction* (C.W. Sharp and M.L. Brehm, eds.), U.S. Government Printing Office, Washington, D.C., 1977.

22. Coulehan, J.L., Hirschl, J.W., Brillman, J., et al. Gasoline sniffing and lead toxicity in Navajo adolescents. *Pediatrics 71*:113–117 (1983).

23. Boeckx, R.L., Postl, B., and Coodin, F.J. Gasoline sniffing and tetraethyl lead poisoning in children. *Pediatrics 60*:140–145 (1977).

24. Nucombe, B., Bianchi, G.N., Money, J., et al. A hunger for stimuli: The psychological background of petrol inhalation. *Br. J. Med. Psychol. 43*:367–374 (1970).

25. Pone, A.K. Sniffing, bagging, huffing. *Emerg. Med. 134*:187–191 (1977).

26. Winek, G.L., Collom, W.D., and Wecht, C.H. Fatal benzene exposure by glue-sniffing. *Lancet 1*:683 (1967).

27. Streicher, H.Z., Gabor, P.A., Moss, A.H., et al. Syndromes of toluene sniffing in adults. *Ann. Intern. Med. 94*:758–762 (1981).

28. King, M.D., Day, R.E., Oliver, J.S., et al. Solvent encephalopathy from toluene inhalation. *Br. Med. J. 283*:663–665 (1981).

29. Giannini, A.J., Black, H.R., and Goettsche, R.C. *The Psychiatric, Psychogenic, and Somatopsychic Disorders*. Medical Economics/Excerpta Medica, Garden City, New Jersey, 1978.

30. DeGowin, R.L. Benzene exposure and aylastic anemia followed by leukemia. *J.A.M.A. 183*:748–751 (1963).

31. Calvert, D.N., and Brody, T.M. Release of catecholamine by carbon tetrachloride. *Am. J. Physiol. 198*:682–685 (1970).

32. Goodard, J.L. Carbon tetrachloride. *Fed. Reg. 33*:3076–3080 (1968).

33. Prockop, L., and Couri, D. Nervous system damage from mixed organic solvents. *Natl. Inst. Res. Monogr. 15*:185–189 (1977).

34. Von Oettingen, W.F. The toxicity and dangers of alaphatic and aromatic hydrocarbons. *Yale J. Biol. Med. 15*:167–184 (1942).
35. Layzer, R.B. Myeloneuropathy after prolonged exposure to nitrous oxide. *Lancet 2*:1227–1230 (1978).
36. Eckenhuff, J.E., and Helrich, M. The effects of narcotics, thiopental and nitrous oxide upon respiration. *Anesthesiology 19*:240–253 (1958).
37. Gawin, F.H. Laboratory assessments in treatments of substance abuse: Utilization and effects on treatment design. *Clin. Chem. 33*(11):953–100B (1987).
38. Nakken, C. *The Addictive Personality*. Pleasant Valley, Minnesota, Hazeldon, 1988.
39. Reilly, D.M. Drug abusing families. (E. Kaufman and P.N. Kaufman, eds.), *Family Therapy of Drug and Alcohol Abuse*. Gardner, New York, 1979.
40. Minuchin, S. Constructing a therapeutic reality (E. Kaufman and P.N. Kaufman, eds.), *Family Therapy of Drug Alcohol Abuse*, Gardner, New York, 1979.
41. Rotter, J.B. Generalized expectancies for interval vs. external control of reinforcements. *Psychol. Mon. Gen. Appl. 80*:1–28 (1966).

23

Benzodiazepines

David E. Smith and Richard B. Seymour
Haight Ashbury Free Clinics, Inc., San Francisco, California

I. INTRODUCTION

Introduced into medical practice in 1960, the benzodiazepines (BZDs) rapidly became one of the most commonly prescribed medications, often replacing short-acting barbiturates and other sedative-hypnotics in treatment. As with lysergic acid diethylamide-25 (LSD) 2 decades earlier, the discovery of the psychoactive properties of BZDs were almost missed. While reordering their laboratory at Hoffmann LaRoche in April, 1957, Earl Reeder pointed out several hundred milligrams of a substance and its hydrochloride salt to Leo Sternbach that they had synthesized in 1955, but had not submitted for pharmacological testing. They sent the hydrochloride salt, later given the generic name chlordiazepoxide and the trade name Librium, to Lowell Randall, head of LaRoche's pharmacology department, for animal testing. Randall reported that the compound possessed interesting psychotropic properties in animals. Shortly thereafter, a second BZD, diazepam with the trade name of Valium, was developed by LaRoche. Since that time, over 3000 different benzodiazepines and heterodiazepines have been synthesized (Sternback, 1983).

Used now for the treatment of anxiety, insomnia, muscle spasticity, convulsive disorders, anesthesia adjuncts, and alcohol detoxication, the BZDs have exhibited what many have seen as significant advantages over the short-acting barbiturates, meprobamate and methaqualone. Methaqualone, a drug with very little molecular resemblance to barbiturates, at first showed great promise, but partly because of an undeserved reputation as a sexual enhancer, became most noted for its abuse and was removed from production in 1984 (Seymour and Smith, 1987, Seymour et al., 1989).

In general, the BZDs have a high lethal/therapeutic ratio, greatly reducing their potential for lethal overdose, and unlike the short-acting barbiturates, meprobamate and other minor tranquilizers, they have not been found to activate liver microsomal enzymes (Smith and Wesson, 1985). Benzodiazepines have been used in alcoholic patients for alcohol detoxification on an inpatient basis, but Newsom and Seymour (1983) warn that they should not be used for this purpose on an outpatient basis.

Benzodiazepines, when they first became clinically available, were viewed by the medical profession as safer alternatives to short-acting barbiturates and other available sedatives. This perception of safety resulted in a liberal physician prescribing attitude, from which BZDs became embroiled in "overmedicated society" concerns in general, and in concerns about the way female patients were treated by a male-dominated medical system. As several observers pointed out, it seemed as though the medical establishment was intent on treating America for a general Valium deficiency.

An unbalanced prescribing of sedative-hypnotic, opioid, and other psychoactive drugs for women was not a new phenomenon, but in the 1960s and early 1970s the uncritical acceptance of medicinal drugs declined when unpredicted side effects to medications became apparent. The frequent failure of high-technology products resulted in heightened legal interest in product failibility and liability. Medicinals evolved as a focus of popular anger and resentment as common human problems failed to yield to technological solutions. Benzodiazepines had increasingly replaced other sedative-hypnotics in treatment and became a primary target for public dismay, especially as concern about the dependence potential of these drugs increased.

In the early 1960s, Leo Hollister, M.D., working at Stanford University, experimentally induced physical dependence in human subjects with benzodiazepines at doses several times the therapeutic levels. These subjects experienced classic sedative-hypnotic withdrawal seizures after the drugs were abruptly withdrawn. This dose-related sedative-hypnotic form of dependency was well established, while increasing data suggested that therapeutic doses of BZDs taken chronically can also produce pharmacological dependence and addiction. As the data hardened, it became apparent that although some persons can take a benzodiazepine drug in therapeutic doses for long periods without withdrawal problems, some persons, particularly those with a predisposition to addiction can develop addiction, pharmacological dependence, and have severe withdrawal symptoms at therapeutic doses. Both the short-acting and long-acting BZDs have pharmacological dependence and addiction potential at therapeutic doses.

II. PHARMACOLOGY

Individual reactions to BZDs taken in doses within the therapeutic range vary substantially. It is unlikely that persons who take BZDs within the therapeutic range for long periods have no significant withdrawal problems. Moreover, persons with a psychobiological predisposition to addiction (often with a personal or family history of alcoholism) who take these drugs in therapeutic doses for more than 1 month but less than 6 months (or for an average of 3 months) may have severe withdrawal psychosis and seizures when the drug is abruptly stopped.

To prevent addiction and dependence, some physicians switch their patients from medium- or long-acting benzodiazepines, such as diazepam, to a short-acting one, such as alprazolam, in the mistaken belief that the shorter-acting drug has less potential for abuse. Also, lowering the equivalent dose can prompt the emergence of the sedative-hypnotic abstinence syndrome (anxiety and insomnia). All benzodiazepines have the same potential for abuse: Thus, shorter-acting benzodiazepines should be used only for their intended therapeutic purpose.

Patients with BZD dependence should enroll in a program of detoxification. Physicians are advised that alternatives to psychoactive medications should be sought for patients with both a dependence on BZDs and a diagnosis of anxiety disorder, as should therapeutically effective medications with a lower potential for dependence, such as imipramine rather than alprazolam for a drug-dependent patient with a history of panic disorder. If alternative drugs, used in conjunction with stress reduction, relaxation training, exercise, and biofeedback, fail and if the patient has major dysfunction, then a BZD can be used, but with extreme caution.

A BZD taken at several times the therapeutic dose for approximately 1 month can produce physical dependence, and abrupt cessation can then induce sedative-hypnotic withdrawal symptoms such as psychosis and seizures (Smith and Wesson, 1983). The signs and symptoms associated with BZD withdrawal are shown on Table 1. These include symptom generation and symptom reemergence, which have specific characteristics, as shown in Figure 1. The physical dependence caused by the BZDs may be a high-dose dependence of the barbiturate type, or a low-dose dependence that can occur with therapeutic doses, as shown in Table 2.

Benzodiazepines suppress alcohol withdrawal and other sedative-hypnotic withdrawal symptoms. The BZDs, alcohol, barbiturates, and other sedative-hypnotic drugs are all cross tolerant. The mechanisms by which central nervous system tolerance and physical dependence on sedative-hypnotics develop are not known. Unlike the effects of BZDs, which are anxioselective to specific receptor sites in many central nervous system nerve cells, whereas other sedative-hypnotic drugs, including alcohol, appear to have a more general effect on the brain. As far as is currently known, these do not have specific binding sites.

Studies conducted more than 25 years ago showed that after diazepam and chlordiazepoxide (Hollister, et al., 1963, 1961) had been taken for 1 month in doses that were two to three times the maximum recommended dose, a withdrawal syndrome of the barbiturate type occurred when the BZD was abruptly stopped. Since meprobamate, glutethimide, methyprylon, alcohol, methaqualone, and other sedative-hypnotic drugs produce a withdrawal syndrome similar to that of the barbiturates, the more general term *sedative-hypnotic withdrawal syndrome* is often used. The time required to develop physical dependence is inversely related to dose. If enough barbiturates are administered to produce continuous sleep, profound pharmacological dependence can be induced in 1 week: for ambulatory persons, dependence will take several weeks of daily dosing to develop. The same is probably true for BZDs.

Sedative-hypnotic withdrawal symptoms are generally divided into major and minor categories. Minor withdrawal symptoms consist of anxiety, insomnia, tremor, and nightmares. A major withdrawal syndrome includes all the symptoms of minor withdrawal and may

Table 1 Comparison of Syndromes Related to BZD Withdrawal

Syndrome	Symptoms	Time course	Responses to reinstitution of benzodiazepine
Sedative-hypnotic–type withdrawal	Anxiety, insomnia, nightmares, seizures, psychosis, hyperpyrexia, death	Symptoms begin one to two days after short-acting BZD is stopped or 2–4 days after long-acting BZD is stopped.	Symptoms reverse 2–6 h after hypnotic-level doses are reinstituted.
Receptor site–mediated withdrawal	Anxiety (including somatic manifestations), insomnia, nightmares, muscle spasm, psychosis	Symptoms begin one day after BZD is stopped. They may continue for weeks to months but improve with time.	Symptoms reverse within 45–90 min after small doses are taken.
Symptom reemergence	Variable, but should be same as symptoms before BZD is taken	Symptoms emerge when BZD is stopped and continue unabated with time.	Symptoms respond within 45–90 min after usual therapeutic doses are taken.

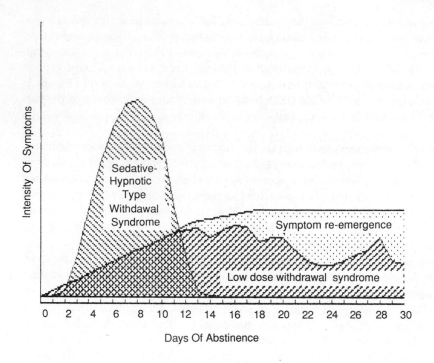

Figure 1 Comparison of relative intensity and time course of BZD withdrawal syndromes.

also include grand mal seizures, psychosis, hyperpyrexia, and death. Untreated, the high-dose sedative hypnotic withdrawal syndrome peaks in intensity as blood levels of the sedative drop, and the patient's signs and symptoms subside over a few days.

Symptoms attributed to BZD withdrawal include anxiety, tension, agitation, restlessness, irritability, tremor, nausea, insomnia, panic attacks, impairment of memory and concentration, perceptual alterations, including hyperacusis or hypersensitivity to touch and pain,

Table 2 High-Dose and Low-Dose Designations of the BZDs

Generic name	Total daily dosage	
	low dose (mg)	high dose (mg]
Alprazolam	0.75– 4.00	> 4.00
Chlordiazepoxide	15.00–100.00	> 100.00
Clonazepam	1.50– 20.00	> 20.00
Clorazepate	15.00– 60.00	> 60.00
Diazepam	4.00– 40.00	> 40.00
Fiurazepam	15.00– 30.00	> 30.00
Halazepam	60.00–160.00	> 160.00
Lorazepam	1.00– 10.00	> 10.00
Oxazepam	10.00– 30.00	> 30.00
Prazepam	20.00– 60.00	> 60.00
Temazepam	15.00– 30.00	> 30.00
Triazolam	0.25– 0.50	> 0.50

paresthesias, feelings of unreality, visual hallucinations, psychosis, tachycardia, and increased blood pressure. Unfortunately, withdrawal has no pathognomonic signs or symptoms, and such a broad range of nonspecific symptoms could be produced by a number of illnesses, including agitated depression, generalized anxiety disorder, panic disorder, partial complex seizures, and schizophrenic disorders.

The validity of a low-dose withdrawal syndrome has been controversial. Many people who have taken BZDs in therapeutic doses for months to years can abruptly discontinue the drug without developing symptoms. Others, taking similar amounts of a BZD develop a physical dependence on the drug and cannot tolerate the symptoms that develop when the drug is stopped or the dosage reduced. Moreover, some physicians believe the symptoms that emerge during the immediate withdrawal period can be explained solely by the return of the symptoms for which the drug was being taken, whereas other physicians propose that at least some of the symptoms are a true withdrawal reaction. At least four possible etiologies could explain the symptoms that begin when BZDs are stopped. These are: symptom reemergence, symptom emergence, symptom overinterpretation, and symptom generation.

III. SYMPTOM REEMERGENCE

According to the symptom reemergence etiology, the patient's symptoms of anxiety, insomnia, or muscle tension abate during benzodiazepine treatment, and the patient forgets how severe they were. Because discomfort in the present seems more real than that experienced in the past, present symptoms may be perceived as more severe when, in fact, they are equal in severity to those experienced before treatment with BZDs.

IV. SYMPTOM EMERGENCE

If the patient's initial symptoms were secondary to a progressive disease, they may have been masked during benzodiazepine therapy. If this is the case, the symptoms that reemerge will be more intense when the drug is stopped, but the intensity will result from the disease's progression.

V. SYMPTOM OVERINTERPRETATION

Most individuals experience occasional anxiety, variations in sleep pattern, and musculoskeletal discomfort and accept these symptoms as reasonable consequences of everyday stresses, overexertion, or minor viral infections. Patients who are stopping benzodiazepines often expect withdrawal symptoms to develop, and may assume that any symptoms occurring during the withdrawal period are caused by drug withdrawal and require medical attention. A study of the frequency with which symptoms attributed to minor barbiturate or low-dose BZD withdrawal actually occurred reported that anxiety, sleep variations, and discomfort were common among untreated, healthy persons who did not use drugs (Merz and Ballmer, 1983).

VI. SYMPTOM GENERATION

According to the final possible etiology, signs or symptoms may develop when BZD treatment is stopped as a result of receptor site alterations caused by the benzodiazepine exposure.

A. Receptor-Site Mediation in BZD Dependence and Withdrawal

Assigning causality to symptoms that emerge after discontinuing a drug is subject to uncertainty, especially when a patient is evaluated after dependence is already established. The time course of symptom resolution is the primary differentiating feature between symptoms generated by withdrawal and symptom reemergence, emergence, or overinterpretation. Withdrawal symptoms subside with continued abstinence, whereas symptoms associated with other etiologies persist.

Such short-acting BZDs as oxazepam, alprazolam, and triazolam have an accelerated time course for the sedative-hypnotic type of withdrawal syndrome, and the peak intensity of withdrawal occurs within 2–4 days. The fluctuation of symptom intensity of the low-dose withdrawal syndrome illustrates the waxing and waning of symptoms that often occurs without apparent psychological cause. This waxing and waning is an important marker distinguishing low-dose withdrawal symptoms from symptom reemergence.

Chronic use, dosage, concurrent drug use, and individual susceptibility all interact in the development of low-dose physical dependence. Moreover, the short-acting BZDs are no less likely to produce physical dependence if taken on a daily basis than are the long-acting BZDs; and once pharmacological dependence develops, the sedative-hypnotic–type withdrawal syndrome produced by short-acting benzodiazepines would be expected to be more intense because of the more rapid drop in tissue levels of these drugs (Hollister, 1980).

Since the reports of finding specific benzodiazepine-binding sites in the rat brain (Mohler and Okada, 1977; Squires and Braestrup, 1977), the character is the BZD receptor site has been the subject of intense research. These receptor sites, localized in synaptic contact regions in the cerebral cortex, cerebellium, and hippocampus, are associated with gamma-aminobutyric acid (GABA) receptor sites and affect their affinity for binding to a specific site, and also modify the cell membrane's permeability to chloride ions. We have hypothesized that low-dose BZD withdrawal is receptor site mediated (Wesson and Smith, 1982). A receptor site–mediated withdrawal syndrome could plausibly explain why BZD withdrawal symptoms take more time to resolve than non-benzodiazepine sedative-hypnotic withdrawal symptoms.

Physical dependence on BZDs may be influenced by exposure to other drugs. Phenobarbital, for example, has been shown to increase the affinity of diazepam to benzodiazepine receptors (Skolnick et al., 1981; Olsen and Loeb-Lundberg, 1981). Pretreatment with a barbiturate may also affect the development of withdrawal symptoms (Covi et al., 1973).

VII. LOW-DOSE BZD DEPENDENCE SYNDROME

The low-dose BZD dependence syndrome is not well understood or well characterized. The dose-response relationship has not been established, and the development of dependence appears to be idiosyncratic. Risk factors include a family or personal history of alcoholism, daily alcohol use, or concomitant use of other sedatives.

Because the time course and spectrum of signs and symptoms of the low-dose withdrawal syndrome are different from those of the sedative-hypnotic–type withdrawal syndrome, the two probably have different mechanisms. Thus, the low-dose benzodiazepine withdrawal syndrome should not be considered a "minor" sedative-hypnotic withdrawal syndrome, but a different syndrome. The BZD syndrome is not completely suppressed by phenobarbital administration; symptoms are rapidly reversed by BZD doses below those that would be expected to be effective; symptom resolution takes much longer with the low-dose withdrawal syndrome than with typical sedative-hypnotic withdrawal (i.e., symptoms usually take 6 months to a year to completely subside); and symptoms are most intense during withdrawal of the last few milligrams of the BZD.

VIII. DETOXIFICATION

There are three accepted protocols for benzodiazepine detoxification. These are reduction of the amount of BZD taken; substitution of a longer-acting BZD; or substitution of phenobarbital. Protocol selection depends on the severity of the BZD dependence, the involvement of other drugs of dependence, and the clinical setting in which the detoxification program takes place.

Given these variables, BZD withdrawal is no more controversial than alcohol withdrawal. As with alcohol detoxification, a minority of BZD users experience medically significant withdrawal. In that detoxification for that minority in both cases may involve life-threatening seizures, care must be taken in all withdrawal situations, and when needed, vital signs monitored during threshold periods of inpatient detoxification.

When a patient develops BZD dependence during treatment of anxiety, the physician must decide whether the patient should undergo detoxification. Abrupt cessation of long-term BZD use can produce severe and even life-threatening withdrawal sequelae.

The graded reduction of BZD protocol is used primarily in medical settings for therapeutic-dose dependence. Substituting a long-acting BZD (such as chlordiazepoxide) can be used to detoxify patients with primary BZD dependence, but it is mainly used to treat patients with alcohol/benzodiazepine combination dependencies, using a fixed-dosage reduction schedule. Substitution of phenobarbital or another long-acting sedative-hypnotic can also be used to detoxify patients with primary benzodiazepine/polydrug dependence; for example, cocaine/benzodiazepine/alcohol combinations. This protocol, which also follows a fixed-dosage detoxification schedule, has the broadest use for all sedative-hypnotic drug dependencies and is widely used in drug detoxification programs. It is particularly valuable for treating high-dose BZD dependence.

If the theory about two BZD withdrawal syndromes, i.e., high-dose dependence of the barbiturate type and low-dose dependence, is correct, drug withdrawal strategies must be tailored to three possible dependence situations. After daily use of therapeutic doses of BZDs for more than 6 months, only a low-dose withdrawal syndrome should be expected. After high-dose use, i.e., doses greater than the recommended therapeutic doses, for more than 1 month but less than 6 months, or for an average of 3 months, a classic sedative-hypnotic withdrawal syndrome should be anticipated. Finally, after daily high doses for more than 6 months, both a sedative-hypnotic withdrawal syndrome and a low-dose withdrawal syndrome should be anticipated.

To treat a low-dose BZD dependence withdrawal syndrome, gradual reduction of the BZD is pharmacologically rational because seizures, hyperpyrexia, and other life-threatening medical complications are not expected. A stepwise reduction of the drug by the smallest unit dose each week is recommended for patients who are pharmacologically dependent but still in control of their medication use. Patients who have lost the ability to control drug use are likely to escalate the dosage again as symptoms emerge, and they require hospitalization.

During withdrawal, psychometric assessment is useful for establishing trends in the multiple, shifting symptoms. A computer can be used to administer a symptom checklist, with the patient sitting at a terminal and entering responses. This interactive method has proved to be more efficient than interviews for tracking symptom changes.

Propanolol has been found to reduce symptom intensity (Tyrer et al., 1981), and the drug is begun at a dosage of 20 mg every 6 hr, starting on the fifth day of withdrawal. This schedule is continued for 2 weeks and then stopped. After withdrawal is completed, propranolol is used as needed to control tachycardia, increased blood pressure, and anxiety. Continuous propranolol therapy for more than 2 weeks is not recommended as propranolol itself may result in symptom rebound when discontinued after prolonged therapy (Glaubiger and Lefkowitz, 1977; Harrison and Alderman, 1976).

To treat the sedative-hypnotic type of benzodiazepine withdrawal, a phenobarbital substitution technique is preferred. At the Haight Ashbury Free Clinics, no patients have had withdrawal seizures when phenobarbital was used, whereas two patients have had seizures during gradual BZD recuction. When treating a patient for drug dependence, it is best not to administer the drug of dependence during treatment.

An estimate of the patient's daily BZD use during the month before treatment is used to compute the detoxification starting dose of phenobarbital, converting the BZD amount to the phenobarbital withdrawal equivalence dosage. These are listed on Table 3. The computed phenobarbital equivalence dosage is given in three or four doses daily. If other sedative-hypnotic drugs, including alcohol, are used, the amount of phenobarbital computed according to the conversion rate for the other sedative-hypnotic is added to the amount computed for the BZD. Regardless of the total computed amount, however, the maximum phenobarbital dosage is 500 mg/day. After 2 days of phenobarbital stabilization, the patient's daily dosage is decreased by 30 mg each day.

Before receiving each dose of phenobarbital, the patient is checked for sustained horizontal nystagmus, slurred speech, and ataxia. If sustained nystagmus is present, the scheduled dose

Table 3 Phenobarbital Withdrawal Conversion for BZDs and Other Sedative-Hypnotics

Generic name	Dose (mg)	Phenobarbital withdrawal conversion (mg)
Benzodiazepines		
alprazolam	1	30
chlordiazepoxide	25	30
clonazepam	2	15
clorazepate	15	30
diazepam	10	30
flurazepam	15	30
halazepam	40	30
lorazepam	1	15
oxazepam	10	30
prazepam	10	30
temazepam	15	30
Barbiturates		
amobarbital	100	30
butabarbital	100	30
butalbital	50	15
pentobarbital	100	50
secobarbital	100	30
Glycerols		
meprobamate	400	30
Piperidinediones		
glutethimide	250	30
Quinazolines		
methaqualone	300	30

of phenobarbital is withheld. If all three signs are present, the next two doses of phenobarbital are withheld and the daily dosage of phenobarbital for the following day is halved.

IX. MEDICAL MANAGEMENT OF DUAL DIAGNOSIS PATIENTS

The medical management of persons with a dual diagnosis of drug addiction and psychiatric disorders requiring medication poses both conceptual and clinical problems. Although psychoactive medications are helpful when properly used, patients with a personal or family history of addiction have a high risk for compulsively using all psychoactive drugs, and these drugs should not be prescribed for them. The question is, what is the appropriate medical response to a person who has addictive disease, or a genetic predisposition to addictive disease, but who is otherwise a good candidate for psychoactive medications?

It is in the best interest of patients with both addictive disease and psychiatric problems to first seek nonpsychoactive therapy alternatives, such as nonpsychoactive drugs, acupuncture, exercise, biofeedback, and other stress-reduction techniques for the alcoholic patient with anxiety. When the severity of the psychiatric problem limits the person's ability to function, and if the use of nonpsychoactive drug alternatives fails, then psychoactive drugs may need to be administered. Unfortunately, these patients will probably then develop compulsivity for the medications, lose control over them, and continue using them in spite of adverse consequences. The physician must exercise the utmost of caution in prescribing for these cases. The fundamentals of good prescribing practices can be thought of as the "six D's," i.e., diagnosis, dosage, duration, discontinuation, dependence, and documentation.

Physicisns make good-faith diagnoses of patients' problems. For an acute problem, such as a brief episode of pain or anxiety, it is within the accepted standard of care to treat that problem based on a tentative diagnosis. As an acute problem lingers and becomes chronic, a firm diagnosis must be made. Because anxiety, insomnia, and pain are invisible disorders, physicians must take the time to find the etiology of the problem.

Once the diagnosis has been made, and a treatment plan outlined, the physician can select the drug that is clinically indicated for the specific problem, prescribing the appropriate drug dosage for the diagnosis, and tailoring the medication schedule to the patient. The treatment goal is to neither undermedicate nor overmedicate, and as symptom severity increases and decreases, the medication should likewise be increased and decreased.

The duration of drug treatment should be planned with the patient, and medication should not be provided in an open-ended fashion. Also, periodic evaluations should be conducted to determine whether the medication should be discontinued: Are there problems with the drug? Has the planned duration of use expired? Has the crisis or problem that prompted use of the drug diminished or disappeared? Has the patient learned alternative ways of dealing with the original problem?

During treatment, the patient should be carefully monitored for developing dependence and toxicity problems. Physicians have a legal and ethical duty to warn the patient about both the side effects of the medications and the potential for developing dependence, which, for a person with addictive disease, can trigger an episode of compulsively taking prescribed and other drugs.

Finally, it is critical to carefully document the patient's initial complaints, eventual diagnosis, course of treatment, and all prescriptions and consultations. Consultations with experts in allied fields can be useful to the primary care physician. Addiction specialists can be consulted for cases of addiction and dependence, much as one would consult a pain specialist or a psychiatrist. These consultations and decisions based on them should also be documented in the patient's file.

X. BZDs AND OTHER DRUG USE

There are many studies that clearly demonstrate that BZDs are often used in combination with other drugs, including alcohol. The studies show the following characteristics of alcohol and other drug use with BZDs; (1) The prevalence of the use of BZDs by alcoholics is between 20 and 40%; (2) The prevalence of use of BZDs by the general psychiatric patient is between 17 and 40%; (3) The prevalence of use of the BZDs is between 9.6 and 16% in the general population; (4) The prevalence of use of BZDs by heroin and methadone addicts is between 25 and 50%; (5) The prevalence of use of BZD is undetermined but probably high in other drug addicts, i.e., cocaine, cannabis, hallucinogens (Chan, 1984; Hu, Reiffenstein, and Wong, 1986; Orzack, Friedman, and Dessain, 1988; Roache and Griffiths, 1986; Sellers et al., 1981).

The use of the BZDs in high-risk populations of alcoholics and drug addicts is due to several reasons, although most studies do not delineate them in systemic and definable ways. The more obvious reasons are that the BZDs in themselves produce addiction, tolerance, dependence, and cross tolerance with other drugs such as alcohol. Whatever the drive for addiction may be, it appears that an alcoholic and a drug addict will at least use and may become addicted to multiple drugs, including BZDs. As with addicition, the addict pursues the drug for the drug effect and continues to use it in spite of adverse consequences. Furthermore, there are times when alcohol and other drugs cannot be conveniently used or obtained and the BZDs may be used as a substitute.

The anxiety syndrome from alcohol withdrawal is common among frequent consumers of alcohol, particularly, alcoholics. The anxiety produced by the alcohol dependence syndrome is similar to that produced by the BZDs, and the two drugs share cross tolerance and dependence so that they can be used interchangeably to suppress the signs and symptoms of withdrawal from their pharmacological dependence. Because alcohol can produce by itself many of the types of anxiety disorders such as generalized anxiety, panic attacks, agoraphobia, and other phobias, the use of BZDs in alcohol use and dependence may be relatively common for these symptoms.

General psychiatric populations contain large percentages of alcoholics and drug addicts as published reports cite the prevalence of alcohol and drug addiction to be between 25 and 50% among "psychiatric patients" (Miller et al., 1988; Schuckit, 1978). Because alcohol and drugs, including BZDs, can produce psychiatric symptoms and mimic psychiatric disorders, the actual numbers of pure general psychiatric patients relative to confirmed alcoholics and drug addicts remain to be determined. Many studies do not clearly differentiate ideopathic psychiatric symptoms from those induced by alcohol and drugs. Some studies suggest that alcohol and drugs frequently produce psychiatric symptoms and syndromes that include affective disorders, anxiety disorders, psychotic states, and personality disturbances which may be transient and remit with abstinence (Laux and Puryear, 1984; Miller et al., 1985, 1988; Schuckit, 1978).

Lastly, the self-administration studies that demonstrate that BZDs have a lower abuse potential in comparison to barbiturates may be misleading in their conclusions. Self-administration by animals and humans of alcohol is usually low; alcohol, of course, is definitely addicting and commonly so (Griffiths et al., 1979, 1980).

XI. THE USE OF BZDs AND COCAINE AS INTOXICANTS

The use of BZDs as intoxicants involves several different types of drug-using behaviors among a diverse population of people. The major patterns of BZD consumption considered here include the use of BZDs alone as intoxicants or as alternatives to other intoxicants, particularly alcohol.

The therapeutic prescription of BZDs can result in pharmacological dependence in two situations: First, some patients increase their daily consumption of a BZD, with or without the concurrence of their physician, to doses beyond the usual therapeutic range. This can result in pharmacological dependence of the classic sedative-hypnotic type that is similar to that of alcohol or BZDs over a period of months to years, even when taken within the accepted therapeutic dosages, can result in addiction and pharmacological dependency. Because the withdrawal syndrome from therapeutic dosages of BZDs produces symptoms that are similar to those for which BZDs are often prescribed, the clinical recognition of the withdrawal syndrome by physicians has been slow. Nonetheless, the therapeutic-dose pharmacological dependency is now accepted by most addiction medicine specialists, and many psychiatrists who prescribe BZDs.

Some discussions of benzodiazepine's use for intoxication include suicide attempts in which BZDs are used. This is particularly the case when discussing emergency room "mentions" of BZDs which occur in the United States' Drug Abuse Warning Network national data base (DAWN). This data base is often used for establishing drug trends. Any sedative medication that is widely available will show a large number of mentions in DAWN for suicidal use. Murphy (1988) and Rich et al. (1986) have pointed out that BZDs and other depressants produce depression of mood through their intoxicating affects. Noting the marked association of BZDs with suicide, Miller and Gold (1990) point out that the association may be more causative than the drugs being merely used as a circumstantial or impulsive method of suicide. While suicide attempts are a significant problem, the low lethality of BZDs when taken alone is actually one of their primary advantages, and this certainly does not constitute use for intoxication as usually defined. Most often, deaths from BZDs result from an "additive effect" when taken in conjunction with other sedative-hypnotics, usually alcohol (Marks, 1985).

Benzodiazepines may be used in combination with heroin or methadone to enhance the sedative effects of opiates. This pattern of intoxicating use has been of substantial concern to directors of methadone maintenance programs.

Benzodiazepines are also used in combination with stimulants, particularly cocaine, in which case they are used to offset unpleasant symptoms of cocaine toxicity. This form of BZD use for intoxication is of great concern to addiction medicine specialists, and the clinical and public health concern over the problem of a BZD and cocaine syndrome led the Haight Ashbury Free Clinics to produce a study, conducted in the United States, in order to better characterize addiction medicine physicians' perceptions of the relationship between BZDs and cocaine, with the focus on patients treated in chemical dependence treatment programs.

The study was conducted by the Training and Education Projects of Haight Ashbury Free Clinics, Inc., in San Francisco in cooperation with the Research Division of the Merritt Peralta Chemical Dependency Recovery Hospital in Oakland, California, as an extension of its physician consultation services. The consultation service had been receiving increasing numbers of requests from physicians about problems of BZD and cocaine addiction.

A questionnaire was mailed to the 3000 members of the American Society of Addiction Medicine and to individual chemical dependence programs that had sought consultation for their patients with benzodiazepine/cocaine use combinations. The mailing collectively yielded 339 responses in the fall of 1987. Geographical distribution of the 339 programs was:

Area	No.	%	Area	No.	%
West Coast	68	20	Southwest	34	10
Northwest	13	4	Southeast	95	28
Mid-West	51	15	Northeast	78	23

Such widespread sampling provides some assurance of generalizability. The following results were obtained from the above programs.

When respondents were asked to give estimates about what drugs were on the increase in patients treated in their programs, cocaine far outstripped all other drugs. Seventy-six percent of the respondents mentioned cocaine as increasing among their treatment sample, whereas all other drugs were reported as increasing by less than 10% (Fig. 2).

Respondents were asked to estimate the direction of change in the number of "crack" users from 1 year ago. About 60% of these respondents reported that crack use was increasing, less than 10% reported a decrease, and about 35% indicated no change. Clearly, drug abuse treatment physicians perceived crack as a continuing and probably growing problem among patients seeking treatment for drug dependency in the United States (Fig. 3).

The addictive use of BZD was often associated with stimulant toxicity, particularly cocaine toxicity. We queried physicians about what drugs their patients were using to self-medicate the cocaine "crash." Almost all programs reported that alcohol was used, about 70% reported that diazepam was used, 60% reported that alprazolam was used, and 40% reported that lorazepam was used. All other BZDs represented less than 30% (Fig. 4).

About 20% of the programs reported that methaqualone, which is no longer available by prescription in the United States, was used to self-medicate cocaine toxicity. Studies at the Haight Ashbury Free Clinics have determined a significant number of methaqualone tablets are drugs of deception and in fact contain a benzodiazepine (Smith, 1985). The distribution was similar in males and females. Thus, we see that use of BZDs in relationship to cocaine toxicity is perceived as common. Shifting the focus directly to BZDs, the respondents were asked if, among their treatment population, BZDs were increasingly being used, decreasingly, or remaining the same. One hundred and forty-two, about 40% of the programs, reported that BZD addiction was increasing, about 20% reported that it was decreasing, and about 35% reported it to be remaining the same (Fig. 5).

The 142 programs that reported BZDs were increasing were asked which of these drugs were increasing. Alprazolam showed the greatest increase with about 60% of the reporting programs (Fig. 6).

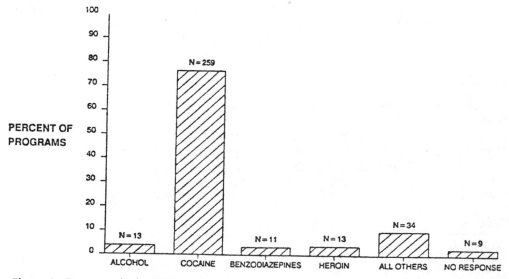

Figure 2 Drugs on the increase.

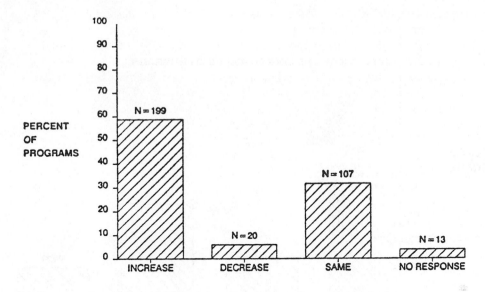

Figure 3 Change in number of crack users from 1 year ago.

Of the 48 programs reporting a decrease in BZDs, diazepam and alprazolam were each reported to be decreasing by about 20% of the programs (Fig. 7).

On the basis of this survey and discussions with colleagues throughout the United States, the following conclusions were drawn:

1. There are several patterns of BZD abuse, misuse, or addiction that are encompassed under the general notion of BZD abuse. Meaningful discussion of BZD addiction must take these into account.

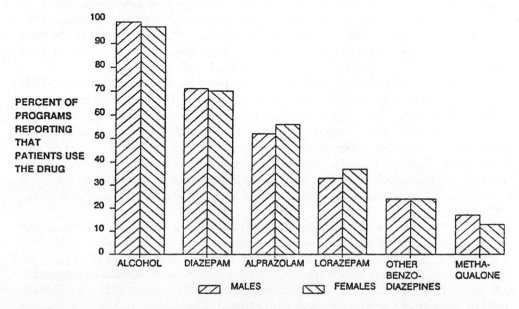

Figure 4 Drugs used to come down from crack.

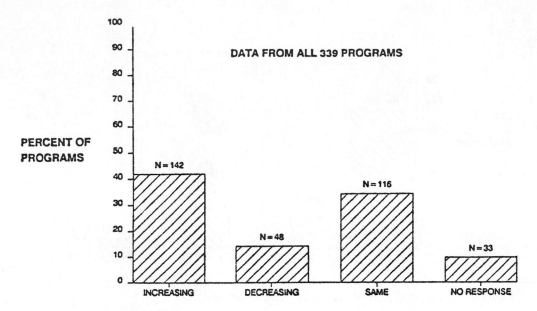

Figure 5 Change in BZD abuse.

2. Primary BZD abuse (or the abuse of a BZD alone for recreational purposes or intoxication) rarely occurs in the United States. Compared with the other available drugs, including alcohol, cocaine, and heroin, primary BZD abuse is rare and is not a major contributor to the United States drug abuse problem.

3. Addiction specialists are concerned about BZD dependence arising from therapeutic applications of the drug. Their concern is justified clinically because many of the patients self-define, or some physician defines the problem as addiction, and the patient is referred for addiction treatment. Usually this is poorly treated in addiction programs for several reasons: (a) the patients do not relate to the patterns of abuse that occur with non-therapeutic drug use, (b) the time course of major withdrawal symptoms are prolonged and exceeds the inpatient treatment limits generally provided in chemical dependency programs, and (c) our treatment technology for treatment of low-dose dependency is poor.

4. Much of the concern of addiction specialists arises from the association between BZD and cocaine addiction. Although we would consider the use of BZDs for this purpose (addiction), the physiological harm that results from this pattern of abuse is probably small. The main risks are behavioral. A cocaine toxic person can tolerate enormous doses of BZDs, which can produce major impairment of judgment. Combining the high-energy levels produced by a stimulant with the added impairment of judgment induced by large doses of sedatives can result in unpredictable, dangerous, and socially disruptive behavior. Sustained, combined use could also result in high-dose benzodiazepine addiction and dependence (Smith et al., 1989b).

The survey lends force to the notion that BZD and cocaine addiction problems are perceived as problematic by addiction medicine specialists in the United States. It is clear that in addiction treatment programs in the United States the biggest increase in BZD use is occurring with multiple-drug addiction patients. This growing pattern of multiple-drug addiction, particularly fueled by the current cocaine epidemic, will continue to have a major impact on chemical dependency programs in the United States.

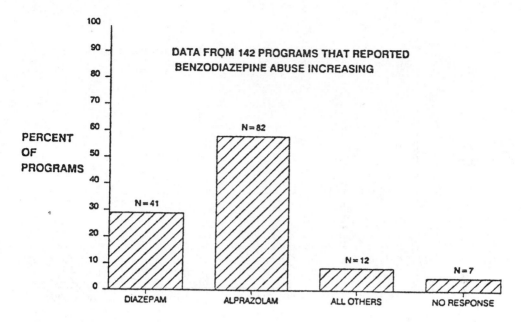

Figure 6 BZDs that are increasing.

XII. ADDICTION AND TREATMENT

In the above section, we focused on the addiction of BZD drugs, primarily in patterns of multiple-drug addicts, wherein the BZDs are being used addictively and to ameliorate the sympathomimetic effects of stimulant addiction, especially prolonged cycles of cocaine intoxication. Many researchers and clinicians are predicting that the next cycle of drug prominance will be dominated by smokeable forms of the current psychoactive drugs. If so, we can expect a deluge of even more virulent and longer-term smokeable stimulants than the current "free base" and "crack" forms of cocaine, such as "ice," the smokeable form of methamphetamine. Given this trend, we may also see the illicit development of both smokeable sedative-hypnotic preparations and smokeable hallucinogenic drugs, the latter along the lines of dimethyltryptamine (DMT), the extremely fast-acting South American hallucinogen that is smoked rather than swallowed.

In discussing the pharmacology of BZDs, we earlier noted some differences between the action of these drugs and others within the general family of sedative-hypnotic drugs. We pointed out that BZDs act through certain specific brain cell receptor sites, whereas other sedative-hypnotics seem to have a more general activity in the brain.

In this section, however, it is germain to discuss the many similarities that exist between not only BZDs and other sedative-hypnotic drugs, but the similarities between BZDs and any other psychoactive drugs that are the object of addiction as well. The first similarity is that BZDs can be the primary object of addictive disease.

High-risk populations for BZD addiction include individuals who have a personal or family history of alcoholism or drug addiction. Individuals may come in contact with BZD in treatment and become addicted through physician misprescribing, or they may be given the drugs by friends, or use them experimentally. Once addicted to BZDs, these individuals may obtain their drugs from the illegal market or by scamming a number of physicians with real or trumped-up ailments, stories of lost prescriptions, etc.

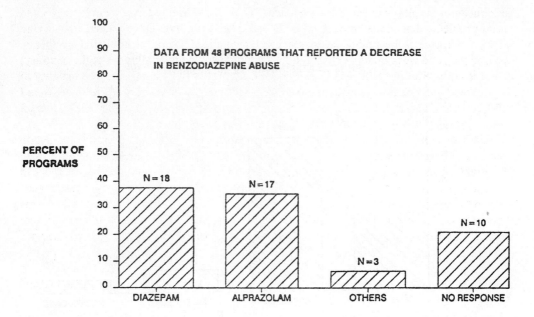

Figure 7 BZDs on decrease.

Addictive disease, including that with BZDs as its focus, is defined here as a disease in and of itself that has its own psychopathology and is characterized by compulsive use of a BZD, loss of control over that use, and continued use in spite of adverse consequences. Pharmacological dependence, characterized by the development of tolerance and the onset of withdrawal symptoms when the drug is abruptly stopped, is a primary component of BZD addiction. The disease is progressive, incurable, and can be fatal if not treated. Although the disease is incurable, it can be brought into remission through treatment, abstinence from all psychoactive drugs, and supported recovery.

Virtually every facet of the above definition calls for and deserves further explication. Although there are cases of use for self-medication of other physical or psychological conditions, as well as to mediate the effects of other drugs, it is now generally recognized that addiction is a primary disease rather than secondary to other conditions. As increasing numbers of addicts experience long-term sobriety and recovery from addiction to BZDs and other psychoactive drugs, it becomes increasingly evident that with the exception of dual diagnosis cases, wherein a patient is suffering from both addiction and a psychiatric disorder, most psychopathology experienced by victims of addictive disease is a result of that disease rather than its cause. As recovering individuals experience years of supported recovery, they often find that what had been originally diagnosed as their underlying psychopathology unravels apparently as a direct result of their recovery and abstinence.

Compulsion, loss of control, and continued use in spite of adverse consequences represent the continuum of active addiction. The pivotal point appears to be the loss of control. Anyone who has lost control over their use of a substance is by definition incapable of returning to controlled use, and any attempt to do so will result in repeated loss of control and addiction. This is what the recovering community means when it says, "A cucumber can remain a cucumber, but once it becomes a pickle, it cannot go back to being a cucumber."

A ubiquitous quality of addiction is the inability of the addict to admit that there is a problem. This quality is often called primary denial, and plays a major role in facilitating continued use in spite of adverse consequences. These consequences may include family and social problems that occur because of BZD and other drug use. Drug-related impairment in the workplace is becoming an increasingly recognized factor in industrial accidents, absenteeism, and work quality deterioration. Despite many popular attitudes to the contrary, denial is not willful disobedience or evidence of a moral failing. It is rather the inability of the addicted individual to recognize the consequences of the disease. Medical diagnosis of BZD addiction and intervention must, in part, break through the addict's denial system if it is to succeed in bringing about effective treatment and recovery.

Unfortunately, all too often physicians themselves are in codenial about the addiction potential of prescribed drugs. This denial is often fed by a lack of clear knowledge as to the nature and interrelationship of the drugs they are prescribing. An example of this can be seen in the response of some physicians to the discovery that diazepam could cause pharmacological dependence within accepted therapeutic dosage ranges. A response to this discovery was to switch patients from diazepam to another BZD, in spite of the fact that all BZDs are cross tolerant and have a basically similar potential for developing both tolerance and pharmacological dependence, as well as becoming a focus for addiction. In crass terms, switching a patient who has developed a pharmacological dependence to diazepam over to another BZD is roughly the same as telling an alcoholic patient whose drug of choice is scotch that everything will be all right if they switch to bourbon (Seymour et al., 1990).

A frequent sign of pharmaceutical dependency on BZDs is the development of tolerance. Tolerance has been defined by Miller and Gold (1990) as a loss of a particular effect at a given dose, or as a need to increase the dose of a drug in order to maintain the same effect. Tolerance can develop more rapidly with short-acting than long-acting BZDs because the interaction between the drug and brain receptors occurs more readily; i.e., the high lipid solubility shorter-acting BZDs are rapidly absorbed and distributed through the brain. The site of action for the BZD molecule is the gamma-aminobutyric acid (GABA) receptor. Because particular functions may depend on the location of receptor sites involved in BZD interactions, tolerance for such functions as sedation, hypnosis, motor activity, euphoria, and others, may develop at different rates and at varying doses. Although tolerance, resulting in a need for increased dosages to achieve desired effects, often accompanies the onset and development of addiction, it is primarily a marker for an adaptation from the interaction between BZDs and their receptors, but not a particularly accurate measure of addictive use.

Addiction in general seems to be progressive whether the disease is active or in remission. That the disease gets worse during its active phase is self-evident. That it continues to get worse during abstinence even though there is no overt symptomatology so long as the addict does not recidivate is a phenomena known primarily to the recovering community. Although there are studies in progress on this dynamic, the observation is clinical and not yet based on hard data. The phenomenon is characterized by the experience of individuals who return to active drug use after a period of abstention, sometimes many years, and find the new active addiction episode marked by rapid development of tolerance and loss of control leading to an active episode more severe than experienced prior to abstinence. Brissette and Seymour (1990) describe this phenomena as "the sleeping tiger." They characterize the addiction as a tiger cub that goes into hibernation when the addict enters abstinence and recovery but continues to grow and can awaken years later as a full-grown tiger.

Addictive disease is considered incurable because, by defintion, an addict cannot return to controlled use without lapsing sooner or later into compulsion, loss of control, and full addictive behavior. Addictive disease can, however, be brought into remission through supported recovery and abstinence from the primary drug as well as any other psychoactive drug.

Treatment for BZD addiction generally begins with detoxification, consisting of a mediated withdrawal of the drug. The substitution and withdrawal method utilizing the long-acting barbiturate phenobarbital is described earlier in this chapter. Because of the anxiolytic relation of BZDs to the GABA receptors, new and effective means for BZD detoxification may soon appear. Specific BZD receptor blocks, represented by Ro 15-1788, have been found and are in clinical trials. These agents are proposed to act as competitive antagonists by binding to the specific domain without inducing a functional change in the receptor. By blocking these binding sites, they block the effects of both agonists and inverse agonists, or substances that reverse the effects of BZDs and BZD agonists (Haefely, 1983).

Besides dealing with the BZD drug withdrawal and concomitant withdrawal symptoms and sequalae, treatment must give due attention to symptom reemergence. In many treatment situations, BZDs are used to manage symptoms, not cure the underlying problems. When the drug is eliminated, therefore, the underlying problems may remanifest themselves and need to be dealt with. Further, they need to be ameliorated without recourse to other psychoactive substances. Fortunately, there are many alternatives to drug therapy that are available to individuals in recovery and abstinence, including various forms of therapy, various forms of exercise, biofeedback, meditation, yoga, and other means developed by the cultures that throughout history have had to cope with the basic human problems that often result in addiction.

Although the disease may be incurable, remission can be achieved through abstinence and supported recovery. Such 12-Step programs as Alcoholics Anonymous and Narcotics Anonymous are playing an increasingly respected role in providing long-term respites from addiction, as are various forms of 12-Step–related group therapy, psychotherapy, and other aftercare and recovery-directed approaches. These can generally be provided on an outpatient basis and can mean the difference between a patient suffering "white-knuckle sobriety" and one enjoying the peace and productivity offered by a life of recovery and abstinence from psychoactive drugs (Seymour and Smith, 1987b).

XIII. A POSTSCRIPT ON PHYSICIAN'S ATTITUDES AND PRACTICES

In a recent article in the *Journal of Psychoactive Drugs*, Miller and Gold (1990) discussed their interpretation of some potentially negative attitudes and practices within the medical profession. They have consented to the presentation as a postscript to this chapter of their comments on physician attitudes and practices vis-à-vis benzodiazepines:

> Physicians in the United States and Europe have traditionally viewed medications and even drugs of abuse or addiction in a way that makes it difficult for them to appreciate the adverse consequences of drug use particularly addictive drug use. Understandably, the physicians's attitude is to find useful and beneficial purposes for medications/drugs. The aim is to ameliorate or eliminate complaints by patients and to improve the patients appreciation of psychiatric and other medical treatments.
>
> Some physicians utilize the self-medication concept, which is fraught with erroneous conclusions, to explain addictive drug use. The self-medication concept purports that drug abuse and addictive drug use are caused by an underlying condition that is alleviated by drugs: the drug user turns to drugs for relief of a depressive or anxiety state. Addictive use by definition is autonomous, with uncontrolled preoccupation to acquire and to use, according to *DSM-III-R* criteria [*Diagnostic and Statistical Manual of Mental Disorders*, 3rd edition–Revised, American Psychiatric Association, Washington, D.C., 1987]. As the depression and/or anxiety from the effects of the drug worsen, the addict continues to use in spite of the consequent depression and/or anxiety from the addictive use. If self-medication were the goal, then at some point during the addictive use, the user would discontinue drug use to avoid the increasing adverse consequences.

In one interesting study (Mayfield, 1979), mood was measured in response to alcohol ingestion in depressed alcoholics, depressed nonalcoholics, and nondepressed nonalcoholics. The depressed nonalcoholics experienced the greatest euphoria from alcohol, followed by the nondepressed nonalcoholics, while the depressed alcoholics benefited the least from the effect of alcohol in improving mood. Paradoxically, it is the alcoholic who will eventually drink to excess despite the low self-medication benefit and the toxicity of the alcohol-induced depression.

Furthermore, physicians rely heavily on a one-to-one doctor-patient relationship for information regarding the effectiveness of a given treatment approach, and they may weigh the risk-benefit ratio for any treatment, particularly pharmacological strategies that have significant untoward effects. Compliance by the patient receiving treatment is a source of gratification to the physician. The physician is trained and imbued with attitudes that drugs are powerful and are frequently indicated to treat illness. Addiction is sometimes viewed by physicians as a minor untoward effect that the patient can live with in order to achieve whatever beneficial effect, even if minor in itself, especially if the patient requests the drug. Moreover, physicians are not usually trained to diagnose and to recognize the syndrome of addiction with its adverse consequences. In fact, the preoccupation with the drug as well as the compulsive and recurrent use seems like almost ideal compliance to the physician, particularly when the patient may prejudiciously report only a favorable response to the drug in order to obtain more. Even if patients express concern over side effects, physicians are geared to de-emphasize it and to encourage continued use of the pharmacological treatment.

The consequences of addiction are sometimes difficult to enumerate if attempted while gathering a history in a one-to-one encounter. Profound alterations in mood, sleep, appetite, energy, attitudes toward self and others, and interpersonal relationships are not easily measured in the usual clinical setting. The level of impairment is often relative to the individual, so absolute standards fail to discriminate with sufficient accuracy the adverse effects of addictive drug use on the patient. The more obvious examples of consequences of addiction can be elusive to the untrained observer. The addicted benzodiazepine user may still persuade the physician that he or she has an underlying anxiety that only responds to more benzodiazepines and prefers to use them to decrease the risk of using other drugs, such as alcohol. The patient may in fact have an anxiety that is induced by benzodiazepines.

Physicians may have difficulty appreciating the power of the reinforcing effects of the drug and may not attempt to remove the benzodiazepines in favor of treating the underlying factors, with the expectation that the addiction will subside. Often in addictive use, specific treatment of addiction is necessary to eradicate the drug use. Sustained moderation of drug use in the context of addiction is extremely difficult, if not impossible, for the drug user. Addiction by definition is loss of control over use of the drug. Finally, the denial that exists in the addict regarding drug effects and consequences make it a formidable task to accurately assess drug use and effect even by knowledgeable and astute physicians.

XIV. DETOXIFICATION FROM BZDs

Outpatient detoxification is possible in the patient who is pharmacologically dependent on BZDs and who can tolerate the protracted and gradual taper over an extended period of time without external support and controls. Also, a more integrated and effective personality and a cohesive social, family and employment support may favor outpatient treatment because it provides some external control for the dependent and implies some adaptive ability and strength in interpersonal relationships. However, a prolonged detoxification may be unrealistic for some because it demands an exercise of control over the drug that the addict and/or pharmacologically dependent sometimes do not possess.

The detoxification from BZDs can be simplified and easily applied if basic principles are observed. First, BZDs have cross tolerance and dependence with each other, alcohol and other sedative/hypnotic drugs. Moreover, BZDs can be substituted for other BZDs and used interchangeably with barbiturates, so that conversion for equivalent doses can be calculated. Second, a long-acting BZD is more effective in suppressing the withdrawal symptoms and producing a gradual and smooth transition to the abstinent state. Greater patient compliance and less morbidity will result from the substitution of the longer-acting BZDs for detoxification from short acting BZDs (Smith and Wesson, 1983; Busto and Sellers, 1986; Perry and Alexander, 1986).

Third, select a BZD with lower euphoric properties such as chlordiazepoxide, avoiding the addiction propensity of diazepam as much as possible. Do not leave prn doses as this will give the addict a choice that can be beyond his or her control and avoid clinically confusing drug seeking behavior.

Withdrawal from BZDs is not usually marked by pronounced and acute hypertension and tachycardia as with alcohol so that prn doses are usually not needed for physiologic parameters. The anxiety of withdrawal should be controlled with the prescribed taper unless objectively it appears that the doses are too low when the standing dose can be increased but not a prn added. Caution is urged at this point as drug seeking behavior needs to be differentiated from anxiety of withdrawal. Only the anxiety of withdrawal when severe, need be treated with increased doses of BZDs although this occurrence is unusual with the long-acting BZDs. The prescriber must be in control of the dispensing of the BZDs for withdrawal as the addict by definition has a loss of control and cannot reliably negotiate in the schedule for tapering.

Fourth, the duration of the tapering schedule is determined by the half life of the BZD that is being withdrawn. For short-acting BZDs such as alprazolam, 7 to 10 days of gradual taper with a long-acting BZD or barbiturate is sufficient; 7 days for low dose use and 10 days for high dose use. For the long-acting BZDs, 10 to 14 days of a gradual taper with a long-acting BZD or barbiturate is sufficient; 10 days for low dose and 14 days for high dose use. Low dose is defined as recommended doses or less, and high dose above and beyond. The doses should be given in a Q.I.D. interval. Exact numerical deductions are not needed as the long acting BZDs accumulate to result in a smooth decline in the blood level of the BZDs over time (Smith and Wesson, 1983; Busto and Sellers, 1986; Perry and Alexander, 1986).

Fifth, the initial starting dose is determined by multiplying 50% of the total dose of BZDs used. Caution is urged because users in medical and non-medical populations often minimize the actual use so that a higher than calculated dose reported by the patient may be used if clinical suspicion warrants it. The conversion of BZDs from short acting to long acting can be employed by reference to Table 3. These conversion factors are interchangeable although recent evidence suggests that alprazolam may not be as stated in the table (Zipursky et al., 1985). However, because of the possibility of under reporting of alprazolam use in this report, an increase in initial dose above what is recalled by the patient may be sufficient. However, other recommendations for detoxification from high doses of alprazolam are the use of phenobarbital in the doses suggested in Table 3, in four divided doses, over the same time period as recommended for a taper with BZDs.

REFERENCES

Brissette, C., and Seymour, R.B. *Beyond the Three Headed Dragon*. Written on the Westwind, Sausalito, California, 1990.

Busto U., Sellers, E. M. Pharmacokinetic determinants of drug abuse and dependence: A conceptual perspective. *Clin. Pharmacokinet. 11*:144-153 (1986).

Covi, L., Lipman, R.S., and Pattison, J.H., et al. Length of treatment with anxiolytic sedatives and response to their sudden withdrawal. *Acta Psychiatr. Scand., 49*:51-64 (1973).

Glaubiger, G., and Lefkowitz, R.D. Elevated beta-adrenergic receptor number after chronic propranolol treatment. *Biochem. Biophys. Res. Commun., 78*:720-725 (1977).

Haefely, W. The biological basis of benzodiazepine actions. *J. Psychoactive Drugs, 15*(1-2):19-39 (1983).

Harrison, D.C., and Alderman, E.L. Discontinuation of propranolol therapy: Cause of rebound angina pectoris and acute coronary events. *Chest, 69*:1-2 (1976).

Hollister, L.E. Benzodiazepines 1980: Current update. *Psychosomatics, 21*:1-5 (1980).

Hollister, L.E., Motzenbecker, F.P., and Degan, R.O. Withdrawal reactions from chlordiazepoxide (Librium). *Psychopharmacologia, 2*:63-68 (1961).

Hollister, L.E., Bennett, J.L., and Kimball, I., Jr., et. al. Diazepam in newly admitted schizophrenics. *Dis. Nerve System., 24*:746-750 (1963).

Marks, J. An International Overview, *The Benzodiazepines: Current Standards of Medical Practice* (D.E. Smith and D.R. Wesson, eds.), MTP Press, Lancaster, England, 1985.

Mayfield, D.G. Alcohol and affect: Experimental studies. *Alcoholism and Affective Disorders* (D.W. Goodwin and D.G. Mayfield, eds.), SP Medical and Scientific Books, New York, 1979.

Merz, W.A., and Ballmer, U. Symptoms of the barbiturate/benzodiazepine withdrawal syndrome in healthy volunteers: Standardized assessment by a newly developed self-rating scale. *J. Psychoactive Drugs, 15*(1-2):71-85 (1983).

Miller, N.S., and Gold, M.S. Benzodiazepines: Tolerance, dependence, abuse, and addiction. *J. Psychoactive Drugs, 22*(1):1-11 (1990).

Mohler, H., and Okada, T. Benzodiazepine receptors: Demonstration in the central nervous system. *Science, 198*:849-851 (1977).

Murphy, G.E. Suicide and substance abuse. *Arch. Gen. Subst. Abuse, 45*(6):593-594 (1988).

Newsom, J.A., and Seymour, R.B. Benzodiazepines and the treatment of alcohol abuse. *J. Psychoactive Drugs, 15*(1-2):97-98 (1983).

Olsen, R.W., Loeb-Lundberg, F. Convulsant and anti-convulsant drug binding sites related to GABA-regulated chloride ion channels. *GABA and Benzodiazepine Receptors* (E. Costa, and G. DiChiari, and G.L. Gessa, eds.), Raven Press, New York, 1981.

Perry, P. J., Alexander, B. Sedative/hypnotic dependence: Patient stabilization, tolerance testing, and withdrawal. *Drug Intell. Clin. Pharm. 20*:532-536 (1986).

Rich, C.L., Young, D., and Fowler, R.C. San Diego Suicide Study: I. Young vs old subjects. *Arch. Gen. Psychiatry, 43*(6):593-594 (1986).

Seymour, R.B., and Smith, D.E. *The Physician's Guide to Psychoactive Drugs*. Haworth Press, New York, 1987a.

Seymour, R.B., and Smith, D.E. *Drugfree: A Unique, Positive Approach to Staying Off Alcohol and Other Drugs*. Facts on File Publications, New York, 1987b.

Seymour, R.B., Smith, D.E., Inaba, D., and Landry, M. *The New Drugs: Look-Alikes, Drugs of Deception and Designer Drugs*. Hazelden Foundation, Center City, Minnesolta, 1989.

Seymour, R.B., Smith, D.E., and Street, P. *Introduction to Addiction Medicine*. Written on the Westwind, Sausalito, California, 1990.

Skolnick, P., Moncada, V., Barker, J.D., et. al., Pentobarbital: Dual action to increase brain benzodiazepine receptor affinity. *Science, 211*:1148-1450 (1981).

Smith, D.E. Look-alike drugs and drugs of deception: Epidemiological, toxicological and clinical considerations. *Phenylpropanolamine: Risks, Benefits, and Conroversies* (J.P. Morgan, D.V. Kagan, and J.S. Brody, eds.), Praeger, New York, 1985.

Smith, D.E., and Wesson, D.R. Benzodiazepine dependency syndromes. *J. Psychoactive Drugs*, *15*(1–2):85–95 (1983).

Smith, D.E., and Wesson, D.R. (eds.). *The Benzodiazepines: Current Standards for Medical Practice*. MTP Press Limited, Lancaster, England, 1985.

Smith, D.E., Wesson, D.R., Landry, M. The pharmacology of benzodiazepine addiction. *Fam. Pract. Recert.*, *11*(9):94–107 (1989).

Smith, D.E., Wesson, D.R., Camber, S., and Landry, M. Perceptions of benzodiazepine and cocaine abuse by U.S. addiction medicine specialists. *Realities and Aspirations: Proceedings of the 35th International Congress on Alcoholism and Drug Dependence, Volume IV*. (R.B. Waahlberg, ed.), National Directorate for the Prevention of Alcohol and Drug Problems, Norway, 1989b.

Squires, R.F., and Braestrup, C. Benzodiazepine receptors in rat brain. *Nature, 266*:732–734 (1977).

Sternbach, L.H. The benzodiazepine story. *J. Psychoactive Drugs, 15*(1):15–17 (1983).

Tyrer, P., Rutherford, D., and Hugett, T. Benzodiazepine withdrawal symptoms and propanolol. *Lancet, 1*:520–522 (1981).

Wesson, D.R., and Smith, D.E. Low dose benzodiazepine withdrawal syndrome: Receptor site mediated. *CA Soc. Treat. Alcohol. Other Drug Depend. News, 9*:1–5 (1982).

Zipursky, R.S., Baker, R.B., Zimmer B. Alprazolam withdrawal delirium unrepressive to diazepan: Case Report. *J. Clin. Psychiatry 46*:344–345 (1985).

24

Amphetamines

Norman S. Miller
Cornell University Medical College, The New York Hospital–Cornell Medical Center, White Plains, New York

I. HISTORY

The amphetamine molecule is chemically simple with a number of intriguing actions. Attempts to refine and emphasize desired effects and minimize the less useful effects have led to the development of derivatives of amphetamines that are of clinical, experimental, and illicit interest [1].

The similarity in chemical structures between amphetamines and the catecholamines is significant for understanding the sympathomimetic properties of amphetamines. The mechanism of action of amphetamines can be inferred from the actions of the catecholamines that are structural analogues [2].

The various sympathomimetic molecules that are chemically related to amphetamine by substitutions in the amphetamine molecule are drugs that include diethylproprion, phentermine, chlorphentermine, fenfluramine, furfenorex, benzphetamine, methylphenidate, and phenmetrazine [2].

Psychostimulants such as mescaline are produced by substitution of the aromatic ring of the amphetamine molecule with one or more methoxy groups. These methoxylated amphetamines appear to act directly on receptors rather than indirectly by release of neurotransmitter. STP 2,5-Dimethoxy-r-methyl-amphetamine (STP) is the most potent methoxylated derivative of amphetamine [2].

The presence of a methyl group in the side chain alpha to the nitrogen results in a molecule that confers inhibitory action on the enzyme monoamine oxidase. This particular chemical modification of the amphetamine molecule has resulted in two clinically useful monoamine oxidase inhibitors, tranylcypromine and pheniprazene.

II. PREVALENCE

A. Estimation of Prevalence

Patterns of use of amphetamines are difficult to determine for a variety of reasons. Estimates of amphetamine use are always significantly low and probably represent only a tip of the iceberg. The indifference of society, the practices of the medical profession, and the denial of the user/addict contribute heavily to the resistance to assess drug use in the United States. The enormous professional pressures to prescribe medicines and the profitability of the manufacture and sales of drugs make surveillance and estimation impractical and even undesirable. Another source of resistance is the reluctance of legislative and medical bodies to pass effective laws regarding drug use. Only a modest amount of literature regarding amphetamine abuse and addiction exists as a result of these factors.

The addictive potential and nature of amphetamines were established in the late 1950s. By the early 1970s, the medical and psychiatric literature contained significant evidence and admonishments of a worldwide epidemic of amphetamine use from Peru and Mexico to Switzerland and France; from Great Britain and Sweden to the United States and Canada. Only recently, studies in Great Britain have found that the availability and the use of amphetamines were second to marijuana as the drug of choice of adolescents.

Amphetamine abuse and addiction gradually increased in prevalence in this country from the 1930s to the early 1960s and accelerated in the mid-1960s until amphetamines were classified as Schedule II drugs by the U.S. government. Even then, various state governments needed to pass "amphetamine acts" to further restrict the prescribing of the drug by physicians for medical and psychiatric disorders.

III. PATTERNS OF USE

Racemic beta-phenylisopropylamine, or amphetamine (Benzedrine), contains two isomers. The dextrorotatory isomer has the greater pharmacological activity. Dextroamphetamine (Dexedrine) was marketed as a more potent form (on a weight basis) of amphetamine. Except for the matter of dosage, no therapeutic distinction can be made between the levo isomer and the dextroisomer, as their pharmacological effects are identical.

Methamphetamine, also known as "speed" and "crystal" (Methedrine), is one of the many amphetamine derivatives that were synthesized by the pharmaceutical industry following the enthusiastic acceptance of amphetamine as a pressor drug, though clearly more potent as a central nervous system stimulant. It has been marketed by many drug companies for pressor and central nervous system stimulatory purposes. The popularity of amphetamine and methamphetamine relative to the other central nervous system (CNS) stimulants does not reflect any great pharmacological difference between these two groups of drugs, rather the highly important factors of their potency, ready availability, low cost, and wide publicity.

Ephedrine occurs naturally in various plants. It was used in China for at least 2000 years before it was introduced into Western medicine in 1924. Its central actions are less pronounced than those of the amphetamines.

Phenylephrine differs chemically from epinephrine in lacking an OH in the 4 position on the benzene ring.

Phenylpropanolamine is available in a wide variety of over-the-counter anorexants in tablets or capsules or in combination with other drugs such as caffeine. Continuation of this central nervous system stimulant as an over-the-counter drug is controversial [3].

Sympathomimetic agents appearing in Schedule IV of the Controlled Substance Act are diethylproprion, mazindol, and phentermine. Diethylproprion possesses pharmacological actions that are similar to amphetamine, although the CNS stimulation is less and the cardiovascular side effects are minimal. Mazindol, an imidazoline derivative, resembles a tricyclic antidepressant. Mazindol is a weaker CNS stimulant than amphetamine, with modest effects on the cardiovascular system. Phentermene is a sympathomimetic agent that is similar to amphetamine only with weaker actions [3].

Drugs introduced in Schedule III of the Controlled Substance Act are benzphetamine and phendimetrazine. These drugs are similar to amphetamines only with less CNS stimulation and cardiovascular effects. Phenmetrazine and methamphetamine are included with dextroamphetamine in Schedule II of the Controlled Substance Act [3].

IV. INTOXICATION

A. Acute Intoxication

The subjective effects of acute amphetamine intoxication were first systematically quantified in 1938 [4]. When amphetamines are taken by mouth, or inhaled as snuff, the user typically experiences sensations of euphoria, anxiety, enhanced self-awareness and self-confidence, heightened alertness, greater energy, and an increased capacity for concentration. Sensations of hunger and fatigue are reduced. The behavior of the user becomes hyperactive, talkative, irritable, and restless. The user moves around frequently with adventitious movements of the body. Judgment is compromised, with decisions and actions that reflect poor discretion. The user may say things or attempt actions that are foolish and hasty. Overt sexual behavior that is out of character may occur. Distortion in thinking and perceptions arise. Suspiciousness and guarded and hypervigilant scanning of the environment characterizes some users. Illusions of movement in space add to the elevated arousal. The emotional affect may appear more or less spontaneous [5–8].

Physiological to amphetamines responses are sympathomimetic. The physiological effects that accompany the psychological effects are those predicted from adrenergic drugs such as amphetamines acting positively on the sympathetic nervous system to mimic effects of norepinephrine and epinephrine. A rise in blood pressure, increase in pulse rate, pupillary dilation, and anorexia are regular concomitants of almost any acute dose of amphetamines. Blood glucose may increase as does blood coagulability. Skeletal muscle tension increases, whereas the smooth muscle contraction in the bronchial tubes and gastrointestinal tract decreases. The cardiovascular effects may manifest themselves not only by an increase in heart rate, but ectopic atrial and ventricular beats such as paroxysmal arterial tachycardias and premature ventricular contractions may occur. An initial increase in cardiac output results from positive chronotropic and inotropic effects, and a later reflexive drop in cardiac output from increased peripheral resistance of the vasoconstrictive effects of the amphetamines occur.

Dry mouth and dysphagia for solid foods may develop. The skin is cool from peripheral vasoconstriction. The pupils are dilated with a gaze that may be fixed or glassy or normal. The deep tendon reflexes are increased and fine tremors may be observable in the hands—especially when held in a position. Urinary retention and constipation result from the inhibitory effect of the sympathetic nerve supply to the bladder and bowel. The physiological effects are dose-related, but tolerance develops over time to some degree to most of the cardiovascular, neurological, and gastrointestinal effects [3,9].

In increasing doses, the mood may be predominantly anxious and the speech rapid, slurred, and incoherent. Stereotypic movements may intermix with fidgetry, jerky, random motions. Teeth grinding may occur. Ataxic gait may be present. The thoughts may be loosely connected, illogical, and tangential. Affect may appear silly and irrelevant. Headache, nausea, vomiting, and malaise may predominate. Frank delusions, especially paranoia, may develop [3,9].

Abstinence withdrawal syndrome from amphetamines that indicates physical dependence follows even small, acute doses. The effects are generally opposite to those of the intoxicating state; the mood may be depressed, thinking and behavior are slowed, movements are deliberate and methodical; fatigue, somnolence, increased appetite, ennui, and perhaps a "craving" or "drive" to use further stimulants may be present [10,11].

These symptoms are more intense and appear sooner with intravenous administration, but otherwise are the same qualitatively for oral and intravenous routes. The oral and intravenous experiences are different because of a faster and greater rise in peak blood levels of amphetamines with the latter.

B. Chronic Administration

Increasingly, with continued use of amphetamines and the passage of time, the pace of the thoughts quicken and concentration is impaired. Abrupt mood changes replace the initial euphoria, to which tolerance develops. Misperceptions and illusions appear and are often disturbing and frightening to the user. Movements, lights, and actions by people in the surroundings are distorted and exaggerated. Frank visual, tactile, olfactory, and auditory hallucinations may follow further amphetamine use. These occur less often with prolonged consecutive oral administrations than with intravenous use. Shadows become people, and the user may see his body as covered with sores and vermin [12,13].

The auditory hallucinations are usually voices that make derogatory statements about the user. The voices may be singular or in groups. The individual may or may not recognize the voices. These voices are frightening and sometimes prompt, aggressive, and violent actions toward the self or others [14,15].

The suspicious and guarded thinking may progress to the frank paranoia of a delusional degree. The delusions may be well formed or vague and often paranoid in content and affect. The individual may act accordingly toward a delusion in a frightened or violent manner. Violent behaviors have been seen to occur in response to the paranoid state toward self and others [16].

The primary characteristics of amphetamine psychosis are ideas of reference, paranoid delusions (delusions of persecution and grandiosity), and auditory and visual hallucinations in the setting of a clear consciousness. Many of these patients with a drug-induced psychosis are diagnosed as acute or chronic paranoid schizophrenics. The similarities between the idiopathic and drug-induced schizophrenia has led to the formulation of a biochemical model of schizophrenia [17–19].

The psychosis is associated with a large individual variation of response, both qualitatively and quantitatively. The psychosis may ensue after administration of a few small doses—or larger doses of amphetamines are required over a longer period of time to induce the psychoses [20,21].

The amphetamine-induced psychosis is antagonized by haloperidol in humans. Haloperidol is a dopamine blocker that neutralizes the effect of dopamine at the postsynaptic site. Haloperidol also is effective in idiopathic schizophrenia in reducing the delusions and hallucinations. Other dopamine blockers such as phenothiazines are also effective in both idiopathic schizophrenia and the amphetamine-induced psychoses.

Amphetamine-derivative psychosis does occur. Phenmetrazine by oral, but particularly intravenous, administration produces a psychosis identical to that produced by amphetamines. Paranoid ideation, stereotyped behavior, hallucinations, and thought disorders all occur from phenmetrazine use. Similarly, other sympathomimetic agents, diethylpropiron and methylphenidate, have also been documented as etiological agents in the amphetamine psychosis.

V. DIAGNOSIS

A simplistic formulation that is useful for conceptualization of drug use is "exposure plus vulnerability" equals use, abuse, and addiction. The supply of amphetamines through legal and illegal production and the prescribing practices of physicians determine the exposure. The vulnerability of individuals and groups to seek out, use, abuse, and become addicted to the amphetamines is derived from psychological and physical predisposition. A complete discussion is complex and outside the range of this chapter. Characterization of the etiology of drug use is at best descriptive at this juncture in our objective understanding, although some sound theoretical formulations have significant support [22–25].

Exposure contributes significantly to abuse and addiction in that an estimated 85% of the population has used some form of an illicit drug by the age of 25. Controversy exists over whether drug use per se is causally related to drug abuse and addiction. The position that addicts have a narrow range of vulnerability is naive. Certainly high-risk populations do exist. These populations may abuse and become addicted to drugs in low levels of exposure. However, higher level exposure may select out less vulnerable populations [22,26,27].

The American pharmaceutical industry has probably been making from 8 to 10 billion doses of stimulant drugs annually. The U.S. Food and Drug Administration (FDA) estimated in 1968 that approximately 4–5 billion conventional doses of amphetamines were sold illegally and diverted into channels of illegal usage. The ease with which distributors of illicit drugs could obtain substantial properties of stimulants in bulk or individual dosage forms made possible the rapid spread of amphetamine abuse in the 1960s. Some diversion of legally manufactured amphetamines to illicit markets may still occur.

Regulation of drug manufacture and sale is not stringent. As a result, some of the "speed" offered for sale, and particularly that in a form suitable for intravenous injection, is now derived from the "basement" chemist [28].

The addictive potential is high with amphetamines. Classification of amphetamines as a Schedule II drug emphasizes that characteristic. The addictive potential, although well established, has not been appreciated by everyone. In a controlled study under double-blind conditions, normal subjects preferred amphetamine's effects over all other drugs, including morphine. Some studies have even demonstrated that amphetamines are preferred over morphine by heroin addicts. These findings suggest the reasons why amphetamines remain prevalent and popular out of proportion to the extent of their chemical utility [29].

Many people find the effects of "uppers" useful and gratifying. Individuals who use "downers" such as alcohol, sedatives, tranquilizers, and hypnotics may use an upper to "get going" in the morning. This downer and upper cycle has been increasingly common with the cocaine and alcohol combination, but is seen with a variety of other stimulants, including amphetamines and amphetamine derivatives prescribed over-the-counter and obtained illicitly. A plethora of possible combinations include "speed balling," in which heroin or a barbiturate is mixed with amphetamines or cocaine. A businessman may use alcohol in the evening and a nasal decongestant in the morning. A housewife may take benzodiazepines or barbiturates during the day and evening and use an amphetamine derivative in the morning.

Frequent entries to amphetamine use are for weight reduction in obesity, as an aphrodisiac to stimulate and prolong sexual pleasure, the emotional "blues," depression, a desire to "to get a kick out of life," and psychiatric diagnoses such as attention deficit disorder in children and narcolepsy in adults. The mode of introduction to these drugs may serve only as an explanation for exposure but not as a sufficient cause for continued use once the adverse consequences have begun to appear. At that point, an addiction may be operative that signals a preoccupation, compulsive use, and recurrent use in spite of costly physical, mental, and emotional consequences.

The treatment of depression with amphetamines is transient and ineffective for the reason similar to the loss of an anorectic effect with the development of tolerance. Dependence develops as well to result in symptoms that worsen the depression as depression is a withdrawal effect of amphetamines. The depression can be profound and worse than the original depression for which amphetamines were prescribed.

The least controversial indications for the use of amphetamines seem to be in the treatment of narcolepsy and attention deficit disorders in children and adults. These conditions are rare and uncommon, respectively, so that the number of legal prescriptions should be minuscule. Amphetamines have been classified as a Schedule II drug in the United States. Since 1969, most of the use of amphetamines has been restricted by voluntary basis on prescribing and by official prohibitions in the United Kingdom.

VI. TOLERANCE AND DEPENDENCE

Tolerance develops to many of the actions of amphetamines and related drugs. Tolerance develops to the euphoria, anorexia, hyperthermia, hypertension, and the increased excretion of norepinephrine. Tolerance implies a relative loss of an effect at a particular dose so that only a transient and less intense euphoria or anorexia may occur in response to amphetamines after chronic administration. Continued use and an increase in dose only produce a short-lived enhancement of an effect that eventually diminishes for that dose [30].

Tolerance to the cardiovascular effects of the amphetamines, and, more specifically, to their vasoconstrictor actions, is strongly suggested by the fact that amphetamine addicts can survive single intravenous doses of 1000 mg or more with only an occasional untoward physiological effect. The risk of a cardiovascular disturbance would be high is a nontolerant user were similarly exposed to amphetamines [25,31].

Little tolerance seems to develop to the "awakening" or "anti-sleep" actions of these drugs. The undiminished effectiveness of amphetamines in the treatment of narcolepsy, and the state of persistent wakefulness during chronic use lend support to this view.

Chronic administration may lead to a depletion of neurotransmitters at the presynaptic site. Less neurotransmitter is available for release into the synaptic cleft to act on the postsynaptic site. A deficiency in the neurotransmitter leads to the development of tolerance to the particular effect produced by the neurotransmitter. Less dopamine for release by the presynaptic neuron is manifested as less euphoria and locomotion [32,33].

Withdrawal states or the expression of physical dependence may be attributable to compensatory postsynaptic changes that occur in response to a depletion in neurotransmitters. Postsynaptic supersensitivity develops from an increased proliferation of receptor sites to compensate for a lack of stimulation from the neurotransmitter. The supersensitivity may underlie the various mood changes and stereotypic behaviors that are seen in the chronic withdrawal states from amphetamine [32–34].

A denervation supersensitivity of postsynaptic sites may develop such as in the caudate nucleus. The increased sensitivity of the caudate nucleus may underlie some of the stereotypic movements. Postsynaptic supersensitivity is similarly an explanation for neuroleptic-induced tardive dyskinesia that may result from a chronic postsynaptic dopamine receptor blockade [32–34].

Often, a significant improvement in mood, energy, and paranoid thinking occurs within days. However, a slow recovery over weeks, months, and perhaps years may be required for complete resolution of the signs and symptoms of withdrawal from chronic amphetamine use. Mood lability, memory loss, confusion, and paranoid thinking and perceptual abnormalities may persist for over a year or perhaps indefinitely.

VII. NEUROCHEMISTRY

Neurons containing dopamine originate in the substantia nigra and the ventral tegmentum in the interpedunclular nucleus. The neurons of the substantia nigra project to the corpus striatum. A feedback pathway from the caudate nucleus to the substantia nigra is mediated by the neurotransmitters acetylcholine (ACH) and gamma-aminobutyric acid (GABA), which inhibit neuronal firing. In addition, presynaptic autoreceptors regulate the release of dopamine by inhibition. Dopamine neurons also project from the ventral tegmentum to the mesolimbic and mesocortical areas of the brain. The "reward" center where reinforcement occurs originates in neurons in the lateral hypothalamus that project in the median forebrain bundle through the septal area to the ventral tegmentum. The presynaptic neurons from the lateral hypothalamus may release opioid peptides because the neurons of the ventral tegmentum contain opiate receptors [34,35]. Amphetamines and related drugs may act on the postsynaptic dopamine neurons of the reward center to enhance drug-seeking behavior.

Norepinephrine-containing neurons originate in the brainstem. The major sites are the locus ceruleus in the pons and the midbrain. The presynaptic neurons from these areas project diffusely to hypothalamic, mesolimbic, and cortical regions. Norepinephrine neurons are involved in both the ascending and descending reticular-activating system and in mediating food reinforcement and promoting satiety effects [36,37].

The action of amphetamines on the dopamine (DA) neurons in the mesolimbic area may be responsible for changes in mood such as euphoria, anxiety, and depression. Similar action on the mesocortical DA neurons may mediate effects on judgment and insight by amphetamines [34,35]. Increased arousal seen with amphetamines may result from amphetamine-enhanced activity of norepinephrine neurons in the reticular-activating system in the midbrain.

Amphetamine and related drugs appear to affect the neurotransmitter systems to enhance their activity by two major mechanisms. The first, and probably the most significant, is promoting release of dopamine and norepinephrine from the presynaptic neurons. The second is to block the reuptake of catecholamines by the presynaptic neuron. Reuptake is the major route of elimination of catecholamines that are released into the synaptic cleft. More catecholamines are present at the postsynaptic site because of their increased release and their termination of action by reuptake by the presynaptic neuron is blocked by amphetamine. A greater sustained action of the catecholamines at the postsynaptic site may be responsible for the behavioral effects of the amphetamines [38,39].

Evidence suggests that amphetamines act on the presynaptic neurons that provide the adrenergic supply to the hunger center in the lateral hypothalamus. Amphetamines may act to block hunger by enhancing catecholaminergic effects at that site. The dopamine innervation to the caudate nucleus is involved in mediating the amphetamine-induced motor stereotypic behavior, perhaps with a contribution from the amygdala. The mesolimbic system and the olfactory tubercle appear to be involved in locomotor activity associated with amphetamine-induced locomotor behavior through effects on dopamine [40–42].

REFERENCES

1. Innes, I.R., and Nickerson, M. (1975). Norepinephrine, epinephrine and the sympathomimetic amines, *Pharmacological Basis of Therapeutics*, 5th ed. (L. Goodman, and A. Gilman, eds.), Macmillan, New York, p. 477.
2. Biel, J.H. (1970). Structure-activity relationships of amphetamine and derivatives. *Amphetamines and Related Compounds* (E. Costa and S. Garattini, eds.). Raven Press, New York, p. 3.
3. Goodman, L., and Gilman, A. (eds.). (1975). *Pharmacological Basis of Therapeutics*, 5th ed. Macmillan, New York.

4. Bahnsen, P., Jacobsen, E., and Thesleff, H. (1938). The subjective effect of beta-phenylisopropylamin-sulfate on normal adults. *Acta Med. Scand. 97*:89.

5. Jacobsen, E., and Wollstein, A. (1939). Studies on the subjective effects of the cephalotropic amines in men. *Acta Med. Scand. 100*:159.

6. Schroeder, D.J., and Collins, W.E. (1974). Effects of secobarbital and d-amphetamine on tracking performance during angular acceleration. *Ergonomnics, 17*:613.

7. Smith, G.M., and Beecher, H.K. (1959). Amphetamine sulfate and athletic performance: Objective effects. *J.A.M.A., 170*:542.

8. Cameron, J.S., Specht, P.G., and Wendt, G.R. (1965). Effects of amphetamines on moods, emotions and motivation. *J. Psychol, 61*:93.

9. Martin, W.R., Sloan, J.W., Sapira, J.D., et al. (1971). Physiologic, subjective and behavioral effects of amphetamine, methamphetamine, ephedrine, phenmetrazine and methylphenidate in man. *Clin. Pharmacol. Ther., 12*:245.

10. Lasagna, L., Von Felsinger, J.M., and Beecher, H.K. (1955). Drug-induced mood changes in man. I. Observations on healthy subjects, chronically ill patients, and post addicts. *J.A.M.A., 157*:1066–1120.

11. Kilbey, M.M., and Ellinwood, E.H. (eds.) (1977). Chronic administration of stimulant drugs: Response modification, *Cocaine and Other Stimulants*. Plenum Press, New York, pp. 410–429.

12. Griffith, J.D., and Cavanaugh, J., Oates (1968). Paranoid episodes induced by drug. *J.A.M.A., 205*:39.

13. Ellinwood, E.H., Jr. (1967). Amphetamine psychosis. I. Description of the individuals and process. *J. Nerv. Ment. Dis., 144*:273.

14. Angrist, B., Sathananthan, G., and Wilk, S. (1974). Amphetamine psychosis: Behavioral and biochemical aspects. *J. Psychiatr. Res., 11*:13.

15. Davis, J.M. (1975). Catecholamines and psychosis, *Catecholamines and Behavior,* Vol. 2 (A.J. Freidhoff (ed.), Plenum Press, New York, Chapter 5.

16. Kalant, O.J. (1966). Abuse of amphetamine-like drugs, *The Amphetamines: Toxicity and Addiction*, Thomas, Springfield, Illinois.

17. Prinzmetal, M., and Bloomberg, W. (1935). The use of benzedrine for the treatment of narcolepsy. *J.A.M.A., 105*:2051.

18. Bell, D.S. (1965). Comparison of amphetamine psychosis and schizophrenia. *Br. J. Psychiatry, 3*:701.

19. Segal, D.S., and Janowsky, D.S. (1978). Psychostimulant-induced behavioral effects: Possible models of schizophrenia, *Psychopharmacology: A Generation of Progress* (M.A. Lipton, A. DiMascok, and K.F. Killan, eds.), Raven Press, New York, p. 461.

20. Connell, P.H. (1958). Amphetamine psychosis. *Maudsley Monograph No. 5*. Oxford University Press, London.

21. Bell, D.S. (1973). The experimental reproduction of amphetamine psychosis. *Arch. Gen. Psychiatry, 29*:35.

22. National Commission on Marijuana and Drug Abuse (March 1973). Drug use in America: Problems in perspective. *Second Report of the National Commission on Marijuana and Drug Abuse*, National Institute on Drug Abuse, Washington, D.C.

23. Mayfield, D.G. (1979). Alcohol and affect: Experimental studies, *Alcoholism and Affective Disorders* (D.W. Goodwin and C.K. Erickson, eds.), SP Medical and Scientific Books, New York, pp. 99–107.

24. Schuckit, M.A. (1983). Alcoholic patients with secondary depression. *Am. J. Psychiatry, 140*(6):711–714.

25. Kramer, J.C., Fischman, V.S., and Littlefield, D.C. (1967). Amphetamine abuse. *J. Am. Med., 201*:305.

26. Grinspoon, L., and Bakalar, J.B. (1980). Drug dependence: Non-narcotic agents, *Comprehensive Textbook of Psychiatry*, 3rd ed. (H.I. Kaplan, A.M. Freedman, and B.J. Sadock, eds.), Williams and Wilkins, Baltimore.

27. Strategy Council on Drug Abuse (1973). Federal strategy for drug abuse and drug traffic prevention, 1973. *Sups. of Docs,* U.S. Government Printing Office, Washington, D.C.

28. Canadian Medical Association (1969). Non-medical use of drugs, with particular reference to youth. Report of the special committee on drug misuse, council on community health care, Canadian Medical Association. *Canad. Med. Assoc. J., 101*:804.

29. Knapp, P. (1952). Amphetamine and addiction. *J. Nerv. Ment. Dis., 115*:406.

30. Rylander, G. (1971). Stereotype behavior in man following amphetamine abuse. *Proc. Eur. Soc. Study Drug Tox., 12*:28.

31. Cox, C., and Smart, R.G. (1970). The nature and extent of speed use in North America. *Canad. Med. Assoc. J., 102*:724.

32. Dominic, J.A., and Moore, K.E. (1969). Supersensitivity to the central stimulant actions of adrenergic drugs following discontinuation of a chronic diet of a-methyltyrosine. *Psychopharmacology, 15*:96.

33. Creese, I., Burt, D.R., and Snyder, S.H. (1977). Dopamine receptor binding enhancement accompanies lesions-induced behavioral supersensitivity. *Science, 197*:596.

34. Dackis, C.A., and Gold, M.S. (1985). Pharmacological approaches to cocaine addiction. *J. Subst. Abuse Treatment, 2*:139–145.

35. Miller, N.S., Dackis, C.A., and Gold, M.S. (1987). The relationship of addiction, tolerance and dependence: A neurochemical approach. *J. Subst. Abuse Treatment*, Vol. 4, pp. 197–207.

36. Ungerstedt, U. (1971). Stereotaxic mapping of the monoamine pathway in the rat brain. *Acta. Physiol. Scand.* (Suppl.)*83*:49.

37. Von Voigtlander, P.F., Moore, K.E. (1970). Behavioral and brain catecholamine depleting actions of U-14.624, an inhibitor of dopamine-B-hydroxylase. *Proc. Soc. Exp. Biol. Med., 133*:817.

38. Chiueh, C.C., and Moore, K.E. (1975). D-Amphetamine-induced release of "newly-synthesized" and "stored" dopamine from the caudate nucleus in vitro. *J. Pharmacol. Exp. Ther., 192*:642.

39. Azzaro, A.J., Ziance, R.J., and Rutledge, C.O. (1974). The importance of neuronal intake of amines for amphetamine-induced release of ^{3}H-norepinephrine from isolated brain tissue. *J. Pharmacol. Exp. Ther., 189*:110.

40. Thornburg, J.E., and Moore, K.E. (1973). The relative importance of dopaminergic and noradrenergic neuronal systems for the stimulation of locomotor activity induced by amphetamine and other drugs. *Neuropharmacology, 12*:853.

41. Russek, M., Rodrigues-Zendejas, A.M., and Teitelbaum, P. (1973). The action of adrenergic anorexigenic substances in rats recovered from lateral hypothalamus lesions. *Physiol. Behav., 10*:329.

42. Hoebel, B.G. (1975). Satiety: Hypothalamic stimulation, anorectic drugs, neurochemical substrates. *Hunger: Basic Mechanisms and Clinical Implications* (D. Novin, W. Wyrujicka, and G. Bray, eds.), Raven Press, New York, p. 33.

25

Nicotine

James Cocores
Fair Oaks Hospital, Summit, New Jersey

I. INTRODUCTION

Nicotine is the deadliest drug used in the world. Cigarette smoking has caused more suffering and death to Americans than World War I, World War II, the Vietnam War, AIDS, heroin addiction, cocaine addiction, and terrorist attacks combined [1]. Tobacco use is linked to over 390,000 deaths each year in the United States alone [2]. But the threat of death is no match for the enormous pleasure derived from tobacco use. Informing patients about the medical consequences of nicotine addiction has proven to be inadequate in motivating many smokers to abstain or seek treatment. Additional measures are needed to engage smokers into treatment.

Tobacco companies are extremely wealthy and politically influential. Even though it has been banned from television, tobacco advertising continues in magazines, movies, and on roadside signs. In addition to commercial advertising, another major force propagating nicotine addiction consists of the example set by relatives and friends. Nicotine addiction continues to flourish even though the disease costs society billions of dollars in health care costs and lost productivity. Public education about the physical hazards of nicotine must continue in order to offset protobacco advertisement. But public education alone is not enough. Additional information must be conveyed to smokers by clinicians of all specialities in order to help reduce the demand for nicotine. Physicians, therapists, and educators must expand their strategy to include information about all aspects of nicotine addiction, especially treatment.

This chapter does not focus on the health consequences, addiction potential, diagnostic criteria, politics, or economics of nicotine addiction. Instead it focuses on the clinical management of nicotine addiction. Smokeless tobacco will first be briefly reviewed in place of cigarette addiction.

II. SMOKELESS TOBACCO

The American Indians introduced Christopher Columbus and Europe to tobacco [3]. Snuff became a popular method of nicotine delivery commonly sniffed or inhaled in cultures such as Great Britain, Bavaria, and South Africa. Oral snuff use later became more popular among Americans, Scandinavians, and North Africans. During the 1800s it was believed that snuff could help combat the plague, and also kill insects which infest house plants and trees. Medicated snuff was used to treat dental, sinus, and stomach problems. The use of smokeless tobacco eventually was viewed as unsophisticated and use persisted primarily in the southern United States. Smokeless tobacco is considered a "gateway" drug leading to cigarettes, alcohol, and other drugs.

One of the fastest growing forms of nicotine addiction among young adults and children is smokeless tobacco [4]. The number of smokeless tobacco users in the United States is estimated at about 12 million [5]. The marked resurgence of smokeless tobacco use among young people is a direct result of marketing by tobacco companies, which use prominent sports figures and entertainers to promote the product. The average consumer of smokeless tobacco is between 18 and 24 years of age [6]. Smokeless tobacco users are primarily male, although one study reported 1% of the adolescent females surveyed used it daily [7]. Over 80% of smokeless tobacco users first experiment with the drug before the age of 15. Most patients treated for smokeless addiction in our suburban clinics are white male athletes in high school or college. They are usually referred by their coach or a parent and comprise about 1% of nicotine patients treated. Smokeless tobacco use is more prevalent in other areas. Thirteen percent of third-grade males and about 22% of fifth-grade males in Oklahoma use smokeless tobacco regularly [8]. Another study of high school students in Oregon found 23% of tenth-grade boys to be daily users [9]. An alarming 21% of kindergarten children in Arkansas have tried smokeless tobacco [10].

There are two basic methods in which smokeless tobacco is used, dipping and chewing. Dipping involves placing moist or dry tobacco between the cheek and gum. Chewing involves the mastication of a wad of tobacco leafs in the cheek area. Manufacturers of smokeless add alkaline materials to snuff and chewing tobacco because large amounts of nicotine enter the buccal mucosa at an alkaline pH. The blood nicotine level achieved using smokeless tobacco can be comparable or even exceed that achieved by smoking cigarettes [11]. Smokeless nicotine blood levels remain higher in comparison to the shorter spiked nicotine blood levels which result from cigarette smoking.

Smokeless tobacco is not safe. It increases the risk of oral and pharyngeal cancer [12]. Gingival blood flow is reduced by smokeless tobacco, resulting in ischemia and necrosis. Epinephrine release is augmented and contributes to hypertension. Other problems include gingival recession, soft tissue alterations, and leukoplakia [4].

Specific personality traits preexist or develop as a direct result of drug addiction. Addiction-prone personality traits such as lacking moderation and difficulty with impulse control both contribute to the etiology of smokeless tobacco addiction. There is also evidence to suggest that smokeless tobacco users have more difficulty trusting others, are more aloof, reserved, detached, tough minded, likely to have used marijuana/alcohol, unsentimental, and more group dependent when compared to nonusers [9]. Dippers are more group dependent than chewers. In addition to personality traits, social factors contribute to the eiology of smokeless tobacco addiction. For example, a nonuser is more likely to begin chewing to-bacco by having more peers or close friends that chew [13]. Parents may perceive smokeless tobacco as less of a health risk and less addicting than cigarettes. Therefore, the image of a chewer may be viewed positively in comparison to cigarette smoking. Genetics also play a role in the development of smokeless tobacco addiction. Personality, environmental, and hereitary factors combined determine the etiology of smokeless tobacco addiction.

There are many similarities between cigarette addiction and smokeless tobacco addiction. The prevention, diagnosis, and treatment of nicotine addiction is similar in all its forms: cigarettes, smokeless tobacco, nicotine gum, or any combination.

III. EDUCATION AND PREVENTION

The prevention of nicotine addiction requires education at home, in school, and by youth groups. Educators should be clinicians experienced in nicotine addiction. The health hazards of all nicotine delivery systems should be discussed. Education on the medical consequences of nicotine addiction can serve as an aversion stimulus with young people who have never used nicotine. Young people who have never used nicotine can be taught to "just say no." Nicotine addiction education should also include progression, the disease concept, and reading assignments.

A. Reading Assignments

Assigning easy to read literature [14,15] is a good first step. A discussion of the reading assignment is necessary to help clarify any misinterpretations. Adolescents are also asked to write a short essay on the reading material. This exercise also helps confirm reading comprehension. Adults also benefit from reading and learning in the privacy of their home. Experience has shown that books are useful in engaging patients with depression [16], panic disorder [17], posttraumatic stress disorder [18], and drug addiction [19,20] into treatment. Reading about nicotine addiction helps prevent experimentation and helps users consider cessation.

B. Progression

Nicotine addiction is a progressive disease. Experimentation slowly progresses to casual use which gradually turns into nicotine addiction. Neophytes have a choice as to whether or not to smoke the next cigarette. People dependent on nicotine have no choice.

The progression of nicotine addiction can be understood in terms of four predictable phases. An understanding of these four phases of nicotine addiction is important for prevention, in understanding progression, when engaging patients into treatment, and formulating a treatment plan. They are the precontemplative, contemplative, action, and maintenance phases [21].

Nicotine users who have not considered cessation are in the precontemplative phase. Adolescents and young adults are commonly in the precontemplative phase. Nicotine users in the precontemplative phase believe, "I can take it or leave it." The germination of defense mechanisms such as denial, rationalization, intellectualization, and minimization begin to sprout during the precontemplative phase of nicotine addiction. The educator's goal is to advance the nicotine user to the next phase of contemplation. This can be accomplished by educating the user about progression—progression in the traditional sense and in the form of understanding these four phases. All nicotine-addicted persons were once capable of controlling their nicotine use. Attempts should be made to weaken the patient's belief of invincibility that sounds like this: "I don't smoke that much," "I won't get hooked," "I am too young," or "it won't happen to me." Scare tactics should be avoided. One lecture or session is usually insufficient when attempting to convert precontemplative users to the contemplative phase. Clinicians and concerned relatives too often try once and then give up. Persistence is necessary in order to succeed. The educator must proceed with confidence, enthusiasm, and empathy. Empathy follows the understanding that nicotine addiction is not a bad habit but a disease. Nicotine addiction is not sought out; it is stumbled upon.

The contemplative phase of nicotine addiction begins with transient thoughts about cutting down or stopping. This phase can begin spontaneously, with education or as a result of accrued nicotine-induced psychosocial stressors. The transition to the contemplative phase may be ushered in by a relatives myocardial infarct or advanced emphysema, the death of a friend, diagnosis of cancer in a relative, shortness of breath, odor on clothing, a dental technician comment, a cough, pregnancy, or the clinician's advice. People in the contemplative stage should be counseled about all treatment programs available. Patients are encouraged to participate in the formulation of their own treatment plan. Nicotine addicts are more likely to make a commitment, follow through, and comply with treatment recommendations when they are involved in designing their treatment plan. This strategy facilitates the transition from the precontemplative to the action phase.

The action phase begins with a commitment to reduce or eliminate nicotine intake. Most patients who have never attempted to stop are usually unwilling to enter a nicotine addiction treatment program. These patients should be encouraged to use will power and gradually reduce nicotine intake by a mutually agreed upon target date. This is a form of nicotine fading. Some smokers stop using will power alone. Those who are unable to stop learn the meaning of nicotine craving, withdrawal symptoms, environmental cues, powerlessness, and relapse. It is difficult to recover without understanding these concepts. The inability to recover using will power also underscores the need for a treatment program. The belief that "I am not hooked," or "I can stop when ever I want" is revised after relapse.

The maintenance phase begins with nicotine abstinence and consists of applying relapse prevention methods to all aspects of daily living. Mourning about nicotine deprivation is gradually replaced by positive reinforcement. The process from feeling deprived without nicotine to feeling content without nicotine takes about 1 year. The process is termed recovery.

C. The Disease Concept

A basic understanding of the disease concept [22] is important in the prevention and treatment of nicotine addiction. The disease concept of addiction can be summarized by one word found in the first step of Nicotine Anonymous [23,24]. "We admitted we were powerless over nicotine—that our lives had become unmanageable." Powerlessness implies that nicotine addiction is foreign, alien, or a physiological disorder. Viewing addiction as a disease removes will power from the picture and helps minimize the stigma of nicotine addiction: A stigma of being bad, lacking intelligence, being evil, weak in character, lacking strength, or having a death wish. Most people believe nicotine addicts can stop using will power alone: "He just doesn't want to stop," or "He is too stupid." Patients are counseled that they are not responsible for the disease, but they are responsible for their own recovery. Nicotine addicts are as powerless over nicotine as cocaine addicts are over cocaine. The disease concept highlights powerlessness and powerlessness is the opposite of will power.

An etiological review also helps strengthen the patient's conceptualization of nicotine addiction as a disease. The cunning disease of nicotine addiction evolves slowly by drawing from three major areas: hereditary, environment, and personality. Studies which support a genetic component to the development of nicotine addiction [25–31] have been proposed. It is believed that all drug addictions result in part from the genetic predisposition. Another equally important etiological factor is environment. Nicotine is readily available in most settings and regions. There is no enforceable age limit; children buy cigarettes from vending machines. The drug is legal, inexpensive, and favorably looked upon. Favorable attitudes are often subliminally shaped by role models who smoke and by advertisements which portray smokers as "smooth characters." The third equally important factor involves aspects of personality. A prevailing personal view that smoking is sophisticated, glamorous, refined, and mature more readily evolves with certain personality traits. The etiology of nicotine addiction depends on specific aspects of the addicts personality, environment, and hereditary. Treatment addresses all three factors.

Prevention entails educating young nonsmokers and neophytes about nicotine addiction. Reading and writing assignments are helpful in preventing the disease. The health consequences of nicotine addiction should be reviewed but should not constitute the focus of discussion. It is more important to focus on the early signs of nicotine addiction, progression, and the disease concept.

IV. DIAGNOSIS

The diagnosis of nicotine addiction is facile to determine using the diagnostic criteria [32,33] or administering tests. Unlike most other drug addicts, nicotine-dependent patients are usually reliable historians.

The Fagerstrom Tolerance Questionnaire (FTQ) is an easy to administer paper-and-pencil test consisting of eight questions that measure nicotine addiction [34]. The FTQ correlates with other measures of nicotine addiction such as carbon monoxide and continine [35]. The questionnaire is commonly used in research and clinical settings. Another self-report test is the Horn's Reason for Smoking Test which measures individual differences in smoking patterns [36].

Making the diagnosis of nicotine addiction requires little skill. Unlike other diseases, efforts to treat the illness are usually minimal or cease after the diagnosis of nicotine addiction is made. Like other diseases, the clinician must do all that is possible to treat the illness. The clinician must be persistent, creative, and innovative even after numerous attempts have been made to motivate the patient. For example, have the resistant patient sign an AMA (Against Medical Advice) form or ally with nonsmoking family member.

V. ENGAGING PATIENTS INTO TREATMENT

Making the diagnosis, counseling users about the disease concept, medical consequences, and progression is sufficient in motivating about 5% of patients to stop on their own without additional professional assistance. The remaining 95% of nicotine addicts require more than education, professional advice, or a health scare. One attempt to persued a patient to enter treatment is usually insufficient. The clinician may have to educate, encourage, and counsel the patient numerous times. The clinician must follow up by keeping the issue of nicotine addiction treatment alive during subsequent sessions. This is essential whether the smoker comes to you for marital counseling, depression, or heart disease. The nicotine addict may stop with education alone, after one counseling session, after numerous counseling sessions, after one treatment attempt, after multiple treatment attempts, or may never stop. The point is to keep trying to engage the nicotine addict into treatment. After the patient has entered treatment the referring clinician should follow up by monitoring compliance with treatment recommendations and relapse prevention.

Table 1 lists levels of cigarette addiction and corresponding treatment methods. The levels in Table 1 are determined by the number of cigarettes smoked and the presence of craving for convenience only. The reader may choose to determine treatment levels in other ways such as replacing the number of cigarettes smoked with Fagerstrom scores, or by substituting the number of cigarettes with the phases of nicotine addiction discussed earlier in association

Table 1 Cigarette Addiction Treatment

Level (No. cigarettes)	Intervention
1 (0–5/wk)	Reading assignment Education Will power
2 (5/wk–10/day)	Set target date Change brands Log cigarettes Fade by 20% every 4 days
3 (10–20/day)	Repeat 1 Review levels 1 and 2 relapses A behavioral and cognitive program —Smokers Anonymous —American Lung Association —Smokenders —Live for Life —Private therapy

4 (> 21/day)	Review 1–3
	Review all relapses
	Plus one: hypnosis
	          acupuncture
	          silver acetate

5 Severe withdrawal	Review 1–4 Review all relapses Nicotine replacement and Clonidine
6 > Three prior treatments	Review 1–5 Review all relapses Scopolamine, antidepressants, or other experimental medicines
7 Difficult to treat patients	Review 1–6 Review all relapses Try a new combination or inpatient treatment

with progression. The levels in Table 1 can also be replaced by the number of treatment attempts. So a smoker who has never tried to stop before should begin treatment at level 1 before going to level 2 or 3.

After the patient becomes familiar with the phases of nicotine addiction, progression, and all the treatment methods have been reviewed the treatment plan is negotiated and developed. The clinician may need to use sales tactics when attempting to engage patients into treatment. She or he must be knowledgeable, secure, persistent, and firm. The clinician must at the same time be pleasant, enthusiastic, nonjudgemental, calm, confident, and emphathetic. Involve a significant other in the process whenever possible. The skill of engaging patients into nicotine cessation treatment requires practice.

Patients with prior treatment attempts should be informed about nicotine cessation treatment programs available which they have not tried. A new target date is negotiated and the new mutually formulated treatment plan is initiated. Each relapse must be reviewed carefully prior to the new stop date. Relapse experience is usually essential to long-term recovery. Patients who have learned from each of their relapses have a good prognosis.

VI. NICOTINE FADING

Nicotine fading involves setting a stop date and gradually decreasing nicotine intake prior to the first day of nicotine abstinence. For example, a stop date is set for 28 days from today and the patient reduces cigarettes smoked by 20% every four days. Fading is the treatment most commonly chosen by smokers contemplating cessation for the first time. If a patient has never tried this method of nicotine cessation, it should be tried along with education and counseling. Smokers are instructed to record the time each cigarette is smoked in a diary or on the back of their physician's business card [37]. A pocket computer is sold commercially that sounds when the smoker may have their next cigarette. The computer is useful for patients who are unwilling to keep a written log of cigarettes smoked during the fading process. Another style of nicotine fading involves the use of a nonpreferred brand. Nonpreferred brands are usually smoked less, less nicotine is obtained when they are smoked [38], and can serve as an aversion stimulus.

VII. BEHAVIORAL AND COGNITIVE THERAPY

A. 12-Step Approaches

The goal of behavioral and cognitive therapy is to change the way in which the drug addict acts and thinks about their drug of choice. Alcoholics Anonymous (AA) has successfully been providing behavioral and cognitive therapy to the public on a large scale since 1935. The 12 Steps of AA [23] have been adopted by other self-help groups such as Narcotics Anonymous. Many hospital-based drug recovery programs use the 12 Steps as part of treatment. Recovery is an on-going process of self-improvement, requiring socialization in a peer group [20]. Addicts use the 12 Steps as a guide to replacing the somber void of drug abstinence with increasing amounts of acceptance, wisdom, freedom, and elevated self-esteem. Addiction and recovery both begin with peer influence.

The more recently founded Nicotine Anonymous is not as available or well attended as AA. The 12 Steps of Nicotine Anonymous are used as an integral part of many nicotine-cessation programs. For example, the second half of the first step highlights the need to identify and explore examples of unmanageability. Identifying specific examples of unmanageability facilitates the acceptance of powerlessness over nicotine. Patients are then better able to accept guidance and follow treatment recommendations.

B. Identifying Defense Mechanisms

Denial, minimization, rationalization, and intellectualization are defense mechanisms essential to the progression of most drug addictions. Nicotine users readily identify these defense mechanisms in others and are not as successful with themselves. Nicotine addicts only begin to identifying these defenses in themselves after the defenses are recognized in others. This process of identification can be accelerated by requiring patients to attend Nicotine Anonymous meetings. Smokers, like other drug addicts, may be resistant to treatment recommendations. Some patients will say, "Thats not for me Doc." Patients should attend at least six Nicotine Anonymous meetings before formulating a conclusion. Nicotine Anonymous helps patients identify the defense mechanisms which fuel progression, provides education, treatment information, and support. If a Nicotine Anonymous meeting is not available in your area call

Nicotine Anonymous World Services at (415) 922-8575 for assistance in establishing a meeting.

C. Understanding Nicotine Craving

It is useful to counsel patients about the difference between craving and the thought of using nicotine. Craving is defined here as an overwhelming obsession with the acquisition and use of nicotine. Craving follows a brief period of nicotine abstinence. Nicotine craving can force a person to leave their comfortable home dressed in night clothes at 1 A.M. to drive in a dangerous storm in search of an all-night convenience store. As recovery time accumulates, the frequency and intensity of craving declines. Craving commonly occurs for about a year and is triggered by environmental and psychological factors and neurotransmitters [39]. It is very difficult to negotiate with a nicotine craving even in the face of a serious health problem. Certain medicines can be helpful in reducing the magnitude and frequency of nicotine craving.

Thoughts of using nicotine are nonreverberating memories of the pleasure associated with nicotine use. Thoughts about smoking transiently enter and leave consciousness. Thoughts are not overwhelming and are not of sufficient magnetic force to make someone drive in a storm in search of nicotine. Thoughts of using nicotine persist a lifetime and are triggered by psychological or environmental cues. Cognitive and behavioral therapy is essential in coping with the life-long pleasurable thoughts of nicotine use.

There are numerous behavioral and cognitive methods of coping with cravings and thoughts. One method involves waiting out the craving by imposing a 10-min delay on any decision regarding the craving. The craving may be minimized by self-assurance that it is not that bad or will not last forever. Distraction is another way of dealing with nicotine craving or thoughts. Patients are encouraged to turn their attention to positive activities such as reading or meditating. Some patients remind themselves of how successful they have been whereas others benefit from listing the benefits already gained from recovery. Some patients mentally review some of the nicotine-induced consequences already experienced while waiting for the craving to pass. Another popular technique involves hypothetically thinking through a relapse and the progression that follows.

D. Environmental Cues

Patients learn to identify specific environmental cues which trigger the desire to use nicotine. Alternate methods of responding or coping are taught and practiced. It may necessitate substituting sugarless gum for a cigarette smoked with a morning cup of coffee. Patients are taught to plan ahead for potentially dangerous situations and how to devise alternate ways of coping with the situation. For some patients getting out of a particular situation or avoiding certain people is useful. Assertiveness training helps prepare the smoker to say "No thank you" to friends and relatives offering nicotine. In addition, practicing assertiveness in other problem situations reduces the small daily frustrations that add up to a stressful day.

E. Flexibility and Alternate Behavior

Nicotine addicts often start out with inflexible personalities or develop them as a result of the addiction. Relapse can be a matter of not being flexible enough to accept alternate thoughts and actions, or insisting on doing things the same way. Sometimes focusing on the progression that follows the smoking of one cigarette results in smoking if the individual has not developed the flexibility of taking an alternate coping route.

Recovering nicotine addicts learn to implement substitute behavior which may include talking to a friend, filing, painting, housework, exercise, bending paper clips, deep breathing, eating almonds or other nutritional substitutes. A self-reward system is developed such as being in a peaceful place, playing a musical instrument, collecting the money usually spent on cigarettes, working on a hobby, going to a movie, or dancing.

F. Stress Management

Involvement in a satisfying job, a less than satisfying job, part-time work, volunteer work, work around the house, or public service helps minimize nicotine withdrawal–related stress. Exercise and improved nutrition is recommended to help reduce stress, and to ward off weight gain. Other stress-management methods include reducing procrastination, dwelling on the past, taking a bath instead of a shower, leaving time for the unexpected, avoiding xanthines, and careful selection of friends [40]. Patients with caffeinism [33] should never stop abruptly, but should be given a fading schedule.

G. Goal Reinforcement

Total abstinence from all nicotine delivery systems is the goal. The goal is reviewed with patients at regular intervals. Recovering nicotine addicts regularly fantasize about smoking one cigarette now and then. Recovering nicotine addicts may be acquainted with a particular "social smoker" who they wish to emulate. Patients are regularly reminded that social smokers become addicted to nicotine; nicotine addicts to not become social smokers. The recovering addict is reminded that tolerance to nicotine is permanent and progression is the rule after smoking one cigarette. A recovering nicotine addict avoids smoking a cigarette, pipe, chewing nicotine gum, chewing tobacco, or smoking one cigar always.

VIII. HYPNOSIS

As many as 50% of nicotine addicts treated using hypnotherapy remain abstinent at the 6- to 12-month follow up [41,42]. Most smoking cessation programs report a success rate of 20% [43]. Claims about the efficacy of hypnosis have not been substantiated in controlled research. But this is true of most other nicotine cessation methods used in clinical practice. Hypnosis, like acupuncture, is viewed by many as a placebo response which leads to cessation through the mystique of the procedure. Uncertainty about its mechanism of action does not negate the fact that many addicts begin long-term nicotine abstinence following hypnosis. Therefore, smokers who inquire about the efficacy of hypnosis should not be discouraged if they have tried other treatments at levels 1, 2, or 3. Clinicians should familiarize themselves with local hypnotherapists and the smoking cessation programs they provide.

IX. ACUPUNCTURE

Oriental medicine includes massage, exercise, herbs, and acupuncture. Some Western physicians reject acupuncture "because it is empirical medicine—developed from experience and observation, but not based on systematic theory or science" [44]. Despite this belief, acupuncturists practice in most cities and towns throughout America. In addition to traditional placement of fine 30- to 36-guage disposable needles, newer more modern applications are available which include low-voltage electropuncture, laser acupuncture, injection of medicines at acupoints, and acupressure. Acupuncture is usually painless. Although there are studies linking acupuncture to endorphins and other neurotransmitters related to pain perception, its mechanism of action is unknown. Patients confirm that acupuncture resolves medical problems ranging from arthritic pain to nicotine addiction. Ear acupuncture is used to reduce or prevent the signs and symptoms of nicotine withdrawal, including craving, restlessness, anxiety, and the sense of deprivation. Acupuncture may also combat weight gain which sometimes accompanies nicotine withdrawal. Like hypnosis, acupuncture is a withdrawal facilitator that should not be used alone but in conjunction with a recovery program.

X. SILVER ACETATE

Silver acetate lozenges containing 2.5 mg of active ingredient are available without a prescription. The cherry flavored lozenge is used approximately every 4 h for about 3 weeks. Silver acetate makes smoke taste bitterly unpleasant at the first puffs of a cigarette. The aversive response serves as a reminder to smokers to extinguish the cigarette. In some cases, the deterrent reaction becomes stronger during cessation. There are a number of anecdotal studies using silver acetate as a smoking deterrent and a few placebo-controlled double-blind studies have been published [45,46]. The lozenges are not to be used more than 6 times per day and no longer than 3 weeks. Silver acetate lozanges are used in conjunction with a comprehensive nicotine addiction treatment program.

XI. NICOTINE REPLACEMENT

Cigarette smoking is reduced following the administration of nicotine intravenously, orally, in a capsule, buccally, nasally, or across the skin [47]. A substitute commonly used in fading is nicotine polacrilex, or nicotine gum. The polacrilex preparation is approved by the Food and Drug Administration. Its alkaline pH permits nicotine absorption across the buccal mucosa.

Nicotine gum is prescribed only after the patient completely understands how to use the polacrilex preparation. Patients should read *How to Use Nicotine Gum & Other Strategies to Quit Smoking* [15]. Correct usage is of paramount importance. Nicotine polacrilex is not chewed like bubble gum; instead it is gently chewed as one would puff on a cigarette and then parked between the teeth and cheek. The amount of nicotine absorbed depends on numerous variables. One is the amount of saliva swallowed while chewing. The majority of swallowed nicotine is not absorbed into the bloodstream because of alteration in the first pass through the liver. Therefore, patients who drink fluids while using nicotine gum may absorb less nicotine than patients who retain nicotine longer in the buccal cavity.

A gum fading schedule is planned after the daily maintenance dose is established. For example, a patient using 15 pieces of 2-mg gum each day during the first week of treatment gradually reduces the number of pieces to 10/day by the end of the first month and to 5/day by the end of the second month. Patients are able to discontinue nicotine gum after 3–6 months of treatment. Patients must be reminded not to smoke while using polacrilex. Patients who use polacrilex for nicotine replacement and fading should be counseled regularly about other aspects of nicotine cessation. Unsupervised patients are more likely to use the gum over an extended period of time and nicotine polacrilex addiction may result [48]. This is especially common with nicotine addicts who also suffer from other drug addictions.

Preliminary research with transcutaneous nicotine patches is promising. Nicotine patches are more likely to deliver a steady, predictable, and measurable amount of nicotine when compared to polacrilex. Nicotine patches are manufactured in different diameters. The transcutaneous system is used by applying the large-diameter patch to skin for the first week, an intermediate-size patch during the second week, and the smallest patch during the third week. A disadvantage of skin patches is the development of contact dermititis.

XII. CLONIDINE

Clonidine is an antihypertensive medication used to treat opiate withdrawal [49]. Two short-term studies, one of which was placebo controlled, showed the efficacy of oral clonidine for smoking withdrawal [50,51]. Oral clonidine reduces the craving, irritability, impatience, anxiety, and restlessness associated with nicotine withdrawal. Some disadvantages of clonidine include its use in hypotensive patients, compliance problems with multiple daily doses, inconsistent blood levels, and side effects. Side effects include orthostatic symptoms, fatigue, dry mouth, and sedation. Clonidine is prescribed only after obtaining a complete medical history and physical. The mechanism of action is unknown, but it is believed that clonidine minimizes nicotine withdrawal symptoms by reversing adrenergic hyperactivity in the locus ceruleus and amygdala.

Transcutaneous clonidine is available in 0.1-, 0.2-, and 0.3-mg patches. A randomized placebo-controlled study found a marked increase in craving, irritability, anxiety, and restlessness in the placebo group when compared to the transcutaneous clonidine group [52]. Hunger and poor concentration persisted in the subjects. Transcutaneous clonidine is preferred to oral clonidine when steady-state blood levels, decreased side effects, and compliance are considered. In severe cases of nicotine withdrawal, it may be necessary to use oral clonidine in combination with the transcutaneous system. Another innovative combination involves the concurrent use of nicotine polacrilex and clonidine [53].

Clonidine is usually prescribed for 3–4 weeks and the dose is gradually reduced over the detoxification period [1]. For example, a transcutaneous patch delivering 0.2 mg of clonidine/day/week is applied. The stop date is set for the third morning after clonidine is started. The 0.1-mg patch is used during the second and third week. If a patient develops contact dermatitis, application of a topical steroid cream often resolves the problem. Clonidine is used in conjunction with a recovery program.

XIII. SCOPOLAMINE

Scopolamine is a belladonna alkaloid used to treat motion sickness. Scopolamine is prescribed in the form of a transcutaneous patch and is used by clinics throughout the United States to facilitate nicotine withdrawal. The use of scopolamine in conjunction with a recovery program is becoming popular. For this reason physicians should be aware of its contraindications and how it is being used to treat nicotine addiction.

The literature surrounding the use of scopolamine as treatment for nicotine addiction is scanty with methodological deficiencies. In 1970, it was reported that mecamylamine and scopolamine reduced puffing in monkeys [54]. A medical protocol using scopolamine was developed later and piloted in humans [55]. Nicotine-dependent patients are treated with one injected dose of scopolamine, atropine, and chlorpromazine. The anticholinergic injection is supplemented with 2 weeks of an oral combination medication containing an anticholinergic and a benzodiazepine. The pilot study reported that 40% of the 500 smokers treated with the anticholinergic protocol remained nicotine free at the end of 1 year [55]. One commercial smoking cessation program has been using this anticholinergic protocol for over 6 years and has treated thousands of patients in dozens of locations across America. The anticholinergic protocol should not be administered by physicians inexperienced with the medicines or the procedure.

A simplified version of the anticholinergic protocol outlined above has been tried and it has been reported that transcutaneous scopolamine alone eliminates nicotine craving and reduces withdrawal symptoms [48,56,57]. One study found 87% of 31 subjects treated with transdermal scopolamine remained nicotine-free at the end of 6 months [56]. Other uncontrolled studies [48,57] report a decrease in nicotine craving and withdrawal symptoms after using transcutaneous scopolamine. Patients who have been medically assessed and found appropriate for scopolamine treatment apply one 1.5-mg transcutaneous patch to the mastoid area for three days. The old patch is discarded after 3 days and a fresh 1.5-mg patch is applied to the opposite mastoid area and worn for three additional days. Transcutaneous scopolamine is not recommended for use beyond 6 days, and is contraindicated in patients with a known hypersensitivity to scopolamine or in patients with glaucoma. Scopolamine should be avoided in patients who are recovering from alcohol or drug addiction [57], with mental disorders [58], cardiac problems, and intestinal problems. Scopolamine is usually reserved for the difficult to treat nicotine addict or multiple relapser.

XIV. TREATING RECOVERING ALCOHOLICS

Recovering alcoholics who smoke cigarettes often smoke more during early recovery. Recovering nicotine addicts often relapse while drinking alcohol. Alcohol users are significantly more likely to smoke cigarettes than nondrinkers. About 29% of Americans suffer from nicotine addiction, whereas over 85% of alcoholics are nicotine dependent. A phenomenological link exists between nicotine and alcohol addiction. It is unknown why the relationship exists, but many theories have been proposed. Psychoanalysts consider smoking an extension of a strong oral drive found in alcoholics. There may be parallel personality traits. Alcoholics commonly lack moderation and have difficulty with impulse control. These two traits coupled with inadequate coping skills also aid in fueling nicotine addiction. In addition, the tendency toward socialization in drinkers may increase their exposure to smokers which increases the drinkers probability of taking up smoking or tobacco chewing. Both addictions may share similar or common underlying genetic and biological family traits. They are the most widespread forms of drug addiction.

Alcohol and drug addicts are one of the most difficult groups of smokers to treat. This is especially true with recovering alcohol or drug addicts. Alcoholics Anonymous has helped millions of people recover from alcohol. Unfortunately, AA has been slow to recognize the need to consider nicotine addiction in treatment even though its founders, Bill W. and Dr. Bob, both died from the disease. Nicotine addiction is also inadequately addressed by most drug and alcohol treatment centers. Many alcoholism counselors believe that alcohol should be treated first and nicotine treatment should not be considered at all prior to a year of alcohol recovery. Many recovering alcoholism counselors are smokers themselves. Their example conveys denial, rationalization, intellectualization, and minimization to newly recovering alcoholics. The most common complaint I have heard from recovering staff members who smoke is, "It is too overwhelming for patients to stop using alcohol, cocaine, marijuana, and nicotine." The implication is that if a drug addict abstains from nicotine they may relapse to alcohol or cocaine. Others say that those who do abstain from nicotine are better able to maintain long-term abstinence from other drugs, including alcohol [59].

Nicotine-dependent staff members present the first obstacle when attempting to address nicotine addiction as part of alcohol and drug treatment. Nicotine-dependent staff members must first begin their own nicotine recovery. This preliminary measure serves as an on-going staff workshop or inservice on the management of nicotine addiction in chemically dependent patients. A drug and alcohol treatment unit can begin to address nicotine addiction only after most of the nicotine-addicted staff members have vintage nicotine recovery. We have already learned this lesson with alcohol and other drugs. It is extremely unwise and poor clinical practice to employ an active marijuana smoker as a drug counselor. It would be similarly impossible for a smoking staff member to counsel patients on nicotine addiction. Recovered alcohol and nicotine counselors make a lasting impression on patients, whereas counselors who use even occasionally are not taken seriously [60]. The herculian process of converting alcohol and drug counseling staff members to a nicotine-free status takes over 1 year when the unit directors are aggressive.

After nicotine-addicted clinical staff members are treated (> 75%), it is reasonable to expect alcohol- and drug-addicted patients to begin complying with nicotine-cessation efforts. Counselors are then able to take treatment methods developed for alcohol and drug addiction and apply them toward the management of nicotine addiction. The nicotine portion of a patients mixed drug addiction can also be used as a hands-on tool for working through drug cravings, dealing with environmental drug triggers, and practicing other relapse-prevention methods, which in turn can be applied to other drug dependencies. It may entail setting a nicotine stop date at the 120th day anniversary of alcohol abstinence, or it may mean abstaining from nicotine along with alcohol. The integration of nicotine addiction treatment into alcohol and drug treatment has started in numerous centers. Preliminary reports suggest that alcoholics are able to abstain from both alcohol and nicotine without jeopardizing their recovery from either.

XV. RELAPSE PREVENTION

Relapse prevention is the most important aspect of recovery. All smoking-cessation treatment plans must include relapse-prevention counseling. Relapse prevention often centers around a delusion shared by many recovering nicotine addicts. The delusion has been stated as, "I can be a social smoker," or "I'll smoke just one cigarette then stop again." It is crucial that the counselor review progression and how one cigarette rapidly leads to many cigarettes. Other guidelines for relapse prevention [20] include:

1. Using all energy and determination to avoid nicotine
2. Planning ahead for hazards and temptations
3. Breaking the pattern of stimulus and response
4. Restoring and strengthening the body
5. Finding alternative interests and pleasures
6. Learning to handle anxiety and depression
7. Dealing with troubled relationships without nicotine
8. Socializing with other recovering smokers
9. Mentally review prior relapses

XVI. PROGNOSIS

Prognosis is a function of commitment, motivation, persistence, and number of relapses. Smokers who have developed social or physical consequences as a direct result of nicotine addiction generally have a better prognosis. But not all smokers diagnosed with lung cancer or myocardial infarct are able to stop smoking. Middle-aged nicotine addicts usually have a better prognosis than younger users. The most guarded prognosis is found in smokers having a major mental disorder and another drug addiction.

A common belief is that prognosis depends on the brand of cigarettes smoked and the amount smoked. The brand or amount smoked is not as crucial as the efficiency with which the nicotine delivery system is used. Variables include the percentage of a cigarette smoked, number of deep puffs per cigarette, or whether the filter air holes are being covered. A patient smoking ultra light cigarettes may reach a higher nicotine blood level than a smoker of regular cigerettes.

Prognosis improves with each treatment attempt and with the knowledge gained from each relapse. Relapse prevention wisdom is strengthened with each treatment attempt and relapse. The experience and knowledge gained with each treatment is cumulative [56]. The following case illustrates this very important point:

Ms. A visited a hypnotherapist 5 years ago and has been nicotine-free ever since. Ms. A recommended hypnosis to her friend, Ms. E. Ms. E visited the hypnotherapist and abstained from cigarettes for 18 h. Ms. E said that hypnosis helped because she resumed smoking only five cigarettes per day instead of 30. Two months later, Ms. E told Ms. A that hypnosis was worthless because her smoking escalated back to 30 cigarettes per day.

Ms. E tried hypnosis as her first smoking cessation effort. Ms. A relapsed after completing Smokenders, attending dozens of Nicotine Anonymous meetings, attending numerous acupuncture sessions, and after 90 days of nicotine gum. Ms. A had made four separate smoking cessation attempts before visiting the hypnotherapist.

Ms. A was finally successful in abstaining from nicotine for 5 years because of the cumulative knowledge gained from each of the five treatment experiences. Ms. E's experience with hypnosis can become very valuable if she studies the relapse and applies the knowledge toward her second treatment attempt. This significantly improves her prognosis.

Relapse is not failure nor is previous treatment a wasted experience when they are carefully examined. Studying prior relapses can lead to highly specific and effective relapse-prevention measures. Relapsers should not be badgered. After a brief "breathing period," the clinician again begins to engage the smoker back into treatment. A new mutually designed treatment plan is formulated and a new target date is set.

XVII. LABORATORY TESTS

Tobacco smoke consumption is measured in a variety of ways, including air, blood, urine, skin [61], and saliva [62]. Laboratory test selection depends on the hypothesis being tested.

Carbon monoxide is eliminated mainly by respiration and is measured via expiration or by measuring carboxyhemoglobin using the spectrophotomotor. The measurement of expired carbon monoxide is inexpensive and noninvasive. Carbon monoxide is a good marker of tobacco smoke consumption and a good indicator of short-term use [63].

Thiocyanate is a metabolite of hydrogen cyanide that takes about 3–6 weeks to reach an individual's presmoking level. Thiocyanate is measured using a spectrophotometer with serum or saliva samples. Because certain foods, such as leafy vegetables, are sources of cyanide, the diet of vegetarians must be carefully assessed. Thiocyanate has relatively good sensitivity and specificity.

Blood nicotine is usually measured by gas chromotography and radioimmunoassay. Measuring nicotine in blood is a direct measure, but the procedure is expensive and the sampling time can be problematic. It is an excellent short-term measure of nicotine with excellent specificity.

The primary metabolite of nicotine is continine. Urinary continine is used as a qualitative indicator, but may not be a good quantitative predictor of blood continine level. Because blood concentrations of continine are stable throughout the day, sampling time is not problematic. Continine is a moderately priced test of tobacco consumption with excellent specificity and sensitivity. Urine continine is commonly used in clinical practice.

For a complete description of various tobacco smoke consumption markers, including absorption, metabolism, and disposition kinetics, see Ref. 63.

XVIII. CONCLUSIONS

Nicotine addiction is the most preventable cause of death. The medical consequences of nicotine addiction are well known, but this knowledge alone has been inadequate in motivating most nicotine addicts to seek treatment. Irregardless of specialty, all clinicians should familiarize themselves with nicotine addiction treatment and take a more aggressive stance in motivating patients to get professional assistance. The clinician may choose to treat nicotine addiction privately, counsel the smoker as the smoker concurrently undergoes a treatment from level 2 to 7, withdraw the smoker with a medicine as the patient attends a behavioral program, or may refer the patient for complete outpatient nicotine addiction treatment [64]. As a minimum, clinicians should be supportive and educate their patients about nicotine addiction treatment with enthusiasm, optimism, and hope. Clinicians have been waiting too long for a "magic bullet" conforming to the scientific method, or for someone else to treat nicotine addiction; sufficient ammunition is already available for each clinician to begin fighting this illogical disease.

REFERENCES

1. Ornish, S.A. (1989). Transdermal clonidine may help reduce craving and withdrawal in smokers. *Psychiatr. Times. 11*:16.
2. U.S. Department of Health and Human Services (1988). *The Health Consequences of Smoking: Nicotine Addiction. A Report of the Surgeon General*. U.S. Government Printing Office, Washington, D.C.
3. Penn, W.A. (1902). *The Soverane Herbe: A History of Tobacco* Grant Richards Co., New York, p. 56.
4. Glover, E.D., Schroeder, K.L., Henningfield, J.E., et al. (1988). An Interpretive Review of Smokeless Tobacco Research in the United States: Part I, *J. Drug Ed., 18*(4):285.
5. U.S. Public Health Service, *The Consequences of Using Smokeless Tobacco A Report of the Advisory Committee on the Surgeon General*, Department of Health, DHEW Publications No. (PHS) 86-2874, U.S. Government Printing Office, Washington, D.C., 1986.
6. Maxwell, J.C. (1980). Maxwell manufactured products report: Chewing stuff is growth segment, *Tobacco Rep., 107*:32.
7. Severson, H.H., Lictensten, E., and Gallison, C. (1985). A pinch instead of a puff? Implications of chewing tobacco for addictive processes. *Bull. Soc. Psychiatr. Addict. Behavior, 4*:85.
8. Glover, E.D., and Edwards, S.W. (1984). Current research in smokeless tobacco, *Annual Association for HPER*, Shangrila, Oklahoma, October.
9. Edmundson, E.W., Glover, E.D., Alston, P.P., and Holbert, D. (1987). Personality traits of smokeless tobacco users and nonusers: A comparison. *Int. J. Addict. 22*(7):671.
10. Young, M., and Williamson, D. (1985). Correlates of use and expected use of smokeless tobacco among kindergarten children. *Psychiatry Rep., 56*:63.
11. Gritz, E.R., Baer-Weiss, V., and Benowitz, N.L. (1981). Plasma nicotine and continine concentration in habitual smokeless tobacco users. *Clin. Pharmacol. Ther., 30*:201.
12. Hoffman, D., and Hecht, S.S. (1985). Nicotine-derived N-nitrosamines and tobacco related cancer. *Cancer Res., 45*:2285.
13. Ary, D.V., Lichtenstein, E.L., and Severson, H.H. (1987). Smokeless tobacco use among adolescents: Patterns, correlates, predications, and the use of other drugs. *Prevent. Med., 16*:385.
14. Henningfield, J.E. *An Old-fashioned Addiction*, Chelsea House Press, Edgement, Pennsylvania.
15. Schneider, N. (1988). *How to Use Nicotine Gum & Other Strategies to Quit Smoking*. Pocket Books, New York.
16. Gold, M.S. (1987). *The Good News About Depression*, Villard Books, New York.
17. Gold, M.S. (1989). *The Good News About Panic, Anxiety, & Phobias*, Villard Books, New York.
18. Slaby, A.E. (1989). *Aftershock*, Villard Books, New York.
19. Gold, M.S. (1987). *The Facts About Drugs And Alcohol*, Bantam Books, New York.

20. Cocores, J.A. (1990). *The 800-COCAINE Book of Drug and Alcohol Recovery*, Villard Books, New York, p. 223.

21. Prochaska, J.O., and Diclemente, C.C. (1983). Stages and processes of self-change of smoking: Toward an integrative model of change. *J. Consult. Clin. Psychol., 51*(3):390–395.

22. Jellinek, E.M. (1960). *The Disease Concept of Alcoholism*, Hillhouse Press, New Haven, Connecticut, p. 139.

23. *Alcoholics Anonymous* (1976). 3rd ed., Alcoholics Anonymous World Services, Inc., New York, p. 58.

24. Jeanne, E. (1984). *The Twelve Steps for Smokers*, Hazeldon Foundation, Center City, Minnesota, p. 3.

25. Fisher, R.A. (1958). Lung cancer and cigarettes. *Nature, 182*:108.

26. Fisher, R.A. (1958). Cancer and smoking. *Nature, 182*:596.

27. Friberg, L., Kaij, L., Denker, S.J., et al. (1959). Smoking habits of monozygotic and dizygotic twins. *Br. Med. J., 1*:1090.

28. Raaschou-Nielsen, E. (1960). Smoking habits in twins. *Danish Med. Bull., 7*(3):82.

29. Shields, J. (1962). *Monozygotic Twins: Brought up Apart and Brought up Together*. Oxford University Press, London.

30. Conterio, F., and Chiarelli, B. (1962). Study of the inheritance of some daily life habits. *Heredity, 17*:347.

31. Pedersen, N. (1981). Twin similarity for usage of common drugs, *Twin Research 3: Epidemiology and Clinical Studies*, Liss, New York, p. 53.

32. American Psychiatric Association (1987). *Diagnostic and Statistical Manual of Mental Disorders*, 3rd ed.–revised, Washington, D.C.

33. American Psychiatric Association (1980). *Diagnostic and Statistical Manual of Mental Disorders*, 3rd ed., Washington, D.C.

34. Fagerstrom, K.-O. (1978). Measuring degree of physical dependence to tobacco smoking with reference to individualization of treatment. *Addict. Behav., 3*:235.

35. Fagerstrom, K.-O. (1989). Measuring nicotine dependence: A review of the Fagerstrom Tolerance Questionnaire. *J. Behav. Med., 12*(2):159.

36. Shiffman, S., and Prange, M. (1988). Self-reported and self-monitored smoking patterns. *Addict. Behav., 13*:201.

37. Rustin, T.A. (1989). Treatment of Tobacco Addiction. *AMSAODD*, 20th Annual Medical Scientific Conference, Atlanta, Georgia.

38. Benowitz, N.L., Hall, S.M., and Herning, R.I. (1983). Smokers of low-yield cigarettes do not consume less nicotine. *N. Engl. J. Med., 390*:139.

39. Pomerleau, O.F., and Rosecrans, J. (1989). Neuroregulatory effects of nicotine. *Psychoneuroendocrinology, 14*(6):407–423.

40. Slaby, A.E. (1988). *Sixty Ways To Make Stress Work For You*, PIA Press, Summit, New Jersey.

41. Crasilneck, H.B., and Hall, J.A. (1975). Hypnosis in the control of smoking, *Clinical Hypnosis: Principles and Applications*, Grune & Stratton, New York, p. 167.

42. Crasilneck, H.B., and Hall, J.A. (1976). Clinical hypnosis: Application in smoking and obesity problems. *Dallas Med. J., 62*(6):296.

43. Kaplan, H.I., and Sadock, B.J. (1988). Caffeine and nicotine dependence, *Synopsis Psychiatry*, 5th ed., Williams & Wilkins, Baltimore, p. 242.

44. Mitchell, E.R. (1987). *Plain Talk About Acupuncture*, Whalehall, New York, p. 5.

45. Rosenberg, A. (1977). An investigation into the effect on cigarette smoking of a new antismoking chewing gum. *J. Int. Med. Res., 5*:68–70.

46. Malcolm, R. (1986). Silver acetate chewing gum as a smoking deterrent. *Chest, 89*:107.

47. Jarvik, M.E., and Henningfield, J.E. (1988). Pharmacological treatment of tobacco dependence. *Pharmacol. Biochem. Behav., 30*:279.

48. Cocores, J.A., Sinaikin, P., and Gold, M.S. (1989). Scopolamine as treatment for nicotine polacrilex dependence. *Ann. Clin. Psychiatry, 1*:203–204.

49. Gold, M.S., Redmond, D.E., and Kleber, H.D. (1978). Clonidine in opiate withdrawal. *Lancet, 1*:929.

50. Glassman, A.H., Jackson, W.K, Walsh, B.T., et al. (1984). Cigarette craving, smoking withdrawal, and clonidine. *Science, 226*:864.

51. Glassman, A.H., Stetner, M.S., Walsh, B.T., et al. (1988). Heavy smokers, smoking cessation, and clonidine. *J.A.M.A., 259*(19):2863.

52. Ornish, S.A., Zisook, S., and McAdams, L.A. (1988). Effects of transdermal clonidine treatment on withdrawal symptoms associated with smoking cessation. *Arch. Intern. Med., 148*(9):2027.

53. Sees, K.L., and Stalcup, S.A. (1989). Combining clonidine and nicotine replacement for treatment of nicotine withdrawal. *J. Psychoactive Drugs, 21*(3):355.

54. Glick, S.D., Jarvik, M.E., and Nakamura, N.K. (1970). Inhibition by drugs of smoking behavior in monkeys. *Nature, 227*:969.

55. Bachynsky, N. (1986). The use of anticholinergic drugs for smoking cessation: A pilot study. *Int. J. Addict.,* 789.

56. Cocores, J.A., Goias, P.R., and Gold, M.S. (1990). The medical management of nicotine dependence in the workplace. *Ann. Clin. Psychiatry, 1*:237–240.

57. Cocores, J.A., and Gold, M.S. (1989). Transdermal scopolamine for nicotine dependence: Use in non-addicts versus recovering addicts, *American Society of Addiction Medicine*, 20th Annual Conference, Atlanta, Georgia, p. 22.

58. Cocores, J.A., and Gold, M.S. (1991). Nicotine dependent psychiatric patients, *The Clinical Management Of Nicotine Dependence* (J.A. Cocores, ed.), Springer-Verlag, New York, p. 420.

59. Bobo, J.K. (1989). Nicotine dependence and alcohol epidemiology and treatment. *J. Psychoactive Drugs, 21*(3):323.

60. Cocores, J.A. (1990). Treatment of the dually diagnosed adult drug user, *Dual Diagnosis Patients* (A.E. Slaby and M.S. Gold, eds.), Marcel Dekker, New York, p. 211.

61. Nanji, A.A., and Lawrence, A.H. (1988). Skin surface sampling for nicotine: A rapid, noninvasive method for identifying smokers. *Int. J. Addict., 23*(11):1207.

62. Noland, M.P., Kryscio, R.J., Riggs, R.S., et al. (1988). Saliva continine and thiocyanate: Chemical indicators of smokeless tobacco and cigarette use in adolescents. *J. Behav. Med., 11*(5):423.

63. Benowitz, N.L. (1983). The use of biologic fluid samples in assessing tobacco smoke consumption. *National Institute on Drug Abuse Monograph No. 48* (J. Grabowski and C.S. Bell, eds.), Bethesda, Maryland, p. 6.

64. Cocores, J.A., and Pottash, A.C. (1991). Outpatient management of nicotine dependence, *The Clinical Management Of Nicotine Dependence* (J.A. Cocores, ed.), Springer-Verlag, New York, p. 331.

26

Hallucinogens

Richard B. Seymour and David E. Smith
Haight Ashbury Free Clinics, Inc., San Francisco, California

I. INTRODUCTION

When the effects of drugs in the group known as the hallucinogens began to be studied in the laboratory, they were first called "psychotomimetic" because they were seen as mimicking the symptoms of psychoses. Studies at that time focused on what these drugs could teach scientists about the nature of mental illness. The psychotomimetic drugs were considered capable of consistently producing short-term changes in thought, perception, and mood without causing major disturbances of the autonomic nervous system or other serious disability. Research with these drugs was considered important for three reasons:

1. It could give the investigator an approximate subjective experience of mental disorder.
2. Model psychoses could be studied in the same way as mental disorders.
3. A study of the drugs' chemical natures could be expected to throw some light on the nature of the hypothetical substances believed to cause mental disorders.

A second term used for many of these substances, and the one we use in this chapter is *hallucinogen*. This means drugs that produce visual, auditory, tactile, taste, and olfactory hallucinations. There has been much disagreement as to just what a hallucination is. There has even been much discussion as to whether or not any of these drugs actually produce hallucinations at all. Some observers maintain that these drugs merely produce visual and temporal distortions. Others mention sensory crossover, such as seeing sounds and hearing colors. Some subjects and scientists postulate that what is seen or experienced via these drugs is there all the time, but that we have been conditioned to be aware of only a small portion of our sensory intake. According to them, when one takes a hallucinogenic drug, that conditioning breaks down and one is aware of a whole new range of sensory material.

Psychedelic, as a term, was coined in the 1960s and means mind manifesting or expanding. In general usage, psychedelic has been generally applied to substances that are used to achieve so-called altered states of consciousness. These drugs were originally referred to as "psychotropic," but that term could be applied to any psychoactive drug.

Hallucinogens came to be called psychedelic when research expanded into areas beyond the approximation of psychoses and the identification of paranormal experience and into the longer term effects the drugs can have on human consciousness.

II. SPRING, AND OTHER MYSTERIES

The history of consciousness-effective drugs is probably as long as that of naturally occurring stimulants, opioids, and sedative-hypnotics. In ancient times, they were used to add a touch of holy wonder to magical and religious ceremonies. The Rites of Spring, actually celebrated with the return of life-enhancing rains in the fall, in classical Greece celebrated the return of Persephone, the daughter of Nature, from her Summer retreat, spent with her husband Pluto in the underworld. Thousands of worshippers would make a pilgrimage to the city of Eleusius, south of modern Athens. There, they gathered at a temple said to cover the entrance to the underworld through which Spring would emerge to bring the world back into flower and fecundity. These pilgrims drank a concoction that gave them a direct perception of the goddess. Ethnopharmacologists, experts on the use of drugs in different cultures, are fairly certain that what these worshippers drank to celebrate the Eleusian Mysteries was a combination of wine, herbs, and ergotomine, a psychoactive mould that grows on rye grain.

Similar substances were used medicinally at the hospital/sanitoriums of Hippocrates' time. Physicians at these aesklepions, named for Aesklepius, the god and father of medicine, gave their patients vision-inducing potions and then based their diagnoses on the hallucination that they described.

Religious and medical practices in less classical parts of the world—our culture refers to them as shamanism and witchcraft—also made great use of hallucinogens. In the pre-Columbian Western Hemisphere, these hallucinogens included a number of plants and fungi, such as the buds of the peyote cactus, South American vines, and various psilocybin mushrooms. Much pre-Columbian "medicine" either went underground or was lost, a victim of the Inquisition, when Europeans reached the New World.

In Europe, hallucinogenic drugs followed narcotic analgesics into disuse during the Middle Ages. When naturally occurring hallucinogens were ingested by accident, the results were seen as cases of demonic possession. On several notable occasions, this happened to entire villages, and may have resulted from ergotomine contamination of village grain supplies. It was not until the nineteenth and twentieth centuries that scientists began to "rediscover" psychedelic drugs and their effects.

III. PEYOTE AND MESCALINE

The first hallucinogenic agent to catch the attention of western scientists was one that had not gone underground—the peyote cactus. Mescaline, 3,4,5-trimethoxyphenylethylamine, a Schedule I drug like most hallucinogens, is the primary active alkaloid in the buttons of the peyote cactus. It is usually taken in capsules or dissolved in water or other liquids and swallowed. Peyote itself is either chewed or steeped in a tea after the white filaments have been removed. They have about one three-hundredth the potency of lysergic acid diethylamide (LSD) and have similar hallucinogenic effects, but the greater visual effects of peyote lead one to believe that the plant probably contains other hallucinogenic elements besides mescaline.

Peyote had been used ceremonially by Indians in northern Mexico and what became the southwestern United States since ancient times. Neither the Spanish Inquisition nor a succession of American governments were able to eradicate its use as a stimulant, general medicine, and ceremonial psychedelic. During the nineteenth century, use of peyote actually increased, spreading through southwestern tribes as an antidote to the despair resulting from the eclipse of their culture by the encroaching white man. Many of these tribes never gave up their fight, and after years of court battles, the ritual use of peyote by the 200,000 or more Native American congregants of the Native American Church was declared legal. In 1990, however, the issue was revived in the courts.

In 1856, the active ingredient in peyote was isolated and named mescaline for the Mescalaro Apaches of northern Mexico. By 1919, it was recognized that the molecular structure of mescaline was related to the structure of the adrenal hormone, epinephrine, which occurs naturally in the human brain. The works of Sigmund Freud, William James, Havelock Ellis, and other scientists stimulated scholarly interest in the drug's effects. Mescaline ingestion served as an introduction to altered states of consciousness of Aldous Huxley and the French artist Henri Michaux, who wrote about its effects. Huxley, a descendant of Sir Thomas Henry Huxley, who popularized the theories of Charles Darwin, wrote a monograph on his subjective experience with mescaline: *The Doors of Perception* became a model for later works and had repercussions beyond his immediate scientific and philosophic circles. The psychological theories of Sigmund Freud and C.G. Jung were coming into vogue with their tantalizing glimpses of libido and the unconscious. The general public was taking an interest in the workings of the human mind. Mescaline provided a doorway into other perceptions, a glimpse at forbidden ground. The rediscovery of ergotomine, in a new and powerful form, opened the next episode in the story of hallucinogenic drugs.

IV. LYSERGIC ACID DIETHYLAMIDE

Lysergic acid diethylamide (LSD) was first synthesized in 1938, but it was not until 1943 that the drug's profound psychological effects were first discovered. In that year, Dr. Albert Hofmann, who was involved in the synthesis of LSD at Sandoz Pharmaceuticals in Basel, Switzerland, accidentally ingested some of the compound and experienced visual alterations and difficulty in riding a bicycle. At the time of initial synthesis, he was looking for an analeptic with stimulant properties similar to those of nikethimide, which LSD resembles in molecular configuration (Wesson and Smith, 1978). Hofmann recognized that the effects he had experienced were due to the LSD and later purposely ingested 250 μg, an amount that he considered to be a small dose. The effects were most profound; later studies confirmed that doses in the range of 30–50 μg were sufficient to produce hallucinations. Hofmann (1970) realized that LSD was one of the most potent psychoactive compounds known.

During the next 2 decades, LSD underwent a social and medical evolution characterized by shifting professional and lay models of the drug's function. According to Metzner (1978), "the first was the *psychotomimetic*, the psychiatric-pharmacological model, that treated the drug experience like a psychosis." This was followed, though not necessarily superseded, by the *hallucinogenic* model that employed LSD as a tool for studying the mechanisms of perception; the *therapeutic* model, which represented rather an about-face for a psychotomimetic; and then the *psychedelic* model that proposed that under proper conditions (Metzner, 1978) "the experience will be enlightening, productive and consciousness expanding."

As each of these models was developed, intriguing information filtered down to the general public. This dissemination of information became a flood when a number of creative people in both the arts and sciences underwent personal psychedelic experiences through a variety of research programs. These included a prolonged study at Harvard University under the guidance of Drs. Timothy Leary, Richard Alpert, and Ralph Metzner, and a reserach program at Stanford University, participated in by the author Ken Kesey, who based portions of his best-selling novel *One Flew Over the Cucoo's Nest* on his experience with LSD and as an orderly in a state mental institution. Many other research participants wrote about their experiences with LSD, mescaline, and other psychedelics in books and articles or discussed them on radio and television.

With the psychedelic model, LSD began to take on a religious-mystical cast, as evidenced by the theme and content of the first manual written by the three principals in the Harvard Project, *The Psychedelic Experience: A Manual Based on the Tibetan Book of the Dead* (Leary, Metzner, and Alpert, 1964). The book was dedicated to Aldous Huxley, the British author who had written extensively on his own experiences with mescaline. There follows a tribute to Walter Yeeling Evans-Wentz, the California-born Oxford anthropologist, who with Lama Kazi Dawa-Samdup, made the first English translation of the Tibetan *Bardo Thodal* as the *Tibetan Book of the Dead*. There are also tributes to Carl Gustav Jung and to Lama Anagorika Govinda, the highly cosmopolitan spokesman for Tibetan Buddhism in the United States.

The Harvard Project's publication of related articles, interviews with and presentations by Leary, Alpert, and Metzner as well as publications by others of like mind undoubtedly added to the shaping of a drug-using subculture centered around the use of LSD and other hallucinogenic drugs. It did not, however, initiate the nonclinical use of LSD. "Acid," as it was now known, was already on the streets by 1964. A variety of other hallucinogenic drugs became available at this time, but never enjoyed the widespread availability of LSD. The most evident of these are described below (Seymour and Smith, 1987).

V. MARIJUANA/CANNABIS

Although marijuana is discussed in depth in Chapter 20 of this book, a brief review of its role as a hallucinogen seems in order. First described in Chinese literature around 2700 B.C., cannabis has been used medically and socially by many human civilizations throughout time. The primary active ingredient in cannabis is tetrahydrocannabinol (THC), and preparations vary in strength depending on the concentration of THC. In the United States, the most common preparations are marijuana, usually composed of the dried leaves and flowers of the male cannabis plant, and hashish, composed of the resin that forms on the mature plant (Smith, 1969).

Declared illegal by national law in 1937, cannabis is classified as a hallucinogen, and as such was placed on Schedule I, along with most other hallucinogenic drugs, in 1970. One of the few psychoactive plants that also has a major industrial use, cannabis has been grown throughout the world as "hemp" for the production of rope. Although there is mention of the plant being cultivated in early America, including its cultivation by George Washington, it is thought that the crops were primarily for their fibers rather than for smoking.

Marijuana can be eaten, smoked, or used in tea. The onset of effects when it is smoked is very rapid, and the effects usually last for several hours. When it is eaten, the onset is slower, but the effects may be of longer duration and more profound. The effects of marijuana and hashish range from euphoria to dysphoria, depending on potency, setting, orientation, expectation, and state of mind. Many of the acute toxic effects of cannabis can be seen as hallucinogenic, including distortion of time, space, and form, and a perceived enhancement of perceptions. Hallucinogenic flashbacks are a relatively common occurrence with marijuana use.

There has been a great deal of controversy concerning marijuana's long-term effects, which are thought to include damage to the nervous system and behavior, the cardiovascular and respiratory systems, the respiratory system and chromosomes, and the immune system. Certain long-term effects have been clinically documented. These include increasing evidence for long-term respiratory problems comparable to those found with tobacco. An amotivational consequence to chronic marijuana use, especially by the young, was first noted by Smith, in studies conducted by the Haight Ashbury Free Medical Clinics in the late 1960s and reported in the *Journal of Psychoactive Drugs* (Smith, 1968), and later discussed by Norman Miller and Gold (1989):

> The amotivational syndrome (overused and non-specific term) described in marijuana addicts includes personality changes that develop over time: diminished drive, decreased ambition, lessened motivation, apathy, shortened attention span, distractibility, poor judgement, impaired communication skills, introversion, magical thinking, derealization and depersonalization, decreased capacity to carry out complex plans or prepare realistically for the future, a peculiar fragmentation in the flow of thought, habit deterioration, and progressive loss of insight.

In their study, Miller and Gold go on to characterize the dependence on and addiction to marijuana in terms of addictive disease, all the characteristics of which are present in marijuana dependence and addiction. As marijuana addiction has become clinically recognized, a variety of treatment approaches have been taken. These include multidisciplinary approaches similar to those taken with other addictive disease manifestations, including the use of 12-step treatment approaches (Miller et al., 1989).

VI. PSILOCYBIN

Psilocybin, found in over 47 varieties of fresh and dried mushrooms, is the phosphate ester of psilocin, or 4-hydroxydimethyltryptamine. The mushrooms can be eaten raw, cooked, steeped into tea, dried, powdered, and taken in capsules, or smoked with such mediums as marijuana. Appearing in a wide variety of shapes, sizes, and potencies, psilocybin-containing mushrooms have been found in most parts of the world. Their ritualistic use has been traced back as far as 1000 B.C. in Pre-Columbian Mexico, and their use continued in secret after its suppression by the Spanish Inquisition. These mushrooms and their effects were considered a myth by Western medicine until they were rediscovered in the mid-1950s.

A derivative of tryptamine, psilocybin and psilocin are classified as "indole" hallucinogens and are similar to LSD and serotonin, an internal neurotransmitter that affects many central nervous system functions. These drugs probably work by stimulating serotonin receptor sites in the brain. Although dosage varies among mushroom types, general potency is about 200 times less than that of LSD. Tolerance develops rapidly, and there is cross-tolerance with LSD and mescaline. Effects are usually apparent within half an hour and may last from 4–8 hs.

WARNING: Some mushroom species thought to be poisonous resemble some psilocybin mushrooms. Someone who has eaten a poisonous mushroom should be taken to an emergency room or poison center with a sample of the mushroom if possible. The staff should be aware that large doses of atropine (an outmoded treatment for mushroom poisoning) can potentiate the effects of muscimole and do damage rather than help.

VII. MORNING GLORY AND HAWAIIAN WOODROSE SEEDS

Two hallucinogenics, ergine (d-lysergic acid aide) and iso-ergine, are found in the seeds of certain morning glory and Hawaiian woodrose vines. These seeds are eaten whole, ground and eaten, or leached with water which is then drunk. The ergot alkaloid–producing morning glories grow in many parts of the world, but their ritual use as drugs was confined to Mexico and Central America. Modern use for hallucinogenic effects began in the late 1950s and peaked in the mid-1960s. In 1959, Hofmann isolated the lysergic acid amides in ololiuqui seeds. The hallucinogenic potential of Hawaiian baby woodrose seeds was introduced to the public in 1965 in a scientific paper crediting these seeds with several times the potency of morning glory seeds. Ingestion of all these seeds has not been extensive. Accompanied by intrinsic nausea and abdominal distress, they served as a poor substitute for LSD when the latter was scarce and more desirable hallucinogen were unavailable.

VIII. NUTMEG AND MACE

Both the hard nut itself, grated and mixed with liquids and best known as a garnish for holiday eggnog and a flavoring in Alfredo sauce, and mace, the orange-crimson network that covers the nut have been used for their hallucinogenic qualities. The visual and tactile hallucinations produced can be intense, up to full psychotomimetic delirium, but the high doses needed produce extreme strain on the kidneys, abdominal spasm, constipation, tachycardia, insomnia, and drowsiness. Usually the long-term kidney pain will discourage any further experimentation with these spices at delerium-producing levels.

IX. METHOXYLATED AMPHETAMINES

Methoxylated amphetamines, or psychotomimetic amphetamines, are a family of drugs that represent an amphetamine subgroup that collectively exhibit the effects of both stimulants and hallucinogenics. The members of family are amphetamine analogues of the drug mescaline. This group contains more than a thousand different but related chemical substances, of which only a few have been used by humans. The more well-known are MDA (methylenedioxyamphetamine), MMDA, DOM (STP), DOET, TMA, DMA, DMMA, and MDMA (methylenedioxymethamphetamine). Methylenedioxyamphetamine and DOM were the representatives most used in the 1960s and 1970s. Methylenedioxymethamphetamine rose in popularity in the 1980s and will be discussed extensively in Section XVI of this chapter.

X. N,N-DIMETHYLTRYPTAMINE

Structurally similar to psilocybin, N,N-Dimethyltryptamine (DMT) is present in hallucinogenic drinks prepared from South American shrubs, including *Mimosa hostilis*. In the United States, it has been smoked after being soaked into parsley or other smokeable substances, taken in liquid form, or injected either intravenously or intramuscularly. The effects are similar to those of LSD, but sympathomimetic effects such as dilated pupils, raised blood pressure, and elevated pulse rate are more pronounced. The most unique quality of this drug is its rapidity of effect. Effects can be experienced within seconds of injection, peak in 5–20 min, and often end within half an hour. The drug molecule bears a close resemblance to a brain enzyme involved in REM sleep, and this may account for its rapid onset and metabolization.

Other hallucinogenic drugs have been observed but rarely used in the United States. These include the *harmala alkaloids*, found in Near Eastern shrubs, and the bark of certain South American vines; ibogaine, from the root of a West African plant; muscimole, derived from the *Amanita muscaria*, or fly agaric mushroom; and the anticholinergic hallucinogens *Atropa belladonna, Mandragora officinarum, Hyoscyamus niger*, and *Datura*. All of these substances can create hallucinogenic changes in consciousness. Most of them, especially the latter grouping, are also highly poisonous and can produce potentially disabling or even fatal consequences. Similar hallucinogenic experiences have been encountered in such states as "dreams, psychosis, starvation, isolation, high fever . . . hypnotic trance, repetitive chanting, prolonged wakefulness, revivalist exhortation, song or dance, fasting, hyperventilation, special postures, exercises and techniques for concentrating attention (Grinspoon and Bakalar, 1979).

XI. STREET AND ILLICIT USE OF HALLUCINOGENS

The nonmedical and nonsanctioned use of LSD did not become illegal until June, 1966. By then its street use was so widespread that, with the exception of cannabis, it was the most commonly available hallucinogenic drug in the United States. Such natural hallucinogenics as peyote and its derivative mescaline, psylocybin mushrooms, and morning glory seeds were available, but these were generally considered "exotic" substances, hard to find, with unclear dosages and often unpleasant side effects. The street use of LSD and other hallucinogenic drugs underwent a transformation from their general introduction through the banning of all hallucinogens in 1970.

At first, there was a general sense of trust in the drug, which was echoed in the LSD culture's mystical trust in the universe itself. Through the summer of 1965, the number of people in the United States who had ingested LSD took a major leap and proceeded to accelerate. The drug was still legal, but commercial LSD, produced by Sandoz Laboratories in Switzerland, became more and more difficult to obtain, but individual entrepreneurs—conscious of the demand—began producing quantities of LSD, often of variable quality. By January, 1967, the "acid" culture had grown large enough to bring together 40,000 people, mostly hallucinogen users, for a Tribal Be-In in San Francisco's Golden Gate Park. By then the culture had its own developing graphic art form, a hybrid of *fin de siècle* art nouveau and optical illusion–oriented op art, and its own newspaper, the *San Francisco Oracle*, which publicized the event. The unprecedented gathering, a foretaste of the massive rock celebrations, such as Woodstock, to come later in the decade, gained equally unprecedented attention in the nation's press, television and magazines. Media and grapevine coverage of the growing subculture in San Francisco's Haight-Ashbury district, where many early LSD users were concentrated, gave rise to soon-to-be-confirmed speculation that the area would be flooded with young people from across the nation by the summer of 1967. This projected influx was labeled the Summer of Love by both media and the evolving counterculture in San Francisco.

It was during this proliferation that the problem of LSD-induced negative reactions became acute. During the clinically supervised stage of LSD's sociopharmacological study, adverse reactions were rare. Cohen (1960), one of the pioneer clinical investigators of LSD, reported that the incidence of psychotic reactions lasting more than 48 h was 0.8/1000 in experimental subjects, and 1.8/1000 in mental patients. However, by June 1967, when the Haight-Ashbury Free Medical Clinic first opened its doors in San Francisco, negative acid trips, or "bummers," as the acid culture called them, were frequent.

Writing in the spring of that year, David E. Smith, M.D. (1967), founder and medical director of the Haight Ashbury Free Medical Clinic, identified the adverse effects of hallucinogenic drugs as "largely psychological in nature," dividing them into acute immediate toxicity and chronic after-effects. This differs from the acute and chronic toxicity designations one finds with opioid and sedative hypnotic drugs in that chronic toxicity usually denotes ongoing physical dependency, whereas the long-term etiology of hallucinogenic drugs usually involves psychological after-effects rather than physical dependency.

The acute toxic effects occurred during the direct drug experience and were commonly called "bad trips." These aberrations could take many forms. Often individuals would knowingly take a hallucinogenic drug and find themselves in a state of anxiety as the powerful psychedelic began to take effect. They were aware that they had taken a drug, but felt that they could not control its effects and wanted to be taken out of their state of intoxication immediately. This condition is similar to that of becoming self-conscious in the midst of a threatening dream, but being unable to awaken from it. Hallucinogenic drug users on a bad trip sometimes try to flee the situation that they are in, giving rise to possible physical danger. Others may become paranoid and suspicious of their companions or other individuals. After eating a number of peyote buttons, one informant spent several excruciating hours firmly convinced that his wife and his best friend, who were in the next room, had plotted for years to kill him while he was helplessly intoxicated on the cactus buds.

Not all acute toxicity is based on anxiety or loss of control. Some people taking hallucinogens display decided changes in cognition and demonstrate poor judgment. They may decide that they can fly, and jump out of a window. Some users are reported to have walked into the sea, feeling that they were "part of the universe." Such physical mishaps have been described within the acid culture as "being God, but tripping over the furniture." Susceptibility to bad trips is not necessary dose related, but does depend on the experience, maturity, and personality of the user as well as the external environment in which the trip takes place. Sometimes the individual will complain of unpleasant symptoms while intoxicated and later speak in glowing terms of the experience. Negative psychological set and environmental setting are the most significant contributing factors to bad hallucinogenic trips.

XII. TREATMENT OF ACUTE TOXICITY

Techniques originally developed in free clinics and community-based self-help programs, as reported by Smith and Shick (1970), are based on the findings that most hallucinogenic bad trips are best treated in a supportive, nonpharmacological fashion through the restoration of a positive, nonthreatening environment. Facilities, such as those occupied by the Haight Ashbury Free Medical Clinic, in a residental setting with little to mark them as *medical*, with a quiet space or calm center set aside for drug crises and with casually dressed staff dedicated to a nonjudgmental attitude were admirably suited for such treatment. Talkdowns of most acute toxicity hallucinogenic reactions may be accomplished without medication or hospitalization. Paraprofessionals with psychedelic drug experience have been particularly effective at such sites as large rock concerts. Amelioration of bad trips has even been accomplished by long-distance telephone calls (Alpert, 1967).

In the talkdown approach, one should maintain a relaxed, conversational tone to assist in putting the individual at ease. Quick movements should be avoided. One should make the patient comfortable, but not impede their freedom of movement. Let them walk around, stand, sit, or lie down. At times, such physical movement and activity may be enough to break the anxiety reaction. Gentle suggestion should be used to divert patients from any activity that seems to be adding to their agitation. Getting the individual's minid off the frightening elements of a bad trip and onto positive elements is the key to the talkdown.

An understanding of the phases generally experienced in an hallucinogenic drug trip is most helpful in treating acute reactions. After orally ingesting an average dose of 100–250 μg, the user experiences sympathomimetic responses, including elevated heart rate and stimulated respiration. Adverse reactions in this phase are primarily managed by reassurances that the observed experiences are normal and expected effects of hallucinogens. This is actually sufficient to override a potentially frightening situation.

From the first to the sixth hour, visual imagery becomes vivid and may take on frightening content. The patient may have forgotten taking the drug, and given acute time distortion, may believe this "retinal circus" (Michaux, 1963) will go on forever. Such fears can be dispelled by reminding the individual that these effects are drug induced, by suggesting alternative images and by distracting the individual from those images that are frightening.

In the later stages, philosophical insights and ideas predominate. Adverse experiences here are most frequently due to recurring unpleasant thoughts or feelings that can become overwhelming in their impact. The therapist can be most effective by being supportive and by suggesting new trains of thought.

The therapist's attitude toward psychedelics and their use is very important. Empathy and self-confidence are essential. Anxiety and fear in the therapist will be perceived in an amplified manner. Physical contact with the individual is often reassuring, but can be misinterpreted. Ideally, the therapist should rely on intuition rather than preconceptions.

Wesson and Smith (1978) noted that medication may be necessary and should be given either after the talkdown has failed or as a supplement to the talkdown process. During the first phase of intervention, oral administration of a sedative, such as 25 mg of chlordiazepoxide or 10 mg of diazepam, can have an important pharmacological and reassuring effect.

During the second and third phases a toxic psychosis or major break with reality may occur, in which one can no longer communicate with the individual. If the individual begins acting in such a way as to be an immediate danger, antipsychotic drugs may be employed. Only if the individual refuses oral medication and is out of behavioral control should antipsychotics be administered by injection. Haloperidol (2–4 mg administered intramuscularly every hour) is the current drug of choice. Any medication, however, should only be given by qualified personnel. If antipsychotic drugs are required, hospitalization is usually indicated. It has been found at the Haight Ashbury Free Medical Clinics, however, that most bad acid trips can be handled on an outpatient basis by talkdown alone.

As soon as rapport and verbal contact are established, further medication is generally unnecessary. Occasionally an individual fails to respond to the above regimen and must be referred to an inpatient psychiatric facility. Such a decision must be weighed carefully, however, as transfer to a hospital may of itself have an aggravating and threatening effect. Hospitalization should only be used as a last resort if all else has failed.

XIII. TREATING CHRONIC HALLUCINOGENIC DRUG AFTER-EFFECTS

Chronic hallucinogenic drug after-effects present situations wherein a condition that may be attributable to the ingestion of a toxic substance occurs or continues long after the metabolization of that substance. With the use of hallucinogens, four recognized chronic reactions have been reported (Seymour and Smith, 1987; Wesson and Smith, 1978); (1) prolonged psychotic reactions; (2) depression sufficiently severe so as to be life threatening; (3) flashbacks; and (4) exacerbations of preexisting psychiatric illness.

Some people who have taken many hallucinogenic drug trips, especially those who have had acute toxic reactions, show what appears to be serious long-term personality disruptions. These prolonged psychotic reactions have similarities to schizophrenic reactions and appear to occur most often in people with preexisting psychological difficulties; primarily prepsychotic or psychotic personalities. Hallucinogenic drug-induced personality disorganizations can be quite severe and prolonged. Appropriate treatment often requires antipsychotic medication and residential care in a mental health facility followed by outpatient counseling.

XIV. FLASHBACKS

By far the most ubiquitious chronic reaction to hallucinogenics is the flashback. Flashbacks are transient spontaneous occurrences of some aspect of the hallucinogenic drug effect occurring after a period of normalcy that follows the original intoxication. This period of normalcy distinguishes flashbacks from prolonged psychotic reactions. Flashbacks may occur after a single ingestion of a hallucinogenic drug, but more commonly occur after multiple hallucinogenic drug ingestions. The flashback experience has also been reported following the use of marijuana (Brown and Stickgold, 1976).

Flashbacks are a symptom, not a specific disease entity. They may well have multiple etiologies, and many cases called flashbacks may have occurred although the individual had never ingested a hallucinogenic drug. Some investigators have indicated that flashbacks may be due to a residue of the drug released into the brain at a later time. Although this is known to happen with phencyclidine (PCP) and its cogeners, there is no direct evidence of retention or prolonged storage of such hallucinogens as LSD.

Individuals who have used hallucinogenic drugs several times a month have indicated that fleeting flashes of light and after-image prolongation occurring in the periphery of vision commonly occur for days or weeks after ingestion. Active and chronic hallucinogenic drug users tend to accept these occurrences as part of the psychedelic experience, are unlikely to seek medical or psychiatric treatment, and frequently view them as "free trips." It is the inexperienced user and the individual who attaches a negative interpretation to these visual phenomena who are likely to be disturbed by them and seek medical or psychiatric treatment. While emotional reactions to the flashback are generally contained with the period of the flashback itself, prolonged anxiety states or psychotic breaks have occurred following a frightening flashback. There is no record of flashback activity specifically attributable to hallucinogenic drug use occurring more than a year after the individual's last use of a hallucinogenic drug.

Flashback phenomena have attracted considerable attention since 1966, and public interest was heightened in 1970 by the widely publicized suicide of Diane Linkletter, daughter of television personality Art Linkletter. Her death was blamed on an LSD flashback and focused public attention on the potential dangers of flashbacks.

XV. A 20-YEAR PERSPECTIVE ON HALLUCINOGENS

For the past 2 decades, since the classification of LSD and virtually all other hallucinogenic drugs in Schedule I, little meaningful research has been conducted on LSD at the clinical level. In contrast to the late 1960s and early 1970s, the clinical treatment of LSD acute toxicity has become a rare occurrence. Smith's contention that the drug community had learned how to handle bad trips without attracting the attention of medical or police authorities (Metzner, 1978) is echoed in data gathered by Newmeyer and Johnson (1979) at rock concerts from 1973 to 1977. Their findings indicated that while treatment incidents involving LSD accounted for only 5.9% of all drug treatment at concert sites, and alcohol accounted for 60.2%, there was a much higher proportion of LSD use without complications. Newmeyer and Johnson stated that:

> . . . for these people, acid-tripping with the Grateful Dead may be an occasional weekend diversion in the time-honored tradition equivalent to tailgate, whiskey-lubricated parties at football games, or six-packs and hot dogs at baseball games. Such public drug use may correspond to what Harding and Zinberg (1977) have identified as rituals of controlled drug use, involving social sanctions which structure and limit the experience.

As we discussed earlier, recent ethnopharmacological and ethnomythological studies, most notably those of Wasson, Ruck, and Hofmann (1978), have indicated that the Hellenic, classical Greek and Roman cultures knew of hallucinogenics, such as ergot, that would have given an experience similar to that of LSD, and used them culturally and ritually as a means to achieve expanded awareness and spiritual fulfillment. Some cultural observers predict a similar development for certain "approved" hallucinogenic drugs in our own culture. Given the nature of the modern world, at least as it appears to us as we near the end of the twentieth century, such applications, if they do come, may come under the apologia of enhanced mental health. Such an approach, i.e., the return of the hallucinogenic as an adjunct to the therapy, is a primary theme of the next drug to be discussed.

XVI. METHYLENEDIOXYMETHAMPHETAMINE

A paradoxical chemical in many ways, MDMA is often thought of as a "new" drug, not as something that was developed in 1914. Perhaps the paper that described its conversion contributed to the drug's long period of obscurity. It was titled, "Verfaren zur Darstellung von Alkyloxyaryl-Dialkytoxyarl-und Alkylendioxarylamino-propanen bzw. deren Stickstoff monoalylierten Derivaten." That Wagnerian pronouncement brought E. Merck and Co. a German patent Number 274,350 for MDMA.

The paper does not discuss the drug's pharmacology, and it seems doubtful that Merck's biochemists had any idea of the drug's psychoactive qualities. The chemical name of MDMA is M-methyl-1-3,4-methylenedioxy-alpha-methylbenzecethanamine-N-alpha-dimethyl-1,3-benzodioxyole-5-ethanomine. That name, or "signature," describes the drug's chemical structure.

Methylenedioxymethamphetamine is a synthetic drug. Similar to MDA, or 3,4-methylenedioxyamphetamine, developed by Merck at about the same time, MDMA is synthesized from molecular components of methamphetamine and safrole, which comes from sassafrass, nutmeg, or another synthetic called piperonylacetone.

Methylenedioxymethamphetamine belongs to a large group of synthetic drugs called the phenylethylamines. These differ in their effects, depending on their molecular structure. Some are relatively inactive; others, including the drugs that we usually think of as amphetamines, produce a stimulant effect coupled with feelings of euphoria. Still others, including MDMA, have consciousness effects similar to those produced by psychedelic drugs and stimulant effects.

These drugs are similar to mescaline, the active ingredient in the psychedelic buttons of the peyote plant found in the southwestern United States and Mexico. Mescaline is a methoxylated phenylethylamine. The first part of this designation indicates that it is chemically related to the amphetamine methoxylated subgroup, or psychedelic amphetamines, which include MDA.

In the early 1980s, health professionals experimented with the use of MDMA in therapy. This use was perfectly legitimate. Before July 1, 1985, a licensed physician could procure MDMA for use as an experimental drug by going to a responsible laboratory and preparing the drug under the guidance of an expert chemist. Any physician doing so needed a peer group of other physicians who were aware of his or her use of the drug and who could be called upon to support such such as responsible medical practice. This and other guidelines for experimental drug use may vary depending on state legislation.

Virtually nothing was published about this research. What information existed was passed from hand to hand in manuscript form, or discussed in very low-profile meetings. The reason for this clandestinicity was a shared knowledge of history and a strong desire not to have it repeat itself. After LSD was declared illegal on June 6, 1966, legitimate research on hallucinogenic drugs came to a virtual standstill and has remained there. These researchers did not want to see the same thing happen with MDMA.

In 1984, when the federal Drug Enforcement Administration (DEA) placed MDMA in Schedule I with MDA and the other hallucinogens, it discovered that there was some medical opposition. Frank Sapienza, a DEA official, commented that he and his colleagues saw MDMA as a rarely used drug that occasionally showed up in drug raids. He said, "We had no idea that doctors were using it for research."

At the request of a coalition of these researchers, who had hired a prestigious Washington, D.C. law firm to represent them, a series of hearings were scheduled to review the status of MDMA prior to scheduling. It appeared that a long, slow process would follow, during which experimental use of the drug would be allowed to continue.

However, just before the hearings were due to begin, the acting administrator of the DEA announced that he had enacted emergency national restrictions on MDMA and placed it in Schedule I of the Controlled Substances Act. This allowed the DEA to move against illicit users, dealers, and manufacturers of the drug, and at the same time, severely restricted research while making experimental treatment illegal. The emergency scheduling was technically in force for 1 year but could be extended if the permanent scheduing of MDMA was still in question.

The authority for this action was an amendment to the Controlled Substances Act, Section 201, which was voted in as part of the Comprehensive Crime Control Act of 1984. In essence, the amendment gives the DEA, as the designee of the United States Attorney General, the authority to place a substance into Schedule I for a period of 1 year if it is found that such action is necessary to avoid an imminent hazard to public safety.

The amendment was enacted by Congress to counter the threat posed by the synthesis and proliferation of illicity synthesized analogues to the powerful narcotic fentanyl. There were very good reasons for enacting the scheduling amendment to deal with these dangerous narcotics. The physicians group, however, questioned its use in the emergency banning of MDMA.

One of the primary factors in the DEA's case for the emergency scheduling of MDMA was a rat study conducted at the University of Chicago. Even though the study involved MDA, methampetamine, and amphetamine, but not MDMA, the DEA drew certain inferences regarding the neurological safety of MDMA use from its findings (Lawn, 1985):

> Of immediate concern to DEA in terms of a hazard to the public safety is a very recent research finding which suggests that MDMA has neurotoxic properties. A paper entitled "Hallucinogenic Amphetamine Selectively Destroys Brain Serotonin Nerve Terminals: Neurochemical and Anatomical Evidence" by G. Ricaurte, G. Bryan, L. Strauss, L. Seiden, and C. Schuster, describes studies which show that single or multiple doses of MDA selectively destroy serotonergic nerve terminals in the rat brain. The serotonergic system which is also present in man plays a role in regulating sleep, mood, sexual activity, and sensitivity to aversive stimuli. Experts have concluded that because of the neurotoxic effects of closely related structural analogs of MDMA (MDA, amphetamine, and methamphetamine) and because both MDA and MDMA cause the release of endogenous serotonin, it is likely that MDMA will produce similar neurotoxic effects to those of MDA. Furthermore, the neurotoxicity of amphetamine and methamphetamine has been shown in 5 diverse mammalian species. This strongly suggests that the substance would be neurotoxic to humans.

A. Scheduling and Neurotoxic Considerations

The above study cited involved research to ascertain the possible long-term effect of a drug. With drugs that have been in general use for a long time, this is relatively easy: You look at the long-time users. That approach is not possible when you have a new drug, or one that has not been in general use. In cases like these, researchers substitute high doses of the drug administered frequently for low doses taken over time.

Admittedly, massive doses of a drug given to a rat perinatally, or by injection may not be the equivalent of periodic low doses of the same substance taken orally over an extended period of time by humans. The possible discrepancies became a major bone of contention in the case of MDMA scheduling. On the other hand, such studies may be the best there are, given the circumstances, and they have doubtless saved us from potentially harmful medicines being marketed prematurely by indicating potential cumulative and idiosyncratic adverse effects.

B. What Is MDMA?

Since its emergency scheduling, MDMA has often been confused with the powerful narcotic fentanyl, and meperidine analogues have been included within the general category of "designer drugs." Because of this confusion, MDMA has been cited in the press as causing many fatal overdoses, actually a consequence of using fentanyl analogues; or parkinsonlike paralysis, actually the result of chemical impurities in meperidine analogues. The narcotic analogues are particularly dangerous drugs that are being synthesized by underground chemists in order to avoid the penalties for manufacture and sale of the narcotics from which they are derived.

Several things distinguish MDMA from the designer drugs. Synthesized in 1914 by a reputable pharmaceutical company, it was not developed as a variation of an existing scheduled drug in order to provide a quasi-legal substance for street sale. Although it bears a resemblance to MDA and other methoxylated amphetamines, the route of action of MDMA and even some of its effects appear to be quite different from these drugs. Therapists who have used it as an adjunct to psychotherapy describe it as a precurser of new therapeutic tools. This does not mean, however, that the use of MDMA and such cogeners as MDE is safe and should be without restraints or controls.

Our own concerns about the nonmedical use of MDMA are twofold. For one, many people who should not be using this or any psychoactive drug may be lured through positive hyperbole presented by well-meaning supporters and out-and-out proselytizers. The potential victims include the young, the drug naive, and those who are vulnerable to addiction.

As a counter to this, responsible researchers and clinicians are working with other concerned groups to get the message across that MDMA is not a toy, and certainly not something that should be used for self-medication, intoxication, or recreation. It is a powerful and untested drug with both a potential for addiction and a potential for medical usefulness.

The second concern is one that MDMA shares with all other popular underground drugs. With no quality control, sociopathic and just plain ignorant manufacturers and dealers can sell just about anything they want to a gullible market and call it MDMA.

C. Actions?

According to psychiatrists who had used MDMA themselves before giving it to patients, the drug is not like LSD, or mescaline, or even MDA. There are no hallucinations. The subject does not experience loss of reality or ego disassociation. None of the effects that caused problems with LSD and other psychedelics occur with MDMA.

Patients who had been given MDMA as an adjunct to therapy praised its efficacy. On a panel discussion broadcast on the *Phil Donahue* television show, one of Dr. Rick Ingrasci's patients, suffering from terminal cancer, pointed out that the MDMA did nothing to cure her cancer or ease its physical symptoms. It does not work that way. What it did was enable her to put death into perspective. It helped her to talk about what was happening to her with her family. Besides patients with terminal disease, MDMA has been used with victims of delayed stress syndrome, childhood and adult trauma such as rape and molestation victims, and in family therapy. Essentially, it is said to have proved useful in cases in which part of the problem involves repression of feelings and experiences.

Even though MDMA bears the street name "ecstasy," which would seem to imply a sexual action, it does not appear to be an aphrodisiac. While it may increase communication and help develop a sense of warmth and understanding between individuals, it neither stimulates sexual activity, nor does it increase physical sensitivity.

D. Abuse Potential

All psychoactive drugs have an abuse potential. This is the studied opinion of many in the drug treatment field and of many in the drug enforcement field. We have seen the cycle over and over again. A "new" psychoactive drug appears with a reputation for providing "safe" treatment. The drug is seen as a panacea. Its use in treatment is called a major medical breakthrough. Prescriptions may come to number in the millions. Then the drug's nonmedical use spreads into the street. It is taken recreationally and addictively at dosages many times those that are clinically recommended. Cases of chemical dependency are reported. Allergic reactions and potentially dangerous side effects begin to appear. Frightening reports of abuse, overdose, addiction, and death stir public action. Legislation outlawing the drug or limiting its use is enacted, and last year's wonder drug becomes this year's front page abuse problem.

If this is the case, one may well ask, why not just outlaw all psychoactive drugs and have done with it? Well, its not that simple. Many of the most dangerous substances in our pharmacopoeia are also the most useful medicines we have. Consequently, a drug's danger must be tempered with its medical usefulness and not even the drugs in Schedule I are totally eliminated from the research pharmacopoeia. The question becomes, just how dangerous is a drug and how stringent need the controls be?

Although they may consider it clinically safe, the responsible researchers and physicians who have worked with MDMA are the first to be concerned with possible abuse potential. They are well aware of the problems that can be posed by psychoactive drugs. They have learned that glowing reports of low toxicity and medical facility attributed to MDMA send mixed signals to the general public. In the street, these signals can be misinterpreted. They can be seen as a green light for recreational use and self-medication.

E. MDMA Research at the Haight Ashbury Free Medical Clinics

Anxiety and other stimulant symptoms were the main side effects of MDMA seen at the Haight Ashbury Free Medical Clinics' Drug Abuse Treatment Program, as described by Darryl Inaba, Pharm. D., director of the program, and Richard B. Seymour at the MDMA scheduling hearings.

Much of the research information generated by the Clinics comes directly from data gathered by the Clinics' own treatment staff. In its 23 years of operation, the Haight Ashbury Free Medical Clinics has had over 1,000,000 patient visits. Today, the drug treatment staff alone sees an average of 460 new clients a month on an outpatient basis. The inference that can be drawn from data concerning MDMA during that period was that whether or not the drug was proliferating on the street, that proliferation was not reflected in treatment figures, at least not at the Clinics or any other reporting treatment facility.

Incidents involving MDMA and methoxylated amphetamines reported in our clinical data include "mentions." This is where a patient may come in with a complaint related to another drug, but states that he or she has been taking MDMA, MDMD, DOM, STP, MDA, Adam, ecstasy, etc. Altogether clients who had problems with or mentioned the use of these drugs at the drug treatment program average about three or four a month. That represents less than 1% of the program's total treatment load. Given that this is an aggregate figure, the percentage of those who were actually treated for MDMA is a fraction of that 1%. These numbers have remained relatively steady since about 1980.

Within the tiny percentage of cases, there are added complications in ascertaining just how many MDMA-related problems are actually being treated. Unless they have been diverted directly from legitimate pharmaceutical sources, most street drugs are synthesized or processed by underground chemists. In the twilight world of illicit or street drugs, things are rarely what they seem. Often easily obtainable substances are disguised to resemble others that are in demand but harder to get. The notion that habitual users can tell the difference between their drug of choice and a counterfeit is often a myth. We learned in an earlier chapter that street cocaine may actually be a mix of caffeine, a couple of other legal stimulants, with a dental anesthetic added for the characteristic tooth and gum numbness associated with the use of cocaine. Often, habitual users will swear that it is the real thing.

Often treatment centers will not know what specific drug a client may have used. It takes sophisticated drug testing equipment to tell the difference between two drugs as similar in structure as MDA and MDMA. The process is also comparatively expensive and unnecessary for symptomatic treatment of stimulant reactions, which are similar for all drugs in the category. In such cases, and if no untoward symptoms are apparent, treatment staff usually takes the word of the client for what they have taken. The client, in turn, has usually taken the word of the person who sold the drug as to what is in it. With MDMA and the methoxylated amphetamines, the acute toxicity symptoms that are usually seen in treatment are similar and result from taking too much of the drug. These dose-related symptoms usually dissipate as the drug wears off, and the patient can be discharged within a few hours.

In treatment data, MDMA is lumped in with the methoxylated amphetamines. The acute toxicity symptoms for all of these involve anxiety, fear reactions usually accompanied by a racing pulse and rapid heartbeat, paranoia—sometimes with delusions—and a sufficient sense of unease to prompt the individual to seek treatment. Treatment usually begins with reassuring the patient that these feelings are a result of taking too much of the drug, are not dangerous, and will wear off as the drug is metabolized. There is some variation depending on the individual. In some cases, these patients come back for a series of counseling sessions. In most cases, a talkdown similar to that used for psychedelic bad trips is sufficient.

F. Severe Toxic Reactions

Severe reactions to what users believed to be MDMA have been reported, including prolonged psychotic reactions. As with any consciousness-effecting drug, these psychotic breaks can happen, especially if the user has underlying psychopathology.

Hayner and McKinney (1986) reported two severe cases involving MDMA. These apparently involved idiosynchratic, life-threatening reactions to the drug.

G. Contraindications

Besides the potential for acute toxicity and the possibility of idiosynchratic side effects, individuals may have existing conditions that make the use of certain drugs especially dangerous for them. These are called contraindications, and such works as the *Physician's Desk Reference* (PDR) provide warnings as to who should not receive a certain drug, and when a certain drug should be prescribed.

There are several contraindications for the use of MDMA. These involve unofficial medical estimates of health conditions that would preclude the use of this drug by certain individuals. Because of its sympathomimetic or stimulant qualities and effects, MDMA should not be taken by people with hypertension, heart disease, seizures, hyperthyroidism, diabetes mellitus, hypoglycemia, glaucoma, or diminished liver function. Because little is known of MDMA's effects in pregnancy, potential to produce birth defects, or effects in a breastfed infant, it should not be taken by a nursing mother, or any woman who even suspects that she might be pregnant.

Although there seems to be no cross tolerance or additive effect between MDMA and MDA or any of the methoxylated amphetamines, all stimulants do have some cumulative effect. Therefore, MDMA should not be used in conjunction with other sympathomimetic drugs. These include cocaine, amphetamine, methamphetamine, caffeine (found in coffee, tea, soft drinks, and many medications), both prescription and over-the-counter diet pills, cold remedies, broncodialators for asthma, hay fever, or other allergies, pep pills, or any preparation containing phenylpropanolamine (PPA) or ephedrine. Methylenedioxymethamphetamine should especially not be taken by anyone using MAO inhibitors, such as Nardil, Parnate, Eutonyl, or any of the tricyclic antidepressants, such as amitriptyline, Amitid, Elavil, Endep, Norpramine, Pertofrane, Adapin, Sinequan, Vivactil, Surmontil, Ludiomil, or Tofranil.

Methylenedioxymethamphetamine is also contraindicated for anyone with a history of panic attacks or who has social or vocational dysfunction from psychological problems that have required 24-h-a-day care by trained personnel because it may cause a recurrence of these problems.

H. MDMA and Addictive Disease

MDMA has addiction potential with the population in general, and a high addiction potential for anyone with or vulnerable to addictive disease. To illustrate this point, Smith cites a communication that took place with a woman who reported that her husband had entered private treatment for chronic cocaine abuse and had been given MDMA. "Now," she said, "he claims that the MDMA has cured his cocaine habit. The only problem is that he now takes MDMA and spends the rest of his time at home drinking and smoking marijuana."

Smith points out that this individual used the MDMA to feed his addiction denial system. This allowed him to change venues and go out of control on his compulsive use of alcohol and marijuana while claiming to have been cured of cocaine addiction.

Our opinion is that everyone is better off not using any psychoactive drugs for so-called recreational or self-medicating purposes. There are many viable alternatives to alcohol and other drugs (Seymour and Smith, 1987).

I. Treatment Issues with MDMA

On May 17 and 18, 1986, the Haight Ashbury Free Medical Clinics' Training and Education Project and the Merritt Peralta Chemical Dependency Recovery Hospital's Institute for Addiction Studies co-sponsored a national conference to MDMA. Co-chaired by David E. Smith, M.D., and Richard B. Seymour, the conference focused on all aspects of the MDMA controversy, including chemistry, pharmacology, therapeutics, abuse treatment, and enforcement. Richard B. Seymour's book *MDMA*, was used as the syllabus, and a selected proceedings was published as the October-December, 1986, issue of *Journal of Psychoactive Drugs*.

During that time, the Training and Education Project became an informational clearinghouse for clinical information on MDMA and related substances. The following material is based on data from the following sources: (1) client visits and telephone inquiries at the Haight Ashbury Free Medical Clinics' Drug Detoxification Project; (2) telephone inquiries and subsequent interviews with MDMA users at the Training and Education Project; (3) inquiries received from and subsequent interviews with drug abuse treatment professionals throughout the country who had encountering MDMA as a drug of abuse; (4) consultations with psychotherapists who used MDMA in their clinical practice; and (5) the collective experience of the Haight Ashbury Free Medical Clinics with MDMA, MDE, and 2-CB; amphetamines, including the methoxylated amphetamines such as MMDA, DOM (STP); and such psychedelics as mescaline, DMT, LSD-25, and psilocybin over the past 20 years.

The Haight Ashbury Free Medical Clinics' Drug Detoxification and Aftercare Project sees more than 400 new drug abuse patients per month primarily for heroin, cocaine, amphetamine, barbiturate, marijuana, and alcohol-related problems. Over the past 6 years, according to the Project's director, Darryl Inaba, Pharm. D., Detox has seen an average of about four patients per month complaining of an MDA or MDMA problem or simply asking questions about these drugs.

J. Acute Toxicity

The first problem area is acute MDMA toxicity, which is essentially the result of taking too much MDMA in too short a period of time. This results in some physical or psychological dysfunction. The symptoms appear to be toxicological in nature, and therefore time/dose related. These symptoms range from a mild caffeinelike toxicity to potentially life-threatening stimulant overdoses.

The second area of concern is prolonged MDMA toxicity, which describes a chronic or regular ingestion of MDMA. Again, the symptoms range in severity from mild dysphoria to frank paranoid psychosis and relate to both acute toxicity, chronicity of use, and secondary drug effects such as sleep and appetite suppression.

The third problem area is the MDMA-induced anxiety syndromes. These are problems related to MDMA's ability to bring unconscious material to consciousness. We have hypothesized that these anxiety syndromes are primarily caused by the lack of resolution and integration of now-conscious and often emotionally potent materials. These anxiety syndromes appear to be psychodynamic in nature and not purely toxicological. They last beyond the period of actual drug intoxication.

Low-Dose Acute Toxicity

Greer and Tolbert (1986) have described some of the low-dose, therapeutic range toxic reactions such as jitteriness, mild anxiety, mild apprehension, and jaw clenching. Because many MDMA users view the MDMA use as a relatively important event and many users even formally ritualize such use, an anticipation and apprehension of the events to come may blend with the sympathomimetic properties of MDMA to further heighten apprehension and perhaps even produce fear in predisposed people. Generally, most of the sympathomimetic reactions are dose related, and are typically mild. Nonmedicinal approaches, such as support, quiet, and reassurance that the symptoms will fade over time, should be successful in reducing this apprehension. In most cases, individuals taking MDMA at the dosages used in therapy, i.e., 50–150 mg, would be aware that problems they may be experiencing are drug related.

Medium-Dose Acute Toxicity

At somewhat higher doses, i.e., 250 mg to 300 mg MDMA, dose and setting-related psychopathology may develop. In a person with low tolerance to stimulants, there may be a Medium Dose Acute Toxicity resulting from ingestion at this level.

Visual distortions have been reported, such as viewing an object that appears to be shimmering, shiny or perhaps moving in a jittery fashion, or with geometric embellishments. There is an awareness that these distortions are drug-induced, and they do not appear to carry any particularly positive or negative content. Also, they do not typically interfere with the therapeutic goals of insight and empathy for most individuals. Some users have reported that they desire to be alone and some report that they become slightly concerned about others noticing their behavior and knowing that they are "high." There can be a slightly paranoid flaver or self-conscious tendency which appears to be dose-related. These feelings of self-consciosness may only occur while inside a building or in crowds, and there may be a tendency to move outdoors.

For many, there may be a fairly distressing depression which may emerge rapidly, especially if there is a sudden shift in consciousness away from the particularly empathic or euphoric stage of the MDMA experience. The subjective aspect of this depression may have to do with returning to a fairly normal consciousness after having experienced often significantly beautiful and/or meaningful feelings.

High-Dose Acute Toxicity

The most obvious and most clinically important acute toxicological problem involves the high dose MDMA toxic reaction. Depending upon personal variables such as prior drug experience (especially with stimulants, hallucinogens and PCP), tolerance to the effects of the drug and setting, the toxic range for MDMA may be as low as 300 mg for some people, but 400 mg or more for others. Toxic symptomatology would be on a continuum ranging from anxiety symptoms and panic with or without tachycardia to psychotic reactions with paranoia and violence. Hypertensive crises and even cerebrovascular accidents and cardiac arrythmias could theoretically occur as with cocaine and the amphetamines.

Some MDMA users may also use other drugs during the same time period. Others may use MDMA in combination with other drugs, such as MDA or marijuana. Other drugs that may have similar properties and effects to those of MDA include 2-CB, or 4-bromo,-2,5-dimethoxyphenethylamine and MDE (Eve) or N-ethyl-3,4-methylenedioxymethamphetamine.

Treatment Considerations for Acute Toxicity

The medical management of acute MDMA toxicity will also be on a contunuum. At the lower doses or at the least severe reactions, the appropriate medical management of the client may simply be a supportive, reassuring interaction with the subject, moving him or her to a perceived safe environment, and reducing stimuli. The person should be told that the distressing symptoms will fade over time. It would be optimal if someone with psychotherapeutic skills were to spend time with the subject, given that potent psychodynamic issues may come forth. It would be best if the person is not left alone, but with someone who is capable of providing psychological support.

For moderately dysfunctional anxiety symptoms which increase with severity, 5–10 mg diazepam may be given orally. For the patient who also experiences tachycardia, propanalol, 10–20 mg, can be given orally, or if given intravenously, administer from 0.5 to 1.0 mg very slowly at a maximum of 1 mg/min up to a total of 6 mg.

If the symptoms are more severe, consideration should be given to containment if (1) anxiety merges into aggressive behavior, (2) evidence of stimulant psychosis with violence to self or to others, or (3) there are suicidal verbalizations or behaviors. If the client has a *stimulant psychosis*, and is markedly anxious, either: (1) Give haloperidol, 2 mg b.i.d., and assess remaining anxiety, treating with diazepam, 5–10 mg iv, if necessary; or (2) Give 5–10 mg diazepam p.o. or i.v. If anxiety is still marked, give diazepam every 1 to 2 h. If anxiety is effectively treated, give diazepam every 4–6 h for a maximum of about 40 mg/24-h period. If stimulant psychosis remains and is an issue relative to violence or danger to self or others, give haloperidol, 2 mg b.i.d. p.o.

For persistent adrenergic crisis, give propanalol orally in doses of 40–60 mg at 4- to 6-h intervals for duration of crisis. A pulse of 90 or less is the goal. Many stimulant psychosis patients will be resistant to haloperidol and may in fact request a sedative-hypnotic to reduce anxiety. Some of these patients may be able to handle the stimulant psychosis if anxiolytic therapy is given. The important diagnosis criterion is: Does the psychotic break represent a clear danger to the client or to others? Also note that the amphetamines and haloperidol both lower seizure threshold, so caution should be used. Also, some patients may be very sensitive to the sedative-hypnotics and proceed into coma with even lower doses than recommended, thus caution is urged. The treatment of stimulant-related problems and treatment concerns is discussed in depth by Wesson and Smith (1979).

Prolonged High-Dose Toxicity

The person who uses high doses of MDMA (or any mood-altering drug) on a daily basis is a person likely to have another addictive disorder. Whereas most people who use MDMA for its psychotherapeutic benefits dislike the stimulant properties of MDMA, some people actively seek out this experience. Clearly, present cocaine problems speak to the fact that stimulant abuse is commonplace. In interviews with MDMA users, it was revealed that some cocaine dealers also sold MDMA as an adjunct to their normal trade, and many cocaine abusers and addicts were introduced to MDMA in this setting. Also, amphetamine addicts who have had access to MDMA may have used MDMA as an alternative to amphetamine, or turned to MDMA as a supplement to their amphetamine use. Because drug switching is a regular part of drug abuse, a regular stimulant abuser might have a tendency to use MDMA at higher doses and for longer periods of time, and to use this drug for its stimulant rather than its empathogenic qualities. These individuals might also exhibit a cross tolerance to MDMA, and thus be able to ingest fairly large quantities of the drug.

The daily or chronic use of a central nervous system stimulant can push a person to the limit and drain their physical and psychological strengths. With the high-dose chronic user, mood swings, emotional lability, and anxiety can increase, trading off with the depression in times of abstinence. In time, stimulant psychosis, paranois, and violence could emerge.

Prolonged LowDose Toxicity

While high-dose chronic use of MDMA suggests stimulant addiction, the lower dose extended use may suggest a different type of drug use. The stimulant addict understands and desires the stimulant effects of amphetamines and cocaine. That is not the case with a number of people we have interviewed. Most often, these are individuals engaged in generalized drug experimentation and their chronic use is usually over a finite period of time, usually a week or two.

The effects of this prolonged MDMA use at lower doses include mild psychopathology. Interviewees describe a lack of mental clarity, being "out of sorts," having mild mental confusion and slight memory impairment. Some mention a lack of motivation, mild disorientation, and forgetfulness. There may be some sleep dysfunction and some nutritional needs may not be met if the pattern continues. They did not report anxiety or hyperactivity, however, and that may be due to titrating or controlling their doses over the day. They also state that cessation of MDMA use returns them to their normal emotions and psychological state.

Treatment Considerations for Prolonged Toxicity

It is important that the existence of addictive disease be assessed. The chronicity of use, as opposed to event-specific use or very rare use, may be a signal of addictive illness. Appropriate treatment for the addiction would include inpatient or outpatient chemical dependency treatment based on an abstinence model of supported recovery. Appropriate referral should be made to such 12-Step programs as Alcoholics Anonymous or Narcotics Anonymous.

MDMA-Induced Anxiety Syndromes

Although it is atypical for a drug user to contact a drug treatment facility to report *positive* drug experiences, we do receive reports of unsupervised, positive psychodynamic facilitation in MDMA users who call, write, or visit the clinics for literatures or questions regarding MDMA. However, the opposite is also true. For some users, MDMA will bring to the surface unconscious material that may manifest itself in a variety of negative ways.

These problems seem unrelated to volume, dose, or duration of MDMA use. We have identified it as a delayed anxiety disorder secondary to MDMA ingestion. In these cases, the MDMA user reports one or more symptoms of anxiety, typically emerging shortly after their initial MDMA experience. These symptoms range from a mild anxiety or concentration difficulties to a full-blown disorder such as panic attack with hyperventilation and tachycardia, phobic disorders, paresthesias, or other anxiety states. In one anecdotal case, the subject self-medicated the MDMA reactions with increasing amounts of MDMA, coupled with other psychoactive drugs, and eventually died.

In some cases, the client will be particularly concerned about a certain part of the body. The client may perceive that a hand is shaking, or that the extremities are cold and clammy. Subjective reactions to these concerns can range from mildly annoying to highly inhibiting. The dysfunction may require psychiatric or psychological intervention.

These clients reported that they took the MDMA for "therapeutic" reasons, though not as an adjunct to therapy. When asked what specific therapeutic goals they had in mind, responses included dealing with family problems, relational difficulties, and high stress patterns in their lives.

Those subjects who have followed up on obtaining therapy have reported feeling either back to normal or better than before taking the MDMA. Most report lasting insights gained from their MDMA experience, insights that they are finally acting upon. They may feel, however, that they should have engaged in psychotherapy first and used the drug as an adjunct to that therapy.

XVII. CONCLUSIONS

Illict and addictive use of hallucinogens continues, and there are periodic outbreaks of hallucinogenic problems requiring medical intervention. Although usually at comparatively low dosages, LSD remains a frequent component of 1960s-style rock concerts and other gatherings. Other hallucinogens are cited from time to time, the most prevalent being psylocybin mushrooms. In groups where these hallucinogens are used, individuals have learned to utilize acute reaction talkdowns. Methylenedioxymethamphetamine is still prevalent with the young, with new wave, and other groups that relate to self-analysis. Its use has also led to the development of "acid houses," i.e., dance clubs and gathering places for young hallucinogenic drug users. Cocaine and other drug dealers see MDMA as a relatively short-fashion drug that does not have the kick of cocaine, heroin, and other "popular" drugs.

The greatest change is that hallucinogenic drugs are no longer the center of a counter- or subculture, as they were in the 1960s. Then, hallucinogenic drugs were seen as a means of achieving cosmic insight and spirituality. Today, the trend is toward seeking and finding spirituality in recovery and through the various 12-Step approaches to abstinence and personal spiritual growth and maturity.

REFERENCES

Alpert, R. Psychedelic drugs and the law. *J. Psychedelic Drugs, 1*(1):7–26 (1967).

Brown, A., and Stickgold, A. Marijuana flashback phenomena. *J. Psychedelic Drugs, 8*(4):275–283 (1976).

Bugliosi, V., and Gentry, C. *Helter Skelter*. Norton, New York, 1974.

Greer, G., and Tolbert, R. Subjective reports of the effects of MDMA in a clinical setting. *MDMA: Proceedings of the Conference* (R.B. Seymour, D.R. Wesson, and D.E. Smith, eds.). *J. Psychoactive Drugs, 18*(4):319–328 (1986).

Cohen, S. Lysergic acid diethylamide: Side effects and complications. *J. Nerv. Ment. Dis., 130*:30–40 (1960).

Grinspoon, L., and Bakalar, J.B. *Psychedelic Drugs Reconsidered*. Basic Books, New York, 1979.

Harding, W.M., and Zinberg, N.E. The Effectiveness of the subculture in developing rituals and social sanctions for controllng drug use, *Drugs, Rituals and Altered States of Consciousness* (B.M. Du Toit, ed.), Balkema, Rotterdam, 1977.

Hayner, G.N., and McKinney, H.E. MDMA: The dark side of ecstasy, *MDMA: Proceedings of the Conference*, (R.B. Seymour, D.R. Wesson and D.E. Smith, eds.), *J. Psychoactive Drugs*, *18*(4):341–348 (1986).

Heinlein, R.A. *Stranger in a Strange Land*. Putnam, New York, 1961.

Hofmann, A. The discovery of LSD and subsequent investigations on naturally occurring hallucinogens, *Discoveries in Biological Psychiatry*. (F.J. Ayd, Jr., and B. Blackwell, eds.), Lippincott, Philadelphia, 1970.

Klein, J. The new drug they call ecstasy. *New York*, May 20, 1985.

Lawn, J.C. Schedules of controlled substances: Temporary placement of 3,4-methylenedioxymethamphetamine (MDMA) into schedule I. *Fed. Reg. 50*(106):May 31 (1985).

Leary, T., Metzner, R., and Alpert, R. *The Psychedelic Experience: A Manual Based on the Tibetan Book of the Dead*. University Books, New Hyde Park, New York, 1964.

Metzner, R. Reflections on LSD—Ten years later. *J. Psychedelic Drugs, 10*(2):137–140.

Michaux, H. *Miserable Miracle* (Trans. L. Varese), City Lights Books, San Francisco, 1963.

Miller, N.S., and Gold, M.S. The diagnosis of marijuana (cannabis) dependence. *J. Subst. Abuse Treat., 6*(3):183–192 (1989).

Miller, N.S., Gold, M.S., and Pottash, A. A 12-step treatment approach to marijuana (cannabis) dependence. *J. Subst. Abuse Treat., 6*(4):241–251 (1989).

Newmeyer, J., and Johnson, G. Drug emergencies in crowds: An analysis of "rock medicine." *J. Psychedelic Drugs, 9*:235–245 (1979).

Rosenbaum, R., Interview: Wavy Gravy. *High Times*, Feb.:36–99 (1979).

Seymour, R.B. *MDMA*. Partisan Press, San Francisco, 1986.

Seymour, R.B. MDMA: Another view of ecstasy. *PharmChem Newsletter, 14*(3):1–4 (1985).

Seymour, R.B., and Smith, D.E. Diagnosis of marijuana dependence (commentary). *Addict. Alert., 3*(9):3–4 (1989).

Seymour, R.B., and Smith, D.E. *Drugfree: A Unique, Positive Approach to Staying Off Alcohol and Other Drugs*. Facts on File Publications, New York, 1987.

Seymour, R.B., Smith, D.E., Inaba, D., and Landry, M. *The New Drugs: Look-Alikes, Drugs of Deception and Designer Drugs*. Hazelden, Center City, Minnesota, 1989.

Shulgin, A.T. What is MDMA? *PharmChem Newsletter, 14*(3):2–3 (1985).

Smith, D.E. Acute and chronic toxicity of marijuana. *J. Psychedelic Drugs, 2*(1):37–45 (1968).

Smith, D.E. Editor's Note. *J. Psychedelic Drugs, 1*(1):1–5 (1967).

Smith, D.E., and Luce, J. *Love Needs Care*. Little Brown, Boston, 1969.

Smith, D.E., Milkman, H.B., and Sunderwirth, S.G. Addictive disease: Concept and controversy, *The Addictions: Multidisciplinary Perspectives and Treatments*. (H.B. Milkman, and H.J. Shaffer, eds.), Lexington Books, Lexington (1985).

Smith, D.E., and Rose, A.J. The group marriage commune: A case study. *J. Psychedelic Drugs, 3*(1):115–119 (1970).

Smith, D.E., and Seymour, R.B. Clinical perspectives on the toxicity of marijuana: 1967–1981, *Marijuana and Youth: Clinical Observations on Motivation and Learning*. National Institute on Drug Abuse, Washington, D.C., 1982.

Smith, D.E., and Shick, J.F.E. Analysis of the LSD flashback. *J. Psychedelic Drugs, 3*(1):13–19 (1970).

Smith, D.E., and Wesson, D.R. Editor's Note. *J. Psychoactive Drugs, 7*(2):111–114 (1975).

Ungerleider, J.T., and Wellisch, D.K. Coercive persuasion (brainwashing), religious cults and deprogramming. *Am. J. Psychiatry, 136*(3):179–181 (1979).

Wasson, R.G., Ruck, C.A.P., and Hofmann, A. *The Road to Eleusis: Unveiling the Secret of the Mysteries*. Harcourt, Brace, Jovanovich, New York, 1978.

Watkins, P., and Soledad, G. *My Life with Charles Manson*. Bantam, New York, 1979.

Weil, A.T. *Marriage of the Sun and Moon*. Houghton Mifflin, Boston, 1981.

Wesson, D.R., and Smith, D.E. *Amphetamine Use, Misuse and Abuse*. Hall, New York, 1979.

Wesson, D.R., and Smith, D.E. Psychedelics, In *Treatment Aspects of Drug Dependence* (A. Schecter, ed.), CRC Press, Boca Raton, Florida, 1978.

27

Sedatives-Hypnotics
(Not Including Benzodiazepines)

Hiten Kisnad
Cornell University Medical College, The New York Hospital–Cornell Medical Center, White Plains, New York

I. INTRODUCTION

The principal use of sedative-hypnotic drugs is to produce drowsiness and to promote sleep. A sedative drug decreases activity, moderates excitement, and calms the recipient. A hypnotic drug produces drowsiness and facilitates the onset and maintenance of sleep, resembling natural sleep, from which the recipient may be easily aroused. This sleep does not resemble hypnosis. The term *tranquilizers* was coined to emphasize a particular characteristic of all sedative-hypnotic drugs, which is to produce tranquility; i.e., to induce calmness without sedation. Barbiturates were referred to as tranquilizers until the introduction of the benzodiazepines, although both can produce sedation. Barring benzodiazepines, the barbiturates are the prototypic drugs and constitute the principal members of the sedative-hypnotic class. Since the advent of benzodiazepines in 1960, the use of barbiturates and other sedative-hypnotic drugs has declined.

II. PREVALENCE

Potions have been used to induce sleep since antiquity. Bromide was the first agent introduced specifically as a sedative (1853) and later as a hypnotic (1864). Chloral hydrate, paraldehyde, urethan, and sulfonal were the only other sedative-hypnotic drugs used before 1900. Barbital was introduced in 1903 and phenobarbital in 1912, whose successes then led to synthesis of 2500 barbiturates, 50 of which were distributed for commercial use [1].

History has repeated itself with the introduction of each new sedative-hypnotic drug. Although the new drug is introduced with unguarded optimism and misguided claims, the essential features of the drug are the same except for some minor improvements in its untoward effects. The toxicities, abuse, addiction, tolerance, and dependence potential persisted for each subsequent drug introduced.

This chapter is dedicated to my late paternal grandfather who encouraged me to pursue a medical career.

Certain populations, i.e., the elderly, chronically ill, those already using or addicted to other drugs, including alcohol, and those who are anxious, depressed, or insomnic are more prone to sedative-hypnotic use and addiction [2].

The exact incidence and prevalence of the use of sedative-hypnotics is difficult to ascertain. Various estimates through surveys are available for the prevalence rates of the use of sedative-hypnotics [3,4].

In 1982, 19% of young adults reported nonmedical use of sedatives, and 15% reported some experience with nonmedical use of tranquilizers, with the incidence being relatively stable in the preceding 5 years.

In 1984, the National Household Survey (1972–1984) and the High School Senior Survey (1981–1984) showed that 14–19% of high school seniors and young adults (18–25 years old) reported past nonmedical use of sedative-hypnotics. But these lifetime prevalence rates were generally below those for other major drug classes except heroin and opioid analgesics: alcohol (93–95%), tobacco (70–77%), marijuana (59–64%), stimulants (18–28%), cocaine (16–28%), and hallucinogens (15–21%) (Table 1).

Data from emergency room visits and medical examiners' reports (1972–1976) indicate that sedative-hypnotics are a major cause of adverse drug reactions (Table 2).

Study of drug-related deaths (1972–1975) in eight large United States cities showed 30% of 924 drug-related deaths were due to narcotics, and 27% were attributable to barbiturates or diazepam (excluding nonbarbiturate sedative-hypnotics). Suicides represent only 8% of narcotic and 15% of sedative-hypnotic–related deaths.

The U.S. population estimate for simultaneous use of alcohol in combination with "sedatives" (use of both drugs simultaneously or on the same occasion) was approximately 3 million, according to the results of a national survey, whereas the concurrent use of both drugs (i.e., during the same time period) was approximately 4 million. Corresponding figures for the simultaneous and concurrent use of alcohol and tranquilizers were both approximately 6 million [5].

Most of these surveys have certain drawbacks: They do not assess the problems with medical use of sedative-hypnotics and they do not use clear and standard definitions for abuse, addiction, tolerance, and dependence.

III. PATTERNS OF USE

The short-acting barbiturates such as pentobarbital (Nembutal) or secobarbital are preferred to long-acting barbiturates such as phenobarbital. The three major barbiturates common in the black market are secobarbital ("reds," "red devils," "seggys," "downers"), pentobarbital ("yellows," "yellow jackets," "nembies"), and a combination of secobarbital and amobarbital ("reds and blues," "rainbows," "double trouble," "tooies"). Other commonly used sedative-hypnotics include meprobamate, gluthethimide, methyprylon, methaqualone, and the benzodiazepines. Paraldehyde and chloral hydrate have been replaced, largely, by other drugs, since the newer sedative-hypnotics have less noxious side effects.

The quality and purity of these drugs are uncertain and depend to a large degree on the extent to which they are adulterated or cut. The amount of hypnotic taken varies immensely, but an average daily dose of 1.5 gm of short-acting barbiturate is not uncommon, and some individuals can tolerate even 2.5 gm/day over several months.

The most common route of administration is oral. Some inject the sedative-hypnotic intravenously, as in "mainlining," whereas a few others inject the drug subcutaneously as in "skin popping"; such patients may develop abscesses or even HIV infection.

Most, if not all, persons with a dependence on barbiturates fall into one of the three major patterns of use. The first pattern of use is episodic intoxication. These users tend to

Table 1 High School Senior Survey: Nonmedical Use of Sedatives and Tranquilizers

Trends in Lifetime Prevalence	Class of 1975 %	Class of 1980 %	Class of 1985 %	Class of 1988 %
Sedatives	18.2	14.9	11.8	7.8
Tranquilizers	17.0	15.2	11.9	9.4

Trends in Annual Prevalence	Class of 1975 %	Class of 1980 %	Class of 1985 %	Class of 1988 %
Sedatives	11.7	10.3	5.8	3.7
Tranquilizers	10.6	8.7	6.1	4.8

Daily Use (in past 30 days)	Class of 1975 %	Class of 1980 %	Class of 1985 %	Class of 1988 %
Sedatives	0.3	0.2	0.1	0.1
Tranquilizers	0.1	0.1	0.0	0.0

Table 1 *(continued)*

National Household Survey: Nonmedical Use of Sedatives and Tranquilizers

Lifetime Prevalence

	Percent Age 12-17				Percent Age 18-25				Percent Age 26+			
	72	77	85	88	72	77	85	88	72	77	85	88
Sedatives	3.0	3.1	4.0	2.4	10.0	18.4	11.0	5.5	2.0	2.8	5.2	3.3
Tranquilizers	3.0	3.8	4.8	2.6	7.0	13.4	12.0	7.8	5.0	2.6	7.1	4.6

Annual Prevalence

	72	77	85	88	72	77	85	88	72	77	85	88
Sedatives	N/A	2.0	2.9	1.7	N/A	8.2	5.0	3.3	N/A	<0.5	2.0	1.2
Tranquilizers	N/A	2.9	3.4	1.6	N/A	7.8	6.4	4.6	N/A	1.1	2.8	1.8

Current Prevalence

	72	77	85	88	72	77	85	88	72	77	85	88
Sedatives	N/A	0.8	1.0	0.6	N/A	2.8	1.6	0.9	N/A	<0.5	0.6	0.3
Tranquilizers	N/A	0.7	0.6	0.2	N/A	2.4	1.6	1.0	N/A	<0.5	1.0	0.6

Source: National Institute on Drug Abuse, Division of Epidemiology and Statistical Analysis.

Table 2 Emergency Room and Medical Examiner Mention. (1975–1986)

DRUG	EMERGENCY ROOM VISITS		DRUG RANK		MEDICAL EXAMINER MENTION		DRUG RANK	
	1985	1986	1985	1986	1985	1986	1985	1988
Phenobarbital	1728	1465	17	20	148	161	11	11
Diphenhydramine	1532	1514	19	17	114	140	13	13
Diazepam	8324	7653	4	4	315	317	6	6
Source:	NIDA				DAWN			

Drug Abuse Statistics: Population Estimate—Nonmedical Usage Sedatives/Tranquilizers

PERCENT

	12-17 years				18-25 years				26 + years				Total			
	Ever Used		Current Use		Ever Used		Current Use		Ever Used		Current Use		Ever Used		Current Use	
	1985	1988	1985	1988	1985	1988	1985	1988	1985	1988	1985	1988	1985	1988	1985	1988
Sedatives	4	2	1	1	11	6	2	1	5	3	1	<0.5	6	4	1	<0.5
Tranquilizers	5	2	1	<0.5	12	8	2	1	7	5	1	1	8	5	1	1

Source: National Institute on Drug Abuse, Division of Epidemiology and Statistical Analysis.

be teenagers or young adults, or psychiatrically disturbed, who take barbiturates to produce a "high" or experience a sense of well-being. Its effect as a sedative or a euphoriant is determined by factors such as the environment in which the abuser takes the drug (setting), the psychological make-up of the person, and, most important, his expectations (set). These young people may become so accustomed to the episodic sense of well-being engendered by the drug that barbiturates become a fairly constant aspect of their lives. Since "sleeping pills" are commonly found in homes, adolescent and youthful polydrug abusers hold "bring your own drug" parties with a variety of sedative-hypnotics from each person's family medicine cabinet.

The second pattern of use of barbiturates that of chronic intoxication, occurs for the most part in middle-aged persons, usually of the middle and upper economic classes, who obtain the drug from their physician rather than from an illegal source (street dealer). They start off taking barbiturates to relieve their insomnia or anxiety, but owing to tolerance, gradually become dependent. They may be unaware of their dependence for months or years until physical signs, such as slurred speech or impairment in thier ability to work, occur. In order to obtain larger supplies of the drug, patients may visit their family physician frequently, visit several different physicians, or even photocopy their prescriptions so that they may be filled at different pharmacies. Like physicians, pharmacists may be unwitting or witting collaborators. When their drug abuse is identified (and confronted), patients typically deny their quest for euphoria. They may present themselves as being depressed or have multiple somatic complaints. They may get temporary relief from sedative-hypnotic use but their general condition seems to deteriorate. The "medical patient" increases the dose to treat his or her insomnia and anxiety gradually, whereas the "addict" may accelerate the dose much more rapidly. Neither the patient nor the physician may recognize the existence of abuse and addiction, especially in the early stages. Both assume the insomnia, anxiety, and tremors that emerge with reduction or cessation of the drug as return of the original symptoms rather than withdrawal, which may be protracted over weeks and months.

The third category/class is that of intravenous barbiturate use, mainly by young adults closely involved in the illegal drug culture. They are often identifiable by the large abscesses in accessible areas of their bodies. They are usually polydrug abusers. They may switch to barbiturates from heroin because barbiturates are less expensive than heroin (it costs approximately $30 for 2–3 gm of injectable barbiturate). These barbiturate addicts, like amphetamine addicts, are loathed by the rest of the drug subculture because of their irresponsible behavior and proneness to violence.

Some people use barbiturates incidentally to their dependence on other drugs. Certain sedative-hypnotic drugs are used in combination with other drugs of abuse to potentiate each other's euphorogenic effects: gluthethimide and codeine (in cough syrup or with acetaminophen) are often combined, taken together, or in intervals of few hours alternately, to produce a better high, but this is particularly dangerous because it can cause fatal respiratory depression. Opioid users combine barbiturate or other sedatives to augment the effects of weak illicit heroin, or to reexperience psychological effects from opioids to which they have developed tolerance. Many heroin or methadone addicts and methadone maintenance patients are physically dependent on both opioids and sedatives. Some alcoholics use these agents to relieve symptoms of alcohol withdrawal, including tremulousness, or to produce intoxication without the odor of alcohol. An amphetamine and barbiturate combined produces more mood elevation than either drug alone. Amphetamine addicts may inject secobarbital as a downer to abort or minimize the paranoia and agitation usually experienced at the end of a trip.

IV. ROLE OF PHYSICIAN AND HEALTH CARE INDUSTRY

Sedatives, unlike heroin, cocaine, amphetamines, marijuana, and many other drugs, are produced entirely by pharmaceutical companies. Diversion of these substances into the drug abuse culture originates primarily from pharmaceutical or medical sources—either by theft or by illegal or careless prescribing practices. Some physicians "sell" drugs or allow themselves to be manipulated by addicts. Many of these physicians are sole practitioners. Although some of these "pill doctors" may be ignorant of the implications of their prescribing practices, others are practicing as much denial as their patients [6,7].

One organized form of sedative-hypnotic distribution was the so-called "stress clinic," which operated in several parts of the United States for several years and dispensed sedative-hypnotics, primarily methaqualone. All such "businesses" have ceased to exist today due to successful prosecution of the proprietors and physicians (U.S. vs Lefkovitz).

Hence, the availability of barbiturates on the street is only part of the problem. For decades, physicians have prescribed barbiturates too willingly and indiscriminately, without keeping track of the number of refills. Many family physicians unwittingly make many patients dependent on barbiturates.

Unlike heroin, but like amphetamines, barbiturates are legitimately manufactured in numerous forms; e.g., the long-acting barbiturate phenobarbital is an ingredient in a large number of different proprietary drugs in combination with other barbiturates, bromides, tranquilizers, analgesics, antihistamines, vitamins, antibiotics, and gastric antacids. Hence, there is little pressure to establish illegal clandestine laboratories to produce the drug. The black market meets its need by diverting shipments of barbiturates from manufacturers to Mexico and back across the border illegally. Additional supplies are obtained by robbing drug warehouses and physicians' offices, medical clinics, and hospitals. Schoolyard dealers who supply marijuana often also carry sedatives.

V. CHEMISTRY

Barbituric acid, the basic building block for all barbiturates, is 2,4,6-trioxohexahydropyrimidine, which lacks central nervous system (CNS) depressant activity, but the addition of alkyl or aryl groups at position 5 confers sedative-hypnotic, among other, activities. The barbituric acid derivatives do not dissolve readily in water, although they are quite soluble in nonpolar solvents. The sodium salts of barbiturates dissolve in water, forming alkaline and often unstable solutions.

Barbiturates with oxygen at C2 are called oxybarbiturates, whereas barbiturates with sulfur at C2 are called thiobarbiturates. Thiobarbiturates are more lipid soluble than oxybarbiturates; lipid solubility, in general, is inversely proportional to latency (onset of action) and duration of action and directly proportional to rate of metabolic degradation and hypnotic potency [8].

VI. INTOXICATION

The acute and chronic effects of mild intoxication with CNS depressants resemble those of alcohol intoxication. Acutely intoxicated subjects show sluggishness, slowed thinking and speech, poor comprehension and memory, compromised judgment, inattention, labile affect and exaggeration of basic personality traits, irritability, quarrelsomeness and moroseness, lack of proper personal hygiene, paranoid ideas, and suicidal tendencies. Subtle distractions of mood and impairment of judgment and motor skills may occur for a day even after just a single dose of 200 mg of secobarbital.

Barbiturates cause drowsiness for a few hours after a hypnotic dose, but it may also cause a hangover effect (residual CNS depression) the following day, along with subtle mood changes, impairment of judgment and fine motor skills (including driving, airplane flying skills), and deteriorating intellectual performance, besides nausea, vomiting, vertigo, and diarrhea. The after-effects may include overt excitement and feelings of being intoxicated, euphoric and energetic, followed by irritability. Barbiturates may induce localized or diffuse pain, and also cause hyperalgesia, especially in neurotic patients. Paradoxical excitement or disinhibition may occur in response to even single low doses of barbiturate sedative-hypnotics, particularly in the very young and old, and in pain states, and particularly with use of phenobarbital and N-methylbarbiturates. Barbiturate abusers tend to be more aware of their mood changes and behavioral impairments than benzodiazepine abusers.

Chronic intoxication has not been studied as well as acute intoxication with barbiturates and related sedative-hypnotics, but their manifestations seem to be quite similar.

Accidents due to impaired coordination and skills can also cause severe bodily injury and death; e.g., motor vehicle accidents, either from being struck or from improper driving. Even single doses of sedatives have been shown to impair driving ability significantly. Essentially, there is increased risk for any accident when one is intoxicated with sedative-hypnotics.

VII. MEDICAL SEQUALAE

In general, the subjective effects of barbiturates and selected sedative-hypnotic-anxiolytic agents are similar to those of alcohol, and the effects vary with the dose, the situation, and the personality of the user.

Sedation, pharmacological hypnosis, and general anaesthesia are usually regarded as increasing depths of a continuum of CNS depression. Most nonbenzodiazepine sedative-hypnotic drugs can induce general anesthesia. Thus, CNS effects range from mild sedation to general anesthesia to coma to death, depending upon the drug, the dose, the route of administration, the extent of tolerance, and the state of excitability of the CNS.

Except for the anticonvulsant actions of phenobarbital and its cogeners, the barbiturates have a low therapeutic index and low degree of selectivity. Hence, it is not possible to achieve a desired effect (sedation, hypnosis) without general CNS depression.

Hypersensitivity reactions may occur in individuals prone to an allergic reaction; e.g., individuals who have a history of asthma, urticaria, and angioedema. Such individuals may develop localized swellings (eyelids, cheeks, or lips) or erythematous dermatitis, or, rarely, exfoliative dermatitis (skin eruptions, fever, delirium, hepatic degeneration, with possible fatal outcome).

Patients lying unconscious for prolonged periods commonly have nerve damage with permanent sequelae, such as peroneal nerve drop, owing to compression and ischemia to a nerve.

Barbiturates may cause hypotensive shock, apnea, laryngospasm, coughing, or even cardiovascular collapse, especially if injected rapidly. Death may ensue owing to cardiac or pulmonary arrest or aspiration of vomitus.

Persistent sedative-hypnotic abuse (unlike alcohol abuse) is not associated with toxic damage to organ systems.

Computed tomographic (CT) scan follow up of sedative-hypnotic abusers has shown an increased prevalence of a widened ventricular system, particularly the third ventricle, indicating atrophy of the central parts of the brain, in two studies, but no such difference in few other studies. Thus, the association between ventricular enlargement and sedative-hypnotic abuse is still unclear.

A. Effects on Sleep and the Electroencephalogram

In hypnotic doses, barbiturates, produce dose-dependent alteration in the stages of sleep. They decrease sleep latency, increase delta bursts and fast EEG activity, and decrease the number of stage shifts to stages 0 and 1 (awakenings), shorten stages 3 and 4 (SWS), and decrease body movement. But it may increase stages 3 and/or 4 sleep in healthy persons, in enuretic and somnambulistic persons, in those with anxiety, and also in barbiturate addicts. The REM latency is prolonged, but length and density of REM sleep is decreased. Nightmares or night terrors may be caused by the deprivation of REM sleep and/or stage 4 sleep. Some tolerance develops to the effects on sleep, as much as 50% after 2 weeks of use. Discontinuation of barbiturate leads to rebound increases in (invariably) all parameters reported to be decreased by barbiturates [9,10].

In small oral or intravenous doses, barbiturates decrease low-frequency electrical activity, and increase low-voltage, fast-activity (15–35 Hz), spreading from the frontal cortex and to the parietal to the occipital cortices. Such EEG activation parallels clouding of consciousness and occasional euphoria. A further increase in dose causes large-amplitude random, slow waves (5 to 12 Hz) in spindle-shaped bursts. The patient loses consciousness but may respond to strong, painful stimuli. The EEG is stable in this and subsequent stages. As the dose is increased further, the wave frequency decreases to 1–3 Hz. Patients do not respond to noxious stimuli. Major surgical procedures are done in this stage. Limbic neuronal firing rates become depressed; there are also occasional brief periods of electrical silence, which eventually progresses to a flat wave.

VIII. PSYCHIATRIC SEQUELAE

The chronic effects of sedative abuse are primarily neuropsychiatric. Persistent sedative abuse and addictive use causes neuropsychological deficits (often permanent), including impairment in memory, coordination, and verbal and nonverbal learning, which persist long after detoxification [11,12]. Prolonged abstinence may decrease the intensity of these deficits.

Persistent sedative-hypnotic abusers are also at an increased risk to develop depressive and anxiety disorders from the drug use. One study showed that 60% of sedative abusers developed significant (secondary) depression by the end of the 6-year follow-up. Chronic hallucinosis may also occur. Changes in personality that simulates significant personality disorders may develop in regular users of sedative-hypnotics. Characteristics of antisocial, histrionic, paranoid, and other personality traits can occur with chronic use of these drugs.

IX. TOLERANCE

Tolerance among sedative-hypnotic abusers can be irregular and capricious even for the most experienced street abuser. Both pharmacodynamic (functional) and pharmacokinetic tolerance to barbiturates can occur [13]. The former contributes more to the decreased effect than does the latter. Acute tolerance occurs earlier than induction of microsomal enzymes. Pharmacokinetic tolerance reaches its peak in a few days.

Pharmacodynamic tolerance refers to adaptation at the receptor level. The cellular membrane becomes more ordered as tolerance develops. Pharmacodynamic tolerance develops both acutely and chronically in response to single or repetitive administration of the sedative-hypnotic drugs. Pharmacodynamic tolerance increases gradually with chronic administration of the drug only if the dose is increased; or else it remains unchanged after reaching a peak in only a few days of drug administration. Tolerance to barbiturates has an upper limit. For example, an addict or patient tolerant to 1.2 gm of pentobarbital/day or 1.2–2.4 gm of secobarbital/day may show little evidence of intoxication on that dose, but addition of even 0.1 gm/day causes prolonged and possibly cumulative toxicity [14]. Although there may be considerable tolerance (adaptation) to the sedative and intoxicating effects, the lethal dose is about the same in addicts as in normal individuals. Hence, acute barbiturate or meprobamate poisoning may be accidentally (drug automatism) or deliberately superimposed on chronic intoxication.

Tolerance to effects on mood, sedation, and hypnosis occurs more readily and greater than that to the anticonvulsant and lethal effects. Hence as tolerance increases, the therapeutic index decreases. The patient may increase the dosage sixfold to produce desired hypnosis, but the enhanced metabolism accounts for only one-third to one-half of this tolerance.

Tolerance to the euphoric effects occurs before tolerance to the respiratory depressant effects, which makes the sedative-hypnotic abuser prone to "accidental" overdoses, leading to serious complications or even death. Tolerance to the hypnotic effects develops faster [1–2 weeks) with short-acting barbiturates compared to several weeks with longer-acting sedative-hypnotics.

Cross-tolerance occurs between barbiturates and other CNS depressant drugs (including alcohol and benzodiazepines) and also to opioids and phencyclidine.

X. ADDICTION AND PHARMACOLOGICAL DEPENDENCE

Use of sedative-hypnotics can result in both addiction and pharmacological dependence. Addiction to nonbarbiturate sedatives and benzodiazepines has the same pathogenic evolution and clinical pathology as barbiturate addiction [15].

The reinforcing properties of barbiturates may be responsible for the development of addiction in humans [16]. Both animal and human models indicate that subjects maintain a high rate of self-administration under given circumstances. Pharmacological dependence (reduction or cessation of withdrawal symptoms with reintroduction of the drug) has been demonstrated experimentally in humans with seco-, pento-, and amobarbital. Daily doses of >400 mg/day of secobarbital or pentobarbital taken over several weeks are normally required to produce pharmacological dependence [17].

A vicious cycle is set when a sedative-hypnotic abuser consumes increasing doses of sedative-hypnotic to avoid or treat the symptoms and signs of withdrawal of sedative-hypnotic with the development of tolerance.

A. Withdrawal

There are marked similarities between the withdrawal syndromes seen with barbiturates and those seen with meprobamate, glutethimide, methaqualone, benzodiazepines, and related sedative-hypnotic drugs. They differ only in severity and temporal onset of symptoms and signs. It resembles the alcohol withdrawal syndrome.

The shorter-acting drugs typically have a more severe, earlier, and abrupt onset of withdrawal compared to longer-acting sedative-hypnotics, which have a milder, later, and more gradual onset of withdrawal. Ultra–short-acting barbiturates used for intravenous anesthesia (thiobarbiturates) ordinarily do not produce a withdrawal syndrome. The barbiturates that do produce a withdrawal syndrome (oxybarbiturates) generally have a short or intermediate duration of action (with half-lives of 10–50 h); e.g., amobarbital, secobarbital, butabarbital, butalbarbital. The severity of the withdrawal reaction varies with the drug, the intensity (daily dose) and the duration of the exposure to the drug, the individual, and the setting.

Since research studies in this field are unethical, the sources of most data are published anecdotal reports. Fraser et al. observed minor withdrawal symptoms and signs in 6% of subjects receiving 400 mg/day secobarbital or pentobarbital for 90 consecutive days, but a 50% minor withdrawal rate and 11% seizure rate in 18 subjects receiving 600 mg/day secobarbital for 35–57 consecutive days. Studies on volunteer prisoners who were formerly addicted to barbiturate drugs reveal that ingestion of a large dose, 900–2200 mg/day, of secobarbital or pentobarbital in divided doses for 32–144 days produced a severe withdrawal reaction. Fourteen of the 18 subjects (75%) developed seizures and 12 (60%) developed delirium. Based on such reports, the patient taking 600 mg/day secobarbital or 60 mg/day diazepam or equivalent for several weeks or months is most likely to experience a withdrawal reaction [18].

The sedative-hypnotic withdrawal symptoms can be classified as minor or major (Table 3). The minor symptoms of withdrawal appear approximately 8–36 h after the last dose of short- to intermediate-acting barbiturate, reaching a peak at 40 h and declining gradually thereafter over 2–15 days. These symptoms, in approximate order of appearance, include anxiety, involuntary twitching of muscles, coarse intention tremors of hands and fingers, progressive weakness, dizziness, distortion of visual perception, nausea and vomiting, insomnia, weight loss, and postural hypotension. There is also a rebound increase of REM sleep and paroxysmal EEG abnormalities. Purposive behavior (drug seeking and pleading) peaks during the second and third day of abstinence from short-acting barbiturates and meprobamate. Withdrawal symptoms with longer-acting barbiturates (and longer-acting benzodiazepines) appear on the second to third day, and peak more slowly and may last 10 days to several weeks.

Individuals withdrawing from 800 mg/day (or more) of secobarbital or pentobarbital taken for 40 days (or more) usually develop psychosis, convulsions, and/or delirum [19]. The delirium resembles alcoholic delirium tremens and is characterized by agitation, delusions, and hallucinations (visual and auditory). Symptoms invariably appear within a day of abstinence. Seizures are usually of the clonic-tonic grand mal type. They generally do not appear until the second or third day. They are often multiple, unlike alcohol withdrawal; most patients do not convulse more than 2–3 days. The psychosis, if it develops, starts on the third to the eighth day and may last as long as 2 weeks. The temporal onset and duration of the major symptoms and signs of withdrawal is earlier and shorter, respectively, with shorter-acting barbiturates compared to longer-acting barbiturates. Agitation and hyperthermia can cause exhaustion, cardiovascular collapse, and death. Hyperpyrexia is an ominous sign. The patient later develops a prolonged sleep, following which the withdrawal syndrome may clear up, treated or untreated, usually by the eighth day. Chronic hallucinosis may ensue.

Babies born to mothers physically dependent on general CNS depressants, including barbiturates and benzodiazepines, manifest a withdrawal syndrome of varying intensity, which is similar in manifestation to the opioid withdrawal syndrome of the newborn. Infants born to mothers dependent on phenobarbital develop barbiturate withdrawal signs approximately 7 days after birth, which peaks at 2–6 weeks of age, and lasts for approximately 2–4 months.

XI. TREATMENT OF WITHDRAWAL

The main goals of treatment are the relief of subjective symptoms, the prevention or treatment of the more serious complications, with minimal risk of direct drug-induced toxicity or introducing dependence on a new drug, and to prepare for long-term rehabilitation. Abstinence is the primary goal of treatment [20].

The type of detoxification recommended is determined by the patient's medical condition

Table 3 Sedative-Hypnotic Withdrawal Symptoms and Signs

Minor Withdrawal Symptoms and Signs
  Insomnia
  Anxiety, restlessness, nervousness, apprehension
  Depression
  Feel tired, weak, or worn out, exhaustion
  Tremors, tremulousness, muscle twitching
  Tachycardia, palpitation, postural hypotension
  Increased temperature
  Dizziness, distortion of visual perception
  Dysphagia, nausea, vomiting, increased appetite, abdominal cramps
  Agitation
  Chills, tearing, yawning, excessive sweating, runny nose
  Frequent urination
  Numbness of extremities, hyperactive reflexes
  Distortion of visual perception
Major Withdrawal Symptoms and Signs
  Seizures, Status epilepticus
  Delirium, psychosis
  Hyperpyrexia, orthostasis
  Cardiovascular collapse, coma
  Death (due to cardiac or respiratory arrest, or aspiration of vomitus)

---

and his or her personal and social circumstances. To adequately deal with potentially sedative-hypnotic dependent patients, the clinician must be able to: (1) diagnose dependent patients by drug history, symptoms, and/or signs, (2) medically stabilize the patient who may be intoxicated or withdrawing from sedative-hypnotics, (3) administer a tolerance test, and if positive, (4) detoxify the patient [21].

1. The sedative-hypnotic–dependent patient may present overtly or covertly. In its overt form, the patient usually presents in the emergency room with symptoms and signs of withdrawal [22]. But the patient may present, covertly, hospitalized for medical, psychiatric, and/or surgical reasons, or as a polydrug abusers where one or more drug dependence may not be accounted for. Caution is urged in interpreting the difference between true withdrawal symptoms and signs and drug-seeking behavior.

2. Many patients are admitted in the middle of the day or at night, in which case tolerance testing is more conveniently begun the following day.

Hence, if a patient is alert and lucid with no signs of withdrawal or intoxication, 20 mg diazepam or 200 mg pentobarbital or 60 mg of phenobarbital p.o. h.s. may be given and the test begun the following morning. If the patient shows signs of intoxication when initially seen, no medication is necessary until the test dose the following morning. If the patient shows withdrawal signs when initially seen, 20 mg diazepam or 60 mg phenobarbital or 200 mg pentobarbital is given po q 2 hourly until the patient is asleep, and then no medication is given until the test dose the next morning. Patients are placed in a low-stimulus environment.

If appropriate and convenient, the patient may be tolerance tested on admission.

3. To perform a tolerance test, Pentobarbital, 200 mg p.o. or phenobarbital, 60 mg p.o., or diazepam, 20 mg p.o., is given to clinically unintoxicated patients, who have been fasted for 2 h to assess the degree of tolerance (Table 4). Two hours following the test dose, if the patient shows signs of intoxication (sleep, dysarthria, ataxia, and a positive Romberg sign),

Table 4 Pentobarbital Challenge Test: Clinical response to 200 mg Oral Test Dose of Pentobarbital

Patients' Condition 2 h After Test Dose	Intoxication (to test dose)	Degree of tolerance	Estimated 24 h Pentobarbital/Phenobarbital Requirement
Asleep, arousable	+ + + +	0/+ (None/Minimal)	None
Drowsy, slurred speech, ataxia	+ + +	+ + (Mild)	400–600 mg/120–180 mg
Comfortable, fine lateral nystagmus	+ +	+ + + + (Marked)	600–1000 mg/180–300 mg
No signs of drug effect, abstinence signs may persist	+	+ + + + + + (Extreme)	1000–1200 mg/300–360 mg

he or she is considered nontolerant and no further medication is needed. If alert, the patient is given additional doses of pentobarbital, 200 mg, or diazepam, 20 mg p.o. q 2 hourly, until he or she exhibits signs of intoxication 2 h after the test dose. The maximum cumulative dose should not exceed 1000 mg of pentobarbital or 100 mg of diazepam. Patients who are intoxicated with one or two doses (< 400 mg pentobarbital or < 40 mg diazepam) are considered nontolerant and require no further medication [23].

Diazepam is preferred by some over pentobarbital because of the greater precision and fewer potential adverse effects at higher doses (e.g., respiratory depression).

4. If the tolerance test is positive, the patient is withdrawn from the sedative-hypnotic with phenobarbital or diazepam. Barbiturates or benzodiazepines (diazepam) can be used interchangeably in treating patients with sedative-hypnotic dependence [24]. The initial daily requirement of phenobarbital is determined by substituting 30 mg of phenobarbital for every 100 mg of pentobarbital administered during the tolerance test.

When the patient has been stabilized on phenobarbital for 48–72 h, a 10%/day dosage reduction schedule is begun. A divided dosage schedule (q.i.d.) is utilized. Doses are held if the patient is sedated excessively until the intoxication subsides and the next dose is adjusted downward. Phenobarbital has a long duration of action; hence excessive sedation may not develop until the second or third day. Patients who develop acute signs of withdrawal (anxiety, tremors, abdominal cramps, increased pulse, agitation, insomnia, orthostasis, hyperthermia) are given 100–200 mg of pentobarbital intramuscularly immediately. This dose can be repeated every hour until signs of withdrawal cease and substitution with oral phenobarbital can be restarted, adjusted at a higher dose, and/or with slower decrements.

For short-acting drugs, 7–10 days is usually sufficient, whereas 2 weeks may be necessary for detoxification for intermediate or long-acting drugs. Patients who are abusing very high doses of a sedative-hypnotic and/or for a long duration (months–years) are withdrawn slowly, occasionally even requiring several weeks (Table 5).

Phenobarbital is preferred to pentobarbital in sedative-hypnotic detoxification because of its rapid absorption, slower elimination rate, longer half-life ($t_{1/2}$ = 80–100 h), smaller fluctuations in serum concentration, lesser potential for abuse (and drug-seeking behavior), larger therapeutic window, more effective anticonvulsant property, and more precision in estimating (and treating) the actual extent of drug abuse.

A continuous intravenous thiopental infusion is an efficacious and safe technique for managing the concomitant problems of drug withdrawal syndrome and a critical illness requiring sedation and mechanical support of ventilation [25].

Table 5 Dose Conversions[a] for Sedative-Hypnotic Drugs Equivalent to Pentobarbital 200 mg/Phenobarbital 60 mg/Diazepam 20 mg

Drug	Dose (mg)
Barbiturates	
amobarbital	200
butabarbital	200
butabarbital (in fiorinal)	200
pentobarbital	200
phenobarbital	60
secobarbital	200
Glycerol	
meprobamate	800
Piperidinedime	
glutethimide	500
Quinazolines	
methaqualone	600
Benzodiazepines	
alprazolam	2
chlordiazepoxide	50
clonazepam	8
clorazepate	30
diazepam	20
flurazepam	30
halazepam	80
lorazepam	4
oxazepam	20
parazepam	20
tenazepam	30

[a]For patients receiving multiple drugs, each drug should be converted to its diazepam or pentobarbital equivalent.

Two approaches are described to treat the neonatal barbiturate withdrawal syndrome [26]. With both approaches the initial dose and all subsequent doses are determined by the severity of symptoms using an abstinence scoring system. The titration approach provides the infant with a total dose of phenobarbital 6–12 mg/kgm body weight/day given in divided doses at 8-hr intervals. The loading dose approach provides the infant with an initial dose of phenobarbital, 20 mg/kgm body weight, followed by maintenance doses sufficient to control the symptoms. Both approaches are effective, but the loading dose method provides more rapid and efficient control.

Patients who are addicted to both sedatives and narcotics need stabilization on both types of drugs before detoxification can occur. Withdrawal of sedative-hypnotics should be accomplished while maintaining the patient on a steady dose of a narcotic (usually methadone). A chronic opiate addict may need transfer to a methadone maintenance program after sedative-hypnotic detoxification.

Patients who are abusing sedative-hypnotics intermittently and who have a reasonable stable living structure can often be treated successfully in an outpatient setting. If the addictive use continues, the patient should be transferred to an inpatient setting for detoxification.

XII. PHARMACOKINETICS

A. Routes of Administration and Absorption

The barbiturates are usually taken orally for hypnotic use, but intravenously for convulsive emergencies or for general anesthesia. The rectal route is used occasionally in infants. Intramuscular injection is avoided because the alkalinity of soluble preparations causes pain and necrosis at the site of injection.

Absorption takes place mainly from the intestine, despite the favorable pH partition in the stomach. Food in the stomach decreases the rate of absorption. The sodium salts are more rapidly absorbed than the free acids because of rapid dissolution.

B. Distribution

Barbiturates are bound to plasma albumin to various extents. Lipid solubility is the primary determinant of this binding; thus about 80% of thiopental is bound compared to only about 5% of barbital. Weak acids can displace barbiturates from albumin. The cerebrospinal fluid (CSF) concentration of drug equals that of unbound barbiturates in plasma.

Highly lipid-soluble barbiturate (thiopental) are rapidly taken by the most vascular areas of the brain such as gray matter (peak within 30 s) and then redistributed into the less vascular areas of the brain and other tissues, which accounts for its ultrashort duration of action. The highly vascular kidney, liver, and heart equilibrate almost as fast as does the brain. The less lipid-soluble oxybarbiturates equilibrate much more slowly, since their uptake is limited by permeability more so than by flow. When the equilibrium is in the direction of the blood compartment, the drug is slowly released back to the blood from tissue storage.

Barbiturates also distribute easily to fetal blood where concentrations approach close to maternal plasma levels.

C. Elimination

The highly lipid-soluble barbiturates are albumin bound, which prevents their excretion by the kidneys and increases their reabsorption by the renal tubules. The barbiturates are transferred by oxidation of radicals at C5 to alcohols, ketones, phenols, or carboxylic acids, which are excreted as such or as glucuronic acid conjugates. Other biotransformations include N-hydroxylation, N-dealkylation of N-alkylbarbiturates to active metabolites, desulfuration of thiobarbiturates to oxybarbiturate, and opening of the barbituric acid ring. Side chain oxidation is responsible for the termination of biological activity.

Barbiturates with low lipid-solubility are significantly excreted unchanged in the urine over a period of several days; e.g., almost 100% of aprobarbital and about 25% of phenobarbital. Alkalinization of the urine hastens excretion of these barbiturates.

Renal impairment retards barbiturate excretion and hepatic disease slows biotransformation of barbiturate, both of which can cause severe CNS and cardiovascular depression [27].

D. Drug Interactions

Barbiturates combined with other CNS depressants such as alcohol and antihistamines augment CNS depression. Isoniazid, methylphenidate, and MAO inhibitors also increase the CNS depressant effects.

Barbiturates induce hepatic microsomal enzymes which accelerates the metabolism and disappearance of corticosteroids, oral contraceptives, testosterone, oral anticoagulants, digoxin, beta-adrenergic antagonists (e.g., propranolol), doxycycline, griseofulvin, sulfadimethoxine, quinidine, phenytoin, and tricyclic antidepressants.

Neonates born to mothers taking phenobarbital may have coagulation deficits because of accelerated metabolism of vitamins D and K and deficiencies of coagulation factors II and VIII. Elderly patients on barbiturates are more prone to fractures because of low plasma calcium levels secondary to accelerated metabolism of vitamin D.

Barbiturates cause endocrine disturbances owing to the accelerated metabolism of endogenous steroid hormones. Barbiturates may facilitate periportal necrosis of the liver owing to increased hepatic generation of certain toxic metabolites.

Barbiturates competitively inhibit the metabolism of certain drugs such as tricyclic antidepressants. Barbiturates compete with, and displace, other weak acids such as thyroxine for binding to plasma albumin. Barbiturates also decrease absorption of griseofulvin and dicumarol [28].

XIII. SITES AND MECHANISMS OF ACTION ON THE CNS

Barbiturates act throughout the CNS, although with different potency in different regions [29]. The mesencephalic reticular activating system (RAS) is exquisitely sensitive to these drugs [30].

Nonanesthetic doses of barbiturates suppress polysynaptic responses preferentially. Inhibition is facilitated and facilitation is inhibited. The synaptic site of inhibition is either postsynaptic, as at cortical and cerebellar pyramidal cells, or presynaptic, as in the spinal cord. This inhibition occurs only at synapses where physiological inhibition is primarily GABA (gamma aminobutyric acid)-ergic and not monoaminergic [31].

Both hypnotic-anesthetic and anticonvulsant barbiturates potentiate GABA-induced increases in chloride ion conductance and reduce glutamate-induced depolarization at about the same concentrations. At higher concentrations, the barbiturates suppress calcium-dependent action potentials, reduce the calcium-dependent release of neurotransmitters, and enhance chloride ion conductance in the absence of GABA.

Although the capacity of the barbiturates to enhance GABA-ergic inhibition resembles that of benzodiazepines, barbiturates to not displace benzodiazepines from their binding sites. Instead they enhance such binding by increasing the affinity for benzodiazepines.

Barbiturates also enhance the binding of GABA and its agonist analogues to specific sites in neural membranes, which is dependent upon the presence of chloride or other anions that are known to permeate through the chloride channels, and they are competitively antagonized by picrotoxin.

Collectively, these findings suggest that a macromolecular complex composed of GABA-ergic receptors, chloride ionospheres, and binding sites for benzodiazepines may be the primary site of action for the CNS depressant barbiturates [32].

Barbiturates also disturb the membrane order of the cells on acute administration but, conversely, the membrane becomes increasingly ordered with chronic administration of the drug. The latter correlates with behavioral tolerance [33].

Barbiturates and dopamine (DA) antagonists both apparently decrease receptor sensitivity and inhibit DA reuptake presynaptically. The supersensitivity to DA antagonists induced by chronic administration of a DA antagonist can be potentiated by barbiturates. Barbiturates appear to block the arousal of postsynaptic DA receptors, though probably not those coupled to adenylate cyclase, and unlike neuroleptics, indirectly. The inhibitory effect of barbiturates on DA receptor arousal possibly accounts for some of the central depressant effects produced by these drugs. Central DA receptors may also play a role in barbiturate withdrawal but its role has not been definitely established [34].

Norepinephrine (NE) seems to play a more important role than DA uptake in the development of tolerance to barbiturates.

XIV. EFFECTS ON ORGAN SYSTEMS

A. Peripheral Nervous System

Barbiturates selectively depress transmission in autonomic ganglia and reduce nicotinic excitation by choline esters, which, in part, explains the hypotensive effect. Pupillary constriction may also occur.

B. Respiration

Barbiturates depress both the respiratory drive and the mechanisms responsible for the rhythmic character of respiration. Increasing toxic doses suppress the neurogenic drives, followed by the hypoxic, and finally the chemoreceptive drives. Toxic doses can cause prolonged hypoxia, leading to brain death.

C. Cardiovascular System

In therapeutic doses, barbiturates produce dose-related slight decrease in the blood pressure and in heart rate (intravenous more so than oral administration). Intravenous barbiturates may cause a decrease in cardiac output, a decrease in renal plasma flow, an increase in peripheral resistance, a decrease in cerebral blood flow, and a fall in CSF pressure. When the cardiovascular system is already compromised as a result of heart failure or hypokalemia, even small doses of sedative-hypnotics can precipitate cardiogenic and peripheral vascular shock. Toxic doses cause direct depression of cardiac contractility and smooth muscle in peripheral vasculature.

D. Gastrointestinal Tract

The oxybarbiturates decrease the tone of gastrointestinal musculature and the amplitude of its rhythmic contractions owing to its peripheral (and partly central) effect, causing constipation, functional paralytic ileus, and intestinal obstruction.

E. Hepatic System

Barbiturates combine with cytochrome P-450, and thus competitively interfere with the biotransformation of certain drugs and endogenous substrates (e.g., steroids).

Barbiturates also increase enzyme, protein, and lipid content of hepatic endoplasmic reticulum; hence inducing metabolism of a number of drugs and certain endogenous substrates, e.g., steroid hormones, bile salts, cholesterol, and vitamins K and D.

Barbiturates induce porphyrin and aminolevulinic acid (ALA) synthesis, which can cause dangerous exacerbations of porphyria in intermittent porphyria patients.

The effect of barbiturates that are themselves metabolized by hepatic endoplasmic reticulum to increase the rate of their own metabolism accounts for part of the tolerance to themselves and cross tolerance with similar drugs, including sedative-hypnotics, anesthetics, and alcohol.

F. Genitourinary Tract

Hypnotic doses do not affect the urinary bladder or ureter or uterus, but anesthetic doses may decrease the force and frequency of contractions and decrease tubular reabsorption, causing oliguria or even anuria.

XV. BARBITURATE POISONING

Ready availability and promiscuous use of barbiturates, and low therapeutic index, cause poisoning which may lead to death (0.5–12.0% of cases). Ingestion could be accidental (children) or deliberate (suicide, especially in drug abusers), or due to drug automatism.

The lethal dose of barbiturates varies multifactorially. Severe poisoning results from ingestion of 10 times the hypnotic dose within short periods of time. Barbiturates with short half-lives and high lipid solubility (amobarbital, secobarbital, and pentobarbital) are more toxic and lethal than the long-acting compounds (phenobarbital and barbital)—6–10 gm of phenobarbital (6 mg/dl plasma level) may prove fatal, whereas 2–3 gm of amo-, seco-, and pentobarbital (1 mg/dl plasma level) may cause death. Concurrent use of other CNS depressants, including alcohol and benzodiazepines, lowers the threshold for poisoning and death.

Barbiturate poisoning is expressed mainly via the CNS and cardiovascular system. Moderate intoxication resembles alcohol inebriation. In severe intoxication, the patient is ataxic, has Babinski's plantar reflex, and develops coma and loses deep tendon reflexes. Pupils may be constricted and react to light, but hypoxic paralytic dilatation may ensue. Breathing may be either slow or rapid and shallow with progression to Cheyne-Stokes rhythm. The blood pressure falls as a result of the central and peripheral (direct and indirect) effects of barbiturates. The patient may succumb to cardiovascular shock, respiratory failure, pulmonary complications, or secondary renal failure. The EEG may be of burst-suppression type with intermittent brief periods of electrical silence.

Appropriate treatment of acute barbiturate intoxication, which includes general supportive measures and the use of dialysis or hemoperfusion, in a sophisticated intensive care unit (without the need of cardiovascular system stimulants as antagonists) reduces the mortality to less than 2%. Gastric lavage or emesis is useful in the first 24 h, especially in the first 4 h. Activated charcoal may adsorb some residual barbiturate. A saline cathartic should be administered repeatedly if bowel sounds are present. A patient airway, artificial respiration, and oxygen assists respiration and prevents pulmonary complications. Dehydration and hypovolemia needs correction so also does hypotension. If the patient develops renal failure, hemodialysis (for long-acting barbiturates) or hemoperfusion (for short-acting, lipidsoluble barbiturates) is indicated, which eliminates the drug faster than by enteric medication.

XVI. THERAPEUTIC USES

Barbiturates and nonbarbiturate sedative-hypnotics are used often for transient or situational insomnia (acute stress, jet lag, acute work shift change) and for chronic insomnia [35].

The use of barbiturates as sedative-hypnotic drugs has declined because of the nonspecificity of its effect on the CNS, lower therapeutic index, rapid and more frequent development of tolerance, more drug interactions, and greater liability for abuse compared to benzodiazepines. However, phenobarbital and butabarbital are still used as "sedatives" in various inefficacious combinations for treatment of functional gastrointestinal disorders, urethral inflammation, hypertension, bronchial asthma, and coronary artery disease. They are combined with analgesic medications (although counterproductive) to treat migraine and other painful conditions. Barbiturates are used to treat the hyperactivity of hyperthyroidism. They may still have valid use as sedatives to decrease restlessness in children suffering from colic, whooping cough, pylorospasm, functional nausea and vomiting, to reduce apprehension prior to minor dental and medical procedures, and to reduce agitated behavior of various origins.

Barbiturates are also used occasionally to antagonize unwanted CNS-stimulant effects of various drugs (ephedrine, theophylline, and dextroamphetamine), for which use they may be superior to benzodiazepines.

Barbiturates are most commonly used as anticonvulsants for epilepsy (including status epilepticus), tetanus, eclampsia, cerebral hemorrhage, and convulsant drug poisonings, although benzodiazepines again are superior in this field. Barbiturates have been largely replaced by benzodiazepines even for preanesthesia medication and basal anesthesia except for certain short-acting and ultra–short-acting barbiturates used as intravenous anesthetics; e.g., for electroconvulsive therapy.

Barbiturates are used diagnostically and therapeutically in narcoanalysis and narcotherapy.

Anesthetic doses of barbiturates also reduce cerebral edema and infarct size (which improve chances of survival) and reduce intracranial hypertension. Phenobarbital (and even the nondepressant barbiturate phetharbital) is used to treat hyperbilirubinemia and kernicterus in the neonate, hemolytic jaundice, and selected cases of cholestasis. It has been used for certain neuromuscular disorders.

XVII. CONTRAINDICATIONS

Barbiturates and nonbarbiturate sedative-hypnotics are contraindicated in patients with primary or secondary sleep apnea. They are best avoided in persons abusing alcohol and/or other CNS depressants. They should not be given to pregnant women, especially in their first trimester owing to its possible teratogenic effects.

Barbiturates should not be used in patients with respiratory insufficiency or compromised cardiovascular state, including cardiac failure and hypovolemia. They are contraindicated in individuals who are hypersensitive to barbiturates and develop allergic reactions, and in patients with acute intermittent porphyria and porphyria variegata because barbiturates enhance porphyria synthesis. If indicated, barbiturates should be used with great caution in elderly patients, in patients with lung, kidney, or liver disease, in persons with drug abuse potential, or persons at suicide risk. Various adverse drug interactions should be considered before giving sedative-hypnotics to patients on other medications [36].

XVIII. NONBARBITURATE SEDATIVE-HYPNOTICS

A. Methaqualone

Methaqualone is a 2-methyl-3-o-tolyl-4(3H)-quinazolinone. It was first introduced in the United States in 1965, as Quaalude. It is a sedative-hypnotic which also has anticonvulsant, antispasmodic, local anesthetic, antihistaminic, and antitussive properties [37]. Although it has been withdrawn from the market, it remains available on the streets as "Mandrakes" (combined with diphenhydramine), "soaps," and "soapers" (taken with alcohol, especially wine). Methaqualone is referred to as "the love drug" or "heroin for lovers." This drug has acquired the street reputation of having aphrodisiac properties, which has increased its popularity in past 15–20 years. It is reported to increase libido, lower sexual inhibitions, and prolong sexual excitement. Methaqualone produces painless pleasant ataxia with feelings of indestructibility and euphoria.

Methaqualone is well absorbed orally in 2 h, highly bound to albumin, and metabolized to 4-hydroxyl methaqualone and the N' oxide. The pharmacokinetics are that of a two-compartment system, with a distribution half-life of less than 1 h and an elimination half-life of 10–40 h. Methaqualone does induce the hepatic microsomal enzymes. It is longer acting than secobarbital and chloral hydrate. The adverse effects include dry mouth, headache, incoordination, ataxia, dizziness, tremors, paresthesia, amnesia, depersonalization, vomiting, diarrhea, urticaria, epistaxis, menstrual disturbance, and hangover. The withdrawal syndrome consists of insomnia, headache, abdominal cramps, nausea, anxiety, irritability, nightmares, and hallucinations. It begins within 24 h and persists for 2–3 days.

Overdose of methaqualone may result in muscle spasms, hypertonia, delirium, convulsions, and even death, more so if combined with diphenhydramine. Coma and cardiovascular and respiratory depression are uncommon and are less severe than with barbiturates.

B. Meprobamate

Meprobamate (Miltown) was first introduced in 1954 as an antianxiety agent, but has been used even as a sedative-hypnotic drug, especially by older physicians. It is a bis-carbamate ester, which is well absorbed orally, with peak plasma levels in 1–3 h. Binding to plasma proteins is minimal. Eighty to ninety percent of the drug is metabolized in the liver, mainly to a side chain hydroxy derivative and a glucuronide, the remainder being excreted unchanged in the urine. Meprobamate can induce some hepatic microsomal enzymes. It suppresses polysynaptic pathways without affecting monosynaptic reflexes. This drug is more selective than barbiturates in its widespread CNS depressant effect; it does not cause general anesthesia. Meprobamate does not appear to affect GABA-ergic activity.

The unwanted effects of meprobamate include drowsiness, ataxia, incoordination, impairment in learning, prolongation of reaction time, mood disturbance, and allergic reactions, even at lower doses, corresponding to blood concentrations of 5–20 mg/ml. Higher doses (blood concentration of 30–100 mg/ml) result in vertigo, ataxia, slurred speech, seizures, stupor, or light coma. Overdoses (12–40 gm/day) (blood concentration of 100–200 mg/ml) can cause hypotension, shock, pulmonary edema, respiratory depression, cardiac failure, coma, and even death. Hemoperfusion is superior to hemodialysis in eliminating the drug. The withdrawal syndrome associated with meprobamate is characterized by insomnia, anxiety, tremors, nausea, vomiting, hallucinations, delusions, and generalized seizures [38].

C. Chloral Derivatives

The pharmacology and uses of the chloral derivatives (Notec, Triclos) that are used clinically are essentially the same because they are all converted in the body to the same active intermediate. The two compounds available in the United States are chloral hydrate and trichlofos sodium. Chloral is 2,2,2-trichloroacetaldehyde and trichlofos sodium is a monosodium salt of the phosphate ester of trichloroethanol, both of which break down to trichloroethanol. Chloral hydrate and trichloroethanol are lipid soluble, permitting its rapid distribution throughout the body. Triclofos is rapidly hydrolyzed to trichloroethanol and comparably distributed. Trichloroethanol is mainly conjugated with glucuronic acid and excreted as such, mostly into the urine. The plasma half-life of trichloroethanol ranges from 4 to 12 h.

Chloral hydrate and triclofos both cause gastrointestinal irritability. Chloral hydrate has a disagreeable taste, unlike triclofos. Chloral hydrate may cause paradoxical excitement in pain states. It cannot be used as a general anesthetic or as an anticonvulsant because of the narrow margin of safety.

In therapeutic doses, chloral hydrate can cause nausea, vomiting, flatulence, epigastric distress, dizziness, ataxia, nightmares, and hangover. Uncommonly, chloral hydrate causes idiosyncratic or allergic reactions, somnambulism, disorientation, and paranoia. Toxic doses produce hypotension, respiratory depression, and cardiac failure. Chloral hydrate and ethanol in combination (the so-called "Mickey Finn") are supraadditive.

The toxic oral dose is approximately 10 gm in healthy adults, although it varies between 4 to 30 gm. Chloral hydrate poisoning can cause gastric necrosis, pinpoint pupils, hepatic necrosis (icterus), and renal irritation (albuminuria). The withdrawal syndrome may consist of delirium and seizures. Death may ensue suddenly owing to a "break in tolerance," partly because of hepatic necrosis.

D. Ethchlorvynol

Ethchlorvynol (Placidyl) is a sedative-hypnotic which has anticonvulsant and muscle relaxant properties. It acts within 15–30 min, peak blood concentration being attained in 1.0–1.5 h. It has an intermediate duration of action and about the same therapeutic index as the barbiturates.

Ethchlorvynol causes a mintlike aftertaste, dizziness, nausea, vomiting, hypotension, facial numbness, vertigo, ataxia, and hangover. It may also cause profound hypnosis, weakness, syncope, nystagmus, or diplopia. An occasional patient may have an idiosyncratic reaction (e.g., excitement) or a hypersensitivity reaction. Ethchlorvynol can cause incoordination, tremors, ataxia, slurred speech, nystagmus, diplopia, toxic amblyopia, dichromatism, scotoma, and reversible peripheral or optic neuritis. Acute intoxication may manifest as hypothermia, hypotension, bullose, pulmonary edema, respiratory depression, and deep coma. The lethal dose usually ranges from 10 to 25 gm. Withdrawal symptoms resemble delirium tremens and a schizophrenic reaction, which are especially severe in elderly patients.

E. Glutethimide

Glutethimide is 3-ethyl-3-phenyl-2,6-piperidinedione. It induces hypnosis without sedative analgesic, antitussive, or anticonvulsant actions. It is absorbed erratically from the gastrointestinal tract. The drug is lipid soluble. About 50% of the drug is bound to plasma proteins. Almost all of glutethimide is metabolized in liver. The half-life of glutethimide ranges from 5 to 22 h, but may exceed 100 h after acute intoxication.

The untoward effects of glutethimide include hangover, excitement, gastric irritation, headache, blurred vision, and skin rashes. Patients on glutethimide tend to show a cyclic variation in the level of intoxication. The symptoms of acute intoxication include its antimuscarimic, anticholinergic effects (dry mouth, ileus, atony of bladder, mydriasis, and hyperpyrexia). It may cause muscle spasms, twitching, and even convulsions. The lethal dose of glutethimide is between 10 and 20 gm. Chronic use may cause osteomalacia. The withdrawal syndrome includes tremors, tachycardia, fever, tonic muscle spasms, and generalized convulsions.

F. Methprylon

Methprylon (Noludar) is 3,3-dimethyl-5-methyl-2,4-piperidinedione. About 97% of methprylon is metabolized. It stimulates hepatic microsomal enzymes. Its plasma half-life is about 4 h but it is longer in acute intoxication. It is best avoided in patients with intermittent porphyria.

Untoward effects, though infrequent, include "hangover," vomiting, epigastric distress, esophagitis, headache, rash, and idiosyncratic excitement. In acute intoxication, methprylon causes hypotension, shock and pulmonary edema, more so, than respiratory depression. The abstinence syndrome is similar to that of barbiturates and include insomnia, confusion, hallucinations and convulsions.

G. Paraldehyde

Paraldehyde is 2,4,6-trimethyl-5-trioxane, a polymer of acetaldehyde. It is a rapidly acting hypnotic with sleep ensuing in 10–15 min after a therapeutic oral dose. Oral paraldehyde is rapidly absorbed. About 75% of paraldehyde is metabolized in the liver, most of the remainder is exhaled. Paraldehyde is depolymerized to acetaldehyde in the liver and then oxidized by aldehyde dehydrogenase to acetic acid, which is ultimately metabolized to carbon dioxide and water. It readily crosses the placental barrier.

It has a strong aromatic odor and a disagreeable taste with associated burning sensation. Orally it is irritating to the throat and stomach; intramuscularly it may cause necrosis and nerve injury; intravenously it may cause cyanosis, cough, pulmonary edema, venous thrombosis, and hypotension. Paraldehyde poisoning may cause acidosis, bleeding gastritis, muscle irritation, azoturia, oliguria, albuminuria, toxic hepatitis and nephrosis, pulmonary hemorrhages and edema, and right ventricular dilatation, besides hallucinations, delusion, and cognitive impairment. Paraldehyde addiction resembles alcoholism and sudden withdrawal may result in delirium tremens and vivid hallucinations.

Paraldehyde has been used extensively in the past to treat alcohol withdrawal delirium tremens. It was also used to treat convulsions arising from tetanus, eclampsia, status epilepticus, and convulsive drug poisoning, and for other abstinence phenomena and psychiatric states characterized by excitement. It is administered preferably as a retention enema, especially in restrained and difficult to manage patients.

H. Ethinamate

Ethinamate is an urethane sedative-hypnotic which has a rapid onset and a short duration of action. It is inactivated by the liver, in part, by hydroxylation, and the resultant product is conjugated and excreted as the glucuronide. Side effects of ethinamate include nausea, vomiting, skin rash, and idiosyncratic excitement. It does cause tolerance and dependence. The withdrawal syndrome is similar to that for the barbiturates. Five hundred milligrams of ethinamate are possibly equivalent to 100 mg of secobarbital.

I. Etomidate

Abroad, etomidate (Amidate) is used as an intravenous anesthetic and also as a sedative-hypnotic drug in intensive care units during intermittent positive-pressure breathing and in epidural anesthesia. It lacks pulmonary and muscular depressant activity, but has a negative inotropic effect on the heart.

J. Clomethiazole

Clomethiazole has sedative, muscle relaxant, and anticonvulsant properties, and used abroad for hypnosis in elderly and institutionalized patients for preanesthetic sedation and for alcohol withdrawal. It has a high therapeutic index, but adverse interactions with alcohol are problematic.

K. Bromisoval

Bromisoval (2-bromo-3-methylbutyryl) is a urea belonging to the bromoureide class. It is debrominated during metabolism in the liver, and is excreted in the bile as glutathione conjugates and in the urine as metacapturates. Bromisoval produces barbituratelike sedative-hypnotic effects and dose-related drowsiness, confusion, and motor incoordination. Prolonged use may cause chronic bromism. Bromisoval causes a possible barbituratelike dependence, which is less severe than with barbiturates. It has a moderate likelihood of abuse and a low therapeutic usefulness. Bromisoval is marketed as a sedative-hypnotic only in a few countries [39].

L. Carbromide

Carbromide, 2-bromo-2-ethylbutyramide, is the primary metabolite of carbromal, which gives it the pharmacological properties of the bromoureide class of nonbarbiturate sedative-hypnotics. It is also debrominated during metabolism, but repeated use causes the symptoms and signs of chronic bromism. It also produces dose-related barbituratelike sedation-hypnosis and related CNS depressant effects. The likelihood of abuse of carbromide is moderate, but the dependence potential is similar to that seen with barbiturates. It has limited therapeutic usefulness; hence it is no longer marketed [39].

M. Nonprescription Sedative-Hypnotic Drugs

Despite the prominent sedative side effects encountered with the use of antihistamines for the treatment of allergic diseases, they have not been consistently effective in the treatment of sleep disorders, partly because of the inadequacy of the doses currently approved and the rapid development of tolerance. Hydroxyzine (Vistaril) antihistamines (10–100 mg tablets) are used as anxiolytic agents and for preoperative and postanesthesia sedation. Diphenhydramine (Benadryl) (25–100 mg) is a commonly used antihistamine for sedation. Promethazine (Phenergan) (25–100 mg) is a phenothiazine without antipsychotic properties marketed as an antihistamine with sedative properties. Pyrilamine maleate (e.g., Compoz) is also a common ingredient in many over-the-counter preparations. Doxylamine, phenyltoloxamine, pyrilamine, and other antihistamines cause significant hangover. They may have a longer than optimal duration of action, except for diphenhydramine which has a half-life of about 4 h.

N. L-Tryptophan

L-Tryptophan is a naturally occurring amino acid found in milk and other food items such as cookies. It used to be available in both drug stores and in health food stores as a dietary supplement either in the pure form or combined with other nutrients, but it has been banned in several states because of its serious adverse effects (unusual blood and muscle disorder) at doses (1–6 gm h.s.) recommended for insomnia.

XIX. SUICIDE AND SEDATIVE-HYPNOTIC DRUGS

Excluding advanced age and depression, alcohol and drugs are the largest risk factor for suicide [40]. Among drugs, abuse and addiction of stimulants (cocaine) and depressants (marijuana) may be more common, but sedative-hypnotics take a heavy toll because their effect on mood (e.g., depression) and cognition (e.g., impaired judgment, disinhibition) renders the user vulnerable and liable to suicidal thinking and action. Polydrug abusers are particularly more prone to suicide.

XX. MULTIPLE DRUG ADDICTION

Use of multiple sedatives is also very common owing to their widespread availability. Recognition of mixed sedative abuse can not only explain perplexing clinical findings, but also help in better overall clinical management. Mixed sedative abuse has a different prognostic significance than abuse of a single drug.

Concomitant use of alcohol and/or benzodiazepines and other sedative-hypnotics can potentiate the CNS depressant effect. Opioids and cannabinoids also have sedative properties, causing an additive CNS depressant effect when combined with a sedative-hypnotic: Almost all cocaine addicts have used marijuana and alcohol. Most marijuana users have used alcohol. About 50–75% of alcohol users and cocaine users have used sedative-hypnotics.

Most of these polydrug users are abusers and addicts and have developed significant tolerance and dependence.

XXI. LONG-TERM TREATMENT

After the detoxification process is completed, patients are referred to either long-term inpatient units or residential drug treatment programs (such as therapeutic communities) or day treatment programs (day hospital) or outpatient clinics, depending on the individual patient's needs. Patients with significant psychopathology tht antedates drug abuse are best treated in (dual diagnoses) psychiatric facilities with strong drug abuse treatment orientation. Provisions should be made for random and frequent urine testing.

Patients may benefit from professional psychotherapy or paraprofessional drug counseling (individual or group setting) and even comprehensive social services. Some select patients may benefit from psychotropic medications; e.g., tricyclic antidepressant for sedative-hypnotic abusers who are severely depressed following detoxification.

XXII. PROGNOSIS

Individuals dependent on sedative-hypnotics for decades are more prone to unnatural deaths (40%), including suicides (11%), serious somatic disease, cerebral trauma, (secondary) psychiatric illness, crime, maladaptive psychosocial functioning, and failure to be gainfully employed [41].

About two-thirds of sedative-hypnotic abusers continue to abuse alcohol or any substance. A pure sedative-hypnotic abuser tends to have a shorter duration of abuse than a polydrug (including alcohol) abuser [42].

Primary psychiatric illness prior to sedative-hypnotic abuse, concomitant alcohol abuse, familial alcohol or drug abuse, and health care access or occupation are poor prognostic indicators.

XXIII. PREVENTION

Patient education about the dangers of drugs and the benefits of health-promoting behaviors is useful. However, physician education can also play a significant role in sedative abuse prevention.

When confronted with a patient complaining of insomnia, a thorough behavioral analysis should be done to consider factors like scheduling of meals, exercise, caffeine or alcohol intake, sleep habits of the spouse, and age-related normal changes in sleep pattern, for which nonpharmacological approaches like environmental manipulation and/or relaxation exercises may help the patient. Underlying causes of insomnia or anxiety, such as a mood disorder (depression), panic disorder, or posttraumatic stress disorder, must be considered and appropriately treated. For example, heterocyclic antidepressants may be useful for select patients. If a sedative-hypnotic is absolutely indicated, it should be used as a temporary, short-term measure. Chronic, open-ended sedative-hypnotic therapy is best avoided. The choice of a particular sedative-hypnotic is also important; e.g., a slower-acting drug is preferred in patients with a known tendency toward overuse.

Denial, minimization, and rationalization about alcohol and drug use is shared by the addict and by those who care for and treat the addict, including family, friends, and health professionals.

REFERENCES

1. Allgulander, C. (1986). History and current state of sedative-hypnotic drug use and abuse. *Acta Psychiatr. Scand.*, *73*(5):465–478.

2. Hay, D., Milne, R.M., and Gilleard, C.T. (1986). Hypnotic drugs, old people and their habits: A general practice study. *Health Bull. (Edinb.)*, *44*(4):218–222.

3. Johnston, L.D., O'Malley, P.M., and Bachman, J.G. *Drugs and American High School Students 1975–1984.* Department of Health and Human Services Publication No. (ADM) 85-1394, U.S. Government Printing Office, Washington, D.C.

4. Miller, T.D., Cisin, I.H., Gardner-Keaton, H., Havrel, A.V., Wirtz, D.W., et al. *National Survey on Drug Abuse. Main Findings 1982.* Department of Health and Human Services No. (ADM) 83-1263, U.S. Government Printing Office, Washington, D.C.

5. Grant, B., and Harford, T. (1990). Concurrent and simultaneous use of alcohol with sedatives and with tranquilizers: Results of a national survey. National Institution on Alcohol Abuse and Alcoholism. *J. Subst. Abuse*, *2*:1–4.

6. Williams, P., Murray, J., and Clare, A.A. (1982). Longitudinal study of psychotropic drug prescription. *Psychol. Med.*, *12*:201–206.

7. Bush, P.J., Spector, K.K., and Rabin, D.L. (1984). Use of sedatives and hypnotics prescribed in a family practice. *South. Med. J.*, *77*(6):677–681.

8. Harvey, S.C. (1985). Hypnotics and sedatives, *The Pharmacological Basis of Therapeutics* (Goodman, Gilman, Rall, and Murad, eds.), Macmillan, New York, pp. 339–371.

9. Hartmann, E. (1976). Long-term administration of psychotropic drugs: Effects on human sleep, *Pharmacology of Sleep* (Williams and I. Karacan eds.), Wiley, New York, pp. 211–223.

10. Kales, A., and Kales, J. (1983). Sleep laboratory studies of hypnotic drugs: Efficacy and withdrawal effects. *J. Clin. Psychopharmacol.* *3*:140–150.

11. Fishman, R.H., and Yanai, J. (1983). Long lasting effects of early barbiturates on central nervous system and behavior. *Neurosci. Biobehav. Rev.*, *17*(1):19–28.

12. Bergman, H., Borg, S., Engelbrektson, K., and Vikander, B. (1989). Dependence on sedative-hypnotics: Neuropsychological impairment, field dependence and clinical course in a 5-year follow-up study. *Br. J. Addict.*, *84*:547–553.

13. Okamoto, M. (1984). Barbiturate tolerance and physical dependence: Contribution of pharmacological factors. *Natl. Inst. Drug Abuse Res. Monogr. Ser.*, *54*:333–347.

14. Okamoto, M., Rao, S., and Walewski, J.L. (1986). Effect of dosing frequency on the development of physical dependence and tolerance to pentobarbital. *J. Pharmacol. Exp. Ther.*, *238*(3):1004–1008.

15. Miller, N.S., Dackis, C.A., and Gold, M.S. (1987). The relationship of tolerance, dependence and addiction: A neurochemical approach. *J. Subst. Abuse Treat.*, *4*:197–207.

16. Ator, N.A., and Griffiths, R.R. (1987). Self-administration of barbiturates and benzodiazepines: A review. *Pharmacol. Biochem. Behav.*, *27*(2):391–398.

17. Allgulander, C. (1978). Dependence on sedative and hypnotic drugs. *Acta Psychiatr. Scand.* (Suppl.) *27C*:1–120.

18. Merz, W.A., and Ballmer, U. (1983). Symptoms of the barbiturate/benzodiazepines withdrawal syndrome in healthy volunteers: Standardized assessment by a newly developed self-rating scale. *J. Psychoactive Drugs*, *15*(1–2):71–84.

19. Gersema, L.M., Alexander, B., and Kunze, K.E. (1987). Major withdrawal symptoms after abrupt discontinuation of phenobarbital. *Clin. Pharm.*, *6*(5):420–422.

20. Sullivan, J.T., and Sellers, E.M. (1986). Treatment of the barbiturate abstinence syndrome. *Med. J. Aust.*, *3*:145(9):456–458.

21. Perry, D.J., and Alexander, B. (1986). Sedative/hypnotic dependence: Patient stabilization, tolerance testing, and withdrawal. *Drug. Intell. Clin. Pharm.*, *20*:532–537.

22. *Diagnostic Criteria from Diagnostic and Statistical Manual of Mental Disorders*, 3rd ed. (1987). American Psychiatric Association, Washington, D.C.

23. O'Brien, C.P., and Woody, G.E. (1986). Sedative-hypnotics and antianxiety agents (A. Frances and R. Hales, eds.). *Am. Psychiatr. Assoc. Ann. Rev.*, *5*:188–199.

24. James, R.T., and Dean, B.C. (1983). Reducing the risk: barbiturate substitution with a benzodiazepine. *Pharmatherapeutica, 3*(7):464–467.
25. Cilip, M., Chelluri, L., Jastremski, M., and Baily, R. (1986). Continuous intravenous infusion of sodium thiopental for managing drug withdrawal syndromes. *Resuscitation, 13*(4):243–248.
26. Finnegan, L.P., Michale, H., and Leifer, B. (1984). The use of phenobarbital in treating abstinence in newborns exposed in utero to psychoactive agents. *N.I.D.A. Res. Monogr., 49*:329.
27. Breimer, D.D. (1977). Clinical pharmacokinetics of hypnotics. *Clin. Pharmacokinet., 2*:93–109.
28. Cushman, P., Jr. (1986). Sedative drug interactions of clinical importance. *Recent Dev. Alcohol., 4*:61–83.
29. Nicoll, R.A. (1979). Differential postsynaptic effects of barbiturates on chemical transmission, *Neurobiology of Chemical Transmission* (M. Otsuka, and Z.W. Hall, eds.). Wiley, New York, pp. 267–278.
30. Ho, I.K., and Harris, R.A. (1981). Mechanism of action of barbiturates. *Ann. Rev. Pharmacol. Toxicol., 21*:83–111.
31. Richter, J.A., and Holman, J.R. (1982). Barbiturates: Their in vivo effects and potential biochemical mechanism. *Prog. Neurobiol., 18*:273–319.
32. Study, R.E., and Barker, J.H. (1981). Diazepam and (-)-pentobarbital: Fluctuation analysis reveals different mechanisms for potentiation of gamma amniobutyric acid responses in cultured central neurons. *Proc. Natl. Acad. Sci., 11*:7180–7184.
33. MacDonald, R.L., and McLean, M.J. (1982). Cellular bases of barbiturate and phenytoin anticonvulsant drug action. *Epilepsia, 23*(1):517–518.
34. Feigenbaum, J.J., and Yanaia, J. (1983). Evidence for involvement of central dopaminergic receptors in the acute and chronic effects induced by barbiturates. *Neuropsychobiology, 9*:(2–3):83–87.
35. Miller, N.S., and Gold, M.S. (1989). Sedative-hypnotics: Pharmacology and use. *J. Fam. Pract., 29*:(6):665–670.
36. *Sedative-Hypnotic Drugs: Risks and Benefits*. National Institute on Drug Abuse, Rockville, Maryland, 1977.
37. Ionescu-Poggia, M., Bird, M., Orzack, M.H., Benes, F., Beake, B. et al. (1988). Methaqualone. *Int. Clin. Psychopharmacol., 3*(2):97–109.
38. Roache, J.D., and Griffiths, R.R. (1987). Lorazepam and meprobamate dose effects in humans: Behavioral effects and abuse liability. *J. Pharmacol. Exp. Ther., 243*(3):978–988.
39. WHO expert committee on drug dependence (1989). Twenty-fifth Report. *WHO Tech. Rep. Ser., 775*:1–48.
40. Berger, F.M. (1967). Drugs and suicide in the United States. *Clin. Pharmacol. Ther., 8*:219–223.
41. Allgulander, C., Borg, S., and Vikander, B. (1984). A 4–6 year follow-up of 50 patients with primary dependence on sedative and hypnotic drugs. *Am. J. Psychiatry, 141*(12):1580–1582.
42. Allgulander, C., Ljungberg, L., and Fisher, L.D. (1987). Long-term prognosis in addiction on sedative and hypnotic drugs analyzed with the Cox regression model. *Acta Psychiatr. Scand., 75*(5):521–531.

28

Alcohol

Donna Yi
Cornell University Medical College, The New York Hospital-Cornell Medical Center, White Plains, New York

I. CHEMISTRY

Wine and spirits have long been valued by man as food and medicinal elixirs with curative, even life-giving powers. Historical references abound in literature, religion, and science about alcohol's effects and consequences, many of which have since been confirmed. The pharmacological effects of alcoholic beverages derive from their common active ingredient, ethanol or ethyl alcohol. A monohydroxylated, 2-carbon chain molecule, ethanol is an aliphatic hydrocarbon of low molecular weight (46.07) [1]. Given to hydrogen-bond formation, ethanol is quite polar and therefore extremely water soluble. With the increasing chain length of the higher weight alcohols, the nonpolar effects of the hydrocarbon chain predominate, leading to a tighter association between molecules by Van der Waals forces. This increases the boiling point and oil/water partition coefficient and decreases the degree of water solubility. Branched-chain alcohols, for example, the primary and tertiary alcohols, resemble the shorter chain structures in that their configuration allows greater hydrogen-bonding capacity [2].

II. ALCOHOLIC BEVERAGES

At room temperature, ethanol is a colorless liquid with a bitter taste and pungent aroma. It occurs as the main product of fermenting raw organic compounds, including grains (e.g., rice, corn, barley, rye, wheat), malt, potatoes, fruit, molasses, cane sugar, or honey with yeast. A by-product of this process is the release of CO_2 as bubbles when the sugars ferment. The distinctive flavor, smell, and appearance of each of the various beverages is then determined not only the ethanol content, but by the type and concentration of congeneric*

---

*The use of the term *congener* is employed here with the dual connotation of components other than ethyl alcohol that are inherently toxic and undesirable. For a more precise description of various constituents of alcoholic beverages see References 1 and 4.

substances. Congeners are present as additives or result as the by-products of preparation, fermentation (yielding 4–10% ethanol), distillation (which increases the ethanol content to 30–95%), or aging. They take the form of methanol, higher molecular weight alcohols also known as fusel oils, aldehydes, ketones, ethers, esters, organic acids, and salts, the high toxicity of each being offset by their presence in alcoholic drinks in appreciably small amounts. Congeneric content does seem to be responsible for the differential effects of beverages with the same ethanol concentration owing to their influence on rates of oxidation and competitive inhibition with ethanol for metabolic pathways [1,3,4].

Additionally, the presence of significant concentrations of toxic compounds different from congeners has been reported in alcoholic beverages. Until the 1960s, arsenic poisoning associated with pesticides used on grape plants was so prevalent it was considered an occupational disease among German wine growers or those ingesting contaminated homemade wines. Lead poisoning from consumption of "moonshine" or illicitly produced whiskey is well known. Hemochromatosis and siderosis can result from direct ingestion of iron in drinks and the indirect effects of altered absorption and metabolism of iron by alcohol. Cobalt toxicity leading to cardiomyopathy has been a consequence of exposure to a cobalt-containing foam stabilizer added to beer. Fluoride, added to wine as a preservative and to arrest fermentation, has been reported as the causative agent in cases of periostitis deformans. There has been increasing speculation about the role of ethanol as a cocarcinogen as well as the presence of alcohol-soluble nitrosaminelike substances in beverages such as Scotch whiskeys, South African spirits (Kachasu), and Japanese rice wines (aflatoxin) [1]. Alcohol has also been implicated less directly as a carcinogen because of its multiple contributions to cirrhosis, gastritis, malnutrition, and avitaminoses.

As a food, alcoholic drinks supply 7.1 cal/gm of ethanol. While small amounts of nutrients such as B vitamins, iron, and carbohydrates are present, alcohol is generally considered to be of no nutritional value.

III. ABSORPTION

Once ingested, absorption of alcohol across membranes takes place via simple diffusion. The most rapid rates of diffusion occur in the small intestine, duodenum, and jejunum; to a lesser degree in the stomach and colon; and only minimally in the mouth.

Rates of absorption are influenced by multiple factors. With increasing concentration, alcohol is absorbed more rapidly. In general, distilled solutions containing 30–50% of ethanol are absorbed more quickly than beer or wine which contain 3–5 and 12% ethanol, respectively. Likewise, as the concentration gradient across the mucosa decreases with more dilute solutions of alcohol, absorption slows. At concentration extremes, however, say less than 10% or greater than 30%, absorption is affected in other ways. Above concentrations of 30%, gastric emptying slows owing to mucosal irritation and the development of small sites of bleeding, inhibition of smooth muscle function, and pylorospasm. The result is slower gastric absorption and delayed entry of the stomach contents into the duodenum. Lower concentrations of 5–10% stimulate excess hydrochloric acid production and as a result delay absorption of water. Still lower concentrations are unable to cause intoxication because of rapid elimination due to water diuresis. Thus, the net absorption of ethanol depends on both the mucosal concentration gradient and the degree of gastric motility. This has been described as the biphasic effect on absorption by ethanol [2].

Volume and rate of consumption are also determinants of ethanol absorption. Ingestion of a constant volume of alcohol vs a constant percentage of ethanol tends to lower the overall effective ethanol concentration and, therefore, the blood alcohol curve. Ingestion of a constant ethanol dose gives rise to a higher total volume of fluid. This speeds gastric emptying and thus duodenal absorption. The rate at which alcohol is consumed will also influence absorption. The same amount of ethanol ingested in divided doses rather than a single dose will give significantly lower blood alcohol levels following each dose vs the one-time peak level reached when the same concentration is consumed all at once as a result of differences in absorption rates. Note, however, that both will be eliminated at the same rate and at the same time [5].

The presence of food will exert an effect on the amount of ethanol that enters the circulation. Dilution of ethanol, slowed passage of stomach contents, and a delayed rise and lower peak in blood alcohol level are the main results of ingesting food with alcohol. The type of food taken can affect absorption as well. Fatty foods tend to slow gastric passage, whereas large quantities of the same can induce nausea, accelerate gastric emptying and ethanol absorption. Milk effectively impedes absorption of alcohol. Interference with gastric motility can be caused by other substances and altered physiological states. Insulin, protein deficiency, hyperthermia, cholinergic drugs, and increased water load before alcohol intake all tend to accelerate rates of ethanol absorption. Stress, hypothermia, sympathomimetics, and anticholinergic agents decrease absorption. Magnesium sulfate, by inducing water retention, lessens the concentration gradient, whereas calcium exerts an inhibitory effect on smooth muscle contractility of the gastrointestinal (GI) tract. Acetylsalicylic acid and aminopyrine (Pyramidon) decrease absorption by inducing pylorospasm and irritation of the gastric mucosa [2].

While oral ingestion is the most common method of administration, alcohol can enter the system by other routes. Inhalation of ethanol vapors or aerosols leads to absorption across alveolar surfaces. In general, the extent to which this occurs is limited by the corrosive effects of ethanol on pulmonary surfaces though intoxication and death from inhalation has been reported.

The amount of ethanol absorbed from injection sites (e.g., subcutaneous, peritoneal) is infuenced by blood supply and absorption surface area available at the site, and is limited by the styptic and pain-provoking actions of locally applied ethanol. Aside from injection, alcohol absorption does not occur through intact skin.

IV. DISTRIBUTION

Following absorption, ethanol is distributed to all organ systems. Further diffusion continues across vessel walls and cell membranes. Depending upon concentration gradients between extracellular and intracellular fluid, tissue equilibration occurs and ethanol is dispersed in the total body water. The high water and low lipid solubility (partition coeficient = 0.1) leads to preferential accumulation of ethanol in those organs with the largest blood supply and tissue fluid volume. Rate of blood flow, vascular permeability, diffusion distances across vessel walls, and consequently total surface area available for exchange further influence equilibration. As might be expected arteriovenous differences in ethanol concentration, which are present until equilibration of the entire body, will disappear first from these tissues. If blood alcohol levels are sustained, the net gradient difference continues to drive ethanol into cells and as blood concentrations decline, the gradient difference falls and absorption slows. Other gradients exist between alveolar air and blood, and along the rostrocaudal axis (e.g., concentrations of ethanol in the ventricles are greater than those in the lumbar spine). Arteriovenous differences in concentration occurring prior to equilibration have led to questions regarding the validity of drug screens. In fact, venous blood samples yield falsely low ethanol concentrations favoring the defendant.

V. BLOOD ALCOHOL LEVELS/CURVE

Graphic representation of ethanol concentration differences accompanying absorption, distribution, and elimination can be seen in the blood alcohol curve. The slope of the ascending initial portion of the curve depends on ethanol concentration absorbed, which in turn reflects the type of alcohol ingested and the presence of food or drugs. For example, meals will slow absorption and give a more gradual, delayed rise in the absorption phase portion of the curve, whereas factors that decrease gastric emptying time increase blood flow and motility are represented by a steeper rise in the initial curve. A flattening of the curve follows the rise during which time absorption and elimination rates are equal. The curve then takes a downward course, reflecting metabolic removal exceeding absorption. Below blood alcohol levels of 10 mg/100 ml, decline proceeds at an exponentially greater rate. Sequestration of ethanol, as might occur with third spacing of fluids, can slow the rate of equilibration.

A quantitative description of the blood alcohol curve in an individual following a given dose of ethanol is provided by the Widmark equation (1932). Widmark's r coefficient represents the volume of distribution as a fraction of body weight [2,6]. In the average adult male Widmark's r is 0.7.

$$A = R + B$$

Where A is the total amount ingested, R the amount still present in the body at any later time, and B the amount that was metabolized or excreted up to that time.

$$R = C_t \times P \times r$$
$$\text{at time}_t$$

Where C_t is the concentration in the blood at time, t, and P is body weight in kilograms. r is then extrapolated back to time, t, when ingestion occurred.

Variations in r can occur with increases in adipose tissue which in turn decrease body water content, and thus the value of r. Further represented is Widmark's factor B in milligrams/ kilograms/hour as the slope of the descending portion of the curve. The rate of disappearance of ethanol from the body is represented by the equation $B \times p \times r$. B is also influenced by changes in body water and distribution, and there is a reciprocal relationship between B and r. Practical application of Widmark's formula lends itself to determining blood alcohol levels at a time after consumption of a known quantity as well as calculating the probable amount consumed if measurement of blood alcohol level at a known time after ingestion is taken [2]. Estimation of hepatic blood flow and total body water have also been derived from these equations.

VI. METABOLISM

Ninety to 98% of the alcohol that enters the body is predominantly broken down in the liver. Normal hepatic functioning is interrupted and metabolism of other substances ceases in favor of ethanol oxidation. A proportional relationship exists between the rate at which this occurs and the size and weight of the individual. With chronic alcohol ingestion, rates can increase by 30–100%. On the average, the body can metabolize 10 ml of alcohol/h, or 4 oz of whiskey, or 1.2 L of beer in 6 h. Amounts greater than this first-pass maximum will exceed the liver's metabolic capacity and contribute to increasing blood alcohol levels.

In the rate-limited first step of ethanol oxidation, H^+ is released from the alcohol and accepted by nicotinamide adenine dinucleotide (NAD) with the formation of the aldehyde and reduced nicotinamide adenine dinucleotide (NADH). The catalyst for this reaction is alcohol dehydrogenase (ADH), a stable, zinc-containing metallo-enzyme, MW 80,000–85,000, high in lysine and arginine content. Though most ADH stores occur in the liver (80–90%), it is found in extrahepatic GI tissues, lungs, kidneys, spleen, omentum, prostate, and brain. Located in the cytosol of cells, ADH has a wide range of substrate specificity. Further variability in metabolic rates is dependent upon an individual's isoenzyme composition (there are eight different isoenzymes known) and the presence of normal or atypical ADH. Atypical ADH, discovered in 85% of post-mortem livers in Japan, has three to five times the activity of normal ADH. More recently, its presence or absence appears to be unrelated to the flushing effect associated with acetaldehyde metabolism. Rather, these individuals may be lacking a different, low K_m isoenzyme.

Initially, ADH joins with the oxidized coenzyme NAD. Alcohol then attaches, forming a ternary complex. During this coupling alcohol conversion to acetaldehyde and hydrid transfer with reduction of NAD to NADH occur. Last, there is release of NADH and dissociation of the enzyme-substrate complex. The reoxidation of NADH and the formation of NAD in the mitochondrial compartment then follow. The strong affinity of NADH for ADH, limits this segment of the first step. However, NADH does not cross the mitochondrial membrane and oxidation is accomplished by coupling with reactions which employ substrates that do penetrate mitochondria. Such shuttle systems include the malate-aspartate cycle and to a lesser degree, the alpha-glycerophosphate and fatty acid oxidation cycles, all of which are capable of hydrogen ion transport. Hydrogen exchange occurs with oxaloacetic acid, catalyzed by malate dehydrogenase, in the cytosol fraction to form malate and regenerate NAD. Malate in turn crosses into the mitochondria where its conversion to oxaloacetic acid makes the latter available to continue reduction of NADH in the cytoplasm.

The first step could be made more efficient by "direct reoxidation" of the reduced complex. Glyceraldehyde, a fructose metabolite, is also a substrate of ADH and can oxidize NADH while it is still bound to the binary complex. Practical application of the enhancing capability of glyceraldehyde is limited by the large quantities of substrate necessary to effect this reaction. Also, stoichiometric amounts yield only a 20–30% increase in alcohol elimination rate, inadequate in a patient suffering from acute ethanol toxicity. Yet another mechanism would be required to handle the excess amounts of acetaldehyde produced.

Competitive inhibition of ADH between ethanol and the various congeners in alcoholic beverages has been employed therapeutically. Ethylene glycol poisoning, marked by renal failure secondary to deposition of calcium oxalate crystals produced by ADH action on ethylene glycol, has been successfully treated by administration of ethanol. Through competitive inhibition, this allows excretion of ethylene glycol in an unmetabolized state. Ethanol has also been employed as a competitive inhibitor in methanol intoxication. Methanol oxidation employs the ADH and catalase enzyme systems. Formaldehyde occurs as a product and is more toxic than methanol. As little methanol is oxidized by ADH, ethanol acts by competing for the catalase system.

While the availability of substrate is the limiting factor behind the first-step reaction, the balance of NAD to NADH exerts great influence. With accumulation of NADH, there is a shift toward excess H^+. To compensate for this, homeostatic shifts favoring reduced metabolites take place in the mitochondria with disruption of the Krebs cycle, increased fatty acid production, lactate production, and increased uric acid.

The interest in finding substrates that can interfere with ethanol metabolism, specifically dehydrogenase activity, and avert intoxication have led to investigations of ADH inhibitors. For example, chelating agents aimed at the zinc content of the enzyme, sulfonylureas which precipitate disulfiramlike reactions, long-term thyroid hormone administration leading to alteration in enzyme-protein synthesis, and fructose have been tried. In vitro use of metronidazole is noted to have augmentative and inhibitory effects on ethanol metabolism. Disulfiram acts as a metal chelator and also inactivates ADH by forming disulfide bonds with enzyme sulfhydryl groups.

The catalase oxidizing system, located in the peroxisomes, like ADH has a wide distribution, including hepatic and renal tissues nd erythrocytes. It is also capable of ethanol oxidation, but to a much less significant degree.

The microsomal ethanol oxidizing system (MEOS) of the endoplasmic reticulum (ER) is similar to the mixed function oxidase system for drug detoxification and reportedly is capable of oxidizing alcohols in normal and alcoholic livers.

Increases in smooth ER and of MEOS activity serve as adaptive mechanisms to chronic alcohol ingestion, utilizing O_2 and the coenzyme nicotinamide adenine dinucleotide phosphate (NADPH). Such induction has been seen in rats given ethanol long term. The extent to which ethanol is handled by MEOS is minor, greater significance being attributed to its role in the metabolism of other drugs and in ethanol-drug interactions.

Following conversion to acetaldehyde, further metabolism leads to acetate formation and entry of acetylcoenzyme A (acetyl-CoA) into the tricarboxylic acid (TCA) cycle, anaerobic and synthetic reactions (cholesterol and fatty acid synthesis). Fortunately, breakdown of acetaldehyde is rapid enough to forestall significant accumulation.

Acetaldehyde, like ethanol, is a colorless, toxic, volatile liquid. Its activity, potency, and lipid solubility exceed that of ethanol. In fact, some metabolic effects that occur during ethanol breakdown such as inhibition of aldehyde oxidation, inactivation of coenzyme A, interruption of mitochondrial oxidative phosphorylation, and hyperglycemia are attributable to acetaldehyde only. Of particular importance are the effects of acetaldehyde on catecholamine metabolism. Vasopressor action from acetylcholine (ACh)–stimulated release of catecholamine stores resulting in central nervous system (CNS) depression or activation at high or low ACh levels, respectively, are among these effects. Catecholamine metabolism is also redirected toward reductive rather than oxidative pathways. Consequently, this makes the biogenic amines available to react with ACh itself in a nonenzymatic fashion. The corresponding aldehydes then react to form products with opiatelike actions [6,7,8].

The similarities between the effects of ethanol and opiates and the cross reactivity with opiates are well known to clinicians. Monoamine oxidase (MAO)–mediated condensation of dopamine and its aldehyde yields tetrahydropapaveroline (THP), a substance employed in the investigation of the endorphin theory's applicability to alcoholism. Tetrahydroxy-papaveroline is a morphine precursor that binds to opiate receptors. When THP is injected into the third ventricle of rats, an increase in ethanol ingestion results. Infusion of THP and salsolinol has also been shown to increase ethanol ingestion, but amounts occurring in vivo seem to be of little clinical significance.

Condensation can also occur between acetaldehyde and the catecholamines to produce tetrahydroisoquinolines, which behave as false transmitters and have been sought as an explanation for alterations seen in chronic alcohol ingestion. This has not been borne out experimentally, however.

Acetaldehyde and dopamine condense to form salsolinol whose opiate actions augment those of morphine, particularly the analgesic effects, and is competitive with naloxone for opiate-binding sites.

Lyases have some involvement in alcohol metabolism, forming condensation products with acetaldehyde which enter into the pentose phosphate shunt and nucleic acid metabolic pathways.

Oxidation of ACh takes place primarily in the mitochondrial fraction via aldehyde dehydrogenase, aldehyde oxidase, and xanthine oxidase enzymes with acetate as the main conversion product. First-order kinetics prevail with rate being concentration dependent.

Aldehyde oxidase and xanthine oxidase are flavoproteins (containing flavin adenine dinucleotide [FAD]) with low affinity (K_m less than 1 mM) for ACh and a wide range of substrates so that they are minimally involved in ACh metabolism. A by-product of their action is H_2O_2, the deleterious effects of which are prevented by rapid metabolism involving the catalase enzyme.

The main pathway for aldehyde oxidation is conversion to acetate via dehydrogenase enzymes, the most important enzyme being the low K_m aldehyde dehydrogenase found in mitochondria. Dehydrogenases have also been isolated from other subcellular fractions, including the mitochondrial outer membrane, microsomes, and cytosomes. In the conversion from acetaldehyde to acetate, NAD is also used as a carrier for H^+ transfer. In the event that the capacity for acetaldehyde oxidation is exceeded, accumulation in the blood will occur, but because zero-order kinetics prevail, this concentration will remain constant.

The role of tetraethylthiuram disulfide (disulfiram, Antabuse) in the treatment of alcoholism is based on its ability to inhibit the actions of aldehyde dehydrogenase, aldehyde oxidase, and xanthine oxidase, leading to acetaldehyde accumulation. The zinc content of alcohol dehydrogenase, and the iron and molybdenum in aldehyde dehydrogenase are chelated by disulfiram. Disulfiram also interferes with catecholamine synthesis by chelating copper, a component of dopamine β-oxidase that converts dopamine to norepinephrine.

Disulfiram was originally used as an antioxidant in the manufacture of rubber and as an antihelminthic. Individuals who were exposed to it were noted to experience marked reactions upon consumption of alcohol. The disulfiram-alcohol reaction is characterized by facial flushing, injection of the sclerae, nausea, vomiting, dyspnea, hyperventilation, tachycardia, headache, and hypotension. Electrocardiographic changes include ST segment depression, flattening of r waves, and a decrease in left-sided predominance. Effectiveness of Antabuse treatment is not only dependent upon the patient's motivation, but on the reinforcing properties of this reaction on behavioral avoidance of alcohol. Acetaldehyde is not an endogenous substance, and in the absence of alcohol disulfiram is ingested without consequence. Though not proven, disulfiram has been suspected of causing side effects such as toxic psychosis, impotence, toxic hepatitis, and fetal malformations, particularly phocomelia.

Accumulation of acetate in the blood occurs as long as ethanol oxidation is taking place. Because of the H^+ overload that occurs, the TCA cycle is interrupted and, therefore, unable to clear excess acetate. Acetate is then handled by other tissues such as skeletal muscle. Acetyl-CoA which results is then routed to pathways for fatty acid, steroids, and ketone synthesis as well as CO_2 and water formation.

VII. EXCRETION

Depending on the amount consumed, 2–10% of ethanol is excreted unchanged in the urine and expired air with lesser amounts being excreted in sweat, saliva, and tears. None is excreted in the feces. The actual percentage excreted varies with consumption as metabolism follows first-order kinetics. Measurement of excreted ethanol has particular value in the forensic setting where it is used to determine blood ethanol levels. Urine provides a less accurate reflection of blood alcohol than does expired air, with the urine concentration of ethanol resulting from an accumulation of the various concentrations entering the bladder over a specific period of time. A more accurate means of calculating blood alcohol level is by breath analysis, the amount of alcohol in expired air being 1/2300 of that in the blood [3]. Results are less valid in the presence of significant lung disease or when residual alcohol is left in the mouth.

VIII. TOLERANCE AND DEPENDENCE

With chronic consumption of alcohol, tolerance, and dependence as manifested by the withdrawal syndrome, and organic brain syndrome occur. The need for increasing amounts of a drug in order to achieve the same degree of effect or a decrease in the effects brought on by a consistent dose define the multidimensional concept of tolerance. Tolerance represents adaptation of the body to the continuous presence of a drug such as alcohol. Target organs contain the receptor sites where adaptation occurs. Adaptation to alcohol primarily involves the brain. Alcohol brings about cellular changes that produce the behaviors and subjective experiences characteristic of intoxication. Adaptation then occurs to offset these effects and maintain homeostatis.

Dependence is manifested by a set of stereotypic, predictable signs and symptoms that constitute the withdrawal syndrome and occur upon cessation of the use of a drug. Dependence and withdrawal represent "deadaptation." Resuming use of the drug can suppress the withdrawal syndrome. The "hangover" is an example of the alcohol dependence syndrome.

Tolerance and dependence are on a continuum, with an increase in the degree of tolerance correlating with an increase in the severity of dependence.

Pharmacokinetic tolerance refers to the metabolic capacity of the individual to dispose of alcohol. This type of tolerance has innate hereditary and acquired components. Following ingestion of a single dose or chronic alcohol intake, acquired tolerance can take acute or chronic forms, respectively. While probably similar to acute tolerance, chronic tolerance is of greater capacity and takes longer to develop. The euphoric effects of alcohol seem to correlate with the degree of tolerance. However, with chronic consumption and aging, individuals can lose this capacity so that sedation without the euphoria may be achieved.

Pharmacodynamic tolerance refers to the effect of alcohol on receptor sites, specifically the cell membrane. Normally the cell membrane, composed of phospholipids and proteins, is aligned so that fatty acids are oriented toward the center. Alcohol causes more fluid movements of these portions and to resist this disruption, the cell membrane increases its intrinsic order. What results is a more rigid cell membrane as has been seen in the red blood cells of alcoholics.

Cross tolerance and competition are properties also attributed to ethanol. Individuals who are tolerant to the effects of alcohol will also be tolerant to effects of drugs that cross react or are cross tolerant with alcohol. Benzodiazepines and barbiturates are two classes of sedative hypnotics that are cross tolerant with alcohol. Thus, benzodiazepines are used in detoxification of alcohol withdrawal. They can also be used to suppress withdrawal signs and symptoms of barbiturate withdrawal. Competition between ethanol and acetaminophen for the same enzyme systems results in potentiation of the acute effects of both drugs.

With cessation of alcohol consumption, reversal, or deadaptation, takes place. This occurs more slowly than the development of dependence and results in central and autonomic hyperexcitability. Mild forms of alcohol withdrawal consist of fluctuations in mood, blood pressure, pulse, sleep, and appetite. The abstinence syndrome can mimic psychiatric illness, including mania, depression, anxiety disorders, and schizophrenia. Severe withdrawal, marked by hallucinations, confusion, and disorientation, may progress to seizures and death.

IX. CNS EFFECTS

Owing to its high solubility of water, ethanol perfuses quickly to the central nervous system. Its action on nervous tissue mimics those of other central depressants. Variability in expression of the acute intoxication state is related not only to the rate of increase in the blood alcohol level, hereditary predisposition and tolerance of the individual, but to the "set" (referring to the psychological state of mind) and "setting" (i.e., environmental influences). Effects are most marked with rising blood levels and lesser once equilibration is achieved.

By altering neuronal membrane permeability, ethanol interferes with transport and conduction systems. Reaction with lipid and protein components disrupts membranes, increasing their fluidity and changing ionic balance of sodium, potassium, and calcium. As a result, decreases in conduction and impulse propagation occur. Observations that sodium influx into neurons declines, that the actions of NA^+, K^+-activated adenosine triphosphatase (ATPase) are inhibited in response to ethanol and that calcium equilibrium is adversely affected by alcohol support the idea that neurophysiological rather than metabolic mechanisms are responsible.

Acute ethanol intoxication manifests with general disinhibition secondary to depression of the integrating and inhibitory functions of the cerebral cortex and reticular-activating system. With loss of inhibition comes increased confidence; slurred and loquacious speech, impaired insight, judgment, and memory; decreased concentration, altered motor skills, and sensory perception, and mood swings. Facial flushing, mydriatic pupils and nystagmus, increased heart rate and respiratory rate, hyperreflexia, and slowing of alpha waves of EEG are present [10]. At low doses stimulatory effects may be experienced, but with continued consumption and increasing levels depressant effects predominate including decreased reflexes and respiration, hypotension, and hypothermia. Progression to a stuporous state can ensue followed by coma and death. The margin between anesthetic (0.45–0.55 g%) and lethal (0.6–0.9 g%) is so small that it prohibits the use of ethanol as a surgical anesthetic agent.

Nervous system diseases in chronic alcoholics are varied. The most common impairments are related to compromised protein synthesis and malnutrition, of which Wernicke-Korsakoff syndrome is the most frequent. Deficiency of thiamine/B_1 is the main etiological factor and symptoms can include confusion, ataxia, ophthalmoplegia, and polyneuropathy [14]. Less common nervous system impairments are cerebellar and cortical degeneration, amblyopia, central pontine myelinosis, Marchiafava-Bignami disease, and pellagra, all of which have nutritional or vitamin-based origins.

X. GASTROINTESTINAL EFFECTS

Frequently substituted for food by many alcoholics, ethanol exerts effects on nutritional status directly and indirectly. By interfering with gastrointestinal functioning, alcohol causes direct injury to tissues and promotes malabsorption. Inhibition of esophageal peristalsis in the distal one-third portion and gastroesophageal sphincter spasm contribute to an increased incidence of reflux esophagitis and possibly cancer in alcoholics [15].

Consumption of ethanol in concentrations of 10% or less leads to reflex stimulation of gastric secretions with greater hydrocholoric acid and lowered pepsin content. Stimulation of gastrin release causes further secretions. Greater than 20% ethanol concentration inhibits gastric secretion and induces pyloric spasm with subsequent delay in the emptying of stomach contents. Still higher concentrations of alcohol, greater than 40%, damage mucosal surfaces by promoting back-diffusion of hydrogen ions, protein loss into the gastric lumen, inflammation, erosion, and hemorrhage. Not surprisingly then do alcoholics have increased rates of acute and chronic gastritis and gastrointestinal bleeding. They are also prone to traumatic tears at the gastroesophageal junction, the Mallory-Weiss syndrome [5,6,15,16].

More commonly, alcoholics have altered bowel function including constipation from a low-fiber diet or diarrhea secondary to gastric irritation.

Impaired absorption in the small intestine of various substances results from ethanol toxicity as well as malnutrition. Malabsorption and subsequent deficiencies in thiamine, folate, B_{12}, and vitamin A are not uncommon. Chronic alcoholic impairments also include alterations in intestinal motility and peristaltic waves.

XI. HEPATIC EFFECTS

The driving of ethanol oxidation toward formation of acetaldehyde generates hydrogen ions and an increase in the NADH/NAD ratio. The redox shift disrupts the Krebs cycle, leading to a rise in lactate/pyruvate ratio, lipogenesis, and decreased glycolysis and gluconeogenesis. Lymphatic outpouring of triglycerides, cholesterol, and phospholipids also occurs. Such altered lipid metabolism contributes to hyperlipemia and fatty infiltration of the liver. Protein deposits also form when their secretion from the liver slows and amino acids are diverted toward handling excess reduced equivalents. Increases in lipolysis and lipogenesis from peripheral sites have been observed in rats [6,11,16–18]. Fat deposition into hepatocytes gives rise to cellular swelling and displacement of cell organelles.

Over time organ damage including hepatomegaly, fatty liver, hepatitis, and cirrhosis occurs. Alcoholic fatty liver also stems from dietary fat deposition, hepatic lipid synthesis, and impaired ability of the liver to clear excess fat. Clinically, manifestations include hepatomegaly, which may or may not be tender, jaundice, and acholic stools. Laboratory evaluation reveals in most cases elevated SGOT, SGPT, GGTP, alkaline phosphatase, and bilirubin. These are usually reversible with cessation of drinking and restored nutrition. Subsequent progression to cirrhosis does not predictably follow. Biopsy and radionuclide liver scanning can provide further diagnostic evidence.

Alcoholic hepatitis, a more severe state of ethanol-induced injury, may present with right upper quadrant pain, fever, anorexia, jaundice, hepatomegaly, and ascites. Histological changes are characterized by polymorphonuclear leukocyte infiltration, steatosis, necrosis, sclerosis, cholestasis, and Mallory or hyaline inclusion bodies. Disruption of organelles, particularly the mitochondria and rough and smooth endoplasmic reticula occurs. To varying degrees, SGOT, SGPT, LDH, and prothrombin time are elevated.

Cirrhosis, occurring in 5–10% of older, chronic alcoholics, results in enlargement of the liver early in the course of the disease and later in a small, shrunken, hard, and fibrotic liver. Hepatocellular injury and impaired outflow from necrotic scarring and nodular regeneration in the lobular structure and portal vein lead to portal hypertension and the development of collateral circulation. Patients present with anorexia, weight loss, and fatigability. They may also complain of nausea, vomiting, hematemesis (in 15–25%), diarrhea or constipation, sexual dysfunction, and menstrual abnormalities. Examination reveals hepatosplenomegaly, or in advanced-stage cirrhosis, a small hardened liver, jaundice, ascites, edema, and pleural effusion. Palmar erythema, spider angiomata, and caput medusae might also be noted. As liver function becomes further compromised, patients may show evidence of demasculinization and feminization marked by body hair loss of the chest and axillae, gynecomastia, and muscle wasting. Dupuytren's contracture of the hands involving hyperplasia of the palmer fascia and nodular formation can also be found. Fever, infection, and peritonitis may arise as complications.

Hepatic dysfunction in cirrhotic patients is reflected in laboratory abnormalities, including liver functions tests as well as hypoalbuminemia and hypergammaglobulinemia, leukocytosis, anemia, and coagulopathy.

In later stages, complications such as ascites, variceal rupture or other GI bleeding, hepatorenal syndrome, hepatic encephalopathy, hepatic failure, coma, and death may occur.

XII. PANCREATIC INJURY

The pancreas also suffers from the effects of alcohol. Exocrine function is stimulated to release enzymes and "autodigestion" results. Ethanol also induces spasm of the sphincter of Oddi. With nutritional abnormalities, fat accumulation, avitaminoses, and iron and calcium deposition there is an overall state of inflammation [11,18–19]. Little agreement exists about the prevalence of pancreatitis in alcoholics, but a large percentage of patients with pancreatitis are alcoholic.

Acute pancreatitis occurs most commonly in males, 30–40 years of age, with a several year history of drinking. With continuing use, attacks increase in number and severity followed by long-term complications. Abdominal pain that may be referred to the back is common. Nausea, vomiting, diaphoresis, and fever may be present. In severe cases, tachycardia, jaundice, and peritonitis may develop and progress with rebound tenderness, guarding, diminished bowel sounds, and distention on physical examination. Prostration, hypotension, and frank shock may follow. Histological changes reveal evidence of interstitial edema, cellular infiltration, necrosis, and hemorrhage. Laboratory analysis can show leukocytosis, hyperglycemia, increased serum amylase, urinary amylase, glycosuria, and proteinuria. Other diagnostic studies such as x-ray, computed tomographic (CT) scan, magnetic resonance imaging (MRI), and ultrasound are helpful in demonstrating intestinal distention, pancreatic enlargement, and pseudocyst. Complications of acute pancreatitis can lead to the development of pulmonary edema, renal failure, pancreatic abscess, pseudocyst, and in 10% of cases, chronic pancreatitis.

Chronic relapsing pancreatitis is marked by necrosis, fibrosis, edema, cellular atrophy, and compensatory dilatation of pancreatic ducts. Obstructive mechanisms are responsible and include cellular infiltration and secretions, stenosis, and metaplasia. Here also, symptoms may include abdominal epigastric pain, nausea, vomiting, anorexia, steatorrhea, and paralytic ileus. Intestinal malabsorption of fat and protein with loss to stool occurs. Increased bilirubin, increased amylase, and calcifications visible on x-ray may be revealed. With recurrent attacks, damage to acinar cells causes insufficiency of the exocrine pancreas and subsequent permanent diabetes mellitus and hyperlipidemia.

XIII. CARDIOVASCULAR EFFECTS

Initial physiological effects of alcohol on the cardiovascular system cause elevation in blood pressure (20–30 mm Hg systolic and 10–20 mm Hg diastolic), and heart rate (10–30 beats/min), following acute administration. With metabolism and oxidation of ethanol, these effects are mediated by catecholamine-induced sympathetic response. These changes not only manifest during the acute intoxication state but with chronic drinking can persist and are also evident during withdrawal from alcohol. The elderly and those with preexisting hemodynamic abnormalities are particularly prone to these effects. With cessation of drinking these parameters normalize over time and frequently will require no further treatment. In the absence of alcohol, premorbid hypertension may be controlled sufficiently with lower doses of medication.

The direct and indirect effects of ethanol on multiple organ systems are compounded by effects exerted by the products of ethanol oxidation, acetaldehyde, and acetate. Peripheral vasodilatation and decreased vascular resistance result from inhibition of the vasomotor center and direct alcohol effects on vasculature. While this appears to be beneficial, ischemic changes are not prevented. Acetaldehyde promotes vasodilatation in the peripheral circulation and stimulates sympathetic response that lead to increased contractility and negative inotropic effects [5,8]. Acetate also causes vasodilatation, increased cardiac output, and positive inotropic effects, which may obscure the depressant actions of ethanol on the myocardium.

Thus, in noncompromised individuals cardiac function may seem to improve. Cerebral blood flow is not altered with low blood alcohol levels, but does increase in severe intoxication (300 mg/dl) in response to oxygen depletion. Lethal doses of ethanol depress respiration and cause cardiovascular collapse.

Alcohol can have multiple consequences on the heart. Disturbances in rhythm such as atrial fibrillation, atrial flutter, and ventricular tachycardia are common. "Holiday heart" syndrome refers to such disturbances following drinking binges.

Alcoholic cardiomyopathy, a disease of the myocardium, is attributed to the direct toxicity of ethanol. It is most common in the fifth decade of life in individuals with a 10-year history of heavy drinking. At a cellular level, respiration of myocardial cells and calcium uptake are inhibited while triglycerides accumulate. Clinically, complaints of shortness of breath are frequent along with other symptoms such as cough, ischemic-type chest pain, palpitations, fatigue, and anorexia. Signs of congestive heart failure, especially right-sided failure, hepatomegaly, and edema may be evident. Cardiac examination is notable for apical pulse displacement laterally, diminished S1, S3 and S4 gallop, ventricular arrhythmias, systolic murmur, and decreased carotid pulse. Electrocardiographic findings include arrhythmias of atrial and ventricular origin, conduction delays, Q waves, and decreased QRS voltage. Radiological evaluation shows evidence of symmetric, four-chamber cardiac enlargement. During end-stage disease there may be progression to pulmonary hypertension, low cardiac output and failure, and sudden death frequently from ventricular arrhythmias and ischemia. While progression can lead to death, abstinence from alcohol arrests the process, and if damage is not extensive, improvement occurs. Notably, cardiomyopathy is all too frequently overlooked as a consequence of alcoholism [5,11].

XIV. NUTRITIONAL DISTURBANCES

Ethanol-mediated metabolic disturbances, the frequent consumption of ethanol in lieu of food, and the lack of nutritive value of ethanol, contribute to the deficiencies in vitamins and minerals frequently seen in alcoholics. Malnutrition and its complications are a common cause of hospital admissions among alcoholics. For lack of funds, the desire to maximize ethanol effect, anorexia, or any number of other reasons, food intake in many alcoholics is significantly curtailed. Alcoholics reportedly substitute up to 50% of their caloric intake with alcohol.

Decreased appetite in alcoholics can stem from different causes. In large amounts, alcohol is anorexigenic. Esophagitis, gastritis, and ulcers also suppress appetite. Actual intake of food can be limited by painful mouth sores and glossitis secondary to deficiencies in vitamins C and B. Zinc deficiency impairs not only appetite, but taste as well [21–23].

A. Thiamine Deficiency

Thiamine, or vitamin B_1, deficiency can also result in anorexia. Thiamine-depleted diet, decreased absorption, and impaired activation of thiamine pyrophosphate may contribute to the thiamine-deficient state common in alcoholics. Decreased hepatic stores of thiamine can result from alcoholic liver damage. The Wernicke-Korsakoff syndrome is marked by encephalopathic changes such as confusion, stupor, memory impairment, ataxia, and ocular abnormalities, including ophthalmoplegia and nystagmus. Treated with replacement of thiamine, this syndrome occurs most frequently in patients 40–60 years of age. If the Wernicke-Korsakoff syndrome is left untreated, it can result in permanent brain damage and death. Necrosis and reactive glial infiltration are seen in the thalamus, specifically the dorsal medial nucleus; mammillary bodies, third nerve nucleus, periaqueductal gray, and the medial vestibular nuclei [13]. Lesions correspond to clinical impairments such as memory, nystagmus, and unsteadiness. Ataxia is associated with vermian atrophy. Thiamine deficiency is also an etiological factor in thiamine-responsive cardiomyopathy and beri-beri.

B. Niacin Deficiency

Lack of niacin contributes to the development of pellagra. It is marked by dermatitis, diarrhea, dementia, with progression to death, the 4Ds. Eating can become painful with the development of glossitis and angular stomatitis. Anorexia, nausea, vomiting, incontinence, diarrhea or constipation, weakness, and delirium may all result.

C. Folate Dificiency

Ethanol's role in deficient levels of folate may stem not only from decreased intake, but possibly from impaired storage, formation and release of circulating folate, decreased small intestine absorption, and an increased rate of excretion. A persistent folate deficient state is associated with peripheral neuropathy, malabsorption, and glossitis. Megaloblastic anemia with bone marrow changes in alcoholics is often due to folate deficiency and can be accompanied by macrocytic anemia, thrombocytopenia, and granulocytopenia. As folate content is higher in beer than other alcoholic beverages, these drinkers are less prone to megaloblastic changes than whiskey or wine drinkers.

D. Pyridoxine Hydrochloride Deficiency

Low levels pyridoxine hydrochloride, vitamin B_6, are associated with peripheral neuropathy and sideroblastic anemia. Alcohol interferes with amino acid transamination and decarboxylation, alters pyridoxal kinase activity, impairs activation of pyridoxine to pyridoxal phosphate, and increases degradation and clearance of pyridoxal phosphate. Acetaldehyde interferes with B_6 levels by displacing pyridoxal phosphate from binding sites and increasing its metabolism. Accelerated breakdown may be due to enhanced activity of pyridoxal–phosphate phosphatase. As liver damage progresses with chronic heavy drinking, these effects are compounded.

E. Hypervitaminosis C

Hypovitaminosis C in alcoholics can often be traced to inadequate intake of dietary sources. Scurvy can result with subperiosteal and gingival bleeding, poor wound healing, and hyperkeratosis.

F. Zinc Deficiency

The most frequently seen mineral deficiencies in alcoholics involve zinc and magnesium. Zinc deficiency affects multiple metabolic pathways that employ this trace element as a cofactor including nucleic acid metabolism, glycolysis, oxidative phosphorylation, and protein synthesis. In alcoholics, renal clearance and excretion of zinc are increased. Zinc is also required as a cofactor for vitamin A dehydrogenase. Lack of this enzyme causes impaired transformation of retinol to retinal, a substance involved in visual adaptation to the dark and when lacking causes night blindness. Other manifestations of zinc depletion are poor wound healing, decreased senses of taste and smell, hypogonadism, dermatitis, hypocalcemia, and hypokalemia.

G. Magnesium Deficiency

Magnesium levels too are adversely affected by poor nutrition and as organ damage takes hold, by renal hyperexcretion, malabsorption, and diarrhea. Deficiency is characterized by CNS and muscular irritability as evidenced by tremors, athetosis, arrhythmias, tetany, seizures, confusion, and hypertension. Magnesium is also an important cofactor and its absence affects enzyme function, particularly enzymes that catalyze phosphate transfer.

H. Deficiencies of Vitamins A, D, and K

Inadequate amounts of fat-soluble vitamins A, D, and K can accompany poor diet, malabsorption, and ethanol-induced organ damage. Loss of vitamin A occurs via decreased absorption, activation, and storage as well as increased metabolism and excretion. Dryness of the skin, hyperkeratosis, keratomalacia, and vision abnormalities, including night blindness, tunnel vision, and xerophthalmia may follow. Unavailability of retinal impairs steroidogenesis in the testes and contributes to hypogonadism. Aggressive treatment warrants caution as vitamin A can be hepatotoxic to the already compromised liver of an alcoholic.

Cirrhosis has particular impact on vitamin D metabolism. The first hydroxylation step toward vitamin D activation takes place in the liver and hepatocellular injury leads to depletion of 25-hydroxy-D3. This predisposes the individual to decreased bone density, osteonecrosis, and fractures. Stores of vitamin D can be compromised by inadequate intake, decreased ultraviolet light exposure, malabsorption related to pancreatic disease and steatorrhea, hypocalcemia, and loss of fat stores. Enhanced vitamin D breakdown may also contribute to deficient states.

Vitamin K depletion leads to defective coagulation from impaired microorganisms synthesis of this vitamin owing to alterations in intestinal flora, malabsorption, steatorrhea, and liver disease. Prothrombin time is prolonged and abnormalities in K-dependent coagulation factors VII, IX, and X occur.

I. Iron

Alcoholics are prone to excess rather than depletion of iron. Increased iron intake from alcoholic beverages (especially wine), increased absorption secondary to gastric acid secretion, pancreatic insufficiency, folate deficiency, and cirrhosis contribute to this. Iron deposition in tissues can lead to multiple organ damage similar to that occuring in hemocrhomatosis. Iron deficiency in alcoholics is often due to hemorrhage from GI bleeding or trauma, or infection.

J. Lipid Accumulation

Alcohol competes with fat and becomes the main energy source in the liver, slowing fat metabolism and causing lipid accumulation. Decreased metabolism and removal along with lipogenesis contribute to the rise in lipids. The decreased oxidative capacity, particularly as hepatocellular injury progresses, enhances this state. Limited secretory functioning of hepatocytes also occurs. Lipogenesis is promoted by the redox shift that comes with ethanol oxidation. Fatty deposition in the liver also has a stimulatory effect on lipoprotein secretion into the bloodstream and on lipogenesis. Alcohol effects on lipoproteins promote an increase in high-density, or alpha lipoproteins, and a decrease in low-density, or beta-lipoproteins [5]. The protective effect of this alcohol-stimulated high-density lipoprotein increase has been noted in several studies showing an inverse relationship between ethanol consumption and risk for coronary heart disease. In fact, the decrease in incidence in heart disease with greater alcohol intake persists even after matching and correction for factors such as smoking and age. However, restraint must be applied in recommending alcohol use therapeutically in such cases as it is also well established that negative consequences such as trauma, liver disease, and cardiac damage of regular drinking far outweigh these benefits [6].

XV. ENDOCRINE EFFECTS

Multiple endocrinological effects occur due to alcohol. Stimulation of the hypothalamic-pituitary-adrenal axis induces adrenocorticotropic hormone (ACTH) and cortisol production and with chronic drinking, a state resembling Cushing's syndrome can occur [5,11,23].

Induction of catecholamine secretions from the adrenal medulla and their altered breakdown favoring reductive rather than oxidative metabolites, with an increase in MHPG (3-methoxy-4-hydroxyphenylglycol) and decrease in VMA (3-methoxy-4-hydroxymandelic acid), is due to the redox shift that accompanies ethanol oxidation. Sympathetic catecholamine release results in a hyperaroused state as part of a stress response to alcohol.

Augmentation of production and decreased degradation are possible mechanisms responsible for increased insulin levels following appropriate stimuli in the presence of alcohol. Inhibition of gluconeogenesis by lessened availability and utilization of precursors (e.g., amino acids), acceleration of glycogen breakdown in the liver by catecholamines and adenyl cyclase, and hypoglycemia mark carbohydrate metabolism changes that occur with alcoholism. Alternately, alcohol can stimulate hyperglycemia from an increase in gluconeogenesis, though the mechanism by which this takes place in unknown. Ketosis from dehydration and malnutrition are not unexpected in alcoholic patients.

Hypothalamic-pituitary axis disruption interferes with the production of sex hormones. There is impaired sexual responsivity in both sexes and decreased levels of follicle-stimulating hormone (FSH), luteinizing hormone (LH), and testosterone. A hyperestrogenic state from the redirecting of androgen precursors, testosterone and androstenedione, to estrogen is seen in cirrhosis with subsequent feminization. This is marked by gynecomastia, proximal muscle wasting, and fat and hair redistribution. Demasculinization from hypoandrogenism further occurs in cirrhotic males as evidenced by decreased levels of testosterone, hypogonadism with testicular atrophy, loss of pubic and axillary hair, and sexual dysfunction. Effects on testosterone occur at multiple levels. Impaired gonadal synthesis of testosterone, decreased hepatic synthesis of testosterone, and increased testosterone inactivation contribute to low levels of the hormone. Additionally, loss of libido and impotence result not only from hormonal abnormalities, but from vascular and neuropathic changes. With chronic drinking, ethanol can cause local injury to the seminiferous tubules, germinal epithelium, and Leydig's cells. This adds to the depletion of testosterone and promotes spermatozoal abnormalities.

Effects on female sexual functioning include loss of libido, fertility and menstrual abnormalities, impaired lubrication, decreased vaginal pressure, and impaired orgasmic function.

Alterations in fluid balance and blood flow are also seen with ethanol intake. Acutely, ethanol induces vasodilatation and while blood alcohol levels are rising inhibits central release of vasopressin from the posterior pituitary, causing greater free-water clearance, less reabsorption, and a net diuresis.

Elsewhere as portal hypertension, cirrhosis, and decreased intravascular oncotic pressure develop, fluid shifts occur, resulting in ascites and edema. Activation of the renin-angiotensin system takes place increasing aldosterone production. Decreased hormone metabolism, venous stasis, and liver damage lead to hyperaldosteronism which further promotes sodium and fluid retention.

XVI. MUSCULOSKELETAL EFFECTS

As with other organ systems, there exists a spectrum of musculoskeletal effects due to alcohol. Decreased myocardial contractility and interruption of uterine contractions results from cardiac and smooth muscle inhibition. Transient enzymatic abnormalities without clinical signs or symptoms and progression to actual myopathic states presenting with pain and tenderness, inflammation, and necrosis of various muscle groups are all ethanol-related clinical syndromes. Tissue destruction can cause persistent laboratory abnormalities, myoglobinuria, renal failure, nerve damage, and electromyographic changes.

XVII. HEMATOLOGICAL EFFECTS

Hematological manifestations related to alcohol include depression of hematopoiesis; decreased survival, number, and functioning of cellular components; bone marrow changes; and impaired hemostasis. Alcohol interferes with pathways for iron metabolism and heme synthesis. Improvement and reversal are seen with cessation of alcohol intake [9,11,24]. Megaloblastic changes along with a loss of cellularity are seen in the bone marrow of alcoholics. Clinical megaloblastic anemia occurs in folate-depleted individuals. Peripheral blood smear changes also tend to arise in the nutritionally compromised; for example, those who are deficient in vitamin B_6 and folate. Further abnormalities include iron deposition and the appearance of ringed sideroblasts.

Anemia in alcoholism develops as a result of depressed hematopoiesis and decreased erythrocyte life span from splenic sequestration and hemorrhage. Changes in erythrocyte morphology can precipitate crises in patients with sickle cell trait or disease.

Likewise, leukocyte formation is depressed secondary to bone marrow suppression and actual cell functioning is impaired, thus contributing to a compromised immune status. Macrophage and lymphocyte functioning are impaired. Granulocyte migration to sites of injury and infection is impeded and with defective hemostasis further slows healing and immune processes. Decreased production of vitamin K–dependent coagulation factors and thrombocytopenia predispose alcoholics to hemorrhagic events, which in turn deplete platelet stores and increase the risk of trauma and complications frequent in alcoholics.

XVIII. CANCER AND TERATOGENIC EFFECTS

The potential carcinogenic and teratogenic effects of alcohol have been attributed to the congeneric substances in alcoholic beverages. While this is mostly speculative, there is greater evidence of an association between alcohol itself and cancer. Alcohol is associated with alimentary cancer and cancer of the respiratory tract, but its exact role or that of one of its metabolites is unknown. It may act alone or synergistically with factors such as smoking, avitaminoses, or preexisting illnesses. Alcoholics have high rates of smoking and in the presence of chronic ethanol exposure, the risk for cancer of the mouth, larynx, pharynx, and upper respiratory tract appears additionally increased. Most hepatomas occur in already cirrhotic livers, but variably so, and the question arises as to whether or not it is the direct damage from alcohol rather than cirrhosis that is the etiological factor.

Multiple abnormalities due to alcohol are seen in fetal alcohol syndrome. It has been reported that chronic heavy drinking during pregnancy is associated with increased rates of miscarriage and stillbirths. Ethanol affects organ system development and overall fetal growth and health. While there may be variation in reports of incidence and prevalence, multiple manifestations have been described including mental retardation, deformities of the cranium, face, heart, and limbs, and impaired resistance of infection.

REFERENCES

1. Lelbach, W.K. Organic pathology related to volume and pattern of alcohol use, *Research Advances in Alcohol and Drug Problems* Vol. 1. (R.J. Gibbins, Y. Israel, et al., eds.). New York, Wiley, 1974.

2. Kalant, H. Absorption, diffusion, distribution, and elimination of ethanol: Effects on biological membranes, *The Biology of Alcoholism*. Vol. 1: *Biochemistry* (B. Kissin and H. Begleiten, eds.). New York, Plenum Press, 1971.

3. Seixas, F.A. Alcohol, *Substance Abuse, Cliical Problems and Perspectives* (J.H. Lowinson, and P. Ruiz, eds.). Baltimore, Williams & Wilkins, 1981.

4. Leake, C.D., and Silverman, M. The chemistry of alcoholic beverages, *The Biology of Alcoholism*, Vol. 1: *Biochemistry* (B. Kissin and H. Begleiter, eds.). New York, Plenum Press, 1971.

5. Ritchie, J.M. The aliphatic alcohols, *The Pharmacologic Basis of Therapeutics* (A.G. Gilman and L.S. Goodman, eds.). New York, Macmillan, 1985.

6. Goldstein, D.B. *Pharmacology of Alcohol.* New York, Oxford University Press, 1983.

7. Von Wartburg, J.P. The metabolism of alcohol in normals and alcoholics: Enzymes, *The Biology of Alcoholism*, Vol. 1: *Biochemistry* (B. Kissin and H. Begleiter, eds.). New York, Plenum Press, 1971.

8. Lindros, K.O. Acetaldehyde—Its metabolism and role in the actions of alcohol, *Research Advances in Alcohol and Drug problems*, Vol. 4 (Y. Israel, F.B. Glaser, H. Kalant, et al., eds.). New York, PLenum Press, 1978.

9. Becker, C.E., and Morelli, H.F. Alcohol and drug abuse, *Clinical Pharmacology* (K.L. Melmon and H.F. Morelli, eds.). New York, Macmillan, 1978.

10. Eidelberg, E. Acute effects of ethanol and opiates on the nervous system, *Research Advances in Alcohol and Drug Problems*, Vol. 2 (Y. Israel, R.J. Gibbins, et al., eds.). New York, Wiley, 1975.

11. Lieber, C.S. *Medical Disorders of Alcoholism*, Vol. XXII. Philadelphia, Saunders, 1982.

12. Grenell, R.B. Effects of alcohol on the neuron, *The Biology of Alcoholism* Vol. 2: *Physiology and Behavior* (B. Kissin and H. Beleiter, eds.). New York, Plenum Press, 1971.

13. McEvoy, J.P. The chronic neuropsychiatric disorders associated with alcoholism, *Encyclopedic Handbook of Alcoholism* (E.M. Pattison and E. Kaufman, eds.). New York, Gardner Press, 1982.

14. Dreyfus, P.M. Diseases of the nervous system in chronic Alcoholics, *The Biology of Alcoholism*, Vol. 3: *Clinical Pathology* (B. Kissin and H. Begleiter, eds.). New York, Plenum Press, 1974.

15. Mezey, E. Effects of alcohol on the gastrointestinal tract, *Encyclopedic Handbook of Alcoholism* (E.M. Pattison and E. Kaufman, eds.). New York, Gardner Press, 1982.

16. Orber, S.H., et al. Diseases of the gastrointestinal tract, *The Biology of Alcoholism*, Vol. 3: *Clinical Pathology* (B. Kissin and H. Begleiter, eds.). New York, Plenum Press, 1974.

17. Feinman, L., and Lieber, C.S. Liver disease in alcoholism, *The Biology of Alcoholism*, Vol. 3: *Clinical Pathology* (B. Kissin and H. Begleiter, eds.). New York, Plenum Press, 1974.

18. Korsten, M.A., and Lieber, C.S. Liver and pancreas, *Encyclopedic Handbook of Alcoholism* (E.M. Pattison and E. Kaufman, eds.). New York, Gardner Press, 1982.

19. Pirola, R.C., and Lieber, C.S. Acute and chronic pancreatitis, *The Biology of Alcoholism*, Vol. 3: *Clinical Pathology* (B. Kissin and H. Begleiter, eds.). New York, Plenum Press, 1974.

20. Knott, D.H., and Beard, J.D. Changes in cardiovascular activity as a function of alcohol intake, *The Biology of Alcoholism*, Vol. 2: *Physiology and Behavior* (B. Kissin and H. Begleiter, eds.). New York, Plenum Press, 1971.

21. Feldman, E.B. Malnutrition in the alcoholic and related nutritional deficiencies, *Encyclopedic Handbook of Alcoholism* (E.M. Pattison and E. Kaufman, eds.). New York, Gardner Press, 1982.

22. Vitale, J.J., and Coffey, J. Alcohol and vitamin metabolism, *The Biology of Alcoholism*, Vol. 1: *Biochemistry* (B. Kissin and H. Beglieter, eds.). New York, Plenum Press, 1977.

23. Axelrod, D.R. Metabolic and endocrine aberrations in alcoholism, *The Biology of Alcoholism*, Vol. 3: *Clinical Pathology* (B. Kissin and H. Begleiter, eds.). New York, Plenum Press, 1974.

24. Chanarin, I. Effects of alcohol on the hematopoietic system, *Encyclopedic Handbook of Alcoholism* (E.M. Pattison and E. Kaufman, eds.). New York, Gardner Press, 1982.

25. Shuckit, M.A. *Drug and Alcohol Abuse. A Clinical Guide to Diagnosis and Treatment*, 3rd ed. New York, Plenum Medical Book, 1989.

29

Anabolic-Androgenic Steroids

Kirk J. Brower
University of Michigan School of Medicine and Alcohol Research Center, Ann Arbor, Michigan

I. INTRODUCTION

Anabolic-androgenic steroids (AASs) refer to the male sex hormone, testosterone, and its synthetic derivatives [1,2]. They are so-named because they have both tissue-building (anabolic) and masculinizing (androgenic) effects [3]. Anabolic-androgenic steroids are indicated and legitimately prescribed in the treatment of a few, uncommon medical conditions such as male hypogonadism, hereditary angioedema, some forms of anemia, and some forms of breast cancer [4].

Increasingly, AASs are sold illicitly for the nonmedical purposes of enhancing physical appearance or athletic performance [5,6]. Although these drugs are presumably taken for their physical effects, the psychological and social reinforcements for successful athletic competition and "looking good" also influence the decision to use AASs [7]. Moreover, numerous psychological effects, including addiction, and adverse physical effects have been associated with using AASs. Therefore, addiction professionals and other clinicians need to be knowledgeable about AASs.

A. Terminology

Anabolic-androgenic steroids are commonly referred to as *anabolic steroids*, or to be even more abbreviated, just as *steroids*. Still, the term *anabolic-androgenic steroid* is technically more correct for several reasons. First, all such compounds have both anabolic and androgenic effects, although any given compound may have a greater degree of either one effect or the other as determined by bioassay [4,8]. Second, illicit users typically combine multiple steroid drugs, some of which may be more anabolic and others more androgenic in their effects. Third, the term *steroid*, by itself, can also denote corticosteroids (such as cortisone, prednisone, and dexamethasone), which are pharmacologically distinct and have very different actions than the AASs. Indeed, steroid refers to a number of pharmacologically different compounds that either are synthesized in vivo from cholesterol or resemble cholesterol in their chemical structure. Nevertheless, for simplicity, steroid and anabolic-androgenic steroid will be used interchangeably for the remainder of this chapter. Common street names for the drugs include "roids" and "juice," although undoubtedly other terms either have been or will be employed.

Drugs that are taken to enhance athletic performance are called *ergogenic drugs*. "Doping" is another term used by the sports world (including the International Olympic Committee) to denote the use of substances for performance enhancement, with connotations of unethical use [9,10]. Anabolic-androgenic steroids are but one example of ergogenic drugs. Other examples are human growth hormone, stimulants, and beta blockers [5,10]. As discussed below, users of AASs typically combine multiple ergogenic as well as nonergogenic drugs.

B. History

Testosterone was first isolated and then synthesized in 1935 [8]. Soon after, the development of synthetic derivatives for therapeutic purposes was prompted *both* by the fact that testosterone itself was rapidly absorbed intramuscularly and quickly metabolized by the liver [2,4], *and* by the desire to create drugs that retained their anabolic effects while minimizing their androgenic effects [8,11]. The use of AASs for their performance-enhancing effects apparently began in the 1940s. Nazi troops were allegedly given AASs to increase their aggressiveness for combat [12], although this claim has been difficult to verify [13]. Bodybuilders also reportedly used AASs in the 1940s [14], although greater consensus exists that Olympic-caliber athletes started to use these drugs during competitions in the 1950s [12,15–17].

Because of widespread concerns of ergogenic drug use by Olympic athletes during the 1960s, drug testing was implemented at the 1968 Olympic Games for various nonsteroidal substances [10]. Not until 1976, however, after a radioimmunoassay technique was developed for processing large numbers of samples quickly, were AASs included in the Olympic drug testing program [18]. Eight positive tests for AASs were confirmed by gas chromatography–mass spectrometry at those games [18]. Anecdotal reports and testimony from former steroid users, however, suggest that 80–100% of competitors in certain events used AASs prior to testing or when testing was not conducted [3]. At the collegiate level, 15% of athletes reported using AASs when surveyed in 1970 [19]. By 1984, the same investigators reported a 20% rate of use.

Despite the nonmedical use of these drugs for approximately 40 years, AASs did not become a household word in this country until recently, when Ben Johnson, the world's fastest runner, tested positive for AASs at the 1988 Olympics [20]. In the same year, a study published in the medical literature received widespread media attention because it reported that 6.6% of male high school seniors in the United States had tried AASs, two-thirds of them before the age of 17 [21]. Over one-third of these students were not even involved in any school sports programs. This study made it clear that the use of AASs was (and is) no longer confined to elite athletes. Accordingly, parents, teachers, coaches, students, and community leaders, in addition to health care professionals, are concerned and need to be knowledgeable.

II. PHARMACOLOGY

The pharmacology of AASs has been reviewed elsewhere [2,4,22] and so only a brief discussion is warranted here. A wide array of AASs have been synthesized and marketed for either human or animal use. Examples of commonly abused AASs are listed in Table 1. The various AASs differ in terms of their chemical structure, route of administration (generally either oral or intramuscular), duration of therapeutic action (with therapeutic dosing ranging from daily to every 2–4 weeks), ease of monitoring in the blood or urine, relative androgenic and anabolic effects, and relative toxicity.

Table 1 Commonly Abused Anabolic-Androgenic Steroids

Generic name	Brand name[a]
Injectables[b]	
Testosterone cypionate[c]	Depo-Testosterone
	(Slang name: Depo-T)
Testosterone enanthate[c]	Delatestryl
Testosterone propionate[c]	Testex, Oreton propionate
Nandrolone decanoate	Deca-Durabolin
	(Slang names: Deca, Deca-D)
Nandrolone phenpropionate	Durabolin
Methenolone enanthate	Primobolan Depot
Bolasterone	Finaject 30[d]
Boldenone undecylenate	Equipoise[d]
Stanozolol	Winstrol V[d]
Oral Agents	
Ethylestrenol	Maxibolan
Fluoxymesterone	Halotestin
Methandrostenolone	Dianabol (Slang name: D-bol, D-ball)
Methenolone	Primobolan
Methyltestosterone	Android, Metandren, Oreton Methyl
Oxandrolone	Anavar
Oxymetholone	Adroyd, Anadrol-50
Oxymesterone	Oranabol
Stanozolol	Winstrol

[a]Representative trade names.
[b]Most injectables are used intramuscularly, although some (like Finaject 30) have been used subcutaneously.
[c]Testosterone esters; metabolized to, and excreted as, testosterone.
[d]Veterinary drugs taken by human steroid users.

Despite these differences, the AASs all share a similar mechanism of action. They bind specific androgen receptors in the cytoplasm of cells. After binding, the steroid-receptor complex diffuses into the nucleus of the cell, where it attaches to chromosomes and activates transcription of specific genes [22]. Cells containing androgen receptors are distributed throughout the brain and body, but are particularly concentrated in male reproductive organs. Androgen receptors in the brain may possibly mediate the psychological and addictive effects of AASs [23].

Testosterone has a four-ring chemical structure with 19 carbon atoms. Synthetic derivatives of testosterone are produced by modifying the structure in three general ways [2]: (1) forming an ester with the 17-beta-hydroxyl group, (2) adding an alkyl group to the 17-alpha-position, and (3) altering the structure at a site other than the 17-carbon position. Usually, esterification or alkylization at the 17-position is combined with altering the structure at a different site.

Most injectable AASs are designed to be released slowly from the injection vehicle, so that they can be administered every 2–4 weeks when used therapeutically. Thus, they are long-acting agents. The oral AASs are designed to be metabolized more slowly by the liver than testosterone, but still need to be administered daily. Thus, they are relatively short-acting agents.

Testosterone esters (testosterone propionate, testosterone enanthate, testosterone cypionate) are administered intramuscularly, released slowly into the circulation, and hydrolyzed to testosterone before becoming pharmacologically active. These agents are generally preferred for treating male hypogonadism, both because they are comparatively less toxic than the alkylated AASs and because therapeutic levels are easily monitored by plasma testosterone assays. When used therapeutically for treating male hypogonadism, a usual dose of testosterone enanthate or testosterone cypionate is 200 mg administered every 2 weeks [4,22]. By contrast, most of the alkylated AASs are effective when administered orally because the alkyl group impedes liver metabolism. However, the alkylated AASs are considered to be more toxic to the liver [2].

Steroid users who are subject to drug testing have generally switched to compounds that either are shorter-acting (those requiring daily administration) or have urinary metabolites that cannot be distinguished from endogenous testosterone (testosterone esters). Drugs like nandrolone decanoate (a long-acting injectable) now tend to be avoided by steroid users who are drug tested because its urinary metabolites are sometimes detectable for 6 months or longer, depending on dose, duration, individual metabolism, and body composition [18].

III. EPIDEMIOLOGY

A. Prevalence

Recent epidemiological studies have estimated that between 250,000 and 700,000 high school students in the United States have tried AASs [21,24], while some experts place the total number of steroid users at 1 million or more [20]. Other studies of high school students reveal prevalence rates for males to range between 4 and 11% and for females from 0.5 to 2.5% [14,25–27]. Even among nonusers, high school males were more likely than females to have heard about AASs, to believe they were effective performance aids, and to consider using them [28]. Among college athletes in this country, rates as high as 20% have been reported [19]. Studies of American weight lifters (including competitive bodybuilders and elite power lifters as well as "recreational lifters") reveal even higher rates of steroid use, ranging from 15 to 55% [29–31]. While these studies differ widely in their methodology, they consistently indicate that steroid use is most common in young, male weight lifters—whether lifting for sports training or other purposes [14,25,32].

Another indicator of increasing illicit steroid use is the growing black market. In 1989, the United States Department of Justice estimated that approximately $300–$400 million worth of these drugs were sold on the black market each year [25], whereas in 1988, a similar estimate by the Food and Drug Administration was $100 million [20]. Studies indicate that between 60 and 80% of nonmedical steroid users purchase their drugs from the black market [2,21].

B. User Types

Although only loosely based on research findings, a proposed model of user types can help clinicians understand the overt reasons for using AASs [29]. The three types of nonmedical steroid users are the athlete, the esthete, and the fighting elite. Certainly, there can be overlap between types.

The athlete seeks to enhance athletic performance. Steroid use is rationalized by the importance placed on winning and by the (sometimes correct) belief that competitors are also taking them. Rewards of use include the glory of victory and money (in the form of college scholarships and professional contracts).

Epidemiological research, however, indicates that steroid use is not confined to athletes. In two different studies of high school students, over one-fourth of steroid users cited appearance, *not* athletic performance, as their main reason for using steroids [21,26]. These are the esthetes who are motivated by having a beautiful body to display. Admiration is their reward. They include bodybuilders, aspiring models and actors, exotic dancers, and those who may seek to increase their perceived social desirability.

The fighting elite strive to enhance their fighting ability. They rationalize their steroid use by the Darwinian concept that only the fittest survive. This group includes soldiers, barroom bouncers, body guards, street gang members, and even policemen. They seek not only muscle size and strength, but also the psychophysiological effect of aggressiveness that has been attributed to using AASs [1].

In contrast to elite athletes, the "recreational athletes" and bodybuilders (including esthetes and fighters) may likely comprise the fastest-growing group of steroid users in this country at present [20]. These are individuals who are trying to play, look, and defend themselves better by getting bigger. They are easily found in America's gymnasiums and health clubs [6], the major sites of distribution for the black market steroids. In addition, they are not ordinarily subject to urine testing (with the possible exception of soldiers and policemen), and they have fewer disincentives to use AASs than the elite athletes, who can be barred from competition.

IV. PATTERNS AND CONSEQUENCES OF USE

A. Performance Enhancement

The scientific community remains divided regarding the efficacy of AASs for enhancing athletic performance. Some experts maintain that the efficacy of these agents has yet to be conclusively proven and may never be because of the difficulties in conducting both blind studies (due to side effects such as testicular atrophy) and studies that employ the high doses of illicit steroid users [2]. In 1977, the American College of Sports Medicine took the position that AASs do not increase muscle size, strength, or performance [33]. In 1984, however, the American College of Sports Medicine revised its position, stating that AASs could increase muscular strength in some individuals, when combined with a proper diet and high-intensity exercise [34]. Other reviews of the literature support the efficacy of the AASs to enhance body size and strength, but not to enhance aerobic performance [1,14]. Regardless of scientific opinion, athletes generally believe that AASs do work *both* to increase size, strength, endurance, and motivation *and* to decrease fatigue and recovery time between workouts. Until further studies are conducted, therefore, it is wise to assume that AASs are effective ergogenic drugs. This assumption facilitates credibility with users, particularly with those users presenting for intervention and treatment. Efficacy, however, does not guarantee safety, especially given the patterns of illicit steroid use.

B. Patterns of Use

Illicit AASs may contain either falsely labeled or veterinary preparations, for which the exact contents and human dose are unknown (see Table 1). Even so, steroid users typically consume between 10 and 100 times the therapeutic dosage [2,35]. To achieve these high doses, two or more steroids are usually taken in combination, a practice known as "stacking." Intramuscular and oral forms of steroids are also combined, and the sharing of needles among steroid users has resulted in reports of infection with HIV (the human immunodeficiency virus that causes AIDS) [36,37].

Nonmedical steroid users typically take AASs in a cyclic fashion, "cycling" on the drugs for a 4- to 18-week period during intensive training, and then stopping the drugs for a period of several weeks to several months [2]. The drugs are stopped both to give the body a pharmacological rest and in time to escape detection at a drug-tested competitive event. During a cycle of use, doses may be increased gradually and then tapered slowly over time in a "pyramid" fashion. When pyramidal dosing is combined with stacking several drugs together, the pattern of use is referred to as "stacking the pyramid" [30]. Cycling for some users does not consist of complete abstinence between cycles, but consists of a low maintenance dosage of AASs between periods of increased dosing [13]. This latter pattern of use may be consistent with pharmacological dependence, inasmuch as users do not completely stop taking AASs because of withdrawal symptoms.

Steroid users are frequently consumers of other drugs, each with their own risks, which are taken either to manage the side effects of steroids, to augment the body-building effects, or to mask the presence of drugs in the urine. For example, estrogen blockers (such as clomiphene or tamoxifen) are taken to prevent gynecomastia, diuretics are taken to eliminate fluid retention [38], human chorionic gonadotropin is taken both to prevent testicular atrophy and to stimulate the testes to produce more androgen [35,38,39], and human growth hormone is taken to increase muscle and body size [5,25]. Diuretics (by producing a dilute urine) and probenicid (by inhibiting the excretion of AASs into the urine) are taken to escape detection by urine testing, but are sometimes tested themselves [10,40]. Moreover, steroid users are not immune from using and developing problems and addictions with more familiar drugs of abuse such as alcohol, cocaine, and marijuana [35,41,42]. In a cross-sectional comparison of users and nonusers, Pope et al. [32] found that steroid users were more likely to use cigarettes, alcohol, and illicit drugs, although the small number of users in their study precluded statistical tests of significance. Another study reported that nearly one-third of a small, convenience sample of 41 steroid users had prior DSM-III-R diagnoses [43] of substance abuse or dependence with cocaine or marijuana [35]. Finally, a recent study found that nine of 20 steroid users were diagnosed with either alcohol abuse or dependence using a structured diagnostic instrument and DSM-III criteria [42]. Further investigation of dual addictions among larger samples of steroid users is needed.

C. Medical and Psychiatric Effects

As illicit sales and the nonmedical use of AASs increase, so do reports of associated morbidity and mortality [2,44]. Anabolic-androgenic steroids have been associated with heart attacks [45], strokes [46], liver disease [47,48], tumors and cancer [48–50], high blood pressure [51], an adverse cholesterol profile [51–53], fluid retention [44], altered immunity [54], and a variety of skin ailments [55]. Men may suffer from sterility, testicular atrophy, enlarged and painful breast tissue, an enlarged prostate gland that makes urinating difficult, and baldness [2,44]. Women can also develop sterility as well as menstrual irregularities and masculinizing features such as a deep voice, an increase in body hair, and an enlarged clitoris [2,44,56].

Psychological effects that have been associated with using AASs include depression [35], suicides [57], marked aggression and homicidal violence (so-called "roid rage") [41,58], mood swings [35,39,59], and psychosis [35,60,61]. Pope and Katz [35] administered a structured diagnostic instrument to a convenience sample of 41 steroid users and found psychotic disorders in 12% and affective disorders (depression or mania) in 22% of the sample. This finding requires confirmation in a larger sample using a control group of weight lifters who do not take AASs.

Adolescents and preadolescents may be particularly vulnerable to the effects of AASs both because they are susceptible to premature epiphyseal closure of their bones [62] and because they may lack the psychological maturity to cope with the sudden changes in mood and physique [39,62]. In addition, adolescence is a time when identity is normally achieved. For some adolescent steroid users, being big becomes their identity, which may adversely affect or delay further psychosocial development [29].

Some of the adverse health effects described above are reversible when steroids are stopped, but others are not. Moreover, some of these effects were reported in medically compromised individuals who were receiving AASs for therapeutic purposes, a group that is not comparable to illicit users of AASs [3]. Indeed, no well-controlled, longitudinal studies of adverse health effects have been conducted with nonmedical steroid users [63], and so the long-term dangers of these drugs are not fully known.

D. Addiction and Pharmacological Dependence

The potential for AASs to lead to both addiction (psychological dependence) and pharmacological (or physical) dependence has special significance. If the abuse of AASs was only a matter of a few individuals freely choosing to enhance their body's performance at their own risk, then the problem might have no more interest to the field of drug abuse than the "abuse" of laxatives to enhance bowel performance. By contrast, there is mounting evidence that AASs are psychoactive drugs, capable of producing addiction as well as reinforcing their own self-administration in part by euphorigenic properties [39,64–69].

The medical opinion that AASs can lead to addiction is a recent one [16,17,70], but not a unanimous one [71]; and evidence for this addiction hypothesis is only beginning to emerge [67]. There are now three case reports of addiction in the medical literature [39,66,68]. These reports documented addictive symptoms such as loss of control and continued use despite adverse consequences as well as pharmacological dependence (withdrawal symptoms and tolerance). Survey research has provided additional evidence of addiction. Yesalis et al. [69], in their survey of high school seniors, described a group of so-called "hard-core users," or heavy steroid users, who responded that they would not stop taking AASs even if it were proven beyond a doubt that AASs caused permanent sterility, liver cancer, or heart attacks. Roughly one-fourth of their sample of 226 steroid users endorsed this response. In other words, up to 25% of these users were willing to continue taking steroids despite adverse consequences, which is consistent with addiction. However, it is indirect evidence of addiction because the consequences were not necessarily or actually experienced.

Our group at the University of Michigan conducted a survey of weight lifters that focused specifically on addictive symptoms and pharmacological dependence with AASs [64,65]. In a pilot sample of 45 steroid users [65], at least one addictive symptom, as listed in DSM-III-R [43], was reported by 93% of the group. Three or more symptoms, consistent with a DSM-III-R diagnosis of dependence, were reported by 58%. More specifically, the following symptoms and their frequencies were: withdrawal (84%), tolerance (20%), continued use despite adverse consequences (47%), more steroids taken than intended (44%), unable to cut down or control use (20%). Thus, symptoms consistent with both psychological addiction and pharmacological dependence were reported. Moreover, one-third of subjects felt "high" on the AASs, suggesting that self-administration may be reinforced in part by euphoric effects.

Frequently reported withdrawal symptoms tended to be depressive in nature and included fatigue, depressed mood, restlessness, anorexia, insomnia, and decreased libido [64,65]. Craving was reported by nearly one-half of the sample, which was as frequently as any depressive symptom [65]. Pope and Katz [35] have reported that major depressions can occur during steroid withdrawal, and completed suicides have also been reported during this period [57]. Clinically, therefore, it is critical to monitor these symptoms.

Other authors have hypothesized that withdrawal from AASs follows a two-phase course [67]. The first phase is characterized by hyperadrenergic symptoms resembling opioid withdrawal [68], whereas the second phase is characterized by the depressive symptoms and craving just described. In the absence of further study, the durations of these phases can only be roughly estimated: phase 1 beginning within 1–2 days and lasting for about 1 week, and phase 2 beginning in the first week and lasting for several months [72]. If substantiated by future research, then phase-specific treatments should optimize outcome.

V. IDENTIFICATION AND ASSESSMENT

A. Clinical Assessment

Addiction professionals and other clinicians may see patients who are addicted to steroids, but miss the diagnosis because patients may deny or hide their use. Thus, the helping professional must be alert to the clinical manifestations of steroid abuse as listed in Tables 2–4. In addition, patients may complain of various subjective effects such as headaches, dizziness, nausea, musculoskeletal pains, urinary frequency, and menstrual irregularities [1,44]. In adolescents, behavioral and school problems may be pronounced, as with other types of drug abuse. In all age groups, sudden increases in body weight and disproportionate increases in muscular development, coupled with obsessive weight-lifting and training activity, should raise concerns. As with other forms of drug abuse, a comprehensive assessment will include a biopsychosocial history from the patient and his significant others as well as a physical, mental status, and laboratory examination.

B. Urine Testing

Identification of steroid use by urine testing involves both the search for synthetic steroids and their metabolites as well as the measurement of endogenous steroid levels and their ratios [18,73]. This two-step identification process is necessary because the commonly administered testosterone esters—such as testosterone cypionate and testosterone enanthate—are metabolized to and excreted as testosterone (Table 1). Thus, they cannot be distinguished from endogenous testosterone except for the hormonal imbalances created by their high-dose administration. Normally, the ratio of testosterone to epitestosterone in the urine of males is 1–2.5 to 1. When the ratio exceeds 6 to 1, then the administration of exogenous testosterone compounds is likely [18] (Table 4). Conversely, anabolic steroids that are not metabolized to testosterone are best identified by their abnormal presence in the urine.

Table 2 Physical Signs of Steroid Use

Vital signs	Increased blood pressure
Skin	Acne
	Oily skin
	Needle track marks in large muscles
	Male pattern baldness
	Hirsutism in females
	Jaundice
Head and Neck	Jaundiced eyes
	Deepening of voice in females
Chest	Gynecomastia in males
	Small breasts in females
Abdominal	Enlarged tender liver
Genitourinary	Testicular atrophy and prostatic hypertrophy in males
	Clitoral hypertrophy in females
Musculoskeletal	Hypertrophy of muscles
Extremities	Edema due to water retention

Source: Derived from Refs. 1, 2, 5, 44, 47.

Table 3 Psychiatric Effects of Anabolic-Androgenic Steroids

Euphoria, hypomania, mania, grandiosity
Dysphoria, depression, irritability, anxiety
Emotional lability, mood swings
Suicidality
Increased energy and motivation during use
Decreased energy and fatigue during withdrawal
Aggression
Changes in libido (increased or decreased)
Paranoia
Psychosis: hallucinations, delusions
Dependence

Source: Derived from Refs. 1, 2, 35, 39, 42, 44, 57–61, 64–69.

Urine testing for steroids by the major sports organizations is widespread [18,40,73], but also controversial because of its potential conflict with civil liberties [74]. By contrast, urine testing in the clinical situation should not generate the same controversy because the only aim is proper diagnosis and treatment, i.e., good medical care, and because the testing occurs within the confidential context of the therapeutic relationship. Unfortunately, most clinicians, unlike sports organizations, do not have access to high-quality laboratories that can test urine for AASs because the technology is new, still evolving, and expensive [18,73]. Factors that contribute to the technical complexity of steroid testing include (1) the need to test for at least 40 different steroid compounds, and (2) the superiority of the expensive and labor-intensive method of gas chromatography–mass spectrometry for both screening and confirmation [18]. Thus, steroid testing is difficult for most clinical laboratories to justify, especially in the absence of much demand for this service. As the steroid epidemic spreads, however, clinical demand will increase and testing should become more widely available for patient care.

When a high-quality laboratory with the capabilities to test for AASs has been identified

Table 4 Abnormal Laboratory Values in Steroid Users

Increased liver function tests[a]
Increased total cholesterol
Increased low-density lipoprotein cholesterol
Decreased high-density lipoprotein cholesterol
Decreased glucose tolerance
Decreased serum luteinizing hormone
Decreased serum follicle-stimulating hormone
Increased serum testosterone (with use of testosterone esters)
Decreased serum testosterone (without testosterone esters or during withdrawal)
Increased serum estradiol (in men using testosterone esters)
Urinary testosterone to epitestosterone ratio > 6
Decreased sperm count and motility; abnormal sperm morphology
Electrocardiograhic abnormalities

Source: Derived from Refs. 1, 2, 5, 44–47, 84.
[a]Because nonspecific liver enzymes such as alanine aminotransferase (ALT) and aspartate aminotransferase (AST) can be elevated with intensive weight lifting alone owing to their presence in skeletal muscle, liver enzymes such as alkaline phosphatase and the liver-specific lactic dehydrogenase (LDH) isoenzyme are preferred [1].

by the clinician, it is important that an adequate sample be obtained. The clinical circumstances will determine whether the process of micturition needs to be directly observed in order to prevent tampering. Measuring the temperature of the urine immediately after collection provides another check against tampering if needed. In all cases, samples should be checked to determine that the urine is concentrated (pH $\geq$ 1.010), acidic (pH $\leq$ 7.0), and of adequate volume (50 ml). Samples should either be collected in or transferred to glass containers. Samples may be stored frozen at $-20\,°C$, but should be analyzed on the day of thawing because of in vitro degradation [75].

When an indication for testing occurs, the patient should be informed on the day of testing that a urine sample is requested and why. Too much advanced notice that testing will occur allows determined users to employ strategies to escape detection. If a patient refuses a urine test, the situation should be handled in the same manner as a refusal of any indicated medical procedure. Underlying fears are discussed, reassurance is given, and the diagnostic indications are stressed. In general, a refusal occurs when the patient either feels threatened by, or lacks trust in, the clinician. Therefore, efforts at establishing and maintaining a therapeutic alliance are always crucial.

In conclusion, urine testing is a valuable tool for detecting steroid use in clinical practice. In deciding when to test, the clinician is guided by knowledge of the signs and symptoms of steroid use (Tables 2–4). Finally, urine testing can be utilized to monitor the course of treatment for steroid addiction.

VI. TREATMENT

Little is known about the optimal treatment of addiction to AASs [29]. A lot is known, however, about the treatment of other drug addictions. Inasmuch as addiction to AASs is similar to other drug addictions, then treatment approaches may accordingly be similar. Indeed, evidence was previously discussed that the same signs and symptoms that are used to diagnose other psychoactive drug dependencies by DSM-III-R criteria, also occur among users of AASs [39,64,65]. Furthermore, steroid users who are concomitantly addicted to other drugs of abuse, such as alcohol and cocaine, may benefit from traditional treatment approaches.

Nevertheless, there are also reasons to expect that users of AASs may differ from other addicted individuals. First, AASs are not *immediately* euphorigenic or reinforcing as are drugs like cocaine, heroin, and alcohol. The effects of AASs—both somatic and psychoactive—take days to weeks to develop, may peak only after months of use, and may not be apparent without concomitantly and strenuously exercising [1]. Thus, patterns of steroid use may involve more delayed gratification than seen with the use of other commonly abused substances. Second, there may be a greater commitment to certain culturally endorsed values (physical fitness, success, victory, "goal-directedness") among steroid users than among other illicit drug users. Third, preoccupation with physical attributes such as body size may distinguish those inclined to use AASs from other drug abusers [29,76].

Therefore, optimal treatment strategies may need to combine proven techniques for other addicted individuals with methods that address the unique needs and characteristics of addicted steroid users [29]. As a supplement to the following discussion, the reader is referred to two recent reviews of the treatment of steroid users [29,72].

A. Intervention

Intervention refers to the process of influencing addicted individuals to accept treatment [77]. In some cases, when a problem with AASs is suspected and either further assessment or treatment is indicated, steroid users may be reluctant to seek help. In particular, the need to see oneself as big and powerful may contribute to denial about having a drug problem. In addition, steroid users may be irritable and aggressive, thereby inhibiting confrontation by concerned friends and family. Denial and other defenses may respond best to the techniques of intervention developed for other drug abusers [78,79].

B. Detoxification

Withdrawal symptoms have been discussed above, and may be severe enough to warrant treatment, as when the patient is depressed and suicidal. Detoxification refers to the treatment of withdrawal from AASs. The goals of treatment are to facilitate initial abstinence by providing relief of distressing withdrawal symptoms, to prevent complications such as suicide, to foster a therapeutic alliance for the next phase of treatment (rehabilitation and relapse prevention), and to restore the functioning of the hypothalamic-pituitary-gonadal axis [72]. As with other drugs of abuse, detoxification may involve both supportive therapy and pharmacotherapy.

Supportive Therapy for Steroid Withdrawal*

Supportive therapy consists of psychological measures such as reassurance, education, and counseling [72]. Patients are most reassured when those treating them are nonjudgmental, understanding, and knowledgeable about AASs and withdrawal. Establishing a therapeutic alliance is of utmost importance, but the treatment staff may be challenged by patients who are aggressive and competitive as a result of pharmacological effects and personality traits. Although an alliance may form quicker with staff members who are either athletes or past steroid users, the underlying therapeutic issue is that the patient needs to feel that he is understood. More specifically, the treatment staff needs to understand the patient's point of view, as the patient perceives both his reasons for taking AASs as good ones and his beliefs about AASs as correct ones. Almost invariably, the illicit steroid user is extremely invested in his physical attributes and body image. When these and other reasons for drug taking are understood by the treatment staff, then the patient can be counseled about finding acceptable alternatives.

Acceptable alternatives for a bodybuilder, for example, may include both nutritional counseling and consultation with an exercise physiologist or other fitness expert, who can assist the patient with setting realistic training goals and provide safe regimens to achieve them. While it is recognized that these substitutes may not provide the same physical gains that AASs can, the psychological benefits of substitutes can be powerful both for engaging patients in treatment and for preventing relapse. Moreover, the selection of appropriate substitutes conveys to the patient that his needs have been understood.

Additionally, users of illicit AASs strongly believe that these drugs work to enhance physical attributes in a variety of ways. Although the scientific literature is conflicted on this point [1-3], attempts to challenge this belief are fruitless and will only undermine the therapeutic alliance. Instead, the treatment staff should agree that these are very potent drugs, only raising concerns about their potential for causing harm.

Patients should be educated about what they may experience during withdrawal, including depressed mood. By anticipating possible symptoms, the patient is reassured by the treatment staff's knowledge if such symptoms should occur. If symptoms have already occurred, then the patient is reassured by the explanation that these are withdrawal symptoms rather than something intrinsically wrong with the patient or his character.

---

*Portions of this section appeared in Ref. 72, and are reprinted with the permission of the publisher.

Supportive therapy is always indicated during withdrawal, because the risks of suicidal depression and relapse are especially high during this period [57]. Patients should be asked if they feel depressed and if they have ever felt so depressed that they thought about killing themselves. They should be encouraged to discuss these feelings if they occur. When the patient is suicidal, consultation with a psychiatrist is advisable.

Pharmacotherapy for Steroid Withdrawal

It is important to emphasize that the pharmacological management of withdrawal from high-dose, illicit steroid use is completely unstudied. At the time of this writing, therefore, pharmacotherapy can be confidently recommended mainly for the treatment of coexisting disorders (e.g., antidepressants when withdrawal is complicated by major depression), or for the relief of specific withdrawal symptoms (e.g., nonsteroidal anti-inflammatory drugs for the treatment of musculoskeletal pains and headache). Possible pharmacotherapy for the treatment of steroid-induced hypogonadotropic hypogonadism [80,81] is best administered in consultation with an endocrinologist. For a more complete description of the varieties of potential pharmacotherapies, along with guidelines for their administration, the reader is referred elsewhere [67,72].

C. Rehabilitation

Rehabilitation is indicated when the assessment reveals that the user is either addicted to AASs or suffers from other adverse health effects. The goals of rehabilitation are complete abstinence from AASs, restoration of health and psychosocial functioning, and the attenuation of factors that might lead to relapse. Abstinence from other drugs and alcohol must also be considered, and is a recommended goal if addiction is present. In terms of factors leading to relapse, addicted steroid users can be expected to experience both strong internal urges and external pressures to resume use. Indeed, craving, defined as the desire to take more steroids, was the most frequently reported withdrawal symptom in a recently studied sample of 45 steroid users [65]. Relapse prevention techniques may be employed to develop alternative coping techniques to manage the urges and pressures to use AASs [82].

An important psychological issue to address during rehabilitation—one that may distinguish steroid users from other drug abusers—is their overreliance on physical attributes for self-esteem [29]. When steroid-induced physical attributes diminish following withdrawal, patients may experience a sense of loss. Treatment must help patients to mourn their loss and find acceptable substitutes. Alternative sources of self-esteem, including a balance of physical and other activities, need to be fostered. Other issues (in addition to body image) that affect self-esteem may also require attention, such as masculinity issues, competitiveness, and the capacity for satisfying relationships. Substituting people who do not use drugs for steroids and steroid-related activities can be implemented by participating in supportive therapy groups.

Finally, steroid users who are also addicted to other drugs or alcohol may benefit from referral to 12-step groups such as Alcoholics Anonymous or Narcotics Anonymous.

VII. PREVENTION

In terms of prevention, strategies need to be based on an understanding of the factors that either contribute to or inhibit the use of AASs. At the present time, these factors are largely unstudied. Moreover, only one steroid prevention study had been published at the time of this writing. It was conducted in the absence of empirical data about risk factors, it provided student athletes only with information about steroids, and—not surprisingly—it had a negative outcome [83]. That is, student athletes expressed greater interest in trying AASs *after* receiving information about them than before. Clearly, potential users need more than information.

As discussed, an important psychological risk factor may be an overreliance on physical attributes for achieving self-worth and other goals. A corollary of this factor is the user's perception that physical attributes provide the best solutions to the challenges of the life cycle. Such goals and challenges, however, almost always occur in a social context. The athletic, good-looking male, for example, especially during adolescence, is socially desirable; and competitiveness, attractiveness, admirableness, and power—traits that are perceived as obtainable through AASs—are meaningful mostly in relation to other people.

If borne out by longitudinal research, then prevention programs might emphasize social skills, including the power and admirableness in refusing AASs. In addition, attention to setting realistic goals that are attainable with a healthy balance of physical means and other activities might be an important aspect of prevention.

Yesalis [7] has argued that successful prevention efforts will require a change, or at least a greater balance, in our social values. Indeed, we may overly value competition in our society, excessively reward the outward winners, practically worship the "beautiful people" through our media coverage, and secretly (if not overtly) envy the big and the powerful. If true, then individuals may become addicted to AASs, but our society is addicted to unbalanced values. As one observer noted, AASs are just the symptom, values such as winning at any cost are the real disease [16].

ACKNOWLEDGEMENT

This work was supported in part by NIAAA Grant 1P50AA07378-03.

REFERENCES

1. Haupt, H.A., and Rovere, G.D. (1984). Anabolic steroids: A review of the literature, *Am. J. Sports Med., 12*:469–484.
2. Wilson, J.D. (1988). Androgen abuse by athletes, *Endocrinol. Rev. 9*:181–199.
3. Lamb, D.R. (1984). Anabolic steroids in athletics: how well do they work and how dangerous are they? *Am. J. Sports Med., 12*:31–38.
4. Murad, F., and Haynes, R.C. (1985). Androgens, *The Pharmacological Basis of Therapeutics*, 7th ed. (A.G. Gilman, L.S. Goodman, T.W. Rall, and F. Murad, eds.), Macmillan, New York, pp. 1440–1458.
5. Council on Scientific Affairs (1988). Drug abuse in athletes: Anabolic steroids and human growth hormone, *J.A.M.A., 259*:1703–1705.
6. Goldstein, P.J. (in press). Anabolic steroids: An ethnographic approach, *Natl. Inst. Drug Abuse Res. Monogr. Ser.*
7. Yesalis, C.E. (1990). Winning and performance-enhancing drugs—our dual addiction, *Physician and Sportsmed., 18*:161–167.
8. Kochakian, C.D. (1988). The evolution from "the male hormone" to anabolic-androgenic steroids, *Ala. J. Med. Sci., 25*:96–102.
9. Strauss, R.H., and Curry, T.J. (1987). Magic, science, and drugs, *Drugs and Performance in Sports* (R.H. Strauss, ed.), Saunders, Philadelphia, pp. 3–9.
10. Wagner, J.C. (1989). Abuse of drugs used to enhance athletic performance, *Am. J. Hosp. Pharm., 46*:2059–2067.
11. Kopera, H. (1985). The history of anabolic steroids and a review of clinical experience with anabolic steroids, *Acta Endocrinol.* (Suppl.) *271*:11–18.
12. Wade, N. (1972). Anabolic steroids: Doctors denounce them, but athletes aren't listening, *Science, 176*:1399–1403.
13. Yesalis, C.E. (January, 1990). Personal communication.
14. Yesalis, C.E., Wright, J., and Lombardo, J.A. (1989). Anabolic-androgenic steroids: A synthesis of existing data and recommendations for future research, *Clin. Sports Med., 1*:109–134.

15. Bergman, R., and Leach, R.E. (1985). The use and abuse of anabolic steroids in Olympic-caliber athletes, *Clin. Orthop. Related Res., 198*:169–172.
16. Goldman, B. (1987). *Death in the Locker Room*, 2nd ed., Body Press, Tuscon.
17. Cowart, V. (1987). Steroids in sports: After four decades, time to return these genies to bottle? *J.A.M.A., 257*:421–427.
18. Hatton, C.K., and Catlin, D.H. (1987). Detection of androgenic anabolic steroids in urine, *Clin. Lab Med., 7*:655–668.
19. Dezelsky, T.L., Toohey, J.V., and Shaw, R.S. (1985). Non-medical drug use behaviour at five United States universities: A 15-year study, *Bull. Narc., 37*(2–3):49–53.
20. Marshall, E. (1988). The drug of champions, *Science, 242*:183–184.
21. Buckley, W.E., Yesalis, C.E., Friedl, K., et al. (1988). Estimated prevalence of anabolic steroid use among male high school seniors, *J.A.M.A., 260*:3441–3445.
22. Griffin, J.E., and Wilson, J.D. (1985). Disorders of the testes and male reproductive tract, *Textbook of Endocrinology*, 7th ed. (J.D. Wilson, and D.W. Foster, eds.), Saunders, Philadelphia, pp. 259–311.
23. Sheridan, P.J. (1983). Androgen receptors in the brain: what are we measuring? *Endocrinol. Rev., 4*:171–178.
24. Terney, R., and McLain, L.G. (1990). The use of anabolic steroids in high school students, *Am. J. Dis. Child., 144*:99–103.
25. *Drug Misuse: Anabolic Steroids and Human Growth Hormone* (1989). U.S. General Accounting Office, Washington, D.C.
26. Johnson, M.D., Jay, M.S., Shoup, B., et al. (1989). Anabolic steroid use by male adolescents, *Pediatrics, 83*:921–924.
27. Johnston, L.D., O'Malley, P.M., and Bachman, J.G. (1990). 15th Annual National Survey of American High School Seniors. University of Michigan News and Information Services, Ann Arbor, Michigan.
28. Krowchuk, D.P., Anglin, T.M., Goodfellow, D.B., et al. (1989). High school athletes and the use of ergogenic aids, *Am. J. Dis. Child., 143*:486–489.
29. Brower, K.J. (1989). Rehabilitation for anabolic-androgenic steroid dependence. *Clin. Sports Med., 1*:171–181.
30. Frankle, M.A., Cicero, G.J., and Payne, J. (1984). Use of androgenic anabolic steroids by athletes, *J.A.M.A., 252*:482.
31. Yesalis, C.E., Herrick, R.T., Buckley, W.E., et al. (1988). Self-reported use of anabolic-androgenic steroids by elite power lifters, *Physician Sportsmed., 16*:91–100.
32. Pope, H.G., Jr., Katz, D.L., and Champoux, R. (1988). Anabolic-androgenic steroid use among 1,010 college men, *Physician Sportsmed., 16*:75–81.
33. American College of Sports Medicine. (1977). Position statement on the use and abuse of anabolic-androgenic steroids in sports, *Med. Sci. Sports, 9*:11–13.
34. American College of Sports Medicine. (1987). Position stand on the use and abuse of anabolic-androgenic steroids in sports, *Med. Sci. Sports Exerc., 19*:534–539. (Republished paper from 1984).
35. Pope, H.G., Jr., and Katz, D.L. (1988). Affective and psychotic symptoms associated with anabolic steroid use, *Am. J. Psychiatry, 145*:487–490.
36. Sklarek, H.M., Mantovani, R.P., Erens, E., et al. (1984). AIDS in a bodybuilder using anabolic steroids (letter), *N. Engl. J. Med., 311*:1701.
37. Scott, M.J., and Scott, M.J., Jr. (1989). HIV infection associated with injections of anabolic steroids (letter), *J.A.M.A., 262*:207–208.
38. McKillop, G. (1987). Drug abuse in body builders in the West of Scotland, *Scot. Med. J., 32*:39–41.
39. Brower, K.J., Blow, F.C., Beresford, T.P., and Fuelling, C. (1989). Anabolic-androgenic steroid dependence, *J. Clin. Psychiatry, 50*:31–33.
40. Gall, S.H., Duda, M., Giel, D., and Rogers, C.G. (1988). Who tests which athletes for what drugs? *Physician Sportsmed., 16*:155–161.
41. Canacher, G.N., and Workman, D.G. (1989). Violent crime possibly associated with anabolic steroid use (letter), *Am. J. Psychiatry, 146*:679.

42. Perry, P.J., Yates, W.R., and Andersen, K.H. (1990). Psychiatric effects of anabolic steroids: A controlled retrospective study, *Ann. Clin. Psychiatry, 2*:11–17.

43. *Diagnostic and Statistical Manual of Mental Disorders* (1987). 3rd ed.–Revised, American Psychiatric Association, Washington, D.C.

44. Kibble, M.W., and Ross, M.B. (1987). Adverse effects of anabolic steroids in athletes, *Clin. Pharm., 6*:686–692.

45. McNutt, R.A., Ferenchick, G.S., Kirlin, P.C., et al. (1988). Acute myocardial infarction in a 22-year-old world class weight lifter using anabolic steroids, *Am. J. Cardiol., 62*:164.

46. Mochizuki, R.M., and Richter, K.J. (1988). Cardiomyopathy and cerebrovascular accident associated with anabolic-androgenic steroid use, *Physician Sportsmed., 16*:109–114.

47. Ishak, K.G., and Zimmerman, H.J. (1987). Hepatotoxic effects of the anabolic/androgenic steroids, *Sem. Liver Dis., 7*:230–236.

48. Creagh, T.M., Rubin, A., and Evans, D.J. (1988). Hepatic tumours induced by anabolic steroids in an athlete, *J. Clin. Pathol., 41*:441–443.

49. Prat, J., Gray, G.F., Stolley, P.D., et al. (1977). Wilms tumor in an adult associated with androgen abuse, *J.A.M.A., 237*:2322–2323.

50. Roberts, J.T., and Essenhigh, D.M. (1986). Adenocarcinoma of prostate in 40-year-old bodybuilder (letter), *Lancet, 2*:742.

51. Lenders, J.W.M., Demacker, P.N.M., Vos, J.A., et al. (1988). Deleterious effects of anabolic steroids on serum lipoproteins, blood pressure, and liver function in amateur body builders, *Int. J. Sports Med., 9*:19–23.

52. Webb, O.L., Laskarzewski, P.M., and Glueck, C.J. (1984). Severe depression of high-density lipoprotein cholesterol levels in weight lifters and body builders by self-administered exogenous testosterone and anabolic-androgenic steroids, *Metabolism, 33*:971–975.

53. McKillop, G., and Ballantyne, D. (1987). Lipoprotein analysis in bodybuilders, *Int. J. Cardiol., 17*:281–286.

54. Calabrese, L.H., Kleiner, S.M., Barna, B.P., et al. (1989). The effects of anabolic steroids and strength training on the human immune response, *Med. Sci. Sports Exerc., 21*:386–392.

55. Scott, M.J. (1989). Cutaneous side-effects of anabolic-androgenic steroid use, *Clin. Sports Med., 1*:5–16.

56. Strauss, R.H., Liggett, M.S., and Lanese, R.R. (1985). Anabolic steroid use and perceived effects in ten weight-trained women athletes, *J.A.M.A., 253*:2871–2873.

57. Brower, K.J., Blow, F.C., Eliopulos, G.A., and Beresford, T.P. (1989). Anabolic-androgenic steroids and suicide (letter), *Am. J. Psychiatry, 146*:1075.

58. Pope, H.G., Jr., and Katz, D.L. (1990). Homicide and near-homicide by anabolic steroid users, *J. Clin. Psychiatry, 51*:28–31.

59. Freinhar, J.P., and Alvarez, W. (1985). Androgen-induced hypomania (letter), *J. Clin. Psychiatry, 46*:354–355.

60. Annitto, W.J., and Layman, W.A. (1980). Anabolic steroids and acute schizophrenic episode, *J. Clin. Psychiatry, 41*:143–144.

61. Pope, H.G., and Katz, D.L. (1987). Bodybuilder's psychosis (letter), *Lancet, 1*:863.

62. Moore, W.V. (1988). Anabolic steroid use in adolescence, *J.A.M.A., 260*:3484–3486.

63. Yesalis, C.E., Wright, J.E., and Bahrke, M.S. (1989). Epidemiological and policy issues in the measurement of the long term health effects of anabolic-androgenic steroids, *Sports Med., 8*:129–138.

64. Brower, K.J., Eliopulos, G.A., Blow, F.C., Catlin, D.H., and Beresford, T.P. (1990). Evidence for physical and psychological dependence on anabolic androgenic steroids in eight weight lifters. *Am. J. Psychiatry, 147*:510–512.

65. Brower, K.J., Blow, F.C., Hill, E.M., and Beresford, T.P. (1990). Symptoms of dependence on anabolic steroids (abstract), *Alcohol Clin. Exp. Res., 14*:135.

66. Hays, L.R., Littleton, S., and Stillner, V. (1990). Anabolic steroid dependence (letter), *Am. J. Psychiatry, 147*:122.

67. Kashkin, K.B., and Kleber, H.D. (1989). Hooked on hormones? An anabolic steroid addiction hypothesis. *J.A.M.A., 262*:3166–3170.

68. Tennant, F., Black, D.L., and Voy, R.O. (1988). Anabolic steroid dependence with opioid-type features (letter), *N. Engl. J. Med., 319*:578.

69. Yesalis, C.E., Vicary, J.R., Buckley, W.E., Streit, A.L., Katz, D.L., and Wright, J.E. (in press). Indications of psychological dependence among anabolic-androgenic steroid abusers, *Natl. Inst. Drug Abuse Res. Monogr. Ser.*

70. Taylor, W.N. (1985). *Hormonal Manipulation: A New Era of Monstrous Athletes*, McFarland, Jefferson, North Carolina.

71. Dreyfus, I.J. (1990). Congress considers restricting steroids, *Physician Sportsmed., 18*:38.

72. Brower, K.J. (in press). Anabolic steroid withdrawal, *Current Therapy in Endocrinology and Metabolism* (C.W. Bardin, ed.), Decker, Philadelphia.

73. Catlin, D.H., Kammerer, R.C., Hatton, C.K., et al. (1987). Analytic chemistry at the Games of the XXIIIrd Olympiad in Los Angeles, 1984, *Clin. Chem., 33*:319-327.

74. Cowart, V. (1988). Drug testing programs face snags and legal challenges, *Physician Sportsmed., 16*:165-173.

75. Catlin, D.H. (January, 1990). Personal communication.

76. Brower, K.J., Blow, F.C., and Hill, E.M. Unpublished data.

77. Rinaldi, R.C., Steindler, M.S., Wilford, B.B., and Goodwin, D. (1988). Clarification and standardization of substance abuse terminology, *J.A.M.A., 259*:555-557.

78. Johnson, V.E. (1986). *Intervention: How to Help Someone Who Doesn't Want Help*, Johnson Institute, Minneapolis.

79. Kaufman, E. (1986). A contemporary approach to the family treatment of substance abuse disorders, *Am. J. Drug Alcohol Abuse, 12*:199-211.

80. Alen, M., and Rahkila, P. (1988). Anabolic-androgenic steroid effects on endocrinology and lipid metabolism in athletes, *Sports Med., 6*:327-332.

81. Alen, M., Reinila, M., and Vihko, R. (1985). Response of serum hormones to androgen administration in power athletes, *Med. Sci. Sports. Exerc., 17*:354-359.

82. Marlatt, G.A., and Gordon, J.R., eds. (1985). *Relapse Prevention*, Guilford Press, New York.

83. Bosworth, E., Bents, R., Trevisan, L., et al. (1988). Anabolic steroids and high school athletes, *Med. Sci. Sports Exerc., 20*(Suppl.):S3.

84. McKillop, G., Todd, I.C., and Ballantyne, D. (1986). Increased left ventricular mass in a bodybuilder using anabolic steroids, *Br. J. Sports Med., 20*:151-152.

30

Opioids

Beth M. Belkin
Cornell University Medical College, The New York Hospital–Cornell Medical Center,
White Plains, New York

Mark S. Gold
Fair Oaks Hospital, Summit, New Jersey, and Delray Beach, Florida

I. INTRODUCTION

Addictive use of opium has been known to occur throughout history and dates back to the time of ancient cultures. The evolution of opioid use in the United States began with fairly unrestricted availability prior to the early twentieth century, and progressed to more vigorous attempts to strictly control use in present society. The distinction between the medical and nonmedical uses of opioids is an artificial one, as the characteritics of the resulting addiction are the same, including the development of tolerance and dependence. However, there may be differences between individuals who use opioids for recreational use and those who use them for medical reasons. In addition, opioid addicts are frequently addicted to other substances, such as alcohol, marijuana, and cocaine. The diagnosis of opioid addiction is made using standard criteria, and the withdrawal syndrome is determined by the half-life, dose, and chronicity of use of a particular opioid. Adverse effects of opioids are consequences of their direct action, the adulterants in the drugs, and the nonsterile practices of intravenous use. Opioid overdose is treated with intravenous naloxone; withdrawal may be treated with either methadone or clonidine. The long-term treatment of opioid addiction may take two basic forms, pharmacological and nonpharmacological.

II. HISTORY

Opium use has been known to have occurred throughout history, probably dating back to the time of the ancient Sumerians. The first undisputed reference to poppy juice is recorded in the writings of Theophrastus in the third century B.C. The term *opium*, derived from the Greek word for "juice," refers to juice from the poppy plant, *Papaver somniferum*. Arabian physicians knew the uses of opium and Arabian traders introduced it to the Orient. By the middle of the sixteenth century, opium use was well established, carrying with it the well-known liabilities of addiction, tolerance, and dependence. In the eighteenth century, opium smoking became popular in the Orient and Europe, although the addictive use of opium was more acceptable among the Orientals than the Europeans and remains so today [1].

Opium contains more than 20 distinct alkaloids. In 1806, morphine was isolated from opium by Serturner and named after Morpheus, the Greek god of dreams. In rapid succession, other derivatives of opium were isolated, including codeine by Rogiquet in 1832 and papaverine by Merck in 1848 [1].

Addictive use of opium in the United States came about as a result of its addictive properties as well as its unrestricted availability up until the early twentieth century. The use of opium was common among immigrating Chinese laborers and also widespread among wounded Civil War soldiers, who had been given the drug to relieve pain, contributing to its addictive use in the United States. Furthermore, because of the addictive potential of the opiates, their use in legitimate medical practice in itself produces a significant prevalence of addiction. Finally, the introduction of the hypodermic needle led to the particularly potent addictive and hazardous practice of parenteral administration of the opiates [2].

Discovery of the opioid agonist-antagonists as well as pure antagonists has led to interesting research findings and important clinical uses. Nalorphine, the first developed, is a mixed agonist-antagonist. It has the analgesic properties of morphine in addition to antagonistic actions. Studies of the properties of nalorphine led to the discovery of pure antagonists, such as naloxone, and the use of these antagonists in conjunction with agonists made possible the discovery of opioid receptors as well as endogenous peptides that bind to these receptors [3–5].

The term *opiate* is used to designate drugs which are derived from opium, such as morphine, codeine and heroin, a semisynthetic congener of morphine. The development of totally synthetic drugs led to the coining of the generic term *opioid* to refer to all the drugs, both naturally occurring opiates and the synthetic opiates with chemical structures and actions similar to morphine. *Narcotic* is a confusing term that, like many other terms in this area, has undergone changes in meaning with continued usage. It is a Greek word meaning "stupor;" it was and still is used to denote drugs that induce sleep. However, the term narcotic has acquired new meanings and now includes drugs which produce tolerance, dependence, and addiction, such as opioids. Narcotic therefore not a particularly useful pharmacological term [6,7].

III. DEMOGRAPHIC PROFILE OF ADDICTION

Opioid addiction has been significantly prevalent for well over 100 years. However, the patterns of use have changed considerably over the years. For example, at the turn of the century most of the opiate-addicted were Civil War Veterans or users of patent medicines which contained a "tincture" of opium.

Many studies of opioid addiction classify the patterns of use as medical or nonmedical. The distinction between medical and nonmedical use is misleading because of the addictive potency of all opioids regardless of whether they are medically prescribed. Consequently, addiction, tolerance, and dependence rapidly occur in medical practice when opioids are used for more than a few weeks. Those at high risk for developing addiction to opioid analgesics in medical practice are individuals with chronic pain syndromes, such as those involving the back and joints, and health professionals, such as physicians, nurses, and pharmacists who have increased access to these drugs [8,9].

Medical opioid addicts typically present initially as individuals with an acute or more frequently chronic pain syndrome for which a less potent but still addicting opioid, such as propoxyphene (Darvon) or pentazocine (Talwin), is prescribed. As the pain persists and/or tolerance and dependence develop, the individual begins to rely on more potent opioids,

Table 1 Opioids

Agonists	Antagonists
Morphine	Naloxone (Narcan)
Methadone	Naltrexone (Trexan)
Meperidine (Demerol)	Mixed Antagonists
Oxycodone (Percodan)	Pentazocine (Talwin)
Propoxyphene (Darvon)	Nalbuphine (Nubain)
Heroin	Buprenorphine (Buprenex)
Hydromorphone (Dilaudid)	Butorphanol (Stadol)
Fentanyl (Sublimaze)	
Codeine	

such as oxycodone (Percodan) and hydromorphone (Dilaudid). The typical pattern is for the addict to obtain the drugs from more than one physician source or from an illicit source, or through self-prescribing. The hallmark of the addicted patient is the unwillingness or inability to consider alternative methods of pain control or relief of symptoms despite adverse consequences of the opioid addiction [10,11].

Opioids which are used for recreational or nonmedical use, such as by the stereotypical "dope" addict, are usually obtained from illicit sources, although physicians may still be reliable sources. The prevalence of heroin addiction in the United States is less than 1%, considerably lower than the prevalence of alcoholism and cocaine addiction, which are approximately at 20 and 5%, respectively. Most heroin addicts are intravenous users, although a minority use the drug intranasally. Before trying heroin, the typical addict uses other drugs, such as alcohol, marijuana, and tobacco, often addictively. The kind of people who become addicts may vary widely, but they tend to be males who live in the inner parts of large cities. An antisocial personality disorder may or may not predate the development of heroin addiction, but such a disorder frequently develops because of the pharmacological effects of heroin addiction combined with the high cost of obtaining it. Once addiction occurs, development in all areas of an individual's life, including education, socialization, occupation, and psychosexual development, is impaired and delayed as a result.

Once a heroin addiction develops, the prognosis is often very poor. At least 25% of opioid addicts will die within 10–20 years of active use, usually as a result of suicide, homicide, accidents, and infectious diseases such as tuberculosis or hepatitis [6,12].

As many as 50–75% of the male and 25–50% of the female opioid addicts have used and continue to use alcohol addictively, and can therefore be diagnosed as alcoholics. In addition, more than half of opioid addicts are also addicted to sedative-hypnotics, usually benzodiazepines, regardless of whether their primary drug of choice is heroin, methadone, or meperidine (Demerol). Other drugs used addictively by heroin addicts include marijuana and cocaine. Monoaddiction to opioids alone is unusual. Among today's drug addicts, multiple drug addiction is the rule [13–15].

Street heroin available in the United States is diluted several times before it reaches the consumer. For example, a typical 100-mg bag bought on the street actually contains only 4–10 mg of heroin. In addition, the potency of the heroin depends on multiple variables, including the supply and factors that determine supply such as police activity and dealer interests. A more predictable source is the occasional unscrupulous physician who sells prescriptions of opioids to an addict. These so called "script doctors" are sometimes difficult to prosecute because they use a front such as a pain or diet clinic to cover their true prescription practices. Finally, the opioid addicts may themselves have gotten hold of prescription pads and false Drug Enforcement Agency (DEA) numbers in order to procure drugs. Some heroin addicts prefer this prescription medication because of its superior quality control as well as the great reliability of the source. For example, experienced heroin addicts examined under controlled conditions cannot distinguish the effects of heroin from those of hydromorphone (Dilaudid), a potent opioid.

A common practice is to use heroin in combination with other drugs to produce certain effects. The additional drug may be an agonist-antagonist such as Talwin, an antihistamine, or a stimulant such as cocaine. The latter combination results in a "speed ball," which is administered intravenously. An additional combination is one in which the weak agonist codeine is mixed with the sedative glutethimide.

IV. DIAGNOSIS OF ADDICTION

The diagnosis of opioid addiction is made using the same criteria that are employed for the diagnosis of any drug addiction. These criteria include a preoccupation with the acquisition of the opioid, compulsive use in spite of adverse consequences, an inability to reduce the amount of use consistently to avoid adverse consequences, and a pattern of relapse to opioids after a period of abstinence. The persistent pursuit of the drug is particularly dramatic in opioid addicts who typically need to obtain financial resources illegally to purchase the illicit drugs, and who generally do this in a vigorous and aggressive manner.

The development of tolerance and dependence with repeated use of the drug is a characteristic feature of all the opioids. Tolerance is defined as the loss of an effect of a drug at a constant dose, or the need to increase the dose of a drug to maintain the same effect. Dependence is the onset of predictable and stereotypic signs and symptoms which result from cessation of a drug and which are suppressed by more of the drug [16].

Tolerance and dependence may develop independently of the addictive use of an opioid. For example, a patient receiving an opioid for analgesia may develop tolerance and dependence initially without becoming preoccupied with acquiring, using, and relapsing to the drug after cessation of its use for analgesia. However, an opioid addict who uses the drug repetitively will almost always develop tolerance and dependence [16].

Another interesting but poorly understood feature of opioid addiction is that at some point, usually after several weeks, the addict reaches a maximum level of tolerance, after which no further increase in dose is observed. However, the level of tolerance reached is often high for the eventual opioid dose may be as much as 10 times that of the original dose.

Studies of animals and humans have shown that even when opiates are available in unlimited supply they tend to be self-administered at a constant dose after a period of increase in dose. This steady rate of self-administration allows the user to avoid both withdrawal symptoms and toxicity. It stands in marked contrast to the typical pattern of cocaine use, as the latter drug tends to be self-administered erratically and excessively, frequently producing toxicity and death after a period of continuous use [16].

V. WITHDRAWAL

The onset of an opioid withdrawal syndrome as well as its intensity and duration are determined by the drug's half-life, its dose, and the chronicity of use. The shorter the half-life, the more rapid the development of tolerance and dependence and addiction. Drugs such as heroin or morphine, which have a short half-life (2–3 h), are characterized by the onset of withdrawal symptoms within 8–16 h after the last dose. The peak withdrawal occurs between 36 and 72 h after the last dose, with resolution of the acute effects of the withdrawal by 5–8 days. However, there is usually a protacted withdrawal syndrome caused by abstinence which consists of milder, persistent symptoms of anxiety and depression, including sleep and appetite disturbances, which lasts weeks to months. A longer-acting drug such as methadone with a prolonged half-life (24 h) typically shows an onset of withdrawal symptoms within 2–3 days after the last use, a peak effect at around 1–2 weeks, and persistent effects for months before resolution occurs [17].

The opioid withdrawal symptoms (Table 2) include nausea, diarrhea, coughing, lacrimation and rhinorrhea, profuse sweating, twitching muscles, piloerection, or "goose bumps," as well as mild elevations in body temperature, respiratory rate, and blood pressure. There may also be yawning, insomnia, and sensations of diffuse body pain. Finally, and perhaps most dramatically, there is an intense drive or craving for more opioids which can be distinguished from the other withdrawal symptoms. The drug-seeking behavior resulting from this drive to use opioids will persist far beyond the acute pharmacological withdrawal period and further medication will only prolong it, making the goal of abstinence more difficult [17].

VI. OVERDOSE

An acute opioid overdose occurs when a user intentionally or inadvertantly injects a much higher dose than usual which is beyond his threshold of tolerance. This may occur when tolerance has been lost after a period of abstinence or when a purer supply of heroin has been used. Furthermore, some overdoses may be due to toxic and allergic reactions which occur in response to adulterants which are used to dilute the heroin. These acute toxic heroin reactions are characterized by a rapid development of pulmonary edema, respiratory distress, cyanosis, and an altered level of consciousness and coma. Fever and leukocytosis may develop as well as increased intracranial pressure and seizures.

Deaths due to overdose of opioids result from direct effects on the brain which cause acute changes in the respiratory and cardiovascular systems. The opioids depress the brainstem response to carbon dioxide to the point of respiratory arrest and cardiovascular collapse. This depressant effect on brain function is synergistic with effects of other drugs such as alcohol and sedative-hypnotics, which also depress the respiratory and cardiovascular systems in the brainstem [20,21].

VII. PHARMACOLOGY

Opioids as a class produce similar pharmacological effects. They cause an intoxication that is characterized by euphoria and a sense of well-being, analgesia, sedation, and somnolence. Other general effects, particularly with chronic use, include lethargy and apathy, anorexia, depression, and anxiety. More specific effects are pupillary constriction, constipation, decreased respirations, hypotension, nausea and vomiting, and depression of the immune system. Tolerance develops at different rates to all of the pharmacological effects.

Opium and morphine are naturally occurring, and are the principal constituents of the poppy plant. The semisynthetic opioids, in contrast, are produced from the basic molecule, morphine. These include diacetylmorphine (heroin), hydromorphone (Dilaudid), codeine, and oxycodone (Percodan). Finally, the purely synthetic opioids which are similar in action to opium and morphine include meperidine (Demerol), propoxyphene (Darvon), diphenoxylate, methadone, and pentazocine (Talwin). All of these drugs produce euphoria, addiction, and tolerance and dependence, but it is the magnitude of the dose as well as the chronicity of use which determine how rapidly and severe these effects develop.

The opioids interact with opioid receptors throughout the brain and body. Endogenous opioid peptides, namely, the enkephalins, endorphins, and dynorphins, are natural ligands which also interact with opioid receptors and have pharmacological properties similar to the exogenously administered drugs. Agonists are opioids which produce pharmacological effects

Table 2 Objective Opiate Withdrawal Signs

1. Pulse 10 beats/min or more over baseline or over 90 if no history of tachycardia and baseline unknown (baseline: vital sign values 1 h after receiving 10 mg of methadone)
2. Systolic blood pressure 10 mm Hg or more above baseline or over 160/95 in nonhypertensive patients
3. Dilated pupils
4. Piloerection, sweating, rhinorrhea, or lacrimation

similar to those produced by opium, whereas antagonists are opioids that block the opioid receptors by binding to them, but producing no intrinsic effects. The mixed agonist-antagonists have both pharmacological properties similar to opium and blocking capacities at the opioid receptor sites. For example, pentazocine (Talwin), a mixed agonist-antagonist, has opioid effects and may displace morphine at the opioid receptor sites, thereby precipitating withdrawal in a morphine addict. All opioid agonists, antagonists, and mixed agonist-antagonists interact with the same opioid receptors [22].

The mechanisms responsible for the development of tolerance and dependence are not precisely known. There is no consistent evidence to support the notion of changes in the opioid receptors or in the levels of endogenous opioid peptides that would result in these events. However, other biochemical systems that may contribute to the development of tolerance and dependence include alterations in intracellular modulators such as adenyl nucleotides, calcium and related substances, and neurotransmitters [22].

Opiates inhibit the gastrointestinal system, resulting in decreased motility with constipation and anorexia. In addition, liver function may be significantly impaired as a consequence of viral hepatitis, which is contracted when the addict engages in needle sharing. Liver damage may also be caused by alcohol, malnutrition, and allergic and toxic reactions to adulterants. Finally, the intravenous injections themselves may produce local arterial occlusion, phlebitis, mycotic aneurysms, necrotizing angiitis, and angiothrombotic pulmonary hypertension [13,18,19].

The direct effects of the opioids on the central nervous system include sedation by suppressing the reticular-activating system in the brainstem; nausea and vomiting by activating the chemo–trigger zone in the medulla; reduced pain perception by suppressing the spinal cord, thalamus, and periaqueductal gray region in the midbrain; and euphoria by stimulating the limbic system. In addition, acute and chronic administration of opioids produce decreases in luteinizing hormone (LH), testosterone, and cortisol, resulting in diminished libido, amenorrhea, impotency and inorgasmia, and reduced sperm count [20,21].

Some of the major adverse effects of opioid use are consequences of the adulterants in the drugs as well as of the nonsterile practices of intravenous use. For example, skin abscesses, cellulitis, and thrombophlebitis are frequent complications. Right-sided endocarditis is often caused by infection with *Staphylococcus aureus*.

Reported neurological complications of heroin use include transverse myelitis, acute inflammatory polyneuropathy, peripheral nerve lesions, toxic amblyopia secondary to quinine, rhabdomyolysis with myoglobinuria, fibrosing chronic myopathy, bacterial meningitis, subdural and epidural abscesses, and tetanus.

Acquired immune deficiency syndrome (AIDS) is probably the most dire consequence of the practice of sharing needles during intravenous drug use. Currently, more than half of all intravenous drug users, many of whom are opioid addicts, are positive for HIV antibodies and will at some point develop AIDS. The rate of death from AIDS in intravenous drug users is high, and this group is a major reservoir for transmission of the AIDS virus to the general population as well.

VIII. PHARMACOLOGICAL TREATMENT

The treatment of opioid overdose includes the intravenous administration of naloxone, 0.4 mg. If the diagnosis of overdose is correct, naloxone should produce an increase in pupillary size and respiratory rate as well as increased alertness within several minutes. Repeated doses every 3–10 min may be necessary. If no response to naloxone occurs, the diagnosis of opioid overdose should be excluded [23].

Opioid withdrawal may be treated with either clonidine or methadone. It is important to remember that while the withdrawal may at times be very uncomfortable for the patient, it is medically benign. Morbidity and mortality from opioid withdrawal almost never occurs. Clonidine has several advantages over morphine in that it is not an opioid. This means that completing the detoxification to an abstinent state is simpler and more likely to engender patient compliance. In addition, because clonidine does not have opioid toxicity, it can be given as needed in order to titrate the severity of withdrawal symptoms. Finally, the addiction liability to clonidine is low. The major disadvantages of clonidine are sedation and hypotension, which are usually dose related [24–26].

Clonidine can be used on an as needed basis with the dose ranging from 0.1–0.3 mg. This can be given up to every 4 h for a total daily dose of 1.0–1.5 mg. The dose should be increased during the peak withdrawal period. For heroin, this peak occurs at 1–3 days; the dose should then be gradually tapered over the next 4 days. In contrast, for methadone the peak occurs at 1–2 weeks, and the dose of clonidine should then be tapered over the ensuing 2 weeks. This tapering is done to ensure that the withdrawal period is not covered by too high a dose of clonidine so that toxicity occurs (Table 2).

Clonidine is an alpha$_2$-adrenergic agonist. It acts centrally in the locus ceruleus on the alpha$_2$ receptors located on the presynaptic neurons which contain norepinephrine. During withdrawal, the opioids release their suppression of the opioid receptors in the locus ceruleus. The locus ceruleus fires a sympathetic discharge. This discharge is inhibited by clonidine, which acts on the alpha$_2$-adrenergic receptors to suppress the release of the norepinephrine-containing neurons during withdrawal [27].

Methadone may also be used to treat opioid withdrawal. However, its use has several drawbacks; namely, it is an opioid with a high addictive and dependence-producing potential, making it difficult to wean during the tapering process. As the dose is lowered, the addict finds it increasingly difficult to comply with detoxification because of the slowly decreasing blood levels of methadone and the continuing protracted effects of withdrawal. Despite clonidine's greater effectiveness, the advantage of methadone is that it may be more effective in relieving the discomfort of the acute withdrawal because it is an opioid [28,29].

In practice, a test dose of methadone, 10 mg, is given for the onset of withdrawal signs and symptoms. This dose is repeated when the withdrawal reappears. The total dose for 24 h is calculated (typically 30 mg for heroin withdrawal) and then given as a standing dose for 2–3 days. Subsequently, the dose is decreased by 5–10% over the next several days. The usual period of methadone administration for heroin withdrawal is 1–2 weeks; and for methadone withdrawal it is 2–3 weeks (Table 3).

The long-term approach to treatment of the opioid addict may take two basic forms, pharmacological and nonpharmacological. The former emphasizes methadone maintenance in conjunction with counseling, and group and individual therapies. The overriding aim is to provide a legal opioid substitute that can be administered orally and monitored closely. The hope is to reduce criminal activity, providing an opportunity for the addicts to return to their

Table 3 Opiate Detoxification

Heroin morphine withdrawal (clonidine)

    Clonidine 20 μg/kg/day in three divided doses or 0.1–2 mg p.o. t.i.d. for 4–5 days and taper over 4–6 days, or:

    Clonidine 0.1 or 0.2 mg p.o. every 4 h p.r.n. for signs and symptoms of withdrawal (peak doses are between 2–4 days).

    Check blood pressure before each dose, do not give if hypotensie (for that individual, i.e., 90/60).

Methadone withdrawal (clonidine)

    Clonidine 20 μg/kg/day in three divided doses or 0.1–0.2 mg p.o. t.i.d. for 14 days.

    0.1–0.2 mg p.o. b.i.d. for 3 days.

    0.1–0.2 mg p.o. every day for 3 days, or:

    Clonidine 0.1–0.2 mg p.o. every 4 h p.o. p.rn.n. for signs and symptoms of withdrawal (18–20 days).

    Check blood pressure before each dose, do not give if hypotensive (for that individual, i.e., 90/60).

Heroin morphine withdrawal (methadone)

    Methadone test dose of 10 mg p.o. in liquid or crushed tablet. Additional 10-mg doses are given for signs and symptoms of withdrawal every 4 h. Average dose is 30 mg in 24 h.

    Next day, repeat total 1st day dose in two divided doses (stabilization dose), then reduce by 3–5 mg a day until completely withdrawn.

Methadone withdrawal (methadone)

    Methadone test dose of 10 mg p.o. in liquid or crushed tablet. Additional 10-mg doses are given for signs and symptoms of withdrawal every 4 h. Average dose is 30 mg in 24 h.

    Next day, repeat total first day dose in two divided doses (stabilization dose) then reduce by 1–5 mg a day until completely withdrawn.

---

family and employment. Methadone also provides an alternative to the high-risk practice of intravenous drug administration with all its attendant medical complications [30].

Methadone is a long-acting opioid that possesses almost all the properties of heroin. The maintenance dose may be as low as 30–40 mg/day, but usually higher doses (e.g., 80–90 mg or higher) are required. Methadone is administered orally in a liquid form. It is given once a day at a program center which is licensed to dispense the drug. Theoretically, the methadone not only decreases the addict's desire to use heroin, but blocks the pharmacological effects of heroin if the latter is used. The major disadvantage of methadone maintenance is that the user remains in a drugged state and is consequently subject to sedation and other adverse effects on cognition and mood. Furthermore, because the addict continues to use an opioid, he or she tends to continue the practice of using multiple drugs such as alcohol, benzodiazepines, and marijuana. In this way, the methadone addict often continues to be an active multiple drug addict. Thus, the effects and consequences of multiple drug addictions continue in the opioid addict who is maintained on methadone, and the original goals of the methadone maintenance are often not attained [31–33].

Another oral opioid antagonist, naltrexone, has not been shown to be of significant value in the treatment of opioid addiction. Naltrexone provides a deterrant to using opioids, and in this respect is similar to Antabuse, which is used in the treatment of alcoholism. Naltrexone blocks the effects of opioids at the receptor site so that the euphoria and other effects of opioids are not experienced. The major problem with this method of treatment is that the naltrexone must be taken every day in order to block the opioid effect. If the addict stops using the naltrexone, he or she can resume the other opioid use and overcome the naltrexone block in about 24 h. The addict can even overcome the block at the same time if the other opioids are taken at high enough doses [34–36].

IX. NONPHARMACOLOGICAL TREATMENT

The nonpharmacological treatment of opioid addiction is based on abstinence and is similar to the treatment of alcohol addiction. The main goal is for the addict to develop a drug-free lifestyle. For those patients who are motivated, an inpatient or outpatient program emphasizing an abstinence approach and based on the principles of Narcotics Anonymous (NA) or Alcoholics Anonymous (AA) may be effective. Furthermore, long-term follow-up in an aftercare program utilizing group and individual therapies enhances the probability of continued abstinence. It is important to emphasize that the recovering addict must remain free from all drugs of addiction. If not, he or she faces a high risk of relapsing to opioids and is almost certain to become addicted to the other drugs, if he or she is not already [37–40].

Continued regular attendance at NA or AA greatly enhances the probability that the addict will be able to maintain abstinence from drugs. Because of the relapsing nature of addiction, the long-term recovery from a drug addiction depends on an ongoing awareness of the nature of addiction which is provided by the 12-Step programs. In addition, the constant association with other addicts who are living a drug-free lifestyle using the 12-Steps provides a supportive milieu as well as role models for identifying both the difficulties and successes in achieving and maintaining recovery.

For those addicts who use opioids ostensibly to treat chronic pain, successful treatment of the addiction often results in a disappearance of the pain as well. This is because one of the major ways that an addiction is perpetuated is by the manifestation of chronic pain. However, the pain—often unconscious—is actually a manifestation of the addiction, serving as a justification for the opioid use. When the addiction is adequately treated, the "need" for opioids to relieve pain frequently disappears.

X. CONCLUSIONS

In summary, opioid addiction is a complex problem that has occurred throughout history. Opioid addicts are frequently addicted to multiple drugs. The progression of opioid addiction usually follows a characteristic course, with adverse effects resulting from a combination of several factors, including effects of the drugs themselves, the adulterants in the drugs, and the nonsterile practices of intravenous use. Opioid overdose is treated with intravenous naloxone; withdrawal may be treated with either methadone or clonidine. The long-term treatment of opioid addiction ideally comprises two basic approaches, pharmacological and nonpharmacological.

REFERENCES

1. Jaffe, J.H., and Martin, W.R. Opiate analgesics and antagonists, *The Pharmacological Basis of Therapeutics* 7th ed. (A.G. Gilman, L.D. Goodman, T.W. Rall, and F. Murad, eds.), Macmillan, New York, 1985, pp. 491–531.
2. Oliverio, A., Castellano, C., and Puglisi-Allegra, S. Psychobiology of opioids. *Int. Rev. Neurobiol.*, 25:277–337 (1984).
3. Croughan, J.L., Miller, J.P., Whitman, B.Y., and Schober, J.B. Alcoholism and alcohol dependence in narcotic addicts: A prospective study with a five-year follow-up. *Am. J. Drug. Alcohol Abuse*, 8:85–94 (1981).
4. Simon, E.J., and Hiller, J.M. The opiate receptors. *Annu. Rev. Pharmacol. Toxicol.*, 18:371–394 (1978).
5. Chang, K.J., and Cuatrecasas, P. Heterogeneity and properties of opiate receptors. *Fed. Proc.*, 40:2729–2734 (1981).

6. Schuckit, M.A. *Drug and Alcohol Abuse: A Clinical Guide to Diagnosis and Treatment*, 2nd ed., New York, Plenum, 1984.

7. Redmond, Jr., D.E., and Krystal, J.H. Multiple mechanisms of withdrawal from opioid drugs. *Annu. Rev. Neurosci.*, *7*:443 (1981).

8. Bonica, J.J. (ed.). *Pain*. New York, Raven Press, 1980.

9. Wallot, H., and Lambert, J. Characteritics of physician addicts. *Am. J. Drug Alcohol Abuse*, *10*:53 (1984).

10. Simpson, D.D., Joe, G.W., and Bracy, S.A. Six year follow-up of opioid addicts after admission to treatment. *Arch. Gen. Psychiatry, 39*(11):1318–1323 (1982).

11. Vaillant, G.E. A 20 year follow-up of New York narcotic addicts. *Arch. Gen. Psychiatry, 29*:237 (1973).

12. O'Brien, C.P., and Woody, G.E. Long-term consequences of opiate dependence. *N. Engl. J. Med., 304*:1098 (1081).

13. Hartman, N., Kreek, M.J., Ross, A., Khuri, E., Millman, R.B., and Rodriguez, R. Alcohol use in youthful methadone maintained former heroin addicts: Liver impairment and treatment outcome. *Alcoholism Clin. Exp. Res., 7*(3):316–320 (1983).

14. Freed, E.X. Drug abuse by alcoholics: A review. *Int. J. Addict., 8*:451–437 (1973).

15. Carroll, J.F., Malloy, M.A., and Kendrick, B.A. Drug abuse by alcoholics: A literature review and evaluation. *Am. J. Drug Alcohol Abuse, 4*:317–341 (1977).

16. Jaffe, J.H. Drug addiction and drug abuse, *The Pharmacological Basis of Therapeutics*, 7th ed. (A.G. Gilman, L.D. Goodman, T.W. Rall, and F. Murad, eds.), Macmillan, New York, 1985, pp. 532–581.

17. Koob, G.F. Neural substrates of opioid tolerance and dependence. *Natl. Inst. Drug Abuse Res. Mongr. Ser., 76*:46–52 (1987).

18. Holaday, J.W. Cardiovascular effects of endogenous opiate systems. *Annu. Rev. Pharmacol. Toxicol., 23*:541–594 (1983).

19. Eckenhoff, J.E., and Oech, S.R. The effects of narcotics and antagonists upon respiration and circulation in man. *Clin. Pharmacol. Ther., 1*:483–524 (1960).

20. Duggan, A.W., and North, R.A. Electrophysiology of opioids. *Pharmacol. Rev., 35*:219–282 (1983).

21. Basbaum, A.I., and Fields, H.L. Endogenous pain control systems: Brainstem spinal pathways and endorphin circuitry. *Annu. Rev. Pharmacol. Toxicol., 19*:245–267 (1979).

22. Akil, H., Watson, S.J., Young, E., Lewis, M.E., Khachaturian, H., and Walker, J.M. Endogenous opioids: Biology and function. *Annu. Rev. Neurosci., 7*:223–225 (1984).

23. Kleber, H.K., and Riordan, C.E. The treatment of narcotic withdrawal: A historical review. *J. Clin. Psychiatry, 43*:30 (1982).

24. Gold, M.S., Redmond, Jr., D.E., and Kleber, H.D. Clonidine blocks opiate withdrawal symptoms. *Lancet, 2*:599–602 (1978).

25. Gold, M.S., Pottash, A.C., Sweeney, D.R., et al. Opiate withdrawal using clonidine. *J.A.M.A.*, 343–346 (1980).

26. Rounsaville, B.J., Kosten, T., and Kleber, H. Success and failure at outpatient opioid detoxification: Evaluation of the process of clonidine and methadone assisted withdrawal. *J. Nerv. Ment. Dis., 173*(2):103–110 (1985).

27. Gold, M.S., Redmond, Jr., D.E., and Kleber, H.D. Noradrenergic hyperactivity in opiate withdrawal supported by clonidine reversal of opiate withdrawal. *Am. J. Psychiatry, 136*:100–102 (1979).

28. Kreek, M.J. Methadone in treatment: Physiological and pharmacological issues. *Handbook on Drug Abuse* (R.I. Dupont, A. Goldstein, and J. O'Donnell, eds.), U.S. Government Printing Office, Washington, D.C., 1979, pp. 57–86.

29. Preston, K.L., and Bigelow, G.E. Pharmacological advances in addiction treatment. *Int. J. Addict., 20*(6/7):845–867 (1985).

30. Senay, E.C., Mieta, C., Dorus, W., Soberu, K., and Baumgardner, M. Comprehensive treatment for heroin addicts: A pilot study. *J. Psychoactive Drugs, 18*(2):107–116 (1986).

31. Strug, D.L., Hunt, D.E., Goldsmith, D.S., Lipton, D.S., and Spunt, B. Patterns of cocaine use among methadone clients. *Int. J. Addict., 20*(8):1163–1175 (1985).

32. Jackson, G., Cohen, M., Hanbury, R., Korts, D., Sturiano, V., and Stimmel, B. Alcoholism among narcotic addicts and patients on methadone maintenance. *J. Stud. Alcohol., 44*:499–504 (1983).

33. Winston, A., Jackson, G., Suljaga, K., Kaswan, M., and Skovron, M.L. Identification and treatment of alcoholics who use opiates. *Mt. Sinai J. Med., 53*(2):90–93 (1986).

34. Kleber, H.D., and Kosten, T.R. Naltrexone induction: Psychologic and pharmacologic strategies. *J. Clin. Psychiatry, 45*:9 (1984).

35. Gold, M.S., Dackis, C.A., Pottash, A.L.C., Sternbach, H.H., Annitto, W.J., Martin, D., and Dackis, M.P. Naltrexone, opiate addiction and endorphins. *Med. Res. Rev., 2*:211–246 (1982).

36. Gritz, E.R., Shiffman, S.M., Jarvik, M.E., Schlesinger, J., and Charuvastra, V.C. Naltrexone: Physiological and psychological effects of single doses. *Clin. Pharmacol. Ther., 19*:773–776 (1976).

37. Peyrot, M. Narcotics anonymous: Its history, structure and approach. *Int. J. Addict., 20*(10):1509–1522 (1985).

38. Woody, G.E., Luborsky, L., McClellan, A.T., and O'Brien, C.P. Psychotherapy for opiate dependence. *Natl. Inst. Drug Abuse Res. Mongr. Ser., 58*:9–28 (1985).

39. Miller, N.S. A primer of the treatment process for alcohol and drug addiction. *Psychiatry Lett., 5*(7):30–37 (1987).

40. Miller, N.S., Gold, M.S., Cocores, J.A., and Pottash, A.L.C. Alcohol dependence and its medical consequences. *N.Y. St. J. Med., 88*(19):476–481 (1988).

VI
Medical Implications

31

Medical Consequences of Alcohol Addiction

David G. Benzer
Milwaukee Psychiatric Hospital, Wauwatosa, Wisconsin

I. INTRODUCTION

Alcoholism is a disease that is frequently encountered in the general medical setting. Alcoholism is present in as many as 20% of patients seen in an ambulatory care setting, and in 30–40% of patients on hospital general medical wards [1,2]. Historically, medicine has effectively recognized, described, and treated the medical complications of alcoholism: Unfortunately, the medical profession has not been so adept at diagnosing and treating the underlying illness. Alcoholism remains greatly underrecognized and underdiagnosed in most medical settings [3]. Barriers to effective diagnosis of alcoholism include inadequate training on the part of the physician, physician discomfort, a judgmental attitude of the physician toward the alcoholic, and denial on the part of the alcoholic. All of these factors may serve to obscure and confuse the diagnostic picture.

Medical complications which develop as a consequence of alcoholism can serve as a starting point from which the physician can begin the process of diagnosing the underlying condition. The medical complications of alcoholism should pique the physician's index of suspicion for this illness. Any treatment for the medical complications of alcoholism must include attempts to motivate the patient to accept treatment for his or her alcoholism. By so doing, the patient can be spared recurring consequences of the disease. Better still is to recognize, diagnose, and treat the alcoholism prior to the appearance of medical complications, thereby protecting the patient from the physical, emotional, and financial costs which are exacted by this chronic and progressive illness.

For those alcoholic patients who present to the medical care system only after the appearance of medical complications, it is imperative that the physician think of the underlying alcoholism in association with the appearance of these complications. While not every patient who presents with gastritis is alcoholic, alcoholism needs to be ruled out in every patient presenting with gastritis. The same can be said for the rest of the medical complications described in this chapter.

II. GASTROINTESTINAL COMPLICATIONS OF ALCOHOLISM

While ethanol is truly a multisystem toxin, no organ system is more dramatically impacted by ethanol than is the gastrointestinal system.

A. Esophageal Complications

After being orally ingested, alcohol first traverses the esophagus. Alcohol significantly lowers the pressure of the lower esophageal sphincter and inhibits peristalsis of the distal esophagus. This enables gastric contents to maintain frequent and prolonged contact with lower esophageal tissues, resulting in reflux esophagitis. Reflux esophagitis can be a source of gastrointestinal (GI) bleeding in the alcoholic patient. Because of alcohol's role in either creating or exacerbating reflux esophagitis, the drinking history of all patients presenting with a complaint of reflux should be scrutinized.

The association between alcohol and esophageal cancer has been clearly established [4]. Tobacco use further increases the risk of developing an esophageal carcinoma in drinkers.

Two additional sources of esophageal bleeding in alcoholics are the Mallory-Weiss syndrome, a longitudinal tear in the esophagus as a consequence of protracted vomiting, and esophageal varices secondary to portal hypertension accompanying alcoholic cirrhosis.

B. Gastric Complications

Alcohol is a toxin which disrupts the integrity of the stomach's mucosal barrier, a finding first noted by Beaumont in 1833 (5). Alcoholic gastritis is a frequent source of GI bleeding in alcoholics, and in one study 50% of the patients with long-standing alcoholism demonstrated histological evidence of either chronic superficial or atrophic gastritis (6). Despite the frequency with which alcoholic gastritis occurs in an alcoholic population, there does not seem to be an associated enhancement of the long-term risk for developing peptic ulcer disease.

C. Small Intestinal Complications

Diarrhea and intestinal malabsorption are the primary medical consequences of alcohol's impact on the small intestine. Alcohol results in the malabsorption of the carbohydrate D-xylose, thiamine, folic acid, vitamin B_{12}, and some fats [7]. Diarrhea is caused by the enhanced osmotic load in the bowel as a result of malabsorption and by alcohol's ability to stimulate jejunal propulsion, resulting in a rapid transit of the intestinal contents. This condition, known as alcoholic diarrhea, generally resolves within 1 week of cessation of drinking.

D. Pancreatic Complications

While there are multiple possible etiologies of pancreatitis, alcoholism is the single most common cause, and is responsible for 30–60% of all cases [8]. The pathogenesis of alcoholic pancreatitis is somewhat unclear, but possibilities include the toxic effect of ethanol on pancreatic acinar cells, precipitation of proteinaceous material in the pancreatic ducts, and subsequent inspissation of the ducts, or, finally, the reflux of biliary and digestive fluids into pancreatic ducts [9].

Whatever the pathogenesis, the clinical spectrum of pancreatic disorders secondary to alcohol includes acute necrotizing, acute edematous, acute relapsing, chronic relapsing, and painless pancreatitis [10]. The clinical presentation is one of abdominal pain, nausea, and vomiting in a patient with a history of alcohol abuse. Acute uncomplicated alcoholic pancreatitis usually resolves with complete restoration of the pancreatic histology and function.

In contrast, chronic alcoholic pancreatitis is often associated with late sequelae of the disease, including calcification of the pancreas, diabetes mellitus, and digestive disorders secondary to exocrine function defects. The mortality rate from acute pancreatitis is generally low, with a high recurrence rate if the alcoholism remains untreated or is refractory to treatment. Unfortunately, the mortality rate from acute necrotizing or hemorrhagic pancreatitis is much higher, ranging from 40 to 85% [10].

E. Hepatic Complications

Alcoholism is responsible for the majority of cases of chronic liver disease in the United States, and cirrhosis of the liver is a major cause of death in males between the ages of 25 and 60 [11].

The pathogenesis of alcoholic liver disease is still not completely understood. There are undoubtedly a multiplicity of factors involved in the etiology of alcoholic liver disease. Among the factors which play a role in the development of this disease are the direct toxic effect of alcohol and/or its metabolite acetaldehyde on hepatic tissue, the individual suspectibility of the patient, the quantity of alcohol consumed, and the duration of alcohol abuse. Also, there is a sex difference involved in the development of alcoholic liver disease, with women at risk for developing alcoholic liver disease at lower ethanol consumption rates than men [12].

There is a variability in the course of the illness in each patient, as well as variability in the pathogenesis. A spectrum of pathology exists in alcoholic liver disease, beginning with fatty infiltration, progressing to alcoholic hepatitis, and finally alcoholic cirrhosis.

The first stage of alcoholic liver disease, alcoholic fatty liver, results from an accumulation of lipids, protein, and water within hepatic cells. Clinically, the patient with an alcoholic fatty liver is often asymptomatic. On physical examination, tenderness or enlargement of the liver may be noted. Laboratory findings include a modest elevation of liver enzymes, and often an increase in the mean corpuscular volume of red blood cells.

Alcoholic hepatitis is a result of inflammation of the liver in response to the continued assault by the ethanol and its metabolites. Clinically, at times, the patient presents virtually asymptomatic, whereas other patients will present with severe right upper quadrant pain, fever, jaundice, leukocytosis, and significantly abnormal liver function studies.

Alcoholic cirrhosis is the process whereby fibrous tissue is deposited within the liver parenchyma in response to tissue damage that occurred during the fatty liver and hepatitis stages. While there are multiple etiologies for cirrhosis of the liver, alcoholic liver disease remains the most common cause. Once again, the patient with alcoholic cirrhosis may present relatively asymptomatic, or may complain of abdominal pain with any one of the many complications of alcoholic cirrhosis. Many of these complications arise as a consequence of portal hypertension, which occurs as a result of the enhanced resistance to the flow of venous blood through the cirrhotic liver. Portal hypertension may result in esophageal varices, which can rupture and bleed, and in the accumulation of ascitic fluid within the abdominal cavity. Other symptoms found in patients with alcoholic liver disease are a result of impaired hepatocellular functioning, and include coagulopathy as a consequence of diminished synthesis of the clotting factors by the diseased liver, and hepatic encephalopathy, which is a toxic brain syndrome caused by the accumulation of nitrogenous waste products that the cirrhotic liver is inefficiently trying to eliminate.

For some patients afflicted with alcoholic liver disease, alcoholic cirrhosis is an end-stage event. In others, the development of hepatocellular carcinoma represents the final stage in the progression of alcoholic liver disease. While alcoholic liver disease is a risk factor in developing hepatocellular carcinoma, it is probably less of a factor than was once thought. Hepatitis B virus is still the leading predisposing factor for risk of developing hepatocellular carcinoma. Many of the patients who have alcoholic liver disease and subsequently develop hepatocellular carcinoma will have serological evidence of previous hepatitis B infection [13].

The diagnosis of alcoholic liver disease is based on physical examination, which may reveal hepatomegaly, jaundice, and signs of portal hypertension such as caput medusae, ascites, and peripheral edema. Additionally, the serological findings in alcoholic liver disease include an elevated bilirubin that generally remains in the range of 1–5 mg/dl. Higher bilirubin levels may be seen in cirrhosis, not infrequently reaching 20–30 mg/dl. Serum glutamate oxaloacetate transaminase (SGOT) and serum glutamate pyruvate transaminase (SGPT) are usually two- to tenfold elevated in alcoholic liver disease. The SGOT level is usually higher than the SGPT and, usually, remains less than 500 IU. Noninvasive imaging, such as computed tomographic (CT) scanning, may demonstrate both enlargement and fatty infiltration of the liver. Magnetic resonance imaging (MRI) and radionuclear scanning may be particularly helpful in assessing portal hypertension associated with alcoholic liver disease. If the diagnosis is still unclear after the above investigations have been accomplished, and the patient's recovery from liver disease is not proceeding satisfactorily in light of documented sobriety, a liver biopsy may be necessary to provide a definitive diagnosis.

Abstinence from alcohol is the cornerstone of treatment for alcoholic liver disease. Mortality from alcoholic liver disease is most impacted by continued drinking [14]. In addition to abstinence, reestablishing a balanced diet and replenishing nutritional deficiencies assist in the healing process.

A number of drugs have been reported to diminish the progression of alcoholic liver disease and limit the development of cirrhotic tissues. Corticosteroids, insulin, glucagon, colchicine, and D-pencilliamine have been tried with equivocal or no success. Propylthiouracil in 300 mg/day dosages has recently been shown to decrease mortality owing to alcoholic liver disease, possibly by reducing hepatic hypermetabolism induced by alcohol [15].

The complications of alcoholic liver disease are of great clinical concern. Some of these complications are:

1. Gastroesophageal varices.
2. The hepatorenal syndrome, which is oliguria with increased creatinine levels in patients with alcoholic liver disease. The prognosis for patients with hepatorenal syndrome is poor.
3. Edema and ascites are commonly seen as sequelae of cirrhosis. These symptoms of portal hypertension are managed by bed rest, sodium restriction, and, in unresponsive cases, a severe fluid restriction.
4. Hepatic encephalopathy is a central nervous system dysfunction resulting from an accumulation of unmetabolized nitrogenous waste products. It is characterized by alterations in consciousness and behavior, and fluctuating neurological signs, including asterixis, which is the characteritic "flapping tremor." Distinct EEG changes and an elevated blood ammonia level are also seen in hepatic encephalopathy. Treatment should focus on eliminating precipitating factors such as GI bleeding and halting the destruction of hepatic tissues by abstinence from alcohol. At the same time, measures to reduce the levels of ammonia and other nitrogenous waste products should be initiated. These include evacuating the bowel with enemas and laxatives, slowing ammonia absorption within the gut with lactulose, and decreasing intestinal bacteria ammonia production of administering the antibiotic neomycin in doses of 500–1000 mg/q.6.h.

The patient with both alcohol withdrawal and actual or impending hepatic encephalopathy presents a therapeutic challenge. Sedatives used to treat the alcohol withdrawal can severely exacerbate the central nervous system (CNS) obtundation, and precipitate a fatal progression of the hepatic encephalopathy. At the same time, untreated withdrawal from alcohol can progress to delirium tremens, which also carries a significant mortality rate if improperly treated. Patients with both syndromes require meticulous monitoring and simultaneous treatment of both conditions. A shorter-acting sedative not dependent upon the liver for biotransformation prior to excretion, such as lorazepam or oxazepam, should be utilized to cautiously manage the withdrawal process.

5. Spontaneous bacteriemia and spontaneous bacterial peritonitis (SBP) occur in cirrhotic patients in whom arteriovenous shunting within the hepatic vascular system allows hepatic reticuloendoethial cells to be bypassed. Increased bacterial colonization of the upper GI tract provides a source of coliform bacteria which shunted away from the hepatic reticuloendoethial system sets the stage for bacteriemia.

    Spontaneous bacterial peritonitis arises within the mileau of severe decompensated liver disease with ascites. Enteric *Escherichia coli* and streptococci are commonly isolated as etiological agents. Impairment in clearing the blood of contaminating organisms from various sites by virtue of intrahepatic arteriovenous shunting, combined with an ethanol-diminished immune response, allows the bacteria to seed the fertile growth medium of ascitic abdominal fluid. The patient with SBP usually presents with fever, and often with abdominal pain. Aggressive antibiotic therapy in response to blood and ascitic fluid cultures is the treatment for patients afflicted with SBP. Unfortunately, patients with late-stage liver disease and multiple complications may not survive this consequence of alcoholic liver disease.

III. CARDIOVASCULAR COMPLICATIONS OF ALCOHOLISM

A. Alcohol and Hypertension

The association between alcohol and hypertension has been demonstrated unequivocally in several large epidemiological studies [16–19]. There is a clear relationship demonstrted between the amount of ethanol consumed and the elevation of blood pressure, with the higher the consumption the greater the elevation of blood pressure, both systolic and diastolic. What has remained unclear is the etiology of this phenomenon. All patients with hypertension should be screened for alcohol consumption rates and the possible diagnosis of alcoholism. Two primary areas of interest are alcohol's effect as a pressor and its ability to provoke an abstinence or withdrawal syndrome as blood levels fall. As a pressor, alcohol may exert its effect upon blood pressure either through a direct action on vascular smooth muscle, or by way of neurohumeral effects via elevation of plasma cortisol, catecholamines, or renin [20].

Hypertension is a primary symptom of the abstinence syndrome precipitated by ethanol. There is a spectrum of severity of the alcohol withdrawal syndrome, ranging from a mild "hangover" with a brief period of elevation of pulse and blood pressure, to a life-threatening syndrome known as delirium tremens.

Alcohol-related hypertension may be caused by either or both of the above mechanisms. What is clear is that in alcoholics, when alcohol consumption ceases, blood pressure levels decline, and if drinking is resumed, blood pressure levels rise again [21,22].

B. Alcoholic Cardiomyopathy

The insidious development of cardiomegaly, particularly left ventricular hypertrophy and dilation, ultimately progressing to symptomatic left ventricular failure, especially in male alcoholics, has been described as alcoholic cardiomyopathy. Physical examination reveals characteristic signs of cardiac decompensation, as do the chest x-ray, ECG, and echocardiogram. Alcoholic cardiomyopathy is still a diagnosis of exclusion made in an alcoholic with all other etiologies for cardiomyopathy having been ruled out. It is not clear, yet, whether the syndrome is produced by alcohol alone, or whether it requires the coexistence of one or more additional factors to produce the pathology [23].

Might the ethanol-induced hypertension, and subsequent increase in afterload, be an accelerator of cardiac hypertrophy? Whatever the precise etiology, it is clear that abstinence from alcohol is essential for a favorable prognosis for those alcoholics suffering from alcoholic cardiomyopathy [24].

C. Cardiac Rhythm Disturbances

Cardiac rhythm disturbances associated with alcohol use, such as the holiday heart syndrome, have been described for decades [25]. However, one large prospective study found a virtually identical percentage of ECG abnormalities in an alcoholic and controlled population [26]. Certainly, alcohol can produce a sinus tachycardia, both directly and as a result of the withdrawal process [27]. Also, alcohol has been shown to be capable of transiently interrupting normal intramyocardial conduction, which may facilitate arrhythmias [28]. In an alcoholic individual, what role alcohol itself plays in producing cardiac rhythm disturbances other than sinus tachycardia and what effect it has in exacerbating other underlying arrhythmogenic conditions such as hypokalemia is uncertain.

D. Coronary Artery Disease

There is an inverse relationship between moderate ethanol consumption (up to 45 ml of ethanol/day), and the risk of developing coronary artery disease and myocardial infarction [29,30]. However, the salutory effect of alcohol on coronary artery disease is outweighed in terms of long-term survival by the enhanced risk for cancer and cerebrovascular accidents in moderate drinkers [31]. There can be no sound rationale for prescribing alcohol for any alleged "medicinal" use.

IV. PULMONARY COMPLICATIONS OF ALCOHOLISM

A. Effect of Alcohol on the Pulmonary System

Even though well over 90% of all alcoholics are also cigarette smokers, there are still pathological consequences of the alcoholism itself on the respiratory system. Ethanol damages the pulmonary system in at least three ways. First, alcohol impairs the "mechanical" respiratory defenses, including tracheal mucociliary action, proper glottic closure, and the cough reflex [38]. Next, alcohol impairs pulmonary bacterial clearance by decreasing surfactant production, and depressing ciliary movement [36]. Finally, diminished cellular immunological defenses, such as macrophage recruitment and hampered leukocyte chemotaxis, complete alcohol's effect on the pulmonary system, thereby making it possible for the alcoholic to be predisposed to a variety of pulmonary infections.

B. Bacterial Pneumonias

The breakdown of the respiratory protective barrier, combined with malnutrition, inadequate dental hygiene, and often intercurrent tobacco addiction, makes the alcoholic particularly prone to bacterial pneumonia. *Streptococcus pneumoniae* remains the most common organism found in bacterial pneumonia in alcoholics as well as in the general population. Pneumonias caused by *Haemophilus influenzae*, *Klebsiella pneumoniae*, and gram-negative organisms can also be found in an alcoholic population.

C. Aspiration Pneumonitis

Impaired respiratory mechanical barriers, especially poor glottic closure, and alterations in the state of consciousness of the alcoholic, can predispose to aspiration of gastric contents. If aspiration pneumonitis occurs as a result of a witnessed aspiration of vomited gastric contents, antibiotic therapy may not be indicated [38]. It is the aspiration of oropharyngeal secretions that sets the stage for the anerogic infections often seen in alcoholics, including pneumonitis, lung abscess, or empyema. *Peptosreptococcus, Fusobacterium*, and *Bacteroides* species are the most commonly occurring pathogens [39].

D. Pulmonary Tuberculosis

Pulmonary tuberculosis is in no way a disease of the past. A recent study demonstrated active tuberculosis occurring in a population of socioeconomically disadvantaged chemically dependent persons with a frequency 28 times that of the general population [40]. However, tuberculosis is not confined to this subset of the population: We recently diagnosed pulmonary tuberculosis in a 50-year-old alcoholic physician who lived and practiced in an affluent suburban area. Treatment of tuberculosis in an alcoholic ideally requires triple drug therapy with meticulous monitoring of liver chemistries, particularly in those patients who have a history of alcoholic liver disease. Abstinence from alcohol and other mood-altering drugs, accomplished through ongoing treatment of the chemical dependency, is crucial before an optimal response to the therapeutic intervention for the tuberculosis.

V. HEMATOLOGICAL-IMMUNOLOGICAL CONSEQUENCES OF ALCOHOLISM

Ethanol's impact on the hematopoietic system is multifactorial, with most of these sequelae representing late-stage medical consequences of alcoholism. Clinicians need to remain vigilant for alcoholism as a possible etiology for a multitude of anemias and infectious diseases. Many of these conditions will properly respond only if abstinence and treatment of the alcoholism is a component of the medical management of the case.

A. Erythrocyte Abnormalities

Ethanol as an Erythrocyte Toxin

Ethanol toxicity leads to direct toxic changes in the hematopoietic system, including vacuolization of marrow precursor cells, decreased cellularity of the marrow, and megaloblastic changes of the erythrocyte not associated with folate deficiency [32]. The first of these changes, the vacuolization of erythroblasts, is identical to that associated with chloramphenicol toxicity, and occurs rapidly with heavy drinking, often in as little as 5–7 days [33]. This toxic effect resolves quickly with abstinence.

The most common toxic effect of ethanol on red blood cells is to produce a macrocytosis. The macrocytosis, with mean corpuscular volumes (MCVs) in the range of 100–110 μm^3 is often the earliest laboratory marker of alcoholism, and is usually not accompanied by anemia. The macrocytosis is a direct toxic effect of ethanol, and occurs even in the absence of folate deficiency or alcoholic liver disease, which are two other etiologies of a macrocytic red blood cell population in alcoholics. Unlike the macrocytosis seen in folate deficiency, which is also quite common in alcoholism, toxic macrocytosis is characterized by the presence of round macrocytes rather than the macro-ovalocytes of folate deficiency [34]. This "alcoholic macrocytosis" resolves slowly, but steadily, over 2–3 months. While the specific mechanism of this macrocytosis is not understood, its presence can serve as a laboratory indicator of alcoholism, and the resolution of the macrocytosis can confirm and demonstrate to both the physician and the patient at least one physiological benefit of abstinence and recovery from alcoholism.

Alcohol-Induced Folate Deficiency

As previously mentioned, folate deficiency with resulting megaloblastic anemia is not uncommon in late-stage alcoholism; in fact, alcoholism is the most common cause of folate deficiency in the United States [35]. Megaloblastic anemia due to folate deficiency is encountered in alcoholics with a history of poor dietary habits and who present with MCVs from 100–140 μm^3. Macro-ovalocytes and hypersegmented neutrophils on peripheral blood smear, and decreased serum and erythrocyte folate levels are diagnostic of the megaloblastic anemia secondary to alcohol-induced folate deficiency. Abstinence and folate replacement form the cornerstone of therapy for such patients.

Iron Deficiency in Alcoholism

Gastrointestinal bleeding is the most common source of iron deficiency anemia in alcoholism. This anemia is easy to overlook in the alcoholic; the decline in mean corpuscular volume that one expects with iron deficiency may not be as dramatic in the alcoholic, who may be experiencing an intercurrent macrocytic process. An MCV in the normal range may be the result, thereby obscuring both pathological processes. Therefore, a serum ferritin level is the laboratory test of choice for the diagnosis of iron deficiency in alcoholism [34].

Other Anemias

Other anemic processes which are occasionally seen in alcoholism include sideroblastic, hemolytic, and spur cell anemias.

B. WBCs and Alcoholism

The alcoholic's propensity for infection is multifactorial; among the contributing factors are malnutrition and liver disease, and the direct toxicity of ethanol on white blood cells (WBCs).

Alcohol inhibits the production of neutrophils (polymorphonuclear neutrophils; PMS) by the marrow, and then interferes with chemotaxis and delivery processes by which PMNs are recruited in response to infection [36]. Both granulocytopenia and impaired PMN functioning decrease the effectiveness of the immune response in the alcoholic. Exacerbating these deficiencies even further is alcohol's impact on T lymphocytes and the system of cell-mediated immunity. Alcohol decreases the number of circulating T lymphocytes as well as the ability of the remaining T lymphocytes to respond to antigenic stimulation [36]. Both malnutrition and liver disease exacerbate this effect on cell-mediated immunity. Finally, there is some evidence that B lymphocytes in the humoral immune system are also negatively effected by alcohol. Particularly impaired is the humoral response to new antigenic stimulation in alcoholics [36].

C. Platelets and Alcoholism

Just as ethanol suppresses the production of erythrocytes, neutrophils, and lymphocytes, so too does it predisose the alcoholic to thrombocytopenia as a direct toxic effect of the drug on platelet production in the marrow. Platelet counts of less than 150,000/ul have been reported to occur in more than 80% of the patients being intoxified in a hospital setting [37].

There is some evidence that alcohol may be able to produce platelet dysfunction at both ends of the spectrum. Thrombocytopenia and decreased platelet aggregation may initially lead to a bleeding diathesis. Later, with abstinence initiated, a rebound thrombocytosis and enhanced platelet aggregation, may result in an increased risk of thromboembolic events [36].

VI. NEUROLOGICAL CONSEQUENCES OF ALCOHOLISM

Alcohol-induced pathology within the nervous system extends from the highest cortical region to the most distant peripheral neurons. Alcohol effects the nervous system through a variety of mechanisms. Malabsorption of thiamine, nicotinic acid, and vitamin B_{12} deprives the neurons of substrate necessary for optimal energy-yielding metabolism. Alcoholic liver disease, with its attendant coagulopathy, may predispose the central nervous system to hemorrhagic events; alcoholic hypertension may further exacerbate this diathesis. Alcoholic seizures and syndromes of dementia and cognitive impairment occur with great frequency in alcoholics, even though the precise mechanism through which alcohol accomplishes these changes is unclear. Some of these conditions, such as the Wernicke-Korsakoff syndrome and hemorrhagic stroke, are grave late-stage consequences of alcoholism, and are accompanied by a worrisome prognosis. Others, such as early alcoholic dementia and alcoholic epilepsy, may completely resolve with abstinence and recovery from alcoholism. As always, the clinician should strive to help the patient work toward the goal of recovery from alcoholism, while at the same time addressing the following neurological complications of the disease.

A. Alcoholic Dementia

In the *Diagnostic and Statistical Manual of Mental Disorders*, 3rd ed.–Revised (DSM-III-R), of the American Psychiatric Association, dementia associated with alcoholism is described as a syndrome of cognitive impairment seen in alcoholics at least 3 weeks after the cessation of ethanol intake, so as to preclude the acute effects of intoxication or withdrawal and which cannot be attributed to any other cause [38]. To make the diagnosis, it is necessary to demonstrate cognitive deficits in areas other than memory alone. Alcoholic dementia is often accompanied by cortical atrophy.

The syndrome of alcoholic dementia can be demonstrated in those recently abstinent alcoholics in whom the clinician notes persistent cognitive deficiencies, which can be documented by neuropsychological testing and through CT scanning to assess for cortical atrophy. Neuropsychological findings may include impaired visuospatial, abstracting, learning, and memory function [39]. Alcoholic dementia and attendant cortical atrophy are not uncommon findings in an alcoholic population; studies have shown more than 50% of alcoholic patients demonstrate cognitive impairment with CT scan–documented cortical atrophy [40,41]. The cognitive deficiencies in alcoholic dementia will improve with time and abstinence, although the period of abstinence during which this improvement occurs is often 6, 12, or even 18 months. Those atrophic changes due to loss of synapses may resolve; atrophy secondary to loss of neurons is most likely permanent [42].

B. Wernicke-Korsakoff Syndrome

The Wernicke-Korsakoff syndrome is a neurological disorder caused by thiamine deficiency. It is most commonly seen in alcoholic patients; however, it may occur in association with other conditions which result in thiamine deficiency, such as upper GI obstruction, hemodialysis, and thyrotoxicosis. The pathological changes seen in the Wernicke-Korsakoff syndrome are symmetric lesions in the thalamus, hypothalamus, mammalary bodies, and the floor of the fourth ventricle [43].

Wernicke's encephalopathy classicly presents with the triad of oculomotor dysfunction, ataxia, and mental confusion. The oculomotor signs including nystagmus, bilateral abducens palsy, other types of gase palsy, or complete opthalmolegia [43].

The patient with Wernicke's encephalopathy may present in a stupor or coma, obfuscating the diagnostic picture, and may result in the correct diagnosis being made only at autopsy [44].

Wernicke's encephalopathy is a medical emergency. Treatment consists of parenteral thiamine, with doses up to 1000 mg given over the first 12 h. It is important for the clinician who encounters acutely ill alcoholics to recognize that administration of intravenous glucose can precipitate or exacerbate Wernicke's encephalopathy syndrome in a patient at risk. In such patients, it is prudent to administer 100 mg of thiamine parenterally prior to glucose loading the patient. Hypomagnesemia, also commonly seen in alcoholics, can hinder an optimal response to a therapeutic intervention with thiamine, inasmuch as magnesium is a cofactor for thiamine transketolase. Treating concommitant hypomagnesemia may be imperative to a successful response to treatment of the patient with Wernicke's encephalopathy.

Most patients treated promptly for Wernicke's encephalopathy will recover within 48–72 h. Those who do not will often evolve into Korsakoff's psychosis.

Korsakoff's psychosis, also called alcohol amnestic disorder, represents the chronic phase in the clinical continuum of the Wernicke-Korsakoff syndrome. Korsakoff's psychosis is characterized by both retrograde as well as antegrade amnesia with relatively spared intellectual functioning [43]. The diagnostic hallmark of Korsakoff's psychosis is confabulation, where the patient invents responses to questions in an attempt to cover-up for profound memory defects. The prognosis for Korsakoff's psychosis is guarded; as many as 50% of the cases do not improve significantly, and may require institutionalization. The most effective approach to Korsakoff's psychosis is preventive; early recognition and prompt treatment intervention by the clinician in patients who are early in the course of their alcoholism will prevent late-stage consequences such as the Wernicke-Korsakoff syndrome.

C. Alcohol and Stroke

The use of alcohol significantly increases the risk for hemorrhagic stroke; the Honolulu Heart Study demonstrated that the risk of hemorrhagic stroke for light drinkers (1–14 oz of ethanol/month) was double that for nondrinkers, and triple for heavy drinkers (40 oz or more of ethanol/month) [45]. The findings of this study are independent of the hypertensive status of the patient. There are a number of correlates of alcoholism that may exacerbate the risk for hemorrhagic stroke in alcoholic patients; a recent report of six patients who experienced intracranial hemorrhage, and who were also diagnosed as alcoholic, noted significant alcoholic liver disease and coagulopathy in all six patients [46].

D. Alcohol and Seizures

The causal relationship between alcohol and seizures has been recognized for many years; Ecchevarria reported in 1881 that 45% of an alcoholic population experienced seizures at some point in time [47]. Seizures in alcoholics may be classified in essentially three categories: (1) those that occur as a result of the alcohol withdrawal syndrome; (2) those that occur in an alcoholic who has intercurrent epileptogenic illness such as head injury, intracranial lesions, or idiopathic epilepsy that predates the onset of the drinking; and (3) those that occur in alcoholic patients who have had either a single or recurrent seizures but do not present during either acute intoxication or withdrawal, and for which no other known epileptogenic foci can be found. The pathogenesis of this final category of grand mal seizures, which occurs in alcoholics, remains obscure. Among the postulated mechanisms are hypomagnesemia, cerebral atrophy, inadequate carbohydrate metabolism, or alcohol-induced disturbances in the cerebral microcirculation [48]. Also uncertain is the therapeutic approach to alcoholic seizures. Obviously, alcoholic patients with other etiologies for their epilepsy require treatment. However, the treatment of seizures secondary to alcoholic epilepsy remains much more controversial. Certainly, abstinence is agreed by all to be essential for a favorable outcome for the patient with alcoholic epilepsy.

E. Alcoholic Polyneuropathy

Alcoholic polyneuropathy is a progressive peripheral neuropathy frequently encountered in late-stage alcoholics as a consequence of nutritional inadequacy. The neuropathy presents as pain, parethesia, and weakness in the lower extremities. As the affliction progresses, motor deficits and, finally, muscular atrophy occurs. Nerve conduction studies and EMGs will usually electrophysiologically confirm the presence of the neuropathy. Treatment of alcoholic polyneuropathy includes abstinence from ethanol, vitamin B complex supplementation, and restoration of general nutritional balance.

F. Alcoholic Cerebellar Degeneration

Alcoholic cerebellar degeneration is not infrequently seen in late-stage alcoholism, with up to 27% of chronic alcoholic patients at autopsy demonstrating cerebellar degeneration [44]. Clinically, the patient with alcoholic cerebellar degeneration presents with a wide-based gait and truncal ataxia. The etiology of this consequence of alcoholism may be a combination of nutritional deficiencies and a direct toxic effect of ethanol, and possibly acetaldehyde. Computed tomographic scanning or magnetic resonance imaging (MRI) will confirm the diagnosis. Treatment of the patient's alcoholism, which would certainly include restoration of nutritional balance, is the treatment for this condition.

G. Rare Neurological Syndromes Attributed to Alcoholism

Tobacco-Alcohol Amblyopia

Tobacco-alcohol amblyopia is an ophthalmological syndrome most often seen in nutritionally deficient tobacco-using alcoholics. This syndrome initially presents as decreased visual acuity, with a progression of symptoms, including difficulty distinguishing colors and scotomas. These ophthalmological defects usually respond to enhanced nutritional and vitamin therapy, particularly the B vitamins.

Central Pontine Myelinolysis

Central pontine myelinolysis is a rare demyelinating disease most often seen in nutritionally debilitated alcoholics. A variety of neurological signs and symptoms may be present, reflecting widespread destruction of pontine and brainstem neurotissue: Quadriplegia, pseudobulbar palsy, dysphagia, ophthalmoplegia, and coma may occur. Hyponatremia or the rapid correction of hyponatremia has been implicated in this syndrome; however, the precise etiology remains obscure. The syndrome is often seen during the recovery phase in patients who are suffering from severe metabolic dysfunction as a consequence of their alcoholism. Magnetic resonance imaging can confirm the presence of the demyelinating lesion in the basis pontis.

Supportive care, continued correction of metabolic deficiencies, nutritional support, and possibly cautious correction of hyponatremia represent the available therapies for this rare disorder, which is often fatal.

Marchiafava-Bignami Disease

Marchiafava-Bignami disease is the final illness in the triad presented here. Demyelination of the corpus callosum results in a wide array of neuropsychiatric symptoms, including impairment in language, gait, and motor skills. Also, confusion, disorientation, hallucinations, and seizures may be present. The etiology is thought to be a nutritional deficiency secondary to late-stage alcoholism. The diagnosis is based on clinical presentation, but may be corroborated by MRI.

VII. ALCOHOL AND CANCER

A significant number of epidemiological studies have conclusively demonstrated that alcohol consumption poses a significant risk for the development of a number of cancers [49,50]. The epidemiological data have come from three major areas of investigation. First are those studies which have linked individual patient histories of alcohol consumption with an enhanced incidence of cancer, especially of the head and neck, liver, and esophagus. The second major category of epidemiological studies centers arouond those particular occupations which have a high exposure to alcohol, such as brewery workers who receive free beer, and also demonstrate higher death rates from cancer. Finally, ethnic and religious groups who demonstrate significantly lower alcohol consumption because of cultural or religious principles also have significantly lower rates of cancer. In contrast, groups with higher consumption have higher death rates from cancer.

A. Possible Mechanisms of Alcohol's Role in Carcinogenesis

The role of alcohol in enhancing cancer risk in persons who use alcohol is not entirely clear. In alcoholic patients, the fact that their nutritional status maybe less than optimal complicates the picture. Also, the fact that most alcoholics use tobacco, a potent carcinogen, further confounds the relationship between alcohol and cancer. Finally, alcohol's action as an immunosuppressant certainly does not diminish the alcoholic's risk of developing cancer. Alcohol has never been shown to be an initiator of cancer; attempts to induce cancer in laboratory animals with alcohol have never been successful [51].

Instead, it is more probable that alcohol acts as a cocarcinogen, either by facilitating penetration of carcinogens into tissues by virtue of alcohol's property as a solvent, or possibly by inducing enzymes, such as the microsomal enzyme system, which can lead to enhanced activation of some carcinogens [51].

Despite the uncertainty that exists as to the precise pathogenesis of cancer in alcoholism, the fact that the incidence of cancer in alcoholics is much greater than the general population remains unquestioned.

B. Specific Cancers Associated with Alcoholism

Head and Neck Cancer

Alcohol and tobacco work synergistically in most cases to promote cancers of the head and neck. This is particularly true of oral cancers, where the effects of alcohol and tobacco are clearly addictive. Both alcohol and tobacco themselves enhance the risk for cancer. However, when both are used the risk becomes multiplicative [51]. Cancers of the larynx and hypopharynx are also enhanced by both alcohol and tobacco consumption. However, the enhancement in these two cancers does not seem to be equal, as in oral cancer. Alcohol seems to be the more significant factor in developing cancer of the hypopharynx, whereas the contribution of tobacco is preeminent in cancer of the larynx [51].

Esophageal Cancer

Alcohol is a major risk factor for the development of esophageal cancer. Even when corrected for the effect of tobacco, the risk of developing esophageal cancer is 20 times greater in heavy drinkers than in the general population [52].

Hepatocellular Carcinoma

Alcohol is not the strong predictor of hepatic carcinoma that was once thought. Prospective studies have indicated that the relative risk of developing hepatocellular carcinoma is about one and a half times greater in alcoholics when compared to nonalcoholics. It appears that intercurrent infection with hepatitis B appears to be a much more significant risk factor: In one study of 20 alcoholic patients with cirrhosis and hepatocellular carcinoma, all 20 had laboratory evidence of previous hepatitis B infection [53].

Other Sites

There is some evidence that alcohol enhances the risk of cancers of the rectum and stomach. Particularly disturbing are recent reports that even social use of alcohol significantly increases the risk of breast cancer in women [54,55].

VIII. NUTRITIONAL AND METABOLIC CONSEQUENCES OF ALCOHOLISM

Ethanol is truly remarkable in its ability to intrude and exert its effect on so very many of the body's metabolic processes. This section will highlight but a few of the nutritional and metabolic consequences of alcoholism. Comprehensive reviews of the biochemical and physiological processes impacted upon by ethanol, in both human and animal subjects, are available and should be consulted for definitive information. Contained herein are some of the more common metabolic and nutritional consequences of alcoholism.

A. Nutritional Consequences of Alcoholism

Ethanol impairs the nutritional well-being of alcoholics in a variety of ways. First, the consumption of ethanol provides the drinker with a significant number of calories, roughly 7 kcal/gm. These calories are often not accompanied by significant quantities of other nutrients. Therefore, the drinking alcoholic is consuming "empty calories." Other nutrient-providing foodstuffs are easily displaced from the alcoholic's diet in favor of the high-energy, mood-altering drug ethanol. Ethanol also impairs the nutritional state of the alcoholic by creating a malabsorption of a number of essential nutrients. Among these nutrients are the carbohydrate D-xylose, thiamine, vitamins A, D, B_6, B_{12}, and folic acid.

Folic acid deficiency may be the most common vitamin deficiency seen in alcoholics. One study of unselected alcoholic patients demonstrated that 38% had low serum folate levels [56]. Clinically, this can lead to megaloblastic anemia, a condition exacerbated by alcoholic liver disease.

Thiamine malabsorption predisposes the alcoholic to a number of serious neurological syndromes, which are discussed in Section VI of this chapter. Thiamine replacement therapy is an important component in the early care of the alcoholic patient.

Alcoholics represent the single largest group of nutritionally impaired patients in the United States. By displacing nutrients, ingesting empty calories, and through malabsorption, alcohol creates nutritional deficiencies in millions of patients afflicted by the disease of alcoholism. One component of a comprehensive approach to recovery for the alcoholic is reestablishing nutritional balance.

B. Carbohydrate Metabolism—Alcoholic Hypoglycemia

Alcoholic hypoglycemia, while not seen with great frequency, is a potentially severe complication of alcoholism. The pathogenesis of this condition begins with the alcoholic patient not consuming adequate quantities of carbohydrates, and subsequently depleting hepatic glycogen reserves. Alcohol further complicates the processes of carbohydrate metabolism by acutely impairing gluconeo-genesis. The net effect is to place the alcoholic at risk for acute hypoglycemia. The clinical presentation of hypoglycemia includes tachycardia, diaphoresis, tremulousness, and agitation. This syndrome is usually seen in patients who have ingested alcohol within the previous 12 h.

Alcoholic hypoglycemia has the potential to cause confusion in the management of the alcoholic patient. The signs and symptoms of alcoholic hypoglycemia are identical to those of the alcohol withdrawal syndrome. Administering sedation to a tremulous, diaphoretic, alcoholic patient who is suffering from alcoholic hypoglycemia may severely compromise that patient. Alcoholic hypoglycemia mimicking the alcohol withdrawal syndrome needs to be considered in each patient who presents with what is presumed to be the alcohol withdrawal syndrome.

Correcting alcoholic hypoglycemia can often be accomplished through initiating a balanced diet and correcting nutritional imbalance. In patients unable to take nutrients orally, intravenous 10% dextrose should be administered until nutrients can be taken by mouth.

C. Alcoholic Ketoacidosis

Like alcoholic hypoglycemia, alcoholic ketoacidosis is a relatively uncommon but potentially life-threatening consequence of alcoholism. The syndrome is most often seen in the alcoholic who has recently been on a drinking binge, and presents with a chief complaint of abdominal pain. The patient usually has not been able to drink for 24–48 h prior to being seen because of the abdominal pain. Consequently, the blood alcohol level is often zero in these patients. In addition to abdominal pain which is often due to alcoholic gastritis or pancreatitis, the patient may also experience nausea, vomiting, and anorexia. Physical findings include tachypnea, diaphoresis, and orthostasis. Mental status may range from normal to coma [57]. The laboratory findings reveal an elevated anion gap, and metabolic acidosis [58]. The patient will be ketotic with an increase in the β-hydroxybutyrate/acetoacetate ratio. This may lead to a falsely low urinary determination of ketones, since the nitroprusside reaction measures only acetoacetate [59].

The pathogenesis of this condition involves alcohol's ability to block ketogenesis, with a resultant rise in serum fatty acids in a nutritionally starved patient. When the alcohol consumption stops, often as a result of abdominal pain from alcoholic gastritis, pancreatitis or severe liver disease, the ketogenic process is unblocked. The ample quantity of free fatty acids that are then metabolized results in the excess of ketones that heralds the syndrome.

Treatment of alcoholic ketoacidosis consists of correcting fluid and nutrient deficiencies. A restoration of carbohydrate balance and recovery from alcoholism will prevent the recurrence of the syndrome.

D. Hypophosphatemia

Inadequate nutritional intake, injudicious use of antacids, diarrhea, and phosphorus wasting secondary to hypomagnesemia are among the causes of hypophosphatemia in an alcoholic population [60]. Indeed, alcoholism is one of the most common etiologies of hypophosphatemia. Many alcoholic patients present for medical care with normal serum phosphorus levels only to experience a profound decline in their serum phosphorus, 2, 3, or even 4 days after treatment is initiated [60]. This may represent a shift of the extracellular phosphorus to intracellular locations, particularly the hepatocytes [60].

Clinically, the symptoms of hypophosphatemia range from the patient being asymptomatic with minimal decline in serum phosphorus levels to disastrous clinical complications, including rhabdomyolysis, red cell dysfunction, cardiac failure, and central nervous system dysfunction [61].

The treatment consists of prompt administration of supplemental phosphorus; in mild cases, oral administration is adequate, whereas intravenous replacement is necessary for the more profound deficiency state.

E. Hypomagnesemia

Like hypophosphatemia, hypomagnesemia is not uncommon in an alcoholic population. The diathesis for hypomagnesemia in alcoholism stems from inadequate nutritional intake, malabsorption, and renal wasting of magnesium [62]. Magnesium depletion presents as muscle cramping, increased tremulousness, and seizures. Because these are also symptoms of the alcohol withdrawal syndrome, it is not surprising that hypomagnesemia can exacerbate the alcohol withdrawal syndrome [63].

Reestablishing nutritional balance will correct mild hypomagnesemia in the alcoholic patient, whereas severe depletion requires parental replacement.

IX. PSYCHIATRIC COMPLICATIONS OF ALCOHOLISM

A. Alcoholism and Psychopathology

Psychopathology and alcoholism interface in three ways. First, there are those psychiatric disorders which occur in alcoholics with no greater frequency than are seen in the general population. An example is schizophrenia, which is not encountered more frequently in an alcoholic population than in the general population. The second manner in which psychopathology and alcoholism relate is by virtue of correlation; some psychiatric disorders are seen more frequently in alcoholics than in the general population. Antisocial personality disorders and affective disorders are psychiatric illnesses which are encountered in alcoholics more frequently than in the general adult population. The fact that these illnesses are correlated does not necessarily imply that one is a consequence of the other. Indeed, while antisocial personality disorder and affective disorders may exacerbate the course of alcoholism and vice versa, there is no evidence that one causes the other.

Finally, alcoholism can cause certain psychiatric disorders, known as organic mental syndromes. DSM-III-R defines several categories of organic mental syndromes that are associated with alcoholism [38].

B. Alcohol Intoxication

Maladaptive behavioral changes, often precipitated by the disinhibiting effect of ethanol, and neuropsychiatric impairment, are the diagnostic hallmarks of acute alcohol intoxication. As tolerance to alcohol develops with the progression of a patient's alcoholism, the blood alcohol concentration required to produce intoxication will increase.

C. Alcohol Withdrawal

As tolerance continues to increase, and as the patient's alcoholism progresses to a pattern of daily drinking, physical addiction to ethanol may occur. Physical addiction is characterized by a withdrawal syndrome that appears as the blood alcohol concentration declines. Signs and symptoms such as tremulousness, diaphoresis, tachycardia, anorexia, insomnia, agitation, and hypertension occur in the alcohol withdrawal syndrome. The milder form of this syndrome does not progress beyond these symptoms. Some patients with late-stage alcoholism may progress beyond this to a more severe form of alcohol withdrawal in which the patient experiences a toxic psychosis, featuring disorientation, hallucinations, and more severe autonomic hyperactivity. This syndrome has been known for years as delirium tremens, and is referred to in DSM-III-R as alcohol withdrawal, delirium.

D. Alcoholic Hallucinosis

Alcoholic hallucinosis is a relatively uncommon syndrome that is seen most often in male alcoholics 24–72 h after the last drink. Unlike alcohol withdrawal, delirium, the hallucinations which occur in alcoholic hallucinosis are seen in a patient who remains oriented to person, place, and time, and usually has insight into the benign nature of the hallucinations. Also, the syndrome is not accompanied by autonomic hyperactivity. The course of alcoholic hallucinosis is generally a few weeks, although a chronic form has been described [41].

E. Alcohol Amnestic Disorder

Also known as Korsakoff's psychosis, alcohol amenestic disorder is a consequence of thiamine deficiency in alcoholics, which has been discussed with the neurological consequences of alcoholism (see Sect. VI.B).

F. Dementia Associated with Alcoholism

Impaired cognition as a consequence of long-standing alcoholism, with subsequent disruption in social or occupational functioning, has been discussed with other neurological consequences of alcoholism (see Sect. VI).

G. Treating Psychopathology in Alcoholic Patients

Alcoholic patients with coexistent psychopathology present a challenge to the clinician. Patients with psychopathology that coexists independent of or correlates with the patient's alcoholism need to be managed so that both their alcoholism and their psychiatric disorder can be kept in remission simultaneously. If either the alcoholism or the psychiatric illness is left unattended, there is little hope that the untreated illness will stay in remission. For example, an actively drinking alcoholic being treated for depression often will not do well. First, the alcohol exacerbates the depression. Then, the depressed alcoholic patient finds it difficult to follow through with treatment direction; appointments with the physician are not kept, medication is not taken as prescribed. This results in a less than optimal course in the treatment of the depression. The alcoholism undermines the therapeutic efforts of the physician and the therapeutic benefit to the patient. On the other hand, a recovering alcoholic who has depression that has not been recognized and treated will find it difficult to maintain sobriety while enduring periods of hopelessness and despair created by the depressive disorder.

Patients with organic mental syndromes secondary to their alcoholism must have treatment initiated for these conditions prior to being treated for their alcoholism. The cognitive impairment that accompanies these disorders, if untreated, makes recovery from alcoholism difficult at best. Promptly initiating treatment for the organic mental disorder, followed by or in conjunction with definitive treatment for their alcoholism, will provide the patient with an opportunity to preclude future complications of their alcoholism.

X. OTHER MEDICAL COMPLICATIONS OF ALCOHOLISM

A. Alcohol-Induced Muscle Disease

Skeletal muscle pathology in alcoholics occurs in two distinct clinical patterns. The first is an acute alcoholic myopathy. This syndrome occurs most often in binging alcoholics, and is thought to be due to an acute toxic effect of ethanol on the muscle tissue. This syndrome is characterized by a spectrum of severity, ranging from an asymptomatic course marked only by a transient rise in serum creatine kinase, to a severe form with pain and swelling of the muscles, myoglobinuria, and some muscle cell necrosis [64]. Rhabdomyolysis can also occur in this severe form of alcoholic myopathy, and can precipitate acute renal failure, which may prove fatal. Most often, however, this relatively uncommon syndrome is self-limited, with recovery occuring over 1–2 weeks [65].

Chronic alcoholic myopathy is an insidious progressive syndrome not infrequently seen in nutritionally deprived patients with late-stage alcoholism. Muscle atrophy, with subsequent weakness, especially of the hips and shoulders, is the usual presentation [65].

Treatment of alcoholic myopathies consists of correcting any coexistent fluid and electrolyte imbalance, reestablishing nutritional balance, and helping the patient begin the process of recovery from alcoholism.

B. Endocrine Effects of Alcohol

Hypothalamic-Pituitary-Gonadal Function

In male alcoholics, serum testosterone levels are depressed by a combination of ethanol's toxic effect on the hypothalamic-pituitary axis and via direct suppression of testicular testosterone production [66]. Additionally, estrogen levels in alcoholic males will rise as a result of the diminished ability of the alcoholic liver to metabolize endogenous estrogens. The hypogonadism induced by alcohol's effect on the endocrine system results in decreased sperm counts, loss of libido, impotence, and testicular atrophy. Rising serum estrogen levels with subsequent feminization is characterized by gynecomastia, spider angiomas, and a more female pattern of fat distribution [67].

Menstrual irregularities, including amenorrhea and menorrhagia, contribute to an increased frequency of gynecologic interventions, especially dilatation and curettage in alcoholic women [68]. The effect of alcohol on the fertility of alcoholic women is equivocal [68].

Abstinence from alcohol will begin to reduce the gonadal consequences of alcoholism in both men and women.

Alcohol's Effect on the Adrenal System

Alcohol is capable of inducing elevated plasma cortisol levels, which may create what is known as the pseudo–Cushing's syndrome [69]. Clinically, the patient presents with a long history of alcoholic drinking and facial edema, elevated blood pressure, truncal obesity, weakness, fatigue, easy bruising, muscle wasting, and hirsutism [67]. In patients with pseudo–Cushing's syndrome, unlike those afflicted with true Cushing's syndrome, abstinence from alcohol will result in resolution of the syndrome over several weeks.

C. Fetal Effects of Alcohol

In 1968, LeMoine described a pattern of growth and developmental retardation, facial, limb, and cardiac anomalies in the progeny of alcoholic women who drank during their pregnancy [70]. These early reports of what is now called the fetal alcohol syndrome have been followed by documentation of a spectrum of alcohol's effect on the unborn child, ranging from the full-blown clinical syndrome of growth deficiency, central nervous system dysfunction, and facial dysmorphia, to a more incidious effect that must be measured longitudinally to demonstrate consistently decreased cognitive performance in children subjected in utero to as little as three drinks per day [71].

The prudent and only recommendation by physicians to women who either are, or are attempting to become pregnant, is to abstain from alcohol. Pregnant women who are advised to abstain but find themselves unable to do so, despite good intentions, may require treatment for alcoholism as a means of assisting them in maintaining abstinence.

D. Dermatological Conditions and Alcoholism

Conclusive evidence that there is a causal relationship between the development of specific dermatological disease and alcoholism is lacking. One dermatological condition that has historically been linked with alcoholism is acne rosacea, a facial eruption characterized by erythema and acnelike lesions. A form of rosacea, known as rhinophyma, is recognized as the stereotypic red bulbous nose of alcoholics. However, while rhinophyma, like rosacea, may be exacerbated by alcoholism, it is not directly caused by alcoholism, and it may occur in nonalcoholic individuals. Other cutaneous changes which may point to alcoholic liver disease include palmar erythema, vascular spiders, Dupuytren's contracture, and white nails. However, it should be remembered that these are cutaneous signs of not only alcoholic liver disease, but also of any significant hepatocellular dysfunction regardless of etiology.

E. Alcohol and Trauma

Traumatic injuries are yet another way in which alcoholics incur medical consequences secondary to their illness. Over half of all motor vehicle fatalities involve alcohol [72,73]. Alcohol markedly impairs cognition, judgment, motor skills, and reaction time, placing the drinking driver at significantly higher risk of experiencing a motor vehicle accident. These same impairments result in other forms of trauma occurring more frequently in drinkers. Burn injuries, drowning, farm accidents, and industrial injuries are often associated with intercurrent alcoholism [74]. Despite the fact that alcohol's association with trauma has been recognized for years, many patients who survive alcohol-related trauma are not evaluated for alcoholism. By not treating the alcoholism in those trauma victims who have experienced alcohol-related trauma, the health care system is acting as an enabler for the patient's alcoholism; mending the consequences of the alcoholism without treating the disease itself allows the alcoholism to progress, and keeps the patient at risk for experiencing more consequences, including future traumatic injury. All trauma victims with a blood alcohol concentration greater than zero at the time of their accident should receive an assessment for alcoholism as a routine component of the medical management of their trauma.

REFERENCES

1. Cyr, M.G., and Wartman, S.C. (1988). The effectiveness of routine screening questions in the detection of alcoholism, *J.A.M.A., 259*:51–58.
2. Barcha, R., Stewart, M.A., and Guze, S.B. (1968). The prevalence of alcoholism among general hospital ward patients, *Am. J. Psychiatry, 125*:681–684.
3. Bowen, O.R., and Sammons, J.H. (1988). The alcohol-abusing patient: A challenge to the profession, *J.A.M.A., 260*:2267–2268.
4. Tuyns, A.J. (1970). Cancer of the esophagus: Further evidence of the relation to drinking habits in France, *Int. J. Cancer, 5*:152–156.
5. Beaumont, W. (1959). *Experiments and Observations on the Gastric Juice and the Physiology of Digestion*, Dover, New York.
6. Dinuso, V.P., Chey, W.Y., and Braverman, S.P. (1972). Gastric secretion and gastric mucosal morphology in chronic alcoholics, *Arch. Intern. Med., 130*:715–719.
7. Roe, D.A. (1981). Nutritional concerns in the alcoholic, *J. Am. Dietary Assoc., 78*:17–21.
8. Sheehy, T.W. (1980). Acute alcoholic pancreatitis, *Cont. Ed. Fam. Physician, 3*:87–109.
9. Malagelada, J.R. (1986). The pathophysiology of alcoholic pancreatitis, *Pancrease, 1*:270–278.

10. Geokas, M.C. (1984). Ethanol and the pancreas, *Med. Clin. North Am.*, 68(1):57-75.
11. Mendenhall, C.L. (1978). What to do for alcoholic liver disease, *Consultant*, 12:23-77.
12. Morgan, M.Y., and Sherlock, S. (1977). Sex-related differences among 100 patients with alcoholic liver disease, *Br. Med. J.*, 1:939-941.
13. Jones, D.P. (1982). Alcohol and the liver, *JOM*, 24:735-740.
14. Borowsky, S.A. (1981). Continued heavy drinking and survival in alcoholic cirrhosis, *Gastroenterology*, 80:1405.
15. Orrego, H.O., Blake, J.E., Blendis, L.M., Compton, K.V., and Israel, Y. (1987). Long-term treatment of alcoholic liver disease with propylthiouracil, *N. Engl. J. Med.* 317:1421-1426.
16. Clark, V.A., Chapman, J.M., and Coulson, A.H. (1967). Effects of various factors on systolic and diastolic blood pressure in the Los Angeles heart study, *J. Chron. Dis.*, 20:571-581.
17. Kannel, W.B., and Sorlie, P. (1975). Hypertension in Framingham, *Epidemiology and Control of Hypertension* (O. Paul, ed.), Stratton Intercontinental, New York, pp. 553-590.
18. Veshima, H., Shimamoto, T., Iada, M., Konishi, M., Tanigaki, M., Doi, M., Tsujioka, K., Nagano, E., Tusuda, C., Uzawa, H., Kojima, S., and Komachi, Y. (1984). Alcohol intake and hypertension among urban and rural Japanese populations, *J. Chron. Dis.*, 37:585-592.
19. Klatsky, A.L., Friedman, G.D., Siegelaub, A.B., and Gerard, M.J. (1977). Alcohol consumption and blood pressure: Kaiser-Permanente multiphasic health examination data, *N. Engl. J. Med.*, 296:1194-1200.
20. Maheswaran, R., Potter, J.F., and Beevers, D.G. (1986). The role of alcohol in hypertension, *J. Clin. Hypertension*, 2:172-178.
21. Saunders, J.B., Beevers, D.G., Paton, A. (1981). Alcohol-induced hypertension, *Lancet*, 2:653-656.
22. Potter, J.F., and Beevers, D.G. (1984). Pressor effect of alcohol in hypertension, *Lancet*, 2:119-122.
23. McCall, D. (1987). Alcohol and the cardiovascular system, *Curr. Prob. Cardiol.*, 12:353-414.
24. DeMakis, J.G., Proskey, A., and Rahimtoola, S.H. (1974). The natural course of alcoholic cardiomyopathy, *Ann. Intern. Med.*, 80:293.
25. Ettinger, P.O., Wu, C.F., DeLaCruz, C., Weisse, A.B., Ahmed, S.S., and Regan, T.J. (1978). Arrhythmias and the "holiday heart": Alcohol-associated cardiac rhythm disturbances, *Am. Heart J.*, 95:555-562.
26. D'Alonzo, C.A., and Pell, S. (1968). Cardiovascular disease among problem drinkers, *J. Occup. Med.*, 10:344.
27. Sereny, G. (1971). Effects of alcohol on the electrocardiogram, *Circulation* 44:558.
28. Greenspon, A.J., and Schaal, S.F. (1983). The "holiday heart": Electrophysiologic studies of alcohol's effects in alcoholics, *Ann. Intern. Med.*, 98:135.
29. Yanu, K., Rhoads, G.G., and Kagan, A. (1977). Coffee, alcohol, and risk of coronary heart disease among Japanese men living in Hawaii, *N. Engl. J. Med.*, 297:405.
30. Klatsky, A.L., Armstrong, M.A., and Friedman, G.D. (1986). Relations of alcoholic beverage use to subsequent coronary disease hospitalizations, *Am. J. Cardiol.*, 58:710.
31. Blackwelder, W.C., Yano, K., and Rhoads, G.C. (1980). Alcohol and mortality: The Honolulu hearty study, *Am. J. Med.*, 68:164-170.
32. Chanarin, I. (1982). Hemopoiesis and alcohol, *Med. Clin. North Am.*, 68:179.
33. McCurdy, P.R., and Rath, C.E. (1980). Vacuolated nucleated bone marrow cells in alcoholism, *Sem. Hematol.*, 17:100.
34. Girard, D.E., Kumar, K.K., and McAfee, J.H. (1987). Hematologic effects of acute and chronic alcohol abuse, *Hematol. Clin. North Am.*, 1:321-333.
35. Herbert, V. (1985). Megaloblastic anemias, *Lab. Invest.*, 52:3.
36. MacGregor, R.R. (1986). Alcohol and immune defense, *J.A.M.A.*, 256:1474-1479.
37. Cowan, D.H. (1980). Effect of alcohol on hemostasis, *Sem. Hematol.*, 17:137.
38. American Psychiatric Association (1987): *Diagnostic and Statistical Manual of Menal Disorders*, 3rd ed.-Revised, Washington, D.C., pp. 123-163.
39. Tarter, R.E., and Edwards, K.L. (1986). Multifactorial etiology of neuropsychiatric impairment in alcoholics, *Alcohol. Clin. Exp. Res.*, 10:128-135.

40. Ron, M.A., Acker, W., Shaw, G.K., and Lishman, W. (1982). Computerized tomography of the brain in chronic alcoholics, *Brain, 105*:497–514.

41. Shaw, G.K., Spence, M. (1985). Psychological impairment in alcoholics, *Alcohol, 22*:243–249.

42. Phillips, S.C., Harper, C., and Kril, J.A. (1987). A quantitative histological study of the cerebellar vermis in alcoholic patients, *Brain, 110*:301–314.

43. Bedi, A.B., Benzer, D.G., and Dries, R.W. (1986). Clinical recognition and treatment of the Wernicke-Korsakoff syndrome as a cause of neuropsychiatric disturbance, *Int. Med. Spec. 7*(4):49–62.

44. Torvik, A., Lindboe, C.F., and Rogde, S. (1982). Brain lesions in alcoholics, *J. Neurol. Sci., 56*:233–248.

45. Donahue, R.P., Abbott, R.D., Reed, D.M., and Yano, K. (1986). Alcohol and hemorrhagic stroke, *J.A.M.A., 255*:2311–2314.

46. Weisberg, L.A. (1988). Alcoholic intracerebral hemorrhage, stroke, *19*:1565–1569.

47. Echevarria, M.G. (1881). On alcoholic epilepsy, *J. Ment. Sci., 26*:489.

48. Brennan, F.N., Lyttle, J.A. (1987). Alcohol and seizures: A review, *J. Roy. Soc. Med., 80*:571–573.

49. Tuyns, A.J. (1982). Incidence trends of laryngeal cancer in relation to national alcohol and tobacco consumption, *Trends in Cancer Incidence* (K. Magnus, ed.), Hemisphere, Washington, D.C.

50. Breslow, N.E., and Enstrom, J.E. (1974). Geographic correlations between cancer mortality rates and alcohol-tobacco consumption in the United States, *J. Natl. Cancer Inst., 53*:631.

51. Tuyns, A.J. (1987). Cancer risks derived from alcohol, *Med. Oncol. Tumor Pharmacother., 4*:241–244.

52. Tuyns, A.J., Pequignot, G., and Abatucci, J.S. (1979). Oesophageal cancer and alcohol consumption. Importance of type of beverage, *Int. J. Cancer, 23*:443–447.

53. Brechot, C., Nalpas, B., and Courouche, A.M. (1982). Evidence that hepatitis B virus has a role in liver-cell carcinoma in alcoholic liver disease, *N. Engl. J. Med., 306*:1384–1387.

54. Le, M.G., Moulton, L.H., Hill, C., and Kramar, A. (1986). Consumption of dairy products and alcohol in a case-control study of breast cancer, *J.N.C.I., 77*:633–636.

55. O'Connell, D.L., Hulka, B.S., Chambless, L.F., Wilkinson, W.E., and Deubner, D.C. (1987). Cigarette smoking, alcohol consumption, and breast cancer risks, *J.N.C.I., 78*:229–234.

56. World, M.J., Ryle, P.R., Jones, D., Shaw, G.K., and Thomson, A.D. (1984). Folate levels in alcoholics, *Alcohol, 19*:281–290.

57. Palmer, J.P. (1983). Alcoholic ketoacidosis: Clinical and laboratory presentation, pathophysiology and treatment, *Clin. Endocrinol. Metab., 12*:381–389.

58. Adams, S.L., Mathews, J.J., and Flaherty, J.J. (1987). Alcoholic ketoacidosis, *Ann. Emerg. Med., 16*:90–97.

59. Williams, H.E. (1984). Alcoholic hypoglycemia and ketoacidosis, *Med. Clin. North Am., 68*:33–38.

60. Knochel, J.P. (1977). The pathophysiology and clinical characteristics of severe hypophosphatemia, *Arch. Intern. Med., 137*:203–220.

61. Knochel, J.P. (1980). Hypophosphatemia in the alcoholic, *Arch. Intern. Med., 140*:613–615.

62. Kaysen, G., Noth, R.H. (1984). The effects of alcohol on blood pressure and electrolytes, *Med. Clin. North Am., 68*:221–246.

63. Fink, E.B. (1986). Magnesium deficiency in alcoholism, *Alcohol. Clin. Exp. res. 10*:591–594.

64. Oh, S.J. (1972). Alcoholic myopathy: A critical review, *Ala. J. Med. Sci., 9*:79–95.

65. Haller, R.G., and Knochel, J.P. (1984). Skeletal muscle disease in alcoholism, *Med. Clin. North. Am., 68*:91–103.

66. Van Thiel, D.H., and Gavalor, J.S. (1982). The adverse effects of ethanol upon hypothalamic-pituitary-gonadal function in males and females compared and contrasted, *Alcohol. Clin. Exp. res., 6*:179–185.

67. Noth, R.H., and Walter, R.M. (1984). The effects of alcohol on the endocrine system, *Med. Clin. North Am., 68*:133–146.

68. Becker, V., Tonnesen, H., Kaas-Claesson, N., and Gluud, C. (1989). Menstrual disturbances and fertility in chronic alcoholic women, *Drug Alcohol Depend., 24*:75–82.

69. Smals, A.G., Kloppenborg, P.W., and Njo, K.T. (1976). Alcohol-induced Cushingoid syndrome, *Br. Med. J., 2*:1298.

70. Lemoine, P., Harousseau, H., and Borteyru, J.P. (1968). Les enfants des parents alcoolques: anomalies observees, *Quest Sem. Log. Med., 25*:476–482.

71. Streissguth, A.P., Martin, D.C., and Barr, H.M. (1983). Intrauterine alcohol exposure and attentional decrements in 4-year-old children, *Alcohol. Clin. Exp. Res., 7*:122.

72. Herve, C., Gaillard, M., Roujas, F., and Huguenard, P. (1986). Alcoholism in polytrauma, *J. Trauma, 26*:1123–1126.

73. Vine, J., and Watson, T.R. (1983). Incidence of drug and alcohol intake in road traffic accident victims, *Med. J. Aust., 44*:17–25.

74. Moessner, H. (1979). Accidents as a symptom of alcohol abuse, *J. Fam. Pract., 8*:1143–1146.

32

Medical Complications of Drug Addiction

Charles J. Engel and David G. Benzer
Milwaukee Psychiatric Hospital, Wauwatosa, Wisconsin

I. INTRODUCTION

The current epidemic of psychoactive drug addiction is entering its fourth decade. The National Institute on Drug Abuse has estimated that during the 1960s, only 5% of the U.S. population used illict drugs [1]. By the 1970s, the figure had risen to 10%, and by the early 1980s, the proportion of those who had ever used an illicit drug had climbed to almost 37%. The 1988 National Institute for Drug Abuse Household Survey found that although the number of "current users"—those who used drugs within the 30 days prior to the study—dropped from 23 million in 1985 to 14.5 million in 1988, other disturbing trends emerged [1]. Of Americans aged 20–40, 22% had used an illegal drug within the past year, while the number of Americans using cocaine at least once per week rose 33% from 1985 to 1988. Applying diagnostic criteria from the *Diagnostic and Statistical Manual of Mental Disorders* of the American Psychiatric Association, the National Institute of Mental Health surveyed adults in three representative cities in the United States in the early part of the 1980s. Based on their data, drug abuse or dependence was projected to affect 3.1 million Americans within the 6 months prior to that survey [2]. Drug dependency disorders were estimated in 1983 to have a direct cost of $2 billion per year, and an indirect cost of $47 billion per year in the United States [3]. There were an estimated 6000 deaths in 1980 due to drug-related causes, including overdose and homicide. The current stimulant epideic has brought with it even more morbidity and mortality owing to overdose and trauma. Chemically dependent patients are well-known overutilizers of the health care system, utilizing approximately twice the health care resources as compared to the non–drug dependent population. In contrast, costs of health care have been shown to be decreased after treatment for chemical dependency. This economic benefit of treating drug addiction is in addition to the obvious sparing of morbidity and human suffering [3].

As the sampling of statistical data from the previous decade indicates, the social and economic cost of drug addiction in the United States is staggering. The level of concern that these costs have evoked at the end of the 1980s gave rise to much military imagery (i.e., the "war on drugs").

Physicians have, for centuries, been familiar with this concept of "fighting" a disease. It is to physicians that many of the complications of drug addiction will first present. It is incumbent upon physicians to not only treat the complications, but also to extend diagnosis and treatment to the underlying illness, i.e., chemical dependency.

II. MEDICAL COMPLICATIONS OF COCAINE ADDICTION

Cocaine use in the United States during the 1970s and 1980s reached widespread, even epidemic, proportions. By the mid-1980s, it was estimated that at least 30 million Americans had used cocaine, with 5 million of those being regular users. At least 1 million Americans were cocaine dependent [4]. In addition to an increased prevalence of usage has come an increasing purity of the drug, from approximately 15% purity in street cocaine several years ago to 80% or more in "crack" cocaine today [5]. With this increased prevalence of use and purity of drug has come an ever-expanding recognition of the morbidity associated with cocaine consumption. The medical literature in the past 5 years has witnessed an explosion of publications detailing the medical complications of cocaine use.

A. Cardiac Complications

Cocaine is a powerful stimulator of central and peripheral adrenergic functions. It appears to act by blocking the presynaptic reuptake of various catecholamines and neurotransmitters, including dopamine, norepinephrine, and serotonin [6]. Chronic use produces postsynaptic receptor hypersensitivity. Cocaine use is associated with tachycardia, hypertension, hyperpyrexia, and tachypnea. The spectrum of cardiovascular consequences of cocaine use is broad, including arrhythmias, ischemia, myocardial infarction, and sudden death.

Arrhythmia

The intranasal insufflation of 100 mg of cocaine, which is a typical recreational dose, produces an elevation of the heart rate of approximately 20 beats/min, with an increase of both systolic and diastolic blood pressure of approximately 20 mm Hg [7]. In studies of normal volunteers, cocaine appears to have relatively modest arrhythmogenic potential. However, a variety of superventricular and ventricular arrhythmias, including ventricular tachycardia and ventricular fibrillation, have been reported as consequences of cocaine ingestion, although some of these reported cases of arrhythmia have occurred in individuals with recent myocardial infarction or ischemic episodes, in which arrhythmias are regularly seen.

Ischemia

The capacity of cocaine to produce chest pain is one commonly encountered in clinical medicine in the 1980s. In a study of patients undergoing cardiac catheterization as part of a work-up for chest pain, intranasal cocaine administration in a dose of 110–200 mg was administered. These doses are equivalent to street doses of cocaine as well as equivalent to doses of cocaine used in otorhinolaryngological procedures. Coronary sinus flow was decreased 17%, coronary vascular resistance was increased 33%, and the diameter of the coronary vasculature was decreased 8–12% [8]. The relationship of cocaine use to acute myocardial infarction is clear, with at least 58 reported cases in the medical literature [5]. Angiographic studies have been performed after myocardial infarction in 45 out of the 58 cases. In most cases, underlying fixed coronary disease was not demonstrated. Pathogenic mechanisms proposed include focal vasoconstriction or spasm, thrombosis, and intimal proliferation of coronary arterioles.

Myocarditis

Leukocytic and eosinophilic infiltrates have been found in cardiac muscle obtained by biopsy or at necropsy in cocaine users [7,9]. Polydrug use, including adulterants in street cocaine, as well as concomitant alcohol use, make a causal relationship unclear. Hypersensitivity to cocaine has been postulated as a possible mechanism.

Contraction Band Necrosis

Contraction band necrosis is a nonspecific histopathological finding, apparently occurring when hyperstimulated myocytes "ratchet" past each other with resultant cell destruction and fibrotic response. This phenomenon may be a reflection of elevated intracytosolic calcium levels, the most common cause of which being elevated catecholamine levels [9].

Chronic Heart Failure

A number of case reports of dilated cardiomyopathy in cocaine abusers have emerged; however, few of these reports have cleanly linked cocaine to this condition [9]. In most cases, the clinical picture is confounded by concomitant use of other drugs, including alcohol. Patients with pheochromocytoma have a cardiac picture which is very similar to that reported in these cases in cocaine addicts. It does make sense to think that long-term use of cocaine could similarly produce a cardiomyopathy. Diffuse contraction band necrosis is seen in pheochromocytoma-related cardiomyopathy, just as it is in cocaine cases.

B. Neurological Complications

Headache

Headache is not an infrequent complaint among cocaine-dependent individuals. Headache is, by now, a well-recognized prodrome of cerebrovascular events. The occurrence of headache after the use of cocaine should prompt the clinician to carry out a work-up for underlying cerebrovascular pathology, including arteriovenous malformations or aneurysms [6]. Migrainelike headache has been reported as occurring after the use of cocaine [10]. These patients developed a pattern of readministration of cocaine in order to forestall the reemergence of the headache. In these cases, work-ups were negative, and the patients subsequently remained headache-free as long as they remained abstinent from cocaine. These findings raise the question of the role of serotinin depletion as a mechanism for headache production. Migraine typically responds to serotonin-enhancing drugs such as ergotamine. The pharmacological effect of cocaine is to increase concentrations of serotinin in the synaptic space, but owing to inhibited reuptake, the serotonergic system is ultimately depleted. The headaches described in these patients can be thought of as withdrawal headaches.

Stroke

Cocaine is recognized as a common cause of cerebrovascular accident (CVA), particularly in young people [11]. Hemorrhagic strokes are approximately two times more common than cerebral infarctions, with the bleed typically taking place from an arteriovenous malformation or aneurysm [11]. The location of the CVAs in these patients includes structures that are rarely involved in young individuals, including thalamic infarctions and occlusions of the spinal artery. The exact mechanism in most cases is uncertain, but hypertension, increased platelet aggregation, vasospasm, cardiogenic emboli, vasculitis, and arterial wall thickening have all been implicated [11,6]. There is at least one report of stroke in a neonate occurring following maternal cocaine use approximately 15 h prior to delivery [12].

Transient Ischemic Attacks

Transient ischemic attacks (TIAs) as a consequence of cocaine use are well described, including involvement of the middle cerebral and vertebrobasilar artery systems [13].

Cerebral Vasculitis

Cerebral vasculitis has been known to be a complication of intravenous methamphetamine use. There is at least one case report of vasculitis of the internal carotid artery secondary to intranasal cocaine use [14]. The angiographic studies demonstrated irregularity and narrowing (beading) of the right internal carotid artery. The patient was treated with steroids with significant improvement.

Seizures

Seizures have long been recognized as a complication of cocaine ingestion. Studies in animals, though not in humans, have demonstrated that the phenomenon of "kindling," or reverse tolerance, occurs, lowering the seizure threshold. Most cases of seizure reported after cocaine ingestion have been generalized, although there have been reports of partial complex seizures as well [13,15]. Additionally, there is a case report of a patient with an adequately controlled seizure disorder who experienced reemergence of her seizure activity after initiation of cocaine use, though still on her anticonvulsant [15]. In a few cases, focal changes have been seen on EEG, and most cases studied have been accompanied by normal computed tomographic (CT) scans. Seizures have resulted from administration of cocaine by all routes. Intravenous diazepam has been useful in the acute management of these seizures. As in alcohol withdrawal seizures, long-term administration of anticonvulsants is not indicated.

C. Pulmonary Complications

Upper airway complications of cocaine dependence are primarily limited to intranasal use, whereas disease of the lower respiratory tract is usually limited to free-base cocaine use.

Pulmonary Function

Free-base cocaine use can result in diminished diffusing capacity (DLCO) [16]. These changes have been found to persist even after cessation of cocaine consumption. How much of this diminution of diffusing capacity is due to cocaine versus the contribution of tobacco or cannabis use is uncertain.

Pulmonary Hemorrhage

There are two reported cases of frank pulmonary hemorrhage in free-base cocaine users [17,18]. In one case, removal of a portion of the lung was necessary in order to control the hemorrhage. The mechanism of hemorrhage in these cases is uncertain. Hermosiderin-laden pulmonary macrophages have been demonstrated in approximately one-third of cases of individuals dying of cocaine-mediated sudden death, suggesting that lesser degrees of pulmonary hemorrhage are fairly common in free-base cocaine users.

Crack Lung

A syndrome of patchy pulmonary infiltrates, airway obstruction, fever, peripheral blood eosinophilia, strikingly elevated immunoglobulin , and pruritus was described in one patient, and was termed the "crack lung" syndrome [19]. This particular patient experienced an exacerbation of her symptom complex on two occasions following relapse to cocaine use. Unfortunately, while no samples of cocaine were available for analysis, the authors made a fairly clear case for cocaine as the causative agent. Pneumothorax, pneumoediastinum, and pneumopericardium have also been reported as a result of free-base cocaine use [6]. These complications seem likely to be due to the pecularities of the smoking technique in freebase cocaine users. These techniques involve deep inspiration of cocaine vapor, followed by a Valsalva maneuver. Sometimes, the technique is modified by the application of positive airway pressure by the drug user's partner, a technique known as "shotgunning." Some of the victims of this smoking technique have required chest tube insertion, but in most cases, they have had complete recovery with conservative treatment. There have also been isolated reports of pulmonary edema secondary to cocaine use.

D. Other Medical Complications

Nasal Septal Perforation

Upper airway morbidity due to cocaine use is primarily related to intranasal insufflation, and includes sinusitis, osteitis, and perforation of the nasal septum [6,20]. Nasal septal perforation is commonly encountered in clinical practice, and probably results from a combination of the traumatic effect of inhaling sharp-edged cocaine crystals at high velocity, repeated cycles of mucosal vasoconstriction and tissue hypoxia, and mucosal anesthesia and trauma. The symptoms of nasal septal perforation include, initially, nasal crusting, bleeding, pain, followed by whistling on inspiration.

Cocaine-Induced Rhabdomyolysis

Along with heroin, amphetamines, phencyclidine, and toluene, cocaine has become increasingly recognized as a cause of rhabdomyolysis [21]. In one large series of 39 cases associated with cocaine use, 28 of the patients had urine toxicology positive for cocaine or its metabolite [22]. The putative mechanism of rhabdomyolysis in these cocaine-related cases include severe trauma, limb compression, and repetitive seizures. Additionally, high tissue catecholamine levels result in elevated intracellular calcium concentrations, which initiates a sequence of events known to result in self-destruction [23].

Acute Renal Failure

Three cases of acute renal failure have been reported in cocaine abusers, all of whom had clear-cut evidence of rhabdomyolysis [24]. The clinical picture was one of acute tubular necrosis with rapid rise of BUN and creatinine, along with normal-sized kidneys and good urinary output.

Endocrinological Effects of Cocaine Dependency

In men, both impotence and gynecomastia have been reported in chronic users of cocaine. Female cocaine-dependent patients may experience amenorrhea, infertility, and galactorrhea. Lactation in a nonparturient female may be a clinical manifestation of cocaine dependency. Prolactin secretion is under dopaminergic inhibitory control. The dopamine depletion which results from chronic cocaine use results in rebound elevation of prolactin levels, thereby stimulating lactation [25].

Hepatic Complications of Cocaine Dependency

The relationship of hepatic disease to cocaine dependency is unclear at the present time. Studies in mice demonstrate a pattern of periportal necrosis and inflammation, whereas the centralobular regions are relatively spared [26]. There is one report in the literature of a case of hepatic disease in a human [27]. In that case, the histopathology was very similar to that reported in the animal studies. Reports of liver function abnormality in cocaine abusers are confounded by concurrent other drug use, notably alcohol.

E. Other Stimulants

The 1970s and 1980s have seen the emergence of stimulant drug combinations, many available without prescription, which have the potential for significant morbidity. Phenylpropanolamine (PPA) is a sympathomimetic drug present in over 100 propriety and prescription drug combinations. In a 1980 survey, it was the fifth most commonly used drug. It is found in anorectics, nasal decongestants, psychostimulants, and premenstrual syndrome agents. Phenylpropanolamine is an agent with relatively potent alpha-adrenergic agonist properties, and is capable of releasing norepinephrine. Its beta-agonist properties are relatively mild, resulting in a typical pattern of hypertension with reflex bradycardia. Commonly, PPA is combined with other stimulants, including ephedrine, pseudoephedrine, and caffeine, which produces a mixed clinical picture. Since 1980, at least 131 adverse reactions involving phenylpropanolamine, including 12 deaths, have been reported to the U.S. Food and Drug Administration (FDA) [28]. Phenylpropanolamine has a low therapeutic index with severe hypertensive reactions produced at doses less than three times the over-the-counter dose of 37.5 mg. Other reported complications of phenylpropanolamine include siezures, intracerebral hemorrhage, rhabdomyolysis, acute renal failure, and a paranoid psychosis, which may persist long after the acute episode [29].

III. MEDICAL COMPLICATIONS OF TOBACCO ADDICTION

The history of tobacco use in the Western Hemisphere dates back to pre-Columbian Indian populations. The epidemic of cigarette smoking in the United States peaked in 1963, and since that time has been gradually declining.

Tobacco smoke is composed of three primary components: nicotine, carbon monoxide, and tar. Tar is that component of the particulate phase which remains after nicotine and water have been extracted, and contains a number of documented carcinogens [30]. Nicotine is a self-reenforcing drug, in that animals will self-administer nicotine, but it appears to be a less potent reenforcer than cocaine or amphetamine [31]. Nicotine stimulates the release of norepinephrine, and may either increase or decrease the release of acetylcholine, depending on the dose administered.

A host of human diseases are related to tobacco dependence, and this section will attempt to highlight only the more salient correlates. For more complete reviews of this subject, the reader is referred to the reports issued by the Surgeon General of the United States in 1988 [32], 1981 [33] and 1979 [34].

A. Cardiorespiratory Complications

In general, the likelihood of medical complications due to tobacco dependency is directly related to dose of tobacco, generally expressed as "pack years." The overall mortality rate in smokers of two packs per day is increased twofold compared to nonsmokers. By age 75, 50% of smokers are dead, compared with only 25% of nonsmokers. Yearly, there are at least 300,000 deaths in the United States due to tobacco-related diseases; 120,000 deaths due to lung cancer alone. There are 170,000 deaths in the United States each year due to coronary artery disease, and 50,000 deaths due to chronic obstructive lung disease, illnesses which are clearly exacerbated by smoking. Thirty percent of the mortality due to coronary artery disease is postulated to be related to tobacco dependence [33]. Cerebrovascular disease and peripheral vascular disease are also tobacco-related diseases. Carboxyhemoglobin levels in smokers are two to 15 times greater than in nonsmokers; carbon monoxide is believed to have a role in the sudden death syndrome.

Cigar smoking is associated with increased mortality, but not to the degree of cigarette smoking [30,31]. Pipe smokers have a slightly increased mortality compared to the nonsmoking population [30]. These differences in mortality, depending on smoking technique, probably relate to the degree of inhalation of smoke which is practiced.

The cessation of tobacco use does bring with it a gradual decrease in the risk of development of smoking related disorders [30]. However, a study of British male former smokers, who had been abstinent for 10–20 years, demonstrated that they still had twice the risk of coronary artery disease as their nonsmoking counterparts [43].

Data from the Berlin-Bremen study indicate that there is a negative time correlation between smoking and high-density lipoprotein (HDL)–cholesterol levels [38]. Even short-term exposure of 1–2 years produced decrements of HDL cholesterol, averaging 0.6 mg/dl in those smoking one to 39 cigarettes per week, and 4.4 mg/dl in those smoking greater than 40 cigarettes per week. This study suggests that even short-term exposure at relatively low levels of tobacco consumption may have atherogenic implications.

The use of tobacco by pregnant women is associated with increased rates of spontaneous abortion, preterm birth, fetal and infant death, and with low birth-weight infants [33]. There is also evidence to suggest an increased risk of sudden infant death syndrome. The mechanism of these deleterious effects in pregnant women and their offspring is unclear at the present time.

B. Cancer

A number of cancers are linked to smoking, including lung (80–90% tobacco-related), larynx, oral cavity, esophagus, bladder, and pancreas [35]. The carcinogenic potential in these cases is, in all probability, related to the components of tar rather than nicotine or carbon monoxide. The risk of bladder cancer in smokers is approximately two times that of nonsmokers, and has been linked to pack years [36]. However, the striking association of smoking with lung cancer is not seen in the case of bladder cancer [37].

The contribution of smoking to the development of chronic obstructive lung disease is mediated through the effects of tobacco smoke on pulmonary immune function, effects on proteolytic enzymes, and disruption of normal ciliary clearance mechanisms. Additionally, smoking acts in a synergistic manner with asbestos exposure to produce lung cancers [30].

C. Smokeless Tobacco

Smokeless tobacco is marketed either as chewing tobacco, moist snuff, or dry snuff, and carries with its use serious medical complications. Sales of smokeless tobacco have increased at the rate of 11%/year since the early 1970s [39]. Currently, there are an estimated 7 to 12 million users, the majority of whom are young men between the ages of 16 and 19. The use of smokeless tobacco may produce oral leukoplakia, some cases of which will show dysplastic changes [40]. Studies of intraoral cancers resulting from smokeless tobacco use demonstrate that cancers tend to occur at the exact site of placement of the tobacco quid [41]. These tumors tend to be verrucous and squamous cell carcinomas of relatively low histological grade. There is also some evidence of increased risk of esophageal carcinoma in users of smokeless tobacco [42]. A less serious complication is that of marked gingival recession in chronic users.

IV. MEDICAL COMPLICATIONS OF MARIJUANA (CANNABIS) ADDICTION

Marijuana remains the most widely used illicit drug in the United States [44,52]. There has been a long-standing controversy regarding the safety and medical consequences of marijuana use. The lack of consensus among medical and scientific experts during the 1960s and 1970s, a time when cannabis usage increased dramatically, contributed to attitudes on the part of a sizable portion of the general population that marijuana is not a particularly dangerous drug; not uncommonly, even in the late 1980s, one encounters patients who see cannabis as being nothing more than an "herb," and describe it as an "organic" product. The Institute of Medicine's Report of 1982 helped to put our understanding of the health consequences of cannabis use into greater perspective [45].

When considering the acute and chronic toxicity of cannabis, it is important to recognize that the potency of cannabis products currently available in the United States is significantly greater than that available several years ago. Since 1975, the potency of marijuana in the United States, as measued by the percentage of delta-9-tetrahydrocannabinol (Δ-9-THC), has tripled from 1.2 to 4.1% [44]. The concentration of psychoactive compounds, particularly delta-9-THC, may range up to 14%.

A. Method of Use

In the United States, the primary route of use of cannabis is by means of smoking. The drug is consumed by other routes, including oral ingestion in foods, capsules, and as a tea; intravenous injection of cannabis products has also been reported. The technique of smoking cannabis is critical for optimal psychoactive effect, and also has implications with regards to the health consequences. Cannabis smokers practice a deep inhalation technique as well as breath holding for 20–30 s, so as to extract as much psychoactive drug as possible. Studies of expired air demonstrate almost complete absorption of delta-9-THC by the pulmonary tissue.

B. Acute Effects

The acute psychoactive and physiological effects of cannabis depend on a number of factors, including the potency of the cannabis product, dose consumed, experience of the drug user with cannabis, and psychological and environmental factors, which have been referred to as the "set and setting" of the drug-using experience. Acute physiological consequences of cannabis use include irritation of the oral pharynx, a hacking cough, tachycardia, and conjunctival injection [44]. The latter may be masked by the use of vasoconstrictive eye-drop preparations. Because of the development of tolerance to the psychoactive effects of cannabis, and the ability of the individual to volitionally overcome the symptoms of cannabis intoxication, it may be difficult, on the basis of physical examination, to detect cannabis usage.

C. Pulmonary Consequences

Since marijuana smoke contains many of the same chemical irritants and toxins that are found in tobacco smoke, concern has emerged that the long-term use of cannabis would result in serious impairment in pulmonary function, including the possible development of pulmonary carcinoma. Although the long-term effects of cannabis smoking await longitudinal studies, an accumulating body of knowledge points toward serious pulmonary complications of cannabis smoking. Compared to smoking tobacco, smoking marijuana results in a four to five times greater increase of carboxyhemoglobin levels, a threefold increase of inhaled tar, and one-third more tar retained in the pulmonary tract [46]. The symptoms of acute and chronic bronchitis occur with approximately the same frequency in users of three to four marijuana joints per day as in people consuming 20 cigarettes per day. In a study of young adults with no respiratory symptomatology, who had been smoking marijuana for at least 5 years in quantities greater than 10 joints per week, important morphological changes were seen in bronchial biopsy specimens [47]. The most significant and common mucosal changes were seen in subjects who smoked both tobacco and marijuana; it appeared that the combination of cannabis and tobacco produced more significant mucosal changes than either substance used alone. The morphological changes noted included squamous metaplasia, stratification of the mucosa, and basement membrane thickening. Studies of both human and animal bronchial epithelial cell cultures, which are exposed to marijuana smoke, demonstrate increased numbers of mitotic figures and cellular dysplasia [48,49]. Although there are case reports in the literature which imply a causal relationship between chronic marijuana smoking and carcinoma of the respiratory tract, the long-term longitudinal studies of cannabis smokers and resultant respiratory pathology remain to be performed [47,50].

D. Cardiovascular Consequences

Smoking marijuana produces peripheral vasodilitation, a sinus tachycardia, and dose-related increases in cardiac load and oxygen requirements [51,52]. The combination of increased cardiac load and elevated carboxyhemoglobin levels could produce a serious imbalance in myocardial oxygen demand and delivery. Although only one report exists in the literature of myocardial infarction associated with cannabis use, the drug has been reported to cause episodes of diaphoresis and chest pain [52]. A variant of cannabis smoking is a substance known as AMP, which is marijuana saturated with formaldehyde. This particular drug combination has been associated with chest pain, tachypnea, tachycardia, hypertension, and diaphoresis.

E. Other Consequences

Cannabis appears to have mild immunosuppressant effects, the clinical relevance of which is uncertain [45]. The amotivational syndrome refers to a cluster of symptoms in chronic cannabis users, including apathy, loss of ambition, difficulty concentrating, impaired memory, and deterioration of school and work performance [53].

V. MEDICAL COMPLICATIONS OF OPIOID DEPENDENCE

The term *opioid* refers to a group of drugs, both naturally occurring and synthetic, with morphinelike activity. Some medical complications of opioid dependency are related to the intravenous route of administration; and, therefore, are discussed in that section. Selected medical complications not entirely related to intravenous administration will be discussed here.

A. Narcotic Bowel Syndrome

The opioids, in general, reduce bowel motility, and severe constipation is a well-documented complication. The narcotic bowel syndrome is an often overlooked clinical entity presenting in a patient who is opioid dependent [54]. The presenting complaint is one of abdominal pain of a chronic nature, but with acute exacerbation. The pain is colicy in nature, typically generalized, and occurs in the context of normal laboratory findings. Intermittent vomiting may occur. Signs of pseudobowel obstruction may be present. X-ray studies disclose evidence of ileus, and may suggest a mechanical small bowel obstruction. The clinical picture is felt to be due to a combination of the direct pharmacological effects of opioids on the gastrointestinal tract, in combination with the gastrointestinal signs of opioid withdrawal. Clonidine has been successfully used to treat this syndrome [55]. Its beneficial effect appears to be due to the ability of clonidine to ameliorate opioid abstinence as well as its direct relaxant effect on gastrointestinal smooth muscle.

B. Heroin-Associated Nephropathy

All types of glomerulonephritis have been reported in intravenous drug users; the term *heroin associated nephropathy* refers to a focal segmental glomerulosclerosis [56]. Patients present with a nephrotic syndrome, and typically have a relentless, progressive course. Actually, heroin-associated nephropathy is a complication of both intravenous heroin or cocaine use [57]. Its pathogenesis is uncertain, and has been speculated to be due to adulterants, such as quinine, which is known to be a cause of acute renal failure. More recent evidence suggests the presence of an immune complex disease due to the finding of immunoglobulin and C-3 deposits in the affected glomeruli [56].

C. Pentazocine

Pentazocine (Talwin) was first marketed in 1967 as a nonaddictive analgesic, and the first reports of its abuse appeared in 1968. There followed an epidemic of pentazocine abuse, particularly localized to major cities in the midwest and south. Typically, 50 mg of pentazocine was mixed with 50 mg of the antihistamine tripelenamine (pyribenzamine, PBZ), and the combination came to be known as T's and blues. Addicts had previously employed mixtures of tripelenamine with morphine or heroin under the street name "blue velvet." It appears that this popularity of T's and blues was stimulated by the poor quality of street heroin and the low cost of the pentazocine/tripelenamine combination. This epidemic of opioid use was particularly destructive in terms of its medical and social complications. A typical user was an unemployed, black male between the ages of 20 and 30. Strikingly high rates of violent, aggressive criminal behavior were associated with this epidemic [58]. Medical complications included severe abscesses and cellulitis, often requiring surgical drainage [59]. Seizures were common, owing to the lowering of the seizure threshold by pentazocine as well as the central stimulatory effect of tripelenamine. Pulmonary foreign body granulomatosis was common in these cases as well as pulmonary arterial and capillary obstruction, resulting in pulmonary hypertension. Ultimately, the manufacturer of Talwin reformulated its product, adding the opioid antagonist naloxone in what appears to have been a successful effort to stem this epidemic of diversion and drug addiction.

VI. MEDICAL COMPLICATIONS OF SEDATIVE-HYPNOTIC ADDICTION

The sedative-hypnotic group of drugs encompasses a variety of agents, including the benzodiazepines, barbiturates, chloral derivatives, ethchlorvynol, glutethimide, methaqualone, and miscellaneous other agents.

A. Benzodiazepines

For the most part, these drugs are quite safe, with a high therapeutic index. The primary medical complications are limited to cases of overdose and withdrawal reactions. There has been considerable debate as to the dependency-producing liability of benzodiazepines; the emergence of withdrawal phenomena is clearly linked to dose nd chronicity of use. This group of drugs, like others in this classification, may result in overdose when combined with other sedative hypnotics, especially ethanol.

B. Barbiturates

The major medical complications of this drug group include overdose and withdrawal states. The barbiturate withdrawal syndrome is the prototype for sedative-hypnotic withdrawal. Use of barbiturates does result in induction of hepatic enzymes, which can affect the metabolic rates of other therapeutic agents, including anticoagulants, digitalis preparations, beta-adrenergic drugs, including propranolol and metoprolol, oral contraceptives, griseofulvin, quinidine, phenytoin, and tricyclic antidepressants [60]. Barbiturates may also competitively inhibit the metabolism of tricyclic antidepressants. Barbiturates increase porphyrin production, and their use will exacerbate acute intermittent porphyria and variegate porphyria.

C. Chloral Derivatives

Chloral hydrate is the prototype of the chloral derivatives. Gastritis may result in chronic users of this drug. Chloral hydrate, in combination with alcohol, has for years been known colloquially as a "Mickey Finn." Sudden reverse tolerance may develop in chronic users of chloral hydrate, resulting in overdose and, possibly, death [60].

D. Ethchlorvynol, Glutethimide, and Methaqualone

The abuse of ethchlorvynol, glutethimide, and methaqualone carries with it the risk of overdose and a barbituratelike withdrawal syndrome. Ethchlorvynol may exacerbate acute intermittent porphyria, and is contraindicated in such patients. Glutethimide has also been used in combination with codeine, and is known colloquially as "doors and fours" or "loads." Methaqualone is no longer available through the legitimate U.S. market, but is still a drug of abuse in the United States.

VII. MEDICAL COMPLICATIONS OF INHALANT ADDICTION

A. The Spectrum of Abused Inhalants

The scope of inhalant use in the United States is unknown, but some surveys have reported as many as one in 10 persons under the age of 17 have experimented with volatile inhalants [53]. The volatile inhalants include a diverse group of drugs, which have in common the capacity to produce a rapid-onset, typically short-acting, intoxication. The depressant, and euphoric effects are similar to alcohol. This group of drugs produce an acute brain syndrome characterized by impaired judgment, amnesia, attentional and concentration difficulties, and, in some cases, an acute psychosis.

The current pattern of inhalant addiction emerged in the 1960s with model-building glue. Since that time, the medical literature has documented the abuse of a panoply of volatile substances. Among these substances are glues containing organic compounds such as toluene, naphtha, benzene, xylene, and chloroform, and cleaning solutions containing carbon trichloroethylene, carbon tetrachloride, and other petroleum distillates. Nail polish remover as a source of acetone, lighter fluids containing naphtha and various aliphatic hydrocarbons, and aerosols, including a group of fluorinated hydrocarbons and nitrous oxide comprise still another group of abusable inhalants. Paints, paint thinners, and lacquers containing toluene, acetone, naphtha, methanol, and ethanol have also been reported in cases of inhalant abuse. Other inhalants, including hair spray, room deodorizers, typewriter correction fluid, and fire extinguisher propellants, have become more commonly abused inhalants in the past decade.

B. The Medical Consequences of Inhalant Addiction

The "sudden-sniffing-death" syndrome appears to result from the development of acute cardiac sensitization to the effects of epinephrine [52]. The result is the development of cardiac arrhythmia, particularly ventricular fibrillation with sudden death. Compounds known to produce this syndrome include benzene, chloroform, tricholorethylene, and tricholorfluoremethane. Toluene in glue has been implicated in the production of sinus brachycardia. Shoe-cleaning fluid containing trichloroethylene has resulted in a dilated congestive cardiomyopathy [61]. Acute hepatic and/or renal failure may be produced, particularly by solvents such as chloroform or carbon tetrachloride. Benzene toxicity includes bone marrow suppression, hepatic necrosis, and fatty infiltration of the liver [62]. Toluene has been reported to produce hepatomegaly, acute and chronic brain syndrome, neuropathy, and renal dysfunction [62]. The common practice of inhaling the fumes of these substances within the confines of a plastic garment bag has resulted in a number of deaths due to suffocation.

VIII. MEDICAL CONSEQUENCES OF HALLUCINOGEN ADDICTION

The hallucinogenic drugs most commonly encountered in clinical practice include lysergic acid diethylamide (LSD) and phencyclidine (PCP). Other hallucinogens include psilocybin, peyote, and psychedelic mushrooms. After an initial popularity in the 1960s, the use of LSD declined in the 1970s and early 1980s, though recently the drug appears to be enjoying a resurgence in popularity. The popularity of PCP appears to have been rather consistent through the past 2 decades [53].

Frequently, exposure to phencyclidine is inadvertent, inasmuch as the drug is commonly sold in the street as tetrahydrocannabinol, the active ingredient in marijuana. Phencyclidine is a member of the cyclohexylamine family, and was initially marketed as a nonnarcotic, nonbarbiturate anesthetic. Severe toxicity, however, soon doomed this drug in the legitimate marketplace in terms of human use. Phencyclidine is capable of producing depressant, stimulant, and hallucinogenic effects, depending on the dose used, the individual's experience with the drug, and the route of administration.

Acute intoxication with hallucinogenic drugs is characterized by loss of contact with reality and bizarre behavior, at times profound. Phencyclidine ingestion is characterized by a vestibulocerebellar syndrome with nystagmus, a sense of weightlessness, vertigo, diplopia, and muscular incoordination [53]. Accidental death, such as drowning or vehicular crashes, may result. The prevalence of phencyclidine-associated death is, in all likelihood, significantly underreported. Rhabdomyolysis may occur after phencyclidine use, presumably as a result of muscular rigidity or extreme muscular exertion. Higher-dose ingestion of phencyclidine can produce a comalike state and seizure activity.

IX. MEDICAL COMPLICATIONS OF DRUG ADDICTION BY ROUTE OF ADMINISTRATION

A. Intranasal

The intranasal insufflation of cocaine in some patients results in progressive mucosal and cartilaginous necrosis with ultimate septal perforation. The treatment for this condition is plastic surgical repair once the patient's addiction is appropriately treated. Intranasal cocaine use is also associated with sinusitis and temporary vocal cord paralysis, resulting in aphonia and a risk of aspiration pneumonitis.

B. Oral

The topical application of cocaine to the gingivae can result in a desquamative gingivitis resembling necrotizing ulcerative gingivitis or erosive oral lichen planus [63]. The body packer syndrome is a peculiar, fatal consequence of the cocaine smuggling trade [64]. Cocaine is packaged in sizes suitable for swallowing; the packaging material may include cellophane, latex, surgical gloves, or condoms, all of which are semipermeable membranes. Leakage or rupture of these packets may result in a fatal cocaine overdose. Bowel obstruction has also been reported [65].

C. Inhalant Use

Suffocation is a reported complication of inhalant drug abuse. Users may place a large plastic bag, such as a garment bag, over their head or upper torso, resulting in suffocation after achieving a state of intoxication from the drug.

D. Smoking

Isolated uvulitis is reported in cannabis smokers, presumably due to the irritant effect of the smoke [66]. Diffuse gingival hyperplasia, chronic dental caries, and periodontal disease have also been reported as complications of cannabis smoking [63]. Cocaine smoking can result in bruxism with abnormal patterns of dental wear [67].

E. Intravenous

Infection with the human immunodeficiency virus (HIV) is a well-recognized consequence of intravenous drug abuse. A recent review of 92 studies of HIV prevalence in intravenous drug users in the United States found a prevalence ranging from 0 to 65% in treatment programs in various parts of the United States [68]. The highest rate, up to 65%, was found in the northeastern part of the country. Risk of HIV infection was most associated with black and Hispanic ethnicity, male homosexual orientation, and several intravenous drug-using practices. These practices include the sharing of needles, particularly at drug "shooting galleries" where drug paraphernalia is either shared or rented. The relative absence of shooting galleries in parts of the United States other than the northeast may explain, to some extent, this diminished risk.

Up through January of 1989, there were 22,025 cases of AIDS reported in intravenous drug users, 27% of all reported adult AIDS cases [69]. Cocaine, in particular, has been implicated as a cofactor in HIV infection in intravenous drug users [70]. This is, perhaps, due to the blatant disregard for any kind of aseptic technique when caught up in the euphoria of cocaine or in the strong preoccupation and urgency of obtaining and using the drug. An additional link appears to be the trading of sex for cocaine, either by prostitutes or, less formally, between intravenous drug using partners [71]. An increase in crack cocaine use has also been correlated with increased rates of venereal disease, particularly gonorrhea and syphilis [72].

Hepatitis is a long-recognized complication of intravenous drug use. Hepatitis A, hepatitis B, non-A, non-B hepatitis and delta agent hepatitis (HDV) can all be transmitted through the parenteral route in intravenous drug users. Antibody to hepatitis A virus appears to be no more common in a population of intravenous drug users than in the general population [73]. In the evaluation of patients with clinically evident liver disease, either on the basis of hepatomegaly, cutaneous stigmata of liver disease, or elevated liver function parameters, etiology should not automatically be ascribed to the obvious drug of addiction. Opioid agents, themselves, are not hepatotoxic [74]. Up to 20% of liver disease in alcoholics has been found to have an etiology other than alcoholism [75]. Similarly, drug-addicted patients may have histological evidence of alcoholic liver disease, even though alcohol consumption may not be emphasized in the patient's history [76]. A careful differential diagnosis needs to be carried out in all chemically dependent patients who present with hepatocellular disease.

A number of complications may occur at the local drug injection site. Postinflammatory hyperpigmentation in olive-skinned or dark-skinned individuals is a common clinical complaint, particularly in those who have enrolled in a drug treatment program. The use of hydroquinone-containing "bleaching creams" is popular in such persons. The combination of pentazocine and tripelenamine (T's and blues) was a popular heroin substitute in the early to mid-1980s. This combination produced a particularly severe necrotizing process involving the skin, subcutaneous tissue, and muscle in intravenous users. Cocaine may also produce necrotizing change of skin and subcutaneum, including fascia, owing to its pronounced vasoconstrictive properties [77,78].

Additionally, localized sepsis, involving unusual, fastidious organisms, such as *Clostridium* species and various fungal species have been reported in intravenous users of cocaine. Granuloma formation may occur at remote organ sites as a result of the injection of materials used to "cut" or dilute drugs marketed for intravenous use. These granulomas may be found in the liver, brain, eyes [79], and lungs, at times producing a syndrome of pulmonary hypertension [80].

Intravenous drug use may also result in a spectrum of serious, potentially fatal, vascular complications involving both the arterial and venous systems [81]. Complications reported include inadvertent intra-arterial injection with distal gangrene, vasculitis, mycotic visceral aneurysms, fungal endocarditis, and combinations of local sepsis with venous or arterial obstruction. Infective endocarditis in intravenous drug users is typically due to *Staphylococcus aureus* [82] or group A *streptococci* [83]. Other unusual organisms have been reported, including *Pseudomonus aeruginosa* in pentazocine and tripelenamine users [84], *Citrobacter freundi* in cocaine addicts, and *Bacillus subtilus* in meperidine addicts. The finding of an unusual causative organism in cases of infective endocarditis mandates that the clinician consider intravenous drug abuse as a potential contributing factor [52].

X. FETAL AND NEONATAL COMPLICATIONS OF DRUG ADDICTION

The past decade has seen increasing attention paid to the problem of the fetal and neonatal consequences of maternal drug addiction. This interest has been given particular impetus by the cocaine epidemic. An estimated 30% of women in the prime childbearing years, ages 18–34, admit to using an illicit drug at some point within the year [85]. Eighteen percent admitted to using such drugs within the month prior to the survey. Most drugs with abuse potential, including alcohol, opiates, cocaine, sedative-hypnotics, and stimulants, are found in significant levels in the fetus if the mother is using the substance. A common misconception among pregnant women is that the placenta filters these substances from the fetal circulation. Additionally, these drugs enjoy a longer half-life within the fetus compared to the adult, owing to the presence of immature enzyme systems (glucuronidation and oxidation). Diminished renal excretion of drug metabolites further contributes to prolonged, potentially damaging drug exposure to the fetus [85]. A disturbing result of these trends is reflected in the fact that Los Angeles County has experienced a doubling every year since 1983 of the number of infants born with illicit drugs in their urine [86].

A. Opiates

There is an increased incidence of low birth weight in infants of opiate-dependent mothers, with approximately 50% of offspring having birth weights less than 2500 gm [87]. Hyperbilirubinemia is reported less frequently than in non–opiate-exposed babies, possibly owing to enzyme induction [88]. Respiratory distress syndrome occurs with increased frequency in children of methadone-maintained mothers, though not in infants born of heroin-addicted mothers [87]. The sudden infant death syndrome is reportedly five to 10 times more common in infants born of opiate-dependent mothers [85]. Neonatal opiate withdrawal is a well-recognized complication of maternal dependency, with 60–90% of infants born of opiate-addicted mothers demonstrating some signs of clinical withdrawal [85]. Neonatal abstinence may not peak until 3–4 days of life, and may persist for 2–3 weeks. The predominant signs of neonatal abstinence include high pitched cry, sweating, tremulousness, gastrointestinal upset, irritability, hyperactivity with excoriations over pressure points, and disturbed sleep patterns. Tachypnea can result in a metabolic alkalosis. Seizures do occur in opiate abstinence, but are more likely a result of a syndrome of polydrug abuse in the mother, including sedative-hypnotics, barbiturates, or cocaine [85]. Because of high caloric expenditure relative to intake, these infants tend to lose weight and have difficulty recovering back to birth weight. Whenever intrauterine drug exposure is considered, both maternal and neonatal urine should be screened for drugs of abuse.

The treatment of the neonatal opiate abstinence syndrome is primarily supportive, and involves swaddling the infant, use of a pacifier, and frequent small feedings. Pharmacotherapy is used only if supportive measures are unsuccessful. Paregoric appears to be the drug of choice in the treatment of neonatal opiate abstinence [85]. Valium and phenobarbital may need to be used in infants who do not respond well to paregoric, and in whom there may be a coincident sedative-hypnotic abstinence syndrome.

B. Tobacco

Maternal tobacco use is clearly associated with increased incidence of low birth weight for gestational age [89]. There is an inverse dose-response relationship between tobacco use and pre- and postnatal growth. Tremors, altered auditory responsiveness, hypertonicity, and exaggerated startle response have all been found in neonates born to smokers when measured at birth and 30 days postnatally compared to controls [90]. Tobacco use in pregnant women is associated with an increased risk of premature delivery, and increased rates of stillbirth and neonatal death.

C. Marijuana

In spite of the widespread prevalence of cannabis smoking in the general population, there is a relative paucity of studies with respect to the effects of cannabis on the fetus and neonate. Marijuana use compared to alcohol or tobacco is the least likely to be reduced by a pregnant female during pregnancy, and the most likely to return to prepregnancy levels 1 year postnatally [91]. Infants born to cannabis-using mothers have an increased incidence of low birth weight, and demonstrate neurobehavioral instability, including irritability and tremulousness as well as deficits in visual function [85].

The ability of cannabis to produce congenital defects in the passively exposed fetus is unclear. A few cases of children born with epicanthal folds and ocular hypertelorism have been reported [91]. In a large study, women who smoked marijuana during pregnancy were found to be five times more likely to have a baby with fetal alcohol syndrome–like anomalies, compared to nonusers of the drug. The rate of occurrence of anomalies in marijuana-exposed offspring in that study was 2% [92].

In the Ottawa study of 47 babies prenatally exposed to marijuana, cannabis use by the mother was associated with the appearance of a fine tremor and exaggerated and prolonged startle response [9]. Testing of these infants at 24 months showed no sign of persistent neurobehavioral effect compared to controls, suggesting either that the effect of marijuana is transient or too subtle to be picked up in young children by the assessment instruments currently available.

D. Cocaine

By 1989, it was estimated that as many as 50 million Americans have tried cocaine, among whom are 8 million regular users of the substance [86]. Maternal cocaine use is capable of producing disastrous obstetrical and neonatal complications. The spontaneous abortion rate in cocaine-using mothers is approximately 23% [86]. There is an increased incidence of placental abruption, and precipitous onset of labor following cocaine use [86]. The increased risk of placental abruption appears to continue in the second and third trimesters, even in women whose cocaine use was discontinued by the end of the first trimester, possibly reflecting cocaine-induced abnormalities in placental vascularity [93]. Cocaine produces increased systolic blood pressure, decreased uterine and placental perfusion, and increased uterine contractility [86].

Cocaine produces intrauterine growth retardation and decreased brain growth [86]. A variety of congenital anomalies have been associated with maternal cocaine use, notably urinary tract abnormalities, including prune belly syndrome, hydronephrosis, and renal agenesis [86,93,94]. Although genital organ anomalies, including hypospadias and pseudohermaphroditism, have been reported, genital defects do not appear to be statistically linked to cocaine exposure [94]. Several case reports document acute cerebral infarction in neonates as well as instances of neonatal myocardial infarction [86,95]. In one study, one-third of 74 infants who were clinically well had ultrasonographic evidence of perinatal cerebral infarction [86]. Generalized seizures may occur in cocaine-exposed neonates, including some in infants who do not have cocaine or its metabolite present in the urine at the time of the seizure episode [93]. Cocaine intoxication has been reported in breast-fed babies whose mothers are cocaine users, and status epilepticus has been reported in a breast-feeding infant whose mother applied cocaine to her nipples to relieve pain [96]. Congenital heart anomalies, including atrial septal defect, ventricular septal defect, and cardiomegaly have been reported to occur ten times more commonly than in controls [97].

Cocaine-exposed newborns demonstrate marked neurobehavioral changes, including irritability, tremulousness, exaggerated startle response, and increased muscle tone. In a study of 38 cocaine-exposed newborns, 17 had abnormal electroencephalograms during the first week of life. Nine out of 17 were abnormal in the second week, but only one remained abnormal between three and 12 months postnatally [98]. Flash-evoked visual potentials were abnormal in 62% of cocaine-exposed infants in the neonatal period, and remained abnormal in 50% at 1 year [86]. Auditory brain stem responses were abnormal as well, suggesting the possibility of cocaine-mediated ischemic insult to brainstem nuclei and impairment of myelination [99].

The incidence of sudden infant death syndrome (SIDS) in cocaine-exposed babies remains equivocal; SIDS has been reported to occur in up to 15% of cocaine-exposed babies on the basis of a retrospective study [100], while a prospective study of cocaine-exposed infants demonstrated no increased in the rate of sudden infant death syndrome [101].

E. Methamphetamine

Methamphetamine, a closely related congenor of amphetamine, known by the street names, "crystal," "crystal meth," "speed," and "ice," is being used with increasing frequency in the United States. Methamphetamine was the most commonly abused drug in San Diego County, accounting for 33–40% of referrals to treatment centers during 1989 [86]. Methamphetamine is pharmacologically similar to cocaine. It appears to cause similar fetal and neonatal consequences, including intrauterine growth retardation, decreased head circumference, preterm delivery with fetal distress, and anemia [86]. Compared to cocaine-exposed infants, methamphetaine-exposed infants appear to be less impaired during their first year of life.

They exhibit lethargy, poor feeding, and severe lassitude. Studies of stimulant-exposed infants at 1 year of age demonstrate diminished fine motor developments as well as decreased visual motor coordination [86]. The long-term developmental consequences of fetal exposure to stimulants remain unclear at this time.

XI. NEUROPSYCHIATRIC COMPLICATIONS OF DRUG ADDICTION

In addition to drug intoxication and withdrawal syndromes, a variety of organic mental disorders can occur as a consequence of psychoactive drug addiction. Psychoactive drugs can mimic many mental disorders, and the use of multiple psychoactive substances simultaneously may create confusing clinical states. Illicit drug consumers are often unaware of the actual content of drug compounds, and, therefore, clinical histories are not always reliable. Toxicology is essential to accomplish adequate differential diagnosis with each case. The defining factors of these mental disorders include brain dysfunction associated with psychological or behavioral disturbances due to a particular psychoactive drug. These disorders are described in detail in the revised *Diagnostic and Statistical Manual of Mental Disorders* (DSM-III-R) of the American Psychiatric Association [102].

A. Organic Delirium

Cocaine, amphetamine, and phencyclidine use, in some instances, can produce an organic delirium. The critical features of this disorder include a diminished ability to maintain attention to external stimuli, a disorganized thought process with an incoherent rambling or irrelevant speech pattern, a diminished level of consciousness, sensory misperception, a disturbed sleep-awake cycle, disorientation, and a fluctuating course. This disorder usually comes on within 1 h of ingestion of the drug, and typically abates within 6 h. Tactile and olfactory hallucinations may occur. The affect is labile, and behavior, at times, may be violent or aggressive, requiring restraint. Excited delerium is reported to be a preterminal state in many cases of fatal cocaine overdose [103].

B. Organic Delusional Disorder

A variety of psychoactive substances, including amphetamine, cannabis, hallucinogens, cocaine, and PCP may produce a delusional state. This condition is characterized by prominent delusions in a patient who is not in a state of delirium. Persecutory delusions are common, particularly with stimulant drugs. Although hallucinations may occur, they are not prominent. Stimulant users may experience formication, which is the sensation of bugs crawling in the skin, resulting in severe excoriation, and there may be body image distortions. This disorder has the potential for a more ominous prognosis; although many cases will clear within a few days, in some instances, particularly related to hallucinogen and cannabis use, the disorder may be very long lasting and be essentially indistinguishable from a functional psychotic disorder.

C. Organic Mood Disorders

In organic mood disorders, the individual develops persistent mood pathology resembling either a manic episode or a major depressive episode as a consequence of psychoactive drug use. Hallucinogens and phencyclidine tend to primarily produce depressive syndromes, with much self-reproach and guilt over the use of the drug. Some individuals experience a preoccupation with thoughts of having permanently damaged their brains as a result of the use of these drugs.

D. Organic Hallucinosis

Organic hallucinosis is defined as the occurrence of prominent, persistent hallucinations due to psychoactive drug use in a patient not in a state of delirium. Hallucinogens are the most common cause of the disorder, and visual hallucinations predominate. The individual may or may not have insight. Although the person may be quite convinced as to the veracity of the hallucinations, this syndrome is not characterized by the presence of a well-developed delusional system.

The set and setting of drug use is important in terms of whether this hallucinatory experience is perceived as pleasant or anxiety provoking. Accidents may occur when the affected individual attempts to flee from an anxiety-producing hallucination.

E. Posthallucinogen Perception Disorder

The occurrence of "flashback" hallucinations in individuals with previous experience with hallucinatory drugs is referred to as the posthallucinogen perception disorder. Typically, these episodes are brief, lasting but a few seconds, but they may become persistent, with the individual experiencing flashback phenomena throughout the entire day for many months. Most commonly, these perceptual disturbances take the form of geometric hallucinations, voices, flashes of color, halos around persons or objects, intensification of colors, and misperception, including macropsia and micropsia. This disorder tends to be triggered by entrance into a dark environment, the use of substances with hallucinogenic capacity, particularly cannabis, and, in some cases, can be willfully induced. This disorder typically remits after several months.

F. Sedative-Hypnotic Amnestic Disorder

The sedative-hypnotic amnestic disorder is characterized by impairment of short-term and long-term memory, at times profound, in individuals with typically long-term or high-dose sedative-hypnotic dependency. Typically, remote events are better recalled than events of the recent past. Immediate recall, however, is not impaired. Affected persons may attempt to cover up their memory deficits by means of confabulation. Prognostically, compared to the alcohol amnestic disorder, sedative-hypnotic amnestic disorder may be expected to fully remit provided the person maintains abstinence from psychoactive drug use.

XII. OVERDOSE

Many cases of drug or alcohol overdose, which present at emergency rooms, represent suicide attempts. After treatment of the acute overdose and stabilization of the patient, evaluation for chemical dependency is indicated in all cases. In this section, the general principles of overdose management will be reviewed as well as the principles of treatment peculiar to specific drug groups.

A. General Principles of Overdose Treatment

Acutely, the chief complication of drug overdose is cardiorespiratory depression. Immediate attention should be directed to the ABCs (airway, breathing, and circulation). The head should be tilted backward, the jaw pushed forward, and the mouth opened, and the upper airway cleared of secretions. In an obtunded patient, an oropharyngeal airway should be inserted with the patient positioned on his side. If respiratory depression is present, a cuffed endotracheal tube should be inserted and respiration assisted, either by means of a bag or by a mechanical ventilator. Pulse, blood pressure, and hemodynamic status are determined, and if compromised, saline is begun through a large-bore intravenous line. Simultaneously, a urinary catheter is inserted and monitoring of intake and output begun. General assessment of the patient is rapidly carried out, including looking for evidence of trauma or needle tracks, checking the patient's clothing for pills or drugs, and obtaining blood and urine samples for toxicology.

An attempt should be made to prevent further absorption of the ingested drug. In the awake patient, syrup of ipecac, 15-20 ml with copious amounts of water should be administered. This may be repeated in 15-30 min, and if not effective, gastric lavage should be carried out. The gastric washing should be saved and sent for toxicological analysis. Obviously, neither induction of vomiting nor gastric lavage should be attempted in an obtunded patient without a cuffed endotracheal tube in place. Activated charcoal should be administered, since it not only inhibits absorption of drugs still in the gastrointestinal system, but also aids removal of drugs already absorbed into the systemic circulation [104].

B. Opiates

The classic triad of depressed level of consciousness, pinpoint pupils, and depressed respiration characterizes opiate overdose. Wheezing and rales may indicate early pulmonary edema, and hypotension may be present as well. Fluid replacement and oxygen therapy will generally correct the hypotension. One must be cautious in the use of oxygen, owing to the fact that opiates depress brainstem sensitivity to carbon dioxide, and the individual, therefore, is increasingly dependent on hypoxic drive [105]. The opioid antagonist naloxone should be administered intravenously in a dose of 0.8 mg (2 ml), and repeated every 3-5 min as needed. No clinical response to a total dose of 10 mg suggests that the overdose is either not due to an opiate agent or may be complicated by drugs other than opiates. The clinician must be mindful of the fact that methadone overdose, owing to the long half-life of the drug, may require repetitive doses of narcotic antagonists.

C. Barbiturates and Sedative-Hypnotic Overdose

The main risk of overdose of barbiturates and sedative-hypnotics is that of depression of the respiratory and brainstem centers, leading to cardiorespiratory collapse. These drugs are especially hazardous when used in combination, particularly with alcohol. Signs of overdose include slurred speech, nystagmus, diplopia, ataxia, and diminished deep tendon reflexes. The clinical picture may progress to somnolence, confusion, coma, respiratory depression, apnea, shock, and death. No antidote is available to the clinician at this time which is useful in reversing a sedative-hypnotic overdose, but naloxone should be given in order to rule out or treat any coexisting opiate effect. Induced emesis or gastric lavage is indicated if the patient presents within 6 h of drug ingestion. The use of activated charcoal and cathartic is also indicated [106]. Forced alkaline diuresis will aid the excretion of phenobarbital [107].

D. Glutethimide

The narrow range between therapeutic and toxic doses has led to many cases of overdose due to the use of glutethimide. Gastric absorption of glutethimide is erratic, decreasing after achievement of a certain blood level, and then increasing again as the blood level declines. Therefore, gastric lavage is indicated up to 24 h after ingestion of this drug.

E. Stimulants

Stimulant overdose is characterized by restlessness, hyperalertness, tremulousness, and certain stereotyped behaviors, such as facial grimacing and bruxism. Violent, assaultive behavior may occur, along with visual or auditory hallucinations. The pupils are dilated and hyperreflexia and tachycardia are present. The major complications of stimulant overdose include hypertheria, seizures, hypertension, and cardiovascular collapse. Minor cases may be treated conservatively with a supportive calming approach. Urinary acidification will aid excretion of amphetamine. Alpha-adrenergic blocking agents are useful for treating hypertension, and beta blockers have been used to treat cocaine-induced arrhythmia [6]. Haloperidol may be used to treat acute psychotic symptoms [108]. Stimulant-induced seizures are best treated with diazepam.

F. Hallucinogens

Hallucinogen use or overdose may produce delusions, hallucinations, and panic reaction. The primary approach is one of using a quiet, nonthreatening, calming environment. Diazepam may be used if needed. This reaction typically resolves spontaneously within 24 h.

G. Phencyclidine

Phencyclidine may have both central nervous system stimulant and depressant effects, depending on the dose used. Physical examination may disclose drowsiness, nystagmus, ataxia, agitation, miotic pupils, and hyperreflexia [105]. Severe hypertensive reactions are possible. Higher doses may be complicated by respiratory depression, apnea, coma, and status epilepticus. Phencyclidine is excreted into the gastric lumen; and, therefore, gastric lavage, activated charcoal, and cathartics are indicated. Acidification of the urine with ammonium chloride and forced diuresis will aid in its removal. When an antipsychotic is needed, a nonphenothiazine such as haloperidol should be employed. Diazepam in small doses, 2–5 mg i.v., is indicated for the treatment of seizures.

H. Marijuana

Manifestations of marijuana use in high doses may include panic reactions with paranoid thinking, progressing to a psychosislike picture. Talking the patient down from the high in a calm, reassuring quiet environment is the treatment of choice. Diazepam may, rarely, be needed. Intravenous cannabis use has been reported, and may produce a severe syndrome characterized by nausea, vomiting, shaking, chills, fever, and tachycardia [109]. This syndrome may be complicated by disseminated intravascular coagulation, rhabdomyolysis, hypotension, and renal insufficiency.

I. Inhalants

Inhalant overdose, apart from the cardiovascular toxicity described in Section VII is primarily characterized by disorientation, at times progressing to coma. Apart from treating those complications, general supportive care is indicated.

XIII. DRUG ADDICTION AND TRAUMA

In the United States, traumatic injury is the fourth leading cause of death after cardiovascular disease, cancer, and stroke. Traumatic injuries are the leading cause of death in the age group 1–44 [110]. Motor vehicle crashes cause 40,000–50,000 deaths per year, and 4 to 5 million injuries per year in the United States. The relationships between increasing blood alcohol concentration and the risk of a highway crash has been well documented for years, both for fatal and nonfatal crashes. Although well understood for alcohol, information available regarding the behavioral correlates of varying levels of other psychoactive drugs is sparse [111]. Although it is possible to measure all psychoactive drugs in body fluid determinations, practical considerations preclude the use of such technology as an initial screening of cases of driving under the influence of drugs (DUID). Current epidemiological evidence suggests that drugs most likely to be associated with impaired driving, other than alcohol, include sedative hypnotics, cannabis, and antihistamines.

The effects of cocaine or other stimulants on driver impairment or driver injury are not well studied. There is some evidence which links the use of sedative-hypnotic agents, particularly benzodiazepines, to the risk of traffic accidents [112]. In a U.S. study of 497 injured drivers, serological tests demonstrated that 25% were positive for alcohol, 10% for marijuana, and 8% for sedative-hypnotics [113]. The sedative-hypnotic group, however, did not differ from the drug-free drivers in the proportion of crashes for which they were deemed to be responsible. In a study of 440 young male drivers, ages 15–44, fatally injured in automobile accidents in California, 81% had one or more drugs present on toxicological analysis [114]. Seventy percent were positive for alcohol, 37% for cannabis, 11% for cocaine, 4% for phencyclidine, and 4% for diazepam. In a study of blood toxicology in 1800 drivers arrested for traffic accidents, 16% had sufficient THC present to constitute intoxication [115].

There is no simple roadside method of determining driver impairment resulting from cannabis or other drugs, other than alcohol, even though combinations of these psychoactive substances clearly lead to serious impairment. Driving simulator studies have found evidence of psychomotor impairment at levels of one cannabis cigarette [116]. In a study of 10 experienced aircraft pilots, a single cannabis cigarette (containing 19 mg of delta-9-THC) reduced the ability of these experienced pilots to perform a simple landing maneuver for up to 24 h [117]. Importantly, these impaired pilots felt subjectively alert, and not under the influence at the time of testing.

A recent study [118] examined the prevalence of cocaine and alcohol use in motor vehicle fatalities, both driver and passenger, in New York City between the years of 1984 and 1987. The years 1984 and 1985 represent a period prior to the crack cocaine epidemic. Cocaine use was detected in 18.2% of the 643 fatalities in the study. Of those who were cocaine positive, 77% were drivers. Cocaine was found in 26% of fatalities aged 16–45, a rate 13 times greater than the other age groups in the study. Importantly, 56% of all drivers killed in these fatal accidents were found to be positive for alcohol, cocaine, or both. Both alcohol and cocaine were found in 10% of the fatalities. This study did not examine the question of cocaine-related driver impairment, and points out the need for further study regarding the etiological role of cocaine in traffic crashes.

Hip fracture is a leading cause of disability and death in the United States, with an estimated 227,000 osteoporotic femoral fractures occurring each year (119,120). Studies have demonstrated that long half-life (greater than 24 h) benzodiazepines are associated with an increased risk of hip fracture compared to short half-life drugs (less than 24 h) [121]. The relative risk of hip fracture was 1.7 times greater for current users of long half-life benzodiazepines than for users of short half-life benzodiazepines. Additionally, the risk of falls in users of long half-life benzodiazepines is increased from 1.8 to 3.1 times the risk in a non–drug-using population [122]. This increased risk appears to be due to the accumulation of the drug, and its psychoactive metabolites with resultant psychomotor impairment. This risk has been demonstrated to be independent of potentially confounding variables, including sex, age, and dementia.

REFERENCES

1. Mason, J. (1990). From the Assistant Secretary for Health (editorial); *J.A.M.A., 263*:494.
2. Meyers, J., Weissman, M., and Tischler, G. (1984). Six-month prevalence of psychiatric disorders in three communities: 1980 to 1982. *Arch. Gen. Psychiatry, 41*:959–967.
3. Kamerow, D., Pincus, H., and MacDonald, D. (1986). Alcohol abuse, other drug abuse, and mental disorders in medical practice, *J.A.M.A., 255*:2054–2057.
4. Abelson, H., and Miller, J. (1985). A decade of trends in cocaine use in the household population, *Natl. Inst. Drug Abuse Res. Monogr. Ser., 61*:35–49.
5. Isner, J., and Chokshi, S. (1989). Cocaine and vasospasm, *N. Engl. J. Med., 321*:1604–1606.
6. Creglar, L., and Mark, H. (1986). Medical complications of cocaine abuse, *N. Engl. J. Med., 315*:1495–1500.
7. Gradman, A. (1988). Cardiac effects of cocaine: A review, *Yale J. Biol. Med., 61*:137–147.
8. Lange, R., Cigarroa, R., Yancy, C., et al. (1989). Cocaine-induced coronary-artery vasoconstriction, *N. Engl. J. Med., 321*:1557–1561.
9. Karch, S., and Billingham, M. (1988). The pathology and etiology of cocaine-induced heart disease, *Arch. Pathol. Lab. Med., 112*:225–230.
10. Satel, S., and Gawin, F. (1989). Migraine-like headache and cocaine use, *J.A.M.A., 261*:2995–2996.
11. Rowley, H., Lowenstein, D., et al. (1989). Thalamomesencephalic strokes after cocaine abuse, *Neurology, 39*:428–430.
12. Chasnoff, I., Bussey, M., Savich, R., and Stack, C. (1986). Perinatal cerebral infarction and maternal cocaine use, *J. Pediatr., 108*:456–459.
13. Mody, C., Miller, B., McIntyre, H., Cobb, S., and Goldberg, M. (1988). Neurologic complications of cocaine abuse, *Neurology, 38*:1189–1193.
14. Kaye, B., and Fainstat, M. (1987). Cerebral vasculitis associated with cocaine abuse, *J.A.M.A., 258*:2104–2106.
15. Choy-Kwong, M., and Lipton, R. (1989). Seizures in hospitalized cocaine users, *Neurology, 39*:425–427.
16. Bates, C. (1988). Medical risks of cocaine use, *West. J. Med., 148*:440–444.
17. Murray, R., Albin, R., Mergner, W., et al. (1988). Diffuse alveolar hemorrhage temporally related to cocaine smoking, *Chest, 93*:427–429.
18. Goodwin, J., Harley, R., Miller, K., and Hefner, J. (1989). Cocaine, pulmonary hemorrhage, and hemoptysis, *Ann. Intern. Med., 110*:843.
19. Kissner, D., Lawrence, W., Selis, J., and Flint, A. (1987). Crack lung: Pulmonary disease caused by cocaine abuse, *Ann. Rev. Respir. Dis., 136*(5):1250–1252.
20. Schwartz, R., Estroff, T., Fairbanks, D., and Hoffman, N. (1989). Nasal symptoms associated with cocaine abuse during adolescence, *Arch. Otolaryngol. Head Neck. Surg., 115*:63–64.
21. Parks, J., Reed, G., and Knochel, J. (1989). Case report: cocaine-associated rhabdomyolysis, *Am. J. Med. Sci., 297*:334–336.
22. Roth, D., Alarcon, F., Fernandez, J., et al. (1988). Acute rhabdomyolysis associated with cocaine intoxication, *N. Engl. J. Med., 319*:673–677.
23. Wrogeman, K., and Pena S. (1976). Mitochondrial calcium overload. A general mechanism for cell necrosis in muscle diseases, *Lancet, 1*:672–673.
24. Singhal, P., Horowitz, B., Quinones, M., et al. (1989). Acute renal failure following cocaine abuse, *Nephron, 52*:76–78.
25. Mendelson, J., Teoh, S., Lange, V., et al. (1988). Hyperprolactinemia during cocaine withdrawal, *Natl. Inst. Drug Abuse Res. Monogr. Ser., 81*:67–73.
26. Kloss, M., Rosen, G., and Rauckman, E. (1984). Cocaine-mediated hepatotoxicity. A critical review. *Biochem. Pharmacol., 33*:169–173.
27. Perino, L., Warren, G., and Levine, J. (1988). Cocaine-induced hepatotoxicity in humans, *Gastroenterology, 93*:176–180.
28. Dilsaver, S., Votolato, N., and Alessi, N. (1989). Complications of phenylpropanolamine, *A.F.P., 39*:201–206.

29. Pentel, P. (1984). Toxicity of over-the-counter stimulants, *J.A.M.A.*, *252*:1898–1903.
30. Jaffe, J. (1985). Drug addiction and drug abuse, *The Pharmacological Basis of Therapeutics* (L. Goodman and A. Gilman, eds), 7th ed., Macmillan, New York, pp. 554–558.
31. Goldberg, A., and Goldstein, D. (1981). Persistent behavior at high rates maintained by intravenous self-administration of nicotine, *Science, 214*:573–575.
32. Surgeon General (1988). *The Health Consequences of Smoking. Nicotine Addiction.* Office of Smoking and Health, eds., Department of Health and Human Services Publication No. (CDC) 88-8406, U.S. Government Printing Office, Washington, D.C.
33. Surgeon General (1981). *The Health Consequences of Smoking: The Changing Cigarette.* Office of Smoking and Health, eds., Department of Health and Human Services Publication No. (PHS) 81-50156, U.S. Government Printing Office, Washington, D.C.
34. Surgeon General (1979). *Smoking and Health.* Office of Smoking and Health, eds., Department of Health, Education, and Welfare Publication No. (PHS) 79-50066, U.S. Government Printing Office, Washington, D.C.
35. Surgeon General (1982). *The Health Consequences of Smoking: Cancer.* Office of Smoking and Health, eds., Department of Health and Human Services Publication No. (PHS) 82-50179, U.S. Government Printing Office, Washington, D.C.
36. Mommsen, S., and Aagaard, J. (1983). Tobacco as a risk factor in bladder cancer, *Carcinogenesis, 4*:335–338.
37. Whitmore, W. (1988). Bladder cancer: An overview, *CA - A Cancer J. Clin., 38*:213–223.
38. Dwyer, J., Rieger-Ndakorerwa, G., et al. (1988). Low-level Cigarette smoking and longitudinal change in serum cholesterol among adolescents, *J.A.M.A., 259*:2857–2862.
39. Squier, C. (1988). The nature of smokeless tobacco and patterns of use, *CA, 38*:26–229.
40. Holmstrup, P., and Pindborg, J. (1988). Oral mucosal lesions in smokeless tobacco users, *CA, 38*:230–235.
41. Sundstrom, B., Mornstad, H., and Axell, T. (1982). Oral carcinomas associated with snuff dipping, *J. Oral Pathol. II*:245–251.
42. Winn, D. (1988). Smokeless tobacco and cancer: The epidemiologic evidence, *CA, 38*:236–243.
43. Cook, D., Pocock, S., and Shaper, A. (1986). Giving up smoking and the risk of heart attacks: A report from the British Regional Heart Study, *Lancet, 2*:1376–1380.
44. Schwartz, R. (1987). Marijuana: An overview. *Pediatr. Clin. North Am., 34*:305–317.
45. Committee to Study the Health-Related Effects of Cannabis and Its Derivatives (1982). Marijuana and Health, National Academy of Sciences, Institute of Medicine, National Academy Press, Washington, D.C.
46. Wu, T., Tashkin, D., Djahed, B., and Rose, J. (1988). Pulmonary hazards of smoking marijuana as compared with tobacco, *N. Engl. J. Med., 318*:347–351.
47. Fligiel, S., Venkat, H., Gong, H., and Tashkin, D. (1988). Bronchial pathology in chronic marijuana smokers: A light and electron microscopic study, *J. Psychoactive Drugs, 20*:33–42.
48. Leuchtenberger, C., and Leuchtenberger, R. (1971). Morphological and cytochemical effects of marijuana cigarette smoke on epithelioid cells of lung explants from mice. *Nature, 234*:227–229.
49. Leuchtenberger, C., Leuchtenberger, R., and Ritter, V. (1973). Effecs of marijuana and tobacco smoke on DNA and chromosomal complement in human lung explants. *Nature, 242*:403–404.
50. Taylor, F. (1988). Marijuana as a potential respiratory tract carcinogen. *South. Med. J., 81*:1213–1216.
51. Beaconsfield, P., Ginsberg, J., and Rainsbury, R. (1972). Marijuana smoking: Cardiovascular effects in man and possible mechanisms, *N. Engl. J. Med., 287*:209–212.
52. Choi, Y., and Pearl, W. (1989). Cardiovascular effects of adolescent drug abuse. *J. Adolesc. Health Care, 10*:332–337.
53. Nicholi, A. (1983). The nontherapeutic use of psychoactive drugs, *N. Engl. J. Med., 308*:925–933.
54. Rogers, M., and Cerda, J. (1989). Editorial: The narcotic bowel syndrome, *J. Clin. Gastroenterol., 11*:132–132.
55. Sandgren, J., McPhee, M., and Greenberger, N. (1984). Narcotic bowel syndrome treated with clonidine, *Ann. Int. Med., 101*:331–334.

56. Sanders, M., and Marshall, A. (1989). Acute and chronic toxic nephropathies, *Ann. Clin. Lab. Sci., 19*:216–220.

57. Cunningham, E., Venuto, R., and Zielezny, M. (1984). Adulterants in heroin/cocaine: Implications concerning heroin-associated nephropathy, *Drug Alcohol Depend., 14*:19–22.

58. Garey, R., Daul, G., Samuels, M., and Egan, R. (1982–83). Medical and sociological aspects of T's and blues abuse in New Orleans, *Am. J. Drug Alcohol Abuse, 9*:171–182.

59. Poklis, A. (1982). Pentazocine/tripelenamine (T's and blues) abuse: A five year survey of St. Louis, MO, *Drug Alcohol Depend., 10*:257–267.

60. Harvey, S. (1985). Sedatives and hypnotics, *The Pharmacological Basis of Therapeutics* (L. Goodman and A. Gilman, eds.), 7th ed., Macmillan, New York, pp. 360–362.

61. Mee, A., and Wright, P. (1980). Congestive (dilated) cardiomyopathy in association with solvent abuse *J.R. Soc. Med., 73*:671–672.

62. Cohen, S. (1977). Abuse of inhalants, *Drug Abuse, Clinical and Basic Aspects* (S. Pradhan and S. Dutta, eds.), Mosby, St. Louis, p. 298.

63. Pallasch, T., and Joseph, S. (1987). Oral manifestations of drug abuse, *J. Psychoactive Drugs, 19*:375–377.

64. Wetli, C., and Mittleman, R. (1981). The body packer syndrome: Toxicity following ingestion of illicit drugs packaged for transportation, *J. Foren. Sci., 26*:492–500.

65. Caruana, D., Weinbach, B., Georg, D., and Gardner, L. (1984). Cocaine packet ingestion—Diagnosis, management and natural history, *Ann. Intern. Med., 100*:73–74.

66. Guarisco, J., Cheney, M., LeJeune, F., and Reed, H. (1988). Isolated uvulitis secondary to marijuana use, *Laryngoscope, 98*:1309–1312.

67. Van Dyke, C., and Byck, R. (1982). Cocaine. *Sci. Am., 246*:128–141.

68. Hahn, R., Onorato, I., Jones, T., and Dougherty, J. (1989). Prevalence of HIV infection among intravenous drug users in the United States, *J.A.M.A., 261*:2677–2684.

69. AIDS Weekly Surveillance Report—United States. (January 2, 1989). AIDS program, Centers for Disease Control, Atlanta, Georgia.

70. Weiss, S. (1989). Links between cocaine and retroviral infection, *J.A.M.A., 261*:607–608.

71. Chaisson, R., Bacchetti, P., Osmond, D., et al. (1989). Cocaine use and HIV infection in intravenous drug users in San Francisco, *J.A.M.A., 261*:561–565.

72. Goldsmith, M. (1988). Sex tied to drugs—STD spread, *J.A.M.A., 260*:2009.

73. Weller, I. (1984). Clinical, biochemical, serological, histological and ultrastructural features of liver disease in drug abusers, *Gut, 25*:417–423.

74. Kreek, M., Dodes, L., Kane, S., et al. (1972). Long-term methadone maintenance therapy: Effects on liver function, *Ann. Intern. Med., 77*:598–602.

75. Levin, D., Baker, A., Riddell, R., et al. (1979). Nonalcoholic liver disease: Overlooked cause of liver injury in patients with heavy alcohol consumption, *Am. J. Med., 66*:429–434.

76. Stimmel, B. (1972). Hepatic dysfunction in heroin addicts: The role of alcohol, *J.A.M.A., 222*:811–812.

77. Fellner, M., and Weinstein, L. (1979). Cutaneous stigmata of drug addiction, *Int. J. Dermatol., 18*:305–306.

78. Jacobson, J., and Hirschman, S. (1982). Necrotizing fasciitis complicating intravenous drug abuse, *Arch. Intern. Med., 142*:634–635.

79. Michelson, J., Whelcher, J., Wilson, S., and O'Connor, G. (1979). Possible foreign body granuloma of the retina associated with intravenous cocaine addiction, *Am. J. Ophthalmol., 87*:278–280.

80. Robertson, C., Reynolds, R., and Wilson, J. (1976). Pulmonary hypertension and foreign body granulomas in intravenous drug abusers, *Am. J. Med., 61*:657–664.

81. Yeagher, R., Hobson, R., Padberg, F., et al. (1987). Vascular complications related to drug abuse, *J. Trauma, 27*:305–308.

82. Tuazon, C., and Sheagran, J. (1975). Staphylococcal endocarditis in parenteral drug abusers: Source of the organism, *Ann. Intern. Med., 82*:788–790.

83. Barg, N., Kish, M., Kauffman, C., et al. (1985). Group A Streptococcal bacteremia in intravenous drug abusers, *Am. J. Med., 78*:569–574.

84. Shekar, R., Rice, T., Zierdt, C., et al. (1985). Outbreak of endocarditis caused by Pseudomonas aeruginosa sterotype OII among pentazocine and tripelenamine abusers in Chicago, *J. Infect. Dis.*, *151*:203–208.

85. Chasnoff, I. (1988). Newborn infants with drug withdrawal symptoms, *Pediatr. Rev.*, *9*:273–277.

86. Dixon, S. (1989). Effects of transplacental exposure to cocaine and methamphetamine on the neonate, *West. J. Med.*, *150*:436–442.

87. Zelson, C., and Green, M. (1977). Progeny and drug abuse, *Drug Abuse, Clinical and Basic Aspects* (S. Pradhan and S. Dutta, eds.), Mosby, St. Louis, p. 433.

88. Zelson, C., Rubio, E., and Wasserman, E. (1971). Neonatal narcotic addiction: Ten year observation, *Pediatrics, 48*:178.

89. Fried, P., and O'Connell, C. (1987). A Comparison of the effects of prenatal exposure to tobacco, alcohol, cannabis, and caffeine on birth size and subsequent growth, *Neurotoxicol. Teratol.*, *9*:79–85.

90. Fried, P., and Watkinson, B. (1988). Twelve and twenty-four month neurobehavioral follow-up of children prenatally exposed to marijuana cigarettes and alcohol, *Neurotoxicol. Teratol.*, *10*:305–313.

91. Fried, P. (1989). Postnatal consequences of maternal marijuana use in humans, *Ann. N.Y. Acad. Sci.*, *562*:123–132.

92. Hingson, R., Alpert, N., et al. (1982). Effects of maternal drinking and marijuana use on fetal growth and development, *Pediatrics, 70*:539–546.

93. Chasnoff, I., Griffith, D. (1989). Cocaine: Clinical studies of pregnancy and the newborn, *Ann. N.Y. Acad. Sci.*, *562*:260–266.

94. Chavez, G., Mulinare, S., and Cordero, J. (1989). Maternal cocaine use during early pregnancy as a risk factor for congenital urogenital anomalies, *J.A.M.A.*, *262*:795–798.

95. Chashoff, I., Bussey, M., Savich, R., and Stack, C. (1986). Perinatal cerebral infarction and maternal cocaine use, *J. Pediatr.*, *108*:456–459.

96. Chaney, N., Franke, J., and Wadlington, W. (1988). Cocaine convulsions in a breast-feeding baby. *J. Pediatr.*, *112*:134–135.

97. Little, B., Snell, L., Klein, V., and Gilstrap, L. (1989). Cocaine abuse during pregnancy: Maternal and fetal implications, *Obstet. Gynecol.*, *73*:157–160.

98. Doberczak, T., Shanzer, S., Senie, R., and Krandall, S. (1988). Neonatal neurologic and electroencephalographic effects of intrauterine cocaine exposure, *J. Pediatr.*, *113*:354–358.

99. Shih, L., Cone-Wesson, B., and Reddix, B. (1988). Effects of maternal cocaine abuse on the neonatal auditory system, *Int. J. Pediatr. Otorhinolaryngol.*, *15*:245–251.

100. Chasnoff, I., Hunt, C., Kletter, R., and Kaplan, D. (1989). Prenatal cocaine exposure is associated with respiratory pattern abnormalities, *Am. J. Dis. Child.*, *143*:583–587.

101. Bauchner, H., Zuckerman, B., McClain, M., et al. (1988). Risk of sudden infant death syndrome among infants with in-utero exposure to cocaine, *J. Pediatr.*, *113*:831–834.

102. *Diagnostic and Statistical Manual of Mental Disorders* (1987). 3rd.–Revised, American Psychiatric Association, Washington, D.C.

103. Fishbain, D., and Wetli, C., (1981). Cocaine intoxication, Delirium, and death in a body packer, *Ann. Emerg. Med.*, *10*:531–532.

104. Levy, G. (1982). Gastrointestinal clearance of drugs with activated charcoal, *N. Engl. J. Med.*, *307*:676–678.

105. Khantzian, E., and McKenna, G. (1979). Acute toxic and withdrawal reactions associated with drug use and abuse, *Ann. Intern. Med.* *90*:361–372.

106. Berg, M., Berlinger, W., Goldberg, M., et al. (1982). Acceleration of the body clearance of phenobarbital by oral activated charcoal, *N. Engl. J. Med.*, *307*:642–644.

107. Mann, J., and Sandberg, D. (1970). Therapy of sedative overdosage, *Pediatr. Clin. North Am.*, *17*:617–628.

108. Smith, D. (1984). Diagnostic, therapeutic, and aftercare approaches to cocaine abuse, *J. Subst. Abuse Treat.*, *1*:5–9.

109. Farber, S., and Huertas, V. (1976). Intravenously injected marijuana syndrome, *Arch. Intern. Med.*, *136*:337.

110. Polen, M., and Friedman, G. (1988). Automobile injury—Selected risk factors and prevention in the health care setting, *J.A.M.A., 259*:77–80.
111. Consensus Development Panel (1985). Drug concentrations in driving impairment, *J.A.M.A., 254*:2618–2621.
112. Honkanen, R., Ertama, L., and Linnoilla, M. (1980). Role of drugs in traffic accidents, *Br. Med. J., 281*:1309–1312.
113. Terhune, K., and Fell, J. (1982). The role of alcohol, marijuana, and other drugs in the accidents of impaired drivers, Technical report DOT HS 806 181. Department of Transportation, National Highway Traffic Safety Administration, Washington, D.C.
114. Williams, A., Peat, M., and Crouch, D. (1985). Drugs in fatally injured young male drivers, Public Health Report, 100:19–25.
115. Reeve, V. (1979). Incidence of marijuana in a California impaired-driver population, California State Dept. of Justice, Sacramento, California.
116. Sutton, L. (1983). The effects of alcohol, marijuana, and their combination on driving ability, *J. Stud. Alcohol, 44*:438–445.
117. Yesavage, J., et al. (1985). Carryover effects of marijuana intoxication on aircraft pilot performance, *Am. J. Psychiatry, 142*:1325–1329.
118. Marzuk, P., Tardif, K., et al. (1990). Prevalence of recent cocaine use among motor vehicle fatalities in New York City, *J.A.M.A., 263*:250–256.
119. Cummings, S., Kelsey, J., Nevitt, M., and O'Dowd, K. (1985). Epidemiology of osteoporosis and osteoporotic fractures, *Epidemiol. Rev., 7*:178–208.
120. Riggs, B., and Melton, L. (1986). Involutional osteoporosis, *N. Engl. J. Med., 314*:1676–1686.
121. Ray, W., Griffin, M., and Downey, W. (1989). Benzodiazepines of long and short elimination half-life and the risk of hip fracture, *J.A.M.A., 262*:3303–3307.
122. Ray, W., Griffin, M., et al. (1098). Psychotropic drug use and the risk of hip fracture, *N. Engl. J. Med., 316*:363–369.

33

Neurological Effects of Drug and Alcohol Addiction

Anne Geller
Smithers Alcohol Treatment Center, New York, New York

I. INTRODUCTION

All drugs which produce euphoria affect the nervous system acutely during intoxication. Chronic use can result in neuroadaptive changes which are the basis for tolerance and dependence. This chapter is not concerned with those effects which are integral to the action of the drug itself, but is focused on neurological impairments which may occur as a consequence of drug use in some individuals. For the most part, the concern will be with structural neurological damage occurring after chronic drug use; however, both transient symptoms and complications arising from a single episode of use will be mentioned when they are of importance for a specific drug. Alcohol is the drug of abuse with the most extensive medical consequences and its adverse effects on the nervous system are both common and diverse. The neurological complications of alcoholism thus constitute the largest segment of this chapter. Because alcohol has such a significant impact on neurological function, it is a potential confounding variable in clinical studies of neurological effects in abusers of other drugs, who are frequently also drinking heavily, if not alcoholically. Head traumas occur more frequently among drug abusers than the general population and may complicate the clinical presentation, as do compression neuropathies, a consequence of prolonged immobility or loss of pain perception in the drugged state. Finally, neurological consequences of poor nutrition and personal neglect may add to the overall picture.

II. ALCOHOL

The traditional picture of central nervous system damage due to alcohol focused, not surprisingly, on striking clinical syndromes. These were often irreversible resulting in death or serious disability, and occurred most frequently in debilitated alcoholics after years of addictive drinking with general neglect of health and nutrition. Wernicke described the acute delirium with opthalmoplegia and ataxia in 1881 [1]. Six years later, Korsakoff (1887) [2] noted the remarkable chronic impairment of memory with relative preservation of other cognitive capacities which occurred in some alcoholics. Around the same time, Maudsley (1879) [3] wrote of a more generalized impairment of cognitive abilities which he had observed in alcoholics resembling the last stages of senile dementia. These three syndromes, Wernicke's encephalopathy, Korsakoff's psychosis, and alcoholic dementia were to constitute the basis of entries in textbooks on brain damage due to alcoholism for almost a century. The work of Peters [4] in the 1930s on the thiamine-deficient pidgeon provided insight into the nature of Wernicke's encephalopathy and the link between Wernicke's encephalopathy and Korsakoff's psychosis became increasingly apparent as more patients survived the acute encephalopathy as a result of thiamine treatment, only to reveal subsequent difficulties with memory.

The nutritional (thiamine deficiency) etiology of Wernicke's encephalopathy having been clearly established, what then of Korsakoff's psychosis and alcoholic dementia? Although deficiency of thiamine and perhaps other vitamins may contribute to the cause of these disorders, a direct toxic action of alcohol itself on the brain has been postulated by a number of workers [5,6]. Long-term alcohol administration to nutritionally supplemented rats has been shown to result in severe neuronal damage [7].

Freund and Ballinger have demonstrated that chronic alcohol abuse (defined as consumption of more than 80 gm of absolute alcohol a day for more than 10 years) results in loss of muscarinic cholinergic receptors in the frontal cortex [8]. They also showed loss of muscarinic receptors and sparing of benzodiazepine receptors in the putamen. This loss of muscarinic receptors occurs in histologically normal brains in the absence of significant atrophy and gross dementia. These findings suggest that alcohol toxicity does not simply result in a random loss of neurons, but in region- and receptor-specific effects. A direct action of alcohol itself, in addition to the nutritional deficits which may occur after long-term alcohol abuse, is consistent with many of the more recent observations regarding alcohol-related brain damage. These observations come from a number of different sources: pneumoencephalograms (PEGs), computed tomographic (CT) scans, magnetic resonance imagining (MRI), positron emission tomography (PET), autopsy material, and event-related potential (ERP) studies in man as well as chronic ethanol treatment (CET) in animals. Alcohol itself appears to produce a continuun of impairments beginning possibly with those which are mild and probably transient in heavy social drinkers [10,11], followed by significant and partly reversible deficits in alcoholics, and ending with the chronic, severe picture of alcoholic dementia. Other events such as acute thiamine deficiency, head trauma, and hepatic failure may be superimposed on this picture.

There are many different factors which are involved in the ways in which drinking alcoholic beverages can adversely effect the brain, which include:

1. Direct action on nerve cells, particularly nerve cell membranes [12].
2. Effects on neurotransmitters, receptors, second-messenger systems [13,14].
3. Chronic changes in membranes, neurotransmitters, or receptors resulting in dependence [15].
4. Poor food intake and malaborption, resulting in vitamin deficiency, particularly thiamine, pyridoxine, niacin [16].
5. Associated metabolic changes.
6. Reduction in cerebral blood flow [17].
7. Damage to other organs indirectly resulting in CNS effects, for example, hepatic enephalopathy.

Undoubtedly as one progresses along the scale from heavy social drinking to severe chronic alcoholism, more factors come into play and the chances of sustaining some degree of nervous system impairment increase. There is, however, considerable individual variability. Some alcoholics suffer severe brain damage, whereas others, at the same age with similar drinking histories and socioeconomic backgrounds, are only minimally impaired. Some evidence exists for genetic factors increasing vulnerability to end-organ damage due to alcohol [18,19].

Table 1 lists for convenient reference the major alcohol-related syndromes with brief summaries of clinical findings, pathological lesions, and etiology when known.

A. Intermediate Brain Syndrome

The intermediate brain syndrome is not technically a diagnosis. It is a term originally coined by Bennett [20] in 1960 to describe the impairment in cognitive abilities observed in many alcoholics coming to treatment. These deficits range from mild, detectable only by neuropsychological testing, to moderate when clinicians can observe defects in memory, thinking, and problem-solving abilities which may interfere with the patient's ability to participate in treatment and to return to work. The impairment is not severe enough, however, to be correctly labeled Korsakoff's psychosis or alcoholic dementia, or to require institutionalization of the patient. Awareness of these impairments is important for the clinician in treatment planning and in return-to-work counseling. Alcoholics toward the more severe end of the cognitive impairment spectrum have been observed to be less able to participate in treatment and to have poorer outcome, but this requires further investigation [21,22].

The particular abilities most affected by excessive alcohol intake have been remarkably consistent over a wide range of studies involving males and females of different socioeconomic and ethnic groups [23,24]. General intelligence and verbal abilities are intact. The IQ as measured on the Wechsler Adult Intelligence Scale (WAIS) is normal. Difficulties occur with abstract thinking and problem-solving abilities as measured on the Halsted Category Test or the Shipley Hartford. Visual spatial and perceptual motor abilities are also impaired. New learning, both verbal and visual, is significantly impaired in alcoholics compared to age-matched controls.

Evidence from CT studies suggest that one-half to two-thirds of alcoholics develop brain atrophy and/or ventricular dilatation [25]. This may occur in some quite early in their drinking careers. Others appear to be unaffected despite long drinking histories. The reasons for these differences are not clear, though genetic factors may play a role. The severity of CT changes and abnormalities in evoked potentials seem to be greater in family history–positive than family history–negative alcoholics [26]. Age is also a factor. In a recent study [27] widened sulci were found, even in younger alcoholics, and appeared to be correlated with lifetime alcohol consumption. Ventricular enlargement, on the other hand, was more prominent in older patients. Measurements of brains at autopsy confirm the CT findings that brain tissue is commonly affected in alcoholics; brain weight tends to be lower, ventricular volume increased, and sulci widened [28,29]. Position emission tomography (PET) and cerebral blood flow (CBF) studies have been conducted to investigate brain pathophysiology in alcoholic patients. Compared with age-matched controls, long-term abstinent alcoholics with memory impairments showed lower glucose use than controls, particularly in the frontal cortex, thalamus, and basal ganglia [30]. Cerebral blood flow studies have shown decrements in blood flow correlated with life-time alcohol consumption [31]. In young (less than 40-year-old), alcoholics, CBF showed abnormal regional patterns [32]. Particularly marked was decreased blood flow to the frontal regions.

Just as a marked improvement in neuropsychological functioning has been noted in some alcoholics who maintain abstinence, certain CT scan parameters have also shown improvement with abstinence. This reversibility of brain atrophy was first shown by Carlen et al. in 1978 [33], and this has subsequently been confirmed by other groups [34,35]. Patients

Table 1 Major Alcohol-Related Syndromes

Syndrome	Clinical Findings	Lesion/Etiology
Intermediate brain syndrome	1. May be difficulty in new learning, some concreteness, lack in mental flexibility 2. Impairment on neuro-psychological testing	Occurs in alcoholics with normal nutritional status. Could be subclinical nutritional deficiency and direct neurotoxic effect of alcohol.
Wernicke's encephalopathy	1. Disorientation 2. Confusion 3. Nystagmus 4. Ocular palsies 5. Ataxia	Mid brain punctate hemorrhages. Nutritional (thiamine) deficiency with or without additional genetically determined enzyme deficiency.
Korsakoff's psychosis	1. Profound deficit in new new learning (recent memory) 2. Some deficits in remote memory 3. Intelligence and verbal abilities usually perserved 4. May confabulate	Mid brain gliosis. Basal forebrain frequently follows Wernicke's encephalopathy. Can occur alone. Permanent syndrome not seen in uncomplicated thiamine deficiency. Only partial responsive to thiamine. Possible neurotoxic component.
Alcoholic dementia	1. Global decline in intellectual functions. Memory affected but not predominantly 2. Apathy, irritability, emotional lability	Etiology unclear. Direct neurotoxic effect of alcohol and possible subclinical nutritional deficiencies, trauma, metabolic.
Central pontine myelinolysis	1. Rapid-onset paraparesis or quadriparesis 2. Dysarthria 3. Dysphagia	Edema of the pons 2° electrolyte disturbance. Hyponatremia.
Marchiafava-Bignami	1. Gradual-onset dementia with psychosis 2. Convulsions 3. Focal symptoms aphasia.	Degeneration of corpus callosum related to alcohol. Etiology unknown.
Alcoholic cerebellar degeneration	1. Acute onset with Wernicke's encephalopathy 2. Subacute onset alone 3. Marked gait ataxia 4. Little arm ataxia or dysarthria	Degeneration of Purkinje cells in cerebellar vermis. Possibly mainly due to thiamine lack. Possibly a direct neurotoxic effect of alcohol. Not dose related. Possibly genetic susceptibility.
Alcoholic polyneuropathy	1. Gradual onset of symmetrical loss of sensation in toes, fingers 2. Symmetrical motor loss beginning distally 3. Loss of reflexes	Degeneration of myelin sheaths of peripheral nerves. Thiamine deficiency.
Optic neuropathy (tobacco-alcohol amblyopia)	1. Acute or subacute onset of impaired vision 2. Central scotomata	Thiamine deficiency.

who remain abstinent show increased brain density and decreased ventricular size. In a 5-year follow-up study [36], alcoholics who had been abstinent for the 5-year period had less brain atrophy, both cortical and subcortical, than they had on initial examination after detoxification. However, they still showed more atrophy than an age-matched control group.

Cerebral blood flow studies have also shown improvements in blood flow with abstinence and treatment [37]. Magnetic resonance imaging of the intracranial cerebrospinal fluid (CSF) volume has shown a highly significant reduction after 5 weeks of abstinence [38]. This reduction could not be accounted for only by de- and rehydration of the brain. Other effects such as the rise of protein synthesis after alcohol withdrawal and a subsequent increase in dentritic growth may be important.

The number of withdrawals from alcohol appears to be related to poorer memory test performance in both males and females [39]. Females showed the same amount of performance errors with a shorter duration of alcohol use and withdrawals than males. Interestingly, Freund in 1970 [40] had showed that shuttle box performance in mice was markedly impaired in a group given 24-h withdrawals four times over a 5-week period compared with mice who were kept continuously alcohol dependent during that period.

Of great concern to clinicians is the extent to which functional deficits observed in most alcoholics in early (up to 1 month) abstinence can be reversed if abstinence is sustained. Parsons [41] reviewed 21 neuropsychological studies in which recovery had been assessed after 1 month to 4 years of abstinence. Eighty percent of the studies indicated that significant improvement is to be expected. Different functions appear to recover at different times. At the end of 1 month, verbal learning and sensory and motor capabilities improve. However, abstracting ability and visual spatial learning remain impaired. Older alcoholics show the least improvement. Abstracting abilities and perceptual motor abilities show improvement between 3 and 6 months of abstinence. Even in the longer studies the alcoholics as a group, though improved from their initial testing, remained impaired relative to controls. For the individual alcoholic it would seem that some are left with no detectable impairment if abstinence is sustained, whereas others, older, and/or with greater initial impairment, show only partial recovery. Alcoholics who resume drinking (even though not at their earlier levels) tend to have more impaired neuropsychological test findings during treatment than eventual abstainers [42]. However, when examined at 6 months or 1 year after treatment, resumers are much more impaired than abstainers.

It is important to recognize that the majority (70%) of alcoholics coming to treatment have some degree of cognitive impairment. It may be mild and transient in some. In others, it may be severe enough to seriously limit the patient's ability to participate in traditional cognitively oriented treatment. In these cases, longer-term residential treatment may be indicated to permit maximum recovery to take place in an alcohol-free environment. In yet others, the degree of cognitive impairment observed requires careful counseling to permit a successful return to work. Cognitive rehabilitation may be productively used with selected patients [43].

B. Blackouts

Although not strictly a consequence of chronic alcohol use, blackouts, episodes of transient anterograde amnesia occurring exclusively during intoxication, would seem to be related in some way to deficits in learning and memory observed in long-term heavy drinkers. Blackouts appear to be associated with a rapid rise in the blood alcohol level and can occur in naive drinkers having their first drinking experience. However, repeated blackouts can be said to be pathognomonic of alcoholic drinking, mainly because to experience such a devastating event as to be totally unable to recall a large segment of one's awake activities, and not to change one's drinking practices to prevent this from ever occurring again, indicates a quite abnormal positive value of intoxication for the individual. Interestingly, blackouts have been little studied since Goodwin's [44] work 20 years ago. Alcoholics were given alcohol and their behavior studied. Five episodes of anterograde amnesia were recorded. There did not appear to be any predictive factors. The alcoholics behaved during the blackout in a "normal" intoxicated manner. Immediate recall was intact, however, no permanent memories were formed. The mechanism for this acute failure of memory consolidation is not known. Clearly in susceptible people the memory system becomes less tolerant than other systems to high blood alcohol concentrations (BACs). (The average BAC in Goodwin's [44] patients was 300 mg %.)

Alcohol's inhibitory effects on the N-methyl-D-aspartate (NMDA) receptor, thought to be involved in long-term potentiation, may be a factor. Long-term potentiation refers to those changes in neuronal biochemistry and physiology which perpetuate brain signals long after those evoked through neurotransmission have decayed [45]. Inhibition of responses at the NMDA receptor may contribute to the cognitive impairments associated with intoxication by preventing transfer from short- to long-term memory processes. The effects of calcium channel blockers on alcoholic blackouts would be interesting to study. Clinically, the alcoholic blackout shares many features with the syndrome of transient global amnesia [46] which is essentially a period of anterograde amnesia occurring in older people without warning. The etiology is not known, but it may be a form of transient ischemic attack in the posterior cerebral circulation. Perhaps the most instructive comparison between an alcoholic having experienced a blackout and a person who had just had an episode of transient global amnesia lies in the affective response to the event. Patients after an episode of transient global amnesia are uniformly terrified. Not to have any recollection of a period of time during which one was walking, talking, and generally acting in the world appears to evoke a radical fear in normal adults. "Who was the I who was acting on the stage while the monitoring self, the remembering self, was absent? "What did I do?" "What might I do?" "Tell me it will never happen again." The alcoholic's calm acceptance of blackouts as an unremarkable part of the drinking experiences, smells of the *belle indifference* of the hysteric. Indeed it is a measure of the intensity of denial in this disease.

C. Wernicke's Encephalopathy

Wernicke described the clinical picture and pathology of the syndrome that bears his name in his textbook of 1881, and it has been little changed since. What is seen is a relatively abrupt onset of a confusional state, accompanied by unsteadiness of gait and visual difficulties. Objectively the patient is confused, disoriented, and often apathetic, and has ataxia of the lower limbs, nystagmus, and partial or complete opthalmoplegia. A tremor may be observed and a peripheral neuropathy is usually present, but may be difficult to test in the acute situation.

Wernicke's encephalopathy is clearly related to thiamine deficiency. This syndrome has been observed not only in alcoholics, but also in malnourished prisoners of war and in intractable vomiting from many causes. Indeed, one of Wernicke's original patients was a seamstress with persistent vomiting following sulfuric acid poisoning.

The mechanism by which thiamine deficiency results in the characteristic lesions in the midline periventricular structures of the brainstem and diencephalon is not yet clear. These regions have been shown to undergo metabolic and histological changes that may not normalize even after prolonged thiamine administration. An episode of severe thiamine deficiency has been shown to result in increased consumtion and accelerated metabolism of alcohol in rats even after 6 months of a normal diet [47]. Furthermore, the previously thiamine-deficient rats showed greater CNS sensitivity to alcohol at a given blood alcohol concentration.

Brain energy metabolism is decreased in chronic alcoholics, as is the rate of formation of thiamine pyrophosphate. Thiamine pyrophosphate, a cofactor for a ketoglutarate dehydrogenase, is reduced in thiamine deficiency, and this is accompanied by decreased aspartate, glutamate, and gamma aminobutyric acid (GABA) [48]. Brain cell death could result from compromised cerebral energy metabolism and local accumulation of lactase. Transketolase may be irreversibly decreased, which may make those with genetically low levels specially vulnerable. An interesting observation with potential therapeutic usefulness is that damage from thiamine deficiency is similar to that seen with excitotoxic amino acids. The administration of an antagonist of NMDA receptors (a subclass of glutamate receptors through which excitotoxic damage is mediated) has been shown to decrease the thalamic damage in thiamine deficient rats [49].

The treatment for Wernicke's encephalopathy is high-dose thiamine (100 mg) given immediately intravenously and twice a day intramuscularly until the patient can take medication by mouth. Improvement in the opthalmoplegia usually occurs within a few hours of thiamine treatment. The acute confusional state clears more slowly over several days. The ataxia may clear completely or partially over a period of days or weeks. Some patients may be left with a permanent residual deficit in coordination. Fifty to eighty-four percent of patients with Wernicke's encephalopathy will be revealed to have Korsakoff's psychosis as their acute confusional state clears. It should be noted that very few, if any, patients with Wernicke's encephalopathy whose etiology is related to alcohol abuse will again regain completely normal cognitive capacity.

In a series from Boston City Hospital, 2.2% of autopsies had lesions in the mid brain, and in a similar study in Australia [50], Wernicke's encephalopathy was diagnosed at autopsy in 2% of the brains examined [51]. This latter study is interesting in that it corroborated earlier observations that patients whose brains showed the characteristic lesions at autopsy had not exhibited the classic Wernicke signs while alive. Indeed, only 14% of the Australian series had been suspected prior to death. Hypotension and lethargy occurred clinically as frequently as did the classic triad of confusion, ataxia, and opthalmoplegia. Twenty percent had died suddenly and unexpectedly. Lishman [52] has suggested that possibly because of widespread use of vitamins the condition has become less fulminating and subclinical forms of the disease might be occurring. Recurrent attacks of subclinical encephalopathy over the years would explain why, in alcoholics, the memory difficulties following Wernicke's encephalopathy tend to remain, whereas in nutritionally depleted prisoners they respond to thiamine.

If lesions do develop in the Wernicke location without being clinically apparent as the autopsy evidence indicates, then high-potency vitamin replacement should be given as often as possible. Indeed, fortification of alcoholic beverages with thiamine, as suggested by Canterwell and Criqui [53], would be a reasonsble idea.

D. Korsakoff's Psychosis

Korsakoff's psychosis is linked to Wernicke's encephalopathy by common pathological findings and common etiology. Victor, whose 1953 paper is the classic of modern clinical studies of the neurological complications of alcohol abuse, entitled his 1971 book *The Wernicke-Korsakoff Syndrome*, and it is frequently referred to by that compound name. Nevertheless, it should be noted that not all patients with Wernicke's encephalopathy develop the amnestic confabulatory psychosis of Korsakoff. Furthermore, many cases of Korsakoff's psychosis develop their amnesic difficulties insidiously without any proceeding history of Wernicke's encephalopathy.

The most striking feature of patients with Korsakoff's psychosis is a severe memory impairment for on-going events. These patients are unable to find their way around the ward or to remember the names of staff and other patients. Memory for remote events, both public and personal, is spotty and vague. Some make up stories, confabulate, to cover the memory gaps, but many do not do this and it is not a necessary part of the syndrome. This devastating memory deficit occurs in some pure cases in the absence of any other clinical signs of intellectual deterioration. Intelligence on the WAIS is preserved. These patients can think, speak, and calculate numbers with customary speed and efficiency. Immediate memory as tested by the digit span is normal, but information can be retained at most for a few minutes after which it rapidly dissipates. Because patients with Korsakoff's psychosis may be articulate, even witty, and may appear superficially intact, the gross memory defect can be overlooked by the casual observer.

Many cases diagnosed as Korsakoff's psychosis are not pure in the sense that though the striking memory impairments are present, so too are other cognitive deficits. Indeed one of the "pure" Korsakoff patients studied so carefully by Mair et al. [55] for 9 years began to show a general intellectual deterioration 2 years before his death. This is not surprising when one considers that patients with Korsakoff's psychosis are subject to the same factors which produce cognitive deficits in other alcoholics. Most cases of Korsakoff's psychosis are found to have, in addition to marked anterograde and retrograde amnesia, less marked visuoperceptive and problem-solving impairments. It has been suggested Korsakoff's psychosis represents one end of a continuum of alcohol damage with the mild often transient memory deficits of most younger alcoholics being near the other end, and perhaps the alcoholic blackout representing the beginning. This does not seem to be case [56]. There is an abrupt discontinuity between the severity of memory impairments of patients with Korsakoff's psychosis and those with similar age and drinking history. Furthermore, alcoholics who do not have Korsakoff's psychosis have predominantly poor visual memory, whereas both verbal and visual memory are severely impaired in affected patients. Patients with Korsakoff's psychosis are exquisitely sensitive to distraction and proactive interference; that is, when trying to remember a current task items from previous tasks keep intruding. Without acute trauma such as thiamine deficiency alcohol results only in mild to moderate memory deficits.

The retrograde amnesia of Korsakoff's psychosis is temporally graded, affecting recent events much more than distant events. This was thought to be a result of anterograde amnesia, much as one sees in a considerably milder form in other alcoholics. That is, events do not get encoded in the permanent memory and thus cannot be recalled. Anyone trying to get a clear, temporally ordered, history from an alcoholic in a detoxification unit knows how fuzzy recollection for events over the recent past can be. However, the situation in Korsakoff's psychosis is different. An unusual clinical opportunity occurred when an eminent scientist developed Korsakoff's psychosis at the age of 65, 2 years after the publication of his autobiography in 1981. He was tested by Butters [57] on events recorded in his own autobiography. He showed a marked retrograde amnesia for his own history with sparing of events only from his remote past. Clearly this could not be due to a deficit in learning, since these events had obviously at one time been known and recorded by him.

In contrast to amnestic syndromes of other etiologies, patients with Korsakoff's psychosis frequently display apathy, lack of initiative, and profound lack of insight, suggesting a cortical component.

Once established, Korsakoff's psychosis in alcoholics is not notably responsive to thiamine. Nevertheless, thiamine and multivitamin supplements should be given to affected patients in order to assist any improvement and attenuate further damage should drinking recur. In Victor's 1971 series [54], one-quarter of the patients showed complete clinical recovery, one-half partial recovery, and the remainder were unchanged. The extent of more subtle nueropsychological deficits in those 25% who recovered clinically is unknown. The time over which recovery may take place can extend beyond 1 year. In an elegant study [55] correlating neuropsychological findings with pathology in patients studied for several years prior to death, the critical lesions for the memory deficit appeared to be bilaterally in the medial nuclei of the mammillary bodies and bilaterally between the wall of the third ventricle and the medial dorsal nucleus of the thalamus. Arendt et al. [58], however, suggest that the critical area affected in alcoholic patients with Korsakoff's psychosis may be the basal forebrain, the major source of cholinergic input to the cerebral cortex and hippocampus. They found that the number of neurons was reduced by 70% in the basal forebrain patients with Korsakoff's psychosis.

Cerebrospinal fluid levels of metabolities of norepinephrine, dopamine, and serotonin have been shown to be reduced in patients with Korsakoff's psychosis. Improvement in memory has been found with the alpha$_2$-adrenergic agonist clonidine [59], and also with the serotonin reuptake blocker fluvoxamine [60]. In neither study could the drug effects be said to be dramatic, but either could be promising leads for therapy in the future.

E. Alcoholic Dementia

Alcoholic dementia has been a rather neglected condition clinically, pathologically, and etiologically. There is no question that a substantial proportion of alcoholics (8% in one series) become demented [52]. This dementia is not clinically distinguishable from dementia due to other causes. There is a progressive deterioration in all cognitive abilities. Acquisition and use of new information is impaired along with general problem-solving abilities. There may be increasing difficulty with remote memory as well. Inappropriate social behavior and personal neglect occur in the later stages. Apathy, irritability, emotional lability, and undue truculence may also be present, as in other dementias. Alcoholic dementia usually develops insidiously against a background of chronic inebriation, and may not be recognized by the patient's family, who attribute the behavior to simple drunkeness. Only when the patient is detoxified may the picture become clear. As mentioned above, cerebral atrophy is a very common finding in CT scans of alcoholics. Computed tomographic scans of patients with alcoholic dementia have not been compared to those of nondementia alcoholics. It would seem likely that cerebral atrophy would be worse among demented alcoholics. Pathological findings have included neuronal degeneration and loss, which are patchy and diffuse throughout the cerebral cortex. The characteristic plaques and tangles seen in the presenile and senile dementias have been rarely observed in the brains of alcoholics with dementia [61].

Alcoholism accounted for 7% of demented patients in three current surveys [52], and was at least as common as multi-infarct dementia. In a series from the Maudsley Hospital, 50 alcoholics had been labeled as having Korsakoff's psychosis and 13 as having alcoholic dementia. Half of the patients with Korsakoff's psychosis had an acute onset. The others had a more gradual and insidious onset. Those patients with Korsakoff's psychosis of gradual onset had global deficits as well as the severe memory impairments, and they resembled the alcoholic dementias in having a later age of onset and also a better prognosis for improvement. Two-thirds of the alcoholic dementias and "gradual-onset" Korsakoff patients showed some improvement.

F. Cerebral Trauma

Alcoholics because of drunkeness are particularly prone to accidents of all kinds. The shrunken brain, fragile blood vessels, and delayed clotting time make them more vulnerable to serious complications of head trauma such as subdural and epidural hematomas. Alcoholics constitute a large percentage of patients admitted to neurosurgical wards because of significant head trauma. The actual incidence of this among alcoholics is difficult to ascertain. Significant head trauma was reported in 7% of alcoholics having seizures. Severe craniocerebral trauma can produce focal deficits such as hemiparesis in addition to more diffuse cerebral dysfunction. Minor degrees of unreported or unnoticed head trauma may contribute to intellectual deterioration in some alcoholics.

G. Hepatic and Other Metabolic Encephalopathies

Alcoholism is the leading cause of cirrhosis of the liver. Some patients with cirrhosis will develop liver failure and subsequent hepatic encephalopathy. Other metabolic derangements such as electrolyte imbalance, hypoglycemia, and respiratory alkalosis are also more common in alcoholics than in the general population. Delirium, particularly if prolonged or repeated, may lead to long-term or permanent cognitive impairments. Again, this may contribute to a picture of intellectual deterioration in the alcoholic.

H. Central Pontine Myelinolysis and Marchiafava-Bignami Disease

In Victor and Laureno's 1978 series [50], central pontine myelinolysis was found in only 0.25% of autopsied cases and Marchiafava-Bignami disease in less than 0.05%. Patients with central pontine myelinolysis are rarely diagnosed before death, though advances in CT scanning now make this a possibility. Clinically, the condition appears as a rapidly evolving paraparesis or quadriparesis in a patient who is confused and usually lethargic. Pseudobular symptoms, dysarthria, and dysphagia are prominent. Severe electrolyte aberrations are found, particularly hyponatremia, which are thought to be the cause of the syndrome [62]. Central pontine myelinolysis occurs in conditions other than alcoholism. The course is usually progressively downhill to death, but with recognition and prompt correction of the electrolyte imbalance, recovery can occur. At autopsy the pons is edematous with central destruction of myelin.

Marchiafava-Bignami disease is rare. It was thought to be limited to Italian males who drank red wine, but one of Victor's cases was a black woman who drank any type of alcoholic beverage. There is a slow onset of mental symptoms which may be manic, paranoid, or delusional, often accompanied by intellectual deterioration. Convulsions and various focal neurological signs are frequent. The course is downhill, usually over several years. The pathology is distinctive with symmetrical necrosis of the corpus callosum. The etiology is unknown and there is no treatment.

I. Deficiencies of Vitamins Other than Thiamine

Deficiencies of niacin, pyridoxine, and pantothenic acid occur in alcoholics and are associated with nervous system disorders [63]. Riboflavin and folic acid deficiency also occur in alcoholics, but the evidence that either deficiency results in nervous system disease is quite flimsy. Niacin deficiency disease (pellagra) is rare in developed countries. However Serdau recently collected 22 cases of alcoholic pellagra in France [64]. The clinical triad of pellagra, i.e., dermatitis, diarrhea, and dementia, consists of erythematous skin lesions, gastrointestinal symptoms of anorexia and diarrhea, and neurological systems, including confusion, hypertonus, and myoclonus. Peripheral neuropathy may also occur. Early symptoms of fatigue, apathy, anorexia, insomnia, and irritability are nonspecific and may be misdiagnosed as depression. In Serdau's autopsy cases, all were neglected, undernourished, and cachectic, and most belonged to the classical category of *clochards*, tramps with no fixed abode. When hospitalized they were given thiamine and pyridoxine but not niacin. These cases emphasize the importance of multivitamin replacement for alcoholics. Pyridoxine and pantothenic acid deficiency give rise to peripheral neuropathies, the latter being associated with the burning feet syndrome (severe dysesthesias manifested by burning pain in the extremities). They occur in conjunction with other B vitamin deficiencies.

J. Alcoholic Cerebellar Degeneration

The unsteady gait, clumsy movements, and slurred speech, manifestations of the acute effects of alcohol on the cerebellar system, are the familiar hallmarks of drunkeness. Alcoholic cerebellar degeneration results in a less diffuse but unfortunately often permanent clinical picture. The gait is primarily affected, being broad based and unstable. Lower limb ataxia is usually severe, but involvement of the upper limbs is minimal. Dysarthia and nystagmus are rare. The ataxia may appear acutely as a component of Wernicke's encephalopathy, or it may evolve more gradually in isolation. When it appears as part of Wernicke's encephalopathy, about 50% of the cases will recover completely from the ataxia [65]; however, a much smaller proportion of those in whom the ataxia occurs alone will demonstrate significant recovery.

The pathology is quite specific, and consists of degeneration of the neurocellular elements of the cerebellar cortex, particularly the Purkinje cells, with an interesting restriction to the anterior and superior parts of the vermis. It should be noted that characteristic lesions have been found in autopsy material from patients who have not manifested the ataxia in life.

In a comparison [66] of ataxic and nonataxic alcoholics there were no differences on measures of coordination such as hand-eye coordination or reaction time. There was also a lack of any dose-response effect with regard to alcohol and ataxia. Indeed, the annual and lifetime consumption of alcohol was actually lower in the ataxic individuals. This suggests either greater variations in individual susceptibility or a nutritional etiology.

The association of cerebellar degeneration with Wernicke's encephalopathy points to a thiamine deficiency etiology. The condition, as Korsakoff's psychosis, is not dramatically responsive to thiamine, which nevertheless should be given for all the reasons outlined above for Korsakoff's psychosis. A direct toxic effect of alcohol on the cerebellum has been suggested and may contribute to the fixed structural lesions [67].

K. Alcoholic Polyneuropathy

Damage to the peripheral nerves may occur in alcoholics either as a result of associated nutritional deficiencies, specifically thiamine, or as a result of trauma, most frequently compression neuropathies. In alcoholic polyneuropathy, the sensory, motor, and autonomic systems may all be affected. There is degeneration of the myelin sheath with resulting impairment of nerve conduction velocities, and there may be direct axonal damage with reduced nerve action potential.

As with other nutritional polyneuropathies, impairment begins distally, is symmetrical, and usually starts with sensory symptoms in the form of abnormal, unpleasant senations; i.e., dysesthesias. The usual progression of symptoms is from dysesthesia, often burning or tingling sensations in the toes and soles of the feet, to actual loss of sensation, numbness, loss of vibratory and position sense, to motor involvement with loss of dorsiflexion of the feet; i.e., bilateral footdrop. Progression marches proximally and slowly over a period of months, with sensation being lost in the classic glove and stocking fashion and motor involvement spreading from the more distal muscle groups to the more proximal. If the condition is severe, cranial nerves may become involved. When involvement is predominantly motor and more proximal than distal, an alcoholic myopathy should be suspected, since both complications may co-exist [68].

L. Autonomic System

Sympathetic

Alcoholism may be associated with sympathetic dysfunction affecting both blood pressure regulation and thermoregulation. The cause of the association between regular alcohol use and hypertension is unclear, but it may in part be due to sympathetic overactivity. During alcohol withdrawal increased sympathetic nerve activity is likely to be responsible for the hypertension, tremor, sweating, and tachycardia. Orthostatic hypotension occurring in some alcoholics during withdrawal may be a consequence of sympathetic nervous system dysfunction. Peripheral sympathetic nerve damage can also affect sweating, which may be lost in a glove and stocking distribution. In a study of thermoregulatory response to heat stress, alcoholics were found to have higher temperatures after heat exposure, with reduced weight loss and impaired distal sweating. Hypothermia conversely can occur in Wernicke's encephalopathy and, as noted previously, the lesions of the latter may be present without the diagnostic clinical signs. This may further contribute to instability of heat regulation in alcoholics.

Parasympathetic

Vagal nerve degeneration has been seen in alcoholic patients manifesting dysphagia and dysphonia, and vagal neuropathy has been shown to result in depressed heart rate responses in alcoholics. Damage to the vagus can be demonstrated by diminished heart rate responses to standing, to sustained hand grip, to atropine, or to Valsalva's manuever. In diabetics, vagal neuropathy has been suggested as a cause of acute death. It is not clear whether this is the case in alcoholics; however, autonomic dysfunction may be related to cardiomyopathy.

Central sleep apnea and hypopnea are common in chronic alcoholics and show associations with central nervous system damage and vagal neuropathy.

Impotence, partial or complete, is quite common in male alcoholics and sacral neuropathy may contribute to impaired sexual function. It is important that this issue be addressed directly. It is usually of much concern to the patient, but is rarely mentioned spontaneously. Reassurance can be offered that with abstinence and daily thiamine some improvement is to be expected though this may require several months.

Alcoholic peripheral neuropathy responds very well to thiamine, the time course for recovery being dependent upon the severity of the condition. Complete recovery can be expected in most patients within several months to a year. Some, however, present with such severe initial deficits that only partial recovery occurs.

Abnormalities in electromyographic studies are often found in alcoholics without clinical signs of peripheral neuropathy, indicating an occult form of the disease [69].

M. Optic Neuropathy

Optic neuropathy is frequently referred to as tobacco-alcohol amblyopia, though there is little evidence for other than a straightforward nutritional etiology, as in alcoholic polyneuropathy. The onset of impaired vision can be acute or subacute. Central scotomata, particularly for red test objects, are found on examination. Dizziness may accompany the visual impairment and symptoms and signs of a general polyneuropathy are frequently present. Treatment and prognosis is as for polyneuropathy.

N. Nerve Trauma

It is good medical practice to inquire closely into the drug and alcohol intake of any patient presenting with a nerve compression syndrome, since chemical dependency is one of the common causes. Most physicians are familiar with "Saturday night palsy," which is a brachial plexus compression. Other nerve compression can result from "passing out" in any number of positions, which can compromise blood flow to peripheral nerves, resulting in ulnar, peroneal, and other nerve palsies. Perhaps the subclinically damaged state [69] of the peripheral nerves contributes to the frequency with which this condition develops in alcoholics. The prolonged ischemia is thought to produce demyelination. Recovery is expected to take place over a few weeks. Thiamine supplements would be prudent in alcoholics with compression neuropathies because of the possibility of underlying nutritional deficiency.

O. Stroke

There is a higher than normal incidence of hemorrhagic stroke and other intracranial bleeding among heavy users of alcohol, with an association of strokes or strokelike episodes within 24 h of a drinking binge. Studies in rats have shown graded contractile responses in cerebral arterioles in an alcohol concentration range of 10–500 mg/ml. Two calcium antagonists, nifedipine and verapamil, were shown to prevent alcohol-induced vasospasm, suggesting a possible therapeutic approach to hypertension and stroke in heavy alcohol users. Moderate alcohol consumption (three to nine drinks a week) was found to be associated with increased subarachnoid hemorrhage in women [72]. The association between alcohol and stroke may be related to hypertension, cerebral artery spasm, and increased bleeding tendency.

P. Seizures

Alcohol and epilepsy have been linked together since the time of Hippocrates. The relationship is complex. The prevalence of epilepsy in the general population ranges from 0.23–2.4% [73] and alcoholism 6.6–10.6% [74]. The increased seizures in alcoholics may be due to withdrawal, to metabolic changes such as hypoglycemia or electrolyte imbalance, or to head trauma and infection for which alcoholics are at greater risk. It is, however, very important to remember that alcoholics may have seizures from non–alcohol-related causes as well. In a series from Denver [75] of 195 cases in seizures in alcoholics, 59% were due to alcohol withdrawal, 20% to head trauma, 5% to vascular disorders, and 2% to tumors. In a prospective study of 250 patients with first alcohol-related seizures, CT scan showed that 6.2% had an intracranial lesion. Most common were subdural hematoma and hygroma. Other conditions included neurocysticercosis, aneurysm, glioma, and cerebral infarction. In 3.9%, the clinical management was changed by the scan results, emphasizing the importance of a complete neurological workup in alcoholics presenting with first seizures. On the other hand, it is also important to be alert to the possible role of alcohol in new-onset seizures in adults. In one series, 23% of adults with new-onset seizures had no other factor but alcohol abuse [76].

In their classic study, Victor and Adams [50] found that i 241 alcoholic patients with seizures carefully selected to exclude those with known other causes (e.g., head trauma), 90% of the seizures occurred within the first 7–48 h of alcohol withdrawal. This tight association between seizures and alcohol withdrawal has recently been questioned by Ng et al. [77], who instead found a relationship between current alcohol intake and seizures. In their study, 16% of the first seizures occurred outside the withdrawal period and the rest exhibited an apparently random timing since the last drink. In spite of this, the preponderance of evidence from both human and animal studies indicates that the period of alcohol withdrawal is one in which there is intense CNS hyperexcitability and an increased propensity for seizures. Devetag [74], in his series, has assigned seizures in alcoholics according to the following categories: (1) solitary convulsive seizures in alcoholics with no prior history of seizures and no other potentially epileptogenic disease *and* no association with withdrawal, 21%; (2) withdrawal seizures, 21%; (3) seizures in alcoholics with other potentially epileptogenic disease, 20%; and (4) recurrent seizures in alcoholics not previously epileptic and not suffering from any other potentially epileptogenic condition *and* not associated with withdrawal, 37%.

Repeated episodes of drinking and withdrawal are thought to predispose to seizures due to a kindling phenomenon [78], though the evidence is conflicting at present. Given the various causes of seizures in alcoholics, it is obvious that no blanket statement can be made about treatment. A complete neurological workup should be done on all first seizures and treatment accordingly planned. In a large series from San Francisco General Hospital [79], the effectiveness of intravenous phenytoin was assessed in a double-blind placebo-controlled study. For patients presenting with seizures in the period of alcohol withdrawal, 1000 mg phenytoin given intravenously was no more effective than placebo in preventing a second seizure.

Seizures are quite rate in detoxification units, and there is no clear evidence that any of the commonly used detoxification agents is better than any other in preventing seizures during the withdrawal period. In one series of 227 patients admitted for withdrawal from alcohol [80], 83 were determined to have risk factors other than alcohol predisposing them to seizures. All were placed on a standard chlordiazepoxide withdrawal regimen. None had seizures.

Anticonvulsant medication is not indicated for those patients whose seizures have been only related to alcohol withdrawal or intake and who have no other risk factors. For patients who, independent of their drinking, have clinical reasons for being placed on an anticonvulsant regimen, careful monitoring is essential. Medication compliance in alcoholics is notoriously poor. Alcohol interferes with drug metabolism through its induction of the microsomal ethanol oxidizing system (MEOS). In an actively drinking alcoholic, drug levels will be unexpectedly high, whereas during periods of abstinence levels may be subtherapeutic.

Q. Anosognosia

Denial or unawareness accompanies many neurological disorders. Anosognosia has been described for right hemiplegia, blindness, loss of memory, hemiballismus, sexual impotence, and incontinence due to central nervous system damage [81]. Schizophrenics treated with neuroleptics may not acknowledge the grossly disturbing movements of tardive dyskinesia [82], and patients with parkinsonian gait and tremor may be unperturbed by their defects. Early stages of dementia are often characterized by poor judgment, lack of concern, and uncharacteristic rudeness, of which the patient is unaware. Confabulation accompanies anosognosia, indeed is part of it. The patient acts as if he can move his limbs, see, or remember normally because he is unaware that he cannot. Patients with Korsakoff's psychosis are usually, at least partially, unaware of their amnesia and may confabulate. It seems possible that the dense denial seen, particularly in some older alcoholics, may have a neurological as well as a psychological basis. Alcoholics near the end of the continuum of central nervous system damage may show evidence of some memory loss, perseveration, unconcern, inappropriate responses, concreteness, loss of volition, or impulsiveness, which are manifestations of cerebral dysfunction. They remain unimpressed by a huge body of evidence demonstrating the consequences of their drinking. They adhere to alternative explanations of events in spite of direct confrontation with the falsity of their beliefs. They seem incapable of changing cognitive set from seeing themselves as normal social drinkers to problem drinkers. They do not respond to the usual therapeutic interventions, nor do they seem capable of responding to the social pressures of a rehabilitation environment with even token verbal compliance. While it is true that they do not present with the gross damage customarily seen in patients with anosognosia, an organic explanation for their intrasigence seems plausible. It certainly reduces staff frustration in these difficult cases.

III. COCAINE

Cocaine use by any route can result during intoxication in a variety of neurological problems. Cocaine is both a local anesthetic and a powerful sympathomimetic and its neurological effects are relate to these properties (Table 2). Of 47 patients in whom stroke followed cocaine use, the mean age was 32 years and all routes of administration were represented [83]. Over half of the patients who were studied, either angiographically or at autopsy, had intracranial aneurysms or anterior venous malformations.

A. Convulsions

The convulsant effects of cocaine are most likely related to its local anesthetic effects and are similar to those of lidocaine [84]. Seizure activity begins in the temporal lobe and then becomes generalized [85]. In single seizures the EEG should be normal soon after the seizure. Multiple seizures and status are associated with high blood levels such as are seen following the internal rupture of a cocaine-filled condom swallowed for smuggling purposes by a body packer. A patient who presents with a cocaine-induced seizure should have a thorough assessment. If no cause other than cocaine use is found, there is no indication for treatment with anticonvulsants, since they do not protect against cocaine-induced seizures, and there is no evidence to suggest that the patient is at increased risk for seizures other than those associated with drug use.

B. Headaches

Headaches in cocaine abusers are common complaints both during intoxication and for several weeks into abstinence. During intoxication the prodromal significance of head pain signalling focal deficits and vascular catastrophes should not be overlooked. There is a report of de novo migrainelike headaches arising during cocaine intoxication and withdrawal [86]. The association of migraine with serotonin dysregulation and the known effects of cocaine as a potent inhibitor of serotonin reuptake present a possible causal link.

C. Dystonic Reactions

Cocaine may lower the threshold for dystonic reactions induced by neuroleptic drugs. Six of seven chronic cocaine users developed dystonic reactions after taking haloperidol [87]. In one case, a dystonic reaction developed in association with withdrawal from cocaine alone without the concommitant use of neuroleptics.

It should be noted that the neurological complications of cocaine are acute effects related to intoxication and withdrawal. Anecdotally, headache has been reported for weeks following abstinence from cocaine. However, there are no formal studies of long-term neurological consequences of cocaine use.

IV. HEROIN

Opinion is divided with regard to whether or not there exist specific damages and deficits resulting from the use of opiates and not as consequences of the method of use, lifestyle, or adulterants mixed with the drug. The following neurological complications have been described [88–92].

Table 2 Acute and Chronic Effects of Cocaine

Condition	Timing	Observations
Stroke	Intoxication	Intracerebral hem: 49% Freq assoc Subarachnoid hem: 29% aneurysms & Cerebral infarction 22% A-V malformations
Seizures	Intoxication	Single Multiple Status epilepticus associated with high blood levels

Transient
  neurological
  symptoms
	Intoxication	Dizziness
		Blurred vision
		Ataxia
		Tinnitus
		Transient hemiparesis

Headache	Intoxication Withdrawal Early abstinence	Can be de novo migraine
Dystonia	Withdrawal	

1. Mononeuropathy
2. Chronic polyneuropathy
3. Brachial and lumbar plexitis
4. Guillain-Barré syndrome
5. Transverse myelitis (from postmortem examinations)
6. Central pontine myelinolysis
7. Delayed postanoxic encephalopathy
8. Diffuse cortical impairment

The pathogenesis of the peripheral nervous system complications remains obscure. It has been considered that the heroin-quinine adulterant mixture may either cause a toxic change in nerve or muscle tissue, or it may stimulate a hypersensitivity response. The question of long-term central nervous system damage from opiates remains open, since in practice it is difficult to find a group of long-term opiate addicts who have been exposed to steady high doses of the opiate in pure form using sterile techniques, who have not contaminated the picture by abusing other drugs, especially alcohol, and have not had a history of head injury. One such study, improbably enough, is available [93]. Seven subjects had been using British pharmaceutical heroin for 17–23 years, were in their fifties at the time of examination, and were using little or no alcohol. Three of the seven had a history of alcohol abuse for periods of 6 months, 1 year, and 17 years. In this group of seven, both greater CT scan abnormalities (similar to alcohol) and neuropsychological deficits were observed compared to age-matched controls. There was, however, no consistent relationship between their intake of heroin and CT changes or neuropsychological impairment.

V. CANNABIS

The data on long-term central nervous system damage in heavy users of cannabis is at present inconclusive. There have been reports of memory impairment, reduced capacity for sustained attention, slower rates of processing, and perceptual motor impairment as well as a number of negative studies [94,95].

In five out of eight controlled studies, persistent short-term memory deficits were detected in chronic cannabis smokers. Two studies involved long-term follow up. In one [96], 30 marijuana-dependent Costa Rican men, compared with 31 matched controls on tests of memory, had scores which were lower, but not significantly, in 1973. When reevaluated 11 years later, they showed significant impairment of short-term memory and attention compared with nonusers. A reevaluation study [97] in India of heavy bhang (marijuana) users, charas (hashish) smokers, and controls was conducted after 11 years. All the users had continued use over this period. The tests of intelligence, memory, and perceptual motor skills, which were used initially, were repeated. Additional deterioration in the users was seen on digit span, speed and accuracy tests, reaction time, and Bender Visuomotor Gestalt Test. In a small but well-controlled study [98] of 10 cannabis-dependent adolescents compared with nine non–drug-abusing adolescents and eight who had abused drugs, but not cannabis, significant differences were obtained on the Benton Visual Retention Test and the Wechsler Memory Prose Passages. Retesting after 6 weeks showed improvement in the cannabis-dependent group, but residual impairment remained.

VI. SEDATIVE-HYPNOTICS

There have been few studies on the long-term effects of prolonged heavy use of sedative-hypnotics alone [99–105]. Bergman and his associates [99] investigated patients using only sedative-hypnotics (barbiturates, benzodiazepines, or mempropamate) but no other drugs and compared them to a pair-wise matched control group from the general population. These 55 sedative-hypnotic users showed a pattern of neuropsychological deficits similar to that seen in alcoholics. Thirty-eight of these patients were reevaluated 5 years later [104]. There was overall neuropsychological improvement; however, half the group showed signs of intellectual impairment at follow-up. Twenty-nine patients had CT scans, which showed an increased prevalence of dilation of the ventricles, but unlike alcoholics, not of widened cortical sulci. There was correlation between impaired neuropsychological status (visual spatial skills) on the initial evaluation and continuing drug abuse at follow-up. Unfortunately, the authors reported that 11 of the patients were showing signs of alcohol abuse at follow-up, but they did not separate this group in the final results. Three studies [100,102,105] have reported neuropsychological impairment in chronic benzodiazepine users. Patients taking high doses of benzodiazepines for long periods of time perform poorly on tests involving visual spatial abilities and sustained attention [105], a pattern of impairment consistent with deficits in posterior cortical function. Unlike alcoholics, these patients function normally on tests of frontal function such as verbal fluency and card sorting. It is not yet known whether these impairments persist after a drug-free period.

VII. VOLATILE INHALANTS

Solvent abuse is rare outside the adolescent population. Unfortunately abuse of volatile inhalants may be associated with permanent central nervous system damage. Most act like general anesthetics with a similar picture of acute intoxication. Chronic central nervous system damage may be a consequence of the euphorigenic substance itself, or of other toxic components in the product, e.g., glue, cement, degreaser, paint, antifreeze, which is being inhaled. Some products also cause peripheral nerve damage. These substances are generally highly fat soluble and diffusely toxic to the nervous system producing a wide array of dysfunctions, including ataxia, myoclonus, chorea, tremor, optic neuropathy, and sensory and motor neuropathies as well as seizures and encephalopathy. Table 3 summarizes some of the consequences of specific inhalant abuse.

Table 3 Chronic Effects of Inhalants

Substance	Source	Symptoms
Gasoline	Fuel	Tremor, ataxia, myoclonus, chorea, encephalopathy [106]
Halogenated hydrocarbons	Degreasers Spot remover Typewriter correction fluid	CNS edema, hemorrhages
h-Hexane	Glues, cements	Peripheral neuropathy
Methanol	Often in solvents	Blurred vision, photophobia, blindness, basal ganglia hemorrhage
Methyl-n-butyl ketone	Paints, inks, resins	Peripheral neuropathy
Nitrous oxide		Sensory disturbances, ataxia, impotence, multiple sclerosislike syndrome [107]
Toluene	Solvents: paint thinners, glues, lacquers	Peripheral neuropathy, optic neuropathy, ataxia, severe muscle weakness, encephalopathy [108]
Trichloroethane	Typewriter correction fluid	Diffuse CNS damage

VIII. CONCLUSIONS

Since euphorigenic drugs have, by definition, their site of action in the CNS and produce their effects by distorting its normal function, it is not surprising that acute and chronic neurological symptoms are common among addicts. As a general rule, the more nonspecific and diffuse the actions of the drug, the more widespread its functional perturbations will be. Alcohol and the inhalants, for example, have effects on nerve cell membranes and on ion transport systems as well as on catecholamine levels and produce diverse pictures of neurological impairment. Opioid drugs whose actions are more targeted toward specific receptor systems have few reported neurological consequences. Stimulant drugs, again, acting more discretely on the CNS, have acute effects which, except for hyperexcitability phenomena, are secondary to their effects on the cardiovascular system and minor, or questionable, chronic direct neurological consequences. Of particular interest are the more subtle effects on memory, problem solving, mental flexibility, curiosity, motivation, and affect which have been studied to some extent in alcoholics but much less with other drug abusers. For the past 100 years, attention has been focused on striking clinical syndromes and the absence of such has been taken to imply a lack of CNS toxicity of the particular drug. In fact, it is chastening to remember that accepted clinical wisdom of 25 years ago was that alcohol did not cause CNS damage provided nutrition was adequate. We need more probing neuropsychological studies than those currently available to be able to say with confidence that a specific abused drug is without long-term effects on the central nervous system.

REFERENCES

1. Wernicke, C. Lehrbuch der Gehirnkrankheiten, Kassel, Berlin, 1881.
2. Korsakoff, S.S. Disturbance of psychic function in alcoholic paralysis and its relation to the disturbance of the psychic sphere in multiple neuritis of non-alcoholic origin, Vestnik Psichiatrii, Vol. IV, fasicle 2, 1887.
3. Maudsley, H. *The Pathology of Mind*, 3rd ed., Macmillan, London, 1879.
4. Peters, R.A. The biochemical lesion in Vitamin B_1 deficiency, *Lancet, 1*:1161–1165 (1936).

5. Freund, G. Chronic central nervous system toxicity of alcohol, *Annu. Rev. Pharmacol.*, *13*:217–227 (1973).

6. Walker, D.W., and Hunter, B.E. Short-term memory impairment following chronic alcohol consumption in rats, *Neuropsychologia, 16*:545–554 (1978).

7. Riley, J.N., and Walker, D.W. Morphological alterations in hippocampus after long-term alcohol consumption in mice, *Science, 201*(4356):646–648 (1978).

8. Freund, G., and Ballinger, W.E. Loss of cholinergic muscarinic receptors in the frontal cortex of alcohol abusers, *Alcohol. Clin. Exp. Res., 12*:630–638 (1988).

9. Freund, G., and Ballinger, W.E. Neuroreceptor changes in the putamen of alcohol abusers. *Alcohol Clin. Exp. res., 13*:213–217 (1989).

10. Parker, E.S., and Noble, E.P. Alcohol consumption and cognitive functioning in social drinkers, *J. Stud. Alcohol, 38*(7):1224–1232 (1977).

11. Parker, E.S., Beirnbaum, I.M., Boyd, R.A., and Noble, E.P. Neuropsychological decrements as a function of alcohol intake in male students, *Alcohol Clin. Exp. Res., 4*:330–334 (1980).

12. Von Wartburg, J.P. Effects of alcohol on membrane structure and function, *Alcoholism, 3*:46–47 (1979).

13. Hoffman, P.L., Tabakoff, B., Szabo, G., Suzdak, P.D., and Paul, S.M. Effects of an imidazobenzodiazepine, Ro 15 4513 on the inco-ordination and hypothermia produced by ethanol and pentobarbital. *Life Sci., 41*:611–619 (1987).

14. Tabakoff, B., Hoffman, P.L., Lee, J.M., Saito, T., Willard, B., and DeLeon Jones, F. Differences in platelet enzyme activity between alcoholics and nonalcoholics, *N. Engl. J. Med., 318*:134–139 (1988).

15. Tabakoff, B., and Hoffman, P.L. Biochemical pharmacology of alcohol, *Psychopharmacology: The Third Generation of Progress* (H.Y. Meltzer, eds.), Raven Press, New York, 1987, pp. 1521–1526.

16. Wollman, H., Smith, T.C., and Stephen, G.W. Effects of respiratory and metabolic alkolosis on cerebral blood flow in man, *J. Appl. Physiol., 24*:60–65 (1968).

17. Berglund, M., and Ingvar, D.H. Cerebral blood flow and its regional distribution in alcoholism and Korsakoff's patients. *J. Stud. Alcohol, 37*(5):586–597 (1976).

18. Blass, J.P., and Gibson, G.E. Abnormality of a thiamine requiring enzyme in patients with Wernicke-Korsakoff syndrome, *N. Engl. J. Med., 297*:1367–1370 (1977).

19. Hrubeck, Z., and Omenn, G.S. Evidence for genetic predisposition for alcoholic cirrhosis and psychosis. Twin concordances for alcoholism and its biological end points, *Alcoholism, 5*:207–214 (1981).

20. Bennett, A.E. Diagnosis of intermediate stage of alcoholic brain disease, *J.A.M.A., 172:1143*–1146 (1960).

21. Leber, W.R., and Parsons, O.A. *Neuropsychological Functioning and Clinical Progress in Alcoholics*. Presented at the Southwestern Psychological Association 26th Annual Meeting, Oklahoma City, April 1980.

22. Gregson, R.A.M., and Taylor, G.M. Prediction of relapse in male alcoholics, *J. Stud. Alcohol, 38*:1749–1760 (1977).

23. Parsons, O.A. Neuropsychological deficits in alcoholics: Facts and fancies, *Alcohol. Clin. Exp. Res., 1*(1):51–56 (1977).

24. Parsons, O.A., and Farr, S.P. The neuropsychology of alcohol and drug use, *Handbook of Clinical Neuropsychology* (S. Filskow and T. Boll, eds.), Wiley, New York, 1981.

25. Lishman, W.A., Jacobson, R.R., and Acker, C. Brain damage in alcoholism: Current concepts, *Acta Med. Scand.* (Suppl.) *717*:5–17 (1987).

26. Begleiter, H., Porjesz, and Kissin, B. Brain dysfunction in alcoholics with and without a family history of alcoholism, *Alcohol. Clin. Exp. Res., 6*:136 (1982).

27. Pfefferbaum, A., Rosenbloom, M., Cousan, K., and Jernigan, T.L. Brain CT changes in alcoholics effects of age and alcohol consumption. *Alcohol. Clin. Exp. Res., 12*:81–85 (1988).

28. Torvik, A., Lindboe, C.F., and Rodge, S. Brain lesions in alcoholics. A neuropathological study with clinical correlations, *J. Neurol. Sci., 56*:233–248 (1982).

29. Harper, C., and Krie, J. Brain atrophy in chronic alcoholics patients: A quantitative pathological study. *J. Neurol. Neurosurg. Psychiatry, 48*:211–217 (1985).

30. Eckardt, M.J., Rohrbaugh, J.W., Rio, D., Rawlings, R.R., and Coppola, R. Brain imaging in alcoholic patients. *Adv. Alcohol Subst. Abuse, 7*:59–71 (1988).

31. Risberg, J., and Berglund, M. Cerebral blood flow and metabolism in alcoholics, *Neuropsychology of Alcoholism* (O.A. Parsons, N. Butters, and P.E. Nathan, eds.), Guilford, New York, 1987.

32. Dally, S., Luft, A., Ponsin, J.C., Girre, C., Mamo, H., and Fournier, E. Abnormal pattern of cerebral blood flow distribution in young alcohol addicts, *Br. J. Addict., 83*:105–109 (1988).

33. Carlen, P.L., Wortzmann, G., Holgate, R.C., Wilkinson, D.A., and Rankin, J.G. Reversible cerebral atrophy in recently abstinent alcoholics measured by computed tomography scans. *Science, 200*:1076–1078 (1978).

34. Artmann, H., Gall, M.V., Hacker, H., and Herrlick, J. Reversible enlargement of cerebro spinal fluid spaces in chronic alcoholics. *Am. J. Neuroradiol., 2*:23–27 (1981).

35. Ron, M.A., Acker, W., Shaw, G.K., and Lishman, W.A. Computerized tomography of the brain in chronic alcoholism: A survey and follow up study, *Brain, 105*:497–514 (1982).

36. Muvroner, A., Bergman, H., Hindmarsh, T., and Telakioi, T. Influence of improved drinking habits on brain atrophy and cognitive performance in alcoholic patients: A 5 year follow up study. *Alcohol. Clin. Exp. Res., 13*:137–141 (1989).

37. Ishikawa, Y., Meyer, J.S., Tanahasi, N., Hata, T., Velez, M., Fann, W.E., Kandula, P., Motel, K.F., and Rogers, R.E. Abstinence improves cerebral perfusion and brain volume in alcohol neurotoxicity without Wernicke-Korsakoff syndrome, *J. Cereb. Blood Flow Metab., 6*:86–94 (1986).

38. Schroth, G., Naegele, T., Klose, V., Mann, K., and Peterson, D. Reversible brain shrinkage in abstinent alcoholics measured by MRI. *Neuroradiology, 30*:385–389 (1988).

39. Glenn, S.W., Parsons, O.A., Sinha, R., and Stevens, L. The effects of repeated withdrawals from alcohol on the memory of male and female alcoholics *Alcohol Alcohol, 23*:337–342 (1988).

40. Freund, G. Alcohol, barbiturate and bromide withdrawal symptoms in mice, *Recent Advances in Studies in Alcoholism* (W. Mello and J. Mendelson, eds.), U.S. Government Printing Office, Washington, D.C., pp. 453–471, 1970.

41. Parsons, O.A., and Leber, W.R. The relationship between cognitive dysfunction and brain damage in alcoholics, *Alcoholism, 5*:326–343 (1981).

42. Fabian, M.S., and Parsons, O.A. Differential improvement of cognitive functions in recovering alcoholic women, *J. Abnorm. Psychol., 92*:87–89 (1983).

43. Goldstein, G. Recovery, treatment and rehabilitation in chronic alcoholics, *Neuropsychology of Alcoholism Implications for Diagnosis and Treatment* (O.A. Parsons, N. Butters, and P.E. Nathan, eds.), Guilford Press, New York, 1987.

44. Goodwin, D.W. Blackouts and alcohol induced memory dysfunction, *Recent Advances in Studies Alcohol* (N.K. Mello, and J.H. Mendelsohn, eds.), National Institute Mental Health, Bethesda, Maryland, 1971.

45. Lister, R.G., Eckardt, M., and Weingartner, H. Ethanol intoxication and memory, *Recent Developments and New Directions* (M. Galanter, ed.), *Recent Dev. Alcohol., 5*:115–125, New York, Plenum, 1987.

46. Fisher, C.M. Transient global amnesia, *Arch. Neurol., 39*:605–608 (1982).

47. Martin, P.R., Impeduglia, G., Giri, P.R., and Karanian, J. Accelleration of ethanol metabolism by past thiamine deficiency. *Alcohol. Clin. Exp. Res., 13*:457–460 (1989).

48. Butterworth, R.F. Effects of thiamine deficiency on brain metabolism Implications for the pathogenesis of the Wernicke-Korsakoff syndrome, *Alcohol Alcohol, 24*:271–279 (1989).

49. Langlais, P.J., Mair, R.G., and McEntree, W.J. Acute thiamine deficiency in the rat: Brain lesions amino acid MK-801 pre-treatment. *Soc. Neurosci. Abstr., 14*:313 (1988).

50. Victor, M., and Laureno, R. Neurologic complications of alcohol abuse Epidemiological aspects, *Adv. Neurol., 19*:603–617 (1978).

51. Harper, C. Wernicke's encephalopathy: A more common disease than realized. A neuropathological study of 51 cases, *J. Neurol. Neurosurg. Psychiatry, 42*:226–231 (1979).

52. Lishman, W.A. Cerebral disorder in alcoholism. Syndromes of impairment, *Brain, 104*:1–20 (1981).

53. Canterwell, B.S., and Criqui, M.H. Prevention of the Wernicke-Korsakoff syndrome. A cost benefit analysis, *N. Engl. J. Med., 299*:285–289 (1978).

54. Victor, M., Adams, R.D., and Collins, G.H. *The Wernicke-Korsakoff syndrome*, Davis, Philadelphia, 1971.

55. Mair, W.G.P., Warrington, E.K., and Weiskrantz, L. Memory disorder in Korsakoff's psychosis. A neuropathological and neuropsychological investigation of two cases, *Brain, 102*:749–783 (1979).

56. Butters, N., and Granholm, E. The continuity hypothesis: Some conclusions and their implications for the etiology and neuropathology of alcoholic Korsakoff's syndrome, *Neuropsychology of Alcoholism: Implications for Diagnosis and Treatment* (O.A. Parsons, N. Butters, and P.E. Nathan, eds.), Guilford Press, New York, 1987.

57. Butters, N. Alcoholic Korsakoff's syndrome: An update, *Semin. Neurol., 4*:229–247 (1984).

58. Arendt, T., Bigl, V., Arendt, A., and Tennstedt, A. Loss of neurons in the nucleus basalis of Meynert in Alzheimer's disease, paralysis agitans and Korsakoff's disease, *Acta Neuropathol., 61*:101–108 (1983).

59. McEntree, W.J., Mair, R.G., and Langlais, P.J. Neurochemical pathology in Korsakoff's psychosis: Implications for other cognitive disorders, *Neurology, 34*:648–652 (1984).

60. Martin, P.R., Adinoff, B., Echardt, M.J., Stapleton, J.M., Bone, G.A.H., Rubinow, D.R., Lane, E.A., and Linnoila, M. Effective pharmacotherapy of alcohol amnestic disorder with fluvoxamine, *Arch. Gen. Psychiatry, 46*:617–621 (1989).

61. Lynch, M.J.G. Brain lesions in chronic alcoholism, *Arch. Pathol., 69*:342–353 (1960).

62. Messert, B., Orrison, W.W., Hawkins, M.J., and Quaglier, C.E. Central pontine myelinolysis. Considerations on etiology, diagnosis and treatment, *Neurology, 29*:147–160 (1979).

63. Victor, M., Adams, R.A., and Collins, G.H. *The Wernicke-Korsakoff syndrome and Related Neurologic Disorders Due to Alcoholism and Malnutrition*, 2nd ed., Davis, Philadelphia, 1989.

64. Serdau, M., Hausser-Hauw, C., and Laplane, D. The clinical spectrum of alcoholic pellagra encephalopathy, *Brain, 111*:829–842 (1988).

65. Dreyfus, P.M. Diseases of the nervous system in chronic alcoholics, *Biology of Alcoholism*, Vol. 3, (Kissin and Begleiter, eds.), Plenum Press, New York, 1974, pp. 265–290.

66. Estrin, W.J. Alcoholic cerebellar degeneration is not a dose dependent phenomenon, *Alcohol. Clin. Exp. Res., 11*:372–275 (1987).

67. Barnes, D.E., and Walker, D.W. Neuronal loss in hippocampus and cerebellar cortex in rats prenatally exposed to ethanol, *Alcoholism, 4*:209 (1980).

68. Johnson, R.H., Eisenhofer, G., and Lambie, D.G. The effects of acute and chronic ingestion of ethanol on the autonomic nervous system. *Drug Alcohol Depend., 18*:319–328 (1986).

69. Lefebre D'Amour, M., Shahani, B.T., Young, R.R., and Bird, K.T. The importance of studying sural nerve conduction and late responses in the evaluation of alcoholics, *Neurology, 29*:1600–1604 (1979).

70. Altura, B.M. Introduction to the symposium and overview, *Alcohol. Clin. Exp. Res., 10*:557–559 (1986).

71. Altura, B.M., Altura, B.T., and Gebrewold, A. Alcohol induced spasms of cerebral blood vessels: Relation to cerebro vascular accidents and sudden death, *Science, 220*:331–333 (1983).

72. Stamfer, M.J., Colditz, G.A., Willett, W.C., Speizer, F.E., and Hennekens, C.H. A prospective study of moderate alcohol consumption and the risk of coronary disease and stroke in women, *N. Engl. J. Med., 319*:267–273 (1988).

73. Chan, A.W.K. Alcoholism and epilepsy, *Epilepsia, 26*:323–333 (1985).

74. Devatag, F., Mandich, G., Zaiotti, G., and Toffolo, G.G. Alcoholic epilepsy: Review of a series and proposed classification and etiopathogenesis, *H. J. Neurol. Sci., 4*:275–284 (1983).

75. Earnest, M.P., Feldman, H., Marx, J.A., Harris, J.A., Biletch, M., and Sullivan, L.P. Intracranial lesions shown by CT scans in 259 cases of first alcohol-related seizures, *Neurology, 38*:1561–5 (1988).

76. Dam, A.M., Fuglsang, Frederiksen, A., Svarre Olsen, U., and Dam, M. Late onset epilepsy:

Etiologies, types of seizures and value of clinical investigation, EEG and computerized tomography scan, *Epilepsia, 26*:227-231 (1985).

77. Ng, S.K., Hanser, W.A., Brust, J.C., and Susser, M. Alcohol consumption and withdrawal in new onset seizures, *N. Engl. J. Med., 319*:666-73 (1988).

78. Post, R.M., Unde, T.W., and Roy Byrne, P.P. Correlates of anti-manic response to carbamazepine, *Psychiatry Res., 21*:71-83 (1987).

79. Simon, R.P., Alldredge, B.K., and Lowenstein, D.H. Alcohol symposium proceedings, *Epilepsia, 29*:492-497 (1988).

80. Lechtenberg, R., and Worner, T.M. *Prospective Study of Seizure Risk Management of Alcoholics During Inpatient Detoxification*, International Symposium on Alcohol and Seizures, Washington, 1988.

81. Fisher, C.M. Neurologic frequents II. Remarks on anosognosia, confabulation, memory and other topics and an appendix on self-observation, *Neurology, 39*:127-132 (1989).

82. Myslobodsky, M.S., Tomer, R., Holden, T., Kempler, S., and Sigal, M. Cognitive impairment in patients with tardive dyskinesias, *J.N.M.D., 173*:156-160 (1986).

83. Klonoff, D.C., Andrews, B.T., and Obana, W.G. Stroke associated with cocaine use, *Arch. Neurol., 46*:989-993 (1989).

84. Rowbotham, M.C. Neurologic aspects of cocaine abuse, *West. J. Med., 149*:442-448 (1988).

85. Matsuzaki, M. Alterations in pattern of EEG activities and convulsant effect of cocaine following administration in the rhesus monkey, *Electroencephalogr. Clin. Neurophysiol., 45*:1-15 (1978).

86. Satel, D., and Gawin, F.H. Migraine-like headache and cocaine use J.A.M.A., 261:2995-2996 (1989).

87. Choy Kwong, M., and Lipton, R.B. Dystonia related to cocaine withdrawal: A case report and pathogenic hypothesis, *Neurology, 39*:996 (1989).

88. Richter, R.W., and Baden, M.M. Neurological complications of heroin addiction *Trans. Am. Neurol. Assoc., 94*:330-332 (1969).

89. Richter, R.W., and Rosenberg, R.N. Transverse myelitis associated with heroin addiction. *J.A.M.A., 206*:1255-1257 (1968).

90. Hall, J.H., and Karp, H.R. Acute progressive pontine disease in heroin abuse, *Neurology, 23*:6 (1973).

91. Rounsaville, B.J., Novelly, R.A., and Kelber, H.D. Neuropsychological impairment in opiate addicts: Risk factors (R.B. Millman, P. Cushman, and J.H. Lowinson, eds.), *Research Developments in Drug and Alcohol Use*, 1981 Annals of the New York Academy of Sciences.

92. Stamboulis, E., Psimaras, A., and Malliara-Loulakaki, S. Brachial and lumbar plexitis as a reaction to heroin, *Drug Alcohol Depend., 22*:205-207 (1988).

93. Strang, J., and Gurling, H. Computerized tomography and neuropsychological assessment in long term high dose heroin addicts, *Br. J. Addict., 84*:1012-1019 (1989).

94. Souief, M.I. Differential association between chronic cannabis use and brain function deficits, *Ann. N.Y. Acad. Sci., 282*:323-43 (1976).

95. Wig, N.N., and Varma, V.K. Patterns of long term heavy cannabis use in North India and its effects on cognitive functions: A preliminary report, *Drug Alcohol Depend., 2*:211-219 (1977).

96. Page, J.B., Fletcher, J., and Tone, W.R. Psychosocial cultural perspectives on chronic cannabis use: The Costa Rican follow up, *J. Psychoactive Drugs, 20*:57-65 (1988).

97. Mendhiratta, S.S., Varma, V.K., Dang, R., Malhotra, A.K., Das, K., and Nehra, R. Cannabis and cognitive functions: A re-evaluation study, *Br. J. Addict., 83*:749-753 (1988).

98. Schwartz, R.H., Grunewald, P.J., Klitzner, M., and Fedio, P. Short term memory impairment in cannabis dependent adolescents, *Am. J. Dis. Child., 143*:1214-1219 (1989).

99. Bergman, H., Borg, S., and Holm, L. Neuropsychological impairment and exclusive abuse of sedatives or hypnotics, *Am. J. Psychiatry, 137*:215-217 (1980).

100. Hendler, N., Cimini, C., Terence, M.A., and Long, D. A comparison of cognitive impairment due to benzodiazepines and narcotics, *Am. J. Psychiatry, 137*:828-830 (1980).

101. Lader, M.M., Ron, M., and Peterson, M. Computed axial brain tomography in long term benzodiazepine users, *Psychol. Med., 14*:203-206 (1984).

102. Petursson, H., Gudjonsson, G.H., and Lader, M.M. Psychometric performance during withdrawal from long term benzodiazepine treatment, *Psychopharmacology, 81*:345-349 (1983).

103. Poser, W., Poser, S., Roscher, D., and Argyrakis, A., Do benzodiazepines cause cerebral atrophy? *Lancet, 1*:715 (1983).

104. Bergman, H., Borg, S., Engelbrektson, K., and Vikander, B. Dependence on sedative hypnotics: Neuropsychological impairment, field dependence and clinical course in a five year follow up study, *Br. J. Addict.,*

105. Golombok, S., Moodley, P., and Lader, M. Cognitive impairment in long term benzodiazepine users, *Psychol. Med., 18*:365-374 (1988).

106. Coulehan, J.L., Hirsch, W., and Brillman, J. Gasoline sniffing and lead toxicity in Navajo adolescents, *Pediatrics, 71*:113-117 (1983).

107. Layzer, R.R. Myeloneuropathy after prolonged exposure to nitrous oxide, *Lancet, 2*:1227-1228 (1978).

108. Streicher, H.Z., Gabow, P.A., and Moss, A.H. Syndromes of toluene sniffing in adults, *Ann. Intern. Med., 94*:758-762 (1981).

VII
Behavior

34

Drug Self-Administration Research in Drug and Alcohol Addiction

John D. Roache and Richard A. Meisch
Substance Abuse Research Center, University of Texas Health Sciences Center at Houston, Houston, Texas

I. INTRODUCTION

Drug addiction is a biobehavioral disorder characterized by repeated instances of drug taking. Definitions of addiction have been a matter of controversy. Early clinical researchers attempted to operationalize the term by describing the state of chronic intoxication that occurred in chronic users of opioids or barbiturates. In these descriptions, some of the most profound effects observed were the physiological signs of withdrawal noted upon cessation of drug use. The presence of such physiological withdrawal signs eventually became entwined with the definition of drug addiction and effectively came to be considered a cardinal sign of addiction. With this definition, drugs like cocaine which do not produce profound physiological withdrawal signs were unfortunately considered by many as being nonaddicting. We now realize that physiological types of drug dependence, characterized by predictable withdrawal syndromes, are neither a necessary nor a sufficient condition to produce addictive behavior. It is now clear that the essential feature of drug addiction is the presence of repeated drug self-ingestion behaviors which occur in a manner considered "compulsive" or "habitual," and which society defines as having deleterious behavioral, medical, or social consequences.

Scientific efforts to examine factors influencing drug addiction have been quite diverse. A number of studies have included laboratory examination of the acute and chronic effects of addictive drugs and surveys or interviews of current users and addicts. These studies have provided information on the pharmacological activity of these drugs and their perceived effects in the user population. However, these techniques are not suitable for a direct experimental analysis of the drug-taking or self-administration behavior. The present chapter describes the basic value of, and information gained from, laboratory studies of drug self-administration in human and nonhuman subjects. Inasmuch as addiction is a socially defined term referring to socially disapproved patterns of drug self-administration, the present chapter will refer only to self-administration behavior.

It should be recognized that many different cultural and socioeconomic factors influence the probability that a particular drug will be self-administered in patterns which become an addictive behavior problem for society. Separate from the consideration of those factors, laboratory studies of drug self-administration typically address specific behavioral and pharmacological variables which influence the probability of drug self-administration. Although research efforts in drug addiction and alcoholism have developed along somewhat separate lines, it should be recognized that alcohol is a drug and there is no evidence that alcohol addiction is a distinct phenomenon from other drug addictions.

II. DRUGS REINFORCE OPERANT BEHAVIOR

All studies of drug self-administration employ techniques in which the subject's own behavior determines the amount of drug delivered. In self-administration studies, therefore, the primary dependent measures of interest are the amount of drug delivered or the amount of behavior engendered when drug delivery depends on that behavior. The latter statement emphasizes the fact that the relevant dependent variable requiring experimental investigation is the drug self-administration behavior itself (i.e., drug-seeking/drug taking behavior). The experimental paradigm which has most successfully examined this variable is the study of operant behavior maintained by drug reinforcement.

In 1962, James Weeks [1] described a technique that permitted rats to self-inject morphine solutions intravenously. The technique involved the implantation of an intravenous catheter which could be chronically maintained in a freely moving animal. The catheter was connected to a pump which infused a small volume of a morphine solution whenever the animal pressed a lever. The experiment showed that rats which were physically dependent on morphine readily pressed a lever if that lever press was followed by an intravenous infusion of a morphine solution. Weeks correctly described this as an instance of operant reinforcement. Operant behavior is behavior that is maintained by its consequences. A *reinforcer* is defined as an event that increases the probability of behavior which leads to its presentation. Thus, this study showed that intravenous morphine delivery could reinforce drug-taking behavior in the same way that food-pellet delivery has been shown to reinforce lever pressing behavior in other experiments.

The basic observation of drug-reinforced operant behavior has been replicated many times, using a variety of drugs, procedures, and species of animals. As an instance of operant behavior, it is now recognized that compulsive drug taking is learned in the same manner as other conditioned behaviors. Laboratory studies have shown that certain drugs produce reinforcing effects and maintain drug-taking behavior under a number of experimental conditions. A discussion of the diverse methods used in these studies is beyond the scope of this chapter. The various methods employed in self-administration research involving human [2] and nonhuman [3] subjects have been recently reviewed. The present chapter outlines the general principles involved in drug self-administration research and the basic factors which influence drug-reinforced behavior.

III. CRITERIA FOR IDENTIFYING DRUG-REINFORCED BEHAVIOR

Drug self-administration must be distinguished from drug reinforcement, since self-administration may occur as a secondary consequence of other nonspecific factors. For example, self-administration may be a consequence of behavior that is maintained by other primary reinforcers. This occurs with fluid-deprived rats who will drink drug solutions made available as their only source of fluid. However, drug ingestion in such cases may be completely incidental to the water repletion which normally follows periods of dehydration. Early studies of alcohol drinking in rodents commonly "forced" alcohol consumption in this manner. Later studies improved upon this by making both water and alcohol solutions concurrently available so that rats could "choose" how much alcohol to drink [4]. In such a choice procedure, specific alcohol drinking can be distinguished from general fluid consumption. Therefore, it should be recognized that all instances of drug reinforcement involve self-administration; however, not all instances of self-administration involve drug reinforcement [5,6].

A. Comparisons to a Vehicle Control

In order to demonstrate that a drug is reinforcing self-administration behavior, it must be shown that the behavior in question is maintained specifically by the consequent delivery of the drug and *not* by any other factors [5,6]. The best way to accomplish this is to demonstrate that self-administration maintained by the drug exceeds that maintained by a vehicle control. The vehicle control must be identical to the drug preparation in every respect except that the drug is not present. Rates of vehicle self-administration can be assessed by presenting the vehicle either sequentially or concurrently with the drug. Sequential presentation involves periods of drug self-administration preceded or followed by comparable periods of vehicle self-administration. When vehicle is substituted for a drug reinforcer, "extinction" of responding should be observed. During extinction, responding may initially continue at the same or at higher levels than that observed with drug solutions. However, if the drug was serving as a reinforcer, vehicle responding will eventually fall off, since the drug is no longer present to maintain the self-administration behavior. Making the vehicle concurrently available with the drug reinforcer is a more powerful procedure, since the vehicle control is present continuously to assess the effects of nonspecific factors.

B. Other Supporting Evidence for Drug Reinforcement

In addition to the examination of vehicle control responding, there are other observations which support the claim that a drug is acting as a reinforcer. One is the use of a unique operant response that is intermittently reinforced [4,5]. Ethanol drinking studies have commonly used water and/or ethanol solution drinking bottles attached to the subject's home cage. In that situation, licking responses and fluid drinking are very natural behaviors which occur with a high probability in the absence of drug reinforcement. However, the same animals, not otherwise fluid deprived, may be required to a press a lever in order to gain access to ethanol reinforcement. In this case, the fact that ethanol (but not vehicle) would specifically maintain this low probability "unnatural" behavior (pressing a lever) is a stronger argument for drug reinforcement. One could be even more confident if multiple (e.g., 16) lever responses were required for each drug delivery so that definite self-administration behavior is required in order to obtain the ethanol reinforcer. The use of such operant techniques also allows one to compare drug self-administration behavior with other conditioned operant behaviors. Thus, one can examine whether drug self-administration shows characteristic patterns of responding which vary as a function of changes in the operant schedule of reinforcement (discussed in following sections).

One final but important observation consistent with drug-reinforced responding is that the self-administration behavior should be an orderly function of drug concentration or dose. If the drug is serving as a reinforcer, then the strength or persistence of the reinforced behavior should vary as a function of the magnitude of the reinforcer. This will be discussed in following sections.

IV. SPECIES GENERALITY

The basic laboratory phenomenon of drug self-administration in laboratory procedures has been widely replicated and extended to include a variety of drugs self-administered by a number of species [2,3,5]. Drugs have been demonstrated to function as reinforcers for mice, rats, rabbits, cats, dogs, rhesus monkeys, squirrel monkeys, and baboons [5,7] as well as humans [2,7]. To date, no mammalian species tested has failed to demonstrate drug-seeking/self-administration behavior.

The species generality of drug self-administration illustrates two important conclusions. First, drug self-administration phenomena are not exclusive to humans and apparently do not require the "higher intellectual" functions sometimes thought to be important in a person's "decision" to abuse drugs. Second, the widespread generality of drug self-administration suggests that it is biologically "normal" for certain drugs to produce reinforcing effects. The latter conclusion leads one to wonder why more people are not drug abusers or addicts. Although it is likely that cultural and social factors serve to limit human drug self-administration, laboratory studies have demonstrated that drug-reinforced behavior in both humans and animals appears to be functionally controlled by many of the same variables [7]. The observation of individual differences in drug self-administration behavior undoubtedly involves many factors, including environmental and historical as well as genetic variables. The species generality of the qualitative observation that drug self-administration occurs does not exclude a role for genetic variables. As will be discussed later, genetic variables clearly have been demonstrated to be factors in individual or strain differences in drug self-administration.

V. PHARMACOLOGICAL VARIABLES

A. Drugs that Serve as Reinforcers

Using a variety of procedures, many different drugs have been demonstrated to function as reinforcers [2,3,5,7,8]. Table 1 lists major classes of drugs and examples of each class which have been reported to maintain drug self-administration. Also listed are drugs and drug classes which have been shown not to maintain self-administration behavior. In general, there is good correspondence between those drugs which are abused by humans and those which maintain self-administration in laboratory procedures [7,8]. This correspondence supports the validity of using laboratory measures of drug self-administration for the empirical analysis of drug addiction phenomena. The correspondence also strengthens the argument that reinforcing effects of drugs are a major, if not the most important, factor determining their addictive potential in humans.

B. Role of Physical Dependence

Physical dependence is a term commonly used to describe the phenomenon which occurs with the chronic administration of certain drugs, most notably morphine-like opiates and barbiturate or alcohol-like central nervous system (CNS) depressants. It is a pharmacological phenomena which is manifested by a characteristic withdrawal syndrome observed upon cessation of chronic drug administration. As previously mentioned, it has its historical roots in the description of physiological signs of withdrawal observed in chronic users of opioids and CNS depressants. In the original study demonstrating intravenous morphine self-administration by rats [1], it was assumed that animals would self-inject morphine only if they were physically dependent on opioids. This assumption was based upon observations that addicted users of opioids and CNS depressants were physically dependent upon these drugs and verbally

Table 1 Drugs and Drug Classes Serving as Reinforcers

Drug class	Examples
Drugs serving as reinforcers	
CNS stimulants	Amphetamine, cocaine
CNS depressants	Ethanol
sedative-hypnotics	Diazepam, pentobarbital
solvents	Toluene
Dissociative	Phencyclidine (PCP)
anesthetics	
Methylxanthines	Caffeine
Nicotine	Nicotine
Opioids	
Opiate-derived	Codeine, heroin, morphine
agonist-antagonists	Pentazocine
Drugs not serving as reinforcers	
Antidepressants	Imipramine
Antipsychotics	Chlorpromazine, haloperidol
Hallucinogens	Lysergic acid diethylamide (LSD)
Opioid Antagonists	Naloxone, naltrexone

described withdrawal as something to be avoided. Researchers of that time interpreted withdrawal avoidance as the cause of continued drug use.

The idea that chronic drug use is due to avoidance behavior persists today. Many consider that drug use is motivated by some kind of relief from the effects of drug absence. This relief may be conceived as an avoidance of the drug withdrawal syndrome in a physically dependent user. Others conceptualize drug use as possibly related to a "self-medication" of some underlying disorder or condition. A laboratory study in rhesus monkeys [9] was the first to show that morphine was self-administered under conditions in which subjects were not physically dependent. Subsequent research has also shown that many drugs can serve as excellent reinforcers when there is no evidence of physical dependence [3,7,8]. Thus, physical dependence is not a necessary and may not be a sufficient condition to maintain drug self-administration [10]. Likewise, self-medication hypotheses have received little empirical support [11]. Clearly, it would not be reasonable to suggest that drug self-administration in a large proportion of animals from a variety of species is due to underlying psychopathology. The few human studies which have examined drug self-administration in psychiatrically or medically ill populations have not demonstrated any increased potential for reinforcing effects or drug addiction in those populations. Thus, it is now understood that certain drugs have direct positive reinforcing effects in the absence of physical dependence and without underlying psychopathology.

The general recognition that physical dependence is not an essential component of drug addiction has come somewhat belatedly, since until recently cocaine was considered by many as being nonaddicting. Now, it is generally understood that drug reinforcers, like cocaine, may maintain quite persistent drug-seeking and drug self-administration behavior. It is this behavioral feature which constitutes socially meaningful definitions of drug addiction. This conclusion has important clinical implications for the treatment of drug addiction which have not yet been fully recognized. It means that detoxifying or withdrawing patients from drugs does not necessarily decrease the probability of relapse. It is virtually certain that detoxification in and of itself does not treat the underlying behavioral disorder of drug addiction.

However, for medical and humanitarian reasons, detoxification is important as a first step in the treatment of physically dependent individuals.

C. Routes of Drug Self-Administration

In laboratory animal studies, procedures have been developed to allow drugs to be self-administered by several routes including oral, intragastric, intramuscular, intraperitoneal, inhalation, intravenous, and intracerebral routes. Human laboratory studies of self-administration mostly have used the oral route, although the intranasal, inhalation, intravenous, and intramuscular routes have also been utilized. The multiplicity of routes used in self-administration studies is consistent with the fact that humans abuse drugs by various routes of administration.

The importance of the route of drug administration is sometimes illustrated by the example of cocaine [12]. Cocaine is generally accepted to have a lesser addictive potential when bucally absorbed from chewing coca leaves as compared to when it is inhaled from smoking "crack." However, in addition to the route of administration, two other pharmacological variables contribute the difference in these two forms of cocaine use. Crack cocaine also is more highly concentrated and is in the free-base form which allows it to get into the brain more readily. Thus, when compared to any other form of cocaine use, crack smoking represents a more rapid and complete delivery to the brain of a more highly concentrated cocaine. Since the effectiveness of a reinforcer depends, in part, on the reinforcer magnitude and also the temporal immediacy of reinforcer delivery, one can see that the development of crack cocaine represents an improved method of addictive drug delivery. Similar developments have recently occurred with "ice," which is a concentrated, smokable, free-base form of methamphetamine.

D. Variations in Drug Reinforcer Magnitude

A fundamental principle of pharmacology is that the effect varies as a function of the drug dose. In self-administration studies, however, the total amount of drug intake (i.e., mg/kg session) is a dependent measure which varies as a function of the subject's behavior. In order to systematically vary drug amount as an independent variable, researchers have varied either the drug concentration, volume, or amount available in each reinforcer delivery. This variation in drug amount per reinforcer delivery effectively varies the magnitude of the reinforcer. Under a wide variety of experimental conditions, the number of drug deliveries self-administered is found to be an inverted U-shaped function of reinforcer magnitude [3,6,7].

The left-hand panel of Figure 1 shows this function for orally delivered pentobarbital solutions in one rhesus monkey. Pentobarbital solutions of approximately 0.6 ml volume were delivered orally upon each completion of 16 mouth contacts on a drinking spout. As pentobarbital concentration was increased, the number of drug deliveries self-administered increased up to a maximum at the 0.5 mg/ml concentration. Further increases in pentobarbital concentration resulted in a decreased number of reinforcer deliveries. However, as shown in the right-hand panel of Figure 1, the total milligram quantity of drug consumed was a direct monotonic function of pentobarbital concentration. These data clearly show that larger amounts of drug were actually self-administered at the higher pentobarbital concentrations despite the decreasing number of reinforcer deliveries on the descending limb of the inverted U-shaped concentration-response function.

The inverted U-shaped concentration-response function usually observed in these studies merits some consideration. First, there is important practical significance to the realization that increased drug concentrations (amount) per delivery may result in an increased total drug amount (dose) self-administered. Second, it is important to recognize that the number of drug

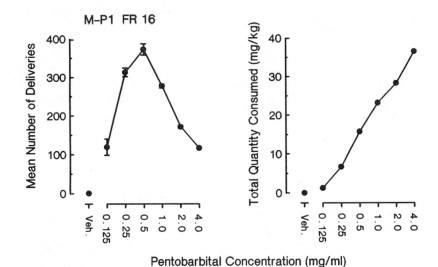

Figure 1 Concentration-response functions for the number of pentobarbital deliveries and the total pentobarbital amount consumed per 3-h session. Data are means from the last five sessions tested at the designated concentration in one rhesus monkey (M-P1). The pentobarbital concentrations were tested sequentially in descending order; Veh. indicates the water vehicle (i.e., 0 mg/ml). Vehicle or pentobarbital solutions were orally delivered in a 0.5-ml volume contingent upon 16 mouth contacts (FR-16) on a drinking spout. Brackets indicate ± SEM; absence of brackets indicate the SEM was within the area of the data point. (These data were excerpted and replotted from Ref. 23.)

deliveries does not necessarily indicate the strength or magnitude of reinforcement. That is to say, the higher concentrations of pentobarbital should not be considered to be "less reinforcing" just because fewer deliveries were self-administered. In order to determine the relative reinforcing effectiveness, or "reinforcing efficacy" of these different drug concentrations, additional experiments must be completed as described in the next section. As will be demonstrated, higher drug concentrations or amounts per delivery consistently have been shown to be more reinforcing than lower concentrations or amounts [3,6,7].

VI. ENVIRONMENTAL VARIABLES

A. Schedules of Reinforcement

The schedule of reinforcement is a description of the contingent relationship between the organism's behavior and stimulus changes in the environment which occur as a consequence. A number of different schedules of reinforcement have been used in self-administration studies [3,7]. Most studies have employed fixed ratio (FR) schedules in which the reinforcer is delivered upon each completion of a specified number of responses. For example, an intravenous drug infusion delivered after every eight lever presses would be described as a FR-8 schedule of intravenous drug infusion.

Figure 2 shows a series of concentration-response functions for the oral pentobarbital-reinforced behavior of one rhesus monkey. Concentration-response functions were separately determined under different FR values. The different FR values indicate the number of mouth contacts required to produce a reinforcer delivery. As can be seen, the shape of the concentration-response function varied as a function of the FR value. Generally, increases

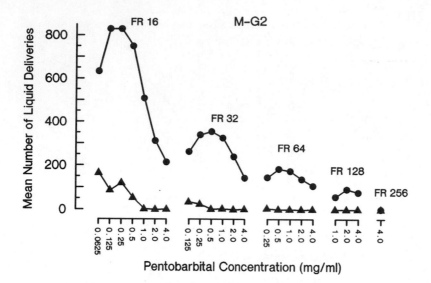

Figure 2 Interactions of pentobarbital concentration and fixed-ratio size on the number of vehicle (triangles) and pentobarbital (circles) deliveries consumed per 3-h session. Data are means from the last six sessions tested at the designated pentobarbital concentration in one rhesus monkey (M-G2). Both vehicle and the designated pentobarbital solution were concurrently available on independently operating fixed-ratio schedules. Various fixed ratio (FR # shown above each set of curves) sizes were tested in an ascending sequence. Each fixed-ratio size was maintained constant while the various pentobarbital concentrations were tested in a descending sequence. (These data were excerpted and replotted from Ref. 24.)

in the FR value resulted in decreases in the number of drug deliveries self-administered at any given concentration. Also noteworthy is the fact that only the higher drug concentrations maintained responding as the FR value was increased. These data illustrate the general findings of behavioral "economic" studies which examine behavioral "cost" factors and their influence on operant behavior. Basically, increasing the cost of obtaining a reinforcer results in decreases in the number of reinforcers obtained. Also, larger costs will be paid for larger magnitude or better reinforcers. These results show that higher drug concentrations are better reinforcers than lower drug concentrations in that self-administration of higher concentrations persists at larger behavioral cost. These data also illustrate that the reinforcing effects of a drug are not a fixed "property" of the drug, but rather depend on multiple factors—in this case, the schedule of reinforcement.

Human laboratory studies also have shown that increases or decreases in behavioral cost result in corresponding decreases or increases in drug self-administration, respectively [2,7]. This may be one of the more effective tools that society has to decrease drug or alcohol use. Studies have reported that decreases in automobile accidents and mortality from cirrhosis have accompanied increases in the price of alcohol [13]. Alternatively, the practice of decreasing the price of alcohol during "happy hour" only serves to increase consumption.

Although fixed ratio schedules of reinforcement have been the most commonly employed, another schedule yielding important information regarding behavioral cost and relative reinforcing effects is the progressive ratio schedule. With progressive ratio schedules, the ratio values are progressively increased in an attempt to determine the ratio or behavioral cost that a subject will pay in order to receive a drug delivery. The conclusions from these studies are that increased drug amounts or concentrations will maintain responding at larger ratio values. Again, these observations indicte that compared to smaller reinforcer magnitudes, larger magnitudes maintain behavior at larger response costs.

B. Concurrent Alternative Reinforcers

As identified in the beginning of this chapter, drugs are one of many reinforcers. Drug addiction can be conceptualized, in part, as the situation in which drugs are one of a few reinforcers maintaining an individual's behavior. Other possible reinforcers such as food, money, family, etc., become less effective in maintaining the addict's behavior. A few laboratory studies of drug self-administration have examined the effects of nondrug reinforcers made concurrently available along with the drug reinforcer. In rhesus monkeys orally self-administering phencyclidine on a fixed-ratio schedule, concurrently available saccharin solutions reduced the amount of phencyclidine self-administered [14]. In human alcoholics, decreased alcohol drinking was observed when hospital ward privileges such as television watching were made mutually exclusive with the decision to drink [15]. Thus, it appears that alternative reinforcers may "compete" with drugs as reinforcers [7]. Understanding this concept of competing reinforcers emphasizes a treatment and prevention strategy in which nondrug alternatives are emphasized and made mutually exclusive with drug use. Such strategies have been remarkably successful in reinforcing abstinence behavior in alcoholics [16].

C. Limitations of Drug Access

Most studies of drug self-administration have employed procedures in which access to drug reinforcers is limited or restricted in some way. Typically, self-administration is limited to a session of a few hours in length [2,3,7]. With these limited access schedules, highly reliable patterns of regular, daily drug self-administration have generally been observed. In contrast, studies allowing relatively unrestricted access to drug (e.g., 24 h/day) often have reported cyclic patterns of alternating periods of high and low drug intake. Human studies with alcoholics given unrestricted 24-h access have noted binge drinking periods in which high blood alcohol levels were achieved that alternate with periods of little or no intake [17]. Studies allowing animals of several different species unrestricted access to intravenously delivered cocaine have also reported cyclic patterns of binge cocaine self-administration [3,12,18]. During the periods of high cocaine intake, the animals eat and sleep very little. Continued unlimited cocaine access may result in death within weeks to months [3,12,18]. The toxicity of cocaine under these conditions is thought to be due to a stimulant-induced disruption of normal eating and sleeping patterns. Whereas mortality has been observed in rats given unrestricted access to heroin, it is less likely than with cocaine, since heroin does not significantly disrupt eating and sleeping behaviors [18]. In contrast to these findings, mortality from cocaine self-administration is not observed in limited-access schedules in which animals eat and sleep between the self-administration sessions. In general, temporal limitations on drug access result in more regular and stable patterns of drug intake which are less damaging to the individual [3].

D. Stimulus Control

Stimuli which become associated with drug reinforcement can also come to control drug-reinforced behavior [3,19]. These stimuli include both external stimuli associated with drug self-administration and also internal stimuli such as the effects produced by the drug. Experimenter administered doses of cocaine can restore self-administration responding which had previously decreased due to extinction. External stimuli such as cue lights previously paired with drug injection can become *conditioned reinforcers* and maintain self-administration behavior even after drug is removed from the vehicle. These conditioned associations between drug reinforcement and drug-related stimuli in the internal and external environments are thought to explain much of the persistence of addictive behavior. In human addicts, it has been suggested that these drug-related conditioned stimuli trigger drug craving and drug-seeking behaviors and are important factors influencing relapse to drug use.

VII. SUBJECT VARIABLES

A. Genetics

All mammalian species so far tested have shown evidence of drug-reinforced behavior. This species generality argues that substantial genetic variation does not affect the fact that drugs can serve as reinforcers. However, there are quantitative differences between subjects in the amount of self-administration behavior observed. Genetic variation within a species almost certainly accounts for some subject variability. Laboratory studies have demonstrated substantial differences in alcohol-reinforced behavior between rodent strains [20]. Family and adoption studies of the children of alcoholics have also demonstrated a genetic influence on the probability of developing alcoholism [21]. Although not yet empirically demonstrated, it is likely that genetics also influences drug-reinforced behavior maintained by drugs other than alcohol.

B. Drug-Reinforcement History

Between subject differences in self-administration also are influenced by the experience ("history") of the individual subject [3,5,7,11]. Clearly drug self-administration is a "learned" behavior. Additionally, the reinforcing effects of a drug may be influenced by the subject's history of drug reinforcement. In both human [11] and nonhuman [3] subjects, the probability and degree of drug-reinforced behavior observed with certain drugs have been shown to increase when subjects have a history of self-administering other drugs. These observations are consistent with the observations that "experienced" human drug abusers often have histories of abusing multiple drugs.

C. Food Deprivation

Food deprivation reliably increases drug self-administration [5,6]. This observation has been reproduced under a variety of conditions. Drug-reinforced behavior increases with food restriction in both rats and rhesus monkeys self-administering drugs by either the oral or the intravenous routes of administration. Many possible explanations for the phenomenon have been ruled out. For example, increased self-administration is not related to increased activity levels or nonspecific increases in drug vehicle self-administration. Although originally observed with alcohol self-administration, it is not related to the caloric value of the drug and has been observed with drugs from a variety of different pharmacological drug classes. The increased self-administration appears to be accounted for by increases in the reinforcing effects of the drug. This effect of food deprivation is rather unique in that it is one of a few variables which may affect drug-reinforced behavior by changing the "internal state" of the organism. This phenomena may also occur in humans since it has been reported that young women with eating disorders often also develop drug and alcohol abuse problems.

VIII. RELATIVE REINFORCING EFFECTS OF DIFFERENT DRUGS

A. Difficulties of Assessment

As mentioned previously, there is a great deal of concordance between drugs which are abused by humans and drugs which are self-administered in laboratory studies [7,8]. That only certain drugs are self-administered indicates qualitative differences between drugs in their ability to serve as reinforcers. There are also quantitative differences between drugs in the patterns of self-administration behavior observed. Whereas researchers are commonly called upon to rank the relative addictive potential of different drugs, such rankings are usually not done based solely upon observations obtained from a single line of research. Considering self-administration procedures alone, methods for clearly demonstrating differences in the effectiveness, or efficacy, of drug reinforcers have not been well established or utilized. Thus, the empirical data demonstrating between drug differences in reinforcing effectiveness are not very conclusive [10]. There are a number of problems inherent in making such comparisons. For instance, the conditions under which a stimulant such as amphetamine serves as a good reinforcer may not be optimal for depressants such as pentobarbital or alcohol. One potentially could say that under a given set of conditions, one drug is a more effective reinforcer than another drug. However, under a different set of conditions, the opposite might be true. Most self-administration research has optimized the conditions for demonstrating the reinforcing effects of a particular pharmacological class of drugs. It clearly has been shown that drugs as diverse as amphetamine, morphine, pentobarbital, alcohol, phencyclidine, and nicotine can each maintain drug-reinforced behavior very robustly. However, different studies examining different drugs have employed different experimental conditions. Other drugs which seem not to maintain self-administration may simply have not been tested under conditions optimal for those drugs. Perhaps, the greatest success in ranking relative reinforcing effects has occurred in comparisons of individual drugs within a pharmacological class where experimental conditions are usually held constant.

B. Indices of Relative Reinforcing Effects

The following indices have been used by researchers in making generalizations regarding the relative reinforcing efficacies of different drugs.

Rates of Self-Administration

As previously identified, the observation of differences in the number of deliveries self-administered is not sufficient in and of itself to conclude that one drug is a better reinforcer than another drug. These data can be supportive of such conclusions only in conjunction with other observations.

Behavioral Cost

Methods considered among the most valid ways to quantify drug differences include the use of progressive ratio schedules or variations of fixed-ratio size. These procedures quantify the behavioral costs that subjects will "pay" for different reinforcers.

Range of Conditions

The range of conditions under which a drug will function as a reinforcer has been used as an indicator of addictive potential. This assessment assumes that there is a greater probability of individuals encountering the addictive effects of those drugs which serve as reinforcers under wider ranges of conditions. Unfortunately, the range of condition factor has not been systematically examined in experimental procedures.

Proportion of Population At Risk

Not all drugs will serve as reinforcers in all subjects tested. Genetic and historical variables certainly affect the probability that an individual's behavior will come under the control of a drug reinforcer. Some researchers have suggested the existence of between drug differences based on the proportion of subjects for whom drugs will serve as reinforcers under a given set of conditions. However, the "nonresponding" subjects have seldom been tested under different conditions to see whether they might then respond.

Stability and Pattern of Self-Administration

The stability and regularity with which drugs maintain self-administration behavior have been suggested to reveal differences between drugs. Certain characteristic patterns of self-administration are reasonably expected if the drug is serving as a reinforcer. However, minor variations in the pattern of responding may relate to the metabolic and dynamic profiles of drug effect more than they relate to differences in reinforcing effects.

C. Relative Reinforcing Effects Within and Between Drug Classes

After noting the limitations and problems related to relative rankings of reinforcing effects, we have attempted to list general conclusions and the basis for those conclusions which some researchers have drawn from drug self-administration research.

CNS Psychomotor Stimulants

Central nervous system psychomotor stimulants, including amphetamine and cocaine, are thought to be among the most effective reinforcers. These drugs have been shown to maintain high rates of self-administration behavior in most subjects tested and under a wide variety of conditions, including large fixed- and progressive-ratio values. However differences among stimulants clearly exist.

Methylxanthines

Methylxanthines, like caffeine, exert a number of stimulant-like effects. However, caffeine is considered to be less reinforcing than stimulants like amphetamine or cocaine in that several studies have failed to demonstrate reinforcing effects of caffeine under conditions in which other stimulants work well. Only recently have there been unequivocal demonstrations that caffeine functions as a reinforcer [22].

Opioids

Opioids, including the naturally derived morphine-like compounds as well as synthetic narcotic analgesics, have been shown to be robust reinforcers. Several of the mixed agonist-antagonist analgesics appear to have reduced reinforcing effects by comparison. There have been suggestions that opioids produce less reinforcing effects than cocaine based upon the patterning and the proportions of the population affected; however, these suggestions have been disputed.

CNS Depressants

Central nervous system depressants, like pentobarbital and ethanol, can serve as strong reinforcers. Benzodiazepines generally have been shown to produce reduced reinforcing effects in comparison to the barbiturates. Depressants sometimes have been considered to be less reinforcing than stimulants or opioids in that there have been fewer conditions under which these drugs have been demonstrated to function as reinforcers, and subject variables such as drug history may play a relatively more important role.

Cannabinoids

Cannabinoids, such as THC, generally have been tested only rarely in nonhuman subjects due to the low water solubility of THC. The lack of demonstrated reinforcing effect in these few animal studies have led some to suggest that cannabinoids produce reduced reinforcing effects in comparison to other drugs. However, human studies have demonstrated self-administration of THC-containing marijuana cigarettes.

Hallucinogens of the LSD Type

In nonhuman subjects, hallucinogens of the LSD type generally have been shown not to function as reinforcers. This observation is discrepant with human abuse data, although hallucinogen use is considered to be minimal in comparison to many other drugs. Possibly, the optimal conditions for hallucinogen self-administration in the laboratory may not yet have been discovered.

Other Drugs

Drugs such as nicotine and phencycline have been shown to be robust reinforcers, but their effects relative to other drugs are difficult to estimate.

REFERENCES

1. Weeks, J.R. (1962). Experimental morphine addiction: Method for automatic intravenous injections in unrestrained rats, *Science, 138*:143.
2. Henningfield, J.E., Lukas, S.E., and Bigelow, G.E. (1986). Human studies of drugs as reinforcers, *Behavioral Analysis of Drug Dependence* (S.R. Goldberg and I.P. Stolerman, eds.), Academic Press, Orlando, Florida, p. 69.
3. Young, A.M., and Herling, S. (1986). Drugs as reinforcers: Studies in laboratory animals, *Behavioral Analysis of Drug Dependence* (S.R. Goldberg and I.P. Stolerman, eds.), Academic Press, Orlando, Florida, p. 9.
4. Amit, Z., Smith, B.R., and Sutherland, E.A. (1987). Oral self-administration of alcohol: A valid approach to the study of drug self-administration and human alcoholism, *Methods Assessing the Reinforcing Properties of Abused Drugs* (M.A. Bozarth, ed.), Springer-Verlag, New York, p. 161.
5. Meisch, R.A. (1987). Factors controlling drug reinforced behavior, *Pharmacol. Biochem. Behav., 27*:367.
6. Meisch, R.A., and Carroll, M.E. (1987). Oral drug self-administration: Drugs as reinforcers, *Methods Assessing the Reinforcing Properties of Abused Drugs* (M.A. Bozarth, ed.), Springer-Verlag, New York, p. 143.
7. Griffiths, R.R., Bigelow, G.E., and Henningfield, J.E. (1980). Similarities in animal and human drug-taking behavior, *Advances in Substance Abuse*, Vol. 1 (N.K. Mello, ed.), JAI Press, Greenwich, Connecticut, p. 1.
8. Johanson, C.E., and Balster, R.L. (1978). A summary of the results of a drug self-administration study using substitution procedures in rhesus monkeys. *Bull. Narc., 30*:43.
9. Schuster, C.R. (1970). Psychological approaches to opiate dependence and self-administration by laboratory animals. *Fed. Proc., 29*:2.
10. Johanson, C.E., Woolverton, W.L., and Schuster, C.R. (1987). Evaluating laboratory models of drug dependence, *Psychopharmacology: The Third Generation of Progress* (H.Y. Meltzer, ed.), Raven Press, New York, p. 1617.
11. Johanson, C.E., and de Wit, H. (1989). The use of choice procedures for assessing the reinforcing properties of drugs in humans, *National Institute on Drug Abuse Research Monograph No. 92: Testing for Abuse Liability of Drugs in Humans* (M.W. Fischman and N.K. Mello, eds.), Department of Health and Human Services, U.S. Government Printing Office, Washington, D.C., p. 171.
12. Fischman, M.W. (1987). Cocaine and the amphetamines, *Psychopharmacology: The Third Generation of Progress* (H.Y. Meltzer, ed.), Raven Press, New York, p. 1543.

13. Seely, J.R. (1960). Death by liver cirrhosis and the price of beverage alcohol, *Canad. M.A.J.*, *83*:1361.

14. Carroll, M.E. (1985). Concurrent phencyclidine and saccharin access: Presentation of an alternative reinforcer reduces drug intake, *J. Exp. Anal. Behav.*, *43*:131.

15. Griffiths, R.R., Bigelow, G.E., and Liebson, I. (1977). Comparison of social time-out and activity time-out procedures in suppressing ethanol self-administration in alcoholics, *Behav. Res. Ther.*, *15*:329.

16. Pickens, R., Bigelow, G., and Griffiths, R. (1973). An experimental approach to treating chronic alcoholism: A case study and one-year follow-up, *Behav. Res. Ther.*, *11*:321.

17. Mello, N.K., and Mendelson, J.H. (1987). Operant analysis of human drug self-administration: Marijuana, alcohol, heroin and polydrug use, *Methods Assessing the Reinforcing Properties of Abused Drugs* (M.A. Bozarth, ed.), Springer-Verlag, New York, p. 525.

18. Geary, N. (1987). Cocaine: Animal research studies, *Cocaine Abuse: New Directions in Treatment and Research* (H.L. Spitz and J.S. Rosecran, eds.), Brunner/Mazel, New York, p. 19.

19. Goldberg, S.R., and Gardner, M.L. (1981). Second-order schedules: Extended sequences of behavior controlled by brief environmental stimuli associated with drug self-administration, *National Institute on Drug Abuse Research Monograph No. 37: Behavioral Pharmacology of Human Drug Dependence* (T. Thompson and C.E. Johanson, eds.), U.S. Government Printing Office, Washington, D.C., p. 241.

20. George, F.R. (1987). Genetic and environmental factors in ethanol self-administration, *Pharmacol. Biochem. Behav.*, *27*:379.

21. Cloninger, C.R. (1987). Recent advances in family studies of alcoholism, *Genetics and Alcoholism* (H.W. Goedde and D.P. Agarwal, eds.), Alan Liss, Inc., New York, p. 47.

22. Griffiths, R.R., and Woodson, P.P. (1988). Reinforcing properties of caffeine: Studies in humans and animals. *Pharmacol. Biochem. Behav.*, *29*:419.

23. Meisch, R.A., Kliner, D.J., and Henningfield, J.E. (1981). Pentobarbital drinking by rhesus monkeys: Establishment and maintenance of pentobarbital-reinforced behavior, *J. Pharmacol. Exp. Ther.*, *217*:114.

24. Lemaire, G.A., and Meisch, R.A. (1984). Pentobarbital self-administration in rhesus monkeys: Drug concentration and fixed ratio size interactions, *J. Exp. Anal. Behav.*, *42*:37.

VIII
Psychiatric Implications

35

Psychiatric Comorbidity in Drug and Alcohol Addiction

Steven M. Mirin and Roger D. Weiss
McLean Hospital, Belmont, Massachusetts, and Harvard Medical School, Boston, Massachusetts

I. INTRODUCTION

The prevalence of additional psychiatric disorders among drug- and/or alcohol-addicted patients has been the subject of considerable interest. Though many investigators [1–5] have reported a high level of psychiatric symptomatology in these patients when they initially present for treatment, the proportion of patients satisfying diagnostic criteria for one or more psychiatric disorders (in addition to drug/alcohol addiction) varies with the population studied, the setting in which the data are gathered, and the methods used to assess such patients. Age, sex, and other demographic characteristics of the patient population affect the relative prevalence of various types of drug/alcohol addiction as well as any other psychiatric disorders which may be present. For example, opiate addiction and alcoholism are far more common among men [6,7], whereas sedative-hypnotic dependence is more common among women [8]. Similarly, with respect to other psychiatric disorders, attention deficit disorder and antisocial personality disorder are primarily diseases of men [9,10], whereas major depression and various types of anxiety disorder are much more prevalent among women [11,12].

With respect to setting, inpatient drug treatment programs generally attract patients with more severe and more varied psychopathology compared to outpatient settings, particularly if the treatment program is located within a psychiatric hospital. Treatment programs with a more medical (i.e., psychiatric) orientation tend to emphasize diagnostic assessment and subtyping of patients with the subsequent application of multiple treatment modalities specific to the various types of psychopathology found. In contrast, settings in which a self-help approach dominates the treatment philosophy evidence less interest in diagnostic specificity, and instead prefer to focus on helping patients develop the motivation and interpersonal skills necessary to lead a drug-free existence.

Even where there is a clinical and/or research interest in exploring the relationship between various types of drug addiction and other forms of psychopathology, the methodology used for assessment of these patients clearly impacts on one's findings and conclusions. For example, structured clinical interviews generally yield more concurrent psychiatric diagnoses in a given patient than standard (nonstructured) interviewing techniques [13]. In addition, both techniques yield different diagnostic findings depending on whether they are applied before, during, or after drug or alcohol detoxification. Moreover, in the case of the latter, the extent and severity of psychiatric symptomatology noted is profoundly affected by how long patients have been drug and alcohol free [14].

Finally, longitudinal studies are needed to differentiate clearly psychiatric syndromes induced by alcohol and drugs from "naturally occurring" psychiatric disorders. Inadequate data exists to determine the extent and duration of drug and alcohol effects during protracted abstinence; i.e., weeks, months, or perhaps years. Correspondingly, the natural history of the development of drug and alcohol addiction in the progression of the mental illness or psychiatric syndrome has not been delineated.

Retrospective analysis of diagnostic data has limitations. Because of patient denial and state-dependent learning, accurate recall of the criterion for diagnostic categories is difficult. Frequently patients forget and distort past histories of psychiatric syndromes and drug/alcohol use.

With these caveats in mind, the following sections will review some of the recent data on the prevalence of various forms of psychopathology found in drug-dependent patients.

II. PREVALENCE OF PSYCHOPATHOLOGY IN DRUG-DEPENDENT PATIENTS

A. Opioid Addicts

Although the settings, patient populations, and evaluative methodologies vary, studies carried out by Rounsaville et al. [3,15] and others [1,2] have consistently found that among opioid addicts, approximately half are suffering from one or more additional psychiatric syndrome at the time they present for treatment. The lifetime prevalence of one or more diagnosable psychiatric syndromes (other than a alcohol/drug addiction) in these patients is even higher [3,15].

In an attempt to develop more reliable methods for evaluating drug addicts for concurrent psychiatric illness, our group [16–18] collected extensive demographic, clinical, and family pedigree data on over 350 consecutive admissions to McLean Hospital's Alcohol and Drug Abuse Treatment Center over a 6-year period. Evaluative techniques included unstructured and structured clinical interviews, serial application of a psychiatric rating scales, and, in patients with presumptive affective disorder, a battery of laboratory tests currently thought to be useful in the evaluation of such patients. Patients were independently assigned a multiaxial DSM-III [19] diagnosis by two psychiatrists after 4 weeks of inpatient treatment. Where diagnostic assessments differed, a consensus diagnosis was assigned. Diagnosis of a comorbid condition (in addition to drug/alcohol dependence) required that the patient manifest signs and symptoms of the disorder both currently and during at least one prior drug-free period in their lifetime, as reported by the patient and verified by collaterals where possible.

In this patient population, we identified 186 individuals for whom opioids were the primary drug of choice, the vast majority of whom were heroin addicts. Within this group, 29.6% received some axis I diagnosis, exclusive of drug or alcohol dependence, and 12.4% were eventually diagnosed as suffering from concurrent major or atypical depression. An additional 5.2% received a diagnosis of bipolar or cyclothymic disorder. Thus, the combined rate of current affective illness in these patients was 17.6%. These data are consistent with the findings of Rounsaville et al. [20], who reported that approximately 17% of opiate addicts entering a multimodality treatment program met research diagnostic criteria (RDS) for current major depression. In yet another study, that group also reported that the lifetime risk for at least one episode of major depression in opioid addicts was as high as 60–70% [21].

Another diagnosis that appeared with a reasonable degree of frequency in our patient population was antisocial personality disorder (approximately 30%). Disorders of impulse control, panic disorder, and generalized anxiety disorder were far less frequent, with a combined prevalence of less than 5%. Diagnostic data on a somewhat larger sample of opioid addicts (n = 533) evaluated by Kosten et al. [22] yielded somewhat similar findings, albeit with some differences related to patients' demographic characteristics, the setting in which the data were gathered, and the diagnostic criteria employed.

In the Kosten study [22] of outpatient opioid addicts evaluated at a community mental health center, 54.7% of the sample received a diagnosis of antisocial personality disorder (ASP), whereas the rate of phobic disorder was 9.2%. As in our studies, ASP was significantly more common among men, whereas major depression, panic disorder, and anxiety disorder were significantly more common among women.

Finally, it should be noted that in our patient population, approximately 50% of opioid addicts presenting for treatment were also found to be suffering from either alcohol abuse or alcohol dependence. Kosten [22] and others [3] have reported somewhat lower rates of concurrent alcoholism in opioid addicts presenting for treatment. In general, the lifetime rate of mixed opioid-alcohol dependence appears to range between 30 and 50% in this population, depending upon the age and socioeconomic status of the patients, the treatment setting, and diagnostic criteria employed.

As will be discussed later, the chronic effects of opiates on mood and anxiety need to be considered before clear, independent Axis I psychiatric diagnoses can be established in a population of chronic opiate addicts, whether heroin or methadone addicts.

B. Cocaine Addicts

Though initially cocaine was thought to be a drug that could be used safely by recreational users (i.e., without the danger of acute medical or psychiatric complications) and without the risk of addiction, recent epidemiological, clinical, and laboratory data suggest quite the opposite. Indeed, over the last decade, the increased prevalence of use, and the availability of more potently addictive forms of the drug (e.g., "crack") has been accompanied by a dramatic increase in drug-related morbidity and mortality, as measured by emergency room visits, cocaine-related deaths, and the number of cocaine addicts enrolling in treatment programs [23,24]. Paralleling the rise in the addictive use of cocaine, its use among general psychiatric patients has also increased dramatically. However, until recently, there have been relatively few studies of the prevalence of comorbid psychopathology among cocaine abusers.

In this context, our group [4,18,25] collected demographic and clinical data on 120 cocaine addicts admited to McLean Hospital between 1980 and 1986. Within this group, the overall prevalence of Axis I psychopathology (exclusive of alcohol abuse/dependence) was 40%. The prevalence of concurrent affective disorder was 26.7%, with 9.2% diagnosed as suffering from major depression and 17.5% receiving a diagnosis of bipolar or cyclothymic disorder. Other Axis I disorders found in these patients included attention deficit disorder, residual type (4.2%), as well as disorders of impulse control and generalized anxiety disorder (less than 2% each).

It should be noted, however, that the prevalence of psychopathology in chronic, heavy users of cocaine is in all likelihood much higher than that found among casual users. Moreover, the distinction between primary and secondary affective disorder, e.g., depression, that preceded, versus that which followed, the development of cocaine addition is often difficult to make; thus, differences in diagnostic criteria can substantially skew estimates of prevalence of primary affective illness not only among these patients, but in drug addicts of all types [26]. Given the chronic effects of stimulant use in inducing manic and depressive syndromes, caution is used in establishing other primary Axis I psychiatric diagnoses in addition to cocaine addiction.

C. Patients Addicted to Central Nervous System Depressants

Although there have been relatively few systemic studies of comorbidity in abusers of central nervous system (CNS) depressants, our group [17] as well as Quitkin et al. [27] have reported that both generalized anxiety and panic disorder are relatively common among such patients. In our ongoing studies [18], we identified 44 patients who preferentially were addicted to CNS depressants (exclusive of alcohol), primarily diazepam and lorazepam. Within this group, almost 60% received some Axis I diagnosis in addition to drug/alcohol dependence. Approximately 25% received a DSM-III [19] diagnosis of generalized anxiety disorder or panic disorder; 13.6% were diagnosed as having major depression, and an additional 6.8% were suffering from bipolar or cyclothymic disorder. In patients with anxiety disorder, panic disorder, or major depression, CNS depressants were used primarily as antianxiety agents, though chronic use of the depressant drugs tended to exacerbate depressive symptomatology in these patients.

D. Alcoholics

Studies of psychopathology in alcoholics reveal an extremely variable prevalence of comorbidity, depending upon the patient population (i.e., inpatient vs outpatient), the rigor of the diagnostic criteria employed, the method of screening (e.g., clinical criteria, rating scale indices), and the time elapsed since the last drink. In most studies that have attempted to quantify the prevalence and severity of depression in these patients, upwards of 70% are moderately to severely depressed at treatment intake [27,28]. However, if patients are followed longitudinally (i.e., a month or longer) the overt level of depressive symptomatology drops sharply. Thus the number of patients who meet DSM-III criteria for major depression at 4–6 weeks postdetoxification is about 10–20% [29]. Among the latter, careful history taking reveals that the majority have experienced major depressive episodes at other points in their lives, including when they have been alcohol free.

In a study of 500 outpatients, Guze and colleagues [30] were able to identify 116 patients (23.2%) who met stringent diagnostic criteria for alcoholism. Among male alcoholics, the diagnosis of secondary depression (i.e., depression occurring after the onset of alcoholism) was made in 52% of patients, compared to a prevalence of 20% in nonalcoholic patients. There was also a significant increase in the prevalence of secondary mania and antisocial personality disorder among these alcoholic males. Among female alcoholics, these investigators found a significant increase in the prevalence of secondary depression, Briquet's syndrome, drug dependence, and antisocial personality disorder when compared to nonalcoholic females. Interestingly, no significant association was found between alcoholism and anxiety neurosis, phobic neurosis, obsessional neurosis, schizophrenia, organic brain syndrome, or primary affective illness in either the male or female patients, nor was there any increase in the frequency of primary affective illness in the first-degree relatives of alcoholics with secondary depression. These findings suggest that while the prevalence of secondary depression is quite high among alcoholics compared to patients with other psychiatric disorders, the prevalence of primary affective illness in these patients and their first-degree relatives is not increased over that found in the general psychiatric population.

In our studies of alcoholics [31], we found that the prevalence of concurrent major depression (with or without melancholia) to be 18.3%. An additional 2.4% were diagnosed as suffering from atypical depression. Bipolar-cyclothymic disorder was found in 10.6% of our alcoholic patients, and an additional 7.7% received some other Axis I diagnosis. Drug abusers with concurrent alcoholism differed from nonalcoholic drug abusers with respect to the prevalence of major depression with melancholia (13 vs 4.8%) and antisocial personality disorder (29.6 vs 12.5%). Alcoholics also tended to have longer histories of both alcohol and drug use and had more alcoholic first-degree relatives. The latter finding suggests that familial and/or genetic factors may have played an important role in the development of alcoholism in these individuals.

Data from the recent Epidemiologic Catchment Area (ECA) Survey also sheds light on the co-occurrence of alcohol abuse/dependence and other psychiatric disorders [32]. In sampling approximately 20,000 persons drawn from the general population in five cities (New Haven, Connecticut, Baltimore, Maryland, St. Louis, Missouri, Durham, North Carolina, and Los Angeles, California), the ECA survey ascertained diagnoses in this group using the Diagnostic Interview Schedule (DIS), which was administered by nonclinician examiners. Although the ECA survey was not designed to yield precise prevalence data for a full range of psychiatric disorders and used less than stringent criteria for the diagnosis of alcohol or drug dependence, the findings do provide a rough estimate of the lifetime (i.e., not necessarily current) prevalence of alcohol and drug abuse/dependence as well as other major psychiatric disorders in the general population.

Thirty-four percent of the individuals in the ECA sample met DSM-III criteria for at least one psychiatric disorder at some point during their lifetime. The lifetime prevalence of alcohol abuse or dependence was 13.7%. Drug abuse or dependence was found in 5.9% of the ECA sample. Among the alcoholics, approximately half had an additional psychiatric disorder, of which the most common was antisocial personality disorder (ASP), which was found in 15% of male alcoholics and 10% of female alcoholics. For both sexes, lifetime prevalence rates for ASP was substantially higher than that found in the general population (i.e., 4% for men; less than 1% for women) [33].

The ECA survey also found an increased prevalence of major depression among alcoholics compared to the general population (19% for females and 5% for males), and in both sexes, depression appeared to predate the onset of alcoholism. The lifetime prevalence of phobic or panic disorder was 38% in female alcoholics compared to 15% of male alcoholics.

III. PSYCHOPATHOLOGY AS A RISK FACTOR FOR DRUG/ALCOHOL ABUSE

A. Prevalence of Drug and/or Alcohol Abuse and Addiction

The literature reflects a growing awareness of the role of drug and alcohol dependence as a complicating factor in patients with other mental disorders [34–44]. As in the case of drug addicts and alcoholics, systematic attempts to assess the prevalence of drug and alcohol dependence in psychiatric patients yield widely divergent findings depending upon the demographic and clinical characteristics of the patients surveyed and the survey methodology employed. Use of multiple indicators of alcohol and/or drug addiction, including structured interviews, patient's self-ratings of "problems" with alcohol or drugs, as well as laboratory indicators of drug or alcohol use (e.g., blood and urine screens, liver enzymes), obviously yield a greater prevalence of drug and/or alcohol problems in these patients than might be discerned through use of any single method alone. In general, lower estimates of prevalence are found when data on drug/alcohol use are derived from patient self-reports, whereas higher estimates are reported when structured clinical interviews coupled with blood and/or urine screening for drugs of abuse are carried out.

Despite the methodological problems inherent in such studies, data from surveys of both inpatients and outpatients reveal that approximately one-third of mentally ill patients in treatment are actively abusing drugs and/or alcohol at the time of intake [34–38]. At McLean Hospital, for example, Eisen et al. [37] used a semistructured interview along with the Michigan Alcoholism Screening Test (MAST) [39] and several questionnaires to assess the point prevalence of alcohol and drug use in 294 psychiatric inpatients.

Using all measures combined, 60% of the men and 44% of the women met at least one set of criteria for drug or alcohol abuse. Twenty-eight percent of the entire sample reported problems with alcohol and/or drug use in the week prior to admission and 11% reported having consumed, on average, more than three drinks per day in the month prior to admission. Using MAST score criteria yielded a higher percentage of patients with alcohol problems than use of a structured interview [34 vs 20%]. Regardless of the instrument used, the prevalence of drug and/or alcohol abuse was substantially higher in these patients than that found in community samples [32,40].

In the above noted study, [37] 26% of the patients surveyed reported use of at least one illicit drug in the month prior to admission. As in the case of alcohol, illicit drug use was significantly more common in men than in women (22 vs 12%). Among men, marijuana and cocaine were the most popular drugs abused, whereas use of central nervous system depressants, hallucinogens, and amphetamines was more common among women, as was the misuse of prescribed medications. Younger patients (i.e., age 30 or younger) had a higher point prevalence of drug or alcohol abuse, were more likely to have used illicit drugs in the month prior to admission, and were more apt to be polydrug users. Similar findings have been previously reported by other investigators [41,42].

With regard to the demographic and clinical characteristics of these psychiatric patients, Eisen and colleagues [37] found that drug abusers were more frequently young, single, and separated or divorced compared to patients without associated drug or alcohol problems. Similar findings were reported by Westermeyer [43], who also found that psychiatric inpatients who were heavy drug users were more likely to have fewer social and occupational resources than their non–drug using peers. Moreover, in the Westermeyer study, drug users were more likely to be diagnosed as suffering from a psychotic disorder than their non–drug using peers.

Finally, though Eisen et al. [37] found that drug/alcohol abusers reported significantly more difficulty with impulsivity, they did not differ from non–drug users with respect to interpersonal functioning, ability to carry out activities of daily living, number of previous psychiatric hospitalizations, their subsequent length of hospitalization, or their condition at discharge. Nor did they differ with respect to the prevalence of various psychiatric disorders. Of patients who met DSM-III criteria for at least one substance use disorder, 70% received a concurrent diagnosis of affective disorder, either bipolar disorder (41%) or unipolar depression (29%). Slightly more than half (52%) also received at least one Axis II diagnosis. Unipolar depression and borderline personality disorder were significantly more prevalent among women, while bipolar disorder, schizophrenia, and other nonaffective psychoses were more common among men.

B. The Self-Medication Hypothesis

The relatively high rate of comorbidity in individuals who abuse drugs or alcohol has given rise to speculation about the role of these agents in the "self-medication" of coexisting, and presumably preexisting, psychiatric illness in these individuals. Specifically, some have hypothesized that in some of these patients, drug and/or alcohol use was initiated in an attempt to alter undesirable mood states, ameliorate intolerable anxiety, or cope with various forms of cognitive disturbance.

Support for the self-medication hypothesis stems mainly from clinical observations gathered in the context of individual, dynamically oriented psychotherapy or psychoanalysis with drug-addicted patients [44,45] rather than well-controlled studies. Not surprisingly, the resulting psychodynamic formulations focus on the interplay between the core conflicts and character problems one often sees in such individuals and the role of drugs and/or alcohol in ameliorating specific problems in intrapsychic or interpersonal functioning. In this context, Khantzian [45] has described the efficacy opioid drugs in helping some users control feelings of anger and aggression. In this paradigm, the narcotizing and tension-relieving effects of opioids are also postulated to compensate for the inability of the users to provide solace or nurturance for themselves, or to successfully obtain it from others. In essence, the subjective effects of opioids are seen as providing a pharmacological "ego glue" for individuals predisposed, by virtue of their developmental and/or psychodynamic heritage, to find them appealing. Similar arguments can be constructed to account for the appeal of CNS stimulants or depressants in certain individuals. Thus, the inhibited individuals who find cocaine both energizing and disinhibiting are more prone to use the drug repetitively than someone without these characteristics. In a similar vein, individuals who experience chronic anxiety may be at increased risk for abuse, and subsequent dependence upon, CNS depressants, including alcohol.

In patients with major psychiatric disorder, the self-medication paradigm takes on more definitive meaning. Thus, patients with major depression who experience intermittent or chronic dysphoria may come to value the powerful, though brief, euphorigenic effects of opioids or cocaine. Patients with bipolar or cyclothymic disorder who use cocaine may discover that the drug can not only bring them out of their depressive episodes, but also enhance their endogenously produced highs. Presumably cocaine-induced changes in both noradrenergic and dopaminergic neuronal transmission play an important role in this regard [46]. Individuals with panic disorder may find that alcohol, benzodiazepines, and other CNS depressants provide immediate, though short-term, relief of anxiety symptoms, whereas those with attention deficit disorder may find that CNS stimulants, including cocaine, including cocaine, help them focus their attention and control their hyperactivity. This appears to be an important factor in their continued use. Both Khantzian [47] and our group [48] have reported successful treatment of such patients with methylphenidate or magnesium pemoline, respectively.

Unfortunately, the usefulness of illicit drugs in the self-treatment of major psychiatric illness is notoriously limited. For example, in a study by Post et al. [49], patients with major depression were allowed to use cocaine in order to assess the effects of this drug on their mood state. At low doses, some subjects experienced elevated mood. At high doses, however, a substantial number of these depressed patients became increasingly dysphoric. Similar findings have been reported in previously addicted individuals given other CNS stimulants, like amphetamine and methylphenidate [50]. In bipolar patients, cocaine use has been reported to exacerbate hypomanic and manic states, with the production of an agitated dysphoric mania with psychotic features after either brief or sustained use.

In assessing the efficacy of illicit drugs in the self-treatment of major psychiatric illness, users also fail to recognize that while some of these agents may provide short-term relief of anxiety or depression, continued use is usually accompanied by exacerbation of the very same symptoms. For example, in a study carried out by our group [51], opioid addicts were allowed to self-administer increasing doses of intravenous heroin in a research ward setting, with and without pretreatment with naltrexone, a potent narcotic antagonist. In those subjects who were allowed to experience opioid effects (i.e., in the absence of antagonist blockade), we observed a profound difference between the acute effects of heroin and those which accompany chronic intoxication in that over a 10-day period, heroin-using subjects developed increasingly dysphoric moods along with a generalized increase in hostility and social withdrawal. Though acute doses of heroin briefly relieved this drug-induced dysphoria, tolerance eventually developed to this effect as well.

Data from clinical studies also suggest that opioid use, particularly when chronic, can produce an organic affective syndrome, with depression as its primary manifestation. In this context, Dackis and colleagues [52] reported that 25% of their detoxified heroin addicts met research diagnostic criteria for major depression. In contrast, among patients recently detoxified from methadone, the point prevalence of major depression was 62%. These investigators postulated that the increased prevalence of major depression among patients previously maintained on methadone was a consequence of a prolonged opioid withdrawal syndrome more common among users of long-acting methadone than among those who are detoxified from heroin. They further suggested that prolonged opiate withdrawal may be accompanied by changes in brain neurotransmitter homeostatis, which in some patients may result in a postwithdrawal depression, and that the latter may constitute an important risk factor for relapse to opiate use in such patients. Other investigators [53] have explored the efficacy of antidepressant treatment in depressed opioid addicts with equivocal results.

The precise relationship between preexisiting affective disorder and risk for the subsequent development of cocaine addiction is unclear. While acute administration of cocaine and other CNS stimulants, particularly in low to moderate doses, produces euphoria and disinhibition, chronic high-dose use is frequently accompanied by dysphoria. Moreover, even after detoxification, some users continue to manifest considerable depressive symptomatology. Though the latter may be temporarily relieved by renewed stimulant use, such use merely perpetuates the cycle of addiction, and in the long run worsens their depressive symptomatology.

Finally, as in the case of the stimulants and opioids, drugs which provide acute relief of anxiety (e.g., alcohol, benzodiazepines) lose their ability to do so when taken repetitively (i.e., tolerance develops). In addition, abrupt withdrawal of these agents often exacerbates those symptoms which provided the initial motivation for their use.

IV. DRUG/ALCOHOL ABUSE AS A RISK FACTOR FOR PSYCHOPATHOLOGY

A wide variety of psychoactive drugs are capable of producing profound changes in cognition, mood, and behavior, which, in some instances, may be indistinguishable from those which accompany "naturally occurring" psychiatric illness. Included among these are CNS stimulants and depresssants (including alcohol), the natural and synthetic hallucinogens, tetrahydrocannabinol (THC) in its various forms (i.e., marijuana, hashish), CNS depressants (including alcohol), and phencyclidine (PCP).

A. The CNS Stimulants

Sequelae of Acute and Chronic Intoxication

In certain vulnerable individuals, low doses of CNS stimulants may produce profound restlessness, agitation, irritability, and dysphoria. There are also reports of stimulant-induced panic episodes, even in individuals with no prior history of panic disorder. The most dramatic untoward effect of stimulant use, however, is the psychosis which may occur, particularly following chronic high-dose use of these drugs. The syndrome is frequently characterized by paranoia, delusions of persecution, auditory, visual, or tactile hallucinogens, parasitosis, (i.e., picking at imaginary bugs under the skin), and compulsive stereotypical behavior [54].

The ability of drugs like cocaine and other CNS stimulants to induce psychosis is consistent with the results of laboratory studies demonstrating their profound effects on noradrenergic and dopaminergic neurons [46]. In addition, the phenomenon of kindling, as it occurs in neuronal systems (including the human brain), may explain why the repetitive use of CNS stimulants poses an incremental risk of affective, cognitive, and behavioral disturbance, even when dosage levels remain relatively constant [55].

Sequelae of Stimulant Withdrawal

The most common form of stimulant-related psychopathology is the abstinence syndrome frequently seen following abrupt withdrawal of these drugs. With regard to cocaine, for example, Gawin and Kleber [26] have described a three-phase syndrome that begins with the "crash," characterized by anxiety, depression, hyperphagia, hypersomnolence, and a rebound increase in rapid eye movement sleep. This state shortly gives way to anergia accompanied by social withdrawal and a clinical state that is difficult to distinguish from "retarded" depression, which may last anywhere from 1 to 10 weeks. In general, the severity of the depressive symptomatology is correlated with the duration and magnitude of prior stimulant use as well as with individual variables, including the presence or absence of an underlying depressive disorder. The withdrawal phase is followed by what these investigators [26] describe as an "extinction" phase of indefinite duration, characterized by euthymic mood and normalization of vegetative functioning, but with intermittent drug craving, particularly in response to conditioned cues which signal drug availability.

B. Alcohol and Other CNS Depressants

Sequelae of Chronic Intoxication

Although alcohol, the benzodiazepines, and the sedative-hypnotic drugs are in extremely wide use, their popularity belies the fact that these drugs can have profound effects on mood, cognition, and behavior, particularly when used chronically. Acute alcohol intoxication has been well described in the literature and is familiar to the vast majority of clinicians [56,57]. Certain aspects of chronic intoxication, however, may be more subtle, particularly when patients are not overtly intoxicated at the time of examination. In addition to the severity and chronicity of depressant abuse, other factors, including age, concomitant drug use, and physiological variables (e.g., ability to metabolize these drugs), also influence the clinical picture. Thus, the chronic alcoholic who presents as apathetic, dysphoric, and intermittently anxious may be variously diagnosed as suffering from maor or atypical depression, dysthymic disorder, or generalized anxiety disorder, with a depressive component that is alcohol induced. In patients with associated neurological sequelae (e.g., Wernicke-Korsakoff disease), deficits in memory and/or overall cognitive functioning may lead the clinician to suspect a primary dementia (e.g., Alzheimer's disease) rather than a drug-induced organic brain syndrome.

Depressant Withdrawal Syndrome

Withdrawal from CNS depressants, including alcohol, can be relatively mild or it can be life threatening, depending upon the extent and severity of prior drug use as well as other variables. Although the depressant withdrawal syndrome has been well described in the clinical literature [8,58], diagnostic confusion is apt to occur in its early stages when anxiety and agitation are most prominent, before more dramatic (i.e., delirium, seizures) sequelae emerge. In this early phase, patients may receive anxiolytic drugs, which briefly alleviate anxiety symptoms, but which perpetuates their drug addiction, or they may receive antidepressants, which increase the risk of seizures as the withdrawal syndrome progresses.

As in the case of stimulant withdrawal, anxiety, depression, and sleep disturbance may continue for months after depressant drugs and alcohol have been discontinued. This coupled with internal and external stressors increases the risk of relapse, particularly in patients who have failed to develop alternative sources of support for remaining drug or alcohol free.

C. Marijuana and the Hallucinogens

Anxiety and Panic Reactions

As mentioned earlier in this section, use of marijuana and the hallucinogens may precipitate acute panic reactions, particularly in inexperienced users, and in individuals whose character structure makes loss of control (due to drug intoxication) extremely frightening. Fortunately, such reactions are usually time limited, although individuals with preexisting generalized anxiety or panic disorder may experience sustained anxiety [59]. Psychosis induced by lysergic acid diethylamide (LSD) and other hallucinogens has also been well described, although the role of preexisting psychopathology (e.g., schizophrenia) in the development of this syndrome is unclear [60].

Sequelae of Chronic Use

Chronic use of marijuana and the hallucinogens may be accompanied by the development of an amotivational syndrome, characterized by chronic apathy, anhedonia, difficulty concentrating, and social withdrawal [61]. Although this syndrome has been linked with chronic, high-dose use of these drugs, the role of preexisting psychopathology, including various character problems and/or underlying depressive disorder, has not been well defined.

D. Phencyclidine

Phencyclidine (PCP) is a veterinary tranquilizer whose addictive liability was first noted in the early 1970s, and for a period of time was a major cause of emergency room visits for drug-related problems. Acute PCP intoxication is accompanied by elated mood, alterations in body image, perceptual distortions, and hypersensitivity to auditory, visual, and tactile stimuli. At higher doses, hyperactivity, delusions, auditory and visual hallucinations, stereotypical behavior, and paranoia may be part of a clinical syndrome that is sometimes difficult to distinguish from an acute exacerbation of schizophrenia or a manic psychosis. However, neurological sequelae (e.g., nystagmus, muscular rigidity, dystonia, tremor, athetosis, and catalepsy) as well as signs of autonomic nervous system hyperarousal are suggestive of PCP intoxication [62]. Chronic, high-dose use, particularly by individuals with preexisting psychotic disorders, appears to be a major risk factor for the development of PCP psychosis.

In summary, while underlying psychopathology is an important risk factor for the subsequent development of drug abuse or dependence, many of these drugs by themselves produce significant alterations in mood, cognition, and behavior in the user. As a result, the clinician is called upon to develop methodologies for distinguishing preexisting (i.e., primary), psychiatric illness from the sequelae of drug intoxication or withdrawal in these patients. This complex task is the subject of the next section.

V. CLINICAL EVALUATION OF THE DUAL DIAGNOSIS PATIENT

A. Initial Assessment

The concurrent presence of two or more psychiatric disorders (including drug and/or alcohol dependence) has important implications for the assessment, treatment, and clinical course of dual diagnosis patients. The following clinical case study illustrates many of the salient issues in the diagnostic evaluation and subsequent treatment of such patients.

Case Report

A 32-year-old white single male presented for outpatient treatment at a local drug treatment facility. The history revealed a 20-year experience with illicit drugs, beginning with marijuana and alcohol at age 12, progressing to hallucinogens and phencyclidine by age 16, and crack, cocaine, oral codeine, and Dilaudid (hydromorphone hydrochloride) by age 18. Since age 20 he had been abusing opioids exclusively on a more or less regular basis, primarily intravenous heroin.

The patient supported his heroin addiction through a variety of illicit activities and had developed a lengthy criminal record. He had dropped out of six prior drug treatment programs and had recently left a residential therapeutic community after 7 days. Also notable in the history were three episodes of drug overdose, two of which necessitated emergency room treatment. Further questioning revealed that on all three occasions he had been aware that both the quantity and quality of the heroin he was injecting might be sufficient to cause an overdose reaction, but that he was "so down at the time I didn't care."

On examination, the patient presented as a disheveled, agitated man who was fearful of impending opiate withdrawal. The history revealed anorexia, with a 20-lb weight loss over the last year, frequent middle of the night awakening, early morning rising, difficulty concentrating, and persistent thoughts of helplessness and hopelessness. There was also occasional suicidal ideation, particularly at times when he was unable to support his heroin habit and during periods of incarceration, accompanied by involuntary opioid withdrawal. Family history revealed a chronically alcoholic father and a mother and maternal grandmother with a history of intermittent untreated depression.

Following a methadone-assisted detoxification, the patient agreed to enter a comprehensive outpatient program which included group and individual counseling, once weekly family therapy, and a vocational rehabilitation program. Two months postdetoxification, however, the patient continued to manifest chronic anxiety and agitation, anhedonia, poor appetite, and sleep disturbance. There was also diurnal variation of mood (i.e., worse in the morning), and despite some positive developments in his life (e.g., being reunited with his girlfriend) he had persistent feelings of low self-esteem, guilt, and hopelessness, which the patient said had been present for as long as he could remember.

A structured clinical interview, using the DIS, yielded a DSM-III-R (DSM-III-Revised, 1987) diagnosis of opioid dependence, chronic, complicated by recurrent major depression. Routine thyroid function tests, a complete blood count, and an SMA-12 were all within normal limits. A 1-mg dexamethasone suppression test yielded a 4:00 p.m. plasma cortisol (16 h postdexamethasone) of 7.8 μg/dl, indicating early escape from dexamethasone suppression. A measure of 24-h urinary free cortisol was 156 μg/24 h, indicative of elevated adrenocortical activity.

The 24-h urinary excretion of 3-methoxy-4-hydroxyphenylglycol (MHPG), the major metabolite of brain-generated norepinephrine, was 3064 μgs/24 h, which is thought to be high (average values usually ranging between 1900 and 2500 μg/24 h). A measure of platelet monoamine oxidase (MAO) activity was also elevated at 11.3 U (normal 4–7 U).

The patient's continuing depression coupled with a positive family history of affective disorder and the above-noted laboratory data led us to recommend a trial of antidepressant medication. However, after 4 weeks of imipramine treatment, the patient was only marginally improved. An imipramine plasma level on a total daily dose of 200 mg/day was 163 µg/ml (combined imipramine and its metabolite desipramine), which was felt to be at the low end of the therapeutic range.

Despite the patient's discouragement (and that of his treaters), imipramine was continued and the dose increased. After 3 additional weeks of imipramine at 300 mg/day, the patient seemed less anxious, his appetite began to improve, and he began to gain weight. His sleep disturbance and anhedonia persisted, however. After 4 additional weeks (total of 12 weeks on imipramine), the patient's sleep had improved and he was substantially less depressed. A repeat dexamethasone suppression test revealed a 16-h (4:00 p.m.) plasma cortisol of 2.8 µg/dl. His urinary free cortisol was 72 µg/24 h, and the urinary MHPG excretion was 2250 µg/24 h. A measure of platelet MAO activity was 9.7 U.

Over the ensuing 8 months, the patient was maintained on imipramine 300 mg/day, with a combined imipramine and desipramine plasma level of 273 µg/ml. During that period, the patient participated in outpatient Narcotics Anonymous (NA) groups, individual counseling, and a vocational rehabilitation program. He remained free of overt depressive symptomatology, though he continued to feel pessimsitic about the future. Random urine screens were occasionally positive for morphine, and the patient admitted to several relapses to intravenous heroin use, particularly on weekends when he frequented neighborhoods where he had previously obtained and used narcotics. He was offered maintenance on naltrexone, a narcotic antagonist (125 mg every three days), which he found useful in suppressing his craving for opioids. On several occasions, the patient appeared intoxicated on alcohol, and though he refused Antabuse (disulfiram), he did agree to attend weekly meetings of Alcoholics Anonymous (AA).

At last follow-up 2 years after the initiation of outpatient treatment, the patient remained employed, though he said he found his current job as a maintenance worker demeaning and boring and occasionally wishes he were "on the street" with his friends, who are still active heroin users. Alcohol addiction continues to be a problem, particularly on weekends. The patient has continued to attend weekly meetings of NA, but stopped going to AA. He is still being maintained on 300 mg/day of imipramine.

Discussion

The above case history illustrates many of the clinical issues which arise in the evaluation of addicts who may have comorbid psychopathology. Typically these patients present with long drug-use histories, and in this respect are indistinguishable from the rest of their drug-addicted peers. As a result, most have experienced the usual psychosocial sequelae of addictive drug use, including loss of relationships, occupational failure, incarceration, multiple attempts at treatment, and repetitive relapse. Their initial drug experience most frequently involves alcohol use followed by use of other drugs, including marijuana, hallucinogens, PCP, and central nervous system stimulants. Opioid use frequently begins with prescription drugs (e.g., Dilaudid) taken orally, which, in some cases, progresses to street drugs (e.g., heroin) taken intravenously.

Characteristically early drug experience involves multiple drugs taken in combination (e.g., alcohol and sedative-hypnotics), or sequentially (e.g., cocaine followed by heroin). Though eventualy a drug of choice emerges, use of other drugs may continue, and may even predominate during periods when the user's drug of choice is unavailable. Progression to addictive use of a particular drug is accompanied by experimentation with more efficient methods of getting the drug into the bloodstream and subsequently into the brain (e.g., intravenous heroin use, cocaine freebasing). For some addicts, these methods become the preferred route of administration and are often associated with a more extreme degree of drug addiction.

As the user works his or her way through the menu of available drugs, drug preference is shaped by a host of factors, including current fashion, drug availability, peer influence, and of course the subjective response of the user to the pharmacological effects of a particular drug. When they present for treatment, such patients have typically experienced multiple episodes of addiction interspersed with periods of unstable abstinence. As a result it is often difficult to discern the precise causal relationship between drug abuse and other psychiatric disorders which may be present. Moreover, given the adverse effects of acute and/or chronic drug use on mood, cognition, and behavior, patients presenting symptoms must be carefully assessed to define the relative importance of drug intoxication or drug withdrawal in the current clinical picture. This often requires prolonged observation of the patient in a drug-free condition. As stated previously, many presenting symptoms resolve once detoxification is completed and illicit drugs are no longer available. Thus, many patients who initially meet diagnostic criteria for major affective disorder, anxiety disorder, or acute organic conditions will improve and will not require specific treatment for these disorders. Similarly, antisocial behavior that occurs in the context of chronic drug use does not imply the presence of a preexisting, and potentially enduring, antisocial personality disorder.

There is, however, a subgroup of drug-addicted patients who also have one or more concurrent psychiatric disorders. These individuals, though drug free, will remain symptomatic. In further evaluating such patients, emphasis should be placed on the chronology of symptom development and particularly on those symptoms experienced during drug-free periods of reasonable duration (i.e., 3 months or more). Unfortunately, drug addicts are often poor historians, their histories being colored by what they perceive to be the expectations of the interviewer and their wish to influence the direction of any proposed treatment. In addition, the problems posed by state-dependent learning, wherein drug-free patients are unable to accurately remember their behavior when intoxicated, whereas intoxicated individuals are unable to accurately remember what they were like when they were sober also complicates the evaluation process.

B. Use of Structured Interviews and Rating Scale Data

In an attempt to improve both the validity and reliability of diagnoses in potentially dual diagnosis patients, some workers in the field have relied on structured interviews like the DIS [13] or the Schedule for Affective Disorders and Schizophrenia (SADS) [63]. In our experience, structured interviews yield more concurrent diagnoses (in addition to drug dependence) than standard clinical interviews. However, in comparing clinical diagnoses derived through use of the DIS with those based solely on clinical assessment, we found that DIS diagnoses in the same individual may change over time and that recently intoxicated patients are assigned many more diagnoses than those interviewed after a 2-week drug-free period [14]. The SADS-L (lifetime version) is particularly useful in assessing patients for chronic and/or recurrent mental disorders which may have been present earlier in life, and which therefore may have played a role in the development and/or maintenance of drug abuse or dependence.

Yet another tool in the assessment of drug addicts whose history and current symptomatology are suggestive of a comorbid psychiatric disorder is the use of rating scales. These may include standard measures of depressive symptomatology like the Hamilton Depression Rating Scale (HDRS) [64] or the Beck Depression Inventory (BDI) [65], as well as scales which measure a broad range of psychopathology like the Symptom Distress Checklist (SCL-90) [66]. Used serially, these scales are useful in both quantitating initial symptoms and measuring symptom change over time.

In studies carried out by our group [4,16,17], serial application of psychiatric rating scales in both dual diagnosis patients and in those with otherwise uncomplicated drug or alcohol dependence reveal that many of these patients, if maintained in a drug-free environment, will, over time (i.e., 4 weeks) manifest a substantial decrease in their measured levels of depression and anxiety, even in the absence of pharmacological treatment. Thus, in our patients, admission ratings on the Hamilton, Beck, and SCL-90 scales documented moderate to severe depression. Over 4 weeks of hospitalization, however, there was substantial symptom reduction, as assessed clinically and as measured by these rating scales. Not surprisingly, however, when we compared patients who eventually received a diagnosis of major or atypical depression (independent of the rating scale data) to a larger subgroup without Axis I depressive disorder, the former had significantly higher depression scores on admission and after the second and fourth week of their hospital stay. Moreover, though both groups improved symptomatically, the differences in depression rating scale scores between the two groups increased over time. Thus, rating scale data coupled with other types of clinical assessment may be useful in identifying who among a large group of depressed drug addicts will eventually receive a diagnosis of major or atypical depression.

C. Use of Family Pedigree Data

In Drugs Addicts with Possible Affective Disorder

Family pedigree studies attempt to ascertain the current and/or lifetime prevalence of various psychiatric disorders in the first-degree relatives (and sometimes second- or third-degree relatives) of patients with an index disorder (e.g., major depression). The prevalence of various illnesses found in the relatives of these patients is then compared with that found in the relatives of normal controls or in the relative of patients who do not have the index disorder but do have other psychiatric disorders (e.g., alcoholism).

In the aforementioned study by Eisen et al. [37], substance abusers reported a higher prevalence of alcohol abuse/dependence among at least one first-degree relative compared to nonabusers. This finding was particularly strong for male substance abusers who were significantly more likely to have an alcoholic father compared to men who did not meet study criteria for substance abuse (30 vs 16%). Substance abusers also had a higher prevalence of heavy drinking and/or alcoholism among their siblings compared to those without an associated alcohol or drug problem (30 vs 15%). It should be noted, however, that even among psychiatric patients without associated drug or alcohol problems, slightly more than half (51%) had at least one first- or second-degree relative with a history of heavy drinking.

In studies carried out by our group [67], family pedigree data were obtained through direct interview of all available first-degree relatives (approximately half of the total) as well as the patients themselves. In looking at the prevalence of affective disorder (i.e., major/atypical depression, bipolar/cyclothymic disorder) in the patients and their relatives, we found that drug abusers with concurrent affective disorder had significantly more first-degree relatives with affective illness compared to drug abusers without affective disorder.

In Drug Addicts Who Are Also Alcoholic

Many patients seeking treatment for alcoholism also are addicted to other drugs [17]. Conversely, there is a high prevalence of alcohol addiction among patients who identify themselves as drug addicts. This frequent co-occurrence of alcohol and drug addiction has led some to suggest that these patients do not descriminate between various drugs of addiction, but simply want to be "high." Alternatively, drug or alcohol intoxication may induce a state in the user that necessitates the use of other (additional) agents. Examples of the latter include the use of alcohol or opiates to modify the activating effects of cocaine, or the use of benzodiazepines to ameliorate symptoms of alcohol withdrawal.

While these explanations for mixed drug/alcohol addiction are applicable to many patients, they do not preclude the possibility that for some the development of one or more of these disorders, particularly alcoholism, may be influenced by familial and/or genetic factors. Supporting this hypothesis are findings from family pedigree studies which reveal that the prevelance of alcoholism in the first-degree relatives of alcoholics is approximately 30–40% compared to 5–10% in the general population [67,68]. Data from twin studies [69] also support a role for familial and/or genetic factors in the development of this disorder in that monozygotic (identical) twins, who share the same genetic heritage, have a significantly higher concordance rate for alcoholism when compared to dizygotic (fraternal) twins. Indeed, the latter have the same concordance rate for alcoholism as nontwin siblings. It should be noted, however, that the concordance rate in identical twins is only 60–70% compared to a rate of 25–35% in fraternal twins, suggesting that other (i.e., psychological, developmental, environmental) factors also play a role in the development of alcoholism in this genetically at risk population.

In Alcoholics with Possible Affective Disorder

Clearly the depressogenic effects of alcohol on mood, and the emotional "fallout" of life as an alcoholic play a role here. In addition, some have suggested that alcoholism and depression are different phenotypic expressions of the same inherited disorder, with alcoholism occurring primarily in males, and affective disorder, especially depression, occurring mostly in females [70,71]. However, in our studies [67] of drug- and alcohol-dependent patients and their first-degree relatives, we found that being alcoholic did not increase the probility that a patient would have a relative with affective disorder. Conversely, having affective disorder did not increase the probability that a patient would have one or more alcoholic relatives. Instead, the prevalence of alcoholism and/or affective disorder among the relatives of our patients was highly correlated with the presence of the same clinical entity in the proband.

D. The Role of Laboratory Tests in Evaluating Drug Abusers for Affective Disorder

A number of investigators have attempted to assess the usefulness of laboratory measures like the Dexamethasone Suppression Test (DST) [72], the 24-h urinary excretion of free cortisol (UFC) [73] and 3-methoxy-4-hydroxy-phenylglycol (MHPG) [74], and platelet monoamine oxidase (MAO) activity [75] in evaluting patients with presumptive affective disorder.

In general, early escape from dexamethasone suppression has proven to be a useful biological marker in patients with severe rather than mild depression (i.e., melancholia) [72]. However, our experience in detoxified drug addicts suggests that the DST is of limited value in this population, in that the vast majority of these patients abuse multiple drugs, some of which (e.g., barbiturates, benzodiazepines, and morphine) induce liver enzymes that rapidly metabolize dexamethasone, yielding false-positive DST findings [76]. However, in depressed drug addicts who have been drug free for an extended period of time (i.e., 4–6 weeks), a positive DST may be useful in supporting a combined diagnosis of depressive disorder, although studies need to be done to assess the long-term effects of drugs and alcohol on the DST.

Elevation of urinary free cortisol (UFC) excretion has also been reported in some depressed patients, suggesting an abnormality in hypothalamic-pituitary-adrenal (HPA) functioning in these individuals with accompanying loss of the normal circadian rhythm of cortisol secretion [77]. At present, however, there are no data on the usefulness of 24-h UFC determinations in the evaluation of depressed drug addicts. Clearly, some drugs of abuse (e.g., heroin) affect the HPA axis [78], but how long these effects persist once patients are drug free is not clear. On the other hand, in our view, elevated levels of UFC in a depressed patient who has been drug free for at least 4 weeks may suggest that part of the patient's symptomatology may be due to a biologically based affective disorder.

Urinary MHPG excretion is thought to reflect, in part, the rate of central nervous system turnover of the neurotransmitter norepinephrine [79] and may in conjunction with other measures of neurotransmitter activity eventually prove useful in subtyping patients with affective disorder [74]. It has been reported that MHPG excretion is low in bipolar depressed patients and high in both manics and some patients with agitated depression [80]. In drug addicts, MHPG excretion has been shown to be dramatically increased during the acute phase of opiate withdrawal, a finding consistent with the excessive central and peripheral noradrenergic activity that characterizes this state [81]. What is unclear, however, is how long noradrenergic hyperactivity persists in these patients and at what point urinary MHPG measurements might be useful in subtyping those who might have concurrent affective disorder.

Though interpretation of urinary MHPG data in recently detoxified drug addicts must be viewed with caution, we have reported [82] that there is a subgroup of opiate addicts with concurrent major or atypical depression and who also have persistently high levels of urinary MHPG (i.e., greater than 3000 μg/24 h) 2–4 weeks after their last dose of heroin. In contrast, among opiate addicts who have been drug free for a comparable period of time, but whose depressive symptoms did not persist beyond the acute withdrawal phase, urinary MHPG values were found to be in mid-range (i.e., between 1950 and 2500 μg/24 h) for this measure.

VI. INFLUENCE OF COMORBID PSYCHOPATHOLOGY ON ASSESSMENT AND RESPONSE TO TREATMENT IN DUAL DIAGNOSIS PATIENTS

In dual diagnosis patients, the concurrent presence of one or more psychiatric syndromes (in addition to alcohol and/or drug addiction) clearly impacts on the assessment and treatment response of these patients.

A. Effects on Assessment

Despite the obvious importance of comprehensive diagnosis in these patients, there are data to suggest that alcohol and drug problems often go unrecognized when patients are evaluated in traditional psychiatric or medical settings. Psychiatric patients who are also alcoholics and drug addicts are just as likely to conceal their alcohol or drug problems as those without additional psychiatric disorders. Moreover, not infrequently, both the patient and the treating clinician share in their wish to deny the existence of an alcohol or drug problem, despite overwhelming social or medical evidence to the contrary (e.g., job loss secondary to alcoholism, multiple convictions for driving under the influence, cirrhosis of the liver). Finally, even when a drug or alcohol diagnosis is made, follow-up, in the form of referral for specialized treatment, does not occur in many instances. Often there is a tacit or explicit assumption that the alcohol and/or drug addiction is the result of an unsuccessful attempt at self-treatment of the underlying psychiatric illness, and that successful treatment of the latter will result in amelioration of the alcoholism or drug addiction. This is a hazardous assumption, since careful attention to the chronology of symptom development may reveal quite the opposite; i.e., alcohol and/or drug use has, by itself, produced a syndrome clinically indistinguishable from naturally occurring psychiatric illness.

B. Effects on Treatment Response

In assessing the impact of comorbidity on the clinical course and treatment response, Stabenau and colleagues [84] found that alcoholics with antisocial personality disorder (ASP) experience an earlier onset of problem drinking and a more rapid downhill course than alcoholics without ASP. There was also evidence that the concurrent presence of other psychiatric disorders, like ASP, may in some cases make both treatment seeking less likely and treatment outcome less positive [84].

It also seems clear that the level of psychiatric symptomatology affects treatment outcome in many patients with drug and/or alcohol problems. Thus, McLellan et al. [85] found that the severity of psychiatric symptomatology is an important predictor of patients' responses to treatment for alcohol or drug problems, in that patients with the most severe psychiatric difficulties do poorly regardless of what modalities are employed. While patients with fewer, and less severe, symptoms do well in almost all forms of treatment. For those patients who fall between these two extremes, however, early diagnosis and appropriate matching of patients' problems to specific treatment modalities appears to have an important impact on prognosis. Similar findings have been reported by Rounsaville et al. [3].

Studies in patients with non–drug related psychiatric disorders also suggest that the concurrent presence of alcohol or drug abuse has an adverse effect of the clinical course and treatment outcome. For example, Safer [86] studied chronic mentally ill outpatients attached to a community mental health center and found that the prevalence of illicit drug and/or alcohol abuse in this population of young schizophrenic and bipolar patients was three to 15 times higher than that found in a survey sample of high school seniors, depending on the drug involved. In a prospective follow-up, the substance-abusing subgroup had a hospitalization rate two and a half times that of other chronic mentally ill patients who were not substance abusers. In many instances, drug use precipitated hospitalization, either as a result of the direct effects of the drugs themselves or the indirect, but persistently adverse, effects of drug and/or alcohol use on medication compliance. Similarly, McCarrick et al. [87] identified a subgroup of chronic mentally ill drug and alcohol abusers in a community support program, and found that these patients evidence more acting out and other problematic behaviors than their drug-using peers.

There is overwhelming evidence that in alcohol and drug addicts with comorbid psychiatric illness, accurate diagnosis and successful treatment requires recognition of, and active intervention for, each of the disorders present. Moreover, failure to do so has an adverse effect on the clinical course, response to treatment, and ultimately on prognosis. Fortunately, growing awareness of this concept has fostered an increasingly multivariate view of the psychopathology found in these patients and the development of more comprehensive, multimodal approaches to their treatment.

C. Effects on Treatment Choices

Because of the large percentage of psychiatric symptoms and syndromes during intoxication and withdrawal, a large number of Axis I psychiatric diagnoses will "clear" with abstinence and treatment of addiction. The clinical findings have an important impact on the choice of treatments. Medications for psychiatric symptoms are often not necessary after the detoxification phase. Also, retrospective recall by the patient alone should not dictate whether another psychiatric disorder requiring medication is present. Historical corroboration and longitudinal follow-up are critically important in accurately assessing addicted patients for other psychiatric disorders and the need for medications and other therapies.

ACKNOWLEDGMENTS

The authors gratefully acknowledge the assistance of Susanne Daley and Claire Ryan in the preparation of this manuscript.

REFERENCES

1. Ross, H.E., Glaser, F.B., and Germanson, T. (1988). The prevalence of psychiatric disorders in patients with alcohol and other drug problems, *Arch. Gen. Psychiatry, 45*:1023–1032.
2. Khantzian, E.J., and Treece, C. (1985). DSM-III psychiatric diagnosis of narcotic addicts: Recent findings, *Arch. Gen. Psychiatry, 42*:1067–1077.
3. Rounsaville, B.J., and Kleber, H.D. (1986). Psychiatric disorders in opiate addicts: Preliminary findings on the course and interaction with program type, *Psychopathology and Addictive Disorders* (R.E. Meyer, ed.), New York, Guilford Press, pp. 140–168.
4. Weiss, R.D., Mirin, S.M., Michael, J.L., and Sollogub, A. (1986). Psychology in chronic cocaine abusers, *Am. J. Drug Alcohol Abuse, 12*(1):17–29.
5. Helzer, J.E., and Pryzbeck, T.R. (1988). The co-occurrence of alcoholism with other psychiatric disorders in the general population and its impact on treatment, *J. Studies Alcohol, 49*:219–224.
6. National Institute of Drug Abuse (1988). *National Household Survey on Drug Abuse*, Rockville, Maryland, National Clearinghouse for Drug Abuse Information.
7. Goodwin, D.W. (1971). Is alcoholism hereditary? A review and critique, *Arch. Gen. Psychiatry, 25*:545.
8. Smith, D.E., Wesson, D.R., and Seymour, R.B. (1979). The abuse of barbiturates and other sedative-hypnotics, *Handbook on Drug Abuse* (R.L. Dupont, ed.), National Institute of Drug Abuse, Bethesda, Maryland.
9. Boreland, B.L., and Heckman, H.K. (1976). Hyperactive boys and their brothers, *Arch. Gen. Psychiatry, 33*:669–675.
10. Cloninger, C., and Reich, T. (1983). Genetic heterogeneity in alcoholism and sociopathy, *Genetics of Neurological and Psychiatric Disorders* (Rowland S. Kety, R. Sidman, et al., eds.), Raven Press, New York, pp. 145–166.
11. Robins, L.N., Helzer, J.E., Weissman, M.M., et al. (1984). Lifetime prevalence of specific psychiatric disorders in three sites, *Arch. Gen. Psychiatry, 44*:949–958.
12. Kashani, J.H., and Orvaschel, H. (1988). Anxiety disorders in mid-adolescence: A community sample, *Am. J. Psychiatry, 145*(8):960–964.
13. Helzer, J.E., Robins, L.N., and McEvoy, L.T. (1985). A comparison of clinical and Diagnostic Interview Schedule diagnoses: Physician reexamination of lay-interviewed cases in the general population, *Arch. Gen. Psychiatry, 42*:657–666.
14. Griffin, M.L., Weiss, R.D., Mirin, S.M., Wilson, H., and Bouchard-Voelk, B. (1987). The use of the Diagnostic Interview Schedule in drug-dependent patients, *Am. J. Drug Alcohol Abuse, 13*:281–291.
15. Rounsaville, B.J., and Kleber, H.D. (1985). Untreated opiate addicts, *Arch. Gen. Psychiatry, 42*:1072–1077.
16. Mirin, S.M., Weiss, R.D., Sollogub, A., and Michael, J. (1984). Affective illness in substance abusers, *Epidemiology of Drug Abuse: Research and Treatment Issues, Community Epidemiology Work Group Proceedings*, Vol. II. NIDA, Rockville, Maryland, pp. 25–52.
17. Mirin, S.M., Weiss, R.D., and Michael, J. (1988). Psychopatholgy in substance abusers: Diagnosis and treatment, *Am. J. Drug Alcohol Abuse, 14*:139–157.
18. Mirin, S.M., Weiss, R.D., Griffin, M.L., and Michael, J.L. (1991). Psychopathology in Drug Abusers and Their Families, (accepted for publication).
19. American Psychiatric Association (1980). *Diagnostic and Statistical Manual of Mental Disorders*. 3rd ed. American Psychiatric Press, Inc., Washington, D.C.
20. Rounsaville, B.J., Weissman, M.M., Crits-Christoph, K. Wilber, C., and Kleber, H. (1982). Diagnosis and relationship to treatment outcome, *Arch. Gen. Psychiatry, 39*:151–156.
21. Rounsaville, B.J., Weissman, M.M., and Kleber, H. (1982). Heterogeneity of psychiatric diagnosis in treated opiate addicts, *Arch. Gen. Psychiatry, 39*:161–166.
22. Kosten, T.R., and Rounsaville, B.J. (1986). Psychopathology in opioid addicts, *Substance Abuse* (S.M. Mirin, ed.), *Psychiat. Clin. North Am., 9*(3):515–532.
23. Fishburne, P.M., Abelson, H., and Cisin, I. (1979). *National Survey on Drug Abuse: Main Findings*, National Institute of Drug Abuse, Publication (ADM) 80-976 U.S. Department of Health, Education, and Welfare, Rockville, Maryland.

24. Helfrich, A.A., et al. (1983). A clinical profile of 136 cocaine abusers, *Problems of Drug Dependence* (L.S. Harris, ed.), National Institute of Drug Abuse Research Monograph; 43, Washington, D.C.

25. Weiss, R.D., Mirin, S.M., Griffin, M.L., and Michael, J.L. Psychopathology in cocaine abusers: Changing trends, *J. Nerv. Ment. Disorders, 176*:719–725.

26. Gawin, F.H., and Kleber, H.D. (1986). Abstinence symptomatology and psychiatric diagnosis in cocaine abusers: Clinical observations, *Arch. Gen. Psychiatry, 43*:107–113.

27. Quitkin, F.M., Rifkin, A., Kaplan, J., and Klein, D.F. (1972). Phobic anxiety syndrome complicated by drug dependence and addiction, *Arch. Gen. Psychiatry, 27*:159–162.

28. Weissman, M.M., and Meyers, J.K. (1980). Clinical depression in alcoholism, *Am. J. Psychiatry, 137*:372–373.

29. Overall, J.E., Reilly, E.L., Kelley, J.T., and Hollister, L.E. (1985). Persistence of depression in detoxified alcoholics, *Alcohol Clin. Exp. Res., 9*:331–333.

30. Guze, S.B., Cloninger, C.R., Martin, R. and Clayton, P.J. (1988). Alcohol as a medical disorder, *Alcoholism: Origins and Outcome*, (Robert M. Rose and James Barrett, eds.), New York, Raven Press, pp. 83–94.

31. Weiss, R.D., Mirin, S.M., Griffin, M.L., and Michael, J.L. (1988). A comparison of alcoholic and nonalcoholic drug abusers, *J. Stud. Alcohol, 49*:510–525.

32. Christie, K.A., Burke, J.D., Regier, D.A., Rae, D.S., Boyd, J.H., and Locke, B.Z. (1988). Epidemiologic evidence for early onset of mental disorders and higher risk of drug abuse in young adults, *Am. J. Psychiatry, 145*(8):971–975.

33. Crowe, R.R. (1974). An adoption study of antisocial personality, *Arch. Gen. Psychiatry, 31*:785–791.

34. Crowley, T., Chesluk, D., Dilts, S., and Hart, R. (1974). Drug and alcohol abuse among psychiatric admissions, *Arch. Gen. Psychiatry, 30*:13–20.

35. Davis, D.I. (1984). Differences in the use of substance of abuse by psychiatric patients compared with medical and surgical patients, *J. Nerv. Ment. Disorders, 172*:654–657.

36. Fischer, D., Halikas, J., Baker, J., and Smith, J. (1975). Frequency and patterns of drug abuse in psychiatric patterns, *Dis. Nerv. Sys., 36*:550–553.

37. Eisen, S.V., Grob, M.C., and Dill, D.L. (1987). Substance abuse in a generic inpatient population, *McLean Hospital Evaluative Service Unit, Report No. 71.*

38. Eisen, S.V., Grob, M.C., and Dill, D.L. (1988). Substance abuse in an inpatient population: A comparison of patients on Appleton and generic units, *McLean Hospital Evaluative Service Unit, Report No. 75.*

39. Selzer, M.L. (1971). The Michigan Alcoholism Screening Test: The quest for a new diagnostic instrument, *Am. J. Psychiatry, 127*:89–94.

40. Weissman, M., Meyers, J., and Harding, P. (1980). Prevalence and psychiatric heterogeneity of alcoholism in a United States urban community, *J. Stud. Alcohol, 41*:672–681.

41. Jekel, J.F., and Allen, D.F. (1987). Trends in drug abuse in the mid-1980's, *Yale J. Biol. Med., 60*:45–52.

42. Clayton, R.R. (1985). The epidemiology of alcohol and drug abuse among adolescents, *Adv. Alcohol Subst. Abuse, 4*(3–4):69–87.

43. Westermeyer, J., and Walzer, V. (1975). Sociopathy and drug use in a young psychiatric population, *Dis. Nerv. Sys., 36*(12):673–677.

44. Rado, S. (1933). Psychoanalysis of pharmacothymia, *Psychoanal. Q., 2*:1–23.

45. Khantzian, E.J. (1985). The self-medication hypothesis of addictive disorders: Focus on heroin and cocaine dependence, *Am. J. Psychiatry, 142*:1259–1264.

46. Wise, R.A. (1984). Neural mechanisms of the reinforcing action of cocaine, *Cocaine: Pharmacology, Effects, and Treatment of Abuse* (J. Grabowski, ed.), National Institute of Drug Abuse Research Monograph 50, Rockville, Maryland.

47. Khantzian, E.J. (1983). An extreme case of cocaine dependence and marked improvement with methylphenidate treatment, *Am. J. Psychiatry, 140*:784–785.

48. Weiss, R.D., Pope, H.G., Jr., and Mirin, S.M. (1985). Treatment of chronic cocaine abuse and attention deficit disorder, residual type with magnesium pemoline, *Drug Alcohol Depend., 15*:69–72.

49. Post, R.M., Kotlin, J., and Goodwin, F.K. (1974). The effects of cocaine on depressed patients, *Am. J. Psychiatry, 131*:511–517.
50. Ellinwood, E.H., Jr. (1979). Amphetamines/anorectics, *Handbook on Drug Abuse* (R.L. Dupont, A. Goldstein, and J. O'Donnell, eds.), National Institute of Mental Health, Washington, D.C., pp. 221–231.
51. Mirin, S.M., Meyer, R.D., and McNamee, B. (1976). Psychopathology and mood during heroin use: Acute vs. chronic effects, *Arch. Gen. Psychiatry, 33*:1503–1508.
52. Dackis, C.A., and Gold, M.S. (1984). Depression in opiate addicts, *Substance Abuse and Psychopathology* (S.M. Mirin, ed.), American Psychiatric Press, Washington, D.C., pp. 20–40.
53. Kleber, H.D., and Gold, M.S. (1978). Use of psychotropic drugs in the treatment of methadone maintained narcotic addicts, *Ann. N.Y. Acad. Sci., 331*:81–98.
54. Ellinwood, E.H., Jr. (1972). Amphetamine psychosis: Individuals, settings and sequences, *Current Concepts on Amphetamine Abuse* (E.H. Ellinwood and S. Cohen, eds.), National Institute of Mental Health, Washington, D.C., pp. 142–158.
55. Post, R.M. (1975). Cocaine psychosis: A continuum model, *Am. J. Psychiatry, 132*:225–231.
56. Sollers, E.M., and Kalant, H. (1976). Alcohol intoxication and withdrawal, *N. Engl. J. Med., 294*:757–762.
57. Liskow, B.I., and Goodwin, D.W. (1987). Pharmacological treatment of alcohol intoxication, withdrawal and dependence: A critical review, *J. Stud. Alcohol, 48*(4):356–370.
58. Brown, C.G. (1982). The alcohol withdrawal syndrome, *Ann. Emerg. Med., 11*(5):276–280.
59. Melges, F.T., Tinklenberg, J.R., and Hollister, L.E. (1970). Temporal disintegration and depersonalization during marijuana intoxication, *Arch. Gen. Psychiatry, 23*:204–210.
60. Vardy, M.M., and Kay, S.R. (1983). LSD psychosis or LSD-induced schizophrenia? A multimethod inquiry, *Arch. Gen. Psychiatry, 40*(8):877–883.
61. Cohen, S. (1981). Cannabis: Impact on Motivation, Part II, *Drug Abuse Alcohol. Newslett., 10*:1–3.
62. Domino, E.F. (1980). Treatment of phencyclidine intoxication, *Psychopharmacol. Bull., 16*:83–85.
63. Endicott, J., and Spitzer, R.L. (1978). A diagnostic interview: The Schedule for Affective Disorders and Schizophrenia, *Arch. Gen. Psychiatry, 37*:837–844.
64. Hamilton, M. (1960). A rating scale for depression, *J. Neurosurg. Psychiatry, 23*:56–62.
65. Beck, A.T., Ward, C.H., Mendelson, M., Mock, J., and Erbaugh, J. (1961). An inventory for measuring depression, *Arch. Gen. Psychiatry, 4*:561–571.
66. Derogatis, L.R., Lipman, R.S., and Covi, L. (1973). The SCL-90: An outpatient psychiatric rating scale, *Psychopharmacol. Bull., 9*:12–28.
67. Mirin, S.M., Weiss, R.D., Sollogub, A., and Michael, J. (1984). Psychopathology in the families of drug abusers, *Substance Abuse and Psychopathology* (S.M. Mirin, ed.), American Psychiatric Press, Washington, D.C., pp. 79–106.
68. Merikangas, K.R., Leckman, J.F., Prusoff, B.A., Pauls, D.L., and Weissman, M.M. (1985). Familial transmission of depression and alcoholism, *Arch. Gen. Psychiatry, 42*:367–372.
69. Partanen, J., Brunn, K., and Markkanen, T. (1966). *Inheritance of Drinking Behavior*, New Brunswick, New Jersey, Rutgers University Center of Alcohol Studies.
70. Hill, S.H., Cloninger, C.R., and Ayre, F.R. (1977). Independent familial transmission of alcoholism and opiate abuse, *Alcoholism (N.Y.) I*:335–342.
71. Winokur, G. (1974). The division of depressive illness into depression spectrum disease and pure depressive illness, *Int. Pharmacopsychiatry, 9*:5–13.
72. Brown, W.A., and Shuey, I. (1980). Response to dexamethasone and subtype of depression, *Arch. Gen. Psychiatry, 37*:747–751.
73. Sachar, E.J., Halbreich, U., Asnis, G., et al. (1981). Neuroendocrine disturbance in depression, *Progress in Psychoneuroendocrinology* (F. Brambilla, G. Racagni, and D. de Wied, eds.), Elsevier, Amsterdam, pp. 263–272.
74. Schildkraut, J.J., Orsulak, P.J., Schatzberg, A.F., et al. (1978). Toward a biochemical classification of depressive disorders. I. Differences in urinary excretion of MHPG and other catecholamine metabolites in clinically defined subtypes of depression, *Arch. Gen. Psychiatry, 37*:747–751.
75. Nies, A., Robinson, D.S., Ravaris, C.L., et al. (1971). Amines and monamine oxidase in relation to aging and depression in man, *Psychosomat. Med., 33*:470.

76. Meltzer, H.Y. (1982). Factors affecting the validity of the dexamethasone suppression test, *Clinical Utility of the Dexamethasone Suppression Test*, Proceedings of a National Institute of Mental Health Workshop, Rockville, Maryland, pp. 54–57.

77. Carroll, B.J. Curtis, G.C., and Mendels, J. (1976). Neuroendocrince regulation in depression, *Arch. Gen. Psychiatry, 33*:1051–1058.

78. Ellingboe, J., Mirin, S.M., Meyer, R.E., and Mendelson, J.H. (1979). Effects of opiates on neuroendocrine function: Plasma cortisol, growth hormone and thyrotropin, *The Heroin Stimulus* (R.E. Meyer and S.M. Mirin, eds.), New York, Plenum Press, pp. 151–175.

79. Chase, T.N., Gordon, E.K., and Ng, L.K.Y. (1973). Norepinephrine metabolism in the central nervous system of man: Studies using 3-methoxy-4-hydroxyphenylethylene glycol levels in cerebrospinal fluid, *J. Neurochem., 21*:581–587.

80. DeLeon-Jones, F., Maas, J.W., Dekirmenjian, H., et al. (1973). Urinary catecholamine metabolite during behavioral changes in a patient with manic-depressive cycles, *Science, 179*:300–302.

81. Gold, M.S., Redmond, D.E., and Kleber, H.D. (1979). Noradrenergic hyperactivity in opiate withdrawal supported by clonidine reversal of opiate withdrawal, *Am. J. Psychiatry, 136*:100–102.

82. Mirin, S.M., Weiss, R.D., Sollogub, A., and Michael, J. (1984). Affective illness in substance abusers, *Substance Abuse and Psychopathology*, American Psychiatric Press, Washington, D.C., pp. 58–77.

83. Schatzberg, A.F., Orsulak, P.J., Rosenbaum, A.H., Toshihiko, M., Kruger, E.R., Cole, J.O., and Schildkraut, J.J. (1982). Toward a biochemical classification of depressive disorders, V: Heterogeneity of unipolar depressions, *Am. J. Psychiatry, 139*(4):471–475.

84. Stabenau, J.R. (1984). Implications of family history of alcoholism, antisocial personality, and sex differences in alcohol dependence, *Am. J. Psychiatry, 141*:1178–1182.

85. McLellan, A.T., Luborsky, L., Woody, G.E., O'Brien, C.P., and Druley, K.A. (1983). Predicting response to alcohol and drug abuse treatments, *Arch. Gen. Psychiatry, 40*:620–625.

86. Safer, D. (1986). *The Young Adult Chronic Patient and Substance Abuse.* Johns Hopkins School of Medicine, Presented at the Annual Meeting of the American Psychiatric Association, Washington, D.C.

87. McCarrick, A.K., et al. (1985). Correlates of acting-out behaviors among young adult chronic patients, *Hosp. Commun. Psychiatry, 36*(8):848–853.

36

Suicide in Drug and Alcohol Addiction

David E. Sternberg
The Kansas Institute, Olathe, Kansas, and Yale University School of Medicine,
New Haven, Connecticut

I. INTRODUCTION

Suicide is likely the leading preventable cause of death. Every year approximately 29,000 Americans commit suicide, making suicide the eighth leading cause of death in the general population and the third among adolescents [1]. In the United States, 12 out of 100,000 people kill themselves every year. This rate has been relatively constant since 1950 [2]. Yet, in the past 20 years, the rate has rapidly increased for young persons, with a concomitant decline occurring for older ones. Several retrospective studies have demonstrated that the vast majority of suicide victims were psychiatrically ill at the time of the death [3–5]. For example, Robbins [5] found that 94% of the suicides were psychiatrically ill at the time of death (47% were suffering from an affective disorder and 25% from alcoholism). Serious psychiatric illness is the most powerful risk factor for suicide, with the suicide rate among such persons being six to 11 times that of sex- and age-match controls [6].

The identification of persons at high risk for commiting suicide is a crucially important life and death task for the clinician. A risk factor is defined as a variable significantly associated with an increased probability of a particular outcome, in this case suicide. A sizable body of research has demonstrated a close association between addiction and suicidal behavior. Addiction to drugs or alcohol is associated with a markedly increased risk of suicide. This relationship has best been described in the case of alcohol, but more recent studies clearly extended it to drug addiction.

This chapter will examine the epidemiological aspects of the association between addiction and suicidal behavior, characteristics of addicts who have suicidal behavior, the relationship of addiction to suicidal behavior in adolescents, methadological problems inherent in studying the association, postulated pathogenesis of suicidal risk with addiction, implications for clinical management, and future directions for research and clinical treatment.

II. THE PROBLEM

Although the relationship between alcoholism and suicide has been studied for many years [3,4,7,8], the extent to which drug addiction contributes to enhanced suicide risk has been recognized only more recently. Indeed, investigations of completed suicides published prior to the early 1970s reported the frequency of drug addiction at 5% or less [3,4,7,9]. The low frequency of suicide classified as alcoholics or drug addicts in studies prior to 1973 [1,2,16,17] may reflect both the use of older and less sensitive diagnostic instruments for evaluating drug and alcohol addiction as well as an actual lower frequency of drug addiction, at the least, in the populations studied at that time.

Furthermore, although the abuse of and addiction to intoxicating substances by a significant proportion of persons who have committed suicide has long been recognized by investigators, usually this observation was considered an epiphenomenon, since the use of intoxicating substances was thought to be expected of persons in the depths of suicidal depression. Earlier studies did not consider the fact that addiction itself can be an independent necessary condition for suicide; that the addiction itself can cause deep and eventually fatal depression.

A. San Diego Suicide Study

The San Diego Suicide Study (SDSS) [10–13] is an extraordinary comprehensive and detailed study of completed suicides, which investigated 283 consecutive suicides in San Diego County between 1981 and 1983. The major finding of this study was the occurrence of more drug addiction than had been reported previously. Overall, addiction was diagnosed in 58% of the San Diego suicides. These studies suggest that drug addiction plays a greater role as a necessary condition for suicides of all ages than had previously been recognized. Although psychiatric diagnoses frequently overlapped with the addiction diagnoses, addiction was reported to be the principal diagnosis in 39% of cases. Thus, this study provides evidence that a sizable proportion of persons who commit suicide have had serious problems with drug addiction. Because the frequency of addiction among suicides is significantly in excess of the 11–18% lifetime prevalence of addictive disorders in the general population, as reported by the Epidemiologic Catchment Survey [14], the 58% rate of drug and alcohol addiction in completed suicides as reported by the SDSS, probably represents an actual increased risk over the general populations' rate. As noted previously, earlier investigations found addiction in 15–39% [4,15] of suicides, and nearly all of which were addiction to alcohol.

The SDSS also found a major shift in the patterns of addiction among suicides over the past 40 years. The data indicated that drug addiction was predominantly found among young suicides. As detailed in a subsequent section, there is a clear parallel between the epidemic of drug addiction among young people in recent years with the recent increase in youth suicides.

It is of note that the SDSS found no significant difference in the rates of alcoholism, drug addiction, or depression between men and women among the consecutive suicides. Yet the Epidemiologic Catchment Survey reported a markedly higher prevalence of addictive disorders, particularly alcoholism, among men (24%) than among women (4%) in the general population [16]. Thus, addictive disorders may be a contributing factor to the well-known higher rate of suicide by men.

B. Other Studies

It is likely that the frequency of drug addiction among completed suicides will vary with differing locations where the frequency of addictive disorders also will vary. In Iowa, for example, follow-up of patients admitted between 1972 and 1981 found that drug addiction was found in only 8.8% of suicides [17]. Nevertheless, the number of completed suicides in this drug- and alcohol-addicted population proved to be 11 times the expected rate. Other investigations found that risk of suicidal death among addicts is as high as 11 to 20 times that of the general population [17–19].

C. Alcoholism and Suicide

It has long been known that the frequency of suicide in alcoholics is considerably higher than in the general population. As early as 1825, Casper investigated 218 suicides and found that 28% could be attributed to "alcoholism debauchery" [20].

The association between alcoholism and suicide can be studied in two manners. First, by studying the drinking habits of suicide victims and suicide attempters; and second, by determining how many alcoholics die by suicide or attempt suicide. Numerous studies reveal that alcoholics kill themselves more often than do nonalcoholics. Although the suicide rate in the general population is less than 1%, between 7 and 27% of all deaths in alcoholics are by suicide [21–25]. Indeed, the lifetime risk for suicide in alcoholics reaches a rate as high as that seen for patients with primary mood disorders [26]. Moreover, 15–25% of all suicides appear to be committed by alcoholics [3,4,7,27]. This rate of alcoholism is much higher than that expected in the general population of the United States (i.e., 5%). Goodwin reviewed 11 studies of the drinking histories of suicide completers and found reported rates of alcoholism to range from 10 to 46% [28]. He related the wide range of alcoholism rates among the studies to the diversity of populations under investigation, and variations in the diagnostic definition of alcoholism.

A proportion of the association between alcoholism and suicide could possibly be explained by alcoholics with concurrent diagnoses of primary affective disorder or primary antisocial personality disorder [29–32], diagnoses which in themselves carry high risks of suicides and suicide attempts. Yet, when Shuckit [33] investigated primary alcoholic men who had no evidence of any preexisting psychiatric disorder, the frequency of suicide attempt continued to be higher than that found in the general population. He found that one in six (16.6%) of primary alcoholic men had attempted suicide, considerably higher than the 1–4% of the general population reporting a suicide attempt [34].

D. Opiate Addiction and Suicide

Heroin addicts kill themselves more frequently than do nonaddicts of similar age groups [35]. Depending upon the population studied, the rates of completed suicide among heroin addicts range between 82 and 350 per 100,000 while the rates of suicide attempts among such addicts range between 7 and 25% [36]. Suicide also occurs at an earlier age among heroin addicts than among alcoholics or the general population. In one study of heroin addicts, all suicides died before the age of 40 [37], and in another, 50% of suicide completers killed themselves before age 28 [38].

E. Suicide Attempts and Addiction

Suicide attempts are far more frequent than completed suicides. In the United States, the annual incidence of suicide attempts is 754 per 100,000 [39] versus 12 per 100,000 completed suicides. Among other populations, the incidence of suicide attempts ranges between 600 to 800 per 100,000 [34,40]. Investigators have found that suicide attempters are at very high risk for an eventual completed suicide. Indeed, persons completing suicide often have a history of suicide attempts, with between 25 and 50% of persons who complete suicide having a previous history of suicide attempts [5,6,41]. Those who attempt suicide have a higher rate of eventual death from suicide than even psychiatric patients without a history of suicide attempts [40,42]. Studies reveal that persons who complete suicide and suicide attempters represent overlapping but separate populations [43]. For example, the attempters are generally younger, are more frequently women, and more often have personality disorders.

Alcoholism is even more common among suicide attempters than among suicide completers. In reviewing six studies on this subject, Goodwin found rates of alcoholism among attempters ranging from 13 to 50% [28]. The wide range in the reported rates of alcoholism were related to the studies' different geographical locations and methodological designs. As noted previously, Shuckit [33] reported that 16.6% of the primary alcoholics without concurrent affective or personality disorder diagnoses that he studied had histories of suicide attempts. In studying a less uniform alcoholic populaton, Hasin and associates [44] reported that 29.2% of their sample had made at least one suicide attempt, and Hesselbrock and colleagues [45] found a lifetime prevalence rate of suicide attempts of 21% in the men and 41% in the women of their sample.

Drug addicts, like alcoholics, also are at higher risk for suicide attempts than is the general population. The lifetime prevalence rate for suicide attempts in selected drug-addict populations ranges between 17 and 30% [18,46].

III. CHARACTERISTICS OF DRUG ADDICTS AND ALCOHOLICS WITH SUICIDAL BEHAVIOR

Obviously, identifying characteristics of persons at high risk for committing suicide is a critically important task for the clinician. The ultimate goal of research in this field is to determine exactly how addicts and alcoholics who commit suicide differ from those who do not. Such knowledge would allow for preventive therapeutic measures to be instituted with the appropriate patients.

A. Demographics

Some characteristics of addicts and alcoholics who commit suicide can be found in demographic trends. Drug addicts who complete suicide are likely to be young—in their 20s to early 30s. For example, the SDSS found that 67% of the suicides under age 30 were diagnosed as addicts, whereas addictive disorders were present in only 46% of those suicides over age 30 [10]. Furthermore, the same study reveals that whereas 60% of suicides between age 30 and 40 were classified as addicts, only 14% of those over age 40 were addicts. Although a recent increase in the suicide rates of young black males has been reported [47], most addicts completing suicide are white males [11].

B. Length of Addictive Disease

The duration of addictive disorder prior to suicide has been studied. Alcoholics appear to be at greatest risk for suicide after 20 years of chronic alcoholism [7]. The SDSS found that among the "pure" alcoholics who committed suicide, alcohol-related problems had occurred for an average 29.3 years. Thus, "pure" alcoholics tend to have alcoholism-related problems for many years before they commit suicide [13]. On the other hand, drug addicts appear to be at greatest risk for suicide at an earlier age and after a shorter duration of addiction than do alcoholics. In the SDSS, the average length of addiction-related problems was significantly shorter for "pure" drug addicts (9.8 eyars) [13]. Interestingly, the average duration of addiction-related problems for persons with mixed alcohol and drug use were similar to the "pure" drug abuse addiction group [13].

C. Multiple Drug Use/Addiction

Among drug addicts, the risk of suicide is significantly correlated with multiple drug use [11,18]. The SDSS reported that the average number of substances used by suicide victims whose principal diagnosis was addiction was 3.6, whereas the group with mixed diagnoses used an average 3.3 substances [11]. Other than alcohol, the drugs most commonly used were cocaine, amphetamine, opiates, and marijuana.

Some studies have reported a high frequency of suicidal behavior among those addicted to sedative-hypnotic drugs [8,46]. Similarly, the additional use of alcohol seems to increase the risk of suicide with other drug use, perhaps by behavioral disinhibition, and perhaps by potentiating the affect of depressants. Indeed, drug addicts at risk for suicide frequently use alcohol [48]. For example, the SDSS found that 84% of the addictive disorder group used both alcohol and drugs, with only 8% being "pure" alcoholics and 8% of that group being "pure" drug addicts [11].

D. Influence of Psychiatric Illness Comorbidity on Suicide Risk

Many studies have noted the importance of the comorbidity of psychiatric symptoms and diagnoses with addictive disorders to suicide risk. There are numerous indications that additional psychopathology can increase the risk for suicide among drug addicts and alcoholics. The most relevant comorbid psychiatric syndromes are the affective disorders, especially depression, and the personality disorders, especially antisocial personality disorder.

E. Depression Comorbid with Addiction

Although previous reports have noted that major depression is not a necessary condition for completed suicide [26], studies of suicide attempts in alcoholics and drug addicts found increased rates of depressive symptoms and/or disorders in those who have attempted suicide [3,4,7,26,27,50]. One study reported that 75% of alcoholics who committed suicide were diagnosed as having an affective disorder [26]. A prospective investigation of alcoholics who later committed suicide reported a very high rate (47%) of depression [51]. Thus, although it was already well known that depressive symptoms are common in alcoholics who commit suicide, this study revealed that depressive symptoms were present at the first admission for alcoholism, many years before the actual suicide.

In the investigations which relate the comorbidity of depression with alcoholism to suicidal behavior, most of the patients studied appear to have had "secondary" depression. That is, alcoholism usually preceded the depressive disorder. Secondary depressive patients tend to have less severe and less consistent depressive symptoms, and are usually evaluated by clinicians as being less symptomatic than "primary" depressive patients. Furthermore, recent experimental studies of intoxication tend to support the impression that chronic intoxication itself may be a crucial factor in suicidal behavior. Tamerin and Mendelson reported that development of severe suicidal depression after 2 weeks of experimental intoxication [52]. Such studies have shown that alcoholics experience increasing anxiety and depression with chronic heavy drinking [53,54]. Such findings suggest that continuous heavy drinking can produce what might be called a "a depressive syndrome of chronic intoxication" [55].

A high incidence of depression has also been described among opiate addicts with suicidal behavior. Murphy and associates reported that 87% of opiate addicts who displayed suicidal behavior had a history of depressive disorders [18]. Indeed, opiate addicts are reported to have a high frequency of coexisting depressive disorders. Rounsaville and colleagues described a 17% incidence of major depression in opiate addicts beginning treatment, and a 48% lifetime prevalence of major depression [56]. Yet, 95% of these patients first experienced a major depression only after the onset of their opiate use. Indeed, opiate drug dependence not only produces a dysphoric organic affective syndrome, but also seems to lead to a protracted withdrawal state following detoxification which can mimic a major depressive disorder [57].

The San Diego Suicide Study also found a large contribution of psychiatric comorbidity to suicide risk in drug addicts and alcoholics [13]. Although addiction coexisted with a wide range of psychiatric disorders, risk for suicides was especially increased in the "mixed" addiction plus affective disorders group. Atypical depression was the most common disorder (29%) found to coexist with the addictive disorders, far more frequent than major depression or dysthymic disorder.

The data from the SDSS suggest that depression in varying degrees is very much present among addicts and alcoholics who commit suicide. Indeed, in these studies, even those classified as "pure" addictive disorder had an average of 4.1 depressive symptoms compared to 6.2 symptoms for those classified "mixed" addiction-affective cases and 7.0 symptoms for pure depressives [12]. Thus, depressive symptoms appear to be ubiquitous among addicts. As Hasin and associates noted, addicts often make suicide attempts in response to sudden, intense feelings of depression which are not of sufficient duration to meet criteria for a major depressive disorder [44].

F. Personality Disorder Comorbid With Addiction

Although many suicide studies have reported a high incidence of personality disorders, few have investigated the influence of personality disorder comorbid with addictive disorders on suicide risk. Of the 15 cases with personality disorders in the San Diego Suicide Study (14 antisocial, one mixed), 14 had histories of addictive disorders [13]. A recent Swedish study of consecutive young suicides reported that drug addiction or alcoholism coexisted with a personality disorder in 81% of cases [58]. Thus, it is likely that the coexistence of personality disorder with an addictive disorder leads to a considerably elevated suicide risk.

G. The Role of Loss in the Suicide of Drug Addicts and Alcoholics

Clinical studies of suicides have found psychosocial stressors in nearly every case, with interpersonal losses and conflicts, medical illness, and economic problems found to be the most common stressors [8]. The relationship between addiction and such stressors in suicide victims was first reported by Murphy and Robbins, who found a greater frequency of interpersonal loss in alcoholics compared to depressives in the 6 weeks prior to their death [59]. Subsequently, Murphy and colleagues confirmed that nearly one-third of the alcoholics who committed suicide had experienced a loss of a close interpersonal relationship within the last 6 weeks of their death [26]. Alcoholism is characterized by chronic disruptions of affectional relationships. Yet in the suicides of alcoholics, the suicidal act appears to closely follow another last incident in what has been a string of disrupted affectional relationships. Similarly, Bergland and associates reported that 36% of alcoholics completing suicide had experienced a significant personal loss during the year preceding the suicide [60]. The most frequent type of object loss reported was marital separation.

Such findings are not restricted to alcoholics, and have been extended to their other kinds of addicts by the SDSS [12]. Drug addicts and alcoholics who commit suicide are especially likely to have a greater than expected frequency of recent interpersonal losses (death, separation, rejection) [12]. Indeed, interpersonal loss occurred more frequently near the time of death (i.e., 6 weeks prior and particularly 1 week prior to death) for addicts than even for persons with "pure" affective disorder.

H. Characteristics of Drug Addicts and Alcoholics Who Attempt Suicide

A history of suicide attempts is a very strong risk factor for completed suicide, carrying even more weight than any specific diagnosis. Patients with a prior history of attempting suicide have a sixfold increased risk of trying again [40]. A combination of addiction and a history of suicide attempts further increases the risk for suicide. An English study reported, for example, that a history of previous suicide attempts was obtained for 67% of alcoholics who committed suicide versus 10% of alcoholics living in that community [4].

Various investigations have compared the demographic and clinical characteristics of alcoholics with and without a history of suicide attempts [33,44,45]. Shuckit [33] explored the clinical correlates of a history of suicide attempts in a consecutive series of primary alcoholics entering treatment. Even among this group of primary alcoholics, he found that one out of six had a history of previous suicide attempts. Those with suicide attempt histories demonstrated more antisocial problems early in life, tended to drink more heavily and to have greater degrees of alcohol-related problems, reported more experience with other drugs of abuse other than alcohol, were more likely to have received psychiatric treatment, and had significantly elevated risks for having first-degree relatives with alcoholism or affective disorders.

Similar results have been reported by other investigators. Hesselbrock and colleagues [45] reported, in their study of hospitalized alcoholics, that suicide attempters as compared to nonattempters were younger, had at least one parent who was alcoholic, tended to have additional psychopathology, and were affected by alcoholism more severely and for a longer period of time. The suicide attempters progressed to problem drinking, attempted to stop drinking, and received their first treatment for alcoholism much earlier than did the nonattempters. In addition, addiction to drugs other than alcohol was significantly more frequent among the suicide attempters (79%) than among the suicide nonattempters (35%). A lifetime diagnosis of major depression was significantly more frequent in the suicide attempters (63%) than in the nonattempters (25%). Similarly, a diagnosis of antisocial personality disorder was significantly more common among suicide attempters (66%) than among nonattempters (44%). Indeed, across all psychiatric diagnostic categories, the mean number of lifetime psychiatric symptoms was significantly higher among suicide attempters than among nonattempters. These results were supported by the study of Hasin and associates [44], who found that younger age was significantly related to suicide attempts, as were addiction to drugs other than alcohol, antisocial symptoms, and greater alcohol-related problems. Although their study found few subjects meeting full criteria for antisocial personality disorder, on average, those with a history of suicide attempts had engaged in significantly more types of antisocial behavior in childhood.

Similar results have been reported for drug addicts. One study of drug addict suicide attempters reported a history of early placement in reform school, childhood hyperactivity, and a maternal history of depression [47]. A comparison of opiate addicts who attempted suicide to those without a history of suicide attempts found that attempters were more likely to have lived in foster homes, to have had juvenile court hearings, to have left home before age 15, to have a history of maternal suicide, and to report depression or alcoholism in a sibling [18].

In summary, all of these investigators suggest that drug addicts and alcoholics who have attempted suicide as compared to those without such a history have more: (1) antisocial problems in childhood and adolescence; (2) severe addictions and alcohol- or drug-related life problems; (3) familial depression or addiction; and (4) multiple drug use.

IV. ADOLESCENT ADDICTION AND SUICIDE

Over the past 25 years, a two- to threefold increase has occurred in suicides among young persons [61]. This increase has been especially concentrated in the 15–24 age group. The suicide rate in the United States among young persons aged 15–24 has risen from 5.2 per 100,000 in 1960 to 13.3 per 100,000 in 1980 [11]. Indeed, the rates of suicide among adolescents and young adults, aged 15–24, have increased since the late 1960s to such an extent that the suicide rate for this age group has approximated that for all age groups combined [62]. In 1985, in the United States, approximately 5121 people in this age group committed suicide [63]. Suicide provided 12.9% of all deaths for this age group, a rate much higher than the 1.4% of deaths caused by suicides in all age groups.

Over the same years, the epidemic of drug addiction and alcoholism among young persons has paralleled the increase in young suicides. A variety of studies now corroborate the association between youth suicide and the epidemic of drug or alcohol addiction among youth.

A. San Diego Suicide Study

Aspects of the SDSS were designed to investigate this disturbing increase in youth suicide. One hundred thirty-three suicides under the age of 30 were compared with 150 suicides aged 30 years and over [10]. The major finding, noted above, was more drug addiction than had been reported in previous studies, and drug addiction occurred significantly more often in the young group. Sixty-six percent of the group under age 30 were diagnosed with drug addiction, compared to only 26% in the group age 30 and over. Few other differences were found between the two groups. For example, alcoholism was as infrequent in the young group (54%) as in the older group (55%).

A second report from the SDSS provided a detailed investigation into the young group. Differences were found between those with addictive disorders and the other young suicides [11]. Seventy (53%) of the young suicides were found to hae a principal diagnosis of an addictive disorder. Thirty-two cases (24%) were found to have an additional principal diagnosis (atypical depression, atypical psychosis, or adjustment disorder with depression), and were categorized as a mixed group. Except for the mixed group having a past history of more therapeutic interventions, the pure and mixed groups were quite similar. The results also indicated that, even among this young group, addiction was usually a chronic condition, present on average for 9 years, and that it produced addiction-related life problems which were quite obvious to the informants interviewed by the investigators.

As noted above, although the young addicts and alcoholics without other principal diagnoses received psychiatric care significantly less frequently than those with additional principal diagnoses (i.e., mixed groups); nevertheless, it was very rare for any treatment to have taken place in the final year of life for those in either group. Evidence for such a lack of treatment among youth suicides is supported by the study of Brent and colleagues [64], who found that only one-third of youth suicide completers had een one lifetime mental health contact, and only 7% were in active treatment at the time of death.

Multiple drug use was usually found in the SDSS. The group with a principal diagnosis of an addictive disorder averaged between three and four substances apiece [11]. The most commonly abused drugs by the young suicides were marijuana (50%), alcohol (41%), cocaine (30%), and amphetamine (23%).

B. Implications

The findings of a large proportion of addictive disorders in a group of youth suicides reported by the SDSS suggest that addictive disorders might be a major factor contributing to the rising rate of suicide among youth. This finding has been supported by other studies. Addictive disorders were found to be twice as prevalent among adolescent suicides compared to matched population controls [65]. The increased frequency of addictive disorders among youth suicides compared with the lifetime prevalence of addictive disorders (11–18%) in the general population [66] strongly suggests that the parallel increases in addictive disorders and suicides among young persons are more than coincidental. In his review of the incidence of suicide among drug addicts, Miles concluded "drug usage may be the most important single factor in the suicide rate increase among youth in the United States" [35].

V. PROBLEMS OF METHODOLOGY

Investigation of the association between an addiction and suicide can be studied in two ways. First, one can study the drug and alcohol use patterns of suicide victims or suicide attempters. Second, one can investigate a population of drug addicts or alcoholics to determine how many attempt suicide or die by suicide. It is only the first method, however, which will specify the degree to which addiction or alcoholism is a risk factor for suicide. Determination of this risk factor obviously requires that both the denominator (i.e., the number of persons in the overall population who have the risk factor of addiction or alcoholism) as well as the numerator (i.e., the number of individuals with the risk factor of addiction or alcoholism who actually commit suicide) be in fact accurate.

Estimates of the denominator, that is, the prevalence of drug addiction and alcoholism in the community are often inaccurate. Accurate estimates of the number of drug addicts in the community are especially rare because many of these drugs are illegal. Even population survey studies often miss that significant proportion of addicts who are homeless or are transients. Furthermore, many epidemiological surveys have inadequately distinguished between drug use or abuse and addiction.

Methodological difficulties also complicate accurately determining the numerator, that is, the number of persons with the risk factor of addiction who attempt suicide or die by suicide. First, even in the general population, there is the problem of determining that suicide is the cause of death. Certainly, many deaths that are ascribed to accidental causes are actually suicides. Cases of death associated with obvious drug addiction or alcoholism are probably even more prone to such bias. For example, a trend exists nationally to not certify death by overdose of illicit drugs as suicide unless the examiner obtains clear evidence of prior suicidal intent.

Finally, many studies leave unclear whether suicide was associated with the addiction or merely with intoxication. Even postmortem positive toxicology results can only establish the use of the drug immediately before death. It does not distinguish between the chronicity of an addiction and recent ingestion. Drug or alcohol use and suicide can clearly be related in two distinctive ways, drugs or alcohol can be involved as a precipitant of the suicidal act; or drug addiction or alcoholism as illness can provide the risk factor for suicidal behavior. Drugs and alcohol are often consumed just prior to suicidal behavior. For example, reports of the prevalence of alcohol consumption prior to suicide have ranged from 21 to 89% [67–69]. Moreover, as noted by Meyerson, alcohol intoxication is likely to increase the chance for a suicide attempt to become successful, regardless of the drinking habits of the attempter prior to the event [70]. Indeed, one report found that although 89% of alcoholics consumed alcohol just prior to successful suicide, so did 38% of nonalcoholics [3].

Nevertheless, despite such problems of methodology, the reports described strongly indicate that drug addicts and alcoholics have a significantly increased risk for attempting suicide and dying by suicide.

VI. PATHOGENESIS OF SUICIDE RISK IN ADDICTIVE DISORDERS

Recent research suggests that suicide is multidetermined and that although there are some consistently observed features associated with suicide risk, the conditions leading to suicide in a specific case may be unique [71]. It is very unlikely that a single theory will adequately explain the process by which addictive disorders enhance the risk of suicide. The drug addict and alcoholic populations marked heterogeneity, and the marked variability in pharmacological action of the different drugs of addiction suggest that the observed increased risk for suicide is caused by a variety of mechanisms.

A. Effects of the Drugs of Addiction on the Brain

The drugs of addiction are powerful mood-altering substances that can cause short-term and perhaps longer-term changes in the central nervous system. Chronic use of stimulant drugs produces marked decreases in brain concentrations of neurotransmitters such as norepinephrine, dopamine, and serotonin [72]. Chronic stimulant use is also associated with dysphoria and a drug withdrawal state consisting of markedly depressed mood [73]. Addiction to central nervous depressants (alcohol, sedative hypnotic drugs, opiates) is reported to be more frequent than any other cases of drugs among addicts who complete suicide [47]. Thus, the drugs of addiction might increase the risk of suicide by directly changing brain chemistry. These neurochemical changes produce organic mental states with characteristic changes in mood. Indeed, studies of subjects chronically given alcohol, heroine, amphetamines, or cocaine reveal that, in contrast to the acute euphoriant affects of these drugs, chronic intake leads to an organic state of affective deterioration characterized by increased depression, belligerance, and anxiety [74–76].

B. Comorbid Psychiatric Disorders

Specific psychiatric disorders which themselves are associated with a high risk for suicidal behavior (e.g., depression and personality disorders) frequently coexist with addictive disorders [77]. Even when a full psychiatric disorder is not present, certain symptoms related to such diagnoses may increase the risk for suicide. For example, the primary alcoholic men studied by Shuckit [33] who made suicide attempts were more likely to demonstrate early life difficulties with parents, school, peers, and police. Even though these problems were not severe enough to qualify for a diagnosis of antisocial personality, the decreased frustration and increased impulsiviity which antedated their alcoholism may have promoted the suicidal behavior. Thus, it is likely that multiple psychiatric symptoms and/or disorders interact with each other to produce a high risk for suicidal behavior.

C. Serotonergic Activity and Disinhibition

Low levels of central serotonergic activity have been linked to persons with a history of violent suicide attempts over a wide range of psychiatric illness, including depression, personality disorders, and alcoholism [78–83]. Impulsive and aggressive individuals have also been shown to have evidence of low levels of serotonergic activity in the central nervous system [84–87]. Furthermore, evidence exists of an increased risk for addictive disorders in individuals with such disinhibitory behavioral disturbances as impulsivity, low frustration tolerance, antisocial behavior, and high risk-taking behavior [88–93]. It is thus possible that the biochemical trait of reduced central serotonergic activity is a common factor linking addiction, behavioral disinhibition, and suicide.

D. Depression as a Final Common Pathway to Suicide

Depressive symptoms are very common among persons with addictive disorders, with the reported prevalence of their depressive symptoms ranging from 30 to 60% [94]. Such depressive symptoms may result from various factors, including psychosocial ones and the direct effects of chronically ingested drugs. The depressive symptoms tend not to remain stable over time, and are not then necessarily indicative of a major depressive syndrome. For example, the development of significant symptoms of depression is nearly ubiquitous at some point in the course of alcoholism [50,95]. Yet, although intense depressive symptoms are very common in alcoholism because they are so transitory, they rarely meet criteria for the diagnosis of a major depressive disorder [96,97]. Nevertheless, such severe dysphoric swings may contribute much to the 10–15% risk of completed suicide sometime in an alcoholic history [51]. Similarly, the SDSS reported that even among the drug addicts and alcoholics who did not display a full depressive syndrome, nevertheless they did have an average of 4.1 depressive symptoms prior to suicide, with symptoms of depressed mood and thoughts of death most common [13]. The drugs by those addicts who commit suicide may themselves have caused or at least significantly exacerbated such depressive symptoms. In such a multidetermined manner, depression may be the final common path to suicide.

VII. CLINICAL MANAGEMENT

A. Overview

Suicide, a major cause of death, is preventable. The assessment of suicide risk is therefore a vital yet difficult task for the clinician. The investigations detailed in this chapter demonstrate that the addictive disorders are associated with a sizable proportion of suicides. Clinicians should thus be alerted that drug addicts and alcoholics are at high risk for suicidal behavior. It should not be difficult are at high risk for suicidal behavior. It should not be difficult to identify persons with addictive disorders, if the right questions are asked with proper techniques. Aggressive treatment of persons with addictive disorders is essential to decrease their suicide risk. Yet, many of the people who eventually commit suicide after having been addicted for many years do so without ever coming to treatment. Indeed, the SDSS noted this dearth of treatment among drug addicts and alcoholics [13]. Only 42% of the drug addicts and alcoholics had ever received any treatment and only 16% of them had received treatment prior to suicide. In contrast, of those with other diagnoses, 75% received some treatment over their lifetime and 58% received treatment in their final year.

B. Problems of Suicide Prediction

Since suicide is usually preventable, good prediction and timely intervention are critical. With proper intervention, most suicidal patients cease wishing to die. One means of facilitating prevention is by further identifying populations at increased risk. Prevention also requires a clinician to accurately estimate the suicide risk at a specific time in a specific person and to then effectively intervene.

It is apparent that suicide rarely occurs in absence of psychiatric illness. Yet, only a small proportion of persons with even such high risk as the addictive disorders ever commit suicide. What is essential is to determine those factors that lead such persons with high-risk disorders to actually commit suicide. Although demographic and other general risk factors can be helpful in estimating the degree of an individual's danger, these are far from infallible predictors. The problem is that of predicting infrequent events. Because of the low base rate for suicide, even specification of sensitive risk factors produces too many false-positive to be practically useful. For example, in an effort to determine the antecedents of suicidal acts, Pokorny [98] followed a sample of 4800 psychiatric inpatients. He identified 67 completed suicides and 179 suicide attempts. Yet, the predictors he derived produced far too many false-positive cases to be practically useful in planning clinical interventions.

Yet, clinical decisions regarding suicide risk are not made only by such statistical predictions. Indeed, suicidal intent tends not to be constant within any individual. It rises, falls, and disppears and, at times, can surface abruptly. Good prediction requires then that the clinician assess the degree of the patient's suicidal intent in the present and project into the immediate future what it is likely to be. Although knowledge of objective risk factors can play an important part in the assessment, it may be even more important for the clinician to elicit the specific person's feelings and thoughts and thereby arrive at appropriate clinical judgments.

C. Suicidal Risk in Persons with Addictions Is Often Minimized

A tendency has been noted among clinicians, when assessing drug addicts and alcoholics, intoxicated individuals, and especially intoxicated drug addicts and alcoholics, to minimize the seriousness of suicide risk. In an effort to describe and analyze the effort of drug addicts and alcoholics to obtain help prior to making a suicide attempt, Wolk-Wasserman conducted interviews with 19 such patients, with their significant others, and with the clinicians whom they contacted [99]. In general, the clinicians did not perceive the patients as depressive, judging that signs of major depression were not present. Furthermore, they often did not even ask whether suicidal thoughts were present. The clinician did not perceive any immediate suicide risk because they assessed the patients as not depressed, but rather as merely dissatisfied, anxious, or irritated with their life situations. Even when the presence of suicidal thought was obvious, the clinicians were inclined to regard them as mere casual thoughts and to consider any past history of suicide attempts as only impulsive actions. At the same time, the patients often did not inform the clincians about their suicidal thoughts, even though these thoughts could be quite pressing. This was the case especially when the patients suspected that such information could produce negative repercussions, such as involuntary hospitalization. The patients were also secretive about suicidal thoughts because of shame and fear of self-exposure.

Clearly, adequate evaluation of the suicidal patient requires the clinician to be aware of any feelings which might interfere with this clinical task. Patients who have addictive disorders and are suicidal are especially likely to complicate the task of evaluation because they can evoke strong feelings in the examining clinician, such as anxiety and anger. The report by Wolk-Wasserman suggests that certain negative countertransference reactions of which the clinicians were unaware (e.g., feelings arising from previous disappointments in treating suicidal addictive disorder patients) led to the patient's risk for suicidal being underestimated or even unexplored.

D. Clinical Assessment

The assessment of suicide risk in drug addicts and alcoholics proceeds much like that of other psychiatric disorders. Suicidal thoughts should always be diligently inquired about and taken seriously, even if they seem manipulative. In addition to asking directly about suicidal thoughts and behaviors, clinicians should inquire into previous attempts, history of drug overdoses and accidents, increasing patterns of drug or alcohol use, and family history of suicide or affective illness. Corroboration of the history and interview is best achieved from friends and family. A history of suicide threats and attempts is the strongest risk factor, increasing the risk of trying again five- to sixfold. It is also vital that clinicians identify such comorbid psychiatric disorders as depression, personality disorders, psychosis, and anxiety disorders.

If such comorbid psychiatric syndromes are present, they must be aggressively treated with psychotherapy and/or psychotropic medications. A positive family history of affective disorders is often helpful in diagnosing a comorbid affective disorder in the suicidal drug addict or alcoholic. Because of their association with suicidal behavior, the clinician should also inquire about any recent interpersonal losses and whether the patient associates these with suicidal thoughts.

In the interview, the patient should be approached in an emphathetic and, at first, circumspect manner, with the clinician remaining calm and uncritical. The clinician should strive to establish sufficient rapport with the patient so that information is not withheld. The patient must be given an opportunity to talk to the clinician alone in a private setting, where he or she can be approached initially by asking how badly, how helpless he or she feels. The goals of the interview are to evaluate the patient for suicidal thinking, suicidal intent, suicidal plans, mental status, and presence or absence of a future orientation.

The choice of treatment and disposition depends on the clincian's impression of the risk for suicide in the near future and the need for treatment of the addictive disorder and any comorbid psychiatric illness. The appropriate clinical judgment should be based on the degree to which the patient wants to commit suicide, the strength of the patient's ability to fight suicidal impulses, the adequacy of the external controls available to a patient, and the risk that the potential for suicide is likely to worsen in the immediate future. If a suicide attempt has been made by an individual who remains intoxicated, such a person must be held until clear and then must be reevaluated. Drug addicts and alcoholics who are suicidal may require constant observation or hospitalization for a period of protection as well as for detoxification. Furthermore, because chronic use of drugs or alcohol increases the risk of suicide, the long-term treatment goal should be abstinence from such substances.

VIII. FUTURE DIRECTIONS

Drug addiction and alcoholism are more prominent causes of suicide than has been previously recognized. Although the addictive disorders are associated with a very sizable proportion of suicides, only a small proportion of drug addicts and alcoholics ever take their own lives. The task of future research thus remains the identification of those persons with addictive disorders who are especially at risk for suicide. Determination of the risk factors for suicide in this population requires longitudinal prospective studies of large numbers of drug addicts and alcoholics. Other areas requiring further research include investigation into the role played by comorbid psychiatric disorders in contributng to suicidal risk, and into the acute and chronic direct actions on the central nervous system of the drugs which may increase suicidal risk.

Because suicide is a late manifestation of the addictive disorders, clinical interventions should be sought earlier in the course of addiction. Similarly, because such large numbers of addicts and alcoholics at risk for suicide are not currently being reached by clinicians, improved education of the general public and media promotion of early treatment could lead to more successful treatment interventions. Finally, it seems likely that to stem the rising tide of suicide secondary to the addictive disorders, a cure will be required for the epidemic of addiction itself.

REFERENCES

1. National Center for Health Statistics, (1986). *Monthly Vital Statistics Report, Annual Summary of Births, Marriages, Divorces, and Deaths: United States, 1985*, 34(13). U.S. Department of Health and Human Services, publication No. (PHS) Washington, D.C., 86.

2. Centers for Disease Control (1985). *Suicide Surveillance, 1970–1980*, U.S. Department of Health and Human Services, Public Health Service, Atlanta, Georgia.

3. Dorpat, T., and Ripley, H.S. (1960). A study of suicide in the Seattle area, *Compr. Psychiatry, 1*:349.

4. Barraclough, B., Bunch, J., Nelson, B., and Sainsbury, P. (1974). A hundred cases of suicide: Clinical aspects, *Br. J. Psychiatry, 25*:355.

5. Robins, E. (1981). *The Final Months*, Oxford University Press, New York.

6. Hirschfeld, R.M.A., and Davidson, L. (1988). Clinical risk factors for suicide, *Psychiatric Ann., 18*:628.

7. Robins, E., Murphy, G.E., Wilkinson, R.H., Gassner, S., and Kayes, J. (1959). Some clinical considerations in the prevention of suicide based on a study of 134 successful suicides, *Am. J. Public Health, 49*:888.

8. Chynoweth, R., Tongs, J.I., and Armstrong, J. (1980). Suicide in Brisbane: A retrospective psychosocial study, *Aust. N.Z. J. Psychiatry, 14*:37.

9. Sanborn, D.E., Sanborn, C.J., and Cimbolic, P. (1973). Two years of suicide. A study of adolescent suicide in New Hampshire, *Child Psychiatry Hum. Dev., 3*:234.

10. Rich, C.L., Young, D., and Fowler, R.C. (1986). The San Diego suicide study: I. Young vs. old subjects, *Arch. Gen. Psychiatry, 43*:577.

11. Fowler, R.C., Rich, C.L., and Young, D. (1986). San Diego suicide study: II. Substance abuse in young cases, *Arch. Gen. Psychiatry, 43*:962.

12. Rich, C.L., Fowler, R.C., Fogarty, L.A., and Young D. (1988). San Diego suicide study: III. Relationships between diagnosis and stressors, *Arch. Gen. Psychiatry, 45*:589.

13. Rich, C.L., Fowler, R.C., and Young, D. (1989). Substance abuse and suicide: The San Diego study, *Ann. Clin. Psychiatry, 1*:79.

14. Robins, L.N., Helzer, J.E., and Weissman, M.M. (1984). Lifetime prevalence of specific psychiatric disorders in three sites, *Arch. Gen. Psychiatry, 41*:949.

15. Hagnell, O., and Rorsman, B. (1979). Suicide in the Lundby study: A comparative investigation of clinical aspects, *Neuropsychobiology, 5*:61.

16. Myers, J.D., Weissman, M.M., Tischler, G.L., Holzer, C.E., III, Leaf, P.J., Orvaschel, H., Anthony, J.C., Boyd, J.H., Burke, J.D. Jr., Kramer, M., and Stolzman, R. (1984). Six-month prevalence of psychiatric disorders in three communities: 1980–1982, *Arch. Gen. Psychiatry, 41*:959.

17. Black, D.W., Warrack, G., and Winokur, G. (1985). The Iowa Record Linkage Study: I. Suicides and accident deaths among psychiatric patients, *Arch. Gen. Psychiatry, 42*:71.

18. Murphy, S.L., Rounsaville, B.J., Eyre, S., and Kleber, H.D. (1983). Suicide attempts in treated opiate addicts, *Compr. Psychiatry, 24*:79.

19. Martin, R.L., Cloninger, C.R., and Guze, S. (1985). Mortality in a follow-up of 500 psychiatric outpatients: II. Cause-specific mortality, *Arch. Gen. Psychiatry, 42*:58.

20. Casper, J.L. (1825). Uber den Selbstmord und seine Zunahme in unserer, *Zeit*, Berlin.

21. Dahlgren, K.G. (1951). On death-rates and causes of death in alcohol addicts, *Acta Psychiatr. Scand., 26*:297.

22. Lemere, F. (1953). What happens to alcoholics? *Am. J. Psychiatry, 109*:674.

23. Mecir, J., Breyinova, V., and Vondracek, V. (1956). The causes of deaths in alcoholics, *J. Stud. Alcohol, 17*:633.

24. Schmidt, W., and deLint, J. (1972). Causes of death of alcoholics, *J. Stud. Alcohol, 33*:171.

25. Thorarinsson, A.A. (1979). Mortality among men alcoholics in Iceland: 1951–74, *J. Study Alcohol, 40*:704.

26. Murphy, G.E., Armstrong, J.W., Jr., Hermele, S.L., Fischer, J.R., and Clendenin, W.W. (1979). Suicide and alcoholism: Interpersonal loss confirmed as a predictor, *Arch. Gen. Psychiatry, 36*:65.

27. Beskow, J. (1979). Suicide and mental disorder in Swedish men, *Acta Psychiatr. Scand., 59*(suppl. 277):1.

28. Goodwin, D.W. (1982). Alcoholism and Suicide: Associated factors, *The Encyclopedic Handbook of Alcoholism* (E.M. Pattison and E. Kaufman, eds.), Gardner Press, New York, p. 655.

29. Gibson, S., and Becker, J. (1973). Changes in alcoholics' self-reported depression, *Q. J. Stud. Alcohol, 34*:829.

30. Schuckit, M.A. (1973). Alcoholism and sociopathy: Diagnostic confusion, *Q. Stud. Alcohol, 34*:157.

31. Fowler, R.C., Liskow, B.I., and Tanna, V.L. (1980). Alcoholism, depression and life events, *J. Affect. Disord., 2*:127.

32. Schuckit, M.A. (1983). Alcoholic patients with secondary depression, *Am. J. Psychiatry, 140*:711.

33. Schuckit, M.A. (1986). Primary men alcoholics with histories of suicide attempts, *J. Stud. Alcohol, 47*:78.

34. Paykel, E.S., Myers, J.K., and Lindenthal, J.J. (1974). Suicidal feelings in the general population: A prevalence study, *Br. J. Psychiatry, 124*:460.

35. Miles, C.P. (1977). Conditions predisposing to suicide: A review, *J. Nerv. Ment. Dis., 164*:231.

36. Galanter, M., and Castaneda, R. (1985). Self-destructive behavior in the substance abuser, *Psychr. Clin. North Am., 8*:251.

37. Vaillant, G.E. (1966). Twelve-year follow-up of New York narcotic addicts: Relation of treatment to outcome, *Am. J. Psychiatry, 122*:727.

38. Bewley, T.H., Ben-Arie, O., and James, J.P. (1968). Morbidity and mortality from heroin dependence, *Br. Med. J., 1*:725.

39. O'Brien, J.P. (1977). Increase in suicide attempts by drug ingestion. The Boston experience, 1964–1974, *Arch. Gen. Psychiatry, 34*:1165.

40. Weissman, M. (1974). The epidemiology of suicidal attempts, 1960–1971, *Arch. Gen. Psychiatry, 30*:737.

41. Roy, A. (1982). Risk factors for suicide in psychiatric patients, *Arch. Gen. Psychiatry, 39*:1089.

42. Rosen, D.H. (1976). The serious suicide attempt: Five-year follow-up study of 886 patients, *J.A.M.A., 235*:2105.

43. Murphy, G.E. (1969). Recognition of suicidal risk: The physician's responsibility, *South. Med. J., 62*:723.

44. Hasin, D., Grant, B., and Endicott, J. (1988). Treated and untreated suicide attempts in substance abuse patients, *J. Nerv. Ment. Dis., 176*:289.

45. Hesselbrock, M., Hesselbrock, V., Szymanski, K., and Weidenman, M. (1988). Suicide attempts and alcoholism, *J. Stud. Alcohol, 49*:436.

46. Ward, N.G., and Schuckit, M. (1980). Factors associated with suicidal behavior in polydrug abusers, *J. Clin. Psychiatry, 41*:379.

47. Marzuk, P.M., and Mann, J.J. (1988). Suicide and substance abuse, *Psychiatric Ann., 18*:639.

48. Murphy, G.E. (1988). Suicide and substance abuse, *Arch. Gen. Psychiatry, 45*:593.

49. Whitters, A.C., Cadoret, R.J., and Widmer, R.B. (1985). Factors associated with suicide attempts in alcohol abusers, *J. Affect. Disord., 9*:19.

50. Weissman, M.M., Pottenger, M., Kleber, H., Ruben, H.L., Williams, D., and Thompson, W.D. (1977). Symptom patterns in primary and secondary depression: A comparison of primary depressives with depressed opiate addicts, alcoholics and schizophrenics, *Arch. Gen. Psychiatry, 34*:854.

51. Berglund, M. (1984). Suicide in alcoholism: A prospective study of 88 suicides: I: The multidimensional diagnosis at first admission, *Arch. Gen. Psychiatry, 41*:888.

52. Tamerin, J.S., and Mendelson, J.H. (1969). The psychodynamics of chronic inebriation: Observations of alcoholics during the process of drinking in an experimental group setting, *Am. J. Psychiatry, 125*:886.

53. McNamee, H.B., Mello, N.K., and Mendelson, J.H. (1968). Experimental analysis of drinking patterns of alcoholics: Concurrent psychiatric observations, *Am. J. Psychiatry, 124*:1063.

54. Nathan, P.E., Titler, N.A., and Lowenstein, L.M. (1970). Behavioral analysis of chronic alcoholism, *Arch. Gen. Psychiatry, 22*:419.

55. Mayfield, D.G., and Montgomery, D. (1972). Alcoholism, alcohol intoxication, and suicide attempts, *Arch. Gen. Psychiatry, 27*:349.

56. Rounsaville, B.J., Weissman, M.M., and Kleber, H. (1982). Heterogeneity of psychiatric diagnosis in treated opiate addicts, *Arch. Gen. Psychiatry, 39*:161.

57.   Sternberg, D.E. (1989). Dual diagnosis: Addiction and affective disorders, *Psychiatric Hosp.*, 20:71.

58.   Runeson, B. (1988). *Major Depressive Episodes and Borderline Personality Disorder in Youth Suicide*. Presented at Second Euoprean Symposium on Suicidal Behavior, Edinburgh, June 1.

59.   Murphy, G.E., and Robins, E. (1967). Social factors in suicide, *J.A.M.A.*, 199:303.

60.   Berglund, M., Krantz, P., and Lundquist, G. (1987). Suicide in alcoholism, *Acta Psychiatr. Scand.*, 76:381.

61.   Holinger, P.C. (1979). Violent deaths among the young: Recent trends in suicide, homicide, and accidents, *Am. J. Psychiatry, 136*:1144.

62.   Taube, C.A., and Barret, S.A. (eds.) (1985). *Mental Health, United States: Suicide in the United States: 1958–1982*, U.S. Department of Health and Human Services publication No. (ADM) 85.

63.   *Monthly Vital Statistics Report* (1987). National Center for Health Statistics Report, 36(5). Washington D.C.

64.   Brent, D.A., Perper, J.A., Goldstein, C.E., and Kolko, D.J. (1988). Risk factors for adolescent suicide, *Arch. Gen. Psychiatry, 45*:581.

65.   Shafii, M., Carrigan, S., Whittinghill, J.R., and Derrick, A. (1985). Psychological autopsy of completed suicide in children and adolescents, *Am. J. Psychiatry, 142*:1061.

66.   Robins, L.N., Helzer, J.E., Weissman, M.M., Orvaschel, H., Gruenberg, E., Burke, J.D., Jr., and Regier, D.A. (1984). Lifetime prevalence of specific psychiatric disorders in three sites, *Arch. Gen. Psychiatry, 41*:949.

67.   Centers for Disease Control (1984). Alcohol and violent death—Erie County, New York 1973–1983, *M.M.W.R., 33*:226.

68.   Haberman, P.W., and Baden, M.M. (1978). *Alcohol, Other Drugs and Violent Death*, Oxford University Press, New York.

69.   Crompton, M.R. (1985). Alcohol and violent accidental and suicidal death, *Med. Sci. Law, 25*:59.

70.   Meyerson, A.T., Schwartz, J.R., and Glick, R.A. (1984). Evaluation and management of suicide, *Clin. Emerg. Med., 4*:111.

71.   Pfeffer, C.R. (1986). *The Suicidal Child*, Guilford Press, New York.

72.   Dackis, C.A., and Gold, M.S. (1985). New concepts in cocaine addiction: The dopamine depletion hypothesis, *Neurosci. Biobehav. Rev., 9*:469.

73.   Washton, A.M., and Gold, M.S. (1984). Chronic cocaine abuse: Evidence for adverse effects on health and functioning, *Psychiatr. Ann., 14*:733.

74.   Tucker, J.A., Vuchinich, R.E., and Sobell, M.B. (1982). Alcohol's effect on human emotions: A review of the stimulation/depression hypothesis. *Int. J. Addict., 17*:155.

75.   Mirin, S.M., Meyer, R.E., and McNamee, H.B. (1976). Psychopathology and mood during heroin use: Acute vs. chronic effects, *Am. J. Psychiatry, 33*:1053.

76.   Griffith, J.D., Cavanaugh, J., and Held, J. (1972). Dextroamphetamine: Evaluation of psychotomimetic properties in man, *Arch. Gen. Psychiatry, 26*:97.

77.   Sternberg, D.E. (1989). Dual Diagnosis, *Drugs of Abuse* (A.J. Giannini and A.E. Slaby, ed.), Medical Economics Press, Oradell, New Jersey, p. 321.

78.   Asberg, M., Traskman, L., and Thoren, P. (1976). 5-HIAA in the cerebrospinal fluid—A biochemical suicide predictor? *Arch. Gen. Psychiatry, 33*:1193.

79.   Banki, C., Arato, M., and Papp, Z. (1984). Biochemical markers in suicidal patients, *J. Affect. Disord., 6*:341.

80.   Ninan, P.T., and van Kammen, D.P. (1984). CSF 5-hydroxyindoleacetic acid levels in suicidal schizophrenic patients, *Am. J. Psychiatry, 141*:566.

81.   Traskman, L., Asberg, M., Bertilsson, L., and Sjostrand, L. (1981). Monoamine metabolites in CSF and suicidal behavior, *Arch. Gen. Psychiatry, 33*:631.

82.   van Praag, H.M. (1982). Depression, suicide, and metabolism on serotonin in the brain, *J. Affect. Disord., 4*:275.

83.   van Praag, H.M. (1983). CSF 5-HIAA and suicide in non-depressed schizophrenics, *Lancet, 2*:977.

84.   Brown, G.L., Goodwin, F.K., and Ballenger, J.C. (1979). Aggression in humans correlates with cerebrospinal fluid amine metabolites, *Psychiatry Res., 1*:131.

85.   Brown, G.L., Ebert, M.H., and Goyer, P.F. (1982). Aggression, suicide, and serotonin: Relationships to cerebrospinal fluid amine metabolites, *Am. J. Psychiatry, 139*:741.

86. Linnoila, M., Virkkunen, M., and Scheinin, M. (1983). Low cerebrospinal fluid 5-hydorxyin-doleacetic acid concentration differentiates impulsive from nonimpulsive violent behavior, *Life Sci., 33*:2609.

87. Bioulac, B., Benezech, M., and Renaud, B. (1980). Serotonergic dysfunction in 47, XYY syndrome, *Biol. Psychiatry, 15*:917.

88. Goodwin, D.W., Schulsinger, F., and Hermansen, L. (1975). Alcoholism and the hyperactive child syndrome, *J. Nerv. Ment. Dis., 260*:349.

89. Schuckit, M.A. (1973). Alcoholism and sociopathy: Diagnostic confusion, *Q. J. Stud. Alcohol, 34*:157.

90. Tarter, R.E. (1982). Psychosocial history, mimimal brain dysfunction and differential drinking patterns of male alcoholics, *J. Clin. Psycol., 38*:867.

91. Cadoret, R.J., O'Gorman, T.W., Troughton, E., and Heywood, E. (1985). Alcoholism and antisocial personality. Interrelationships, genetic and environmental factors, *Arch. Gen. Psychiatry, 42*:161.

92. Zuckerman, M. (1972). Drug usage as one manifestation of a "sensation seeking trait," *Drug Abuse: Current Concepts and Research* (W. Keup, ed.), Thomas, Springfield, Illinois, p. 154.

93. Adlaf, E.M., and Smart, R.G. (1983). Risk-taking and drug use behavior an examination, *Drug Alcohol Depend., 11*:287.

94. Dorus, W., and Senay, E.C. (1980). Depression, demographic dimensions, and drug abuse, *Am. J. Psychiatry, 137*:699.

95. Mirin, S.M., Weiss, R.D., and Sollogub, A. (1984). Affective illness in substance abusers, *Substance Abuse and Psychopathology* (S.M. Mirin, ed.), American Psychiatric Press, Washington, D.C.

96. Schuckit, M.A., Zisook, S., and Mortola, J. (1985). Clinical implications of DSM-III diagnoses for alcohol abuse and alcohol dependence, *Am. J. Psychiatry, 142*:1403.

97. Laskow, B., Mayfield, D., and Thiele, J. (1982). Alcohol and affective disorder: Assessment and treatment, *J. Clin. Psychiatry, 43*:144.

98. Pokorny, A.D. (1983). Prediction of suicide in psychiatric patients: Report of a prospective study, *Arch. Gen. Psychiatry, 40*:249.

99. Wolk-Wasserman, D. (1987). Contacts of suicidal alcohol and drug abuse patients and their significant others with public care institutions before the suicide attempt, *Acta Psychiatr. Scand., 76*:394.

37

The Psychotherapy of Dually Diagnosed Patients

Edward Kaufman
University of California, Irvine, California

I. INTRODUCTION

Dually diagnosed patients consist of substance abusers with substantial psychiatric disorders and psychiatric patients in whom substance abuse is a significant problem. The psychotherapy of dually diagnosed patients deals with both groups. Although there are similarities in the treatment of both types of patients, there are also considerable differences with more distinctions in the early phases of therapy than later. The commonality of dual diagnoses has been well documented and will not be reviewed in detail in this chapter. (For a thorough review of this subject see Meyer, 1986).

The psychotherapy of dually diagnosed patients can be divided into three phases (Bean-Bayog, 1986): (1) achieving sobriety, (2) maintaining abstinence and early recovery, and (3) advanced recovery. To outline these: The phase of achieving sobriety includes: assessing psychopathology and the extent and consequences of substance abuse, developing methods to establish and maintain a drug-free state, diagnosing and beginning treatment of other disorders, enlisting participation of significant others, and finally, developing a therapeutic contract. The phase of early recovery involves a supportive, directive psychotherapeutic approach that focuses on the disease of substance abuse and the goal of abstinence as well as on adequate treatment for concomittant psychiatric disorders. In this phase, defenses are redirected and psychodynamic psychotherapy is used mainly to reinforce methods of maintaining abstinence. Therapy during the advanced recovery phase uses a more traditional reconstructive psychotherapeutic approach that explores underlying issues (Kaufman and Reoux, 1988). Of course, when the psychiatric diagnosis is a major psychotic illness such as schizophrenia or bipolar disease, therapy is directed more towards prevention of recurrence of psychosis through understanding of psychosocial stressors, facilitating medication

Adapted with permission from The Psychotherapy of Dually Diagnosed Patients Edward Kaufman *J. of Substance Abuse Treatment*, Vol. 6, pp. 9–18, Copyright 1989, Pergamon Press.

compliance, and family education. With personality disorders and anxiety disorders, the goal is insight and personality change using an integration of psychodynamic psychotherapy and cognitive behavioral methods. Defenses and underlying issues are explored while a firm identity and control of substance abuse is maintained.

II. PHASE I: ACHIEVING SOBRIETY

A. Substance Abuse Assessment

The first step of Phase I is to assess the extent of substance abuse and its physical, vocational, social, and familial consequences. Medical examination which delineates the specific physical effects of the substance(s) involved and a detailed psychosocial evaluation are also obviously important.

The pattern of use of every type of abusable substance is assessed. Some important specifics are quantity, quality, duration, expense, how intake was supported and prevented, physical effects, tolerance, withdrawal, and any drug-related complications, particularly psychopathology. A clinical approach for assessment of substance abuse emphasizing comprehensive evaluation and management of the multiple physical, mental, and behavioral manifestations has been outlined by Pattison (1986) and will not be repeated in detail.

The consequences of substance abuse pervade all biopsychosocial spheres. Assessment should include the specific events and situations that are the consequences of the problem, which are identified and labeled as part of the disease. The disease is given a specific name such as the disease of alcoholism or, depending on therapeutic context, drug dependence or chemical dependence. This early approach focuses on the disease as the problem, not the person. This helps provide a reduction of the guilt, shame, and stigma associated with substance dependence.

A decidedly different approach may be necessary when assessing substance use in psychiatric patients in whom a substance abuse problem has not been previously recognized than in established substance abusers. The latter will most often be quite candid if the diagnosis of substance abuse is already well established, particularly if they are hospitalized and have little to gain by exaggeration of substance abuse or related consequences. Previously undiagnosed substance abuse in psychiatric patients may have to be elicited cautiously and without confrontation. Their substance use history should be evoked with nonpejorative, nonlabeling questions such as, "How do you use alcohol?" "When do you smoke marijuana?," or "Do your family or friends ever complain about your use of alcohol or drugs?" Intervention techniques can only be used with great care in severe mentally ill patients, if at all.

B. Assessment of Psychopathology and Psychodynamics

The second step is a careful evaluation of psychopathology with specific attention paid to the determination of whether signs and symptoms of mental illness are primary or secondary. We must keep in mind that essentially all substance abusing patients (SAs) have some psychopathology, particularly acute and chronic cognitive deficits and personality disorders.

Although the final determination of psychopathology should be postponed until a week or two after detoxification, this assessment should begin in the initial evaluation. Postponement is necessary because so many substance abusers present with apparent psychopathology that is secondary to substance abuse that dissipates as drugs and alcohol leave the body. These common symptoms of mental illness include depression, which is very common in the first week after detoxification, cognitive dysfunction, and personality disorders. Most cognitive dysfunction resolves in the first three weeks after detoxification, but lingering dysfunction persists and only resolves slowly after two to three years of sobriety (Grant and Reed, 1985).

Personality disorders are so common in opiate dependents that Craig (1988) found at least one personality disorder in everyone of the 121 male addicts he studied by the use of the Millon Inventory.

Depression, cognitive dysfunction, and personality disorders occur so frequently in substance abusers that several dilemmas are presented. Should a patient presenting with one or more of the ubiquitous diagnoses in this triad on admission, be considered as a dual diagnostic problem? What quantitative level of mental disturbance should be considered problematic? And finally, should the diagnosis always be postponed until several weeks after detoxification?

Evaluation of psychodynamics during this phase is interesting and presents a paradoxical problem. Psychodynamic constructs like dreams, fantasies (particularly during intoxification), primitive transference, and regressive behavior are often readily available to the newly withdrawing substance-dependent person, yet their level of cognition and/or psychosocial maturity do not permit them to utilize this type of material appropriately. Their tendency to form intense transferences with rapid swings from clinging attachment to hostile rejection must be foremost in the therapist's mind. However, these transferences must be interpreted at this phase in a manner that helps to dissipate rather than to foster them, since either the intense dependency or the hostility when needs are not met can drive the patient out of treatment. In general, an evaluation of the psychodynamics of drug use, intoxication, and independence is helpful at this stage, although the content of the psychodynamic formulation will be used minimally.

C. Family Assessment

The third step is family assessment. The therapist should insist that the entire family participate in the diagnostic assessment. The patient may or may not be more honest about use and abuse in the presence of the family, and family members can often provide more accurate information. The family's pattern of reactivity to drug use and psychopathology should be observed as well as discussed.

Each family member and the entire family system is evaluated for their participation in substance abuse and related behaviors as well as their own substance abuse and psychopathology. While always holding the substance abuse SA ultimately responsible for all substance use and related behaviors, we examine the role of the family's interactional patterns in substance use and abuse. We look at the family's need to maintain the SA's behavior in order to, for example, create excitement, triangulate conflicts, avoid intimacy, or keep an eternal, pseudoindividuated baby in the household forever. We evaluate active substance abuse in other family members as well as their enabling behaviors and the extent of their own suffering as a result of the SA's problems (codependency). Family assessment is directed toward a treatment plan that involves every family member in the effort to achieve new behaviors that help not only the substance abuser but themselves as well.

D. Detoxifications

The method employed for detoxification will depend on the severity and duration of dependence as well as on the existence of concomitant disorders, including polydrug abuse, medical conditions, and psychiatric disorders. Patients with severe problems in the above three areas will require hospital detoxification as will those physically dependent on depressant drugs. Patients on heroin without other problems may be detoxified in outpatient methadone detoxification programs or in a private office using clonidine. Most experts in substance abuse are unwilling to distribute any habituating drugs to SAs in a traditional outpatient setting. Exceptions to this rule of thumb are only in closely monitored community settings which monitor other routes of supply as well as the home environment. Prescribed sedative drugs are at risk for mixed intoxication, dependence, or overdose as well as dangerous withdrawal complications, particularly seizures. Nonhabituating substances to relieve anxiety such as Buspar, Vistaril, Benadryl, or L-tryptophane are occasionally helpful. However most SAs are not fond of these agents, complaining that they provide no relief.

Antidepressants have been used to block cocaine highs and relieve rebound depression, so they may be helpful in interrupting cocaine abuse (Gawin and Kleber, 1984). Effective parental limit setting may be sufficient for some adolescents to stop drug abuse. Awareness through education of the physical and psychosocial consequences of substance abuse may motivate some abusers to stop. Moderately severe or binge substance abusers may need brief hospitalization to initiate a drug-free state. If the abuse pattern is severe, that is, if intake is excessive, social or vocational functioning grossly impaired, or physical dependence present, hospitalization may be set as a requirement early in therapy. Other complications requiring inpatient treatment were described above. Inpatient treatment offers an intensive orientation to a comprehensive approach that may provide the impetus for abstinence, particularly if effective, comprehensive aftercare programs are initiated and followed.

Detoxification from substances of abuse is absolutely necessary to determine if psychiatric illness is primary or secondary to substance abuse. No matter how fully described a history of diagnosed mental illness, there cannot be certainly that illness is primary until an individual has been observed off drugs and alcohol for several weeks (e.g., cocaine and stimulant abusers may appear as manic-depressives; alcoholics, tranquilizer abusers, and opiate addicts as depressives; hallucinogen users as schizophrenics, etc.).

Once detoxification is accomplished, it is best to treat dually diagnosed patients in units where staff is either sufficiently qualified or trained to deal with the problems of both substance abuse and mental illness. If a specialized unit is available, it is best to emphasize the treatment of mental illness first (after detoxification). However, caution should be maintained when hospitalizing hard core substance abusers on a traditional psychiatric ward regardless of psychiatric diagnosis. This point is even more valid when they are antisocial personalities. Such individuals can disrupt psychiatric care in these units, particularly if staff is not trained to deal with this type of manipulative behavior. Once psychiatric illness is stabilized, then the patient can benefit from care on a specialized chemical dependency unit. When psychiatric illness is primary, such as alcoholism secondary to bipolar affective disorder, appropriate medication (e.g., lithium) may provide sufficient stabilization in some patients so that they can achieve sobriety on lithium without intensive participation in a chemical dependency program. However, most patients with secondary substance dependence require a stay on a chemical dependence unit as well as a psychiatric unit in order to reinforce a method for maintaining abstinence, unless the psychiatric unit has provided this.

E. Beginning Abstinence

Patients who have been dependent or have serious complications of substance abuse are informed by this author that he has only been successful in treating individuals at their level of chemical abuse when they have agreed to undertake a program to ensure abstinence. They are given their choice of programs (Antabuse, methadone maintenance, naltrexone, etc.) but told that in the author's personal experience and review of the literature that the 12-Step programs of Alcoholics Anonymous, Cocaine Anonymous, Narcotics Anonymous (AA, CA, NA, respectively), etc., have the best track records in providing a method of abstinence which works well in stabilizing them while psychotherapy takes place. A lifetime commitment to abstinence is not required. Rather the one-day-at-a-time approach is recommended; the patient establishes a method of maintaining abstinence in which he or she commits to it for only one day at a time, but which is renewed daily using the basic principles of 12-Step programs. With patients who continue to resist AA, a comprehensive alternative program is suggested such as combining individual, group, couple, and family therapy.

The concept of abstinence needs a very different interpretation with most chronic mental patients although some are chemically dependent, requiring the same handling of their substance abuse as primary drug abusers and alcoholics. The majority of chronic mental patients are not substance abusers. However, they often encounter many serious problems with drugs and alcohol. Bipolar patients may augment or attenuate cycles with stimulants or sedatives. Schizophrenics may quiet down auditory hallucinations with alcohol or may use hallucinogens and marijuana as part of peer culture. For some of these psychiatric patients, a single use of lysergic acid diethylamide (LSD) or even marijuana can precipitate a psychotic episode. Such individuals, even though they may never have been chemically dependent, require a commitment to total abstinence as desperately as any heroin addict or physically debilitated alcoholic. On the other hand it may be difficult to require a commitment to abstinence early in their treatment, and the demand for total abstinence may have to evolve more gradually.

The establishment of a method for maintaining abstinence is made a condition of the psychotherapeutic contract. The therapist engages in psychotherapy only if the patient has chosen to participate in a program for staying drug-free. Patients attending AA (or related meetings) may have to try different groups and shop around for the most appropriate type of meeting. Initially, patients may find that larger, passive meetings with speakers are more comfortable and provide successful role models for identification. Once a patient engages with a program, smaller 12-Step study groups and male or female stag groups, requiring a more active role by participants, are often extremely beneficial. Patients are also encouraged to obtain a sponsor.

With dually diagnosed patients who require psychotropic medication, it is essential that the patient find a sponsor who is supportive of such treatment or personally trusting of the psychiatrist who prescribes the medication. Alcoholics Anonymous groups supportive of necessary psychotropic drugs can also be found but with difficulties because so many non-psychotic members have abused a wide variety of prescribed and illicitly obtained psychotropic drugs. Regular or random urines or breathalyzer checks for substances of abuse may be extremely helpful to some individuals in maintaining early abstinence.

It is of interest that over the past 10 years most psychotherapists working with chemically dependent patients have become more and more insistent on maintenance of abstinence as a *prerequisite* for psychotherapy. Although each cities different psychodynamic reasons for this insistence, Bean-Bayog (1986), Brown (1985), Khantzian and Schneider (1986), Vaillant (1987), Wallace (1985), and Zimberg (1985) all agree on this requirement. Their reasons will be discussed under Phase II of the treatment process.

F. Treatment Contract

In the final phase of the assessment, a treatment contract is developed with the substance abuser and family which covers the following components:

1. Agreement on method of detoxification and completion of same.
2. Commitment to abstinence.
3. Commitment to a comprehensive method for continuing abstinence after or instead of hospitalization including:
   (a) Number of weekly 12-step meetings (2–7)
   (b) Number of weekly educational meetings (1–2)
   (c) Number of weekly group therapy sessions (1–2)

    (d) Extent of modification of diet, exercise, relaxation techniques
    (e) Weekly family and couple therapy
    (f) Urines for analysis of drugs of abuse and/or breathalyzer
 4. Commitment by each family member to a comprehensive family program, including speci-
     fying number of self-help support groups such as Al-Anon, Cocanon, etc., significant-
     other groups, couple and family therapy, adolescent and latency peer groups, and ACA
     groups (1–7 weekly).
 5. When there is major psychiatric illness requiring medication such as lithium, major tran-
     quilizers or antidepressants, the patient agrees to take the medication as prescribed.
 6. The therapist may choose to list his/her own desired therapeutic behaviors as part of
     the contract, e.g., listen carefully, not act as a critical judge, avoid enabling behaviors, etc.

If the patient or his family do not follow the contract and the patient continues to abuse
substances, I prefer to terminate treatment until the patient either enters hospital or shows
evidence of reimplementing the required behaviors as specified in the contract. Many patients and families who do not commit to workable contracts and who are asked to leave
therapy return in the future agreeing to participate in a workable program.

III. PHASE II: EARLY RECOVERY

Initial treatment focuses on methods for maintaining a drug- and alcohol-free state. The first
6 months to 2 years of psychotherapy should be supportive and should utilize more directive
therapies such as cognitive-behavioral. However, the psychodynamic assessment performed
in Phase I should always be kept in mind and further developed as the patient demonstrates
unconsciously motivated behavior in the transference, dreams, fantasies, and maladaptive
daily activities. These are used in this phase to help the patient understand self-destructive
behaviors and the meaning of stressors that trigger them so that they can avoid these stressors
or deal with them without regression. Maintaining sobriety is still the goal of therapy in early
recovery. Interventions are directed at the cognitive and behavioral aspects of substance abuse.
The focus should be on how the patient abuses a substance, not on why, when reviewing
the history or immediate stressors. Examining how (behavioral causes and effects) allows
the suggestion of alternative behaviors that can avoid triggering relapse. Encouraging and
presenting opportunities to practice drug-free behavior provides coping strategies for the sober
patient. Focusing on why should only be done when it facilitates rapid abandonment of destructive behaviors. Why questions should be avoided when they provoke excuses and the need
to defend oneself as a good person. Replacing maladaptive and dysfunctional activities with
behavior that maintains sobriety is a treatment goal of early recovery. Healthy substitute objects and behaviors of all kinds are helpful and should not be confronted (smoking is usually
addressed much later). The therapist may encourage active alternatives like regular exercise
or education. Object substitution may also prevent or at least lessen the grieving that substance
abusers sometimes experience while mourning the loss of the drug with its associated activities and people.

    Psychotherapy during early recovery does not confront defenses too rapidly or remove
them prematurely. These defenses are instead redirected and supported to help maintain
abstinence and continued treatment. Wallace (1985) states that if long-term sobriety is to be
maintained, defenses must ultimately be removed, but only gradually over periods of time
often ranging from 2 to 5 years of abstinence. Therapy is a time-dependent process. Therapeutic
interventions appropriate later may be inappropriate during early sobriety.

    Denial is a prominent defense used by substance abusers and can serve a self-destructive
purpose when used to continue addictive behavior. However, most denial should not be

confronted early in therapy. As described by Wallace (1985), deliberate denial tactically used as a temporary coping device of certain life difficulties or problems can be extremely valuable. Denial can be employed for adjusting to or coping with former triggers of substance use. This method of handling stress and anxiety is very familiar to the substance abuser. Wallace (1985) notes that in the alcoholic, increments of self-awareness and disclosure are often associated with increased anxiety. Premature reduction of denial hinders defenses against this anxiety which may trigger a return to drinking (Wallace, 1985). Denial should be worked on gradually, titrating any anxieties that arise from confronting it and that threaten a return to substance abuse.

Substance abusers also frequently employ projection and rationalization as mechanisms to defend against anxiety. Uncomfortable and undesirable self-qualities are attributed to others. Blaming others arouses resentment in them, which can trigger anger and recurrent or continued substance abuse by many SAs who find themselves in self-destructive alternatives (e.g., self-blame vs blaming others) (Wallace, 1985). A tendency to get others to take responsibility is characteristic of many substance abusers. Projection and rationalization are shifted to help attain and maintain abstinence. Previous dysfunctional behavior is attributed (by projection and rationalization) to the disease rather than to others or the self. Wallace (1985) describes assimilative projection (assuming that others are like oneself and perceiving them as such) as the most outstanding characteristic of both drinking and sober alcoholics. Therapeutically, this preferred defense allows identification with alcoholics and alcoholism, enabling the patient to explain past behavior and to learn the new behavior of sobriety through identification with sober alcoholics. Once sober, the patient has a lifetime to gradually recognize that not all difficulties can be explained by alcoholism (Wallace, 1985). In the same discussion of the alcoholics' preferred defense structure, Wallace (1985) cautions against a shift from rationalizing drinking behavior to using sobriety to rationalize other behavior. Needing to stay sober can be justification for avoiding stressful situations and emotional cues that previously triggered drinking. It can also be overused in that it becomes a rationalization for avoidance of most growth behaviors.

The therapist should recognize and therapeutically redirect defenses to help accomplish the primary goal of early recovery: staying sober. Prematurely reducing or removing preferred and effective means of coping with anxiety can result in relapse of substance abuse or in the patient's terminating therapy. Confronting and interpreting defenses, as well as owning of more responsibility by the patient, comes later in successful psychotherapy of substance abusers.

During the early supportive phase of psychotherapy with substance abusers, psychodynamic therapy definitely has a place. At least partial resolution of certain intrapyschic conflicts is helpful in reinforcing the principles of Alcoholics Anonymous or other 12-Step groups. For example, unresolved omnipotence, narcissistic entitlement, and power/dependency conflicts may prevent a patient from obtaining a sponsor or using AA fully, or may result in the patient's continuing patterns of grossly unsatisfying relationships. Psychodynamic therapy of such conflicts may help the patient to accept the principles of AA and to build more mutually satisfying relationships. However, intimate relationships are fraught with danger at this phase and should be discouraged.

Any tendency toward a dependent, regressive and/or angry, sadistic transference should be avoided by rapid interpretations aimed at curbing this behavior. Intense, hostile, or dependent reactions outside of the therapy can also be interpreted. Again, the goal is not insight or intimacy but avoidance of relationships with destructive persons or of destruction in relationships as a result of experiencing overwhelming closeness.

Brown (1985) integrates psychotherapy with Alcoholics Anonymous. She likens the period of early sobriety to infancy and states that it is characterized by extreme dependency and a corresponding need and reliance on external structure and support. She reminds us that alcohol (or drugs) becomes the primary object to the SA, providing constant support without disappoint, yet gratification is under the SA's control. This object cannot be relinquished without primitively gratifying object replacements, like AA, cigarettes, coffee, food, soft drinks, and temporary relationships. A selection of these should be permitted to each SA, as they will evolve out of this dependent phase over time (Khantzian and Schneider, 1986) and give up these objects only very gradually.

Khantzian and Schneider (1986) are found that addicts are especially conflicted in regard to interpersonal dependency. He observes that addicts alternate between distant, supercilious postures of self-sufficiency and self-destructive dependency. Transference manifestations of intolerable anxiety about dependency feelings could easily be misinterpreted as resistance to the therapy. Defenses against this anxiety should not be confronted as resistance, but supported as allowing the patient to continue in treatment. The conflicts about dependency which threaten to end treatment prematurely should be addressed directly (Brown, 1985).

Other substitutes for the lost object should include active replacement with a new repertoire of habit patterns and behaviors. In this phase, identification with AA, NA, etc., helps them develop away from using action as a means of establishing control. As they deal with and grasp their dependency, these patients need to feel some sense of control over their environment. They can be given control over therapeutic hours (time of meetings, content of sessions) as well as their input into how many and what kind of and where and when they attend AA meetings (Brown, 1985). Alcoholics Anonymous lore states that 90 meetings in 90 days are essential at first. After this period, the quality of the program is more important than the number of meetings.

In this phase, SAs are coached and supported in moving out of friendships, patterns, and environments that were triggers for substance abuse. Alcoholics Anonymous tells the newly sober member to stay away from slippery places if they are to avoid slipping. A new environment that does not contain all these cues to substance use provides a sense of safety, if the anxiety about the newness of it can be overcome (Brown, 1985).

This phase also requires a dual shift for the average therapist, (e.g., from confronter of denial to motivate the SA into treatment, the therapist shifts to supporter; from nondirective listener, the therapist shifts to active teacher of new strategies and coping behaviors [Brown, 1985]).

Khantzian and Schneider (1986) emphasize early developmental impairment in the ego structure of substance abusers. These impairments predispose an individual to need to use drugs or alcohol as protection for defective ego defense mechanisms. Substances are used to mute or to contain threatening and potentially overwhelming affects. Thus in early recovery the therapist should provide a secure environment that places a premium on safety and adequate control of affects such as depression, rage, anger, and anxiety. Khantzian and Schneider (1986) state that the need to find external sources of narcissistic sustenance can be gradually transferred into intrapsychic resources. The therapist can initially meet some of this need while taking care to avoid indiscriminate overgratification. Extremes of being too withholding or too giving are avoided. Narcissistic needs are partially gratified in order to improve the patient's sense of self-esteem and self-stability. The therapist provides care and security until patients can obtain these on their own. Identification with the therapist facilitates the patient's sense of self. The therapist should be willing to share helpful self-disclosure and to be much more involved than any "neutral screen." The patient is provided with direct assistance and information. When the patient is involved with a therapeutic team, manipulative and splitting activities must be kept to a minimum so that the patient learns newer and more adaptive ways to get needs met. The treatment team must be consistent and cohesive while providing a safe environment that is neither too giving nor too withholding (Khantzian and Schneider, 1986).

Bean-Bayog (1986) suggests that alcoholism itself is a traumatic experience that produces psychopathology in the same way that war experiences cause a posttraumatic stress disorder. Bean-Bayog's model implies a treatment approach that first stops the trauma from continuing and then prevents recurrence by teaching the SA how to be sober. In early recovery, the damage from the trauma is repaired and healed. She emphasizes several issues that should be dealt with during this phase, including coping with the effects of stopping drinking (e.g., acute and protracted withdrawal), slowly healing dementia, family uproar and outrage, grief over loss of alcohol, conscious realization of ungrieved losses, and the onslaught of shame (Wallace, 1985).

Zimberg (1985) considers the core issue to be conflict between dependence needs (from repressed feelings of inadequacy) that cannot be met and the compensatory needs for control, power, and achievement (reactive grandiosity). Zimberg also states that the central problem in psychotherapy with alcoholics is breaking through the reactive grandiosity that defends against profound feelings of inferiority and dependency. He points out that alcohol served not only to tranquilize anxiety but to artificially induce feelings consistent with a grandiose self-image. Zimberg observes that when the effects of the alcohol wear off, feelings of worthlessness intensify and the cycle spirals progressively downward, reinforced by continued alcohol use. Unresolved grandiosity may also interfere with accepting the principle of a "higher power" in 12-Step programs. Dependence on others and admitting powerlessness over a substance are not compatible with an SAs reactive grandiosity and feelings of omnipotence. These conflicts can be approached with psychodynamic therapy in this phase.

Paradoxically, the need for grandiosity can be met by a group such as Alcoholics Anonymous. This need is sublimated through the program and the goal of helping other substance abusers. The group can become the "higher power;" the patient identifies with this power, substituting it for his grandiosity or for his omnipotent projections onto the therapist. The group also provides a forum for demonstrating verbally and behaviorally the power and control possessed through the group's principles. Unresolved dependency needs can also be met through meetings and sponsors. By becoming a sponsor or speaker oneself, the advanced AA member enhances self-esteem and reduces anxiety through helping others, using the more mature defense of altruism.

Kernberg (1975) has not written specifically about the psychotherapy of substance abusers, but has developed a method of psychotherapy for borderline patients which has much in common with the methods we are proposing at this stage of therapy, e.g., limit setting to block acting out, interpretation of negative transference and related defenses, staying in the here and now only, and not interpretating primitive positive transference in order to enhance the development of the therapeutic alliance.

It is interesting that each of the therapists who have written about long-term, intensive psychotherapy of substance abusers have emphasized the need for sobriety and a method for sustaining this state, regardless of how diverse their therapeutic and theoretical orientation. Patients with psychiatric diagnoses of major psychotic disorders, including severe depressions, will need even more of a supportive and holding environment. This can be difficult because of their propensity for a strong dependent transference. The need for these patients to continue to take their psychotropic medications on a regular basis is as essential as the need for a substance abuse–free environment. Patients with the dual diagnoses of borderline personality and substance dependence will require even more structure. Antisocial personalities do not do well in long-term psychotherapy unless there is concurrent depression. They are best referred to a long-term therapeutic community (TC) for the entire middle phase of therapy, 12 to 18 months. Following graduation from a TC, formerly diagnosed antisocial personalities can benefit from exploratory psychotherapy. Dually diagnosed patients with severe psychopathology do not do well in TCs unless there is substantial professional input into treatment.

Although the tricyclic antidepressants have little or no abuse potential with most patient groups, they are surprisingly often abused by SAs, particularly methadone-maintained patients and alcoholics. This is mainly true of sedating antidepressants like Elavil and Doxepin, which cause a sedated oblivion in high doses, particularly in combination with alcohol, narcotics, or benzodiazepines. Caution should also be exercised in viewing alprazolam as helpful for panic disorders in primary subsance abusers, as it tends to reinforce polydrug abuse in these patients. In anyone with a history of prior drug or alcohol abuse or dependence, Xanax is, in my experience, contraindicated. Nonsedating antidepressants should be used first, and if not successful, followed by MAOIs for panic disorders in substance abusers. There are research findings that demonstrate the need for and efficacy with psychotherapy for dually diagnosed patients. This work was done by McLellan (1986). utilizing psychiatric severity as a predictor of treatment outcome for heroin addicts. He found that a global estimate of psychopathology (psychiatric severity) was the single best predictor of outcome (e.g., low-severity patients improve in any treatment program, and high-severity patients do not improve in any program with the notable exception of methadone maintenance with the addition of professional psychotherapy).

IV. PHASE III: ADVANCED RECOVERY

Advanced recovery involves more traditional in-depth psychotherapy that gradually shifts from supportive to reconstructive. This is done with patients with personality and anxiety disorders, but rarely with those with psychoses. The therapist may even demarcate an actual transition by explaining to the patient the needed changes in both the patient's and therapist's behavior. Explaining that the therapist will be less directive will help the patient understand noticeable changes in the therapy. The therapist will at this point interpret transference more, structure the therapy around psychodynamic themes, and examine dreams in more detail and depth.

Once the core identity as an alcoholic is firmly in place, a shift occurs from external behavioral control to internalization of control through identification, expansion of focus, and the use of uncovering psychotherapy (Brown, 1985). Brown acknowledges this as a difficult time for patients, since they must simultaneously maintain an alcoholic identity, applying cognitive-behavioral controls over abuse, while exploring underlying issues contributing to the alcoholism or hindering a satisfying sobriety. Wallace (1985) states that after teaching the alcoholic to use preferred defenses to achieve and maintain sobriety in the early stage of treatment, directly addressing these defenses to achieve real changes in personality is a task of later therapy after years of abstinence. He further states that to establish secure and comfortable sobriety, the learned defensive coping strategies are gradually exchanged for nondefensive authentic relationships; both the therapist and the patient must risk a heightened but manageable anxiety for insight into self and others to increase.

Intense anxiety or anger often erupts as defenses are lowered and uncovering psychotherapy continues. For the patient to tolerate the anxiety necessary for insight, his or her identity as an alcoholic or substance abuser must first be solid. Controls on substance abuse might be intact and ready for reimplementation as needed. During all phases of therapy the patient and therapist must be constantly aware of the centrality of drugs and alcohol. Specific triggers can be identified and explored in therapy and the focus can be shifted to underlying issues. Desires to use substances may be warning signals to stop uncovering or, when interpreted as such, may permit the reconstructive psychotherapy to continue.

A critical area in implementing full recovery is the capacity to tolerate meaningful intimacy. Because these patients have not developed adolescent and young adult maturational relationship patterns, they must begin from the beginning in forming adult relationships.

Thus, they may not be capable of even beginning to deal with meaningful intimacy until several years into this phase of advanced recovery. The incorporation of the therapist as capable of intimacy facilitates this process, but the development of intimacy also depends on a good deal of practice. During this time the therapist should be supportive of continued relationship trials while exploring the underlying fears and should maintain a continued role as teacher of the gradual steps and frustrations of achieving intimacy.

The final step in advanced recovery is working through termination. This work is not done with finality in substance abusers, since the door should always be left open for their return. In addition, they are encouraged to continue in a 12-Step group at varying levels of intensity as needed for the rest of their lives.

V. THERAPIST COUNTER TRANSFERENCE

Countertransference is a complex, multidetermined issue in dealing either with patients who abuse substances or with those who are mentally ill. When one individual carries both diagnoses, countertransference feelings become even more complicated. The initial definitions of countertransference in psychoanalytic psychotherapy focused on the therapist's unconsciously determined reactions to the patient's transference, particularly those caused by reacting to the patient as if he or she were an important figure from the therapists's own past. The concept of countertransference has been broadened to include the therapist's uncontrolled reactions to who the patient is as a person (MacKinnon and Michels, 1971) (angry, depressed, paranoid, competitive), the type of material the patient is dealing with (incest, violence, greed, victimization), or the concept of the superiority of the therapist over the patient. Countertransference is in evidence whenever the therapist cannot recognize or will not acknowledge his or her own role in producing or provoking behavior in the patient. In the field of substance abuse treatment, countertransference is often relabeled as therapist codependency or enabling and is one of the most frequent causes of "burnout."

One problem with the use of the term codependency is that it covers only a minority of countertransference reactions, and a focus on the former concept can blind therapists to looking for other types of unconsciously determined personal reactions. On the other hand, the concept of codependency can greatly enhance our understanding of many different forms of countertransference. The concept of codependency gives the therapist a frame of reference for changing his or her antitherapeutic countertransference reactions, for example, the overprotective, overcontrolling, or overinvolved therapist can relate these behaviors to codependency and change them through self-knowledge as well as through Al-Anon or, where appropriate, Adult Children of Alcoholics groups. (The Chemical Dependency Treatment staff at Cambridge Hospital in Massachusetts are all required to attend Al-Anon meetings regularly because it is felt that codependency issues are so common in hospital staff working regularly with substance abusers [SAs] [Vaillant, 1981].

Still another way to view the therapist's out-of-control responses to patients is from a systems point of view in which the therapist replays unresolved issues from his or her own family of origin with the patient and the patient's family. When these patients are dealing with more than one therapeutic person at the same time, as in hospital settings, they will frequently play one therapist off against the other in much the same way as they manipulated their parents. The therapist's ability to avoid being drawn into recreating this system depends on knowledge of their own families and development as well as having a mechanism for not being drawn into such "splitting" and manipulative behaviors.

Substance abusers tend to evoke strong emotions in therapists, either of overinvolvement/rescuing or of distancing/rejection. Some therapists may alternate between the two depending, respectively, on the patient's compliance or defiance. These therapist behaviors are intensified in dually diagnosed patients, particularly in patients with borderline, histrionic, or passive-aggressive personalities, or with manic depressive disease, all of whom invariably also provoke a great deal of therapist overinvolvement and/or rejection. On the other hand, patients with antisocial personalities may be very successful at seducing a therapist for personal gain; depressive patients may foster the therapist's sense of powerful healing omnipotence; and obsessive compulsives may evoke the therapist's competitiveness, boredom, or rejection.

A contemporary concept of countertransference includes the therapist's tuning into his or her own unconscious feelings and fantasies about patients in order to learn aspects of the patient's behavior that are not consciously obvious. The more the therapist is aware of his or her own underlying feelings, the less they will be acted out in a manner that is harmful to the patient. Thus, a therapist can learn by tuning into his or her own positive or negative feelings that the patient is provoking loving or angry feelings (Levin, 1987). Rather than expressing these feelings directly, the therapist should understand to what extent the patient is provoking these feelings versus tapping the therapist's own issues. Self-knowledge then permits the therapist to emotionally understand what the patient is experiencing. As therapists understand their own feeling states, they will identify patients' conflicts and feelings before they become overt. Thus, the therapist uses countertransference in this context as an extremely helpful tool.

Strong countertransference feelings are often provoked in the early phases of therapy as the dually diagnosed SA provokes, tests, fuses with, and rejects the therapist. In beginning therapy, the therapist does not share the majority of countertransference feelings with dually diagnosed patients, but must tune in to them in order to understand the patient's true commitment to treatment and vulnerability to certain stressors which can trigger relapse and/or return to substance abuse. In later stages of therapy, the therapist can share certain countertransference responses as a way of facilitating, uncovering, and enhancing the patient's self knowledge.

VI. CONCLUSIONS

Guidelines for the successful psychotherapy of dually diagnosed substance abusers are presented which are synthesized from several approaches and have been used by the author for several years. Although this individualized method of comprehensive psychotherapy is successful in the hands of the therapists cited, the style and personality of each individual therapist is also an important variable in predicting treatment outcome (Woody et al., 1986). Likewise, patients with more severe psychopathology do better with therapists who are professionally trained (Woody et al., 1986). Each individual therapist should utilize these guidelines as a basis upon which to graft their own individual therapeutic style and personality. Each patient must be understood as a unique individual who will require flexibility and special modifications of the basic approach.

REFERENCES

Bean-Bayog, M. (1986). Psychopathology produced by alcoholism, R.E. Meyer (ed.), *Psychopathology and Addictive Disorders*. Guilford, New York.

Brown, S. (1985). *Treating the Alcoholic, a Developmental Model of Recovery*. Wiley, New York.

Craig, R.J. (1988). A psychometric study of the prevalence of DSM-III personality disorders among treated opiate addicts. *Int. J. Addict., 23*:115–124.

Gawin, F.H., and Kleber, H.D. (1984). Cocaine abuse treatment: An open pilot trial with lithium and desipramine. *Arch. Am. Psychiatry, 41*:903–910.

Grant, I., and Reed, R. (1985). Neuropsychology of alcohol and drug abuse, A. Alterman (ed.), *Substance Abuse and Psychopathology*. Plenum, New York.

Kaufman, E., and Reoux, J. (1988). Guidelines for the successful psychotherapy of substance abusers. *Am. J. Drug Alcohol Abuse, 14*:199–209.

Kernberg, O.F. (1975). *Borderline Conditions and Pathological Narcissism*. Jason Aronson, New York.

Khantzian, E.J., and Schneider, R.J. (1986). Treatment implications of psychodynamic understanding of opioid addicts, R.E. Meyer (ed.), *Psychopathology and Addictive Disorders*. Guilford, New York.

Levin, J.D. (1987). *Treatment of Alcoholism and Other Addictions*. Jason Aronson, Northvale, New Jersey.

MacKinnon, R.A., and Michels, R. (1971). *The Psychiatric Interview in Clinical Practice*. Saunders, Philadelphia.

McLellan, A.T. (1986). Psychiatric severity as a predictor of outcome from substance abuse treatments, R.E. Meyer (ed.), *Psychopathology and Addictive Disorders*. Guilford, New York.

Meyer, R.E. (ed.). (1986). *Psychopathology and Addictive Disorders*. Guilford Press, New York.

Pattison, E.M. (1986). Clinical approaches to the alcoholic patient. *Psychosomatics, 27*:762–770.

Vaillant, G.E. (1987). *Alcoholism and Drug Dependence: Harvard Guide to Modern Psychiatry*. Belknap, Cambridge, Massachusetts.

Vaillant, G.E. (1981). Dangers of psychotherapy in the treatment of alcoholism, M.H. Bean and N.E. Zinberg (eds.), *Dynamic Approaches to the Understanding and Treatment of Alcoholism*. Free Press, New York.

Wallace, J. (1985). Critical issues in alcoholism therapy, S. Zimberg, J. Wallace, and S. Blume (eds.), *Practical Approaches to Alcoholism Psychotherapy*, 2nd ed. Plenum, New York.

Wallace, J. (1985). Working with the preferred defense structure of the recovering alcoholic, S. Zimberg, J. Wallace and S. Blume (eds.) *Practical Approaches to Alcoholism Psychotherapy* 2nd ed. Plenum, New York.

Woody, G.E., Luborsky, L., McLellan, A.T., and O'Brien, C.P. (1986). Psychotherapy as an adjunct to methadone treatment, R.E. Meyer (ed.), *Psychopathology and Addictive Disorders*. Guilford, New York.

Zimberg, S. (1985). Principles of alcoholism psychotherapy, S. Zimberg, J. Wallace, and S. Brown (eds.), *Practical Approaches to Alcoholism Psychotherapy*, 2nd ed. Plenum, New York.

IX
Genetics

38

Biological Vulnerability to Alcoholism

Marc A. Schuckit
Veterans Affairs Medical Center, and University of California, San Diego, California

I. INTRODUCTION

The adequate definition of alcoholism is an important concern for all studies of etiology in alcoholism. Briefly, the ideal rubric would offer unambiguous and objective criteria that are easy to apply in research and treatment settings (Goodwin and Guze, 1984). Although no perfect definition of alcoholism exists, most diagnoses require individuals to have been drinking heavily over an extended period of time and to have subsequently suffered multiple major life problems. This usually entails daily drinking with an inability to stop for long periods, along with repeated efforts to control intake, and consumption often meets or exceeds a fifth of spirits or its equivalent in wine or beer per day. This pattern, often present for years before diagnosis, is accompanied by evidence of impaired social or occupational functioning and is often associated with evidence of tolerance or physical symptoms of withdrawal from alcohol (American Psychiatric Association, 1980).

Because research concerning the biological factors involved in the predisposition toward alcoholism is in the early stages, most investigators have chosen to focus on relatives of severely alcoholic individuals with the hope that genetic factors may be most obvious and easy to identify. Thus, alcoholism in relatives often requires not only that they fulfill the definition but also that the alcoholic family member have suffered severe alcohol-related consequences, such as job loss or divorce, or have received treatment for alcoholic detoxification or rehabilitation. Future work will have to determine the generalizability of results to relatives of less severely alcoholic individuals. Thus, the present focus of studies is on a biological vulnerability toward relatively severe alcoholism. Most investigations do not analyze biological influences in the decision to begin drinking during teenage years or in the occurrence of temporary

Adapted from Biological Vulnerability to Alcoholism, Marc A. Schuckit, *J. of Consulting and Clinical Psychology*, 1987, Vol. 55, No. 3, pp. 301–309.

and relatively mild problems that might be observed as part of growing up in a heavy-drinking society (a problem in perhaps 40% or more of young men) (Cahalan and Cisin, 1968; Fillmore and Midanik, 1984).

Another issue of importance in the definition of alcoholism is the distinction between primary and secondary illness. In primary alcoholism, the severe life problems associated with heavy and persistent drinking develop in individuals with no major preexisting psychiatric illness (Schuckit, 1983a, 1984a). Thus, alcoholics who develop their alcohol-related life problems after the emergence of manic depressive disease or antisocial personality disorder (i.e., secondary alcoholics) are usually excluded from these investigations for fear that genetic factors influencing the primary disorder (e.g., manic depressive disease) might obscure the genetic factors that predispose the subject toward alcoholism. There is evidence from longitudinal follow-up studies that primary alcoholics demonstrate significantly different clinical histories and 1-year outcomes than secondary alcoholics (Schuckit, 1985c).

II. IMPORTANCE OF GENETICS

Regardless of the definition of alcoholism that is used, there is evidence that alcoholism is a genetically influenced disorder. This conclusion is supported by work from family, twin, and adoption studies in humans as well as in animals. Family studies have revealed a threefold to fourfold increased risk for this disorder in sons and daughters of alcoholics, without clear evidence of a heightened vulnerability toward other primary psychiatric diseases (Cotton, 1979; Schuckit, 1986). However, demonstrating the familial nature of alcoholism does not clearly support the contribution of genetics because most children are raised by their biological parents.

Research with twins evaluates the relative contributions of genetics and environment by comparing the risk for alcoholism in identical and fraternal twins of alcoholics (Schuckit, 1981). Because both types of twins share major childhood environmental events, an alcoholism risk closely related to environment would show identical twins and fraternal twins of alcoholics to be at equally high risk. However, because identical twins share 100% of their genes and fraternal twins share only 50%, alcoholism that is genetically influenced should be significantly higher in the identical twin of an alcoholic than in the fraternal twin.

Several twins investigations have examined the similarity of drinking quantity and frequency in twins in the general population. Two of these studies have concluded that genetic factors appear to contribute to drinking patterns but, perhaps reflecting the emphasis on a "normal" population, do not contribute to adverse consequences (Jonsson and Nilsson, 1968; Partanen, Bruun, and Markkanen, 1966). Other investigators have demonstrated that genetic factors might be important in the rate of absorption or elimination of alcohol, with a high level of heritability shown for the alcohol elimination rate (0.8–0.98) and for the appearance and destruction of its first breakdown product, acetaldehyde (0.6–0.8) (Radlow and Conway, 1978; Vesell, Page, and Passancanti, 1971). However, pointing out how the rate of alcohol metabolism can be affected by the use of other drugs, by dietary and drinking habits, and by smoking history, another study reported a heritability level of 0.57 for the absorption and 0.46 for the elimination of alcohol (Kopun and Propping, 1977).

There is a series of anecdotal reports of the adult drinking habits of monozygotic (MZ) twins separated sometime early in life. Because of their retrospective and anecdotal nature, these studies offer few definite conclusions, and most of the data relate to drinking practices rather than to alcoholism. A review of the literature shows as many as 100 studied cases of separated twins in which the authors have noted a level of similarity in the separated twins' choice to drink, experience of life problems related to alcohol intake, and usual drinking patterns (Jonsson and Nilsson, 1968; Newman, Freeman, and Holzinger, 1937; Shields, 1962).

Several twins studies have directly addressed the concordance rate for alcoholism in MZ versus dizygotic (DZ) twins. Kaij studied 174 male twin pairs containing at least one twin who was registered with an alcohol problem at a temperance board. As many as 90% of the twins were interviewed, and zygosity was established by anthropological markers and blood typing (Kaij, 1960). Under relatively crisp criteria for alcoholism, the concordance rate was 58% in MZ twins and 28% in DZ twins. In addition, a Veterans Administration twin register study also reported a higher MZ than DZ concordance rate (26 vs. 12%; Hrubec and Omenn, 1981), but a recent British investigation of 61 twin pairs revealed no MZ/DZ differences in concordance as measured by the Schedule of Affective Disorders and Schizophrenia (SADS-L) (Gurling, Oppenheim, and Murray, 1984; Murray et al., 1983).

In summary, twins studies offer some evidence of heritability in the decision to drink and in the frequency and quantity of alcohol imbibed. Most studies dealing directly with alcoholism have also shown a significantly higher level of concordance for this disorder in MZ twins versus DZ twins, and studies of MZ twins separated early in life have been anecdotally consistent with the importance of genetic factors.

The third type of genetic study of humans evaluates the risk for alcoholism in biological children of alcoholics who were adopted out and raised separately from their real parents (i.e., adoption studies). Whether using a half-sibling methodology or actual adoption records, these investigations have also consistently revealed a threefold to fourfold higher risk for alcoholism in adopted-out sons of alcoholics, even when they were raised by nonalcoholic adoptive parents (Cadoret, Cain, and Grove, 1980; Goodwin, 1985; Schuckit, Goodwin and Winokur, 1972). In one of the most frequently cited studies, Goodwin et al., (1973) documented an 18% rate of alcoholism among 55 Danish adopted-away sons of alcoholics by the age of 30 compared with a 5% rate of alcoholism among 78 adopted-away control subjects. Further evaluation showed that the amount of alcoholism in the offspring of alcoholics did not differ significantly whether they were raised by an alcoholic parent or not (Goodwin et al., 1974). Using a similar approach, Bohman, Sigvardsson, and Cloninger (1981) also noted a fourfold higher rate of alcoholism in Sweden among 29 adopted-away daughters of alcoholic mothers (10.3%) than among 577 control subjects (2.8%).

Human research is also attempting to identify important subgroups among primary alcoholics. For example, one preliminary series of studies has identified at least two possible subtypes. The first is likely to be more severe, to be seen in men, and to be closely allied with criminality (i.e., male-limited type), whereas the second is equally likely to be seen in either sex and appears to be more responsive to environmental factors (i.e., milieu-limited type) (Cloninger, Bohman and Sigvardsson, 1981; Cloninger et al., 1984). Although the results of these investigations must be considered preliminary, they highlight the probability that not all alcoholics are likely to be equally sensitive to the same genetic influences. These studies also demonstrate how much work still needs to be done and emphasize how the search for markers of a predisposition to alcoholism is likely to identify multiple factors that are differentially relevant in different alcoholic subgroups. These results also point out the importance of environmental factors in alcoholic problems.

Cloninger and colleagues have used family, twin, and adoption studies to estimate the rate of heritability for alcoholism. Utilizing some earlier twin and family studies, they have estimated an overall heritability rate of about 64%, but the figure may actually be as high as 90% for the hypothesized male-limited subtype (Cloninger et al., 1983, 1984).

Animal studies have also contributed to our understanding of how biological factors might influence the decision to drink, the level of central nervous system (CNS) sensitivity to the effects of ethanol, and the voluntary intake of enough alcohol to cause intoxication (Deitrich and Spuhler, 1984; Meisch, 1982). At least one recently developed animal model addressed biological factors that might interact to yield enough voluntary oral intake to cause intoxication, tolerance, and physical dependence (Li, 1984; Schuckit et al., 1985). Although the focus in this article is on human research, these studies have demonstrated that factors important to alcohol consumption and subsequent problems can be genetically influenced, even in subhuman mammals. These models may be important in future attempts to increase our knowledge of neurochemical and physiologic systems that contribute to specific markers for the alcoholism risk.

Thus, one can conclude that there is generally consistent evidence supporting the importance of genetic factors in the development of alcoholism. Alcoholism is probably a polygenic and multifactorial problem, with genetically influenced biological factors that interact with environmental events (Cloninger, Reich, and Yokoyama, 1983) to contribute significantly to the risk for development. There is little direct documentation of the environmental factors mediating the risk, but Cloninger's work indicates the possible importance of early-life home instability, a relatively low-status occupation for the father, and the subject's need for an extended neonatal hospital stay. Additional factors that, by common sense, might be important include the availability of alcoholic beverages in society (e.g., the price of liquor and number of liquor outlets), social attitudes toward drunkenness, and peer pressures toward excessive drinking.

The studies outlined here have searched for trait markers of a vulnerability toward alcoholism (Schuckit, 1985d). These markers should be easily measured properties that are present before the illness develops and can be observed during remission from active problems. The markers might be fortuitous and indirectly associated with a predisposition, perhaps because the genes influencing the marker are located on the same chromosome, relatively close to the genes influencing the development of alcoholism. On the other hand, it is possible that the trait markers observed will actually be directly involved in the mechanisms that increase the alcoholism risk.

III. STUDIES OF MEN WITH A VULNERABILITY TOWARD ALCOHOLISM

Trait markers are observable either before alcoholism develops or while the illness is in remission. Unfortunately, heavy drinking and its associated lifestyle (with the increased risk for trauma and nutritional deficiencies) is capable of producing in some people biological, physiological, and emotional or cognitive changes that might continue for extended periods of time after abstinence (Schuckit, 1984a). Thus, observing alcoholics even after 20 years of abstinence could reveal cirrhosis, brain damage, evidence of a peripheral neuropathy, or other problems that did not predate the alcoholism and are not appropriate trait markers of a vulnerability toward this disorder. As a result, most investigators have attempted to identify trait markers by observing individuals at high risk for the future development of alcoholism but who have not yet developed major alcohol-related life problems.

A. Methodological Considerations

There are at least three possible approaches to the study of populations at high risk for the development of alcoholism. First, and most important, are studies of children of alcoholics who have been adopted out and reared by nonalcoholic adoptive parents. These children are then followed with repeated evaluations over time to observe differences from control subjects on the way hypothesized markers actually associate with alcoholism. Unfortunately, such detailed evaluations of the adopted-away children of alcoholics are expensive and difficult to carry out because few appropriate groups have been made available for study. Two such cohort investigations of the offspring of alcoholics have reported limited data: One studied children who were adopted out between 1924 and 1927 in Copenhagen, and another used adoption records in Iowa (Cadoret, Cain and Grove, 1980; Jacobsen and Schulsinger, 1981; Utne et al., 1977).

The second approach is to intensively study a limited number of families of alcoholics, searching for markers that are present in alcoholic relatives but are absent in nonalcoholic relatives. Such investigations can provide useful information about the probable pattern of inheritance in alcoholism. However, these studies often require personal interviews and the testing of multiple generations within families, and results must be interpreted while controlling for the effects of prior drinking patterns, age, and so on. As a result, these expensive and time-consuming investigations rarely gather data from more than a limited number of families. Therefore, this approach is probably best reserved for use after preliminary data have identified the markers that are most appropriate for future investigation.

Most studies of populations at high risk for alcoholism have utilized cohorts or groups of normal individuals chosen because of their date of birth, their educational institution, or their use of public resources or contact with police agencies. The goal has been to identify and study individuals at high risk for future alcoholism before the disorder has actually developed. One large cohort of 9000 children from complication-free, full-term births (some with an alcoholic biological parent) in Copenhagen between 1951–1961 is presently being evaluated (Gabrielli and Mednick, 1983; Pollock, Volavka, and Goodwin, 1983; Schulsinger, 1972). In a related approach, U.S. investigations of populations at elevated risk for alcoholism have evaluated biological sons of alcoholics who were identified at various ages. In most cases, sons were chosen so higher risk and lower risk groups could be followed over time to observe the actual development of alcoholism. The selection of men reflects the expectation that men will show higher rates of vulnerability to alcoholism (Schuckit and Morrisey, 1979) and the possibility that results from ethanol challenges could vary with the phase of the menstrual cycle or with the consumption of birth control pills, which could jeopardize study results if women were used (Jones and Jones, 1976).

Some studies of populations at high risk for alcoholism have evaluated perpubertal boys in order to observe them before actual exposure to ethanol, but these have risked missing the markers that appear only after puberty or follow the exposure to modest drinking (Begleiter et al., 1984; Behar, Berg, and Rapoport, 1983). Other investigations have selected older subjects, usually in their late teens to midtwenties, populations that offer investigators the opposite pattern of assets and liabilities (Schuckit, 1985b).

In the approach used in our laboratory since 1978, a mailed questionnaire has been used to identify young, drinking but not yet alcoholic men at elevated risk for the development of alcoholism. The questionnaire utilizes a highly structured format to gather information on demography and pattern of alcohol and drug intake as well as on associated problems; personal, medical, and psychiatric histories; and family history of major psychiatric disorders, including alcoholism and drug abuse. The definition of psychiatric illness follows the *Diagnostic and Statistical Manual of Mental Disorders* (DSM-III; American Psychiatric Association, 1980), with modifications of alcoholism and drug abuse criteria that require evidence of major life problems related to substances (Schuckit, 1984a). From these mailings, the sons of primary alcoholics who were themselves drinkers but who had not experienced major life problems from alcohol or drugs and who had no past history of medical or psychiatric disorders were selected as higher risk or family history positive (FHP) subjects. Each FHP man was matched with a lower risk family history negative (FHN) individual on age, sex, race, educational level, quantity and frequency of drinking, substance intake history, height-to-weight ratio, and smoking history.

Men selected for study were subsequently tested individually in the laboratory on three occasions, where they consumed placebo, 0.75 ml/kg of ethanol, or 1.1 ml/kg of ethanol.

The subjects were unaware of the hypotheses being tested, and the two family history groups had very similar scores on the effects they expected from three drinks (Schuckit, 1984c). The ethanol was given as a 20% by volume solution (for active beverages) in a sugar-free, noncaffeinated beverage, which was drunk over a 10-min period. Before the challenge, laboratory personnel determined the subject's baseline level of functioning on a variety of cognitive and psychomotor tests, mood and anxiety scales, and hormonal levels. After drinking the beverage, individuals were observed over a 4 h period, during which their reactions to the two doses of ethanol and the placebo were established.

Other studies of high-risk populations have used slightly different methods. For example, Tarter et al., (1984) evaluated cognitive and psychomotor test performance without ethanol challenges in a series of boys in their midteens who were in trouble with the law. A group in Oklahoma utilized labor unions, social organizations, and churches to identify both male and female children of alcoholics (Schaeffer, Parsons, and Yohman, 1984). In another series of studies, Begleiter et al. (1984) utilized community volunteers in their preteen years to study the electrophysiological attributes of young sons of alcoholic fathers, and a similar approach was used by Behar et al. (1983). As a result, children of various ages and socioeconomic groups with alcoholic parents have been identified through a variety of methodologies and have been studied either at baseline or after an ethanol challenge.

B. Populations at Elevated Risk for Alcoholism

Preliminary findings have indicated several potential trait markers of a vulnerability toward alcoholism. However, even after a potential marker has been identified and replicated in other laboratories, there are many important research steps that must be taken. First, the association between the marker that has been identified in sons of alcoholics and the future development of alcoholism must be established through follow-up investigations. Second, the genetic basis of the biological marker must be established. Third, the actual mechanism for the expression of the vulnerability needs to be studied. Despite these caveats, early work has identified at least one possible behavior trait marker (a decreased intensity of reaction to ethanol) and several electrophysiological markers that may prove to be important.

Decreased Intensity of Reaction to Ethanol

Our investigations, as well as the results from two laboratories in the United States and Denmark, have documented the ethanol reactions of sons of alcoholics and carefully matched control subjects. Subjective levels of intoxication were measured on an analogue scale at baseline and again at several intervals after drinking. Subjects were required to rate the intensity of different aspects of intoxication, including overall drug effect, dizziness, nausea, level of "high," and so on.

Before challenges, the FHP and FHN subjects expressed similar expectations of the effects of ethanol; after drinking, both groups developed similar patterns of blood alcohol concentrations over time (Mednick, 1983; O'Malley and Maisto, 1985; Schuckit, 1980, 1984c, 1985a). Despite these similarities and identical self-reports for the two groups following placebo, the FHP men rated themselves as significantly less intoxicated than did the FHN men after drinking 0.75 ml/kg of ethanol (Fig. 1). A similar but nonsignificant trend was noted after subjects drank a 1.1 ml/kg ethanol dose (Fig. 2). Overall, FHN subjects scored 39% higher on the "drug effect" item over the 4 h after the lower dose challenge and scored 24% higher after the higher dose. In both settings, the maximum group difference was observed 60–120 min after the drinking had been consumed.

In our own laboratory, FHP subjects also demonstrated smaller increments in cognitive and psychomotor performance after drinking. For example, to measure the level of sway in the

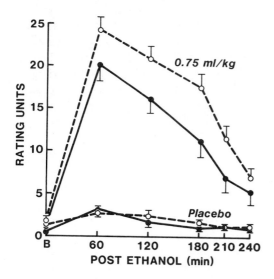

Figure 1 Mean self-ratings on a 0 (none) to 36 (great) scale measuring the drug effect of placebo and 0.75 ml/kg of ethanol for 23 matched pairs with positive (closed circles) and negative (open circles) family histories. (Bars indicate standard errors and B indicates baseline. (From M.A. Schuckit (1984). Subjective responses to alcohol in sons of alcoholics and controls. *Arch. Gen. Psychiatry, 41*:879–884. Copyright 1984 by the American Medical Association. Reprinted by permission.)

upper body, we asked subjects to stand still, with hands at the sides and feet together. Although there were no group differences at baseline or after consuming placebo (Fig. 3), the FHN subjects showed significantly greater increase in body sway after drinking the 0.75 ml/kg dose of ethanol (Schuckit, 1985a). Using the raw data, we found a significant time × family history interaction, $F(3, 197) = 3.84$, $p = 0.01$, although the family-history effect alone was not quite significant ($p = 0.06$). Similarly, preliminary analyses of changes in hormones sensitive to an ethanol challenge have revealed a less intense response in FHP subjects for cortisol and prolactin after drinking although these data analyses were carried out without placebo controls, and attempts to replicate these findings have not yet been published (Schuckit, 1984b; Schuckit, Parker, and Rossman, 1983).

If we speculate on the meaning of the results, we may assume that a decreased intensity of reaction to low doses of ethanol would make it more difficult for individuals to discern when they are becoming drunk. However, the greater similarity in levels of intoxification after higher doses of alcohol showed that men in both family groups were capable of experiencing a similar drug effect. An impaired ability to fully experience the effects of moderate alcohol doses could make it harder to know when to stop drinking during an evening; it may be more difficult to use relatively subtle cues to learn when to quit before becoming too drunk. This is an example of a biologically influenced factor that might not cause alcoholism but, in conjunction with a heavy drinking milieu, could predispose an individual toward a higher risk for alcohol-related life problems.

Possible Electrophysiological Markers

Studies of sons of alcoholics have tentatively indicated two types of brain waves as markers associated with a predisposition toward alcoholism. The first, event-related potentials (ERPs), are computer-averaged brain waves measuring electrophysiological brain reactions to stimuli (Porjesz and Begleiter, 1983). One part of the ERP, a positive wave observed at approximately

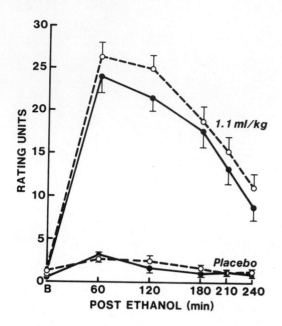

Figure 2 Mean self-ratings on a 0 (none) to 36 (great) scale measuring the drug effect of placebo and 1.1 ml/kg of ethanol for 23 matched pairs with positive (closed circles) and negative (open circles) family histories. (Bars indicate standard errors and B indicates baseline. From M.A. Schuckit (1984). Subjective responses to alcohol in sons of alcoholics and controls. *Arch. Gen. Psychiatry, 41*:879–884. Copyright 1984 by the American Medical Association. Reprinted by permission.)

300 ms after a stimulus (the P300), occurs in normal individuals after they experience an anticipated but rare event. The P300 is thought to correlate with an individual's ability to selectively attend to an anticipated stimulus. Following up on observations of a nonreversible flattened amplitude of P300s in alcoholics, Begleiter et al. (1984) documented a similarly decreased P300 wave in the preadolescent sons of alcoholics. Our own laboratory has recently replicated this trend for a lower amplitude P300 wave, and an earlier study with Elmasian et al., (1982) questioned whether FHP and FHN subjects might demonstrate P300 amplitudes that respond differently to ethanol and placebo challenges. Another study evaluated other possible ERP differences between family history groups (Schmidt and Neville, 1984).

In a second finding, alcoholics have been shown to demonstrate relatively low levels of slow waves (e.g., alpha waves) on background cortical electroencephalograms (EEGs) before ethanol, and they might show a greater increase in this wave after an ethanol challenge (Gabrielli et al., 1982; Pollock et al., 1983; Volavka et al., 1982). Following up on these results, studies of populations at high risk for the development of alcoholism have revealed similar EEG patterns in the sons of alcoholics. Thus, it is possible that ethanol has different reinforcing properties in individuals at high risk for alcoholism: Perhaps it corrects for a lower level of alpha activity and, thus, produces more feelings of relaxation (Schuckit et al., 1981).

In summary, follow-up studies on electrophysiological differences between alcoholics and control subjects have identified two possible trait markers for alcoholism in the sons of alcoholics. Some of these findings, however, are preliminary and require replication. Future investigations must evaluate the relations between physiological findings and other potential

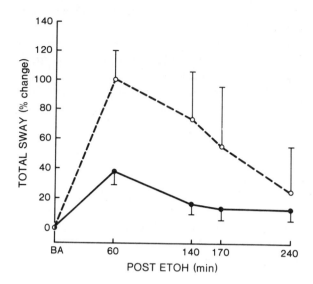

Figure 3 Percent increase in body sway or standing steadiness following 0.75 ml/kg of ethanol for 23 matched pairs with positive (closed circles) and negative (open circles) family histories. (Bars indicate standard errors and B indicates baseline. ETOH = ethanol.)

markers of a predisposition toward alcoholism, including the apparently decreased reaction to ethanol in these young men.

Cognitive and Psychomotor Impairment

The series of studies carried out in our laboratory has documented no major cognitive or psychomotor differences between sons of alcoholics and control subjects before an ethanol challenge. However, our subjects have been highly functioning young men, and it is possible that some sons of alcoholics may show cognitive or psychomotor deficits but that these individuals were not a part of our sample (i.e., our sample contained students or university employees). Therefore, it is of interest to examine the results of studies using sons of alcoholics who have been identified at a younger age through their associations with juvenile authorities. Comparisons of FHP and FHN subjects from this population have shown lower verbal IQs for the FHP subjects as well as decreased auditory word span performance, lower levels of reading comprehension, a higher number of errors on the Categories Test of the Halstead-Reitan Neuropsychological Test battery, and problems with constructional praxis and abstract problem-solving (Gabrielli and Mednick, 1983; Knop et al., 1984; Schaeffer et al., 1984; Tarter, et al., 1984).

A related finding has associated the risk for alcoholism with signs of hyperactivity or impulsivity during childhood (Goodwin et al., 1975; Knop et al., 1984; McCord, 1981; Mednick, 1983). However, childhood hyperactivity can reflect nonspecific stressors, such as living with an alcoholic parent, and might be temporary and distinct from a true hyperactive child syndrome or from attention deficit disorder (Schuckit, Petrich, and Chiles, 1978). A number of other studies following cohorts over time have not demonstrated a close association between impulsivity or hyperactive child syndrome and the future development of alcoholism (Tarter, Hegedus, and Gavaler, 1985; Vaillant, 1984; Vaillant and Milofsky, 1982). In addition, in our own laboratory, FHP subjects were no more likely to have demonstrated hyperactivity in childhood or to have shown more signs of impulsivity on personality tests than FHN subjects (Saunders and Schuckit, 1981).

In summary, some men may show an association between cognitive and psychomotor test performance problems, signs of hyperactivity in childhood, and the future development of alcoholism. However, these behavior problems are not apparent in the sons of alcoholics who function moderately well, and the relation between these variables and future alcoholism may not be strong enough to be identified through prospective cohort studies of the general population.

B. Personality Profiles and the Future Development of Alcoholism

During the course of heavy drinking and the months following recovery, alcoholics are likely to show many abnormalities on personality tests (Schuckit and Haglund, 1982). However, many of these results may reflect the actions of ethanol as well as the mood swings and life crises inherent in an alcoholic lifestyle, and abnormal results may become normal with continued abstinence. In addition, some personality traits that remain after drinking may reflect other primary psychiatric diagnoses, such as antisocial personality disorder, and not alcoholism per se (Schuckit, 1973).

It is, thus, not surprising that observations of personality attributes in young men at high risk for the future development of alcoholism show few consistent results. In our own laboratory studies of highly functioning young men, few baseline group differences were observed on scores of neuroticism, extraversion, state anxiety, or locus of control; on scales of the Minnesota Multiphasic Personality Inventory (MMPI); or on indirect measures of personality, such as the portable Rod Frame Test (Morrison and Schuckit, 1983; Saunders and Schuckit, 1981; Schuckit, 1982, 1983b; Schuckit and Penn, 1985). However, no definitive answers are available because of limitations in the number of pairs studied, because of the difficulty of proving an absence of a significant difference between groups, and because of the highly select nature of some of the populations investigated. The personality differences between alcoholics and control subjects (MacAndrew, 1979) do justify further evaluations.

C. Biochemical Markers

A number of unique patterns of blood proteins can be observed in alcoholics even after continued abstinence. These include at least one major enzyme of ethanol degradation, enzymes important in the metabolism of brain neurotransmitters, and some blood antigens.

Most ethanol in the body is broken down by the enzyme alcohol dehydrogenase (ADH) to acetaldehyde, a psychoactive substance that is subsequently destroyed by the enzyme aldehyde dehydrogenase (ALDH) (li, 1977). The patterns of form (or isoenzymes) for both ALDH and ADH are genetically controlled. Although the pattern might change in normal individuals with age and although the amount of enzyme can be strongly influenced by drinking, the types of isoenzymes are not likely to be significantly altered by drug intake.

There are at least four isoenzymes of ALDH in the human liver, each with different biochemical properties (Greenfield and Pietruszko, 1977). The ALDH isoenzyme most sensitive to low doses of acetaldehyde varies markedly in different ethnic groups and is missing in 30–50% of Orientals (Harada et al., 1983; Suwaki and Ohara, 1985). In the absence of this isoenzyme form, ethanol oxidation results in significantly higher levels of blood acetaldehyde after drinking, with a subsequent syndrome of facial flushing, palpitations, and nausea that resembles a mild ethanol-disulfiram interaction. Orientals missing this enzyme are less likely than their cohorts to drink heavily and appear to have a lower rate of alcoholism (Suwaki and Ohara, 1985). Thus, one genetically controlled enzyme does influence the chance of developing alcoholism within Oriental subgroups, although this finding may have limited applicability to non-Oriental populations. There is little evidence of significant differences among Occidental groups on their ALDH isoenzyme pattern.

Second, monoamine oxidase (MAO), an enzyme important in the degradation of brain neurotransmitters, has been reported to have abnormal activity levels in people with a variety of psychiatric disorders and personality types. The activity level of this enzyme is said to be low in alcoholics, although it is not clear whether it returns to normal after an extended period of abstinence (Sullivan et al., 1979). There is preliminary evidence that sons of alcoholics may also demonstrate lower levels of MAO activity, although most studies have demonstrated only a trend and not a significant difference from control populations (Scher, 1983; Schuckit, Shaskan, and Duby, 1982).

Finally, based on comparisons of alcoholic and control subjects, a number of other blood proteins are of interest. These include the brain protein Ptl-Duarte (Comings, 1979) and a possible linkage in repulsion between the D gene of the Rh system, the SS phenotype for complement C3, and alcoholism (Hill et al., 1980). Each of these potential markers requires further evaluation in relatives of alcoholics as well as in populations at high risk for the development of alcoholism before definitive conclusions can be drawn.

IV. CONCLUSIONS

This article has reviewed information on the biological vulnerability toward alcoholism. Most of the work is based on the premise that alcoholism is a genetically influenced disorder. In evaluating the studies, however, it is important to remember the likelihood that biological factors explain only one important part of the risk for alcoholism. The final development of this disorder probably depends on the interaction between biological and environmental factors. The emphasis on biology in this article reflects both the discipline of the author and the ease with which biological factors can be measured and thus identified early in the course of a series of studies.

At this point in the research, the methodologies being used are of as much interest as the results themselves. In general, researchers have taken advantage of persistent differences between alcoholic and control subjects to identify foci for studies of populations at high risk for the development of alcoholism. Potential trait markers of greatest interest are those that not only differentiate alcoholic from control subjects but also retain their efficacy with extended abstinence. It is these measures that are generally used to compare the children of alcoholics with the children of control subjects.

The results of any of the studies of populations at high risk for alcoholism are affected by research approach. Different markers might be identified in young prepubertal children than in older or highly functioning children of alcoholics. Results may also be affected by the definition of alcoholism used and by whether children of primary or secondary alcoholics were evaluated.

Despite the diversity of methodologies, several important leads toward identifying the trait markers associated with a vulnerability toward alcoholism are apparent. Sons of alcoholics appear to show a decreased intensity of reaction to modest doses of ethanol, to have lower amplitude ERP P300 brain waves, and to show unusual patterns of wave form frequencies on background cortical EEGs. Other interesting and potentially important findings require further evaluation.

Once a behavior or test result is accepted as being significantly different in populations at high risk for alcoholism than in control subjects, much work remains before the actual presence of a trait marker for alcoholism can be established. Thus, this article has described a series of research projects that are in their infancy, and much important work remains to be done.

These findings contain a number of clinical and research implications. First, the studies outlined in this article underscore the probability that biological and genetic factors are important in a vulnerability toward alcoholism. Taken together with family, twins, and adoption studies, the results can be used to highlight the importance of biological influences and to emphasize the probability that alcoholism is not just a moral weakness.

Second, the series of studies contains implications for the prevention of alcoholism. The fourfold increased risk for alcoholism in children of alcoholics emphasizes how vulnerable this particular group is to the development of alcohol-related life problems. These individuals might be chosen as the focus of some intensive prevention efforts in the future.

Third, the present results hold a number of implications for the future. It is the hope of many investigators that identification of the biological factors associated with a vulnerability toward alcoholism will help clinicians develop more specific and effective prevention and treatment efforts. Further progress will also help to identify those sons and daughters of alcoholics who have inherited the traits that increase their vulnerability. These individuals can then be followed over time in order to identify the social and cultural factors that maximize the chances for expression of the vulnerability and the factors that provide protective action.

In conclusion, interesting and important research is now being carried out to help identify the biological vulnerabilities to alcoholism. Recent years have witnessed great progress in this field, and research strategies appear to be bearing fruit. Although no generally accepted biological marker of a vulnerability toward alcoholism has yet been identified (with the possible exception of the ALDH isoenzyme pattern), the results of research have been most promising. We recognize the deficiencies inherent in any brief overview and encourage the reader to reexamine our references and to follow the literature in this field as it unfolds further in the coming years.

ACKNOWLEDGMENTS

Special appreciation is expressed for the invaluable work done by Eric Gold, Karen Croot, and Patti Finn, without whose efforts in this series of studies could never have been accomplished. This work was supported by National Institute on Alcohol Abuse and Alcoholism Grant #05526-03, by the Research Service of the Veterans Administration, by a grant from the Joan B. Kroc Foundation, and by the Alcoholic Beverage Medical Research Foundation.

REFERENCES

American Psychiatric Association (1980). *Diagnostic and Statistical Manual of Mental Disorders*, 3rd ed. Washington, D.C.

Begleiter, H., Porjesz, B., Bihari, B., and Kissin, B. (1984). Event-related brain potentials in boys at risk for alcoholism. *Science, 227*:1493–1496.

Behar, D., Berg, C.J., and Rapoport, J.L. (1983). Behavior and physiological effects of ethanol in high-risk and control children: A pilot study. *Alcoholism Clin. Exp. Res., 7*:404–410.

Bohman, M., Sigvardsson, S., and Cloninger, C.R. (1981). Maternal inheritance of alcohol abuse: Cross-fostering analysis of adopted women. *Arch. Gen. Psychiatry, 38*:965–969.

Cadoret, R.J., Cain, C.A., and Grove, W.M. (1980). Development of alcoholism in adoptees raised apart from alcoholic biologic relatives. *Arch. Gen. Psychiatry, 37*:561–563.

Cahalan, D., and Cisin, I.H. (1968). American drinking practices: Summary of findings from a national probability sample. *Q. J. Stud. Alcohol, 29*:130–151.

Cloninger, C.R., Bohman, M., and Sigvardsson, S. (1981). Inheritance of alcohol abuse: Cross-fostering analysis of adopted men. *Arch. Gen. Psychiatry, 36*:861–868.

Cloninger, C.R., Bohman, M., Sigvardsson, S., and von Knorring, A.L. (1984). Psychopathology in adopted-out children of alcoholics, M. Galanter (ed.), *Recent Developments in Alcoholism*. Plenum Press, New York, pp. 37–51.

Cloninger, C.R., von Knorring, A.L., Sigvardsson, S., and Bohman, M. (1983, March). *Inheritance of Alcohol Abuse*. Presented at the International Conference on Pharmacological Treatments for Alcoholism: Looking to the Future, organized by the Alcoholism Education Centre and the Institute of Psychiatry, University of London, England.

Comings, D.E. (1979). The genetic heterogeneity of human brain proteins and their diagnosis in living patients. *Nature, 277*:28–32.

Cotton, N.S. (1979). The familial incidence of alcoholism: A review. *J. Stud. Alcohol, 40*:89–116.

Deitrich, R.A., and Spuhler, K. (1984). Genetics of alcoholism and alcohol actions, R. Smart and E.M. Sellers (eds.), *Research Advances in Alcohol and Drug Problems*, Vol. 8. Plenum Press, New York, pp. 47–98.

Elmasian, R., Neville, H., Woods, D., Schuckit, M.A., and Bloom, F. (1982). Event-related brain potentials are different in individuals at high risk for developing alcoholism. *Proc. Nat. Acad. Sci., U.S.A., 79*:7900–7903.

Fillmore, K.M., and Midanik, L. (1984). Chronicity of drinking problems among men: A longitudinal study. *J. Stud. Alcohol, 45*:228–236.

Gabrielli, W.F., and Mednick, S.A. (1983). Intellectual performance in children of alcoholics. *J. Nerv. Ment. Dis., 171*:444–447.

Gabrielli, W.F., Mednick, S.A., Volavka, J., Pollock, V.E., Schulsinger F., and Itil, T.M. (1982). Electroencephalograms in children of alcoholic fathers. *Psychophysiology, 19*:404–407.

Goodwin, D.W. (1985). Alcoholism and genetics. *Arch. Gen. Psychiatry, 42*:171–174.

Goodwin, D.W., and Guze, S.B. (1984). *Psychiatric Diagosis*. Oxford University Press, New York.

Goodwin, D.W., Schulsinger, F., Hermansen, L., Guze, S., and Winokur, G. (1973). Alcohol problems in adoptees raised apart from alcohol biological parents. *Arch. Gen. Psychiatry, 28*:238–243.

Goodwin, D.W., Schulsinger, F., Hermansen, L., Guze, S.B., and Winokur, G. (1975). Alcoholism and the hyperactive child syndrome. *J. Nerv. Ment. Dis., 160*:349–353.

Goodwin, D.W., Schulsinger, F., Moller, N., Hermansen, L., Winokur, G., and Guze, S.B. (1974). Drinking problems in adopted and nonadopted sons of alcoholics. *Arch. Gen. Psychiatry, 31*:164–169.

Greenfield, N.J., and Pietruszko, R. (1977). Two aldehyde dehydrogenases from human liver: Isolation via affinity chromatography and characterization of the isoenzymes. *Biochem. Biophys. Acta, 483*:35–45.

Gurling, H.M.D., Oppenheim, B.E., and Murray, R.M. (1984). Depression, criminality and psychopathology associated with alcoholism: Evidence from a twin study. *Acta Genet. Med. Gemellol, 33*:333–339.

Harada, S., Agarwal, D.P., Goedde, H.W., and Ishikawa, B. (1983). Aldehyde dehydrogenase isozyme variation and alcoholism in Japan. *Pharmacol. Biochem. Behav., 18*:151–153.

Hill, S.Y., Goodwin, D.W., Cadoret, R., Osterland, C.K., and Doner, S.M. (1980). Association and linkage between alcoholism and eleven serological markers. *J. Stud. Alcohol, 36*:981–989.

Hrubec, Z., and Omenn, G.S. (1981). Evidence of genetic predisposition to alcohol cirrhosis and psychosis: Twin concordances for alcoholism and its biological end points by zygosity among male veterans. *Alcoholism Clin. Exp. Res., 5*:207–212.

Jacobsen, B., and Schulsinger, F. (1981). The Danish adoption register, S.A. Mednick and A.E. Baert (eds.), *Prospective Longitudinal Research: An Empirical Basis for the Primary Prevention of Psychosocial Disorders*. Oxford University Press, Oxford, England, pp. 225–230.

Jones, B.M., and Jones, M.K. (1976). Women and alcohol: Intoxication, metabolism, and the menstrual cycle, M. Greenblatt and M.A. Schuckit (eds.), *Alcoholism Problems in Women and Children*. Grune & Stratton, New York, pp. 103–136.

Jonsson, E., and Nilsson, T. (1968). Alcoholism in monozygotic and dizygotic twins. *Nord. Hyg. Tidskr., 49*:21.

Kaij, L. (1960). *Studies on the Etiology and Sequels of Abuse of Alcohol*. University of Lund, Department of Psychiatry, Sweden.

Knop, J., Goodwin, D., Teasdale, T.W., Mikkelsen, U., and Schulsinger, F. (1984). A Danish prospective study of young males at high risk for alcoholism. D.W. Goodwin, D. Teilmann Van Dusen, and S.A. Mednick (eds.), *Longitudinal Research in Alcoholism*. Kluwer-Nijhoff, Boston, pp. 107–122.

Kopun, M., and Propping, P. (1977). The kinetics of ethanol absorption and elimination in twins and supplementary repetitive experiments in singleton subjects. *Eur. J. Clin. Pharmacol., 11*:337–344.

Li, T.K. (1977). Enzymology of hyman alcohol metabolism, A. Meister (ed.), *Enzymology of Human Alcohol Metabolism*. Wiley, New York, pp. 19–56.

Li, T.K. (1984, December). *An Animal Model of Alcoholism*. Paper presented at the American College of Neuropsychopharmacology, San Juan, Puerto Rico.

MacAndrew, C. (1979). On the possibility of the psychometric detection of persons who are prone to the abuse of alcohol and other substances. *Addict. Behav., 4*:11–20.

McCord, J. (1981). Alcoholism and criminality: Confounding and differentiating factors. *J. Stud. Alcohol, 42*:739–748.

Mednick, S.A. (1983, May). *Subjects at Risk for Alcoholism: Recent Reports*. Paper presented at the 14th Annual Medical Scientific Conference of the National Alcoholism Forum, Research Society on Alcoholism, Houston, Texas.

Meisch, R. (1982). Animal studies of alcohol intake. *Br. J. Psychiatry, 141*:113–120.

Morrison, C., and Schuckit, M.A. (1983). Locus of control in young men with alcoholic relatives and controls. *J. Clin. Psychiatry, 44*:306–307.

Murray, R.M., Clifford, C., Gurling, H.M.D., Topham, A., Clow, A., and Bernadt, M. (1983). Current genetic and biological approaches to alcoholism. *Psychiatr. Dev., 2*:179–192.

Newman, H.H., Freeman, F.N., and Holzinger, K.J. (1973). *Twins: A Study of Heredity and Environment*. University of Chicago Press, Chicago.

O'Malley, S.S., and Maisto, S.A. (1985). The effects of family drinking history on responses to alcohol: Expectancies and reactions to intoxication. *J. Stud. Alcohol, 46*:289–297.

Partanen, J., Bruun, K., and Marrkanen, T. (1966). *Inheritance of Drinking Behavior: A Study on Intelligence, Personality, and Use of Alcohol of Adult Twins*. Finnish Foundation for Alcohol Studies, Helsinki, Finland.

Pollock, V.E., Volavka, J., and Goodwin, D.W. (1983). The EEG after alcohol administration in men at risk for alcoholism. *Arch. Gen. Psychiatry, 40*:857–861.

Porjesz, B., and Begleiter, H. (1983). Brain dysfunction and alcohol, B. Kissin and H. Begleiter (eds.), *The Pathogenesis of Alcoholism*. Plenum Press, New York, pp. 415–483.

Radlow, R., and Conway, T.L. (1978, August). *Consistency of Alcohol Absorption in Human Subjects*. Paper presented at the American Psychological Association, Toronto, Canada.

Saunders, G.R., and Schuckit, M.A. (1981). Brief communication: MMPI scores in young men with alcoholic relatives and controls. *J. Nerv. Ment. Dis., 168*:456–458.

Schaeffer, K.W., Parsons, O.A., and Yohman, J.R. (1984). Neuropsychological differences between male familial and nonfamilial alcoholics and nonalcoholics. *Alcoholism Clin. Exp. Res., 8*:347–358.

Scher, K.J. (1983). Platelet monoamine oxidase activity in relatives of alcoholics. *Arch. Gen. Psychiatry, 40*:466.

Schmidt, A.L., and Neville, H.J. (1984, June). *Event-Related Brain Potentials (ERPs) in Sons of Alcoholic Fathers*. Paper presented at the meeting of the International Society for Biological Research, Santa Fe, New Mexico.

Schuckit, M.A. (1973). Alcoholism and sociopathy—diagnostic confusion. *J. Stud. Alcohol, 34*:157–164.

Schuckit, M.A. (1980). Self-rating alcohol intoxication by young men with and without family histories of alcoholism. *J. Stud. Alcohol, 41*:242–249.

Schuckit, M.A. (1981). Twin studies on substance abuse, L. Gedda, P. Parisi, and W. Nance (eds.), *Twin Research 3: Epidemiological and Clinical Studies*. Liss, New York, pp. 61–70.

Schuckit, M.A. (1982). Anxiety and assertiveness in sons of alcoholics and controls. *J. Clin. Psychiatry, 43*:238–239.

Schuckit, M.A. (1983a). Alcoholism and other psychiatric disorders. *Hosp. Commun. Psychiatry, 34*:1022–1027.

Schuckit, M.A. (1983b). Extroversion and neuroticism in young men. *Am. J. Psychiatry, 140*:1223–1224.

Schuckit, M.A. (1984a). *Drug and Alcohol Abuse: A Clinical Guide to Diagnosis and Treatment*, 2nd ed.) Plenum Press, New York.

Schuckit, M.A. (1984b). Differences in plasma cortisol after ethanol in relatives of alcoholics and controls. *J. Clin. Psychiatry, 45*:374–379.

Schuckit, M.A. (1984c). Subjective responses to alcohol in sons of alcoholics and controls. *Arch. Gen. Psychiatry, 41*:879–884.

Schuckit, M.A. (1985a). Ethanol-induced changes in body sway in men at high alcoholism risk. *Arch. Gen. Psychiatry, 42*:375–379.

Schuckit, M.A. (1985b). Studies of populations at high risk for alcoholism. *Psychiatric Dev., 3*:31–63.

Schuckit, M.A. (1985c). The clinical implications of primary diagnostic groups among alcoholics. *Arch. Gen. Psychiatry, 42*:1043–1049.

Schuckit, M.A. (1985d). Trait (and state) markers of a predisposition to psychopathology, L.L. Judd and P. Groves (eds.), *Physiological Foundations of Clinical Psychiatry*, Lippincott, Philadelphia, pp. 1–19.

Schuckit, M.A. (1986). Alcoholism and affective disorders: Genetic and clinical implications. *Am. J. Psychiatry, 143*:140–147.

Schuckit, M.A., Engstrom, D., Alpert, R., and Duby, J. (1981). Differences in muscle-tension response to ethanol in young men with and without family histories of alcoholism. *J. Stud. Alcohol, 42*:918–924.

Schuckit, M.A., Goodwin, D.A., and Winokur, G.A. (1972). A study of alcoholism in half siblings. *Am. J. Psychiatry, 128*:1132.

Schuckit, M.A., and Haglund, R.M.J. (1982). An overview of the etiologic theories on alcoholism, N. Estes and E. Heinemann (eds.), *Alcoholism: Development, Consequences, and Interventions*. Mosby, St. Louis, pp. 16–31.

Schuckit, M.A., Li, T.K., Cloninger, E.R., and Deitrich, R.A. (1985). Genetics of alcoholism. *Alcoholism Clin. Exp. Res., 9*:475–492.

Schuckit, M.A., and Morrisey, E.R. (1979). Psychiatric problems in women at alcoholic detoxification. *Am. J. Psychiatry, 136*:611–617.

Schuckit, M.A., Parker, D.C., and Rossman, L.R. (1983). Prolactin responses to ethanol in men at elevated risk for alcoholism and controls. *Biol. Psychiatry, 18*:1153–1159.

Schuckit, M.A., and Penn, N.E. (1985). Performance on the rod and frame for men at elevated risk for alcoholism and controls. *Am. J. Drug and Alcohol Abuse, 3*:113–118.

Schuckit, M.A., Petrich, J., and Chiles, J. (1978). Hyperactivity: Diagostic confusion. *J. Nerv. Ment. Dis., 166*:79–87.

Schuckit, M.A., Shaskan, E., and Duby, J. (1982). Platelet MAO activities in the relatives of alcoholics and controls: A prospective study. *Arch. Gen. Psychiatry, 39*:137–140.

Schulsinger, F. (1972). Psychopathy: Heredity and environment. *Int. J. Ment. Health, 1*:190–206.

Shields, J. (1962). *Monozygotic Twins*. Oxford University Press, London.

Sullivan, J.L., Cavenar, J.O., Maltbie, A.A., Lister, P., and Zung, W.W.K. (1979). Familial biochemical and clinical correlates of alcoholics with low platelet monoamine oxidase activity. *Biol. Psychiatry, 14*:385–389.

Suwaki, J., and Ohara, H. (1985). Alcohol-induced facial flushing and drinking behavior in Japanese men. *J. Stud. Alcohol, 46*:196–198.

Tarter, R.E., Hegedus, A.M., and Gavaler, J.S. (1985). Hyperactivity in sons of alcoholics. *J. Stud. Alcohol, 46*:259–261..

Tarter, R.E., Hegedus, A.M., Goldstein, G., Shelly, C., and Alterman, A. (1984). Adolescent sons of alcoholics: Neuropsychological and personality characteristics. *Alcoholism Clin. Exper. Res., 8*:216–222.

Tarter, R., Hill, S., Jacob, T., Hegedus, A., and Winsten, K.J. (1984, June). *Neuropsychological Comparison of Sons of Alcoholic Depressed and Normal Fathers*. Paper presented at the meeting of the International Society for Biological Research Association, Santa Fe, New Mexico.

Utne, H.E., Hensen, F.V., Winkler, K., and Schulsinger, F. (1977). Alcohol elimination rates in adoptees with and without alcoholic parents. *J. Stud. Alcohol, 38*:1219–1223.

Vaillant, G.E. (1984). The course of alcoholism and lessons for treatment, L. Grinspoon (ed.), *Psychiatry Update*. American Psychiatric Press, Washington, D.C., pp. 311–319.

Vaillant, G.E., and Milofsky, E.S. (1982). Natural history of male alcoholism. *Arch. Gen. Psychiatry*, *39*:127–133.

Vesell, E.S., Page, J.G., and Passancanti, G.T. (1971). Genetic and environmental factors affecting ethanol metabolism in man. *Clin. Pharmacol. Ther.*, *12*:192–201.

Volavka, J., Pollock, V., Gabrielli, W.F., and Mednick, S.A. (1982). The EEG in persons at risk for alcoholism, in M. Galanter (ed.), *Currents in Alcoholism*, Vol. 8. Grune & Stratton, New York, pp. 116–123.

39

Genetic and Clinical Implications of Alcoholism and Affective Disorder

Marc A. Schuckit
Veterans Affairs Medical Center, and University of California, San Diego, California

I. INTRODUCTION

Alcoholism and affective disorder are two highly prevalent psychiatric problems [1,2]. The symptom patterns of sadness and excessive drinking frequently occur in the same patient, but the prognoses and treatments of primary alcoholism and primary affective disorder are quite different [3–5]. To understand the relationship between these disorders, it is important to distinguish between drinking, alcohol problems, and alcoholism on the one hand and sadness, grief, and affective disorder on the other.

Between 80 and 90% of the population of the United States drink at some time during their lives, and 30–40% of these may develop some temporary alcoholic-related problems [5–8]. This is distinct from the 8–10% of men and 3–5% of women who go beyond temporary alcohol difficulties and meet the criteria for alcoholism, a diagnosis indicating pervasive and persistent alcohol-related life problems [2,4,6]. Similarly, sadness is a normal reaction to stress and is experienced by almost everyone at some point in his or her life. Grief is a temporary but more intense sadness that is time-limited and related to a recent loss. A major affective disorder, however, is a life-threatening psychiatric problem carrying high risks for morbidity and mortality that must be aggressively treated [3].

The diagnostic criteria for alcoholism and major affective disorder rest with the constellation or grouping of symptoms and their time course [3,4]. A problem arises, however, when a single patient presents with two or more clinical syndromes [9]. One way to increase understanding of the relationship between any two disorders is to distinguish between primary and secondary illness. The approach presented by the Washington University group [3,10,11] makes this differentiation by focusing on the chronology of symptom development, using the primary label as the one that fulfilled research criteria at the youngest age. For example,

This chapter was reprinted from the *Am. J. Psychiatry, Vol. 143*:2, 1986. Copyright © 1986 American Psychiatric Association. Reprinted by permission.

a patient who met criteria for alcoholism at age 33 and who fulfilled research criteria for affective disorder at age 40 would be diagnosed as having primary alcoholism and secondary affective disorder. Alternative approaches to the primary/secondary distinction include giving a primary lavel to the most severe disorder or using equal but independent labels if a second symptom picture develops during a period of remission from the first disorder [12,13]. No matter which approach is used, most investigations evaluating patients with alcoholism and affective symptoms [14–16] have concluded that an attempt at establishing a hierarchy is worthwhile.

The primary/secondary dichotomy, at a minimum, implies that the future clinical course of an illness is likely to be complicated if a secondary disorder is present. In some instances the diagnostic approach might indicate that the future course is likely to follow that of the primary problem [4,17–19]. In either case, researchers or clinicians looking at the natural history or genetics of diseases should focus on patients with primary diagnoses so that the second constellation of symptoms does not obscure the outcome [19].

These diagnostic events caveats are especially important when dealing with patients with primary or secondary substance abuse. Alcoholism can be considered a great mimicker in psychiatry because persistent heavy drinking is likely to precipiate symptoms of anxiety, depression, confusion, or psychosis [17]. It makes little prognostic sense, for example, to assume that the auditory hallucinations and/or paranoid delusions seen in the midst of an alcoholic psychosis indicate that a patient has independent schizophrenia [20]. Psychoses secondary to alcoholism are likely to clear within several days or weeks of abstinence, but the diagnosis of schizophrenia indicates that the patient will likely have lifelong, persistent psychotic symptoms requiring antipsychotic medications [3,4,21–23]. Similarly, depressive symptoms are not unique to major affective disorders and are common during cocaine abuse, methadone maintenance, or alcoholism [14,17]. These secondary affective syndromes are also likely to disappear within days or weeks of abstinence. The sadness probably reflects the combination of life stresses, symptoms of withdrawal, and/or pharmacological alterations induced by drug actions.

The confusion between primary alcoholism with secondary depression and primary affective disorder with secondary alcoholism might be partly resolved with valid and reliable biological diagnostic tests. One possible candidate is the dexamethasone suppression test (DST), which identifies an abnormality in the body's sensitivity to exogenously administered cortisone-like drugs in about 50% of patients with severe primary affective disorders [24]. Unfortunately, heavy doses of alcohol can also disturb cortisol regulation, and as many as a third of alcoholics show abnormal response in the DST, at least during their first 1–4 weeks of abstinence [25–27; unpublished 1984 paper of Castro et al.]. Because alcohol-induced depressions are likely to clear spontaneously within several weeks, an abnormal DST during the first week of abstinence is of little diagnostic importance at the time when such clinical distinctions can be most difficult [5,28–32].

In the following sections of this chapter I will review some of the reasons behind the diagnostic confusion between primary alcoholism and primary affective disorder and present data indicating that these are two separate and distinct psychiatric disorders, with little evidence of genetic overlap. Finally, I offer some thoughts on the clinical implications of these findings.

II. REASONS FOR DIAGNOSTIC CONFUSION

At least five factors contribute to the confusion between alcoholism and affective disorder: (1) alcohol can cause depressive symptoms in anyone, (2) signs of temporary serious depression can follow prolonged drinking, (3) drinking can escalate during primary affective episodes in some patients, especially during mania, (4) depressive symptoms and alcohol problems occur in other psychiatric disorders, and (5) a small proportion of patients have independent alcoholism and affective disorder.

As few as two or three drinks of ethanol are likely to have a biphase effect on mood. During rising blood alcohol concentrations, people are likely to feel stimulated and happy, but when the blood alcohol level is falling these feelings tend to change to sadness and irritability [30–33], problems that may carry over to the next day [34]. The degree of sadness varies with the individual but is likely to be longer lasting and more profound following higher blood alcohol levels and longer periods of drinking. Therefore, even modest doses of alcohol are likely to cause temporary emotional discomfort.

A. Signs of Temporary Serious Depression Can Follow Prolonged Drinking

The exact percentage of alcoholics who experience clinically significant depression during drinking bouts is still debated. This is, in part, because most surveys sample patients who have actually entered treatment, and someone with two symptom patterns (in this case severe alcohol problems and signs of depression) is more likely to seek care than someone with only one problem [35; unpublished 1984 paper of Weissman]. The reported prevalence of depressive symptoms also changes with the diagnostic criteria used: higher rates result when symptom checklists are used systematically than when global impressions are recorded [1]. Also, some studies relate only the presence of depressive symptoms in alcoholics at the time they enter care, while others give histories of significant depression at any time during the alcoholic's clinical course.

In view of all of these methodological problems, it is estimated that between one-quarter and two-thirds of alcoholics have had depressive symptoms severe enough to interfere with functioning during their alcoholic careers. The rate of severe depression during alcoholism is between 30 and 40%, but, when less stringent criteria are applied, the figure may be almost 70% [23,36]. As is true in the population in general, depressive symptoms are probably more likely to be reported by female alcoholics than male alcoholics [27,37; unpublished 1983 paper of Hesselbrock and Hesselbrock]. Regardless of sex, the quality of the depressions seen in the course of heavy drinking can be quite similar to the symptom profile noted during primary affective episodes [14,17,38]. This underscores the conclusion of Martin et al. [15] that phenomenologically defined major depressions are heterogeneous, with diverse prognoses and treatment needs.

Although periods of sadness are common in alcoholics, they do not usually last long enough (i.e., 2–4 weeks) to meet research diagnostic criteria for secondary affective disorder. Accurate documentation of the severity and chronicity of the affective disturbance probably requires face-to-face structured interviews with patients and resource persons. Using this approach in interviews with 577 consecutive male patients along with two relatives for each, another laboratory found that about 30% of the primary alcoholics had at least one secondary affective episode sometime during their heavy drinking years [5,22,29]. Similarly, in a careful community survey [2] almost a third of the alcoholics were found to have experienced affective disorders (perhaps while drinking) at some time in the past.

The results of several prospective studies [39–42; unpublished 1982 paper of Vaillant) are also consistent with the conclusion that, especially for men, the label of primary alcoholism is usually appropriate for alcoholic patients reporting associated depressions; i.e., alcoholism preceds the affective disorder. These investigations did not demonstrate a high prevalence of severe depressions antedating alcoholism, nor were there early-life elevations in the Minnesota Multiphasic Personality Inventory (MMPI) depression subscale in men who later became alcoholics, when compared with control subjects.

Clinical observations of alcoholics with secondary affective disorder indicate that the severe depressions occurring during heavy drinking rarely run the course of primary affective episodes. Although the intensity of symptoms can be severe, the affective disturbances are likely to be transitory, showing greater improvement or disappearance of symptoms within several days or weeks of abstinence [5,28,29,43]. Also, a 4-year follow-up of a group of alcoholics who were able to maintain abstinence [44] showed little evidence of significant depression. Finally, comparisons of alcoholics with and without secondary affective disorders reveal that the former more closely resemble alcoholics than patients with primary affective disorder. This is true for sociodemographic characteristics [10,36,38,45], for family histories of alcoholism [23; unpublished 1984 paper of Weissman], and for early-life social problems as well as for the adult course of alcoholism [3,16,23,36,46,47].

The high rate of depressive symptoms among primary alcoholics has led some authors to question if postabstinence depressions could contribute to the return to drinking [37,48]. A definitive answer to this question will come only through careful longitudinal studies of large numbers of patients, but mood swings are often seen in the months following abstinence. These mood swings, however, are not likely to meet criteria for affective disorder. Even when affective episodes are seen [48], the rate of serious depressions per year must be compared with the rate among an adequate control group to be properly interpreted. Higher-than-expected rates of psychopathology following abstinence, for some patients, may be a consequence of having already returned to drinking. There is little evidence that the occurrence of depressive episodes is a significant direct contributor to the loss of sobriety [37,44,49].

In summary, symptoms of depression are common during heavy drinking, and temporary intense depressions are often seen during the course of alcoholism. For about 90% of the men and women who have symptoms of alcoholism and depression together, the primary diagnosis is alcoholism, not affective disorder [28,50,51]. Several clinical studies [28,29,46,47] have indicated that patients with primary alcoholism and secondary affective disorder more closely resemble alcoholics than patients with primary affective disorder and can be expected to have a clinical course of alcoholism, not major depression. Affective disturbances developing during alcoholism can be severe but are likely to clear within several days or weeks of abstinence alone.

B. Drinking Can Escalate During Primary Affective Episodes

Impaired judgment is often a problem during mania and depression, and some patients with affective disorder change their drinking habits while ill. It is possible that a few patients use alcohol to "self-medicate" their symptoms, taking advantage of the heightened spirits and feelings of relaxation which can be seen during rising blood alcohol levels but paying the price of intensified symptoms when blood levels fall.

An increase in drinking is seen in as many as two of three manic patients [43,52]. However, drinking to the point of actually precipitating some sort of life problems is noted in only about 20%, and labels of secondary alcoholism are justified for only about 5% [53–55]. These data underscore the importance of distinguishing between drinking, temporary alcohol-related problems, and alcoholism.

Only 20–30% of patients with severe depressions escalate their alcohol intake [56]. When criteria for alcoholism are invoked, only 5–10% of depressed patients with primary affective disorder have secondary alcoholism, although the concomitance of the two problem pictures may indicate a worse prognosis for the depressive symptoms [22,50,53,57].

C. Depressive Symptoms and Alcohol Problems Occur in Other Psychiatric Disorders

There are at least four primary psychiatric labels that carry an increased risk for both depression and drinking problems. First, patients with antisocial personality disorder demonstrate a pattern of impulsiveness, difficulty learning from mistakes, and multiple antisocial problems in many life areas beginning at a young age [3,4,17,58,59]. They also have problems moderating behavior, and 60–80% have alcohol-related life problems serious enough for them to be diagnosed as secondary alcoholics [17,59]. The course of antisocial personality disorder also involves frequent temporary affective disturbances, which can precipitate suicide attempts and completions [17,58,60,61]. Patients with primary antisocial personality disorder experiencing alcohol and depressive problems as part of the usual course of their primary problem might be mislabeled as having primary affective disorder or primary alcoholism. However, their prognosis is that of antisocial personality. This adds to the confusion between major depressive episodes and severe, persistent alcohol-related problems.

Second, a similar case can be made for somatization disorder, also called Briquet's disease [22]. This syndrome, diagnosed by the early onset of somatic complaints and conversion symptoms in multiple body systems, is often accompanied by affective disturbances. Fifteen percent or more of patients with somatization disorder may also fulfill criteria for secondary alcoholism [22]. Third, primary drug abusers, especially heroin addicts on methadone, frequently abuse alcohol as a substitute for their primary drug and (with or without concomitant alcohol abuse) are also likely show depressive disturbances [62,63]. Finally, many individuals with characterological depression relate histories of alcohol misuse [64], adding to an already confusing picture.

Each of these four primary disorders has a different course and distinct treatment needs. Although patients with these disorders often develop alcohol problems and depressive symptoms, they do not usually have the prognosis of alcoholism or primary affective disorder.

D. A Small Proportion of Patients Have Independent Alcoholism and Affective Disorder

In the absence of valid and reliable biological tests, the establishment of primary and secondary labels rests with gathering the best historical information possible. Unfortunately, the system is not perfect. Until a better approach is developed, primary and secondary disorders are distinguished by the chronology of development of symptoms or notation of the most severe or incapacitating disorder. Even after interviewing patients and resource persons it can still be difficult to detect the simultaneous onset of two illnesses. By definition, therefore, with our present approach it can be problematical to determine that a patient has two primary illnesses. Because so many secondary psychiatric syndromes are seen in the course of substance abuse, this problem can be especially important for these disorders [4,17,38].

Alcoholism and affective disorder are among the most prevalent disorders in the general population and in groups in treatment [2; unpublished 1984 paper of Weissman]. Unless the presence of one primary illness protects a patient from developing a second problem, it is likely that at least 5–10% of the patients who have primary affective disorder could also have alcoholism—they have the same risk for alcoholism as the general population. According to this logic, the approximately 10% risk for primary alcoholism multiplied by the roughly 10% risk for major affective disorder would indicate that about 1% of the population might really have both illnesses independently.

Compounding the problem is the possibility that there could be assortative mating between patients with alcoholism and those with affective disturbances. If, for example, alcoholic men were more likely to marry women with psychiatric disorders, including affective disorder, than women from the general population, the children of these parents could be at elevated risk for both problems. Consistent with this contention are data generated by a group of scientists at Yale. They found that although the overall rate of affective disorders in first-degree relatives of primary alcoholics was not significantly higher than that of the general population, alcoholics who showed both alcoholism and affective disorder themselves were significantly more likely than other alcoholics to have first-degree relatives with affective disorder as well as first-degree relatives with alcoholism [16; unpublished 1984 paper of Weissman].

In summary, it is likely that at least 5–10% of alcoholics have independent affective disorder. At various times these men and women could develop temporary depressions secondary to heavy drinking, as well as more persistent affective episodes both when abusing alcohol and when abstinent. Limitations in our present diagnostic methods make it difficult to identify these people. Therefore, the careful clinician must be alert for the small percent of patients who appear to have primary alcoholism but whose affective disturbances do not remit after 2 or more weeks of abstinence. It is also necessary to identify those alcoholics who develop severe depressive disorders during periods of nondrinking. Although there are no data on the best treatment for these men and women, it makes sense that they may require the same therapies that are appropriate for any major or minor primary affective disorder.

Thus, in this section I have demonstrated that there are many reasons for the present confusion between alcoholism and affective disorder. These problems can be minimized, however, if clinicians and researchers carefully distinguish between symptoms and diagnoses and do their best to identify the primary illness.

III. LACK OF GENETIC RELATIONSHIP

Both alcoholism and the major affective disorders are genetically influenced [40,65]. The risk of depressive disorder in close relatives of patients with primary affective disorder is 20%, compared with 5–10% for the general population [66], and at least six twin studies carried out since 1930 show an affective disorder concordance of about 70% for identical twins and 15% for fraternal twins [67]. In addition, several adoption studies [19,68] concluded that there is an increased risk for affective disorder in adopted-away children of affectively ill biological parents, a rate that is not changed by the presence of affective illness in the adoptive parents.

Many studies support the importance of genetic factors in alcoholism. The familial nature of this disorder is amply documented [69]. as is the higher alcoholism concordance rate for identical than for fraternal twins [70], although one 1984 paper [71] disagreed. Adoption studies have revealed a fourfold increased risk for alcoholism in the adopted sons and daughters of alcoholics compared with adopted children of control subjects, with no evidence that being reared by an alcoholic adoptive parent further increases the risk [65,72,73].

There are some reasons to ask of alcoholism and affective disorder might be genetically related to each other [74,75]. First, alcoholism is more often seen in men and affective disorder is more prevalent in women [74; unpublished 1984 paper of Weissman], leading Winokur et al. [74] to raise the possibility that they may represent a single disorder with different manifestations in the two sexes. Supporting this conclusion are reports that there may be an increased rate of alcoholism among male relatives of women with affective disorder and an increased risk of depressive episodes in female relatives of male alcoholics [43,74].

If a true genetic relationship exists, one would expect a consistent increased prevalence of the second illness in relatives of patients with the first disorder [unpublished 1984 paper of Weissman]. However, there is a disagreement about elevated risks for affective disorder in relatives of primary alcoholics. Several investigations from our own laboratory [5,23,29] have shown no higher prevalence of carefully defined affective disorder in first-degree relatives of alcoholics, and Goodwin et al. [72] reported no higher rate of affective disorder in adopted-away sons of alcoholics. Goodwin et al. [76] found a trend for an increased risk for depressive disorder among daughters of alcoholics, but this occurred only if they had been reared by an alcoholic adoptive parent. It is also possible that some cases of affective disorder in relatives of alcoholics may reflect situational sadness in the spouse and/or affective disorder in the spouse's family through assortative mating.

The other side of the question is even clearer. Although some studies have reported an increase in alcoholism among relatives of patients with affective disorder (especially if their depressive illness had an early onset) [77–79], most have found no close relationship. At least two groups of investigators [57,80] have noted no increased risk for alcoholism in families of manic depressive (bipolar) patients, and others [22,81] have reported that the risk for alcoholism in close relatives of unipolar patients is no higher than for normal control subjects. In a series of studies of probands in the general population, Weissman et al. [13; unpublished 1984 paper] reported the prevalence of illness in 2003 first-degree relatives of 335 probands with major depressive disorders of bipolar illness. Although alcoholism was noted in about 8% of close relatives of control subjects, it was seen in only 6–12% of relatives of people with various types of affective disorders. The only patients with major affective disorder likely to have alcoholic parents, siblings, or children appear to be those who themselves show secondary alcoholism, although not all authors agree even with this [53; unpublished 1984 paper of Weissman]. Supporting the conclusion that affective disorder and alcoholism are genetically distinct problems are studies by Angst [82] and by Cloninger et al. [83]. The latter concluded that although the relationship is complex, the two disorders appear to aggregate in different families and show little evidence of genetic linkage.

It is still possible that there is an association between the two disorders within some subtypes of affective disorders or that the two problems may be genetically linked in some families but not in others. One important subgroup of patients with affective disorder could be those with depressive spectrum disease: individuals distinguished by the presence of close family members with alcoholism or antisocial personality disorder as well as, perhaps, relatives with depression [84–87]. However, a major problem with the concept of depressive spectrum disease is the heterogeneous nature of the sample outlined. Combining together into one subgroup patients who have relatives with antisocial personality disorder and patients who have alcoholic relatives may be ill-advised because these two disorders are probably not genetically linked and do not have similar prognoses [83,88; unpublished 1982 paper by Vaillant]. In another approach, Akiskal et al. [64,89] proposed a spectrum of personality problems, some subgroups of which are likely to have both alcohol problems and incapacitating affective symptoms. This might be another example of severe sadness and alcohol problems occurring as a complication of a third illness.

In summary, there is little consistent evidence supporting an increased risk for alcoholism in the relatives of patients with primary affective disorder. A similar answer probably applies to the risk for serious affective distrubances in the relatives of primary alcoholics, but the data are less conclusive. The findings from adoption studies, however, taken together with the other evidence presented in this section, do not support a close genetic association between primary alcoholism and primary major affective disorder.

IV. IMPLICATIONS FOR TREATMENT AND FUTURE RESEARCH

The general conclusion of this review is that alcoholism and affective disorder are probably distinct illnesses with different prognoses and treatments. However, symptoms of depression are likely to develop in the course of alcoholism, and some patients with affective disorder increase their drinking when ill, with perhaps 5–10% fulfilling criteria for secondary alcoholism.

While the following thoughts use the available data to generate some clinically useful suggestions, the incomplete nature of the information outlined above must be stressed; there is much important research yet to be done. Work in our laboratory has focused on the primary/secondary diagnostic approach based on chronology, but the usefulness of other attempts to establish a hierarchy of concomitant clinical syndromes must also be explored in future research. In addition, the emphasis on searching for relatively pure groups with either affective disorder or alcoholism ignores potentially important clinical subgroups with less distinctive pictures (e.g., patients with personality disorders). Finally, in placing the comments into perspective the reader must recognize that although I have emphasized careful descriptions of symptoms and their time course, social and psychological factors that might cluster within families and contribute to the overlap between depression and alcohol problems [16] are also potentially important. Despite all those caveats, we can begin to look at the clinical implications of what we do know.

First, the mood-disturbing properties of alcohol indicate that patients with major affective disorder should not drink when ill. This conclusion is strengthened by the potentially dangerous pharmacological interactions between ethanol and antidepressant medications or lithium [90; unpublished 1984 paper of Subhan and Hindmarch).

Second, the majority of primary alcoholics have severe mood swings in the course of active drinking, and for perhaps 20–30% this disturbance may last long enough to be labeled secondary affective disorder. Even short-lived depressions in actively drinking alcoholics must be taken seriously because there is a 10–15% risk of suicide completion during alcoholism [91]. There are also some data to indicate that, no matter which disorder is primary, the concomitant appearance of alcohol problems and depressed mood may identify patients with exceptionally high suicide risk [15,91]. The presence of two problems might also increase the chance for relapse for both [unpublished 1984 paper of Weissman]. Therefore, all alcoholics should be asked about depressive symptoms and suicidal ideas, and those with the latter may require hospitalization until the suicidal thoughts disappear. The overlap between depressive symptoms and alcohol problems is so great that Weissman [unpublished 1984 paper] advised clinicians always to look carefully for the second problem when a patient presents either one.

Third, the ideas presented in this paper raise the question of the appropriate use of antidepressants or lithium in patients with primary alcohol abuse and secondary affective disorders. Unfortunately, there is still much debate in the literature on these issues. Studies are made difficult by the usual delay between beginning medication and achieving maximal clinical effects as well as by the trend for substance-associated affective disorders to clear spontaneously within several weeks of abstinence. In addition, many alcoholics have significant organ damage, including cardiac abnormalities, and the careful clinician is hesitant to administer antidepressants or lithium to such patients unless there are clear justifications for doing so.

The data on lithium are of interest and show some potential promise. Pharmacologically, this drug may help alcoholics by attenuating the euphoria incurred during drinking [92]. Also, several small controlled studies [93,94] indicated that, compared with alcoholics given placebo, lithium-treated alcoholics may be more likely to decrease their drinking and require fewer hospital admissions on follow-up. The drug might be especially useful in alcoholics who still demonstrate severe mood impairments after 3–4 weeks of abstinence [94]. Unfortunately, not all studies are in agreement about efficacy, a majority of patients who start taking lithium may not take the drug regularly, and there are potential dangers if a patient on lithium should return to drinking and subsequently change his or her salt intake or develop nausea, vomiting, or diarrhea. Until more data are generated, it is probably unwise to give lithium to the average primary alcoholic.

A literature review reveals even less evidence that tricyclic antidepressants are appropriate to deal with the affective disturbances in the average primary alcoholic, nor is there much evidence that these drugs help prevent a return to active drinking [95,96]. Although results from uncontrolled studies have been promising, careful comparison of outcome following administration of tricyclics versus placebo do not indicate any treatment efficacy for the active drug in primary alcoholism. Further research is justified by animal studies [97] indicating that some of these agents might attenuate drinking in rodents. Until more data to the contrary are generated, however, these drugs have little place in the treatment of the usual primary alcoholic.

Fourth, patients with major affective disorders who demonstrate severe, persistent alcohol problems may require alcohol detoxification and should be carefully evaluated for concomitant medical problems that might have been caused or exacerbated by the alcohol. It might also be advisable to consider alcoholism rehabilitation for such patients, if only because concomitant drinking is likely to worsen the affective disturbances and interfere with effective treatment. In other words, when alcohol and affective problems coexist, the careful clinician must evaluate the possibility that both problems need to be addressed.

Finally, the small number of alcoholic patients demonstrating severe affective disturbances unrelated to their heavy drinking or whose major depressive episodes persist after 2 or 3 weeks of abstinence may have two independent disorders. It is also possible that these people may have been misdiagnosed as alcoholics and might require lithium (for bipolar illness) or other antidepressant medications [94]. These men and women can be best identified by gathering a careful history and by monitoring their clinical course.

All of the recommendations made in this section are empirical. I hope that the future will bring more intensive research into the natural history and optimal treatment of primary alcoholics with secondary depression and patients with primary affective disorder and secondary alcoholism. In any such work, however, it will be necessary to control carefully for the possible importance of different definitions of illness; the impact of outpatient versus inpatient versus general population case-finding techniques; the time since last drink; and the possible effect of withdrawal symptoms, the history of use of drugs other than alcohol, socioeconomic factors, and so on.

Future research might address the neurochemical and psychological mechanisms of depression seen during heavy drinking and examine why only a minority of alcoholics develop affective disturbances severe enough to fulfill criteria for secondary affective disorder. Because the depression that occurs during heavy drinking can look identical to an episode of primary affective disorder, it may be possible to exploit this clinical picture as a model for studying affective disorder. The biochemical indexes and electrophysiological patterns observed in alcoholics with secondary depressions may help us to better understand the pathophysiology of major affective disorder. Finally, it is also possible to look forward to the day when new research tools, such as restriction gene mapping [unpublished 1984 paper of Kidd et al.], can help us to use trait markers to better distinguish between primary alcoholism and primary affective disorder.

ACKNOWLEDGMENTS

Supported by grants 05526 and 04353 from the National Institute on Alcohol and Alcohol Abuse and by the Veterans Administration Research Service.
The author thanks Cristiana Motet-Gregorias for help in preparing the manuscript.

REFERENCES

1. Weissman, M.M., Meyers, J.K., and Harding, P.S. Psychiatric disorders in a U.S. urban community: 1975–1976. *Am. J. Psychiatry, 135*:459–462 (1978).
2. Weissman, M.M., Meyers, J.K., and Harding, P.S. Prevalence and psychiatric heterogeneity of alcoholism in a U.S. urban community. *J. Stud. Alcohol, 41*:672–681 (1980).
3. Goodwin, D.W., Guze, S.B. *Psychiatric Diagnosis*, 3rd ed. Oxford University Press, New York, 1984.
4. Schuckit, M.A. *Drug and Alcohol Abuse: Clinical Guide to Diagnosis and Treatment*. Plenum, New York, 1984.
5. Schuckit, M.A. The clinical implications of primary diagnostic groups among alcoholics. *Arch. Gen. Psychiatry, 42*:1043–1049 (1985).
6. Haglund, R.M.J., Schuckit, M.A. The epidemiology of alcoholism, *Alcoholism: Development, Consequences, and Interventions*. N.J. Estes and M.E. Heinemann (eds.). Mosby, New York, 1982.
7. Cahalan, D., Cisin, I.H. American drinking practices: summary of findings from a national probability sample. *Q. J. Stud. Alcohol, 29*:130–151 (1968).
8. Fillmore, K.M. Relationships between specific drinking problems in early adulthood and middle age. *J. Stud. Alcohol, 36*:892–907 (1975).
9. Moses, L.E., Emersons, J.D., and Hosseini, H. Analyzing data from ordered categories. *N. Engl. J. Med., 311*:442–448 (1984).
10. Winokur, G. Family history studies, VIII: secondary depression is alive and well, and . . . . *Dis. Nerv. Syst., 33*:94–99 (1984).
11. Guze, S.B., Woodruff, R.A., and Clayton, P.J. Secondary affective disorders: a study of 95 cases. *Psychol. Med., 1*:426–428 (1971).
12. Winokur, G. Types of depressive illness. *Br. J. Psychiatry, 120*:265–266 (1972).
13. Weissman, M.M., Gershon, E.S., Kidd, K.K., et al. Psychiatric disorders in the relatives of probands with affective disorders. *Arch. Gen. Psychiatry, 41*:13–21 (1984).
14. Schuckit, M.A. Alcoholism and affective disorderr: Diagnostic confusion, in *Alcoholism and Affective Disorders*. D.W. Goodwin and C.K. Erickson (eds.). SP Medical and Scientific Books, New York, 1979.
15. Martin, R.I., Cloninger, C.R., and Guze, S.B. Alcohol misuse and depression in women criminals. *J. Stud. Alcohol, 46*:65–71 (1985).
16. Menkangas, K.R., Leckman, J.R., Prusott, B.A. et al. Familial transmission of depression and alcoholism. *Arch. Gen. Psychiatry, 42*:367–372 (1985).
17. Schuckit, M.A. Alcoholism and other psychiatric disorders. *Hosp. Community Psychiatry, 34*:1022–1027 (1983).
18. Weissman, M.M., and Klerman, G.L. Sex difference and the epidemiology of depression. *Arch. Gen. Psychiatry, 34*:98–111 (1977).
19. Schuckit, M.A. Trait (and state) markers of a predisposition to psychopathology, *Psychiatry*, Vol. 3. L.L. Judd and P. Groves (eds.). Lippincott, Philadelphia, 1985.
20. Goodwin, D.W., Alderson, P., and Rosenthal, R. Clinical significance of hallucinations in psychiatric disorders. *Arch. Gen. Psychiatry, 24*:76–80 (1971).
21. Schuckit, M.A. The history of psychotic symptoms in alcoholics. *J. Clin. Psychiatry, 45*:53–57 (1982).
22. Lewis, C.E., Helzer, J., Cloninger, C.R. et al. Psychiatric diagnostic predispositions to alcoholism. *Compr. Psychiatry, 23*:451–461 (1982).
23. Schuckit, M.A. Alcoholic patients with secondary depression. *Am. J. Psychiatry, 140*:711–714 (1983).

24. Carroll, B.J., Feinberg, M., Greden, J.F., et al. A specific laboratory test for the diagnosis of melancholia: standardization, validation, and clinical utility. *Arch. Gen. Psychiatry, 38*:15–22 (1981).
25. Dackis, C.A., Bailey, J., Pottash, A.L.C. et al. Specificity of the DST and the TRH test for major depression in alcoholics. *Am. J. Psychiatry, 141*:680–683 (1984).
26. de La Fuente, J.R., Rosenbaum, A.H., Morse, R.M., et al. The hypothalamic-pituitary-adrenal axis in alcoholics. *Alcoholism Clin. Exp. Res., 7*:35–37 (1983).
27. Newsom, G., and Murray, N. Reversal of dexamethasone suppression test nonsuppression in alcohol abusers. *Am. J. Psychiatry, 140*:353–354 (1983).
28. Schuckit, M.A. A short-term follow up of women alcoholics. *Dis. Nerv. Syst., 33*:672–678 (1972).
29. Schuckit, M.A., Zisook, S., and Mortola, J. Clinical implications of DSM-III diagnoses for alcohol abuse and alcohol dependence. *Am. J. Psychiatry, 142*:1403–1408 (1985).
30. Gibson, S., and Becker, J. Changes in alcoholics' self-reported depression. *Q. J. Stud. Alcohol, 34*:829–836 (1973).
31. Mayfield, D.G. Psychopharmacology of alcohol: affective change with intoxication, drinking behavior, and affective state. *J. Nerv. Ment. Dis., 146*:314–321 (1968).
32. Mayfield, D.G. Psychopharmacology of alcohol: affective tolerance in alcohol intoxication. *J. Nerv. Ment. Dis., 146*:322–327 (1968).
33. Tamerin, J.S., Weiner, S., and Mendelson, J.H. Alcoholics' expectancies and recall of experiences during intoxication. *Am. J. Psychiatry, 126*:1697–1704 (1970).
34. Birnbaum, I., Taylor, T., and Parker, E. Alcohol and sober mood state in female social drinkers. *Alcoholism Clin. Exp. Res., 7*:362–368 (1983).
35. Berkson, J. Limitations of the application of the 4-fold table analysis to hospital data. *Biometrics, 2*:47–53 (1946).
36. Cadoret, R., and Winokur, G. Depression in alcoholism. *Ann. N.Y. Acad. Sci., 233*:34–39 (1974).
37. Hatsukami, D., and Pickens, R.W. Posttreatment depression in an alcohol and drug abuse population. *Am. J. Psychiatry, 139*:1563–1566 (1982).
38. Weissman, M.M., Pottenger, M., Kleber, H. et al. Symptoms patterns in primary and secondary depression. *Arch. Gen. Psychiatry, 34*:854–862 (1977).
39. Kammeier, M., Hoffman, H., and Loper, R. Personality characteritics of alcoholics as college freshmen and at the time of treatment. *Q. J. Stud. Alcohol, 34*:390–399 (1973).
40. Schuckit, M.A. Studies of populations at high risk for alcoholism. *Psychiatry Dev., 3*:31–63 (1985).
41. McCord, J. Alcoholism and criminality. *J. Stud. Alcohol, 42*:739–748 (1981).
42. Vaillant, G. The etiology of alcoholism. *Am. Psychol., 37*:494–503 (1982).
43. Liskow, B., Mayfield, D., and Thiele, J. Alcohol and affective disorder: assessment and treatment. *J. Clin. Psychiatry, 43*:144–147 (1982).
44. Pettinati, H.M. Sugerman, A.A., and Maurer, H.S. Four year MMPI changes in abstinent and drinking alcoholics. *Alcoholism Clin. Exp. Res., 6*:487–494 (1982).
45. Woodruff, R.J., Jr., Murphy, G.E., Herjanie, M. The natural history of affective disorders, I: symptoms of 72 patients at the time of index hospital admission. *J. Psychiatr. Res., 5*:255–263 (1967).
46. Woodruff, R.A., Guze, S.B., Clayton, P.J. et al. Alcoholism and depression, *Alcoholism and Affective Disorders*. D.W. Goodwin and C.K. Erickson (eds.). SP Medical & Scientific Books, New York, 1079.
47. Woodruff, R.A., Guze, S.B., Clayton, P.J. et al. Alcoholism and depression. *Arch. Gen. Psychiatry, 28*:97–100 (1973).
48. Behar, D., Winokur, G., and Berg, C.J. Depression in the abstinent alcoholic. *Am. J. Psychiatry, 141*:1105–1107 (1984).
49. Polich, J.M., Armor, D.J., and Braiker, H.B. *The Course of Alcoholism: Four Years After Treatment*. Santa Monica, California, Rand Corp., 1980.
50. Keller, M.B., Lavon, P.E., Lewis, C.E. et al. Predictors of relapse in major depressive disorder. *J.A.M.A., 250*:3299–3304 (1983).
51. O'Sullivan, K., Willans, P., Daly, M., et al. A comparison of alcoholics with and without co-existing affective disorder. *Br. J. Psychiatry, 143*:133–138 (1983).

52. Morrison, J.R. Bipolar affective disorder and alcoholism. *Am. J. Psychiatry, 131*:1130–1133 (1974).

53. Dunner, D.L., Hensel, B.M., and Fieve, R.R. Bipolar illness: factors in drinking behavior. *Am. J. Psychiatry, 136*:583–585 (1979).

54. Sherfey, M.J. Psychopathology and character structure in chronic alcoholism, *Etiology of Chronic Alcoholism*. E. Diethelm (ed.). Thomas, Springfield, Illinois, 1962.

55. Stenstedt, A. A study in manic-depressive psychoses. *Acta. Psychiatr. Neurol. Scand.* (Suppl.)*79*:3–11, 1952.

56. Mayfield, D.G. Alcohol and affect: experimental studies, *Alcoholism and Affective Disorders*. D.W. Goodwin and C.K. Erickson (eds.). SP Medical & Scientific Books, New York, 1979.

57. Robins, E., Gentry, K.A., Munoz, R.A. et al. A contrast of the three more common illnesses with the ten less common in a study and 18-month follow-up of 14 psychiatric emergency room patients, II: Characteristics of patients with the three ore common illnesses. *Arch. Gen. Psychiatry, 34*:269–281 (1977).

58. Robins, L.N. Sturdy childhood predictors of adult antisocial behavior. *Psychol. Med., 8*:611–622 (1978).

59. Schuckit, M.A. Alcoholism and sociopathy—diagnostic confusion. *Q. J. Stud. Alcohol, 34*:157–164 (1973).

60. Maddocks, P.D. A five year follow-up of untreated psychopaths. *Br. J. Psychiatry, 116*:511–516 (1970).

61. Robins, L.N. *Deviant Children Grown Up*. Williams & Wilkins, Baltimore, 1966.

62. Green, J., and Jaffe, J.H. Alcohol and opiate dependence. *J. Stud. Alcohol, 38*:1274–1293 (1977).

63. Moore, J.T., Judd, L.L., Zung, W.W.K. et al. Opiate addiction and suicidal behaviors. *Am. J. Psychiatry, 136*:1187–1189 (1979).

64. Akiskal, H.S., Rosenthal, T.L., Gatjak, R.F., et al. Characterological depressions: clinical and sleep EEG findings separating "subaffective dysthymias" from "character spectrum disorders." *Arch. Gen. Psychiatry, 37*:777–783 (1980).

65. Schuckit, M.A. Genetic and biochemical factors in the etiology of alcoholism, *Psychiatry Update: The American Psychiatric Association Annual Review*, Vol. III. L. Grinspoon (ed.). American Psychiatric Press, Washington, D.C. 1984.

66. Gershon, E.S., Bunney, W.E., Jr., Leckman, J.F., et al. The inheritance of affective disorders: A review of data and of hypotheses. *Behav. Genet. 6*:227–261 (1976).

67. Gershon, E.S., Targum, S.D., Kessler, L.R., et al. Genetic studies and biologic strategies in the affective disorders. *Prog. Med. Genet., 2*:101–164 (1977).

68. von Knorring, A.L., Cloninger, C.R., Bohman, M., et al. An adoption study of depressive disorders and substance abuse. *Arch. Gen. Psychiatry, 40*:943–950 (1983).

69. Cotton, N.S. The familial incidence of alcoholism: a review. *J. Stud. Alcohol, 40*:89–116 (1979).

70. Kaij, I. *Studies on the Etiology and Sequelae of Abuse of Alcohol*. University of Lund Department of Psychiatry, Sweden, 1960.

71. Gurling, H.M. Genetic epidemiology in medicine—recent twin research. *Br. Med. J., 288*:3–5 (1984).

72. Goodwin, D.W., Schulsinger, F., Hermansen, L., et al. Alcohol problems in adoptees raised apart from alcoholic biological parents. *Arch. Gen. Psychiatry, 28*:238–243 (1973).

73. Bohman, M., Sigvardsson, S., and Cloninger, R. Maternal inheritance of alcohol abuse. *Arch. Gen. Psychiatry, 38*:965–969 (1981).

74. Winokur, G., Retch, T., Rimmer, J., et al. Alcoholism, III: Diagnosis and familial psychiatric illness in 259 alcoholic probands. *Arch. Gen. Psychiatry, 23*:104–111 (1970).

75. Winokur, G. Alcoholism and depression. *Subst. Alcohol Actions Misuse, 4*:111–119 (1983).

76. Goodwin, D., Schulsinger, F., Knop, J., et al. Psychopathology in adopted and non-adopted daughters of alcoholics. *Arch. Gen. Psychiatry, 34*:1005–1009 (1977).

77. Winokur, G., and Clayton, P. Family history studies, II: Sex differences and alcoholism in primary affective illness. *Br. J. Psychiatry, 113*:973–979 (1967).

78. Winokur, G., Cadoret, R., Dorzab, J., et al. Depressive disease: a genetic study. *Arch. Gen. Psychiatry, 24*:135–144 (1971).

79. Angst, J. Genetic aspectsd of depression, *Depressive Illness*. P. Kielholz (ed.). Hans Huber, Berne, 1972.
80. James, J., and Chapman, C. A genetic study of bipolar affective disorder. *Br. J. Psychiatry, 126*:449–456 (1975).
81. Gershon, E.S., Hamovit, J., Guroff, J.J., et al. A family study of schizoaffective, bipolar I, bipolar II unipolar, and normal control probands. *Arch. Gen. Psychiatry, 39*:1157–1167 (1982).
82. Angst, J. *Zur Aetiologie und Nosologie endogener depressiver Psychosen*. Springer-Verlag, Berlin, 1966.
83. Cloninger, C.R., Reich, T., and Wetzel, R. Alcoholism and affective disorders: familial associations and genetic models, *Alcoholism and Affective Disorders: Clinical, Genetic, and Biochemical Studies*. D.W. Goodwin and C.K. Erickson (eds.). SP Medical & Scientific Books, New York, 1979.
84. Behar, D., Winokur, G., Van Valkenberg, C., et al. Familial subtypes of depression: a clinicl view. *J. Clin. Psychiatry, 41*:52–56 (1980).
85. Winokur, G., Morrison, J., Clancy, J., et al. The Iowa 500: familial and clinical findings favor two kinds of depressive illness. *Compr. Psychiatry, 14*:99–106 (1973).
86. Winokur, G., Cadoret, R., Baker, M., et al. Depression spectrum disease versus pure depressive disease: some further data. *Br. J. Psychiatry, 127*:75–77 (1975).
87. Winokur, G. Unipolar depression: is it divisible into autonomous subtypes? *Arch. Gen. Psychiatry, 36*:47–52 (1979).
88. Crowe, R.R. An adoption study of antisocial personality. *Arch. Gen. Psychiatry, 31*:785–791 (1974).
89. Akiskal, H.S., Hirschfeld, R.M.A., and Yerevanian, B.I. The relationship of personality to affective disorders. *Arch. Gen. Psychiatry, 40*:801–810 (1983).
90. Knoben, J.E., and Anderson, P.O. *Handbook of Clinical Drug Data*, 5th ed. Drug Intelligence Pub., Hamilton, Illinois, 1983, pp. 109–127.
91. Berglund, M. Suicide in alcoholism. *Arch. Gen. Psychiatry, 41*:888–894 (1984).
92. Judd, L.L., Hubbard, R.B., Huey, L.Y., et al. Lithium carbonate and ethanol induced "high" in normal subjects. *Arch. Gen. Psychiatry, 34*:463–467 (1977).
93. Kline, N.S., Wren, J.C., Cooper, T.B., et al. Evaluation of lithium therapy in chronic and periodic alcoholism. *Am. J. Med. Sci., 268*:15–22 (1974).
94. Merry, J., Reynolds, C., Bailey, J., et al. Prophylactic treatment of alcoholism by lithium carbonate. *Lancet, 2*:481–482 (1976).
95. Halikas, J.A. Psychotropic medication used in the treatment of alcoholism. *Hosp. Commun. Psychiatry, 34*:1035–1039 (1983).
96. Viamontes, J.A. Review of drug effectiveness in the treatment of alcoholism. *Am. J. Psychiatry, 128*:1570–1571 (1972).
97. Daoust, M., Saligaut, C., Chaldelaud, M., et al. Attenuation by antidepressant drugs of alcohol intake in rats. *Alcohol, 1*:379–383 (1984).

X
Neurochemistry

40

A Neuroanatomical and Neurochemical Approach to Drug and Alcohol Addiction: Clinical and Research Considerations

Norman S. Miller
Cornell University Medical College, New York Hospital–Cornell Medical Center, White Plains, New York

Mark S. Gold
Fair Oaks Hospital, Summit, New Jersey, and Delray Beach, Florida

I. HISTORY

A. Confusion in Terms

Confusion surrounds the definitions and uses of the concepts of tolerance, dependence, and addiction to alcohol and drugs. Although in standard medical texts the definitions appear relatively straightforward, the relationship between them is not nearly as clear [1,2].

This confusion is a result of a number of factors. The first is a lack of definitive knowledge regarding alcohol and drug addiction. The term *addiction* is largely a descriptive one. The terms *tolerance* and *dependence* have firm physiological foundations. The second factor is that personalized usage, additions, and subtractions by both specialists and laymen have led to misleading alterations and misconceptions for these terms.

The third factor is that various disciplines have different criteria for establishing tolerance and dependence and defining addiction. Psychologists and behavioralists describe these phenomena as certain observable behaviors. Physiologists record measurable variables such as blood pressure, pulse, and brain wave activity. Clinicians determine the meaning of these terms through the acquisition of historical information and the clinical relevance is judged. The fourth factor is that the relevance of tolerance and dependence to the clinical course and prognosis of drug addiction is not well understood [2].

A neurochemical approach for defining addiction, tolerance, and dependence may be helpful in clarifying the confusion. The following discussion is an attempt to provide a model or models for a uniform basis for considering neurochemical addiction, tolerance, and dependence to alcohol and drugs. The models are in part speculative and derived from available, current neuroanatomical and neurochemical concepts underlying brain function.

II. DIAGNOSIS

A. Definition of Alcohol and Drug Addiction

Alcohol or drug addiction may be defined by three major behavioral characteristics: (1) preoccupation with the acquisition of alcohol or a drug, (2) compulsive use, and (3) relapse [1,3]. Pervasive to the three requisites is the phenomena of loss of control. The World Health Organization (WHO) concludes that the cardinal manifestation of addiction is loss of control of the use of a particular substance. The definition proposed by WHO for a drug dependence syndrome is a cluster of cognitive, behavioral, and physiological phenomena that include a compulsion, desire to stop, a stereotypical drug-taking habit, evidence of tolerance and withdrawal, use of drug to alleviate withdrawal symptoms, high priority of drug-seeking behavior, and rapid reinstatement of the syndrome after a period of abstinence. These criteria are essentially similar to the definition of drug addiction. Tolerance and dependence are additional concepts that may or may not be important in drug-seeking behavior [4]. These behaviors of addiction do not necessarily, but probably do, imply a physiological basis. Our inadequate methods of measurement and disagreement regarding what to measure make elucidation of the neurochemical variables difficult [2].

Preoccupation

Preoccupation with the acquisition of a drug suggests that the drug has a high priority in the user's mental and affective states [5]. The drug occupies a central importance in the addict's life; in a hierarchy of priorities, the acquisition of the drug ranks at or near the zenith. Even drive states such as hunger, sex, and survival may become subordinated and sacrificed for the pursuit of the drug or alcohol.

Compulsion

Compulsivity is often, but not always, indicated by regular and frequent use. More significant is that the use of a particular drug continues in the presence of the untoward consequences. Compulsivity is dramatically illustrated when the addict uses a drug in spite of compelling reasons to abstain. It is critical to recognize that the individual is using a drug because of its addictive nature, and not because of its consequences. The consequences are the result of and not the cause of the compulsive use [5]. The consequences are often psychological, such as anxiety, depression, and disturbed interpersonal relationships. The major areas of the addict's interpersonal life which are affected adversely as a result of the addiction, include family, friends, employment, and legal.

Relapse

Relapse is an informative criterion, as addicts can and often do discontinue their drug use for varying periods of time. The rule, and not the exception, is that there are periods of abstinence intermingled with prolonged abnormal drug use. If an accurate corroborative history can be obtained, the time for drug use is often greater than admitted by the addicts. The true episodic, or binge user, is not as common as may appear by clinical histories for the same reasons of denial. Relapse is a state in which there is a voluntary return to drug and alcohol use, or regardless of conscious resolve and apparent commitment to abstain, the addict inexplicably returns to the use of alcohol or drugs. This relapse often occurs without apparent recollection, or at least a defiant disregard of the aversive consequences of the drug use in the past [6].

B. Physiological Basis for Tolerance and Dependence to Alcohol and Drugs

Alcohol

Although a physiological basis for addiction to drugs and alcohol almost certainly exists, the underlying neurochemical events have not been fully elucidated. Alcohol and drugs clearly do initiate addictive behavior. The interaction between the drug and brain is most likely responsible for the initiation of the addictive process [7]. Subsequent and sequential neurochemical communications and changes ensue for the development of the actual addictive process. The mechanism of action for alcohol is to disturb the membrane fluidity of the cells. Ethanol acutely disorders the membranes to make them more fluid [8,9]. The development of tolerance is manifesed by changes in the brain neuronal membranes to a less fluid or more rigid form [10–12,13,14–18]. This adaptive change in membrane fluidity is to maintain homeostasis for normal physiological functioning in the presence of the drug. Behavioral tolerance correlates with the development of the adaptive change in membrane fluidity [13].

Cocaine

Cocaine addiction may serve as a model for neurotransmitter changes in the development of addiction. A major pharmacodynamic effect of cocaine is to block the reuptake of dopamine into the presynaptic neuron [19]. Reuptake is a major mechanism for termination of dopamine action. Degradation by intraneuronal enzymes and uptake into storage vessels are the subsequent routes of elimination for dopamine. If reuptake is prevented, then greater concentrations of dopamine remain in the synaptic cleft and more dopamine is available at the postsynaptic site for stimulation of specific receptors in the cell membrane. Many of the signs and symptoms produced by cocaine can be attributed to the enhanced dopaminergic activity that results from the increased dopamine-receptor interaction. Mood, appetite, thought (delusions) and perceptual disturbances (hallucinations), and increased mental and motor activity are subserved by dopamine neurons [20].

Tolerance that develops to the signs and symptoms produced by cocaine in the intoxicated state is accompanied by these adaptive changes in the neurons in the central nervous system. Dependence is manifested by signs and symptoms opposite to those to which tolerance is developed to the presence of cocaine and a reversal of the neuroadaptive changes. Cocaine can produce euphoria, insomnia, anorexia, delusions and hallucinations, and increased mental and motor activity to which tolerance develops. Withdrawal from cocaine is marked by depression, hypersomnolence, hyperphagia, and slowness of mental and motor activity [21,22]. Depletion of dopamine from storage sites and a reduction in subsequent release from presynaptic neurons may occur in the development of tolerance during chronic cocaine usage. The dopamine agonist bromocriptine can reverse or prevent the onset of these withdrawal syndromes that result from development of cocaine dependence [23]. The suppression of withdrawal symptoms by bromocriptine suggests that dopamine depletion is operative in the development of dependence.

C. Tolerance and Dependence as Criteria for Alcohol and Drug Addiction

Connection Between Tolerance, Dependence, and Addiction

The connection between tolerance and dependence and addiction is controversial. Tolerance and dependence to narcotics, and even to alcohol, can occur without developing addictive behavior. Larger doses may be required to achieve the same effect and a predictable withdrawal syndrome on cessation of the drug may ensue without a demonstrable preoccupation with acquisition, compulsive use, and relapse to the drugs. Examples are abundant in patients who receive potent analgesics such as morphine and meperidine in hospitals for pain. Most patients do not continue to seek these drugs even though they have become tolerant and dependent pharmacologically. Addiction, on the other hand, may recur in the absence of the development of tolerance and dependence. Finally, addiction, tolerance, and dependence coexist frequently, although the causal temporal relationship between them is not clear.

There are many drugs that produce addiction, although the development of tolerance and dependence is not clinically obvious and easily measurable. Examples of this phenomenon are alcohol and marijuana. The popular conception is that tolerance and dependence do not develop to marijuana use. This is also the current claim for cocaine [24]. This lack of acceptance for marijuana and cocaine in producing tolerance and dependence may be a problem of definition and accurate measurement and observation. Addiction to alcohol frequently occurs in the absence of significant tolerance and dependence if the criteria are measured by changes in vital signs. The chief manifestations of cocaine and amphetamine intoxication are mood elevation, hyperactivity, anorexia, hallucinations, delusions, and increased blood pressure [25,26]. Increasing doses are required to maintain these effects as tolerance to cocaine/amphetamines occurs regularly. Doses of amphetamines up to 30,000 mg intravenously per day have been reported, and cocaine addicts regularly report the development of tolerance [2]. Marijuana intoxication leads to a distortion of perceptions, particularly time and space, mood fluctuations, decreased motor activity, and increased appetite. Tolerance to these effects of marijuana and cocaine may be difficult to measure and quantitate clinically and experimentally.

The withdrawal from cocaine/amphetamines can be dramatic and is manifested by severe depression, decreased motor activity, increased appetite, intense craving for more drug, disordered thinking, and delusions of persecution [27]. Blood pressure and other vital signs are usually normal. This withdrawal syndrome is distinct, although not unique in the symptomatology; variations of these withdrawal symptoms can be seen in a number of other drugs, such as alcohol [27]. The withdrawal from marijuana is subtle and marked by restlessness, intense craving for more drug, mood changes, mailise, and nausea. There are nonspecific symptoms that are present in other drug withdrawals as well.

Prototypes for Tolerance and Dependence

The prototypes for tolerance and dependence are alcohol and morphine. These drugs have been used as a gold standard for unclear reasons [2]. Curiously, morphine withdrawal is most remarkable for the craving which is more behavioral than any observable physiological measurements. Nausea, vomiting, myalgias, and piloerection may be present, but otherwise the physical signs and symptoms of withdrawal are uncomplicated and benign [28]. Morphine, however, is accepted without question as producing physical dependence.

Alcohol dependence is marked by a spectrum of signs and symptoms. All or, more often, only a part of the spectrum is evident in the withdrawal period. This spectrum of signs and symptoms includes anxiety, depressions, insomnia, tremors, malaise, hallucinations, disordered thinking, delusions, seizures, hypertension, fever, and tachycardia.

The more common symptoms in alcohol withdrawal of anxiety and depression are not used as hard criteria for dependence. For unclear reasons, dependence as a deadaptation to alcohol by the body is determined by only hypertension and tachycardia, and only of a severe and abnormal degree. If careful measurements are made during withdrawal in regular users of alcohol, a transient elevation of blood pressure and pulse rate over baseline frequently occurs to both acute and chronic alcohol administration. These elevations may or may not be in the abnormal range. The vascular changes are attributable to the sympathetic nervous system discharge that occurs during the deadapation of the body from alcohol during acute onset of abstinence. Anxiety is now accepted as a manifestation of the sympathetic nervous system function. The same autonomic nervous system response underlies the symptoms of anxiety from different states, including withdrawal from alcohol and drugs or an apparently spontaneous or provoked mood change.

Addiction

Tolerance and dependence probably occur regularly in alcohol and drug addiction. Our operational definitions may not include sufficient criteria to describe the manifestations of tolerance and dependence in addiction. There is a need to redefine the criteria for tolerance and dependence to include more manifestations of the adaptation and deadaptation by the body to the presence and absence of a drug. More signs and symptoms are needed to be inclusive of the abstinence syndrome. More commonality than difference will then be found for various drugs; cross tolerance, dependence, and addiction will be more fully explained. The central nervous system response to drug intoxication and withdrawal may be less specific than our theories and suppositions suggests. Development of tolerance and dependence by the central nervous system (CNS) may be nonspecific with only clusters of variations that are secondary and determined by each drug.

III. TOLERANCE AND DEPENDENCE

A. Definition of Tolerance and Dependence to Alcohol and Drugs

The pharmacological and physiological definitions of tolerance to alcohol or a drug specify that an increasing dose is necessary to maintain the safe effect or the effect is less at a particular dose. Tolerance may develop to the hypothermic effect of alcohol after repeated exposure, such that a particular dose fails to lower temperature and a larger dose is needed to produce hypothermia. A behavioral definition of tolerance is an observable adaptation of a particular behavior to a specific dose of drug. Tolerance to a drug has developed if more drug is needed than previously in order to reach the same expected state of intoxication or impairment in a behavior [2].

The definition of dependence is the onset of a predictable and stereotypic set of signs and symptoms upon the cessation of the use of a particular drug. The continued use of the drug is necessary to suppress the development of those signs and symptoms, which tend to be constant and specific for a given drug. For instance, alcohol has a predictable array of signs and symptoms as part of the abstinence/withdrawal syndrome [29]. The withdrawal syndrome is a spectrum that includes anxiety, insomnia, tremor, headache, nausea, seizures, and other objective and subjective parameters. Not all components need be present, and frequently are not, to confirm withdrawal from alcohol or other drugs.

B. Relationship Between Tolerance and Dependence to Alcohol and Drugs

The relationship between tolerance and dependence is controversial, although there are empirical evidence and theoretical considerations to support the view that the two form one entity on a continuum.

Tolerance

Tolerance is an expression of adaptation of a particular organism or cell to a continued presence of a foreign substance such as a drug. This homeostatic response represents the body's (cell's) adjustment to maintain a normal physiological function [30]. The cellular membrane's response to alcohol can be measured on a biochemical level [13]. An increase in order (or a decrease in fluidity) of the bilipid layer of the cell membrane in the continued presence of ethanol occurs during the development of tolerance [31,32]. The greater rigidity of the cell membrane is a homeostatic response to the persistent disordering or fluidizing effect of alcohol.

Tolerance to cocaine may involve changes in dopamine presynaptic terminals that may occur as a result of chronic blockade of reuptake. A supersenitivity of the dopamine postsynaptic receptor may result from an upregulation in response to low dopamine release. Presynaptic depletion and postsynaptic supersensitivity of dopamine neurons may represent the adaptive changes that occur during the development of tolerance.

Dependence

Dependence, on the other hand, is an expression of the deadaptation of the organism or cell to the absence of a drug. Symptoms accompany the movement from the "adaptive" pharmacodynamic set point in the presence of alcohol to the original pharmacodynamic set point in the absence of alcohol [30]. The final effect is to maintain homeostasis for normal physiological functioning. The fluidity or order parameters of cell membranes and dopamine stores and receptor sensitivity may return from the tolerant state to normal baseline values during withdrawal from alcohol and cocaine [20,23,33].

Relationship Between Tolerance and Dependence

Tolerance and dependence appear to be inversely related in the clinical setting. The greater the tolerance is to a drug, the less severe is the dependence syndrome. Conversely, the less the tolerance, the more severe the signs and symptoms of dependence. Alcoholics with increased tolerance to alcohol have milder withdrawal symptoms. As alcoholics progressively lose tolerance to alcohol, the severity of the dependence syndrome increases. This loss of tolerance is also seen in the effect of aging on the response to alcohol. Tolerance to alcohol decreases with increasing age in animals and humans. The severity of the dependence or withdrawal signs and symptoms also increases correspondingly with increasing ages [34].

Dependence alternatively may be viewed as a failure of the homeostatic mechanisms of adaptation to a drug. The signs and symptoms of withdrawal may represent the lack of the organism or cell to change further or reach a maximum point of adaptation in response to the presence of a drug. The pharmacodynamic set point is not at a state for normal functioning. Dependence may be an expression of a physiologically abnormal set point for functioning [30].

IV. NEUROCHEMISTRY OF ADDICTION: MODELS

A. Preoccupation

Cocaine Model

Preoccupation, compulsivity, and relapse have an identifiable neurochemical basis, and a more correct description of an addiction may be psychological and behavioral manifestations which are drug induced and drug sustained.

The addict often appears preoccupied with the drug even after prolonged periods of abstinence. This recall, or recurrence of obsessional thoughts about the drug, probably has a neurosubstrate that is located in the hippocampus of the limbic system. The hippocampi are responsible for registration and recall of recent experiences. The left hippocampus stores verbal memory and the right hippocampus stores nonverbal memory. Deficits in neuronal discharging in the hippocampus result in disturbances in the acquisition and storage of new information or memories. An enhancement of neuronal discharges in these same areas of the limbic system might lead to excessive or obsessional recall of previously registered experiences, particularly those associated with drug use. Stimulation of depth electrodes placed in the hippocampus or temporal lobe in humans results in recall of a series of "forgotten" or stored experiences. Addicts appear to have an increased amount of obsessional thinking regarding a variety of mental and physical experiences, including those pertaining to drugs.

A change in presynaptic or postsynaptic function might account for involuntary recall present in the preoccupation. A supersensitivity of the postsynaptic receptors with increased neuronal firing in the hippocampus could lead to spontaneous and enhanced recall of events. Dopamine-binding sites are increased after chronic exposure to cocaine. Dopamine (DA) toxins such as 6-hydroxydopamine that destroy presynaptic neurons lead to increased postsynaptic DA-binding sites. This type of "denervation supersensitivity" appears to represent a compensatory response to the destruction of DA neurons by 6-hydroxydopamine and subsequent reduction of presynaptic release of dopamine [20].

The development of persistent alteration in the postsynaptic receptor activity in cocaine stimulation may be similar to what is observed in tardive dyskinesia. Neuroleptic blockade of dopamine postsynaptic receptors apparently leads to a supersensitivity of dopamine-related function. Dopamine is a major neurotransmitter responsible for motor activity that is controlled by the basal ganglia. The supersensitivity of the dopamine receptors leads to spontaneous and enhanced activity of the neurons in the substantia nigra. Overactivity of basal ganglia function is manifested by hyperkinetic motor behavior such as orolingual buccal dyskinesias. Cocaine addicts can be extremely sensitive to extrapyramidal side effects from neuroleptic blockade in early withdrawal from cocaine. The increased reactivity to neuroleptics indicates a postsynaptic supersensitivity due to the presynaptic dopamine deficiency [23].

A "dyskinetic" recall may occur in the hippocampus as a result of chronic depletion of dopamine by cocaine that is in effect of functional or chemical blockade. Dopamine postsynaptic receptors in the hippocampus may be overactive analogously to that which recurs in the basal ganglia. An increased recall may produce recurrent or obsessional thoughts about drug use. This recall may be more sensitive to environmental cues or simply arise spontaneously as impulses motivating drug use from the reverberating circuits in the hippocampus. The recall from supersensitive postsynaptic dopamine neurons in the hippocampus may underlie relapse that appears to occur with or without external stimuli and cues.

B. Compulsivity

Cocaine Model

Dopamine Reward System.   The dopamine reward system may play a role in the neurochemical basis of compulsive use of drugs. The endogenous reward system has a neuroanatomical location. Olds discovered discrete brain regions in the hypothalamus that he termed "pleasure centers" [23]. Electrical stimulation of these pleasure centers in animals lead to rewardlike behavior. The circuit of the reward system includes descending fibers from the lateral hypothalamus that project to the ventral tegmentum via the medial forebrain bundle. The ventral tegmental area is the location of major dopamine neurons. Interruption of dopamine neurotransmission decreases the reward behavior produced by electrical stimulation of the lateral hypothalamus.

Central stimulants that are readily self-administered appear to activate dopamine neurons in the reward center. The ventral tegmentum projects to several other dopamine areas in the striatum, limbic system, and cerebral cortex. Lesions in the nucleus accumbens, located in the limbic system, result in a decrease in the self-administration of cocaine in animals [20,23].

Limbic System.   Electrodes implanted in the septal area of the limbic system in humans have provoked subjective sensations of intense pleasure similar to organsm [35,36]. The subjects continue to ask for repeated stimulation because of unusually strong positive, rewardlike reinforcement received.

Cocaine is considered to be an extremely reinforcing drug that is used compulsively; a monkey, if given an unlimited supply of cocaine, will continue to press the bar that releases the drug until the point of self-destruction [1]. Cocaine may act on the dopaminergic nerve endings in the reward center to produce dramatic enhancement in the reward states and reward behavior.

Dopamine agonists, such as apomorphine and piribedil, have amphetamine reward–reinforcing properties. Selective dopamine antagonists reduce both electrical and central stimulant self-administration by animals. Noradrenergic receptor antagonists have no such effect. In humans, amphetamine-induced euphoria is blocked by dopamine receptor antagonists. Acute administration of cocaine induces euphoria that appears to result from increased dopamine neurotransmission. Chronic cocaine administration may lead to a depletion of neuronal dopamine in the brain and an inhibition of dopamine function. Reuptake blockade prevents the recycling and reuse of dopamine in the presynaptic sites, resulting in brain dopamine levels falling after repeated administrations of cocaine. In humans, dopamine inhibits prolactin secretion, and hyperprolatinemia occurs in a number of chronic male and female cocaine addicts that may be an expression of dopamine depletion. The hyperprolactinemia peaks about 10 days after the cessation of cocaine use and thereafter gradually returns to normal over 2 weeks [20,23].

The intense depression that occurs with cocaine use may also be related to the chronic dopamine depletion. Decreased dopamine activity may be the neuronal basis for the subjective experience of drug craving. Administration of the dopamine agonist bromocriptine may ameliorate the intense craving that occurs in acute withdrawal from cocaine. Cocaine addicts report increased craving after administration of dopamine antagonists. Neuroleptic treatment may increase drug craving in cocaine addicts [20,23].

Alcohol Model

Dopamine System.   The dopamine reward system may play a role in the neurochemical basis of addiction to alcohol. Rats that are implanted with slow-release pellets containing the stimulants amphetamine or nicotine show a dramatic increase in ethanol self-selection. This appears to represent a selective dopamine effect on alcohol consumption because it does not occur with a variety of other drugs (hallucinogens, depressants) [37].

The administration of thioridazine and dihydroergotoxine (DHET) in combination reduced ethanol intake in rats. Either chemical alone did not significantly reduce ethanol intake. Dihydroergotoxine counteracts the activation of dopamine neurons by the postsynaptic blockade of thioridazine. This suggests that the drug combination exerts a synergistic effect on reducing dopaminergic transmission in the central nervous system. These results support an important role of dopaminergic transmission in the rewarding effect of ethanol [38].

Intravenous ethanol preferentially stimulated the firing rate of dopamine neurons in the ventral tegmental area which project to limbic and cortical areas of the forebrain over that of dopamine neurons in the substantia nigra. Intravenous ethanol was more effective in stimulating the firing rate of dopamine neurons in the ventral tegmental area in high than low ethanol–preferring rats. Also, under the same conditions, the dopamine content was decreased and the dihydrophenylacetic acid (DOPAC) content increased in the prefrontal cortex of the high, but not low ethanol preferring rats [39].

Other neurotransmitters play a role in the compulsive use of alcohol. The neurotransmitter gamma-aminobutyric acid (GABA) has been implicated in alcohol use in humans and animals. Stimulation of GABA B main receptors by calcium bis-acetylhomotaurine (Ca AOTA) or of noradrenergic receptors by metapromine reduces the voluntary intake of ethanol in rats. The effect of metapromine was opposed by a treatment with (+)bicuculline and not by a treatment with bicuculline metobromide (does not cross the blood-brain barrier). Baclofen, a GABA B agonist, reduces voluntary intake of ethanol [40].

Serotonin System.   Clinical and animal studies suggest that ethanol consumption is influenced by 5-dihydrotryptamine (5-HT) transmission. The treatment with a selective 5-HT receptor agonist, 8-OH DPAT caused a significant reduction in ethanol consumption in high-preference ethanol rats. This finding suggests that activation of the central 5-HT system reduces ethanol intake. Neurochemical studies have shown that ethanol-preferring P rats have lower levels of serotonin (5-HT) in cerebral cortex and hippocampus and higher levels of norepinephrine in the cerebral cortex in comparison to ethanol-nonpreferring rats. Additionally, significantly higher receptor numbers for 5-HT in the frontal cortex and hippocampus of preferring rats have been found. No difference in receptor numbers of alpha$_1$, and alpha$_2$, and adrenergic receptors in cortical membranes between preferring and nonpreferring rats was observed [41].

In severe, dependent alcoholics abstinent from alcohol for 2–20 days, [^{3}H]serotonin uptake loss was significantly lower than in nonalcoholic controls and in former dependent alcoholics (1–12 years).

Human and animal studies suggest a role for neurotransmitters in alcohol preference. Dopamine appears to play a role in enhancing or rewarding compulsive alcohol consumption. Serotonin, GABA, and norepinephrine appear to decrease compulsivity of alcohol intake.

Opiate Model

The locus coeruleus is a pontine nucleus densely populated with noradrenergic neurons and opiate receptors [56–58]. The latter receive input from B-endorphinergicneurons whose cell bodies are located in the hypothalamus [59]. Microiontophoretic studies have demonstrated that opiate agonist application decreases the firing rate of noradrenergic locus ceruleus neurons, and reversal of this inhibition is obtained with naloxone administration [60,61]. Ultrastructural and electrophysiologic studies also suggested that presynaptic α_2-noradrenergic receptors on locus ceruleus neurons decrease cellular firing rates when stimulated [62,63]. With chronic opiate exposure, an increase in postsynaptic noradrenergic receptors has been demonstrated and probably reflects the development of tolerance [64]. Simultaneous endogenous opiate down-regulation with chronic narcotic administration is suggested by animal and human studies which demonstrate diminished endorphin, enkephalin, and adrenocorticotropin levels, and diminished response to provocative testing with naltrexone [65,66]. Upon cessation of exogenous opiates, withdrawal symptoms appear, firing rates of individual noradrenergic locus ceruleus neurons increase, and brain and plasma MHPG (3-methoxy-4-hydroxy-phenylglycol) levels increase [67]. With subsequent administration of either methadone or clonidine, withdrawal symptoms abate and MHPG levels normalize [68], and one group has reported normalization of endorphin levels with clonidine treatment of opiate withdrawal [69]. In hypertensive patients clonidine treatment results in lowering of endorphin and adrenocorticotropin levels [70]. These data are all consistent with the dual inhibitory control of locus ceruleus activity.

The successful use of clonidine was followed by successful trials of other α_2 agonistic medications like aldomet and lofexidine to treat narcotic withdrawal [71,72]. The successful use of clonidine also suggested that treatment which upregulates the endogenous opiates would relieve narcotic abstinence symptoms. Most recently, Vescovi, Jones, and Cashman have independently reported the successful use of intravenous lysine acetylsalicylate to relieve narcotic abstinence symptoms [73]. They believe its effectiveness is based upon its ability to increase the production and release of endogenous opiates.

Alcohol and Opiates

A relationship between ethanol and opiate dependence was first suggested by Davis and Walsh [74] who reported that dopamine-derived tetrahydroisoquinoloine alkaloids (certain of which are intermediates in the biosynthesis of morphine in the opium poppy) may be formed during ethanol metabolism in rats. These workers theorized that such alkaloids may play a role in the development of tolerance and physical dependence on ethanol. The presence of acetaldehyde blocks the normal conversion of the amine-derived aldehyde to the corresponding acid. The inhibition of the nicotinamide-adenine dinucleotide (NAD)-linked aldehyde dehydrogenase after ethanol ingestion may result in localized elevated concentrations of aromatic aldehydes in tissues rich in biogenic amines. These intermediate aldehydes are highly reactive compounds. A possible alternate route for the metabolism of these aldehydes is condensation with the parent amine. In the case of condensation of dopamine and its aldehyde (3,4-dihydroxy-phenylacetaldehyde) the product is a benzyltetrahydroisoquinoline alkaloid, tetrahydropapaveroline (THP) [75]. Tetrahydropapaveroline (norlaudanosoline) is the requisite intermediate in the biosynthesis of morphine in the opium poppy (Papaver somniferum) [76].

The successful use of clonidine for the treatment of opiate withdrawal has been followed by trials of clonidine for other abstinence syndromes which resemble the opiate withdrawal syndrome in some way. Clonidine has also been found useful for amelioration of alcohol withdrawal symptoms [77], benzodiazepine withdrawal [78], and tobacco withdrawal [79]. These trials were based on clinical evidence of noradrenergic hyperactivity associated with other withdrawal syndromes.

The use of alcohol by narcotic addicts, especially when narcotics are not available, is well documented [80,81]. It has been reported that approximately 20% of a sample of methadone maintenance patients had been discharged from a program as a consequence of alcohol abuse [82]. It is also known that in clinical practice, the effects of alcohol are potentiated in patients on tranquilizer or narcotic analgesic therapy [83]. However the presence of alcoholism in drug-intoxicated patients is often overlooked [84]. Outpatient use and abuse of alcohol has also rendered the results of outpatient detoxification studies less valid.

C. Relapse

Current Research

The literature regarding relapse is quite diverse. A variety of personality, demographic, cognitive, physiological, environmental, and behavioral variables have been investigated, and many different conceptual systems have been employed to explain relapse. The majority of studies fall within one of two general classes: (1) studies that attempt to identify predictors of relapse over time, or that assess variables between groups of relapsed and nonrelapsed subjects; and (2) studies that investigate specific events surrounding discrete relapse episodes. The available evidence suggests that studies of the latter type are more likely to yield informative generalizations about the determinants of relapse [42–49].

Neurochemical Model

A neurochemical model does not fully explain why some individuals may relapse, whereas others may not. A variety of personality, demographic, cognitive, environmental, and behavioral factors play important roles in determining relapse.

Relapse is perhaps more difficult to understand on a neurochemical basis than preoccupation and relapse. Preoccupation with the acquisition of a drug, especially while the addiction is active, and compulsive use during the time of the development of tolerance and dependence to a drug may be evident because of concurrent drug-brain interactions. A motivation for drug acquisition and use may be to offset the onset of incipient withdrawal symptoms, which can be unpleasant. The mood of depression that immediately occurs as a withdrawal effect of cocaine use, especially chronic use, is described as very intense and severe by users; more cocaine will temporarily relieve the depression, however. The anxiety and depression that accompany acute alcohol withdrawal appear to be motivating factors for repeated alcohol consumption as alcohol can be an antidote for these aversive mood states.

The self-treatment or self-administration of drugs for the withdrawal symptoms with more drugs is not always a sufficient explanation for repetitive and compulsive use because the addict is aware that these aversive effects from chronic drug use will subside spontaneously with abstinence. The distress and discomfort may be less to endure the short-term unpleasant withdrawal symptoms than to continue to "medicate" symptoms that only worsen with repeated use. Also, relapse must explain why an addict returns to drug use after long periods of abstinence during which symptoms of withdrawal have subsided.

Craving

Craving is a term that has been used to describe the intense desire to use more drug. Craving is a drive that appears to supersede the anguish of the adverse symptoms of intoxication and withdrawal that inevitably follow the return to drug use. The craving occupies a preeminent position in the acute and prolonged periods of withdrawal in alcohol and drug addiction. The basis of the craving in cocaine addiction may be crucial in the reward pathways. Decreased dopamine availability at the synapse or supersensitivity of the dopamine postsynaptic neurons may be experienced as craving by the cocaine addict. The dopamine neurons in the reward system may be sent in an undercompensated state that signals an increased need for reward sensation [20,23].

Alcohol may produce persistent changes in membrane fluidity that result in craving. A more ordered neuronal membrane may lead to subjective experiences that create a drive state for more alcohol use. The altered cellular membrane fluidity may affect dopamine presynaptic or postsynaptic function in the reward area. Acute alcohol administration enhances dopamine transmission similarly to cocaine [37,39]. Chronic alcohol use may result in a persistent decrease in dopamine activity similarly to cocaine by producing a more rigid cell membrane [13].

The addict's return to the use of alcohol or a drug after weeks or perhaps months and years of abstinence may be explained in part by a physical alteration in brain neuronal membranes that persists. The clinical effect of dopamine deficiency may remain owing to a relative permanent exhaustion of presynaptic dopamine stores or a supersensitivity of postsynaptic receptor sites. This relative neuronal dopamine lack may manifest itself in a psychological state manifested by craving that may signal a relapse [23]. The postsynaptic dopamine deficient neurons in the hippocampus may be supersensitive and fire spontaneously at low levels of stimulation similarly to what occurs in tardive dyskinesia to provoke relapse to alcohol and drugs.

Hippocampus

The hippocampus in the limbic system contains the memory function of recall. Drive states located in the limbic system such as sex, hunger, or mood may be associated directly with recall mechanisms, so that recall is linked to the instincts. The effect of the drug on the instincts becomes a stored memory that can be recalled such that the drive states become permanently associated with the drug. Persistent neurotransmitter changes such as supersensitivity may underlie these larger and more functional alterations in the drive states. The reward and the memory centers in the limbic system may become associated with the drive states that were provoked by the drug alterations in dopamine function. Relapse may involve spontaneous firing of dopamine neurons in the hippocampus that serve recall of the drive states that become linked to the drug and alcohol. Alcohol and drugs are then used in response to the stimulus from the drive states that are augmented by the reward center. The alcohol and drug use become entrained by the drives for survival, sex, food, and mood.

Frontal Lobe

Drugs have effects on the brain that enhance the uninhibited expression of the instincts. Alcohol and cocaine affect important frontal lobe function that ordinarily inhibits the drive states in the limbic system. The frontal lobe subserves psychological and behavioral functions such as judgment, motivation, ethical conduct, propriety, impulse control, planning, and initiation that are significantly affected by alcohol and drugs. Behaviorally and neurophysiologically, there is a suppression or slowing of these important functions, and subsequently the instincts are allowed uninhibited, freer, and more complete expression. Individuals with frontal lobe impairment frequently show persistent, repetitive, perseverating behavior similar to that present in the automatic and stereotypic behavior of an addiction. The powerful motivation to use alcohol and drugs associated with the drive states reinforced by the reward center is relatively unabated and uninhibited by the higher cortical centers such as the frontal lobe.

D. Drive States and Addiction to Alcohol and Drugs

Instincts

Mood, appetite, survival, and sexual reproduction are drive states that are located in the limbic system [50]. Relatively discrete neuroanatomical designations exist for each of the drives. Electrode stimulation experiments in these various areas have demonstrated that a particular sensation in humans and a behavior in animals reflecting these drive states can be provoked. Electrodes implanted in the septal area of the limbic system in humans have aroused subjective sensations of intense pleasure similar to sexual orgasm. The subjects vigorously seek repeated stimulation because of the apparently strong positive reinforcement received [51]. These sensations and pleasure-seeking behaviors are similar to those described by cocaine users [2].

Drug Effects

Drive states, particularly sex and hunger, are understandably, enormously potent, and are responsible for the survival of a species. Any alteration or provocation of these drive states can result in powerful and incorrigible behavior such as manifested in an addiction. A persistent association may develop between the drive states that are essentially instincts and the alcohol and drug that stimulated them [50]. Drugs such as alcohol and cocaine may be altering and redirecting the instincts; in a sense the alcohol and drugs are overtaken and orchestrated by the drive states. These changes in the instincts by the drugs are subserved by the neurotransmitter systems in the brain. Dopamine, GABA, serotonin, and norepinephrine may undergo alterations in synaptic function to enhance or diminish the neurochemical functions underlying the behavioral changes that result from the addiction to alcohol and drugs.

E. Other Addictions

Other nonchemical addictions such as gambling, sex, and eating may share common underlying neuroanatomical and neurochemical mechanisms. The same drive states and instincts may form the bases of all the addictions. Eating disorders, particularly bulimia and gambling disorders, are associated with a particularly high prevalence of alcohol and drug addictions.

Psychological and behavioral phenomena are similar in all of these disorders. Bulimics and gamblers are preoccupied with the acquisition and compulsive use, and frequently relapse to stereotypic food behaviors and to risk taking, respectively. The obvious difference is that an exogenous drug-brain interaction occurs with alcohol and drug addiction to initiate addictive behavior. In regard to eating and gambling, other endogenous interactions appear to take place to initiate the additive behavior.

F. Genetics

The reasons that some individuals become addicted to alcohol and drugs and others do not have received considerable attention in research in the past 10–20 years. Genetic research, namely, adoption, twin, familial, and high-risk studies, has demonstrated that a predisposition to alcoholism may be inherited. The children of alcoholics may carry an increased risk of becoming alcoholic, whether or not they are raised by the alcoholic. Environmental factors appear to play a secondary role if the genetic predisposition is present.

A neurochemical explanation for this inherited vulnerability has not been confirmed, although one probably exists in the form of genetic alterations. The genetic basis for nonalcohol, drug addiction has not been as discretely and specifically studied as it has been for alcoholism. Drugs appear to have common characteristics with alcohol as presented in the neurochemical models. The susceptibility to develop an addiction to drugs appears to overlap significantly with that of alcohol. More than 50% of alcoholics under the age of 30 have an addiction to at least one additional drug. Increased exposure through availability may be only a partial explanation. The genetic neurochemical predisposition may be similar for alcohol and drugs.

V. SUMMARY

A. Basis of Addiction

The basis of alcohol and drug addiction may involve distortion and redirection of drive states by the drug. The preoccupation, compulsive use, and relapse in behavioral terms is descriptive and confirmatory. Tolerance and dependence may only be incidentally associated with addiction as a result of a nonspecific cellular adaptation by the body to the drug. The cellular adaptation may be similar in all organs, including the neurons in the brain.

Tolerance and dependence may have no specific relationship to alcohol and drug addiction. Tolerance and dependence can occur in the absence of observable addiction. Addiction is probably more complex than tolerance and dependence, since it may involve the lower brain stem and higher cortical functions. Tolerance and dependence may be largely limited to universal cellular alterations. Addiction is difficult to study because of the variability of behavioral phenomena and the underlying intricacies of the neurosubstrates.

Tolerance and dependence are still useful as they are indicators of alcohol and drug use. However, it is a misconception that long-term chronic use is necessary for tolerance and dependence to develop [2,1]. Some studies have shown that tolerance can develop within hours and days to a single dose of alcohol or a drug [52,53]. It is known that anxiety, depression, and insomnia can occur after a single dose of ethanol in humans, and that they are considered to be symptoms of withdrawal from ethanol [54]. The common term for this is "hangover." Redefining our criteria for tolerance and dependence to alcohol and other drugs may be in order [55].

B. Importance of Diagnosing Addiction

Although tolerance and dependence are useful in assessing drug effect, the key to a diagnosis of a primary problem with alcohol or drugs is *addictive behavior*. The components of addiction are preoccupation with the acquisition of the drug, compulsive use, and relapse. Once these key behaviors regarding alcohol and drugs are identified as an addiction, then the consequences of an addiction can be more clearly identified. If the essential nature of the addiction is not extracted, confusion that the consequences lead to the "addictive use" of alcohol and drugs may result.

REFERENCES

1. Jaffe, J.H. (1985). Drug addiction and drug abuse, (A.G. Gilman, L.S. Goodman, T.W. Rall, and F. Murad, eds.). *The Pharmacological Basis of Therapeutics*, 7th ed. Macmillan, New York, pp. 532–581.

2. Hoffman, F.G. (1983). *A Handbook on Drug and Alcohol Abuse: The Biomedical Aspects*, 2nd ed. Oxford University Press, New York/Oxford.

3. Vaillant, G.E. (1983). *The Natural History of Alcoholism*. Harvard University Press, Cambridge, Massachusetts.

4. Edwards, G., Auf, A., and Hodgson, R. (1981). Nomenclature and classification of drug and alcohol-related problems: A WHO memorandum. *Bull. W.H.O.*, *59*:225-242.

5. Jellinek, E.M. (1060). *The Disease Concept of Alcoholism*. Hillhouse Press, New Brunswick, New Jersey.

6. Tucker, J.A., Vuchinich, R.E., and Harris, C.V. (1985). Determinants of substance abuse relapse, (M. Galizio and S.A. Maish, eds.). *Determinants of Substance Abuse*. Plenum, New York, pp. 383-424.

7. Siegel, R.K., Albers, R.W., Agranoff, B.W., et al. (1981). *Basic Neurochemistry*, 3rd ed. Little, Brown, Boston.

8. Goldstein, D.B., Chin, J.H., and Lyon, R.C. (1982). Ethanol disordering of spin-labeled mouse brain membranes. *Proc. Nat. Acad. Sci. U.S.A.*, *79*:4321-4323.

9. Lieber, C.S. (1982). *Medical Disorders of Alcoholism Pathogenesis and Treatment*. Saunders, Philadelphia.

10. Beauge, F., Subler, H., and Borg, S. (1985). Abnormal fluidity and surface carbohydrate content of the erythrocyte membrane in alcohol patients. *Alcoholism Clin. Exp. Res.*, *9*:322-326.

11. Chin, J.H., and Goldstein, D.B. (1977). Effects of low concentrations of ethanol on the fluidity of spin-labeled erythrocyte and brain membranes. *J. Pharm. Pharmacol.*, *13*:435-441.

12. Chin, J.H., and Goldstein, D.B. (1984). Cholesterol blocks the disordering effects of ethanol in biomembranes. *Lipids, 19*:929-935.

13. Goldstein, D.B. (1984). The effects of drugs on membrane fluidity, (W.M. Cowan, E.M. Shooter, C.F. Stevens, and R.C. Thompson, eds.). *Ann. Rev. Pharmacol.*, *24*:43-64.

14. Grieve, S.J., Littleton, J.M., Jones, P., et al. (1979). Functional tolerance to ethanol in mice: Relationship to lipid metabolism. *J. Pharm. Pharmacol.*, *31*:737-742.

15. Ingram, L.O. (1976). Adaptation of membrane lipids to alcohols. *J. Bacteriol.*, *125*:670-678.

16. LaDroitte, P. (1984). Sensitivity of individual erythrocyte membrane phospholipids to changes in fatty acid composition in chronic alcoholic patients. *Alcoholism Clin. Exp. Res.*, *9*:135-137.

17. Lee, N.M., Friedman, H.J., and Loh, H.H. (1980). Effect of acute and chronic ethanol treatment on rat brain phospholipid turnover. *Biochem. Pharmacol.*, *29*:2815-2818.

18. Littleton, J.M., Geryk, J.R., and Grieve, S.J. (1979). Alterations in phospholipid composition in ethanol tolerance and dependence. *Alcoholism Clin. Exp. Res.*, *3*:50-56.

19. Feldman, R.S., and Quenzer, L.F. (1984). *Fundamentals of Neuropsychopharmacology*. Sinauer, Sunderland, Massachusetts.

20. Dackis, C.A., and Gold, M.S. (1985). New concepts in cocaine addiction: The dopamine depletion hypothesis. *Neurosci. Biobehav. Rev.*, *9*:469-477.

21. Mule, S.J. (1984). The pharmacodynamics of cocaine abuse. *Psychiatr. Ann.*, *14*:724-727.

22. Siegel, R.K. (1984). Cocaine smoking disorderrs: Diagnosis and treatment. *Psychiatr. Ann.*, *14*:728-732.

23. Dackis, C.A., and Gold, M.S. (1985). Pharmacological approaches to cocaine addiction. *J. Subst. Abuse Treat.*, *2*:139-145.

24. Schuckit, M.A. (1984). *Drugs and Alcohol Abuse*. Plenum, New York.

25. Green, A.R., and Costain, D.W. (1981). *Pharmacology and Biochemistry of Psychiatric Disorders*. Wiley, New York.

26. Gold, M.S., and Verebey, K. (1984). The psychopharmacology of cocaine. *Psychiat. Ann.*, *14*:724-727.

27. Goodwin, D.W., and Guze, S.B. (1984). *Psychiatric Diagnosis*. Oxford University Press, New York/Oxford.

28. Melium, K.L., and Morrelli, H.F. (1978). *Clinical Pharmacology*, 2nd ed. Macmillan, New York.

29. Majchrowicz, E., and Noble, E.P. (1979). *Biochemistry and Pharmacology of Ethanol*, Vol. 1. Plenum, New York.

30. Hill, M.A., and Bangham, A.D. (1975). General depressant drug dependency: A biophysical hypothesis. *Adv. Exp. Med. Biol.*, *59*:1-9.

31. Chin, J.H., Parsons, L.M., and Goldstein, D.B. (1978). Increased cholesterol content of erythrocyte and brain membranes in ethanol-tolerant mice. *Biochim. Biophys. Acta, 513*:358–363.

32. Vanderkooi, J.M. (1979). Effect of ethanol on membranes: A fluorescent probe study. *Alcoholism Clin. Exp. Res., 3*:60–63.

33. Johnson, D.A., Lee, N.M., Cooke, R., and Loh, H.H. (1979). Adaptation to ethanol-induced fluidization of brain lipid bilayers: Cross tolerance and reversibility. *Molec. Pharmacol., 17*:52–55.

34. Kates, M., Manson, L.A. (1984). *Biomembranes: Membrane Fluidity.* Plenum, New York.

35. Beach, F.A. (1974). A review of physiological or psychological studies of sexual behavior in mammals. *Physiol. Rev., 27*:240–305.

36. Cox, A.W. (1979). Control of "sex centers" in the brain. *Med. Aspects Hum. Sexual. April*: 113.

37. Ellison, G., Levin, E., and Potthoff, A. (1986, June). Ethanol intake increases during continuous stimulants but not depressants. *Third Congress International Society for Biomedical Research on Alcoholism Abstracts* 31, Helsinki.

38. Fadda, F., Franch, F., and Gessa, G.L. (1986, June). Inhibition of voluntary ethanol consumption in rats by a combination of dihydroergotoxine and thioridazine. *Third Congress International Society for Biomedical Research on Alcoholism Abstracts* 32, Helsinki.

39. Gessa, G.L., and Fadda, F. (1986, June). Ethanol stimulates mesocortical dopaminergic system in ethanol preferring rats. *Third Congress International Society for Biomedical Research on Alcoholism Abstracts* 107, Helsinki.

40. Boismare, F., Daoust, M., Lhuintre, C., et al. (1986, June). Noradrenaline and GABA brain receptors are co-involved in the voluntary intake of ethanol by rats. *Third Congress International Society for Biomedical Research on Alcoholism Abstracts* 30, Helsinki.

41. Lumeng, L., Wong, D.T., Threlkeld, M., et al. (1986, June). Neuronal receptors of alcohol-preferring (p) and non-preferring (NP) rats. *Third Congress International Society for Biomedical Research on Alcoholism Abstracts* 33, Helsinki.

42. Hunt, W.A., Barrett, L.W., and Branch, L.G. (1971). Relapse rates in addiction program. *J. Clin. Psychol., 90*:586–600.

43. Marlatt, G.A. (1980). Craving for alcohol, loss of control, and relapse: A cognitive-behavioral analysis, (P.E. Nathan, G.A. Marlatt, and T.L. Berg, eds.). *Alcoholism: New Directions in Behavioral Research and Treatment.* Plenum, New York.

44. Schachter, S. (1982). Recidivism and self-cure of smoking and obesity. *Am. Psychologist, 37*:436–444.

45. Cummings, C., Gordon, J.R., and Marlatt, G.A. (1980). Relapse: Prevention and prediction, (W.R. Miller, ed.). *The Addictive Behaviors.* Pergamon Press, Elmsford.

46. Marlatt, G.A., and Gordon, J.R. (1980). Determinants of relapse: Implications for the maintenance of behavioral change, (P. Davidson and S. Davidson, eds.). *Behavioral Medicine: Changing Health Lifestyles.* Brunner/Mazel, New York.

47. Lichtenstein, E. (1982). The smoking problem: A behavioral perspective. *J. Consult. Clin. Psychol., 6*:804–819.

48. Miller, W.R., and Hester, R.K. (1980). Treating the problem drinker: Modern approaches, (W.R. Miller, ed.). *The Addictive Behaviors.* Pergamon Press, Elmsford, New York.

49. Ogborne, A.C. (1978). Patient characteristics as predictors of treatment outcomes for alcohol and drug abusers, (Y. Israel, R.B. Glaser, R.E. Kalant, et al., eds.). *Recent Advances in Alcohol and Drug Problems,* Vol. 4. Plenum, New York.

50. Pincus, J.R., and Tucker, G.J. (1985). *Behavioral Neurology,* 3rd ed. Oxford University Press, New York/Oxford.

51. Heath, R.G. (1972). Pleasure and brain activity in man. *J. Nerv. Ment. Dis., 154*:3–18.

52. Tahakoff, B., and Rothstein, J.B. (1983). *Medical and Social Aspects of Alcohol Abuse.* Plenum, New York.

53. Wilson, J.R., Erwin, G., McClearn, G.E., et al. (1984). Effects of behavior: II. Behavior sensitivity and acute behavioral tolerance. *Alcoholism, 8*:4.

54. Victor, M., and Adams, R.P. (1953). The effect of alcohol on the nervous system. *Res. Publi., Assoc. Res. Nerv. Ment. Dis., 32*:526–573.

55. Millam, J.R., and Ketchum, K. (1981). *Under the Influence.* Madrona, Kirkland, Washington.

56. Vogt, M. (1954). The concentrations of sympathin in different parts of the central nervous system under normal conditions and after the administration of drugs. *J. Physiol. 123*:451–458.

57. Levitt, P., Moorve, R. Y. (1974). Origin and organization of brainstem catecholamine innervation in the rat. *J. Comp. Neurol. 186*:505–528.

58. Pert C. B., et al. (1976). Opiate receptor: Autoradiographic localization in rat brain. *Proc. Natl. Acad. Sci. 73*:3729–3733.

59. Bloom, F. E., et al. (1978). Beta-Endorphin: cellular localization, electrophysiological and behavioral effects. *Adv. Biochem. Psychopharmacol. 18*:89–109.

60. Aghajanian, G. K. (1978). Tolerance or locus coeruleus neurons to morphine and suppression of withdrawal response by clonidine. *Nature 276*:186–188.

61. Bird, S. J., Kuhar, M. J. (1977). Ioncophoretic application of opiates to the locus coeruleus. *Brain Res. 122*:523–533.

62. Langer, S. Z. (1980). Presynaptic receptors and the modulation of neurotransmission: Pharmacological implications and therapeutic relevance. *Trends Neurosci. 3*:110–112.

63. Swanson, L. W. (1976). The locus coeruleus: A cytoarchitectonic, golgi and immunohistochemical study in the albino rat. *Brain Res. 110*:39–56.

64. Gold, M. S., Kleper, H. D. (1979). A rationale for opiate withdrawal symptomatology. *Drug and Alcohol Dep. 4*:419.

65. Pickworth, W. B., et al. (1982). Morphine-like effects of clonidine on the EEG, slow wave sleep and behavior of the dog. *Eur. J. Pharmacol. 81*:552.

66. Gold, M. S., et al. (1981). Opiate detoxification with lofexidine. *Drug and Alcohol Depend. 8*:307–315.

67. Crawley, J. N., et al. (1979). Clonidine reversal of increased norepinephrine metabolites during morphine withdrawal. *Eur. J. Pharmacol. 57*:247–250.

68. Redmond, D. E., Charney, D. S. (1980). The locus coeruleus norepinephrine connection with clonidine. Presented at the Neuropsychopharmacology of Clonidine Symposium ACNP Annual Meeting, San Juan, Puerto Rico, December 16, 1980.

69. Gil-Ad, I., et al. (1985). Effect of clonidine on plasma B-endorphin, cortisol, and growth hormone secretion in opiate-addicted subjects, *Isr. J. Med. Sci. 21*:601–604.

70. Yasunari, K., et al. (1985). Central alpha-activation by clonidine reduces plasma level of B-endorphin in patients with essential hypertension. *Life Sci. 37*:1461–1467.

71. Gold, M. S., et al. (1981). Evidence for an endorphin dysfunction in methadone addicts: Lack of ACTH response to naloxone. *Drug Alcohol Depend. 8*:257.

72. Gold, M. S., et al. (1982). Anti-withdrawal effects of alpha methyl dopa and cranial electrotherapy. *Society for Neuroscience Abstract 133*:22.

73. Vescovi, P., et al. (1984). Heroin detoxification by lysine acetylsalicylate. *Current Therapeutic Research 35*:826–831.

74. Davis, V. E., Walsh, M. D. (1970). Alcohol, amines and alkaloids: A possible basis for alcohol addiction. *Science 167*:1005–1007.

75. Holtz, P., Heise, R. (1938). *Arch. Exp. Pathol. Pharmakol. (Naunyn-Schmiedebergs):191*:87.

76. Leete, E. (1959). *J. American Chem. Soc. 81*:3948.

77. Manhem, P., et al. (1985). Alcohol withdrawal: Effects of clonidine treatment on sympathetic activity, the renin-aldosterone system, and clinical symptoms. *Alcoholism: Clinical and Experimental Research 9*:238–243.

78. Keshavan, M., Crammer, J. (1985). Clonidine in benzodiazepine withdrawal. *Lancet i*:1325–2326.

79. Glassman, A. H., et al. (1984). Cigarette craving, smoking, withdrawal and clonidine. *Science 226*:864–866.

80. Brown, B. S., et al. (1973). Use of alcohol by addict and non-addict populations. *Am. J. Psychiatry 130*:599–601.

81. Perkins, M. E., Bloch, H. I. (1971). A study of some failures in methadone treatment. *Am. J. Psychiatry 128*:47–51.

82. Gearing, F. R. (1969). Read at the Second Annual Conference on Methadone Treatment, New York, October 26–27, 1969.

83. Mehar, G. S., et al. (1974). Interaction between alcohol, minor tranquilizers and morphine, *Int. J. Clin. Pharmacol. 9*:70–74.

84. Hirsch, C. S., et al. (1973). Unexpected ethanol in drug-intoxicated persons. *Postgrad Med. 54*(2):53–57.

41

The Pharmacokinetics and Pharmacodynamics of Alcohol and Drugs of Addiction

Lawrence E. Hoeschen
University of Manitoba, Winnipeg, Manitoba, Canada

I. INTRODUCTION

This chapter will describe the pharmacology of addiction, and will focus on two main areas of pharmacology; namely, pharmacodynamics and pharmacokinetics. Pharmacodynamics is the study of biochemical and physiological affects of drugs and their mechanisms of action. Pharmacokinetics deals with the absorption, distribution, biotransformation, and excretion of drugs (Benet and Sheiner, 1985). The term *dependence*, synonymous with addiction, is defined by the World Health Organization (WHO) as

> a socio-psycho-biological syndrome manifested by a behavioral pattern in which the use of given psychoactive drug (or class of drugs) is given a sharply higher priority over other behaviors which once had significantly greater value (i.e., drug use comes to have a greater relative value) (Edwards et al., 1981).

This definition avoids the old distinction between psychological dependence and physical dependence, where compulsive drug-seeking behavior characterized the psychological aspect and a recognizable withdrawal syndrome characterized the physiological aspect. This distinction is no longer valid, particularly with the recent discovery of the neuroanatomical and neuropharmacological mechanisms of stimulant addiction (Dackis and Gold, 1985; Miller et al., 1987). However, in the following discussion the old distinctions will be alluded to when the pharmacodynamic properties of a drug are described with reference to the drug's ability to reinforce drug-taking behavior (psychological dependence), and when the pharmacokinetic properties are described (elimination kinetics) with reference to the development of a withdrawal syndrome, (physiological dependence).

In the subsequent discussion of the pharmacodynamic and pharmacokinetic properties of the various classes of drugs, the emphasis will be on the manner in which these properties contribute to the addictive process. The pharmacodynamics discussion will focus on the mechanisms of action at the cellular level. For more detailed descriptions, the reader will be referred to the appropriate literature where it exists.

II. CONDITIONING FACTORS

The factors influencing the motivation to take mood-altering drugs are complex and varied (Edwards et al., 1981; Jaffe, 1985; Nurco, 1979), but this discussion will be limited to the pharmacological properties of the drug itself. Having taken a mood-altering drug at first, a person may continue to use that drug if the experience is pleasurable; hence reinforcing (Haefely, 1986; Jaffe, 1985; Wise, 1980, 1988). If physiological addiction should develop, the person will continue to take the drug to avoid the unpleasant sensation of withdrawal (Haefely, 1988; Wikler, 1980). These two events vividly demonstrate the well-known principles of conditioned behavior (Pavlov, 1927; Skinner, 1938). Further, there are factors which influence the ability of a drug to produce and maintain the drug-taking behavior. First, the stimulus-response time; i.e., the faster the drug reaches its target organ, the central nervous system (CNS), after it is taken, the more likely it is to maintain the drug-taking behavior (if it is pleasurable). Second, the magnitude of the response (the potency); i.e., some drugs have a greater inherent ability to produce pleasure than others.

This can be objectively assessed in animal studies (Brady and Lukas, 1984). Third, there is a combination of the first two factors, in the production of the withdrawal syndrome. If the withdrawal is extremely unpleasant and occurs fairly quickly after cessation of the drug, then continued use or resumption of the drug is more likely (Busto et al., 1989; Griffiths et al., 1981).

III. PHARMACODYNAMIC FACTORS

The cellular mechanisms of action have been described for most of the drugs of addiction (Jaffe, 1985; Koob and Bloom, 1988; Wise, 1988) and will be discussed in detail later. The mechanisms are varied. There are general membrane "solvent" effects, e.g., ethanol (Goldstein, 1983); indirect effects on receptors, e.g., barbiturates (Ho and Harris, 1981); and specific receptor interactions, e.g., opiates (Koob et al., 1986; Pert and Snyder, 1973) benzodiazepines (Mohler and Okada, 1977; Squires and Braestrup, 1977), and more recently phencyclidine (Sonders et al., 1988). However, whatever the cellular mechanisms may be, the end result, i.e., the physiological effect, is the addictive behavior. This behavior has been well studied and quantitated in animal studies (Brady and Lukas, 1984). For certain drugs, specific anatomical locations have been found which mediate the drug-seeking behavior; i.e., a reward system of connecting neurons and neurotransmitters (Koob and Bloom, 1988; Miller et al., 1987; Wise, 1980). This has been particularly well described for the stimulant drugs (Dackis and Gold, 1985), and has been suggested for the opiates as well (Mucha and Herz, 1985).

Ethanol-preference studies have linked this phenomena to serotonin neurotransmitters in the CNS (Zabik, 1989), despite the fact there is no known specific receptor site of action for ethanol. Although the correlation between a cellular mechanism of action and the physiological effect, i.e., drug-taking behavior, is not always consistent (with the exception of the stimulant drugs) (Koob and Bloom, 1988; Liebman, 1985; Woods et al., 1987), there is reasonably good correlation between animal behavior and human behavior in drug-preference studies (Griffiths et al., 1979).

IV. PHARMACOKINETIC FACTORS

The pharmacokinetic properties of a drug influence the development of addiction in two areas; namely, reinforcement of drug-taking behavior, and emergence of the withdrawal syndrome.

A. Reinforcement

The route of administration of a drug is a key factor in the rapidity of onset of its effects (Benet and Sheiner, 1985; Rowland, 1978). Drugs taken by inhalation reach the CNS in high concentrations most quickly, because of the large surface area for absorption (lungs) and the short circulatory route to the brain. In descending order of rapidity of onset, the routes are intravenous, intranasal, and oral. The rapidity of onset of the mood-altering effect of inhaled drugs may partially explain the current epidemic of "crack" (see pg. 756) (Gawin and Ellinwood, 1988), and the long-standing widespread addiction to nicotine (Benowitz, 1988). Even with drugs taken by the oral route, there have been differential effects in preference related to their different absorption rate (Griffiths et al., 1984b), although there is not a great deal of documentation of this phenomenon.

The distribution of a drug may also be a determinant in reinforcement. The theory seems attractive, but research in this specific area of reinforcement is lacking. Drugs that are not highly protein bound will be delivered to the target organ, the CNS, more readily, and high lipid solubility will assure rapid entry into the brain as well. However, high lipid solubility will also shorten the duration of action in the CNS as the drug is distributed rapidly to other sites in the body. This latter property may mitigate against the development of physiological dependence.

B. Withdrawal

It has been demonstrated with CNS depressants that the withdrawal intensity and rapidity of onset is related to its elimination rate for barbiturates (Boisse and Okamoto, 1978) and benzodiazepines (Busto et al., 1986). Furthermore, it has been shown that the drugs with the shorter elimination rates produce greater drug-taking or drug-seeking behavior (Busto et al., 1986; Griffiths et al., 1981). These phenomena are likely to be demonstrated only in the case of barbiturates and benzodiazepines, as they are the only two groups of addictive drugs that have individual drugs within the groups with differing elimination rates.

There is a seemingly paradoxical effect that the elimination rate has on the development of physiological dependence. On the one hand, a slow elimination rate ensures a milder, more gradual withdrawal, and thus may not produce a powerful desire to resume taking the drug once it has been stopped. However, a slow elimination rate is required to produce a long-lasting effect on the CNS, and hence produce tolerance and physiological dependence (Busto and Sellers, 1986; Hollister, 1961). Drugs with fast elimination rates would produce a harsher, less gradual withdrawal state, but their rapid elimination rate may preclude any development of physiological dependence. However, if a drug with a relatively fast elimination rate were taken at frequent intervals, to ensure a constant CNS effect, then cessation of the drug would produce a more severe withdrawal (Robinson and Sellers, 1981). This concept has provided the rationale for the present treatment of CNS depressant withdrawal syndromes (Robinson and Sellers, 1981).

For an excellent discussion of the pharmacokinetic factors in drug addictions the reader is referred Busto and Sellers (1986).

V. CNS DEPRESSANTS

A. Ethanol

Ethanol, nicotine, and caffeine are the most widely used drugs in North America (Schuckit, 1989), and alcoholism is present in approximately 7% of the adult population, regardless of which definition is used to define alcoholism (Bissell, 1988). Its chemical effects have been known for centuries and have been well described. In some people, ethanol produces feelings of self-confidence, relaxation, expansiveness, gregariousness, and joviality. In others, it produces depression and hostility. At higher concentrations it interferes with cognitive processes, impairs judgment and concentration, and can produce coma (Jacobs and Fehr, 1987; Schuckit, 1989). Ethanol has acute and chronic effects on every organ system in the body (Geokas, 1984; Jaffe, 1985), but this discussion will be restricted to the CNS effects, specifically to the addictive process. For detailed descriptions of the pharmacology of ethanol, the reader is referred to Majchrowitz and Noble (1979), Goldstein (1983), and Pohorecky and Brick (1988).

Mechanism of Action

The literature has much conflicting data on the mechanism of action of ethanol, and it is extremely difficult to synthesize data obtained from different animal species, routes of administration, concentrations of ethanol, durations of exposure, and then try to extrapolate to a human model of behavior.

Membrane Effects.   Ethanol is a small molecule without protein moieties or other convenient components that would enable it to attach to specific receptors or membranes. In fact, there is very little evidence that ethanol exerts its effects through any receptor system (Goldstein, 1983). It has been well documented that ethanol and the other primary alcohols "dissolve" in membranes to exert their effects, and that there is a good correlation between the degree of solubility in the cell membrane, the carbon chain length, and the potency of the particular alcohol (Goldstein, 1983; Rang, 1960; Seeman, 1972). Because this is such a generalized, nonspecific biophysical effect, it has a myriad of consequences within the neuron itself; e.g., ion fluxes, enzymes systems, and neurotransmitters.

Recent research has shown that ethanol dissolves in the cell membrane and "disorders" it. The process is called *fluidizing* the membrane and has been demonstrated with electron spin resonance techniques (Goldstein, 1983). When the ethanol is given chronically it can actually change the lipid composition of the membrane, thus creating a neuroadaptation (Chin et al., 1979), and a physical basis for tolerance and dependence.

Neurotransmitter Effects.   Acute ethanol ingestion has a biphasic effect on noradrenergic neurons in the brain. Small doses increase norepinephrine, whereas large doses decrease it. Chronic ethanol ingestion increases the overall turnover of epinephrine. However, there are no studies correlating norepinephrine turnover with tolerance or dependence (Pohorecky and Brick, 1988). There is some evidence that acute ethanol intake increases dopamine release and turnover in mesolimbic neurons, but dopamine receptor–binding studies are inconclusive (Pohorecky and Brick, 1988). There has been considerable research recently on the relationship between serotonin-containing neurons and ethanol consumption (Pohorecky and Brick, 1988). Although there is no question that the seritonergic system can influence ethanol consumption (Zabik, 1989), the true mechanism is not known and there are many other confounding factors (Gill and Amit, 1989). Acute exposure to ethanol has been shown fairly conclusively to depress acetylcholine release (Pohorecky and Brick, 1988). The evidence for the effect of ethanol on gamma-aminobutyric acid (GABA) transmission is inconsistent (Kulonen, 1983; Pohorecky and Brick, 1988) as with all the other neurotransmitters, with the exception of acetylcholine. It is important to note that none of the research in neurotransmitter metabolism shows any correlation with addictive behavior.

Enzyme Systems.   Acute ethanol decreases Na-K-ATPase (adenosine triphosphatose) activity in neurons as well as decreasing cyclic adenosine monophosphate (AMP) levels acutely. However, tolerance to the acute effect occurs with chronic ethanol treatment (Pohorecky and Brick, 1988).

Ion Channels.   Ethanol has been shown to inhibit brain calcium channels, but the molecular mechanism is not known. After chronic ethanol administration, these calcium channels develop tolerance (Leslie, 1987). Sodium channels are inhibited by in vitro ethanol treatment, but tolerance develops very rapidly; i.e., within 24 h (Mullin and Hunt, 1987). Acute exposure to ethanol enhances the opening of chloride channels mediated by GABA, but there may be a direct ethanol effect as well (Allan and Harris, 1987). There is not enough data at present to develop a clear understanding of ethanol's effect on potassium channels (Carlen, 1987). Once again, it is important to note that none of this research has been correlated with addictive behavior.

The cellular mechanism of the effect of ethanol is multifactorial, and studies aimed at specific mechanisms have generally been unrewarding. Furthermore, the question arises as to whether ethanol is even capable of being self-administered; i.e., reinforcing, irrespective of the knowledge of the mechanism. The self-administration studies have also been inconclusive (Kornetsky et al., 1988).

Pharmacokinetics

The pharmacokinetic properties of ethanol have been extensively studied, but many uncertainties still exist. Essentially the only way ethanol is used and/or abused is by oral administration (Goldstein, 1983; Holford, 1987). Absorption of ethanol takes place in the stomach and small intestine, the latter site producing more rapid absorption (Erickson, 1979, Goldstein, 1983). Absorption takes place by passive diffusion, and therefore the higher the concentration of ethanol, the more rapid the rate of absorption should be. However, the mucosal barrier is a rate-limiting factor, and high (greater than 30% V/V) concentrations of ethanol decrease gastric motility, and thus reduce entry of ethanol into the small intestine, thereby reducing the rate of absorption (Erickson, 1979; Goldstein, 1983; Holford, 1987; Pitchie, 1985). Ethanol is most rapidly absorbed when its concentration is between 15 and 30% (Kalant, 1971). The time to peak concentration in the blood has ranged from 0.49 to 1.14 h in various studies (Halford, 1987). Any factor which alters gastric motility, including food, will influence the rate of ethanol absorption (Ritchie, 1985). Ethanol is evenly distributed throughout total body water, both intracellularly and extracellularly. The average volume of distribution calculated from several studies was 37.3 L in a 70-kg person (Holford, 1987), which approximates the amount of total body water.

Ninety percent of ethanol is metabolized in the liver, almost entirely by the enzyme alcohol dehydrogenase. A small percentage is metabolized by catalase, and by the microsomal ethanol-oxidizing system (MEOS) (Lieber, 1977). The latter system is said to play a slightly larger role in ethanol metabolism in chronic alcoholics (Korsten et al., 1975).

The metabolism of ethanol was originally thought to follow zero-order kinetics; i.e., a rate of oxidation constant with time, at approximately 150 mg/L/h. However, there is evidence that the rate may be dose dependent (Martin et al., 1984).

In spite of many attempts to find a drug to hasten ethanol metabolism only one has been shown to do this consistently; i.e., fructose (Holford, 1987; Tygstrup et al., 1965). Ethanol is fascinating in that there are not a lot of consistent data about its pharmacology that would predict its prominent position in the addictions field. It is taken orally, which increases the time of onset of its mood-altering properties. With the exception of its membrane effects, which may be the definitive mechanism, a specific mechanism of action is not well defined. The animal studies on reinforcement are inconsistent. The blood levels required for its effect are an order of magnitude higher than any other drug of abuse. However, its elimination rate is just slow enough to allow constant CNS exposure if taken frequently enough, and just rapid enough to produce a significant withdrawal syndrome, which would contribute to continued consumption.

B. Benzodiazepines

Benzodiazepines were first used in clinical medicine in 1960. The first benzodiazepine to be used was chlordiazepoxide (Harvey, 1985). Within a year, a physiological withdrawal syndrome was noted to be associated with the use of chlordiazepoxide (Hollister, 1961), but this issue was controversial until appropriate placebo-controlled trials were done (Busto et al., 1986; Fontaine et al., 1984; Tyrer et al., 1981).

Benzodiazepines are safe and effective for the treatment of short-term anxiety and show little cardiac or respiratory depression when given in moderate doses (Harvey, 1985; Jacobs and Fehr, 1987). They produce relaxation and calmness, as their intended effects, and mild motor incoordination, drowsiness, and disinhibition as well. They can also produce impaired cognition and memory, slurred speech, confusion, and depression. Some benzodiazepines have been known to produce euphoria (Jacobs and Fehr, 1987). As of 1988, there were approximately 50 different benzodiazepines in clinical use throughout the world (Haefely, 1988). The following discussion will not focus on the anticonvulsant or muscle relaxant properties of the benzodiazepines.

Mechanism of Action

The discovery of benzodiazepine receptors in mammalian brain in 1977 (Mohler and Okada, 1977; Squires and Braestrup, 1977) ushered in a new and exciting era of benzodiazepine research. Since that time, much has been learned about the mechanism of action of the benzodiazepines. The benzodiazepine receptor is actually three receptors, or one receptor which can have three different conformations (Haefely, 1986, 1988; Oreland, 1987). The three receptors accommodate (1) agonists, (2) inverse agonists (opposite but active effects), and (3) antagonists (block agonists and inverse agonists. It is part of a larger protein complex which also contains the GABA receptors ($GABA_A$ and $GABA_B$). When activated, this complex opens up the chloride channel in the membrane, which in turn hyperpolarizes the membrane and produces its inhibitory effect. Most of these GABA receptor–benzodiazepine receptor–complex neurons are more appropriately termed *interneurons*, which are strategically placed throughout the CNS to exhibit their inhibitory function on other neurons, and to exert their clinical effects as sedatives, anxiolytics, anticonvulsants, and smooth muscle relaxants.

In spite of the ability of benzodiazepines to produce a physiological dependence, as demonstrated by the emergency of a withdrawal syndrome (Busto et al., 1986; Fontaine et al., 1984), there has been no consistent evidence that the drugs have any ability to be self-administered (Woods et al., 1987). However, there is some evidence that people who have a history of previous sedative abuse or dependency will self-administer benzodiazepines, as opposed to naive users (Senay, 1989; Woods et al., 1987).

Pharmacokinetics

All benzodiazepines essentially act in the same manner and their major differences are in their relative potencies and their pharmacokinetics. For the purposes of abuse and dependency, the oral route is by far the most common method of administration. All benzodiazepines absorbed poorly and erratically by intramuscular injection, except lorazepam (Greenblatt et al., 1979, 1982). Lorazepam is unique in that it is also well absorbed sublingually (Greenblatt et al., 1979, 1982). For detailed reviews of the pharmacokinetics of benzodiazepines the reader is referred to Bellantuono et al., 1980 and Greenblatt et al., 1983.

Benzodiazepines are very well absorbed from the gastrointestinal tract, and are thus excellent oral sedatives and anxiolytics. This feature is offset in some of the benzodiazepines by a first-pass hepatic metabolism effect. Maximum absorption of benzodiazepines varies from 30 to 180 min, the shortest times to peak plasma concentration being recorded, although not consistently, for diazepam, chlordiazepoxide, alprazolam, and midazolam (Bellantuono et al., 1980; Greenblatt et al., 1983). The longest absorption times are for oxazepam, prazepam, and halazepam (Busto, et al., 1989; Greenblatt et al., 1981). All benzodiazepines are extensively protein bound, and, at physiological pH, highly lipid soluble and readily distributed in the body (Bellantuono et al., 1980; Busto et al., 1989). The bioavailability of the benzodiazepines is generally very good after oral absorption, with the exception of midazolam because of its first-pass effect (Busto et al., 1989; Greenblatt et al., 1983). The average volume of distribution for the benzodiazepines as a group is 1 L/kg (Busto et al., 1989), but there is a large variation (0.26–1.83 L/kg) (Bellantuono et al., 1980; Greenblatt et al., 1983).

The elimination half-lives of the benzodiazepines are quite variable and are an important feature in their clinical usage (Greenblatt et al., 1981). However, it is important to point out that the half-life of a drug does not necessarily correlate with its duration of clinical effect after single doses, but assumes more importance after multiple doses when a steady state has been reached.

The volume of distribution, determined by lipid solubility, and protein binding seems to be a more important determinant of the duration of action (Greenblatt et al., 1983). The shortest half-lives belong to midazolam (1–4 h) and triazolam (1.5–5.0 h), whereas the longest half-lives belong to diazepam (20–70 h), N-desmethyl diazepam (51–120 h), and flurazepam (51–120 h) (Bellantuono et al., 1980; Greenblatt et al., 1983). If there is basically no difference in the mechanism of action among the various benzodiazepines, then one would not expect any particular benzodiazepine to be abused more than another. However, the pharmacokinetic differences have been shown to influence drug preference. Preference for diazepam (a rapidly absorbed drug) over oxazepam (a slowly absorbed drug) has been shown (Griffiths et al., 1984a, 1984b), and the subjects cited this as a reason for preference (Griffiths, 1984b). The elimination kinetics also influence drug-seeking behavior. Patients taking short-acting benzodiazepines, when cut off their drug, were shown to resume their drug use 7 days earlier than those patients who were cut off their long-acting benzodiazepine (Busto et al., 1986). It is this latter phenomenon that has served as the basis for the pharmacological treatment of sedative withdrawal (Marks, 1988; Busto et al., 1989).

Benzodiazepines are addictive drugs, the evidence for this being in the emergence of a well-described physiological withdrawal syndrome.

C. Barbiturates

The barbiturates are classed as sedative-hypnotics and are derived from barbituric acid. Barbituric acid was first synthesized in 1864 and its anticonvulsant and hypnotic properties were discovered shortly after 1900 (Richter and Holtman, 1982). There are three subclasses of barbiturates, loosely based on their duration of action. Ultra–short-acting barbiturates are used to induce anesthesia, and are mostly given intravenously, whereas short- to intermediate-acting barbiturates are used orally, and are prescribed as sedative-hypnotics. This latter group is the one most frequently abused. Last, the long-acting barbiturates are used as anticonvulsants (Schuckit, 1989), and are prescribed for oral ingestion. There are also barbiturate-like drugs such as methaqualone, ethchlorvynol, methyprylon, and glutethimide, which act very similarly to the barbiturates. These latter drugs, as well as meprobamate, a carbamate ester, will not be discussed here, and the reader is referred to Harvey (1985).

Barbiturates are usually taken orally and are rarely used intravenously. Low doses produce tranquility, relaxation, and mild euphoria, with some motor incoordination. Moderate doses produce a pleasurable state of intoxication, but can produce oversedation, confusion, hostility, slurred speech, and impaired judgement (Jacobs and Fehr, 1987).

Mechanism of Action

Barbiturates are known to interact with a lipid component of neuronal membranes (Ho and Harris, 1981), and increase membrane fluidity. However, this effect may not occur until anesthesia is produced (Olsen, 1988), and hence may not be applicable to its initial euphoric effects. Barbiturates may not have a specific receptor site, but they demonstrate a nonspecific physical interaction with hydrophobic molecules in the membrane and have an effect on several ion channels; namely, sodium, potassium, calcium, and chloride. In particular, research has shown a consistent effect on chloride channels. Because of this fairly generalized effect, it is not surprising to learn that barbiturates affect many neurotransmitter systems; namely, acetylcholine, norepinephrine, dopamine, and GABA, and serotonin (Ho and Harris, 1981; Richter and Holtman, 1982). The most consistent findings have been in the relationship of barbiturate action to GABA (Harvey, 1985; Ho and Harris, 1981; Richter and Holtman, 1982).

The current theory on the mechanism of the sedative-hypnotic action of barbiturates is that the barbiturate binds to the post synaptic neuronal membrane specifically at the site of the GABA receptor–chloride channel protein complex to exert its inhibitory effects (Olsen, 1988). There is evidence that this is a specific barbiturate receptor site, as demonstrated in binding studies, and there is correlation between the binding affinity and the biological activity (Olsen et al., 1988).

In contrast to benzodiazepines, for which the evidence is weak, the barbiturates have consistently exhibited reinforcing properties (i.e., self-administration properties in animal studies) (Ator and Griffiths, 1987; Griffiths et al., 1981).

Pharmacokinetics

The barbiturates that are administered intravenously for anesthesia will not be discussed, as the major form of barbiturate drug abuse is by the oral route. The use of barbiturates, both by prescription and on the street, has been largely supplanted by benzodiazepines (Harvey, 1985), and their decline in popularity has paralleled an increase in the popularity and sophistication of the science of pharmacokinetics. Therefore, there has been little detailed research done on the pharmacokinetics of barbiturates since 1975 (Breimer, 1977; Harvey, 1985), except perhaps in the field of anesthesia (Olsen, 1988). For details of the individual barbiturate drugs, the reader is referred to Breimer (1977).

Barbiturates are absorbed mainly from the intestine, and the sodium salts are absorbed more rapidly than the free acid (Breimer, 1977; Breimer and de Boer, 1975; Harvey, 1985). The thiobarbiturates are more lipid soluble than the oxybarbiturates, and hence will distribute to tissues more rapidly and to a greater extent than the oxybarbiturates. The barbiturates are well absorbed, but there is a significant first-pass metabolism effect in the liver for some of them. The goal in producing barbiturates for the treatment of insomnia was a rapid absorption, rapid onset of action, and a short duration of action to avoid daytime sedation. There is considerable variation among the individual drugs in this class and not many of them achieved the latter goal (Breimer, 1977). The absorption rates vary from drug to drug, achieving peak serum levels anywhere from 20 min to 2 h (Breimer, 1977). The volume of distribution ranges from 0.51 L/kg (cyclobarbital) to 1.52 L/kg (secobarbital). The elimination half-life ranges from a mean of 1.6 h (methohexital, an intravenously administered drug), to 29.6 h (pentobarbital) (Breimer, 1977). Phenobarbital was not studied in the experiments cited above, but it is known to have a half-life of approximately 100 h (Rall and Schleifer, 1985).

The pharmacokinetic factors that would be important in producing addiction are: rate of absorption, degree of distribution, redistribution, and rate of elimination. Reinforcing properties have been demonstrated for oral preparations in animals (Ator and Griffiths, 1987), but there are no details on the differential rates of absorption. There is, however, some evidence of the effect of the differences in the elimination rates of various barbiturates on the addictive process, specifically on the production of physiological dependence and withdrawal (Boisse and Okamoto, 1978). This concept has been used as the rationale in treating barbiturate withdrawal with phenobarbital (Jacobs and Fehr, 1979; Robinson and Sellers, 1981).

Generally speaking, the barbiturates are quite addictive drugs, based on self-administration studies and the known propensity for acute withdrawal reactions. However, they have been largely replaced by the benzodiazepines.

D. Solvents

Although the effects of solvent inhalation have been studied for years, there is little pharmacological data in the area of substance abuse. The vast majority of the research literature concerning the pharmacological actions of inhaled solvents is in the field of industrial and occupational exposure. Information from this field should not be used to extrapolate to substance abuse. Although the method of exposure is the same in both areas, i.e., inhalation, the duration and intensity of exposure are quite different (Cohen, 1981; Klaassen, 1985). Industrial exposure is more chronic, less intense, whereas abuse is intense and periodic.

The effects of inhalation are rapid in onset, after the first few inhalations. There is a sensation of euphoria, dizziness, numbness, weightlessness, and dissociation from the environment. Similar to ethanol, there may be giddiness, disinhibition, slurred speech, impaired judgment, and perceptual distortion. There is considerable variation among individuals, partly because of the different chemical constituents of the various solvents (Jacobs and Fehr, 1987). For detailed lists of the solvents of abuse and their chemical composition, the reader is referred to Jacobs and Fehr (1987) and Schuckit (1989). Briefly, the more common chemicals are toluene, hexane, benzene, chloroform, acetone, Freons, and nitrites. These are contained in glues, cleaning solutions, nail polish removers, lighter fluids, paints, paint thinners, and aerosols (Jacobs and Fehr, 1987; Schuckit, 1989).

Mechanism of Action

Because of the diversity of compounds, it is impossible to give a detailed discussion of the mechanisms of action of the solvents. All the solvents are highly lipid soluble and distribute well to all tissues, especially the CNS. The mechanisms of action are not known, but their mode of action resembles that of other general anesthetics (Cohen, 1981), and clinically they can produce a state similar to stage 1 or 11 levels of anesthesia (Glaser, 1974). There is some evidence that animals will self-administer some of the solvents (Sharp and Brehm, 1977), but very few have been studied.

Pharmacokinetics

The interesting feature of all the inhaled solvents is rapid onset and short duration of action; i.e., approximately 45 min (Schuckit, 1989). Because of the high lipid solubility, there is rapid distribution, which contributes to the short duration of action (Watson, 1980). There has not been a well-documented description of a physiological withdrawal syndrome (Cohen, 1981; Jacobs and Fehr, 1987).

The rapidity of onset of effects and the demonstration of the reinforcing properties in animals support the conclusion that solvents are addicting.

E. Opiates

The psychological effects of opium, the juice obtained from the plant *Papaver somniferum*, have been known for well over 2000 years, and the earliest recorded references occurred in the third century B.C. (Jaffe and Martin, 1985). Morphine was first isolated from opium in 1806, and codeine in 1832 (Jaffe and Martin, 1985). Interestingly, the most common method of opium administration in the nineteenth century was by inhalation, but this was eventually surpassed in popularity by the intravenous route with the invention of the hypodermic needle (Jaffe and Martin, 1985). In addition to the naturally occurring opiates such as opium, morphine, and codeine, several semisynthetic opiates have been produced by minor chemical alterations in the basic product; e.g., heroin, hydromorphine, and oxycodone (Schuckit, 1989). Heroin was first introduced in the 1980s (Gold and Rea, 1983).

The opiates as a group all have the same clinical effects, and the differences among them occur in their potencies, route of administration, and duration of action (Jaffe, 1985; Wikler, 1980). They produce analgesia, drowsiness, euphoria, relaxation, and a clouding of mental functioning, and in higher doses can produce stupor, coma, shock, and respiratory arrest (Jacobs and Fehr, 1987; Schuckit, 1989). Classically, the rapid intravenous administration of heroin is said to produce a "rush" or "kick" similar to sexual orgasm, and lasts about 45 s (Jaffe, 1985).

Mechanism of Action

Progress in the search for a mechanism of action of the opiates was greatly enhanced by the discovery of the opiate receptor in the CNS (Pert and Snyder, 1973). Since then, four subclasses of receptors have been discovered; i.e., mu, kappa, sigma, and delta. Mu and kappa receptors are associated with analgesia, whereas psychotomimetic effects are associated with the sigma receptor, and alterations in affective behavior are associated with delta receptors. Opiate receptors are widely distributed throughout the central and peripheral nervous systems (Carr, 1988; Koob et al., 1986), but are concentrated in certain areas of the central nervous system which subserve the various clinical effects; e.g., analgesia, and euphoria. The periaqueductal gray area is one of the major areas mediating analgesia (Jaffe, 1985), and is distinct from another area of opiate receptor concentration, the medial forebrain bundle, which is associated with positive reinforcement (Wise, 1988).

Self-administration studies in animals have demonstrated that only certain subtypes of opiate receptors mediate the reinforcing properties of opiates. Mu and delta receptors have been shown to be the most likely candidates (Koob et al., 1986; Mucha and Herz, 1985).

Thus, there is ample evidence that the opiates act on several discrete areas in the CNS where there is a concentration of opiate receptors, and have differential effects on subsets of receptors in order to produce their various clinical effects. In particular, part of the medical forebrain bundle, the dopamine-containing mesolimbic system, has been shown to mediate the reinforcing properties (Koob and Bloom, 1988; Wise, 1988). The two areas involved are the nucleus accumbens and the ventral tegmental area (Koob and Bloom, 1988; Wise, 1988), although there is some suggestion that the opiates have a more powerful effect on the nucleus accumbens (Koob et al., 1986). The opiates have been shown to have powerful reinforcing properties in self-administration studies (Brady and Lukas, 1984).

In addition to having reinforcing properties to aid in the development of addiction, the opiates produce a distinct, unpleasant withdrawal syndrome, which, interestingly enough, is not mediated by the mesolimbic reward system, but through the periaqueductal gray area (Koob and Bloom, 1988).

Pharmacokinetics

Opiates are taken in all the usual route of administration; i.e., oral, intranasal, inhalation, and intravenous. There has been very little research done on the pharmacokinetics of the opiates, especially the opiates that are abused. The more sophisticated pharmacokinetic studies have been done on the newer synthetic opiates used for anesthesia (Davis and Cook, 1986).

Only a few of the opiates are effectual orally because the majority of them are diminished by the first-pass effect of hepatic metabolism. Codeine, levorphanol, and oxycodone are the major drugs that are effective orally (Jaffe and Martin, 1985). Codeine is approximately two-thirds as effective orally as parenterally, whereas the bioavailability of oral morphine preparations varies from 15 to 59% (Sawe et al., 1981). The bioavailability of oral meperidine is approximately 56% (Edwards et al., 1982).

Opiates that are taken intravenously act within minutes, but there is some variation in onset of action because of differing lipid solubilities. Heroin's euphoriant effects are felt almost immediately because it is rapidly converted to monoacetylmorphine, which is highly lipid soluble and more potent than morphine (Busto and Sellers, 1986). The duration of action is similar for all opiates, being approximately 2–4 h, with the exception of methadone. Methadone's half-life is to 1.5 days. Protein binding of the opiates is variable, being 60–80% for meperidine (Edwards et al., 1982) and 33% for morphine (Jaffe and Martin, 1985).

Because the duration of action is relatively short, and because the opiates are taken at frequent intervals, either orally or intravenously, significant physiological dependence develops and a withdrawal syndrome is produced which is severely distressing to the patient, but not life threatening in any way. The use of methadone, both for maintenance of the addict, and for treatment of withdrawal, are examples of a drug with a long half-life that protects the use from an acute severe withdrawal.

Very few opiates are inhaled, the chief ones being opium itself, which contains over 20 distinct alkaloids (Jaffe and Martin, 1985), and therefore would produce a complex pharmacokinetic profile; and heroin, which is very rapidly metabolized to monoacetylmorphine (Boerner et al., 1975; Busto and Sellers, 1986). The volume of distribution of morphine ranges from 1.6 L/kg in the elderly to 2.12 L/kg in the young (Owen et al., 1983).

The opiates, generally speaking, are highly addictive, having significant reinforcing properties, and the ability to produce a significant withdrawal syndrome.

VI. CNS STIMULANTS

A. Amphetamines and Cocaine

The active ingredient in the leaf *Erythoxylon coca* has been used for centures as a stimulant and anorexiant (Kleber, 1988; Schuckit, 1989). Cocaine was first isolated in 1857, and amphetamine was first synthesized in 1887 (Schuckit, 1989). The two drugs are essentially indistinguishable clinically and neuropharmacologically (Gawin and Ellinwood, 1989). Presently, cocaine is the more popular drug, and we are in the midst of our fifth and largest epidemic of cocaine abuse, the previous ones occurring in the 1890s, 1920s, early 1950s, and late 1960s (Gawin and Ellinwood, 1988). The other major stimulants are methylphenidate, methamphetamine, and caffeine, and various diet pills (Schuckit, 1989).

The clinical effects of the above-named drugs are similar in quality, but differ greatly in potency (Jacobs and Fehr, 1987; Schuckit, 1989). As an example, cocaine produces a feeling of euphoria, well-being, increased alertness, garrulousness, decreased appetite, and a decreased need for sleep.

Mechanism of Action

Amphetamine and cocaine act by acutely increasing synaptic levels of dopamine in specific areas of the brain (Koob and Bloom, 1988; Miller et al., 1989; Wise, 1980, 1988). Both amphetamine and cocaine block the reuptake of dopamine into the presynaptic neuron, its normal method of removal. In addition, amphetamine causes release of dopamine from the presynaptic neuron. The immediate "high" that is felt is said to be due to this flood of dopamine in the synapse which stimulates the postsynaptic receptors, and it is this mechanism that is responsible for the well-documented powerful reinforcing properties (Koob and Bloom, 1988; Wise, 1988).

After chronic stimulant usage, the dopamine synthesis mechanism is said to be exhausted and the postsynaptic dopamine receptors are "supersensitive" so that discontinuation of the stimulant then produces a dopamine depletion syndrome that is responsible for the symptoms of anhedonia and craving (Dackis and Gold, 1985; Gawin, 1988; Wise, 1988). The dopamine-containing neurons that are particularly influenced by the stimulant drugs are concentrated in the medial forebrain bundle, which constitutes the "reward" system (Gawin, 1988; Miller et al., 1989; Wise, 1980, 1988). The ventral tegmental area and the nucleus accumbens are the two major collections of such neurons in the pathway, but the precise input and output paths have not been fully elucidated (Gawin, 1988; Wise, 1988). This system, and its manipulation by cocaine, amphetamine, and dopamine agonists and antagonists, is responsible for the extremely powerful reinforcing properties of the stimulant drugs (Aigner and Balster, 1978; Wise, 1988).

Pharmacokinetics

The stimulants are taken by a variety of routes. Amphetamines are usually taken orally or intravenously, whereas cocaine can be taken intranasally, intravenously, or by inhalation (Busto et al., 1989; Jacobs and Fehr, 1987; Schuckit, 1989). Caffeine is taken orally, but in many forms; e.g., in coffee, chocolate bars, tablet forms (Busto et al., 1989). Amphetamine, when taken orally, reaches a peak plasma concentration in 1.25 h, and the peak levels can be lowered by acidifying the urine (Anggard et al., 1970; Busto et al., 1989). Plasma protein binding is only 20%, while the volume of distribution is fairly large; i.e., 6.1 L/kg in drug users (Anggard et al., 1970). In animals, there is rapid distribution into tissues after intraperitoneal administration and peak brain concentrations are reached after 30 min (Maickel et al., 1969). The elimination half-life is 4.2 h in drug users, slightly shorter in naive subjects, and considerably longer when the urine is basic (Anggard et al., 1970).

Caffeine is rapidly and completely absorbed, with peak plasma levels being reached in 30–60 min (Blanchard and Sawers, 1983a). It is only 15–30% protein bound, and its volume of distribution varies between 0.54 and 0.70 L/kg (Blanchard and Sawers, 1983b). The elimination half-life of caffeine is quite variable, ranging from 2.7 to 9.9 h (Blanchard and Sawers, 1983a).

Cocaine is lipophilic and is obtainable in two forms, cocaine hydrochloride (salt form) and cocaine base. Cocaine hydrochloride can be taken orally, intranasally, or intravenously. Cocaine base is derived from the salt by extraction with solvents and exists in the form of a paste, or it is extracted with baking soda to form a more solid form called "rock" or "crack" (Jacobs and Fehr, 1987). Both of these forms are of much higher potency than the salt form (40–70% pure vs 0–25% pure), and are inhaled (Busto et al., 1989; Gawin and Ellinwood, 1988; Hogberg and Schnoll, 1983; Paly et al., 1982).

When taken orally, peak levels are reached in 50–90 min, and when taken intranasally, time to peak levels is dose dependent and ranges from 35 to 160 min (Busto et al., 1989). When smoked, peak plasma levels of cocaine are reached in 3 min (Paly et al., 1982). Inhalation is said to be a more effective route of delivery than the intravenous route because a larger amount is absorbed more rapidly through the large surface area of the lungs, and the inhalable form of the drug is far more concentrated than the intravenous form (Busto et al., 1989; Gawin and Ellinwood, 1988).

Cocaine is rapidly distributed to the tissues and has a short elimination half-life, ranging from 31 to 82 min (Busto et al., 1989). The clinical effect lasts for approximately 20–40 min (Busto et al., 1989; Jaffe, 1985). Plasma protein binding is 35% (Busto et al., 1989), and the volume of distribution is 1.98 L/kg (Chow et al., 1985).

The key features of the addicting properties of the stimulants (cocaine and amphetamines) are their inherent reinforcing properties, and, if smoked (cocaine), the rapid delivery to the CNS. They are taken in binges and are very short-acting. These latter properties would lead one to predict that there would be no physiological withdrawal. However, with the "discovery" of the proposed neuropharmacological mechanisms of anhedonia and craving, after cessation of drug use, the distinction between physiological dependence and psychological dependence becomes blurred. Nevertheless, the stimulants are extremely addictive drugs.

B. Nicotine

Nearly 30% of adult Americans smoke (Benowitz, 1988), and when they try to quit, there is a 70% relapse rate after 3 months (Hunt et al., 1971). This gives us some indication of its addictive properties. Although the practice of ingesting tobacco was present before the discovery of America (Janiger and de Rios, 1973), nicotine was not isolated from tobacco until the 1820s (Henningfield and Goldberg, 1988a). Research in the 1920s showed that nicotine was the active ingredient to which smokers were responding (Henningfield and Goldberg, 1988a). More recently, the reinforcing properties of nicotine have been well established (Henningfield and Goldberg, 1983).

Nicotine is a stimulant with effects on many organ systems (Benowitz, 1988), but this discussion will be limited to the effects on the central nervous system. It produces arousal, improvement in attention, and learning. Smokers also report pleasure and reduced anger and tension, but these latter effects may be due to relief of withdrawal symptoms (Benowitz, 1988). for more detailed descriptions of the pharmacology of nicotine, the reader is referred to Benowitz (1988) and Grenhoff and Svensson (1989).

Mechanism of Action

There are three main sites of physiological action that involve the nicotine receptors in the body: the neuromuscular junction, the autonomic ganglia, and the central nervous system, and this discussion will focus on the latter area.

There have been certain subtypes of nicotine receptors discovered in the CNS which account for the behavioral effects of nicotine, and these effects can be blocked by the appropriate centrally acting pharmacological tools (e.g., mecamylamine) (Kumar et al., 1987; Morrison and Stephenson, 1969). In addition, activation of these receptors, when located on presynaptic neurons, causes release of norepinephrine, dopamine, and acetylcholine (Grenhoff and Svensson, 1989). One specific area of the brain in which this effect is found is the locus coeruleus, an area known to mediate arousal, vigilance, and stress reactions (Svensson and Engberg, 1980). Nicotine also acts on the mesolimbic dopamine system (Pert and Chiueh, 1988), which is involved in the brain reward system (Wise, 1980, 1988). This somewhat analagous to effects of other stimulants; e.g., cocaine (Dackis and Gold, 1985; Miller et al., 1987).

The action of nicotine on the brain reward system, specifically the ventral tegmental area (Pert and Chiueh, 1988) could explain the drug's reinforcing properties (Henningfield and Goldberg, 1983).

Pharmacokinetics

Nicotine is absorbed by inhalation most commonly, but it is also absorbed through the mucous membranes. It is highly ionized in cigarette smoke, which has an acidic pH of 5.5, but in spite of this, it is rapidly absorbed through the lungs. Tobacco smoke from pipes and cigars and some European cigarettes is alkaline (pH 8.5), and thus contains nicotine in a primarily unionized state which further enhances its absorption (Benowitz, 1988; Busto et al., 1989). Chewing tobacco, snuff, and Nicorette gum are all buffered to an alkaline pH to facilitate absorption through the mucous membranes (Benowitz, 1988). Most low-tar cigarettes contain 0.8 mg of nicotine (Guerin, 1980), and experienced smokers can absorb up to 80–90% of the nicotine in the mainstream smoke. Under experimental conditions, higher amounts have been used where the average absorption was about 1 mg (Benowitz, 1984; Feyerabend et al., 1985). The absorption of nicotine from 2.5 gm of oral snuff was 3.6 mg, and from 7.9 gm of chewing tobacco was 4.6 mg in the studies cited above. Peak nicotine levels from smoking area reached within 15 min after smoking 1.5 cigarettes for 9 min, whereas peak levels after smokeless tobacco occur after 30 min (Benowitz, 1984). Being a lipophilic base, nicotine is rapidly and widely distributed to tissues. Its volume of distribution is quite large and variable: In one study, it was 79 ± 45 L by one method of calculation, and 173 ± 623 L by another method in a 70-kg man (Feyerabend et al., 1985). Nicotine is metabolized primarily in the liver (Busto et al., 1989). The elimination half-life of nicotine is approximately 2 h (Feyerabend et al., 1985), but the range is 1–4 h (Benowitz et al., 1982). However, with repeated dosage, there may be an increase in the half-life as the nicotine accumulates (Feyerabend and Russell, 1978).

In spite of a relatively short half-life, nicotine will accumulate in the body because of the manner in which it is consumed; i.e., repeated doses over the day. Therefore, nicotine exposure is a 24-h-long event (Benowitz et al., 1982).

It is apparent from the widespread use of the drug, as well as the difficulties encountered in trying to quit, that nicotine is an addictive drug. When one examines the research done on nicotine, it becomes even more obvious. Its stimulus response time is short; i.e., by inhalation. Its reinforcing properties have been demonstrated in animal studies. There is 24-h exposure to the drug because of the way in which it is consumed; i.e., frequent doses. There is a significant withdrawal syndrome occurring 24–48 h after cessation because of its relatively short half-life (Benowitz, 1988). In summary, it is a very addictive drug.

VII. HALLUCINOGENS

A. Cannabinols

Cannabinols are the major ingredient of marijuana and hashish. The three principal cannabinols are delta-9-tetrahydrocannabinol, or, delta-1-tetrahydrocannabinol (THC), a cannabidiol (CBD), and cannabinol (CBN), although there are over 60 known cannabinols in the plant *Cannabis sativa* (Busto et al., 1989). The pharmacologically active compound, in terms of its psychotomimetic properties, is THC. Cannabidiol is devoid of psychotomimetic properties, whereas CBN has about one-tenth the potency of THC if given intravenously (Agurell, 1986). The active drug is therefore THC, and it has been used in some form or another for at least 4000 years (Schuckit, 1989).

The user usually experiences euphoria, relaxation, sleepiness, and increased sexual arousal. There is a distorted sense of time, mild paranoia, and short-term memory difficulties. At higher doses, hallucinations and vivid paranoid delusions can occur. Panic attacks can also occur, and are more common in a first-time user (Jacobs and Fehr, 1987; Schuckit, 1989). Interestingly, the psychotomimetic effects occur slightly later than the time of peak plasma concentration (Agurell, 1986). It was originally thought that the effect was due to its active metabolite, but this was subsequently disproven. There has been an extensive amount of research on THC, and for a more detailed description of its pharmacology the reader is referred to Dewey (1986), Hollster (1986), Agurell et al. (1986), Razdan (1987), and Pertwee (1988).

Mechanism of Action

As stated before, the principal active ingredient of cannabinols is delta-9-THC. However, a metabolite, 11-OH-delta-9-THC is equally potent, but its concentration after intravenous administration or smoking is only one-tenth of that of delta-9-THC after oral administration. However, the hydroxy metabolite assumes equal importance in the psychotomimetic effect after oral doses (Agurell, 1986; Bristo et al., 1989).

The mechanism of action of THC is very complex, and there are not a lot of firm conclusions about a specific site of action (Pertwee, 1988). Cannabinols are very lipid soluble, and as a result are difficult to isolate in extraction procedures and binding studies. This has been postulated as a reason for the conflicting evidence in the neuropharmacological research. Electrophysiological studies have shown that THC appears to have a biphasic effect on neuronal transmission; i.e., excitatory at low doses and inhibitory at high doses. However, the evidence is not conclusive. There has been extensive research on the effect of THC on neurotransmitter levels, turnover, uptake, and storage, but once again the data is inconclusive as the reports are conflicting: The principal neurotransmitters that have been studied are norepinephrine, dopamine, 5-hydroxytryptamine, acetylcholine, gamma-aminobutryic acid, histidine, and spermidine. Binding studies have shown that THC can alter binding to adrenoceptors, dopamine receptors, and opioid receptors. The effects are biphasic and concentration dependent, and differ in different preparations (Pertwee, 1988). Studies on the intracellular enzyme systems, ATPase, adenylate cyclase, and guanylate cyclase, have also been inconclusive. However, there is slightly more consistent evidence showing THC's ability to stimulate phospholipase A_2, and thus alter prostaglandin metabolism (Martin, 1986). It has been shown to alter membrane fluidity, but this is dependent on both the concentration of THC and the lipid composition of the membrane (Pertwee, 1988).

It is important to note that in addition to the research findings in the cellular mechanisms giving no clear consensus, there is no correlation with THC's psychotomimetic properties (Pertwee, 1988). The only exception to this general conclusion is that there is a weak correlation with THC's ability to "fluidize" membranes (Hillard et al., 1985; Lawrence and Gill, 1975).

Pharmacokinetics

Although THC can be taken orally and has been taken intravenously, by far the most common route of administration is by inhalation (Agurell et al., 1986; Jacobs and Fehr, 1987). The concentration of THC in a marijuana "joint" is 1–3%, and in hash oil it is 2–5%, but can be as high as 15%. Hashish is usually 10–20% THC, but 70% concentrations have been found. A 500-mg joint typically contains 5 mg of THC, but more potent preparations may contain 20–30 mg (e.g., Californian sinsemilla) (Jacobs and Fehr, 1987). However, the actual amount delivered to the lungs is highly variable because of the individual variations in smoking technique (Agurell et al., 1986). Under experimental conditions, with a marijuana cigarette containing 19 mg of THC, experienced smokers reached their desired high having absorbed 13 mg of THC by inhalation (Agurell, 1986). Comparable doses by other routes of administration in kinetic studies were 5 mg intravenously and 20 mg orally (Agurell et al., 1986; Ohlsson et al., 1980).

Three minutes after a 5-mg intravenous infusion, the plasma concentration of THC is approximately 160–315 mg/L, and declines rapidly to 15 mg/L. Smoking produces a peak concentration of THC at 3 min as well, 30–120 mg/L (Ohlsson et al., 1980). Oral ingestion produces a peak concentration of 6 mg/L 1 h after ingestion (Perez-Reyes et al., 1982). Delta-9-THC is rapidly transferred from blood to various tissues and accounts for the short subjective effects of the drug relative to its long elimination half-life (Busto et al., 1989).

It has an extremely large volume of distribution, approximately 10 L/kg (Agurell et al., 1986; Busto et al., 1989), which is typical for a highly lipophilic drug. The drug is 95% bound to plasma lipoproteins (Wahlqvist et al., 1970).

Delta-9-THC, the parent compound, is metabolized firstly to 11-OH-delta-9-THC, which is equally potent but in very small concentration relative to delta-9-THC. However, after oral ingestion the metabolite concentration is clinically important relative to the parent compound because of the first-pass effect.

The elimination half-life of the drug is approximately 20–30 h (Hunt and Jones, 1980; Ohlsson et al., 1982), and a difference has been noted between chronic (28 h) and naive (57 h) users (Lemberger et al., 1970).

Delta-9-THC is an addictive drug, but only moderately so. Because it is inhaled, it reaches the central nervous (CNS) rapidly. However, its psychotomimetic effects are milder than the other hallucinogens. It has a long elimination half-life, which allows it to produce some "neuroadaptation," but its rapid distribution to other tissues negates some of this effect. The long elimination half-life of THC also moderates the withdrawal, which is known to be mild, if present at all (Hollister, 1986).

B. Lysergic Acid Diethylamide

Lysergic acid diethylamide (LSD) is a psychotomimetic whose psychodelic properties were discovered in 1943, and its popularity as a psychedelic drug peaked in the late 1960s (Jaffe, 1985).

Clinically, the drug produces an increased awareness of sensory input, of enhanced mental activity, altered body images, sensory distortions, and hallucinations. The usual street dose range that will produce these effects ranges from 20 to 500 μg (Jacobs and Fehr, 1987; Schuckit, 1989).

Mechanism of Action

Lysergic acid diethylamide is the most potent of the hallucinogenic drugs and produces a picture similar to other hallucinogens such as dimethyltryptamine (DMT), diethyltryptamine (DET), mescaline, and 2,5-dimethoxy-4-methylamphetamine (DOM or STP) (Schuckit, 1989).

Recent research in animals (Titeler et al., 1988) and in human cadaveric brain tissue (Sadzot et al., 1989) has shown that LSD binds with high affinity to a subpopulation of 5-hydroxytryptamine receptors in the brain; namely, 5-HT2 receptors. Further, it was shown that there is a very strong correlation between binding affinity and clinical potency (Sadzot et al., 1989). The drug is not known to have reinforcing properties that produce repetitive use (Jaffe, 1985; Schuckit, 1989).

Pharmacokinetics

Lysergic acid diethylamide can be taken orally, subcutaneously, intravenously, or by inhalation. The drug is well absorbed when taken orally. The actual high lasts 6–12 h (Longer than most other hallucinogens; i.e., 2–4 h), but the elimination half-life is approximately 3 h (Jaffe, 1985). The drug is not known to be highly addictive (Jacobs and Fehr, 1987; Jaffe, 1985).

C. Phencyclidine

Phencyclidine (PCP) is an arylcyclohexylamine that was first synthesized in 1926 and introduced into practice in 1958 was a potent, rapid-acting anesthetic with no respiratory depressant effects (Sonders et al., 1988). However, its psychotomimetic side effects caused it to be withdrawn from clinical use in 1965, and it became popular as a hallucinogen in the 1970s.

The behavioral toxicity of PCP is dose related. Doses of 1–5 mg of PCP produce incoordination, a floating feeling of euphoria, and heightened emotionality. There is also an increase in sweating and lacrimation. Toxic symptoms are noted at 10-mg doses and consist of a drunken state, numbness of the extremities, and perceptual illusions. Above 10 mg, the clinical picture can progress to catalepsy, mutism, coma, and convulsions (Schuckit, 1989). A typical high lasts 4–6 h (Jaffe, 1985), but the psychosis can last from 24 h to 1 month (Schuckit, 1989).

Phencyclidine is unique as a hallucinogen in that animal studies have shown that it can be self-administered, whereas other hallucinogens have not demonstrated this property in convincing fashion (Schuckit, 1989).

Mechanism of Action

Phenylcyclidine is a complex drug and its clinical effects exhibit involvement with different neurotransmitter, e.g., catecholemines, acetylcholine, serotonin (Schuckit, 1989), glutamate, and dopamine (Cho et al., 1989).

Recently, animal studies with PCP have demonstrated two separate and specific PCP receptors in the brain. One, the PCP receptor, binds PCP with more affinity than the other, a sigma-type opiate receptor. Benzomorphan drugs, such as cyclazocine, which also produce a schizophrenialike effect in humans similar to PCP, also bind to these receptors (Sircar and Zukin, 1984; Sonders et al., 1988).

Pharmacokinetics

Phenylcyclidine can be inhaled, snorted (intranasal), injected (intravenous), or ingested (oral). The usual methods of taking the drug are oral and inhalation (Schuckit, 1989). The kinetics have been investigated in man (Busto et al., 1989), but the doses used in the two major studies, for eithical reasons, were not high enough to produce significant clinical effects (Cook et al., 1982a, 1982b). After oral ingestion of PCP peak plasma concentrations were attained approximately 1.5 h later. After inhalations of PCP, peak levels were achieved between 5 and 22 min. The volume of distribution is very large, being 6.2 L/kg body weight, and indicates extensive tissue distribution. The drug is approximately 65% protein bound with slightly smaller values for females. The elimination half-life of PCP is 16 h after intravenous dosing, 27 h after oral dosing, and 24 h after inhalation.

With respect to the development of addiction, there seems to be some inherant reinforcing property of the drug (Schuckit, 1989), but the cellular mechanisms are not known at this time. Furthermore, elimination kinetics (Cook et al., 1982a, 1982b) are consistent with the fact that there is no withdrawal from the drug, although "psychological dependence" could develop (Jacobs and Fehr, 1987).

One could speculate that inhalation of the drug could contribute to its addiction potential but it is not known to be a highly addictive drug (Jacobs and Fehr, 1987).

VIII. DISCUSSION

It is not within the scope of this chapter to discuss the nonpharmacological factors in the development of addiction, but one must acknowledge that they are as important as the pharmacological factors (Edwards et al., 1981; Nurco, 1979; Wikler, 1980). Although the evidence is controversial in many of these areas (Edwards, 1981), there are some factors that promote or retard drug-taking behavior; e.g., health hazards (immediate and long term), ease of administration, ease of access to the drug, legalization of the drug, genetic predispostion, cultural influences, societal acceptance of the drug, cost of the drug, and perhaps personality of the

Table 1 Factors in Addiction

Pharmacological characteristics of drug	Nonpharmacological characteristics of user/society
Potency of high	Legality
Quality of high	(e.g., legal: ethanol, nicotine, caffeine,
(pain relief; relief of anxiety; drowsiness; excitement; euphoria; perceptual	prescribed narcotics and sedatives)
distortion)	Accessibility
Reinforcing properties	Ease of administration
(animal studies)	(i.e., trauma to body)
Rapidity of onset	Cost
(lipid solubility; protein binding; route	Acceptance in society/culture
of administration)	Health hazards
Duration of action	(immediate: psychosis, cardiovascular and
(volume of distribution; lipid solubility;	respiratory accidents)
protein binding; metabolism and excretion;	(remote: AIDS, hepatitis, cirrhosis,
i.e., half-life)	dementia, bronchitis, cancer)
Withdrawal phenomena	Genetic factors
(half-life; frequency, quantity, duration of	Psychological make-up
dosage)	Socioeconomic factors

user. The pharmacological factors consist of the pharmacodynamic and pharmacokinetic characteristics of the individual drugs (Table 1).

When one looks at all of these factors, it is possible to devise a theoretical composite "score" for each drug, on the basis of how it is used in today's society. At the very least, one could use this score to explain an individual drug's abuse prevalence. Table 1 is not exhaustive, but it can serve as a guideline to judge how prevalent the addiction to any drug might be.

For example, the highly reinforcing properties that are inherent in the opiates and stimulants are offset by the fact that they are illegal, (i.e., street drug usage), not readily accepted by society as a whole, and not as readily available. Obviously these last three factors are interrelated. In addition to its inherent reinforcing properties, cocaine can be inhaled. This method of extremely rapid delivery adds to its addictive potential and appears to be a major factor in the cocaine epidemic. However, ethanol, which is not a potent euphoriant, does not exhibit impressive reinforcing properties, and causes more organ damage than any other drug, but is widely accepted by the public, and is legal and accessible. Nicotine is interesting in that it has demonstrable reinforcing properties, is easy to administer, and has a rapid onset of action, is accepted by society (less so than before), is legal, and is accessible. This likely explains why it is one of the most abused drugs in society. One could take any drug that is known to cause addiction and explain its use in the manner just described. There will always be exceptions, but conceptualizing the drugs of addiction in this way may help the student, counsellor, nurse, researcher, or physician understand the process of addiction.

REFERENCES

Agurell, S., Halldin, M., Lindgren, J.E., Ohlsson, A., Widman, M., Gillespie, H., and Hollister, L. Pharmacokinetics and metabolism of delta-1-tetrahydrocannabinol and other cannabinols with emphasis on man. *Pharmacol. Rev., 38*(1):21–43 (1986).

Aigner, T.G., and Balster, R.L. Choice behavior in rhesus monkeys: Cocaine versus food. *Science, 201*:534–535 (1978).

Allan, A.M., and Harris, R.A. Involvement of neuronal chloride channels in ethanol intoxication, tolerance, and dependence, *Recent Developments in Alcoholism*, Vol. 5 (M. Galanter, ed.). Plenum Press, New York, 1987, pp. 313-325).

Anggard, E., Gunne, L.M., Jonsson, L.E., and Niklasson, F. Pharmacokinetic and clinical studies on amphetamine dependent subjects. *Eur. J. Clin. Pharmacol.*, *3*:3-11 (1970).

Ator, N.A., and Griffiths, R.R. Self-administration of barbiturates and benzodiazepines: A review. *Pharmacol. Biochem Behav.*, *27*:391-398 (1987).

Bellantuono, C., Reggi, V., Tognoni, G., and Garattini, S. Benzodiazepines: Clinical pharmacology and therapeutic use. *Drugs*, *19*:195-219 (1980).

Benet, L.Z., and Sheiner, L.B. Pharmacokinetics: The dynamics of drug absorption, distribution, and elimination, *The Pharmacological Basis of Therapeutics*, 7th ed. (A.G. Gilman, L.S. Goodman, T.W. Rall, and F. Murad, eds.). Macmillan, New York, 1985, pp. 3-34.

Benowitz, N.L. Pharmacologic aspects of cigarette smoking and nicotine addiction. *N. Engl. J. Med.*, *319*(20):1318-1330 (1988).

Benowitz, N.L., and Jacob, P. Daily intake of nicotine during cigarette smoking. *Clin. Pharmacol. Ther.*, *35*:499-504 (1984).

Benowitz, N.L., Kuyt, F., Jacob, P. Circadian blood nicotine concentrations during cigarette smoking. *Clin. Pharmacol. Ther.*, *32*:758-764 (1982).

Bissell, L. Diagnosis and recognition, *Alcoholism. A Practical Treatment Guide*, 2nd ed. (S.E. Gitlow and H.S. Peyser, eds.). Grune & Stratton, 1988, pp. 19-35.

Blanchard, J., and Sawers, S.J.A. The absolute bioavailability of caffeine in man. *Eur. J. Clin. Pharmacol.*, *24*:93-98 (1983a).

Blanchard, J., and Sawers, S.J.A. Comparative pharmacokinetics of caffeine in young and elderly men. *J. Pharmacokinet. Biopharm.*, *11*(2):109-126 (1983b).

Boerner, U., Abbott, S., and Roe, R.L. The metabolism of morphine and heroin in man. *Drug Metab. Rev.*, *4*(1):39-73 (1975).

Boisse, N.R., and Okamoto, M. Physical dependence to barbital compared to pentobarbital. IV. Influence of elimination kinetics. *J. Pharmacol. Exp. Ther.*, *204*(3):528-540 (1978).

Brady, J.V., and Lukas, S.E. Testing drugs for physical dependence potential and abuse liability. *National Institute of Drug Abuse Research Monograph 52*. U.S. Department of Health and Human Services, Bethesda, Maryland, 1984, pp. 1-28.

Breimer, D.D. Clinical pharmacokinetics of hypnotics. *Clin. Pharmacokinet.*, *2*:93-109 (1977).

Breimer, D.D., and de Boer, A.G. Pharmacokinetics and relative bioavailability of heptabarbital and heptabarbital sodium after oral administration in man. *Eur. J. Clin. Pharmacol.*, *9*:169-178 (1975).

Busto, U., and Sellers, E.M. Pharmacokinetic determinants of drug abuse and dependence. A conceptual perspective. *Clin. Pharmacokinet.*, *11*:144-153 (1986).

Busto, U., Sellers, E.M., Naranjo, C.A., Capell, H., Sanchez-Craig, M., and Sykora, K. Withdrawal reaction after long-term therapeutic use of benzodiazepines. *N. Engl. J. Med.*, *315*(14):854-859 (1986).

Busto, U., Bendayau, R., and Sellers, E.M. Clinical Pharmacokinetics of non-opiate abused drugs. *Clin. Pharmacokinet.*, *16*:1-26 (1989).

Carlen, P.L. The electrophysiology of potassium channels, *Recent Developments in Alcoholism*, Vol. 5 (M. Galanter, ed.). Plenum Press, New York, 1987, pp. 347-357.

Carr, D.B. Opioids. *Int. Anesthesiol. Clin.*, *26*(4):273-287 (1988).

Chin, J.H., Goldstein, D.B., and Parson, L.M. Fluidity and lipid composition of mouse biomembranes during adaptation to ethanol. *Alcoholism Clin. Exp. Res.*, *3*(1):47-49 (1979).

Cho, A.K., Hiramatsie, M., Pechnick, R.N., and Di Stefano, E. Pharmacokinetic and pharmacodynamic evaluation of phencyclidine and its decaderitero variant. *J. Pharmacol. Exp. Ther.*, *250*(1):210-215 (1989).

Chow, M.J., Ambre, J.J., Ruo, T.I., Atkinson, A.J., Bowsher, J.J., and Fischman, M.W. Kinetics of Cocaine distribution, elimination, and chronotropic effects. *Clin. Pharmacol. Ther.*, *38*(3):318-323 (1985).

Cohen, S. The Intentional inhalation of volatile substances. *Adv. Subst. Abuse*, *2*:123-143 (1981).

Cohen, S. The hallucinogens and the inhalants. *Psychiatr. Clin. North Am.*, *7*(4):681-688 (1984).

Cook, C.E., Brine, D.R., Jeffcoat, A.R., Hill, J.M., Wall, M.E., Perez-Reyes, M., and Di Guiseppi, S.R. Phencyclidine disposition after intravenous and oral doses. *Clin. Pharmacol. Ther.*, *31*(5):625–634 (1982a).

Cook, C.E., Brine, D.R., Quin, G.D., Perez-Reyes, M., and Di Guiseppi, S.R. Phencyclidine and phenylcyclohexene disposition after smoking phencyclidine. *Clin. Pharmacol. Ther.*, *31*(5):635–641 (1982b).

Davis, P.J., and Cook, D.R. Clinical pharmacokinetics of the newer intravenous anesthetic agents. *Clin. Pharmacokinet.*, *11*:18–35 (1986).

Dackis, C.A., and Gold, M.S. New concepts in cocaine addiction: The dopamine depletion hypothesis. *Neurosci. Biobehav. Rev.*, *9*:469–477 (1985).

Dewey, W.L. Cannabinoid pharmacology. *Pharmacol. Rev.*, *38*(2):151–178 (1986).

Edwards, G., Arif, A., and Hodgson, R. Nomenclature and classification of drug and alcohol-related problems: A WHO memorandum. *Bull. WHO, 59*(2):225–242 (1981).

Edwards, D.J., Svensson, C.K., Visco, J.P., and Lalka, D. Clinical pharmacokinetics of pethidine: 1982. *Clin. Pharmacokinet.*, *7*:421–433 (1982).

Erickson, C.K. Factors affecting the distribution and measurement of ethanol in the body, *Biochemistry and Pharmacology of Ethanol*, Vol. 1 (E. Majchrowitz and E.G. Noble, eds.). Plenum Press, New York, 1979, pp. 9–26.

Feyerabend, C., and Russell, M.A.H. Effect of urinary pH and nicotine excretion rate or plasma nicotine during cigarette smoking and chewing nicotine gum. *Br. J. Clin. Pharmacol.*, *5*:293–297 (1978).

Feyerabend, C., Ings, R.M.J., and Russell, M.A.H. Nicotine pharmacokinetics and its application to intake from smoking. *Br. J. Clin. Pharmacol.*, *19*:239–247 (1985).

Fontaine, R., Chorinard, G., and Annable, L. Rebound anxiety in anxious patients after abrupt withdrawal of benzodiazepines treatment. *Am. J. Psychiatry, 141*:7 (1984).

Gawin, F.H. Chronic neuropharmacology of cocaine abuse. Progress in pharmacotherapy. *J. Clin. Psychiatry, 49*:511–517 (1988).

Gawin, F.H., and Ellinwood, E.H. Cocaine and other stimulants. *N. Engl. J. Med., 318*(18):1173–1182 (1988).

Gawin, F.H., and Ellinwood, E.H. Cocaine dependence. *Ann. Rev. Med., 40*:149–161 (1989).

Geokas, M.C. Symposium on ethyl alcohol and disease. *Med. Clin. North Am., 68*(1): (1984).

Gill, K., and Anit, Z. Serotonin uptake blockers and voluntary alcohol consumption: A review of recent studies, *Recent Developments in Alcoholism*, Vol. 7 (M. Galanter, ed.). Plenum Press, New York, 1989, pp. 225–250.

Glaser, F.B. Inhalation psychosis and related states, *A Treatment Manual for Acute Drug Abuse Emergencies* (P.G. Bourne, ed.). Government Printing Office, Washington, D.C., 1974, pp. 95–104.

Gold, M.S., and Rea, W.S. The role of endorphins in opiate addiction, opiate withdrawal, and recovery. *Psychiatr. Clin. North Am., 6*(3):489–520 (1983).

Goldstein, D.B. *Pharmacology of Alcohol*. Oxford University Press, New York, 1983.

Greenblatt, D.J., Shader, R.J., Franke, K., MacLaughlin, D.S., Harmatz, J.S., Allen, M.D., Werner, A., and Woo, E. Pharmacokinetics and bioavailability of intravenous, intramuscular, and oral lorazepam in humans. *J. Pharmaceut. Sci., 68*(1):57–63 (1979).

Greenblatt, D.J., Shader, R.I., Divoll, M., and Harmatz, J.S. Benzodiazepines: A summary of pharmacokinetic properties; *Br. J. Clin. Pharmacol., 11*:115–165 (1981).

Greenblatt, D.J., Divoll, M., Harmatz, J.S., and Shader, R.I. Pharmacokinetic comparison of sublingual lorazepam with intravenous, intramuscular, and oral lorazepam. *J. Pharmaceut. Sci., 71*(2):248–252 (1982).

Greenblatt, D.J., Divoll, M., Abernethy, D.R., Ochs, H.R., and Shader, R.I. Clinical pharmacokinetics of the newer benzodiazepines. *Clin. Pharmacokinet., 8*:233–252 (1983).

Grenhoff, J., and Svensson, T.H. Pharmacology of nicotine. *Br. J. Addict., 84*:477–492 (1989).

Griffiths, R.R., and Balster, R.L. Opioids: Similarity between evaluations of subjective effects and animal self-administration results. *Clin. Pharmacol. Ther., 25*(5):611–617 (1979).

Griffiths, R.R., Lukas, S.E., Bradford, L.D., Brady, J.V., and Snell, J.D. Self-injection of barbiturates and benzodiazepines in baboons. *Psychopharmacology, 75*:101–109 (1981).

Griffiths, R.R., McLeod, D.R., Bigelow, G.E., Liebson, I.A., and Roache, J.D. Relative abuse liability of diazepam and oxazepam: Behavioral and subjective dose effects. *Psychopharmacology, 84*:147–154 (1984a).

Griffiths, R.R., McLeod, D.R., Bigelow, G.E., Liebson, I.A., Roache, J.D., and Nowowieski, P. Comparison of diazepam and oxazepam: Perference, liking and extent of abuse. *J. Pharmacol. Exp. Ther., 229*(2):501–501 (1984b).

Guerin, M.R. Chemical composition of cigarette smoking, *A Safe Cigarette?* (Gori, G.B. and Bock, F.G., eds.). Cold Spring Harbor Laboratory, Cold Spring Harbor, New York, 1980, pp. 191–204.

Haefely, W. Biological basis of drug-induced tolerance, rebound, and dependence. Contribution of recent research on benzodiazepines. *Pharmacopsychiatr., 19*:353–361 (1986).

Haefely, W.E. Benzodiazepines. *Int. Anesthesiol. Clin., 26*(4):262–272 (1988).

Harvey, S.C. Hypnotics and sedatives, *The Pharmacological Basis of Therapeutics*, 7th ed. (A.G. Gilman, L.S. Goodman, T.W. Rall, and F. Murad, eds.). Macmillan, New York, 1985, pp. 1628–1650.

Henningfield, J.E., and Goldberg, S.R. Nicotine as a reinforcer in human subjects and laboratory animals. *Pharmacol. Biochem. Behav., 19*:989–992 (1983).

Henningfield, J.E., and Goldberg, S.R. Progress in understanding the relationship between the pharmacological effects of nicotine and human tobacco dependence. *Pharmacol. Biochem. Behav., 30*:217–220 (1988a).

Henningfield, J.E., and Goldberg, S.R. Pharmacologic determinants of tobacco self-administration by humans. *Pharmacol. Biochem. Behav., 30*:221–226 (1988b).

Hillard, C.J., Harris, R.A., and Bloom, A.S. Effects of the cannabinoids on physical properties of brain membranes and phospholipid vesicles: Fluorescence studies. *J. Pharmacol. Exp. Ther., 232*:579–588 (1985).

Ho, I.K., and Harris, R.A. Mechanism of action of barbiturates. *Ann. Rev. Pharmacol. Toxicol., 21*:83–111 (1981).

Holford, N.H.G. Clinical pharmacokinetics of ethanol. *Clin. Pharmacokinet., 13*:273–292 (1987).

Hollister, L.E. Health aspects of cannabis. *Pharmacol. Rev., 38*(1):1–20 (1986).

Hollister, L.E., Motzenbecker, F.P., and Degan, R.O. Withdrawal reactions from chlordiazepoxide. *Psychopharmacology, 2*:63–68 (1961).

Horberg, L.K., and Schnoll, S.H. Treatment of cocaine abuse. *Curr. Psychiatr. Ther., 22*:177–187 (1983).

Hughes, T.L. Models and perspectives of addiction. Implications for treatment. *Nurs. Clin. North Am., 24*(1):1–12 (1989).

Hunt, C.A., and Jones, R.T. Tolerance and disposition of tetrahydrocannabinol in man. *J. Pharmacol. Exp. Ther., 215*:35–44 (1980).

Hunt, W.A., Barnett, L.W., and Branch, L.G. Relapse rates in addition programs. *J. Clin. Psychol., 27*:455–456 (1971).

Jacobs, M.R., and Fehr, K. *Drugs and Drug Abuse*, 2nd ed. Addiction Research Foundation, Toronto, 1987.

Jaffe, J.H. Drug addiction and drug abuse, *The Pharmacologic Basis of Therapeutics*, 7th ed. (A.G. Gilman, L.S. Goodman, T.W. Rall, and F. Murad, eds.). Macmillan, New York, 1985, pp. 532–581.

Jaffe, J.H., and Lukas, S.E. Testing drugs for physical dependence potential and abuse liability. *National Institute on Drug Abuse Research Monograph 52*. U.S. Department of Health and Human Services, Bethesda, Maryland, 1984, pp. 1–28.

Janiger, O. and de Rios, M.D. Suggestive hallucinogenic properties of tobacco. *Med. Antrophol. Newslett., 4*:1–6 (1973).

Kalant, H. Absorption, diffusion, distribution, and elimination of ethanol: Effects on biological membranes, *The Biology of Alcoholism*, Vol. 1 (B. Kissin and H. Begleiter, eds.). Plenum Press, New York, 1971, pp. 1–62.

Klaassen, C.D. Nonmetallic environmental toxicants: Air pollutants, solvents and vapors, and pesticides, *The Pharmacological Basis of Therapeutics*, 7th ed. (A.G. Gilman, L.S. Goodman, T.W. Rall, and F. Murad, eds.). Macmillan, New York, 1985, pp. 1628–1650.

Kleber, H. Cocaine abuse: Historical, epidemiological, and psychological perspectives. *J. Clin. Psychiatry,* (Suppl.) *49*(2):3–6 (1988).

Koob, G.F., and Bloom, F.E. Cellular and molecular mechanisms of drug dependence. *Science, 242*:715–723 (1988).

Koob, G.F., Vaccaino, F.J., Amalric, M., and Bloom, F.E. Neurochemical substrates for opiate reinforcement. *NIDA Res. Monogr. Series, 71*:146–164 (1986).

Kornetsky, C., Bain, G.T., Unterwald, E.M., and Lewis, M.J. Brain stimulation reward: Effects of ethanol. *Alcohol Clin. Exp. Res., 12*(5):609–616 (1988).

Korsten, M.A., Matsuzaki, S., Feinman, L., and Lieber, C.S. High blood acetaldehyde levels after ethanol administration in alcoholics. *N. Engl. J. Med., 292*:386–389 (1975).

Kulonen, E. Ethanol and GABA. *Med. Biol., 61*:147–167 (1983).

Kumar, R., Reavill, C., and Stolerman, I.P. Nicotine are in rats: Effects of central administration of ganglion-blocking drugs. *Br. J. Pharmacol., 90*:239–246 (1987).

Lawrence, D.K., and Gill, E.W. The effects of delta-1-tetrahydrocannabinol and other cannabinoids on spin labelled liposomes and their relationship to mechanisms of general anesthesia. *Mol. Pharmacol., 11*:595–602 (1975).

Lemberger, L., Silberstein, S.D., Axeliod, J., and Kopin, I.J. Marijuana: Studies on the disposition and metabolism of delta-9-tetrahydrocannabinol in man. *Science, 170*:1320–1322 (1970).

Lieber, C.S. Metabolism of ethanol, *Metabolic Aspects of Alcoholism*, (C.S. Lieber ed.). University Park Press, Baltimore, Maryoand, 1977, pp. 1–30.

Liebman, J.M. Anxiety, anxiolytics and brain stimulation reinforcement. *Neurosci. Biobehav. Rev., 9*:75–86 (1985).

Leslie, S.W. Calcium channels: interactions with ethanol and other sedative-hypnotic drugs, *Recent Developments in Alcoholism*, Vol. 5 (M. Galanter, ed.). Plenum Press, New York, 1987, pp. 289–302.

Maickel, R.P., Cox, R.H., Miller, F.P., Segal, D.S., and Russell, R.W. Correlation of brain levels of drugs with their behavioral effects. *J. Pharmacol. Exp. Ther., 165*:218–224 (1989).

Majchrowitz, E., and Noble, E.P. (eds.). *Biochemistry and Pharmacology of Ethanol*, Vols. 1 and 2. Plenum Press, New York, 1979.

Marks, J. Techniques of benzodiazepine withdrawal in clinical practice. *Med. Toxicol., 3*:324–333 (1988).

Martin, R.B. Cellular effects of cannabinoids. *Pharmacol. Rev., 38*:45–74 (1986).

Martin, P.R., Kapur, B.M., Whiteside, E.A., and Sellers, E.M. Intravenous phenobarbital therapy in bariburate and other hypnosedative withdrawal reactions: A kinetic approach. *Clin. Pharmacol. Ther., 26*(2):256–264 (1979).

Martin, E., Moll, W., Schmid, P., and Dettli, L. The pharmacokinetics of alcohol in human breath, venous and arterial blood after oral ingestion. *Eur. J. Clin. Pharmacol., 26*:619–626 (1984).

Miller, N.S., Dackis, C.A., and Gold, M.S. The relationship of addiction, tolerance, and dependence to alcohol and drugs: A neuro-chemical approach. *J. Subst. Abuse Treat., 4*:197–207 (1987).

Miller, N.S., Millman, R.B., and Gold, M.S. Amphetamines: Pharmacology, abuse, and addiction. *Adv. Alcohol Subst. Abuse, 8*(2):53–69 (1989).

Mohler, H., and Okada, T. Benzodiazepines receptor: Demonstration in the central nervous system. *Science, 198*:849–851 (1977).

Morrison, C.F., and Stephenson, J.A. Nicotine injections as the conditioned stimulus in discrimination learning. *Psychopharmacology, 15*:351–360 (1969).

Mucha, R.F., and Herz, A. Motivational properties of kappa and mu opioid receptor agonists studied with place and taste preference conditioning. *Psychopharmacology, 86*:274–280 (1985).

Mullin, M.J., and Hunt, W.A. Effects of ethanol on the functional properties of sodium channels in brain synaptosomes, *Recent Developments in Alcoholism*, Vol. 5, (M. Galanter, ed.). Plenum Press, New York, 1987, pp. 303–311.

Nurco, D.N. Etiologic aspects of drug abuse, *Handbook on Drug Abuse*, (R.I. Dupont, A. Goldstein, J. O'Donnell, and B. Brown, eds.). National Institute of Drug Abuse, U.S. Government Printing Office, Washington, D.C., 1979.

Ohlsson, A., Lindgren, J.E., Wahlen, A., Agurell, S., and Hollister, L.E. Plasma delta-9-tetrahydrocannabinol concentrations and clinical effects after oral and intravenous administration and smoking. *Clin. Pharmacol. Ther., 28*:409–418 (1980).

Ohlsson, A., Lindgren, J.E., Wahlen, A., Agurell, S., Hollister, L.E., Gillespie, H.K. Single dose kinetics of deutenium labelled delta-1-tetrahydrocannabinol in heavy and light cannabis users. *Biomed. Mass Spectrum,* 9:6-10 (1982).

Olsen, R.W. Barbiturates. *Int. Anesthesiol. Clin.,* 26(4):254-261 (1988).

Oreland, L. The benzodiazepines: A pharmacological overview. *Acta Anesthiol. Scand.,* (Suppl. 88) 32:13-16 (1987).

Owen, J.A., Sitar, D.S., Berger, L., Brownell, L., Duke, P.C., and Mitenko, P.A. Age-related morphine kinetics. *Clin. Pharmacol. Ther.,* 34(3):364-368 (1983).

Paly, D., Jetlow, P., Van Dyke, C., Jeri, F.R., and Byck, R. Plasma cocaine concentrations during cocaine paste smoking. *Life Sci.,* 30(a):731-738 (1982).

Pavlov, I.P. *Conditioned Reflexes,* Oxford University Press, New York, 1927.

Perez-Reyes, M., Di Guiseppi, S., Davis, K.H., Schindler, V.H., and Cook, C.E. Comparison of effects of marijuana cigarettes of three different potencies. *Clin. Pharmacol. Ther.,* 31:617-624 (1982).

Pert, A., and Chiueh, C.C. Effects of intracerebral nicotinic agonists on locomotor activity: involvement of mesolimbic dopamine. *Soc. Neurosci. Abstr.,* 12:917 (1986).

Pert, C.B., and Snyder, S.H. Opiate receptor: Demonstration in nervous tissue. *Science, 179*:1011-1014 (1973).

Pertwee, R.G. The central neuropharmacology of psychotropic cannabinoids. *Pharmacol. Ther.,* 36:189-281 (1988).

Pohorecky, L.A., and Brick, J. Pharmacology of ethanol. *Pharmacol. Ther.,* 36:335-427 (1988).

Rall, T.W., and Schleifer, L.S. Drugs effective in the therapy of the epilepsies, *The Pharmacological Basis of Therapeutics,* 7th ed. (A.G. Gilman, L.S. Goodman, T.W. Rall, and F. Murad, eds.). Macmillan, New York, 1985, pp. 1628-1650.

Rang, H.P. Unspecific drug action. The effects of a homologous series of primary alcohols. *Br. J. Pharmacol.,* 15:185-200 (1960).

Razdan, R.K. Structure-activity relationships in cannabinoids: An overview. *NIDA Res. Monogr. Ser.,* 79:1-210 (1987).

Richter, J.A., and Holtman, J.R. Barbiturates Their in vivo effects and potential biochemical mechanisms. *Prog. Neurobiol.,* 18:275-319 (1982).

Ritchie, J.M. The aliphatic alcohols, *The Pharmacological Basis of Therapeutics,* 7th ed. (A.G. Gilman, L.S. Goodman, T.W. Rall, and F. Murad, eds.). Macmillan, New York, 1985, pp. 1628-1650.

Robinson, G.M., Sellers, E.M., and Janecek, E. Barbiturate and hypnosedative withdrawal by a multiple phenobarbital loading dose technique. *Clin. Pharmacol. Ther.,* 30(1):71-76 (1981).

Rowland, M. Drug administration and regimens, *Clinical Pharmacology. Basic Principles in Therapeutics,* 2nd ed. (K.L. Melmon and H.F. Morelli, eds.). Macmillan, New York, 1978, pp. 25-70.

Sadzot, B., Barabar, J.M. Glennon, R.A., Lyon, R.A., Leonhardt, S., Jan, C.R., and Titeler, M. Hallucinogenic drug interactions at human brain 5-HT receptors: Implications for treating LSD-induced hallucinogenesis. *Psychopharmacology,* 98:495-499 (1989).

Sawe, J., Dahlstrom, B., Paakzow, L., and Rane, A. Morphine kinetics in cancer patients. *Clin. Pharmacol. Ther.,* 30:629-635 (1981).

Schuckit, M.A. *Drug and Alcohol Abuse: A Clinical Guide to Diagnosis and Treatment,* 3rd ed. Plenum Press, New York, 1989.

Seeman, P. The membrane actions of anesthetics and tranquilizers. *Pharmacol. Rev.,* 24(4):583-655 (1972).

Senary, E.C. Addictive behaviors and benzodiazepines: 1. Abuse liability and physical dependence. *Adv. Alcohol Subst. Abuse,* 8(1):107-124 (1989).

Sharp, C.W., and Brehm, M.L. (eds.). *Review of Inhalants: Euphoria to Dysfunction.* National Institute on Drug Abuse. U.S. Department of Health, Education, and Welfare Publications No. (ADM) 77-553, U.S. Government Printing Office, Washington, D.C., 1977.

Sircar, R., and Zukin, S.R. Further evidence of phencyclidine/sigma opioid receptor commonality. *NIDA Res. Monogr. Ser.,* 64:14-23 (1986).

Skinner, B.F. *The Behavior of Organisms*, Appleton-Century-Crofts, New York, 1938.

Sonders, M.S., Keana, J.F., and Weber, E. Phencyclidine and psychotomimetic sigma opiates: Recent insights into their biochemical and physiological sites of action. *Trends Neurosci.*, *11*(1):37–40 (1988).

Squires, R.F., and Braestrup, C. Benzodiazepine receptors in rat brain. *Nature, 266*:732–734 (1977).

Svensson, T.H., and Engberg, G. Effect of nicotine on single cell activity in the noradrenergic nucleus locus coeruleus. *Acta Physiol. Scand.*, (Suppl. 479) *108*:31–34 (1980).

Titeler, M., Lyon, R.A., and Glennon, R.A. Radioligand binding evidence implicates the brain 5-HT2 receptor sits as a site of action for LSD and phenylisopropylamine hallucinogens. *Psychopharmacol, 94*:213–216 (1988).

Tyrer, P., Rutherford, D., and Huggett, T. Benzodiazepines withdrawal symptoms and propranolol. *Lancet, 1*:520–522 (1981).

Tygstrup, N., Winkler, K., and Lundquist, F. The mechanism of fructose effect on the ethanol metabolism of the human liver. *J. Clin. Invest., 44*(5):817–830 (1965).

Wahlquist, M., Nilsson, I.M., and Sandberg, F. Binding of delta-1-tetrahydrocannabinol to human plasma proteins. *Biochem. Pharmacol., 19*:2579 (1970).

Watson, J.M. Solvent abuse by children and young adults. A review. *Br. J. Addict., 75*:27–36 (1980).

Wikler, A. *Opioid Dependence: Mechanisms and Treatment*, Plenum Press, New York, 1980.

Wise, R.A. Action of drugs of abuse on brain reward systems. *Pharmacol. Biochem. Behav.*, (Suppl. 1) *13*:213–223 (1980).

Wise, R.A. The neurobiology of craving: Implications for the understanding and treatment of addiction. *J. Abnorm. Psychol., 97*(2):118–132 (1988).

Woods, J.H., Katz, J.L., and Winger, G. Abuse liability of benzodiazepines. *Pharmacol. Rev., 39*(4):251–413 (1987).

Zabik, J.E. Use of serotonin-active drugs in alcohol preference studies, *Recent Developments in Alcoholism*, Vol. 7 (M. Galanter, ed.). Plenum Press, New York, 1989, pp. 211–223.

XI

Education

42

Alcohol and Drug Addiction in the Psychiatric Curriculum

Joseph Westermeyer
University of Oklahoma, Oklahoma City, Oklahoma

I. INTRODUCTION

A. Rationale: The Pandemic in Alcohol-Drug Addiction

Addiction epidemics are not new. The well-described gin epidemic occurred over three centuries ago in the United Kingdom [1]. Two hundred years ago, epidemics of opium smoking began in several Asian countries. The last century has seen epidemics of sedatives, stimulants, hallucinogens, and opioids, involving both synthetic and naturally occurring drugs [2,3]. Especially in the 4 decades since World War II, the number and severity of these epidemics has increased over previous levels [4]. Over the last 2 decades, alcohol and drug epidemics have increased to a point at which national as well as international offices, agencies, and organizations have been established in order to deal with them. Increasing alcohol abuse in the United States during the 1800s and early 1900s led to federal prohibition against commercial beverage alcohol production and sales. Despite the Narcotic Act of 1914, passed to limit widespread opiate addiction, several opiate epidemics have afflicted the United States. Since the 1950s waves of amphetamine, hallucinogen, cannabis, phencyclidine, and cocaine epidemics have occurred and recurred, initially in urban areas and later in rural areas.

It is difficult to determine one or a few particular causes to these epidemics, and to the more recent alcohol-drug pandemic. However, certain general precursors or correlates can be identified, beginning with the gin epidemic. None of these factors is absolutely necessary for an epidemic, but several have accompanied most epidemics. These contributing or causal factors are as follows:

1. Introduction of a new drug into the society (e.g., tobacco in fifteenth century Asia and Europe, cocaine in twentieth century Europe and North America).
2. Introduction of a new, more effective, or more intoxicating method of administration (e.g., smoking used to consume opium in seventeenth century Asia, invention of the syringe and needle in the nineteenth century).

3. Purification of naturally occurring drugs, so that a more potent drug results, or so that a more purified compound may be smoked, sniffed or injected (e.g., cocaine from coca leaf, morphine or heroin from opium).

4. Development of synthetic drugs, which are (when compared to naturally occurring drugs) more potent, less expensive, or liable to diverse routes of administration (e.g., barbiturates, benzodiazepines, amphetamines and other stimulants, fentanyl and other synthetic opioids, phencyclidine).

5. Cheaper and more rapid forms of commerce, so that drugs may be transported more easily, either licitly or illicitly (e.g., clipper sailing vessels, steam engine, gasoline engine, turbine, airplane).

6. Increasing disposable income after providing food, shelter, and clothing, so that alcohol and drugs may be regularly purchased; more disposable income has resulted from high-yield crops, irrigation, fertilizers, pesticides, synthetic clothing materials.

7. Decreasing cost of alcohol and drug production (e.g., excess carbohydrate available for alcohol manufacture, inexpensive industrial chemicals, more efficient production of tobacco and cannabis).

8. Wide distribution of requisite chemical-pharmaceutical skills and necessary base products, equipment, and chemicals around the world, together with new and easily manufactured compounds (e.g., availability of acetic acid for heroin, "designer drug" manufacture).

9. Worldwide sociocultural change from more traditional societies (i.e., primarily rural, agrarian, illiterate, strongly influenced by religion and traditional mores, barter economy) to more modern societies (i.e., large urban populations, secular separation of occupational and personal and recreational lives, ascendency of the nuclear family over the extended family, impersonal transactions in a money economy, loss of tribal identities) [5]; traditional cultural taboos against drug use diminish [6] while exposure to new forms of drug use expands.

10. Evolution of a new multinational, peer- and youth-oriented, individualistic cultural value system that supports drug experimentation and use (e.g., drug-oriented music, jargon, lifestyle).

11. Sequential use of substances to counter the adverse effects of psychoactive substances abuse has increased. A typical pattern is daytime or worktime use of stimulant drugs (e.g., caffeine, amphetamines, cocaine). In order to relax after work, induce sleep, or counter hypervigilance, sedative drugs are then consumed (e.g., alcohol, opiates, sedatives).

12. Concurrent use of drugs has fostered problems, as one drug reinforces another, or as combined drug use produces greater pathological effects at the neuroneural junction. Examples include nicotine and caffeine, alcohol and cannabis, and heroin and cocaine.

A major cause for concern is the high potential prevalence rates for alcohol-drug addiction. With most psychiatric disorders, the maximum lifetime prevalence rates are relatively low (e.g., around 1% for schizophrenia, 15–20% for major depression). However, in certain subgroups lifetime prevalence rates for substance abuse among males range up to 20–25%, with a lifetime risk of 50% for adult males (i.e., will develop substance abuse before their death) [3,7].

In this social context, medical facilities are increasingly concerned with education and training in the addictions [8,9]. Without special education and training, physicians neglect the assessment and care of substance abusers, and indeed sometimes contribute to its development and maintenance [10]. On the contrary, training can prove beneficial to patient care, thereby improving the efficacy of physicians' clinical work [11].

B. Psychiatry as a Context for Teaching Substance Abuse

Alcohol-drug addiction is too diverse a field to be taught only in psychiatry. In the basic science years as well as in the clinical years, various facets of alcohol and drug abuse are appropriately taught in other fields. Examples include the following:

Biochemistry: the metabolism of alcoholism

Pharmacology: absorption, action, metabolism, and excretion of the drugs of abuse as well as the drugs used to treat addiction (e.g., disulfiram, naltrexone, methadone); first-order and zero-order kinetics; hepatic first-pass effect; biliary-intestinal recirculation, addiction, tolerance, withdrawal

Public health: epidemiology of alcoholism and addiction; primary and secondary prevention approaches; social consequences and economic costs

Social, behavioral and psychological sciences: use of psychoactive substances in sociocultural context; effects of alcohol and drug use on psychological and social processes

Neurosciences: sites of alcohol and drug action in the central nervous system (CNS); neurotransmitter effects of drugs that are liable to abuse; modes by which substances of abuse can exacerbate or mimic psychopathological conditions

Genetics: research data on substance abuse from monozygotic/dizygotic twins and half sibs; family studies linking substance abuse with depression and other disorders; adoption studies evaluating genetic, constitutional, and environmental factors

Immunology: suppressant effects of various drugs on body defenses (e.g., alcohol and the bone marrow, certain solvent-inhalants and lymphoid tissue)

Pathology: diseases related to specific modes of administration or drugs (e.g., smoking and cardiopulmonary diseases, alcohol and CNS and gastrointestinal diseases) as well as general or nonspecific consequences of chronic drug abuse (e.g., nutritional deficiencies, trauma, infections)

Pediatrics: fetal alcohol/tobacco/solvent-inhalant syndromes; ill, neglected or abused children of addicted parents (e.g., failure to thrive); newborn opioid-sedative-alcohol withdrawal; childhood hyperactivity and paternal alcoholism; childhood and adolescent onset of alcohol and drug abuse

Medicine: overdose, alcohol- and drug-related neoplasms/inflammation/atrophy

Emergency room medicine: acute intoxication, trauma, suicide attempt, rapid identification and referral to treatment resources

Neurology: dementias, central cerebellar atrophy, myelitis, peripheral neuropathy

Psychiatry as a field also has its particular contributions to medical education and training in alcohol-drug addictions. The argument has been made that psychiatrists should initiate and guide curricular changes in the addictions [12]. Reasons for its inclusion in the psychiatric curriculum include the following:

1. Diagnostic criteria for alcohol-drug addiction are classified under psychiatric disorders in the *International Classification of Disease*. These criteria are not likely to be taught adequately if psychiatrists fail to teach them.
2. Alcohol and drug addiction resembles other psychiatric disorders in its neurotransmitter aspects, genetic-familial components, effects on psychological function and behavior, resultant social impairment, need for biopsychosocial assessment, combinations of somatotherapies/psychotherapies/sociotherapies, long-term rehabilitation and recovery process, tendency for relapse, case management and multidisciplinary approaches.
3. There is a high prevalence of alcohol and drug disorders in psychiatric patients (up to 40–60% among psychiatric inpatients, and 15–25% in psychiatric outpatients) [13–15].

4. Addicted patients manifest high rates of psychopathology during their recovery (e.g., depression, generalized anxiety, panic or phobic disorders, paranoia, sociopathy, dementia, alcohol- and drug-related psychoses) [16].

5. Many of the research advances made in the addictions have been accomplished by psychiatrists [17]. Psychiatric journals and texts publish new developments in the field.

In order to cover essential features of the addictions, and not needlessly to repeat content, a task force or curriculum committee subgroup should assess, direct, and monitor the alcohol-drug curriculum over the years of medical education [18].

II. PSYCHIATRIC CONTRIBUTIONS TO INFORMATION ON SUBSTANCE ABUSE

A. Definition

Like other psychiatric diagnoses, there is no one set of internationally accepted diagnostic criteria for the addictions. Some classifications are so broad and general as to be difficult to apply, especially in forensic cases (e.g., early World Health Organization [WHO] criteria) [19]. Other systems are so complex and specific as to defy and practical application in the clinical context [20]. Depending on the classification used, the focus may be on the drug or alcohol use, its physiological concomitants, its social or psychological repercussions, the duration of the disorder, and/or the resistance to treatment [21]. Subgroups of addicted persons have been suggested, based on the presence of familial substance abuse, age at onset, associated mental disorders, pattern of use, or type of drug [22].

This lack of agreement over definition complicates the teaching task, but does not make it impossible. These classificatory problems reflect our struggles in attempting to integrate our knowledge regarding multicausal disorders, with varying courses and manifestations, and a wide range of therapeutic responses (which are not always related to severity or duration or psychopathology). Other fields of medicine have similar problems with degenerative, collagen, atopic, and psychophysiological disorders. Students need to start with a list of criteria for the addictions that are currently employed in the field. The DSM-III-R (*Diagnostic and Statistical Manual of Mental Disorders*, 3rd ed.–revised, American Psychiatric Association, 1987) criteria for various manifestations of alcohol and drug addiction are excellent for this purpose; these criteria show strong agreement with other criteria when tested in patients. Since diagnostic criteria for the addictions have changed regularly in recent years, and will probably continue to change over the students' professional careers, it is important to prepare them for these changes. This involves exposure to the history and diverse functions served by our diagnostic categories.

B. Pathological Courses and Pathways to Recovery

The natural course of addiction varies with the drug, the age at onset, genetic loading, and access to treatment [23]. Even when these variables are held constant, there is still considerable variability in course. Some individuals recover and make outstanding contributions to their communities, some have recurrences over many years, some maintain abstinence but never resume their former level of social competence, and some continue to deteriorate and die prematurely of alcohol- and drug-related problems despite intensive treatment. The neophyte physician must learn that addiction courses are widely variable and difficult to predict at our current state of knowledge.

The usual time frame for recovery, along with its associated psychodynamics and social changes, should be taught. Students should learn that the first several weeks to several months are a crucial time during which the recovering patient requires much support and frequent clinic visits. Treatment can even produce emotional distress, social isolation, and anomie by excluding fellow substance abusers from the patient's social network [24]. Sleep, endocrine, and vital sign abnormalities can persist for up to a year [25]. Vocational adjustment may be required [26]. Even in optimal cases, recovery to a level of functioning may take a few years. Recovery can follow a highly erratic path over several years.

C. Epidemiology

From an epidemiological perspetctive, alcohol-drug addiction shares certain common attributes with other psychiatric disorder. As a chronic and sometimes recurrent problem, addiction tends to show a high prevalence (i.e., number of cases in the population at any one point in time) but low incidence (i.e., number of new cases appearing over a particular time span, such as a year). Epidemiological studies of alcohol-drug problems often involve methods similar to those of other psychiatric epidemiology (i.e., establishing rapport, skilled interviewing, confidentiality) rather than the methods used for other disorders, such as infectious diseases or cancer. Subjects may not be aware, or wish to divulge (even to themselves), that they have a substance abuse problem—a situation similar to that sometimes observed in other major and disabling psychiatric conditions.

Psychiatrists teaching the epidemiology of addiction should be aware of certain differences from the epidemiological study of other psychiatric disorders. Special methods do exist for investigating the distribution of alcohol-drug addictions in populations. These include, but are not limited to the study of body fluids in selected groups (e.g., arrestees, accident victims in morgues, the military, emergency room patients) and the study of certain tissue abnormalities highly correlated with alcoholism and addiction (e.g., hepatic cirrhosis). Familiarity with the nuances of these methods facilitates the task of the academic psychiatrist charged with education in this field. Students should know that, unlike schizophrenia and affective disorder, the crude rates of addiction can fluctuate from almost nil to over 10% of an entire population, or 20% of all adults [3,7,21]. Recent federal data obtained in the national U.S. Epidemiological Catchment Area (ECA) project demonstrated alcohol-drug disorders to be the most prevalent psychiatric condition.

D. Pharmacology

Psychiatrists offer several advantages over other disciplines in educating medical students about the central nervous system (CNS) effects of the substances of abuse. These drugs act principally at the neuroneural junction, acting as neurotransmitters or affecting the usual actions of neurotransmitters. Psychiatrists are qualified for teaching in this area by virtue of their familiarity with neurotransmitter theories of psychiatric disorder, the neurotransmitter effects of psychiatric medications, and the growing literature on CNS neurotransmitter substances and maps.

This is not to infer that psychiatrists should replace the pharmacologist in providing basic information on the drugs of abuse. Such is obviously not the case. However, psychiatrists can build upon the students' basic pharmacology through their clinical observations and scientific readings. Students must learn that animal data from laboratories do not always extrapolate to man in society. Pharmacokinetics and pharmacodynamics when drugs are given in moderate or therapeutic doses to naive human subjects can differ markedly from the metabolism and actions of high doses in alcohol or drug addicts. For example, the half-life of a drug with typical first-order kinetics may change with massive dosage (e.g., methadone), or a drug with zero-order kinetics can have some superimposed first-order kinetics with addiction (e.g., muscle enzyme induction with alcohol) [21]. Certain pharmacodynamic actions, such as the biliary-intestinal recirculation of certain drugs, have no special relevance for ordinary medical prescribing, but are highly relevant to clinical observations in certain forms of drug abuse (e.g., phencyclidine, glutethimide).

E. Diagnosis

Many medical and surgical conditions can be defined in terms of abnormal tissue, pathological laboratory findings, or physical examination. Although some psychiatric conditions can be defined by such methods, most conditions which we treat cannot be so defined. Diagnosis depends upon history of the clinical problem, mental status examination, family and social history, collateral sources of information, observations of the patient over time, course of the disorder over weeks or months (and sometimes years), the patient's social competence, and response to treatment (including therapeutic trials). In the addictions, as with many other psychiatric disorders, no one physical finding, laboratory test, or tissue abnormality is pathognomonic. Instead we must obtain information in many ways, from many sources, and over a period of time in order to assess whether the patient fits the criteria for a psychoactive substance use disorder.

Academic psychiatrists must appreciate the reliability and validity of self-reports among addicted persons as well as the factors which augment or undermine these. The educator in the addictions must know the various excretion times of heroin, amphetamines, opium, and tetrahydrocannabinol in chronic heavy users, so that blood or urine tests can be interpreted. The importance of conducting psychiatric reassessment following a period of abstinence should be emphasized. Students should learn the methods of regular monitoring over time, such as self-report, observation, collateral sources of information, improvement of associated medical problems, supervised administration of medications (e.g., disulfiram, methadone, naltrexone), and body fluid monitoring for drug-alcohol use (e.g., urine screens, breathylyzer, blood levels).

F. Treatment

Psychiatrists teaching addiction psychiatry must convey concepts and information regarding the care and management of addicted patients. These include recognition and acute interventions for overdose, recognition and management of withdrawal and other acute drug-related emergencies, and concomitant treatment of alcohol-drug abuse in the presence of medical, surgical, or other psychiatric conditions. The risks of concurrent administration of certain psychotropic medications along with drug or alcohol abuse should be appreciated.

Treatment approaches often not familiar to psychiatrists should be studied. These include special medications (e.g., disulfiram, clonidine, naloxone, naltrexone, methadone), special procedures (e.g., withdrawal regimens, overdose regimens), and special resources for psychosocial recovery (e.g., Alcoholics Anonymous, Narcotics Anonymous, halfway house, therapeutic communities). Students should be aware of the goals and methods of family therapy, group therapy, and self-help groups as these relate to substance abuse [21].

G. Prevention

Primary and secondary prevention of substance abuse is facilitated by learning to use therapies other than opioids and sedatives in managing chronic pain, chronic anxiety, and chronic dysphoria, while not avoiding appropriate medication for acute, time-limited conditions. Safe prescribing practices for drugs of potential abuse can be taught. As citizens of their respective societies, physicians can assume leadership roles in guiding drug laws and law enforcement policies against dangerous recreational drugs.

There are many opportunities for early recognition of substance abuse in virtually all fields of medicine, but especially in the primary care fields and in psychiatry. Physicians should learn the signs associated with the addictions (e.g., venous scars or tracks, acne rosacea) as well as becoming aware of high rates of the addictions with certain disorders (e.g., diabetes, lower respiratory infection, trauma). Psychiatric syndromes often associated with substance abuse should serve as a stimulus for special diagnostic screening (e.g., depression, panic, phobias, acute psychosis, sociopathy, hysteria).

III. ACQUIRING CLINICAL SKILLS RELEVANT TO SUBSTANCE ABUSE

A. Interviewing

Psychiatrists acquire skills in establishing a doctor-patient relationship with a diverse group of patients in a variety of contexts. They become adept at discussing a highly personal problem with an embarrassed executive, in dealing with the anger and grief of a mother distraught at her sons' violent behavior in the home, and in observing and listening to a disorganized patient whose speech and behavior are incomprehensible and perhaps frightening or repulsive to others [27]. These skills stand psychiatrists in good stead when serving patients who present with alcohol-drug addictions. In addition to practicing this skill, psychiatrists also learn to teach it by role modeling, by observing and critiquing students, and by showing films and videotapes of doctor-patient interactions. Psychiatrists emphasize the key roles of rapport, building trust, and mutual cooperation in undertaking diagnosis and treatment. It is feasible to teach certain aspects of effective interviewing to nonpsychiatrist generalists [28–30].

Although most physicians do conduct interviews with patients, psychiatrists devote the kind of attention to interview techniques that the internist devotes to palpation, percussion, and auscultation. In the midst of conducting interviews, psychiatrists consider whether to facilitate, clarify, support, educate, confront, interpret, suggest, or make recommendations to the patient [31,32]. They make decisions regarding how to proceed with interviewing a confused, paranoid, demented, dependent, aggressive, angry, disinterested, or hallucinating patient as well as how to understand the meaning of symptoms. Tact, it has been said, involves the ability (within limits) to read minds. Psychiatrists pay attention to verbal as well as nonverbal communications, manifest content as well as the process of communicating, conflict between apparent affect and verbal content, relating the patient's current statements to past behavior, and so forth [33]. A "third eye" screens for reliability and validity regarding the patient's self-reports [34]. All of these skills have special relevance in curing for addicted patients.

B. Phasing Assessment-Reassessment, and Response to Treatment

Much modern medical assessment is carried out rapidly, over hours or a few days. Patients and families increasingly have little tolerance for uncertainty. In the midst of such urgency, psychiatrists must often counsel positive expectancy, benign neglect and watchful waiting. This approach is especially apropros to alcohol-drug addictions owing to the following factors:

1. Thorough detoxification over days or a few weeks (and sometimes a few months) is needed to assess the patient free of drug effect.
2. Subacute withdrawal symptoms may persist over several weeks to several months, mimicking depression, panic attacks, generalized anxiety, and somatoform disorders, especially with opioids, sedatives, and alcohol [35].
3. Pathological findings on psychological tests, the electroencephalogram, and computerized axial tomography may not return to normal for several months, especially with alcohol [25,36].

4. The untoward effects of nutritional deficiency, social isolation, family alienation, physical inactivity, or other disabilities may not improve for 1–2 years [26].
5. Brief episodes of alcohol or drug abuse often recur during the early stages of recovery [37]. These relapses must be distinguished from treatment failure with its subsequent need for more extensive and/or intensive treatment.

In light of these changes over weeks or months, initial assessment must often continue over weeks or months. There is no sense in merely evaluating drug effect or withdrawal consequences (say in a psychological test) if these do not relate to the patient's eventual status. By the same token, major depression, panic attack, hypomania or mania, social phobia, paranoia, or other disorders may appear or recur within the first few weeks or months of abstinence [15,38].

C. Confrontation, Crisis Management, Contingency Contracting

Of all the medical specialties, psychiatrists especially develop skills in relationship-based and verbal therapies. Interviewing provides a continuity between assessment and therapy, as one flows almost indistinguishably into the other and back again [39]. Within the doctor-patient relationship, the physician becomes a therapeutic modality [40]. Psychiatrists are well trained in applying the three Cs of substance abuse treatment: confrontation, crisis management, and contingency contracting. Whenever possible, these modalities are applied within a family context. General physicians can be taught these methods under close supervision.

Confrontation

Confrontation is sometimes misconstrued by students as mere angry verbal assault on the patient. Rather it involves pointing out the consequences of the individual's substance use, along with any inconsistency among what the patient thinks, feels, says, and does. It is an important step in allying the patient with family, therapists, and others who are emphasizing these two points: (1) a problem exists, (2) something must be done about it.

Crisis Management

Confrontation, threatened loss of family or job, acute illness, suicide attempt, arrest, or other drug-related problems results in a crisis for the patient. Handled properly, the crisis can be the first step toward treatment and eventual recovery. We have the opportunity in such cases to teach medical students and residents the nuances of crisis management. This involves aiding the patient and family in assessing the situation, considering alternatives and resources, and making therapeutic and other appropriate decisions.

Contingency Contracting

The family, school, employer, or parole officer may be willing to negotiate certain assistance or resources in return for certain commitments or behaviors from the patient. The physician can serve as a broker in this process, which is sometimes called contingency contracting. The experienced clinician can help all sides strike an agreement which is feasible, fair, incremental (rather than all-or-none), and on-going.

D. Pharmacotherapy

Psychiatrists are familiar with many drugs used for certain alcohol- and drug-related conditions. These conditions include the following:

1. Acute, subacute, and chronic withdrawal from opioids, sedatives, and alcohol
2. Delusional disorders associated with abuse of cannabis, amphetamines, and other stimulants, hallucinogens including phencyclidine

3. Organic affective disorder associated with drug abuse

4. Hallucinosis, delirium tremens, and withdrawal seizures associated with alcohol, benzodiazepines, and other drugs

5. Appearance of psychopathological conditions during abstinence (e.g., major depression, mania, panic) [41]

Management of these disorders depends on the skilled and timely use of methadone or other opioids, benzodiazepines and other antiseizure medications, and blocking agents such as clonidine.

There are additional pharmacotherapies used primarily for the treatment of substance abuse. These include disulfiram, naltrexone, and methadone maintenance. While these drugs are usually prescribed only by specialists in substance abuse, medical students should know about these medications and their actions, since they may encounter patients who are being treated with them.

Even as withdrawal treatment is proceeding, reassessment is called for. Withdrawal can be precipiated or kindled by a variety of problems: sepsis, pylorospasm, blood loss, head injury, psychosocial stressors, psychopathology, and other complicating factors [42].

IV. ATTITUDES TOWARD ADDICTED PATIENTS

Attitudes toward patients affect the quality of care which is rendered [43,44]. This fact has particular relevance for substance abuse care, since medical students come with a range of attitudes toward drug abusers which reflect the general attitudes of their society [45]. Generally, these attitudes are negative: the drug abuser, alcoholic, or addict is often judged automatically as poor, weak, evil, deceitful, incapable of change, irresponsible, immoral, egocentric, and passive-aggressive [46,47]. These attitudes deteriorate further during medical school, often reaching a low point during residency training and continuing at that level later during practice [48–51]. Negative attitudes among medical students are not unique to addicted patients; they frequently also exist with regard to the elderly, homosexuals, patients with venereal disease, criminal patients, and schizophrenic patients [52]. There is a difference, however. Although medical students are mostly not elderly, homosexual, or schizophrenic, many students do use the psychoactive substances accepted in their societies [53]. This latter fact may reinforce the notion that substance abusers are hedonists or weak since they cannot retain control over use like the medical students. Such negative attitudes appear especially apt to develop in medical students, since this group has typically had fairly extensive nonmedical drug use [54–57]. Nurses and other health professionals also share these antitherapeutic attitudes [58–61].

The notion of addressing student attitudes is frightening to some, especially to students themselves. However, medical educators are in the business of guiding students in exchanging nontherapeutic attitudes for therapeutic ones. Physicians cannot bolt from the emergency room at the sight of blood, or refuse to examine a crying infant or an agitated elderly patient, or abandon a paranoid patient in need of medical care.

Examples of information and experiences which are conductive to developing positive or at least therapeutic attitudes regarding substance abuse include the following:

1. Addicted persons do not manifest their ordinary personality while under drug effect.

2. It is important to treat the alcohol-drug addiction itself, and not just its medical or surgical complications.

3. Addicted persons can and often do recover from their disorder.

4. Recovery from addiction is facilitated by early intervention and treatment [62].

5. The addictions comprise a disorder with many manifestations of other disease states (e.g., genetic and constitutional factors, epidemiological disturbutions, deteriorating course, diagnostic criteria, response to treatment).

Fundamental attitudinal change cannot be mandated, or tested for on an examination, although instruments are available to monitor attitudinal change [62]. Change can be facilitated and assessed, however [63]. This can be accomplished in various ways. One effective means consists of having students examine and reconsider their own attitudes toward the addictions before and after a learning experience [64]. Such experiences might include a didactic course, learning to interview and assess addicted patients, or serving a clinical clerkship in a unit which assesses and treats addicted patients. This process may also be helped along by having the patients consider and reassess their attitudes toward their own psychoactive use (including caffeine, tobacco, alcohol), as well as that of their peers, friends, and family. Positive attitude changes can also develop solely from positive clinical experiences with substance-abusing patients during training [65].

V. GOALS AND PHASING OF TRAINING IN THE ADDICTIONS

Timing, duration, and content of training in the addictions depends on the objectives of the training. Objectives in turn depend on priorities, since all physicians cannot become experts in this field. And the priorities must be determined by the health needs of the population and the health care system.

One of the first needs is to be able to recognize alcohol and drug abuse, ideally at an early phase. In part this depends on the clinician's knowing what symptoms or problems are apt to be associated with substance abuse (e.g., depression, headache, falls, vehicular accidents, child abuse). Also in part the clinician must be able to acquire relevant clinical data to make a diagnosis (e.g., interviewing skills, taking a substance use history, interpreting laboratory tests, informant sources). Depending upon when this occurs in the course of training, it may require as long as a few weeks (e.g., in the second or third year of medical school), or as short as a few days (e.g., during residency in psychiatry). General physicians must also learn to make referrals of identified cases to persons who can conduct further assessment and undertake treatment. These educational and training goals should ideally be accomplished by the time medical school is completed. This requires a alcohol- and drug-related curriculum throughout the 4 years of medical school. A model curriculum might include the following:

First year: alcohol and drug use in various societies over time; biopsychosocial factors supporting alcohol-drug use (e.g., economic factors, advertising); biochemistry of alcohol
Second year: pharmacology of drugs of potential abuse in both naive and addicted persons; pathophysiology of drug- and alcohol-related diseases; diagnostic criteria, psychodynamics, sociodynamics, and epidemiology of substance disorder
Third year: interviewing patients for alcohol-drug use and abuse, making the diagnosis of a psychoactive substance use disorder
Fourth year: identifying alcohol-drug abuse in patients presenting with other problems, conveying the diagnosis, motivating the patient to seek treatment, working with the family, referring the patient to treatment

Since some medical schools do not yet provide this education and training, then training may be addressed in residency or in continuing education courses.

A more advanced level of training can involve pretreatment asessment, which goes beyond mere diagnosis. What are the patient's current resources, therapeutic needs, and past successes or failures in treatment? This requires greater clinical sophistication and more training time (i.e., full time over several weeks to a few months). It may also be possible to educate the trainee about the processes of and approaches to treatment, so that the trainee can then select particular treatment approaches for the patient. This approach is feasible during the later stages of medical school but is usually pursued during residency. It requires several weeks to a few months [66].

Subspecialty training in the addictions requires a 1-2 years of fellowship training, to occur later during residency (i.e., PGY 4) or following psychiatric residency. Those completing such a course should be able to assess all substance abuse patients, including forensic, multiple disordered, polydrug abuse, complex, and treatment-failure cases. Fellows should be able to apply and/or supervise a wide variety of treatment modalities. Graduates at this level should be able to establish, develop, direct, administrate, and evaluate services for substance abuse. Given adequate supervision, psychiatric fellows in the addictive disorders can learn to conduct clinical supervision of trainees who are at more elementary levels [67]. For those pursuing an academic career, two fellowship years are required to acquire research and teaching skills.

REFERENCES

1. Rodin, A.E. (1981). Infants and gin mania in 18th-century London, *J.A.M.A.*, *245*:1237.
2. Chopra, R.N. (1928). The present position of the opium habit in India, *Indian J. Med. Res.*, *16*:389.
3. Westermeyer, J. (1983). *Poppies, Pipes and People: A Study of Opium and Its Use in Laos*, University of California Press, Berkeley.
4. Cameron, D.C. (1968). Youth and drugs: A world view, *J.A.M.A.*, *206*:1267.
5. Lurie, N.O. (1970). The world's oldest on-going protest demonstration: North American Indian drinking practices, *Pacific Historical Rev.*, *40*:311.
6. Lebeer, G., and Orenbuch, J. (1985). A contribution to the study of young people's attitudes towards drug use and users, *Bull. Narcotics*, *37*:99.
7. Whittaker, J.O. (1982). Alcohol and the Standing Rock Sioux Tribe: A twenty-year follow-up study, *J. Stud. Alcohol, 43*:191.
8. Pokorny, A., Putnam, P., and Fryer, J. (1978). Drug abuse and alcoholism teaching in U.S. medical and osteopathic schools, *J. Med. Ed.*, *53*:816.
9. Clare, A.W. (1984). Alcohol education and the medical student, *Alcohol Alcohol.*, *19*:291.
10. Lisansky, E.T. (1975). Why physicians avoid early diagnosis of alcoholism, *N.Y. State J. Med.*, *75*:1788.
11. Spickard, W.A., and Tucker, P.J. (1984). An approach to alcoholism in a university medical center complex, *J.A.M.A.*, *252*:1894.
12. Drew, L.R.H. (1977). Alcohol and medical practice—the role of the psychiatrist in instituting change, *Aust. N.Z. Journal Psychiatry, 11*:241.
13. Crowley, T.J., Chesluk, D., Dilts, S., and Hart, R. (1974). Drug and alcohol abuse among psychiatric admissions: A multidrug clinical-toxicologic study, *Arch. Gen. Psychiatry, 30*:13.
14. McLellan, A.T., Druley, K.A., and Carson, J.E. (1978). Evaluation of substance abuse problems in a psychiatric hospital, *J. Clin. Psychiatry, 39*:425.
15. Westermeyer, J. Studying drug abuse in psychiatric populations: A reanalysis and review, *Psychiatry and Drug Abuse* (R. Pickens and L. Heston, eds.), Grune & Stratton, New York, 1979, p. 47.
16. McNamee, H.B., Mirin, S.M., Kuekule, J.C., and Meyer, R.E. (1976). Affective changes in chronic opiate use, *Br. J. Addict.*, *71*:275.
17. Madden, J.S. (1984). Psychiatric advances in the understanding and treatment of alcohol dependence, *Alcohol Alcohol.*, *19*:339.
18. Coggan, P.G., Davis, A.K., and Hadac, R. (1984). Alcoholism curriculum development: An examination of the process, *J. Fam. Pract.*, *19*:527.

19. WHO Expert Committee on Drugs Liable to Produce Addiction (1951), Third Report, WHO Technical Report Service 57, Geneva, WHO.

20. Criteria Committee, National Council on Alcoholism (1972). Criteria for the diagnosis of alcoholism, *Am. J. Psychiatr., 129*:127.

21. Westermeyer, J. (1986). *A Clinical Guide to Drug and Alcohol Problems*, Praeger, New York.

22. Schuckit, M.A. (1984). Relationship between the course of primary alcoholism in men and family history, *J. Stud. Alcohol, 45*:334.

23. Anderson, B., Nilsson, K., and Tunving, K. (1983). Drug careers in perspective, *Acta Psychiatr. Scand., 67*:249.

24. Favazza, A.R., and Thompson, J.J. (1984). Social networks of alcoholics: Some early findings, *Alcoholism Clin. Exp. Res., 8*:9.

25. Johnson, L.C., Burdick, A., and Smith, J. (1970). Sleep during alcohol intake and withdrawal in the chronic alcoholic, *Arch. Gen. Psychiatry, 22*:406.

26. Waldo, M., and Gardiner, J. (1984). Vocational adjustment patterns of alcohol and drug misusers following treatment, *J. Stud. Alcohol, 45*:547.

27. Hollister, W.G., and Edgerton, J.W. (1974). Teaching relationship-building skills, *Am. J. Public Health, 64*:41.

28. Waldron, J. (1973). Teaching communication skills in medical school, *Am. J. Psychiatry, 130*:579.

29. Werner, A., and Schneider, J.M. (1974). Teaching medical students interactional skills: A research-based course in the doctor-patient relationship, *N. Engl. J. Med., 29*:1232.

30. Verby, J.E. (1976). The audiovisual interview: A new tool in medical education, *J.A.M.A., 236*:2413.

31. Froelich, R.E. (1969). A course in medical interviewing, *J. Med. Ed., 44*:1165.

32. Enelow, A.J., Adler, L.M., and Wexler, M. (1970). Programmed instruction in interviewing: An experiment in medical education, *J.A.M.A., 212*:1843.

33. Kimball, C.P. (1969). Techniques of Interviewing, I. Interviewing and the meaning of the symptom, *Ann. Intern. Med. 71*:147.

34. Cline, D.W., and Garrard, J.N. (1973). A medical interviewing course: Objectives, techniques, and assessment, *Am. J. Psychiatry, 130*:574.

35. Adamson, J., and Burdick, J.A. (1973). Sleep of dry alcoholics, *Arch. Gen. Psychiatry, 28*:146.

36. Sherer, M., and Haygood, J.M. (1984). Stability of psychologial test results in newly admitted alcoholics, *J. Clin. Psychol., 40*:855.

37. Milkman, H., Weiner, S.E., and Sunderwirth, S. (1984). Addiction relapse, *Adv. Alcohol and Subst. Abuse, 3*:119.

38. Cadoret, R., and Winokur, G. (1974). Depression in alcoholism, *Ann. N.Y. Acad. Sci., 233*:34.

39. Kimball, C.P. (1970). Interviewing, diagnosis and therapy, *Postgrad. Med., 47*:88.

40. Rogers, D.E. (1974). The doctor himself must become the treatment, *Pharos, 37*:124.

41. Pickens, L.R.W., and Heston, L.L. (eds.). *Psychiatric Factors in Drug Abuse*, Grune & Stratton, New York, 1979.

42. Ballenger, J.C., and Post, R.M. (1978). Kindling as a model for alcohol withdrawal syndromes, *Br. J. Psychiatry, 133*:1.

43. Gulledge, A.D., and Litin, E.M. (1968). Attitude and its influence on the doctor-patient relationship, *New Physician, 17*:77.

44. Chappel, J.N., and Schnoll, S.H. (1977). Physician attitudes: Effect on the treatment of chemically dependent patients, *J.A.M.A., 237*:2318.

45. Kilty, K.M. (1975). Attitudes toward alcohol and alcoholism among professionals and nonprofessionals, *J. Stud. Alcohol, 36*:327.

46. Chappel, J.N. (1973). Attitudinal barriers to physician involvement with drug abusers, *J.A.M.A., 224*:1011.

47. Engs, R.C. (1982). Medical, nursing, and pharmacy students' attitudes towards alcoholism in Queensland, Australia, *Alcoholism Clin. Exp. Res., 6*:225.

48. Fisher, J.C., Mason, R.L., Keeley, K.A., and Fisher, J.V. (1975). Physicians and alcoholics: The effect of medical training on attitudes toward alcoholism, *J. Stud. Alcohol, 36*:949.

49. Fisher, J.C., Keeley, K.A., Mason, R.L., and Fisher, J.V., (1975). Physicians and alcoholics: Factors affecting attitudes of family-practice residents towards alcoholics, *J. Stud. Alcohol, 36*:626.

50. Rock, N.L., and Silsby, H.D. (1975). The attitudes of American physicians stationed with the United States Army, Europe, in regard to alcohol and drug abuse, *Milit. Med., 140*:781.

51. Smith, C.M., and Barnes, G.M. (1977). Physicians' perspectives on alcohol and drug problems, *N.Y. State J. Med., 77*:2140.

52. Viukari, M., Rimon, R., and Soderholm, S. (1979). Physicians' perspectives on alcohol and other patients, *Acta Psychiatr. Scand., 59*:24.

53. Sparks, R.D. (1976). Attitudes in medicine toward alcoholism, *Man Med., 1*:173.

54. Mechanick, P., Mintz, J., Gallagher, J., Lapid, G., Rubin, R., and Good, J. (1973). Nonmedical drug use among medical students, *Arch. Gen. Psychiatry, 29*:48.

55. Laporte, J.R., Cami, J., Gutierrez, R., and Laporte, J. (1977). Caffeine, tobacco, alcohol, and drug consumption among medical students in Barcelona, *Eur. J. Clin. Pharmacol., 11*:449.

56. Rochford, J., Grant, I., and LaVigne, G. (1977). Medical students and drugs: Further neuropsychological and use pattern considerations, *Int. J. Addict., 12*:1057.

57. Thomas, R.B., Luber, S.A., and Smith, J.A. (1977). A survey of alcohol and drug use in medical students, *Dis. Nerv. Syst., 38*:41.

58. Mogar, R.E., Helm, S.T., Snedeker, M.R., Snedeker, M.H., and Wilson, W.M. (1969). Staff attitudes toward the alcoholic patient, *Arch. Gen. Psychiatry, 21*:449.

59. Soverow, G., Rosenberg, C.M., and Ferneau, E. (1972). Attitudes towards drug and alcohol addiction: Patients and staff, *Br. J. Addict., 67*:195.

60. Brink, P.J. (1973). Nurses' attitude toward heroin addicts, *J.P.N. Ment. Health Serv., 11*:7.

61. Lemor, A.V., and Moran, J. (1978). Veterans Administration Hospital staff attitudes toward alcoholism, *Drug Alcohol Depend., 3*:77.

62. Chappel, J.N., Veach, T.L., and Krug, R.S. (1985). The Substance Abuse Attitude Survey: An instrument for measuring attitudes, *J. Stud. Alcohol, 46*:48.

63. Chappel, J.N., Jordan, R.D., Treadway, B.J., and Miller, P.R. (1977). Substance abuse attitude changes in medical students, *Am. J. Psychiatry, 134*:379.

64. Rezler, A.G. (1976). Methods of attitude assessment for medical teachers, *Med. Ed., 10*:43.

65. Powell, B.J., Mueller, J.F., and Schwerdtfeger, T. (1974). Attitude changes of general hospital personnel following an alcoholism training program, *Psychol. Rep., 34*:461.

66. Harris, I., and Westermeyer, J. (1978). Chemical dependency education within medical schools: Supervised clinical experience, *Am. J. Drug Alcohol Abuse, 5*:59.

67. Westermeyer, J. (1985). Fellowship in chemical dependency, *Am. J. Drug Alcohol Abuse, 11*:349.

43

Education of Primary Care Physicians

David C. Lewis
Brown University, Providence, Rhode Island

I. INTRODUCTION

The primary physician has a specific role to play where substance abuse is a problem or potential problem (see Fig. 1). We must change both our institutions and our curricula in order to improve the training of primary care physicians to perform that role. Many of the specific examples of such changes which will be given in this chapter come from the experience of developing the new Project ADEPT (Alcohol and Drug Education for Physician Training in Primary Care) medical curriculum at Brown University, and from establishing a comprehensive alcohol intervention program at the Roger Williams Hospital. Sample materials from the new curriculum are included.

First, there has to be a focus on ambulatory care. Improving the effectiveness of teaching in the ambulatory care setting is an important need for all of medical education [1,2]. What is true of ambulatory care teaching in general is also true of teaching and learning about alcohol and other drug problems in particular. Dr. Kelly Skeff of the Stanford University School of Medicine has described seven factors that enhance the effectiveness of faculty as ambulatory care teachers [3,4]. Here are Dr. Skeff's categories expanded with commentary about their relevance to teaching and learning about alcohol and other drug problems.

II. ESTABLISHING A POSITIVE LEARNING CLIMATE

Negative attitudes on the part of instructor and student have played an important role in undermining a positive learning climate [5–7]. Stereotyped perceptions of alcoholics as skid-row bums prevail among medical students [8]. The patients are stigmatized as "difficult" because their behavior is self-injurious and their illness, chronic. Since much medical training takes place in inpatient settings, students see alcoholic patients in the acute phase of their illness or with the intractable, chronic, physical sequelae of alcoholism rather than when they are recovering and doing well. This experience reinforces the erroneous impression that alcohol

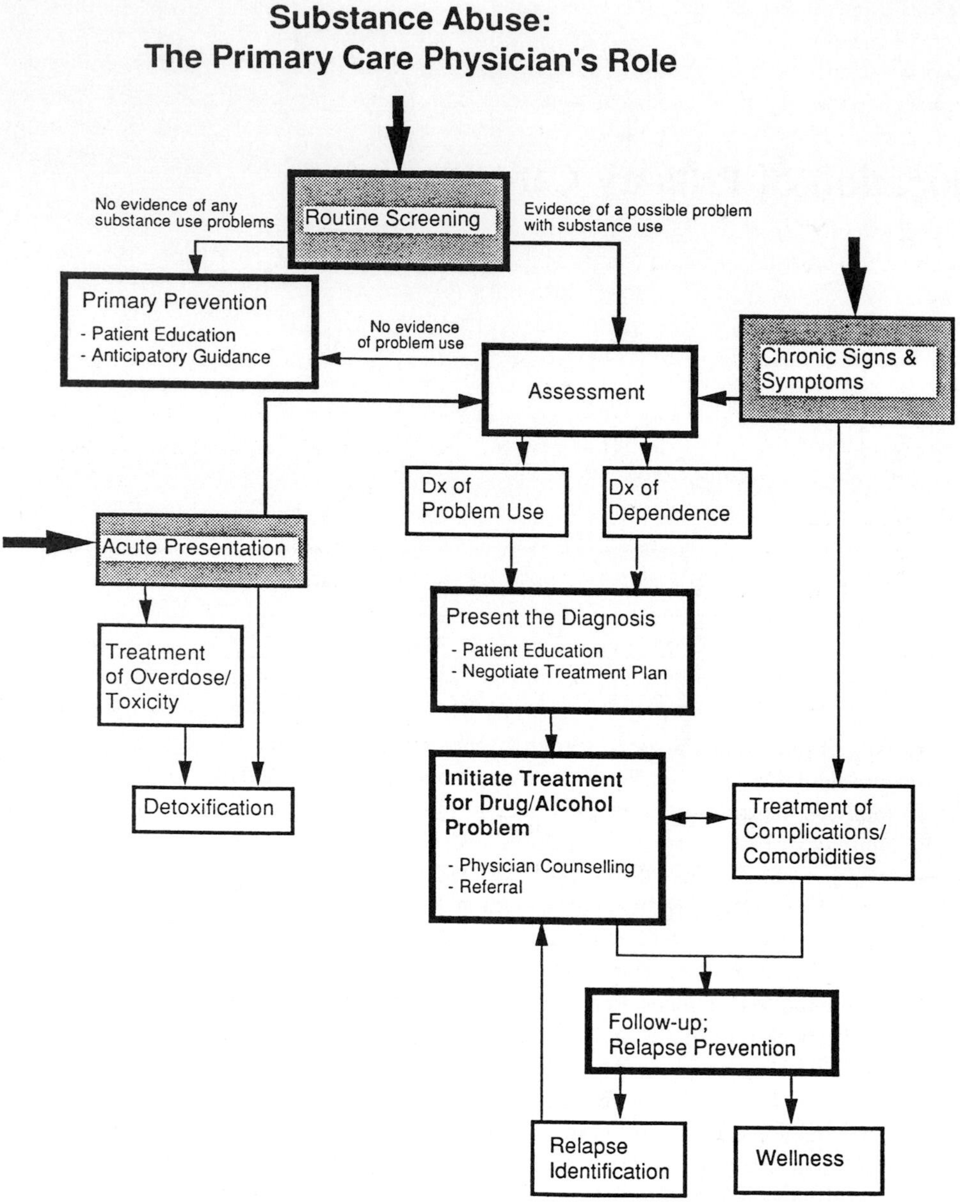

Substance Abuse:
The Primary Care Physician's Role

```
                                    │
                                    ▼
No evidence of any          ┌──────────────────┐      Evidence of a possible problem
substance use problems      │ Routine Screening │      with substance use
                            └──────────────────┘
```

Figure 1 Role of the physician. (From Goldstein, M.G., and Liepman, M.R. [1989]. Introduction and overview, *Project ADEPT Curriculum for Primary Care Physician Training*, Vol. I, Brown University, Providence, Rhode Island, p. 42.)

problems occur only with severe physical and social complications. Negative attitudes toward alcoholic patients deepen as students move on to internship and residency.

The new emphasis on educating primary care physicians provides some hope in countering this negative outlook [9–11]. Primary care physicians are usually the first to see patients with medical problems associated with alcohol use [12]. Therefore, they are in an ideal position to encourage prevention, make early diagnoses, provide immediate treatment, and refer patients for more specialized services. In fact, the evidence is mounting that when intervention occurs before a drinking problem gets out of hand, much less intense and costly treatment is necessary and a good deal of personal and family agony can be prevented. Training opportunities are enhanced when the patients manifest a variety of problems with alcohol/drugs ranging from problems of episodic intoxication to severe dependence, and also include those who have been dependent and have recovered.

Without an appropriate institutional setting, quality teaching will be undermined no matter how thoughtful the training design or how informed and free of negative attitudes the trainee. For effective learning, the institutional environment is at least as important as the attitudes that instructors and students bring to the learning process [13,14].

While most hospitals today deal in a very sophisticated way with the complications of drinking, they manage to an extraordinary extent to avoid dealing with the existence of the drinking behavior itself [15]. As a result, although drinking is involved in the illness of 10–20% of ambulatory and 25–50% of the general hospital patients, only a handful receive a diagnosis for their alcohol problem while they are in the hospital. This discrepancy requires an institution-wide approach and change.

The author's experience over more than a decade at The Roger Williams General Hospital, 238 bed community teaching hospital of the Medical School at Brown University, illustrates one model of how the general hospital can be responsive to patients with alcohol problems and in doing so create a more positive training model [16,17]. While this illustration is not limited to an ambulatory setting, the general hospital with its inpatient, ambulatory and emergency services is at the core of the currently constituted medical training system and thus deserves special attention.

The alcohol intervention program at Roger Williams General Hospital was implemented in 1977. A five-member interdisciplinary team staffs the intervention program. The "A (Addiction) team" consists of a physician, nurse-counselor, alcoholism counselor, social worker, and an intake secretary. The presence of a team comprised of professionals with varied backgrounds offering consultation makes the hospital staff aware of the variety of skills and personnel that can be brought to bear on the problems of these patients.

From the very beginning, hospital-wide communication was stressed because the entire hospital organization was regarded as a potential constituency for the fledgling program, a series of formal and informal education programs was held with hospital trustees, administrators, and all personnel. In addition to the professional staff, A team members made presentations to dietary, maintenance, secretarial, and administrative units of the hospital. An Employee Assistance Policy which emphasized rehabilitation rather than dismissal for drinking problems was begun. Once the alcohol intervention program was in place, the A team provided formal consultative services to the personnel department and informal advice to many employees. The formal orientation of every new employee at Roger Williams Hospital includes a session about the approach to and the assessment and management of the alcoholic as well as details about the hospital's program for patients and employees. In-service training for all professional staff is an ongoing part of the program.

Nurses have become the key staff people. The nurse member of the multidisciplinary A team meets with head nurses on every nursing unit, not only for continuing in-service education, but also to help identify those patients who might be approached about their drinking problems. Nurses take the initiative in identifying patients with drinking problems and in urging house staff and practicing physicians to request a consultation from the A team.

Medical students and residents join the A team for 1-month rotations. Their contacts with other residents and medical students serve to increase access to patients throughout the hospital. The addition of social work and nursing students has had a similar effect in widening our patient contacts. The positive response by the trainees has gained credibility for the alcohol program with the sponsoring departments at the hospital.

In working with patients throughout the hospital, our clinical approach is nonjudgmental, open, and persistent. Typically, the staff introduce themselves as follows: "We are the group in the hospital that's interested in drinking" (and wait for the response), or "Your physician wanted me to stop by and chat with you about drinking," or "I have been asked to stop by to see if you have any concerns about your drinking."

Since about 10% of admissions can be identified with drinking- and drug-related problems, the inpatient consultation level of the A team has risen from one or two consults a month to two to three each day. When formal treatment is indicated, about half these patients are referred to an ambulatory follow-up clinic and the remainder to other community programs. Periodic chart reviews point to the impact of the screening program. Before the program began, only 12% of pancreatitis patients were identified in a discharge diagnosis as having a serious drinking problem. After the program was underway that percentage tripled at the Roger Williams General Hospital, whereas remaining at 12% in other general hospitals in Rhode Island.

The lack of continuity of care was a major issue. To a great extent, the problem was resolved by instituting an ambulatory clinic at the general hospital to provide care beginning with the initial intervention. Patients can visit the clinic while they are inpatients, thereby lessening resistance to the first ambulatory visit. After discharge, ongoing outpatient treatment is provided in group, family, or individual sessions with the A team staff at the hospital or in one of several community-based counseling services. As an alternative to this approach, a close liaison between the general hospital and a specialized community-based treatment facility can be established.

The existence of an ambulatory clinic at the general hsopital presents a second important advantage. It provides the setting where hospital staff can see patients who were formerly under their care in the emergency room or inpatient service. After effective treatment, these patients can appear to be totally different people from the acutely ill individuals that the hospital staff remember. For many staff members, this exposure dramatically counters a negative view of alcoholics and alcohol abusers and a pessimism about their recovery.

Learning the limitations of the professional role is important in educating care givers at all levels. Fortunately, the growth of treatment programs has helped health professionals to understand they are not on their own. It has been very reassuring to learn they have help available and that community resources like Alcoholics Anonymous (AA) and Al-Anon have grown at the same time as organized professional treatment programs. AA and Al-Anon groups hold meetings at the hospital, thereby facilitating the link between professional services and self-help.

The program at the Roger Williams General Hospital involved institutional changes: changes in staff roles, new hospital services, and greater involvement at every staff level in the care of patients with drinking problems. The end result has been better care for patients and an improved learning climate for the trainees [18].

III. CONTROL OF THE TEACHING SESSION

Control here refers to the teacher's role; getting your "teaching act" together. If you are going to stand up and give a lecture, it has to be a well-organized lecture with good audiovisual support. If you are going to do a demonstration with a patient, it has to be pertinent, efficient, and pay attention to the time constraints in teaching settings.

As far as content is concerned, alcohol and drug medical education has to exhibit the same scientific rigor as does training in diabetes, rheumatoid arthritis, or any other chronic illness. We are not teaching folk medicine but psychopharmacology, family dynamics, genetics, the identification of populations at risk, the variety of treatment approaches and self-help groups, and the occurrence of recovery and relapse. The teaching is based on a wealth of empirically based information and skills directed at improving medical care for these very common medical problems.

IV. COMMUNICATION OF GOALS

When medical students, residents, or practicing physicians know the goals of the teaching, it enhances their motivation and ability to learn. Organizing training experiences in this way is not difficult, but implementation may be. Typical of most alcohol/drug education is that teaching goals far exceed what can be practically accomplished. One approach toward the effective and realistic achievement of teaching goals is to carefully define the competencies that are to be taught as well as the methods and preferred format for teaching them.

There are several examples of the definition of competencies. A 1985 Consensus Conference was oriented toward the task of reaching agreement concerning what physicians in training and practicing physicians needed to know to diagnose and care for patients with alcohol and other drug abuse problems. At the Consensus Conference a process was followed in which small groups selected the essential knowledge and skills that were needed by psychiatry, pediatrics, family medicine, and internal medicine. A report of the conference consensus statements was published [19]. The exercise of the Consensus Conference has been repeated by several national professional societies and medical schools [20–24].

V. ENHANCING UNDERSTANDING AND RETENTION

Effective training of any sort takes into account attitudes of the instructors and students, and attends to learning both in the area of knowledge and skills. Medical training is no exception, and is further enhanced when the skills that have been acquired can be practiced under supervision.

Several fundamental issues need to be addressed in organizing the training. How do you decide what to teach? At what intensity and depth? How much time is given to a particular topic? Clearly, the standard for primary care education is different than the standard for specialist education. What are the skills you need for screening, making a diagnosis, and making an appropriate referral?

The experience of Project ADEPT at Brown University illustrates one approach to the setting and communicating of goals and the methods by which a new curriculum can be developed to enhance understanding [25,26]. It is an approach that has been effective. Project ADEPT has already developed and published two volumes containing 10 new teaching modules on subjects such as prevention, assessment and diagnosis, treatment, and adolescent substance abuse [27,28]. A third volume on AIDS (acquire immune deficiency syndrome) and substance abuse is also being published. In addition, in cooperation with the American Medical Association and the American Society of Addiction Medicine in this project, plans are now underway to modify ADEPT materials for continuing medical education for phsicians in practice.

At the outset, the faculty members who authored it agreed that the final curriculum would reflect the following characteristics:

The health professional and patient in the primary care setting are the focus of training.
The content emphasis (e.g., alcohol, cocaine, cigarette smoking, etc.) is based on the prevalence of the health problem in the patient population.
The learning is competency based. The essential knowledge and skills needed by the primary care physician are specified. The learning objectives of imparting knowledge and skills and exploring of attitudes are explicit as are the educational format and methods used to improve competencies.
Skills training is emphasized. This includes careful attention to the quantity and quality of feedback from the instructor and peers in the learning process.

In fact, skills training has emerged as the focus of the new curriculum. While both attitudes and knowledge are important, the greatest perceived deficit in physicians is the skill to interact with patients and their families concerning the prevention, diagnosis, intervention and referral in regard to alcohol and other drug problems. By teaching the skills necessary to interact with drug and alcohol patients we were able to change physicians' attitudes as well as to increase their effectiveness with their patients.

Finding the most effective way to teach the skills is challenging. Assuming that fundamental interviewing skills have been acquired, role playing both with other students/residents and with simulated patients with feedback are very effective practice exercises. One technique that we have found to be helpful is the skill checklist. Examples of this approach will be given below with samples from the curriculum.

In analyzing this effort to change the way an institution teaches its students/residents, key elements in the process deserve attention. Although part of the process that facilitates and sustains these activities at Brown University may be unique to our institution, it is likely the basic elements are common to other institutions of medical education.

Role models can not be minimized as part of the effectiveness in teaching. For primary care training and the teaching of basic skills, addiction specialists are not the only or even the most desirable role models. Teachers have to be credible to the students they are teaching. The adolescent pediatrician, for instance, can be a more credible teacher to the pediatric residents than an expert psychiatrist who is imported to teach pediatric residents. The methods and content of the skills training can be organized so that teachers need not be addiction experts. In Project ADEPT the material has been "boiled down" to a central core of knowledge and skills (as distinct from what one would teach a specialist) and prepared in a way that is supportive of primary care teaching. Paying attention to the role model and the credibility of the teacher is essential.

Attention to process has been a central feature of introducing real change into our training programs [29]. Two key staff members who helped organize and energize faculty participation were the project's Faculty Development Coordinator, trained in Psychiatry and Internal Medicine, who paid careful attention to the needs of the faculty to become more informed and effective teachers. The second key staffer, with an doctorate degree in education in Instructional Design, collaborated in the creation and evaluation of the new approaches and materials. While there are but a handful of curriculum designers who have experience with medical education, a strong recommendation is that if medical schools and national professional societies are serious about improved training, they would benefit from making a priority of creating positions for such individuals. While each institution will need to take its own approach, at Brown University we have been able to sustain an energetic and productive faculty group interested in improving training about alcohol and other drug problems by attending in a methodical way to both student and faculty needs.

VI. EVALUATION

The body of research on training outcomes is abysmal. We do not know enough about what kind of educational process will lead to a particular type of result. We need to find out what works effectively in terms of the behavioral payoff from teaching. Research methods are available to conduct the types of training evaluations we need. The methods are most similar to treatment outcome research and particularly research on the effectiveness of brief interventions. In addition, a new method, the use of standardized patients, has great promise as an evaluation tool [30]. Given renewed interest in prevention and treatment outcome research, perhaps some of these researchers will specialize in evaluating both short- and long-term training outcomes.

VII. FEEDBACK

The opportunity to practice under supervision and get good feedback from an experienced instructor is an underutilized experience in medical education generally and a tremendously weak spot in continuing medical education. Influencing physicians already in practice may require different strategies from teaching medical students and residents. Whatever the approach, the quality and the quantity of feedback is probably the single most powerful reinforcer of what people learn.

VIII. SELF-DIRECTED LEARNING

We all talk about self-directed learning, but it is not easy to promote. Medical students do not want any homework assignments and neither do practicing physicians. Practicing physicians want it all delivered at a single 1-h Grand Rounds. There has to be a way in which we can continue to learn over time in the practice setting. Several of the national professional societies have developed elaborate self-teaching materials (e.g., the American College of Physicians MKSAP course). When they are used, they are very instructive. The chart audit program of the Board of Family Practice provides an innovative approach to learning and quality assessment.

As we examine continuing medical education (CME), there is some cause for optimism. Several interesting and thoughtful papers have appeared over the last few years [31–34]. In the future, changes in communication fostered by technology will have a profound effect on education and training. The technology is such that eventually knowledge retention will not be any problem at all. The premium on the ability of the health professional or anyone else to remember a fact will diminish in importance. Knowledge will be readily accessible. You will probably ask your question to a machine verbally and the answer will come back in any form you direct. Factual knowledge will be taken care of, but the skills development and practice will not. Providing that part of training is going to remain a unique challenge for the medical profession.

We have to develop better ways to teach, whether it be interactive video, simulated patient exercises, or teleconferencing. Interactive video is now being developed by the Library of Medicine and the Board of Medical Examiners. The teleconference is another technological innovation with interactive capability. Patient interviews can be conducted before the audience. The audience can call-in using a toll-free 800 number and converse with expert panelists. It is a practical approach since the requisite satellite dishes are becoming more common in universities and teaching hospitals. Many innovations like these will make the process of education for practicing physicians and for physicians-in-training more efficient and helpful.

IX. PERSONAL SIGNIFICANCE OF SUBSTANCE ABUSE TO THE LEARNER

Connected with any of the seven educational approaches discussed above, the importance of the alcohol/drug subject in student's lives deserves special attention. Many medical students and residents have grown up in families troubled by a significant alcohol or drug abuse problem. Also, personal alcohol and drug use by medical students and residents can also be an important consideration and worthy of attention [35–37]. Several surveys indicate the vulnerability of this population [38–47]. Unless some of the attendant personal feelings of these trainees can be dealt with, both effective learning and patient care can be compromised. The author routinely lets third-year medical students confront and share their personal feelings about the subject at the onset of clinical clerkship training. Students are remarkably forthcoming and candid in this discussion, and invariably rate this session highly in their evaluation of the course.

Fortunately, there is now a supportive program in some medical schools for students in trouble with alcohol/drugs [48–53]. The most highly developed version of the support program is called AIMS (Aid for the Impaired Medical Student). Started in 1982 at the University of Tennessee College of Medicine at Memphis, there are as of this writing some 20 schools who have joined in a Consortium for Student and Professional Well-Being. Currently in draft form but under active consideration by the AAMC (American Association of Medical Colleges) are *General Guidelines for the Development of Chemical Impairment Programs in Medical Schools.** Less well developed are support programs for residents. A handful of schools and teaching hospitals have addressed this issue. One example is a *Policy on Resident and Faculty Impairment* adopted by the Department of Medicine at the University of Oklahoma College of Medicine in Tulsa.**

In addition to programs supportive of personal problems in students and residents, the way in which undergraduate and graduate medical education is conducted is itself perceived as a problem. Isolation, stress, and unrealistic expectations still pervade physicians-in-training [54–56]. The humanizing of medical training is still more discussed than practiced [57].

In general, the developments of the past few years in the training of primary care physicians give cause for optimism [58,59]. There is renewed interest in the routine education of all health professionals concerning alcohol/drug problems. The reemergence of primary care as a viable career choice has generated an energetic core of new faculty who will, along with their specialist colleagues, provide the training leadership for the future.

X. THE PROJECT ADEPT CURRICULUM: EXAMPLES OF TRAINING MATERIALS

The Project ADEPT curriculum materials are now being used in over half of the U.S. medical schools and several hundred teaching hospitals. Unlike a book format, the materials are modular (e.g., prevention, assessment and diagnosis, presenting the diagnosis and initiating treatment, treatment) and in a form ready for faculty use (e.g., lecture outlines, student handout materials, graphics for making overhead films of slides, role play exercises, skill checklists, bibliographies, test materials).

---

*For more information about the AIMS project, contact Hershel P. Wall, M.D., Associate Dean, University of Tennessee College of Medicine, 800 Madison Ave., Memphis, TN 38163.
**For more information about the Policy on Resident and Faculty Impairment, contact Ronald B. Saizow, M.D., Tulsa Medical College, 2815 S. Sheridan, Tulsa, OK 74129.

Table 1, a student handout, and accompanying preface, summarizes problems of chronic substance abuse that are encountered in primary care settings.

Figures 2 and 3 are skill checklists. In Project ADEPT a checklist is incorporated into each module at the point where the teaching centers on clinical skills. Both trainee and instructor become familiar with the skill checklist as a specific guide to learning, teaching, and practicing the skills to be acquired. Students can be rated by other students outside of formal class time using these skill checklists. Figure 2 contains the Skill Checklist from the module on Presenting the Diagnosis and Initiating Treatment. Figure 3 is the Skill Checklist from the module on Prevention.

Numerous role play scenarios are presented with information for the patient and physician role. These are preceded by instructions for the instructor about conducting a role play session. Two such role play exercises with the instructions appears below.

DIAGNOSING CHRONIC SUBSTANCE USE PROBLEMS IN THE PRIMARY CARE SETTING:

Related Physical Problems, Psychological Problems, Physical Findings, and Relevant Labs

The table on the following pages is designed to give the primary care provider a summary of related findings that may accompany chronic substance use as well as relevant laboratory tests to aid in diagnosis. The data presented here is intended for use in conjunction with screening questions and history taking to provide a complete picture of certain chronic substance use disorders. This data is *not* intended as a substitute for skillful patient interviewing.

For several substances and classes of substances, the following information is provided:

Related Physical Problems: Listed here are some of the major physical problems that either accompany chronic use or are a result of chronic substance use. These complaints represent a sample of medical problems that the patient may present to the physician when a chronic substance use problem exists or that may be apparent in the past medical history.

Related Psychological Problems: Here, major psychological problems accompanying or resulting from chronic substance use are listed. The patient may present these as problems to the physician, they may be directly observed or detected by the physician, or they may be disclosed in the past medical history.

Possible Physical Findings: This category of data provides the common physical findings that may accompany chronic substance use.

Relevant Laboratory Tests: Laboratory studies that will contribute to your diagnosis are listed in the final column. Also provided are detection times for toxicology screens.

Signs and symptoms of intoxication, overdose, and withdrawal are not addressed here. See "Assessment and Management of Intoxication and Overdose" and "Assessment and Management of Withdrawal" modules for this information.

Table 1 The Primary Care Setting—Problems of Chronic Substance Use: Related Physical Problems, Psychological Problems, Physical Findings and Relevant Lab Tests

Substance	Related physical complaints	Related psychological problems	Possible physical findings	Relevant lab studies
Alcohol	Frequent injuries; abdominal pain, nausea, vomiting (gastritis, pancreatitis); diarrhea; headaches; insomnia; myopathy; vague physical complaints; impotence; peripheral neuritis; convulsions; congestive heart failure, palpitations, insomnia	Depression (esp. bipolar disorder), anxiety, sudden unexplained mood changes, paranoia, memory loss, lying, unreliability	Hypertension, injuries e.g., bruises, cigarette unexplained burns, etc.; enlarged liver, cutaneous stigmata of liver disease (i.e., spider angioma, plmar erythema); ecchymoses on legs, arms or chest; smell of alcohol on breath	CBC ($\uparrow$ MCV $\uparrow$ MCH or cytopenias), $\uparrow$ liver function test (GGT, SGOT > SGPT), $\uparrow$ uric acid, $\uparrow$ triglycerides, rib fractures on CXR
Cocaine	Fatigue, sinusitis, sore throat, horseness, persistent fever, chest pain, sexual problems, bronchitis, weight loss, nausea and vomiting, headaches, muscle jerks and spasms, convulsions, arrhythmia	Acute paranoid ideation, mania, depression, sociopathy, anxiety, panic, anhedonia	Rhinitis, rash around the nasal area, perforation of the nasal septum, hypertension, tachycardia. Crack: Hoarseness; parched lips, tongue and throat; singed eyebrows or eyelashes; IV stigmata	Immunoassays, chromatography/mass spectroscopy, urine tox screen (up to 12–48 hr after use)
Stimulants	Skin ulcers, insomnia, weight loss	(Same as cocaine)	Worn down teeth (from tooth grinding) scratches, skin ulcers, dyskinesia	Urine toxicology screen (up to 24–48 hr after use)
Inhalants (hydrocarbons)	Weight loss, breathing difficulties, fatigue, nose bleeds, weakness, stomach upset, intellectual changes	Anxiety, depression, personality/intellectual changes, impaired performance	Halitosis, rash around nose or mouth; mental status changes	CBC, liver function tests, kidney function tests

Category				
Cannabis	Chronic dry cough, bronchitis, sinusitis, pharyngitis, laryngitis	Memory loss amotivational syndrome, anxiety	Conjunctival suffusion; distinct odor of burnt leaves on breath and clothes; dilated, poorly reactive pupils	Urine toxicology screen (occasional user, 1–3 days; chronic heavy users may have a positive screen for 1 month or more after cessation)
Opioids	Complaints of severe pain (to attain drugs), infections (esp. cellulitis, abscess, pneumonia, SBE)	Depression, panic reactions, lethargy, sociopathy or ASP disorder	Track marks, skin lesions, constricted pupils, swollen nasal mucosa, thrombosis, lymphadenopathy	Urine tox screen[a] (up to 2–4 days after use)
Depressants	Insomnia, restlessness, convulsions, pneumonia	Depression, anxiety paranoia, psychosis	Slurred speech without the odor of alcohol; "track" marks if IV user (esp. barbiturates); pupillary constriction with glutethimide (Doriden®)	Urine tox screen[b] (Detection time after last use: up to 1 week; barbiturates, chronic users, up to several weeks; long-acting benzodiazepines, chronic users, weeks–months)
Hallucinogens	Palpitations, chest pain (esp. in older users); convulsions with PCP	Panic reactions, anxiety, depersonalization, paranoia, confusion, psychosis, OBS, mania	Myopathy; renal failure with PCP	Urine tox screen (Detection time after last use: PCP several days to several weeks; LSD, up to 12 hr; LSD metabolites, 2 days) myoglobinuria, elevated CPK creatine/BUN with PCP

[a] If a screening assay is positive for opioids, a confirmatory test specific for morphine or codeine is necessary. Illicit versus clinical use of these substances cannot be determined by test results alone. Further, it is impossible to distinguish whether heroin, codeine, or morphine has been taken when low concentrations of morphine or codeine are found in the urine. Ingestion of a large quantity of poppy seeds will produce a positive immunosasay result up to 60 hr after ingestion. To distinguish between poppy seed ingestion and heroin use, use GC/MS to test for 6-O-acetylmorphine (a heroin metabolite). Methadone must be analyzed separately; Fentanyl and its analogues are not detected by routine methods.

[b] Xanax (alprazolam) may not be detected in routine assays. If suspected, the laboratory test should be instructed to use GC/MS for specific testing for alprazolam.

Source: Text and table by Wartenberg, A., Dubé C.E., Lewis, D.C., and Cyr, M.G. (1989). In Cyr, M.G., Assessment and diagnosis, Project ADEPT Curriculum for Primary Care Physician Training, Vol. I, Brown University, Providence, Rhode Island, pp. 38–40.

PRESENTING THE DIAGNOSIS AND INITIATING TREATMENT
SKILL CHECKLIST

Establish a Supportive Relationship:
P.E.A.R.L.S.

_____ Partnership: Makes a statement of partnership; e.g., "We'll work together on this."

_____ Empathy: Makes empathic comments; e.g., "This seems upsetting to you."

_____ Assurance: Makes statements that predict a positive outcome, e.g., "Our past experience has shown a high success rate."

_____ Respect: Makes a respectful comment; e.g., "You seem to be dealing with this problem very well."

_____ Legitimation: Makes a legitimating comment; e.g., "Giving up your substance use is very difficult to do."

_____ Support: Makes a supportive statement; e.g., "I'll be available to you during treatment."

Educate the Patient (Explanatory Model):
E.M.E.R.A.L.D.S.

_____ Explains implications and consequences of future use.

_____ Misunderstandings corrected

_____ Education: Provides valid, factual information about related substance use.

_____ Reviews the patient's understanding of information provided.

_____ Allows the patient to describe his/her understanding of the problem.

_____ Links substance use to specific signs/symptoms over time. (How substance use is related to the patient's symptoms or complaints; e.g., "The stomach problems you've been having are due to your drinking.")

_____ Describes the importance of abstinence/cutting down.

_____ Steers clear of pejorative (i.e., negative) labeling; e.g., "You are an addict/alcoholic."

Negotiate the Treatment Need/Plan and Contract with the Patient:
D.I.A.M.O.N.D.S.

_____ Defines problematic substance use as a condition that can be treated or addressed.

_____ Identifies and provides clear definite treatment recommendations.

_____ Allows the patient to express his/her own solutions, concerns and fears.

_____ Makes reasonable compromises in the treatment plan to insure acceptance (IF NECESSARY).

_____ Organizes and reviews details of the negotiated treatment plan.

_____ Needs the patient's verbal agreement to begin treatment. Solicits agreement.

_____ Decides if arrangements are needed to start treatment. Makes arrangements (IF APPROPRIATE)

_____ Schedules a follow-up appointment.

Figure 2 Presenting the diagnosis and initiating treatment skill checklist. (From Cyr, M.G. (1989). Presenting the diagnosis and initiating treatment, *Project ADEPT Curriculum for Primary Care Physician Training*, Vol. I, Brown University, Providence, Rhode Island, p. 40.)

PREVENTION SKILL CHECKLIST

Low-Risk Patients: *When routine screening reveals no problematic substance use and risk factors are few.*

_____ Express interest in working with the patient to prevent the problems of alcohol or drug abuse.

_____ Ask the patient to express his/her understanding of the problems of alcohol and drug use.

_____ Correct misunderstandings.

_____ Provide valid, factual information about alcohol and drug use. Provide pamphlets.

_____ Reinforce positive attitudes expressed by the patient regarding avoiding problematic alcohol and drug use.

_____ Suggest strategies for avoiding problems with alcohol and drugs and try to get patient's agreement.

High-Risk Patients: *When routine screening reveals moderate to heavy use of alcohol or experimental use of other substance and/or multiple risk fctors.*

> —*Problems with substance use may be beginning to develop*
> —*CAGE: May be negative or may have only one positive response*
> —*May have a history of psychosocial problems related to substance use in the past*
> —*Has not been diagnosed for substance abuse or dependence in the past (See Relapse Prevention...)*
> —*Does not currently meet the DSM-III-R criteria for dependence or abuse because symptoms are not repeated or continuous*

_____ Express concern regarding the potential health effects of continued substance use/experimentation.

_____ Ask the patient to express his/her understanding of potential for developing problems with substance use.

_____ Correct misunderstandings.

_____ Provide valid factual information about the effects of substance use. Provide pamphlets.

_____ Determine the patient's reasons for continued substance use/experimentation.

_____ Review risk factors (e.g., family history of substance abuse, ethnicity, high-risk occupation, etc.)

_____ Review with the patient his/her developing problems and link them to substance use.

_____ Personalize the benefits of avoiding/eliminating/cutting back on substance use.

_____ Negotiate a plan: Determine the patient's plan, describe options, negotiate a compromise.

_____ Identify social supports.

_____ Make a referral and/or follow-up appointment.

Figure 3 Prevention skill checklist. (From Goldstein, M.G., and Dubé, C.E. (1989). Substance abuse prevention, *Project ADEPT Curriculum for Primary Care Physician Training*, Vol. I, Brown University, Providence, Rhode Island, pp. 26–27.)

Tertiary Prevention: *When routine screening reveals problematic substance use.*

> —*CAGE: One or more positive responses*
> —*Has developed problems associated with substance use*
> —*Evidence of psychosocial consequences exists*
> —*Medical consequences may be apparent or may be absent*
> —*Meets the DSM-III-R cirteria for substance* abuse *or* dependence

For tertiary prevention, use the skills listed in the "Presenting the Diagnosis and Initiating Treatment" skill checklist.

Treat medical, psychiatric complications, comorbidities and/or refer.

Relapse Prevention: *For those who were previously diagnosed and treated and are in partial or full remission. (NOTE: If the patient has relapsed, use the "Presenting the Diagnosis and Initiating Treatment" checklist.)*

_____ Express an interest in working with the patient to maintain sobriety or abstinence

_____ Current treatment status: Are you currently in any kind of treatment or self-help group (e.g., NA, AA)?

Ask the patient to describe his/her current relationship with drinking/drugs:

_____ How have you been doing with your abstinence from alcohol/drugs?

_____ How do you feel about drinking/using drugs now?

_____ Do you ever miss drinking/taking drugs? What do you do when you feel this way?

_____ Ask the patient to describe his/her understanding of the risk of relapse.

_____ Correct misunderstandings.

_____ Provide valid factual information about the risk of relapse.

Assess refusal skills:

_____ Since treatment, have you been tempted to drink/use drugs? What were the circumstances? What made you decide not to drink/use drugs?

_____ What would you do when/if someone offers you a drink/drugs?

_____ When was the last time you took a drink/used drugs? What were the circumstances? What could you have done differently that would have stopped you?

_____ "Slips" = Opportunities to learn (Use "slips" as an opportunity to learn new skills and to learn more about high risk situations.)

_____ "Slips" = Failure (Avoid viewing slips as indicative of failure.)

_____ Reinforce existing strategies. Help the patient to identify his/her own strategies and suggest new strategies for avoiding high risk situations in which the patient may relapse.

_____ Identify social supports and stress their usefulness.

_____ Provide a realistic appraisal of the risk of relapse emphasizing the need for continued self-monitoring and follow-up.

_____ Make a follow-up appointment or referral if necessary.

Figure 3 *Continued*

A. Presenting the Diagnosis and Initiating Treatment Role Play Materials*

The role play cases documented on the following pages are a continuation of four role play cases in the Assessment and Diagnosis module. If you have recently presented Assessment and Diagnosis, participants will be familiar with many aspects of these cases and be able to discuss them in greater detail.

The Presenting the Diagnosis and Initiating Treatment role plays given here are intended to provide an opportunity for session participants to practice skills on the related Skill Checklist. Four cases from Assessment and Diagnosis are provided illustrating different levels of problem severity. Sample problems associated with use of three different substances (alcohol, cocaine and marijuana) are also illustrated in these cases. (For further issues regarding these cases, please see the Assessment and Diagnosis module).

Each set of role play materials include two elements:

1. Patient Information: This information is intended for use by the person playing the patient. It provides relevant background information, which may or may not come up in the interview but is nevertheless important in describing the patient, his/her psychosocial background and related family issues. Also provided are instructions on how to react to the diagnosis of substance abuse and conditions under which the patient will accept treatment.

   The individual playing the patient should be encouraged to improvise responses consistent with the Patient Information whenever additional information is requested in the interview.

2. Physician Fact Sheet: This sheet details all of the information already known to the physician about each case prior to the interview. It is intended to provide relevant background information and to set the stage for the interview. This sheet should be given as preparation for the role play physician prior to the role play. Copies may be distributed to role play observers as well.

B. Using Role Play Materials

Role play cases may be performed by session leaders to model interviewing skills. Session participants may use the role plays for practicing interviewing skills or as simulated patient cases. When performing role plays in a teaching session, we recommend the process outlined below:

1. Select individuals to play the physician and patient roles. Give a copy of the Patient Information sheet to the role play "patient." Give a copy of the Physician Fact Sheet to the role play "physician" and to all observers. Allow a few minutes for preparation.
2. Review the Physician Fact Sheet with all participants.
3. Discuss the details of the case as they relate to Presenting the Diagnosis and Initiating Treatment:
   What important data from the history and physical exam would be helpful in explaining the diagnosis to the patient?
   a. What substances are currently being used in a problematic way?
   b. What specific signs and symptoms are associated with substance use?
   c. What are the risk factors associated with the possibility of future problems?
   d. What are the possible complications of future use?

---

*From Cyr, M.G. (1989). Presenting the diagnosis and initiating treatment, *Project ADEPT Curriculum for Primary Care Physician Training*, Vol. I, Brown University, Providence, Rhode Island, pp. 42–44.

What treatment options are appropriate for this patient?
What the goals of the interview?

4.   Distribute copies of the Skill Checklist to all participants. Review key points on the Skill Checklist, and inform all observers to listen for and make note of skills used.

5.   Start the role play. (NOTE: Both the "physician" and the "patient" may elect to keep their respective handouts during the role play should they need to refer to them.)

6.   Once the role play is complete, review the Skill Checklist. First, ask the role play physician to give an overall impression of the interview and then to assess his/her own skills using the Skill Checklist. Next, ask the role play patient to give his/her impression of the interview. Finally, ask for feedback from the group and provide feedback yourself on the effectiveness of skills used.

7.   Use selected discussion questions. (Depending on the group you are teaching, you may pose selected discussion questions, or draw discussion points from the group. Either way, discussion questions provide some direction regarding potential issues surrounding the case.)

Patient Information—Role Play: Tom S.*

Age:	45
Reason for Visit:	Low back pain; Needs disability form filled out
Health Concern:	No other health concerns
Past Medical History:	Has been in excellent health; has not seen doctor in "a long time" except for treatment of several minor injuries at work over the past 2 yrs. (twisted ankle, bruises from 2 separate falls, cuts, etc.)
Cigarettes:	1 pack per day
Alcohol:	2–9 beers on most days. Has been drinking in this way "as long as I can remember." Started drinking at age 16.
Drugs:	None. Takes no prescription or nonprescription drugs.
CAGE:	Never tried to *cut down*.
	Occasionally gets *annoyed* at his wife's criticism of his going out with the boys after work. She "nags" him about driving home drunk when he feels he can "drive just fine" never having had an accident.
	Denies any *guilt* or ever having an *eye-opener*.
Family:	Wife works as a nurse's aid, part time in the evenings. His drinking has been a source of arguments for them. They have one grown son (25 yrs.).
Parents:	Father drank heavily all of his life and died at 74 of renal failure. Mother never drank at all. She is living at age 72, but suffers from adult-onset diabetes and a "heart condition."
Friends:	Most are heavy drinkers
Occupation:	Construction worker

You have scheduled this appointment with your new physician in order to have your disability form filled out. (You are unable to work because of your back pain.) You are not taking any medication for your back, and request Darvon® because you've heard that it helps. You do not believe that your drinking is a problem, and will discuss it openly.

Reaction to Diagnosis:	You are surprised to hear that your drinking may be a problem. However, when medical evidence is provided, you begin to realize that perhaps you should drink less. You agree that you should try to quit smoking.

---

*From Cyr, M.G. (1989). Presenting the diagnosis and initiating treatment, *Project ADEPT Curriculum for Primary Care Physician training*, Vol. I, Brown University, Providence, Rhode Island, pp. 45–47.

Treatment: You do not believe you need treatment. Will agree to a trial of controlled drinking and a follow-up visit. You will "think about" the possibility of attending AA in the future. You will try to cut back on your smoking but refuse a referral.

Physician Fact Sheet—Role Play: Tom S.

Age:	45
Reason for Visit:	Low back pain; Needs disability form filled out
Health Concern:	No other health concerns
Past Medical History:	Has been in excellent health; has not seen doctor in "a long time" except for treatment of several minor injuries at work over the past 2 yrs. (twisted ankle, bruises from 2 separate falls, cuts, etc.)
Cigarettes:	1 pack per day
Alcohol:	2–9 beers on most days. Has been drinking in this way "as long as I can remember." Started drinking at age 16.
Drugs:	None. Takes no prescription or nonprescription drugs.
CAGE:	Never tried to *cut down*.
	Occasionally gets *annoyed* at his wife's criticism of his going out with the boys after work. She "nags" him about driving home drunk when he feels he can "drive just fine" never having had an accident.
	Denies any *guilt* or ever having an *eye-opener*.
Family:	Wife works as a nurse's aid, part time in the evenings. His drinking has been a source of arguments for them. They have one grown son (25 yrs.).
Parents:	Father drank heavily all of his life and died at 74 of renal failure. Mother never drank at all. She is living at age 72, but suffers from adult-onset diabetes and a "heart condition."
Friends:	Most are heavy drinkers
Occupation:	Construction worker

He has requested that you complete a disability form for work. (He is unable to work because of back pain.) He has requested Darvon® for his back pain.

Physical Exam Results:

Robust, tanned man in no acute distress

BP	150/90
HR	88 reg
Skin	no changes
lungs	clear
heart	normal
abdomen	slightly obese, no hepatomegaly
neuro	normal

Normal physical except for paraspinal muscle tenderness and straight leg raising which is limited by back pain.

Laboratory Results:

CBC	MCV elevated
SGOT/SGPT	Normal
GGT	2x normal
Bili	Normal
alk phos	Normal

LDH	Normal
Uric acid	Elevated
BAL	0

This is Mr. S.'s first visit to your office. You have collected the above data. Based on this data, present your diagnosis concerning his substance use. Negotiate a treatment plan. This interview should take about 15 minutes.

Patient Information—Role Play: Karen S.*

Age:	28
Reason for Visit:	Recurrent sore throats
Health Concern:	Wants to make sure she doesn't have an infected throat. Requests a throat culture.
Past Medical History:	No serious past medical problems
Cigarettes:	None
Alcohol:	None
Drugs:	Admits to smoking marijuana daily (first joint shortly after wakening and several joints before work at night)
CAGE:	CAGE questions are all negative for alcohol.
	Has never really thought about *cutting down* on marijuana use since she is convinced that smoking it isn't the least bit harmful.
	Her parents frequently criticize her behavior and she gets *annoyed* because they are so "straight."
	She has never felt particularly *guilty* about her smoking.
	She has an *eye opener* (marijuana first thing in the morning) nearly every day.
Family:	Unmarried; in a long-term relationship with a man she met in college; no children; one older brother (30), an engineer.
Parents:	Both parents are in their 50's, light social drinkers and in good health
Friends:	Most friends smoke marijuana, especially at social gatherings
Occupation:	Although trained as an elementary school teacher, she works as a waitress with no plans to pursue teaching
Hobbies, etc:	When asked about hobbies and interests, she is very evasive and states that she "likes to get together with friends"

This is your first visit with the doctor. You didn't have a physician, and obtained this doctor's name from a friend. You have been having sore throats on and off for the past several weeks and would like a throat culture.

Reaction to Diagnosis:	You are defensive about your marijuana use and don't believe that it in any way effects your health. With specific evidence of health effects from your physician, however, you will concede that excessive marijuana use might be harmful.
Treatment:	Refuses treatment. Refuses referral to counselling. Will agree to try to cut down on marijuana use, but "won't make any promises." Agrees to a follow-up visit.

---

*From Cyr, M.G. (1989). Presenting the diagnosis and initiating treatment, *Project ADEPT Curriculum for Primary Care Physician Training*, Brown Universiy, Providence, Rhode Island, pp. 54–56.

Physician Fact Sheet—Role Play: Karen S.

During the routine history, you discovered the following information:

Age:	28
Reason for Visit:	Recurrent sore throats
Health Concern:	Wants to make sure she doesn't have an infected throat. Requests a throat culture.
Past Medical History:	No serious past medical problems
Cigarettes:	None
Alcohol:	None
Drugs:	Admits to smoking marijuana daily (first joint shortly after wakening and several joints before work at night)
CAGE:	CAGE questions are all negative for alcohol.
	Has never really thought about *cutting down* on marijuana use since she is convinced that smoking it isn't the least bit harmful.
	Her parents frequently criticize her behavior and she gets *annoyed* because they are so "straight."
	She has never felt particularly *guilty* about her smoking.
	She has an *eye opener* (marijuana first thing in the morning) nearly every day.
Family:	Unmarried; in a long-term relationship with a man she met in college; no children; one older brother (30), an engineer.
Parents:	Both parents are in their 50's, light social drinkers and in good health
Friends:	Most friends smoke marijuana, especially at social gatherings
Occupation:	Although trained as an elementary school teacher, she works as a waitress with no plans to pursue teaching
Hobbies, etc:	When asked about hobbies and interests, she is very evasive and states that she "likes to get together with friends"

Ms. S is a new patient who has made an appointment with you because she has been experiencing recurrent sore throats over the past several weeks. She has requested a throat culture.

Physical Exam Results:

Normal except for:
   erythema of the posterior pharynx
   lungs ronchi, clear with cough

Laboratory Results:

CBC   normal

This is the first time you've seen Ms. S. She didn't have a physician and obtained your name from a friend. You have collected the above data. Based on this data, present your diagnosis concerning her substance use. Negotiate a treatment plan.

This interview should take around 15 minutes.

ACKNOWLEDGMENTS

To the working committee of faculty at Brown University who created the Project ADEPT curriculum, and especially to Drs. Catherine Dubé and Michael Goldstein who guided the process.

REFERENCES

1. Rosenblatt, R.A. (1988). Current successes in medical education beyond the bedside. *J. Gen. Intern. Med., 3*:S44–S61.
2. Schroeder, S.A. (1988). Expanding the site of clinical education: Moving beyond the hospital walls. *J. Gen. Intern. Med., 3*:S5–S14.
3. Skeff, K.M. (1988). Enhancing teaching effectiveness and vitality in the ambulatory setting. *J. Gen. Intern. Med., 3*:S26–S33.
4. Skeff, K.M. (1988). An educational framework for the Analysis of teaching, *Subst. Abuse, 9*:61–75.
5. Clark, W.D. (1981). Alcoholism: Blocks to diagnosis and treatment. *Am. J. Med., 71*:275–286.
6. Chappel, J.N., Jordan, R., and Treadway, B. (1977). Substance abuse attitude changes in medical students. *Am. J. Psychiatry, 134*:379–384.
7. Chappel, J.N., Veach, T.L., Krug, R.S. (1985). The Substance Abuse Attitude Survey: An instrument for measuring attitudes. *J. Stud. Alcohol, 46*:48–52.
8. Kinney, J., Bergen, B.J., and Price, T.R.P. (1982). Perspective on medical students' percepton of alcoholics and alcoholism. *J. Stud. Alcohol, 43*:488–496.
9. Cotter, F., and Callahan, C. (1987). Training primary care physicians to identify and treat substance abuse. *Alcohol Health Res. World., 11*(4):70–73.
10. Kamerow, D.B., Pincus, H.A., and Macdonald, D.I. (1986). Alcohol abuse, drug abuse, and other mental health disorders in medical practice. *J.A.M.A., 255*:4–7.
11. Bowen, O.R., and Sammons, J.H. (1988). The alcohol-abusing patient: A challenge to the profession (commentary). *J.A.M.A., 260*(15):2267–2270.
12. Lewis, D.C. (1989). Putting training about alcohol and other drugs into the mainstream of medical education, *Alcohol Health Res. World, 13*(1):8–13.
13. Lewis, D.C. (1986). Medical education in alcohol and drug abuse. *Sub. Abuse, 7*:7–14.
14. Ross, R.S., Heyssel, R.M., and Stokes, E.J. (1986). An approach to education about alcohol. *Sub. Abuse, 7*:18–22.
15. Moore, R.D., Bone, L.R., Geller, G., Mamon, J.A., Stokes, E.J., and Levine, D.M. (1989). Prevalence, detection, and treatment of alcoholism in hospitalized patients. *J.A.M.A., 261*(3):403–407.
16. Lewis, D.C., and Gordon, A.J. (1983). Alcoholism and the general hospital: The Roger Williams Intervention Program. *Bull. N.Y. Acad. Med., 59*(2):181–197.
17. Williams, C.N., and Lewis, D.C. (1985). Overcoming barriers to identification and referral of alcoholics in a general hospital setting: One approach, *R.I. Med. J., 68*:131–138.
18. Lewis, D.C. (1989). The need for alcohol intervention programs in general hospitals, *Trustee, 42*(6):8–27.
19. National Institute of Alcohol Abuse and Alcoholism (1985). *Consensus Statements from the Conference on Alcohol, Drugs and Primary Care Physician Education: Issues, Roles, Responsibilities*, November 12–15, 1985, Rancho Mirage, California. U.S. Department of Health and Human Services, Rockville, Maryland.
20. Bigby, J., and Englund, S. (1986). *Identification and Assessment of Alcohol and Drug Abuse Medical Education Products/Approaches in General Internal Medicine* (ADM 281-85-0013). National Institute of Alcohol Abuse and Alcoholism, Rockville, Maryland.
21. Society for Teachers of Family Medicine (1986). *Identification and Assessment of Alcohol and Drug Abuse Medical Education Products/Approaches in Family Medicine* (ADM 281-85-0012). National Institute of Alcohol Abuse and Alcoholism, Rockville, Maryland.
22. American College of Obstetricians and Gynecologists (1987). *Identification and Assessment of Alcohol and Drug Medical Education Products/Approaches in Obstetrics and Gynecology* (ADM 281-86-007). National Institute of Alcohol Abuse and Alcoholism, Rockville, Maryland.
23. Ambulatory Pediatric Association (1986). *Identification and Assessment of Alcohol/Drug Medical Education Products/Approaches in Pediatrics* (ADM 281-85-0014). National Institute of Alcohol Abuse and Alcoholism, Rockville, Maryland.
24. American Psychiatric Association (1986). *Minimum Knowledge and Skill Levels of Alcohol and*

Drug Use Curricula in Psychiatry (ADM 281-0011). National Institute of Alcohol Abuse and Alcoholism, Rockville, Maryland.

25. Goldstein, M.G. (1988). A faculty development model for a curriculum in alcohol and substance abuse. *Subst. Abuse, 9*:119–128.

26. Dubé, C.E., Goldstein, M.G., Lewis, D.C., Cyr, M.G., and Zwick, W.R. (1989). Project ADEPT: The development process for a competency-based alcohol and drug curriculum for primary care physicians, *Subst. Abuse, 10*(1):5–15.

27. Dubé, C.E., Goldstein, M.G., Lewis, D.C., Myers, E.R., and Zwick, W.R. (eds.) (1989). Project ADEPT, Curriculum for primary care physician training, *Core Modules*, Vol. I, Brown University Center for Alcohol and Addiction Studies, Providence, Rhode Island (300 pp. and videotape).

28. Dubé, C.E., Goldstein, M.G., Lewis, D.C., Myers, E.R., and Zwick, W.R. (eds.) (1980). Project ADEPT, Curriculum for primary care physician training, *Core Modules*, Vol. II, Brown University Center for Alcohol and Addiction Studies, Providence, Rhode Island (306 pp. and videotape).

29. Lewis, D.C. (1989). Educating physicians to help patients who have alcohol and other drug problems, *Natl. AHEC Bull., 7*:2.

30. Stillman, P.L., Swanson, D.B., Smee, S., Stillman, A.E., Ebert, T.H., Emmel, V.S., Caslowitz, J., Greene, H.L., Hamolsky, M. Hatem, C., Levenson, D.J., Levin, R., Levinson, G., Ley, B., Morgan, G.J., Parrino, T., Robinson, S., and Willms, J. (1986). Assessing clinical skills of residents with standardized patients. *Ann. Intern. Med., 105*:762–771.

31. Felch, W.C. (1987). Continuing medical education in the United States: An enterprise in transition. *J.A.M.A., 258*(10):1355–1357.

32. Lawrence, R.S. (1988). The goals for medical education in the ambulatory setting. *J. Gen. Intern. Med. 3*:S15–S25.

33. Manning, P.R., and Petit, D.W. (1987). The past, present, and future of continuing medical education: Achievements and opportunities, computers and recertification. *J.A.M.A., 258*(24):3542–3546.

34. Miller, G.E. (1987). Continuing education: What it is and what it is not (special communication). *J.A.M.A., 258*(10):1352–1354.

35. Herrington, R.E., Benzer, D.G., Jacobson, G.R., and Hawkins, M.K. (1982). Treating substance-use disorders among physicians, *J.A.M.A., 247*:2253–2257.

36. Marchand, W.R., Palmer, C.A., Gutmann, L., and Brogan, W.C., III (1985). Medical student impairment: a review of the literature, *West Va. Med. J., 81*:244–248.

37. Morse, R.M., Martin, M.A., Swenson, W.M., and Niven, R.G. (1984). Prognosis of physicians treated for alcoholism and drug dependence, *J.A.M.A., 251*:743–746.

38. Kory, W.F., and Crandall, L.A. (1984). Nonmedical drug use patterns among medical students. *Int. J. Addict., 19*:871–884.

39. McAuliffe, W.E., Wechsler, H., and Rohman, M. (1984). Psychoactive drug use by young and future physicians. *J. Health Soc. Behav., 25*:34–54.

40. Maddux, J.F., Hoppe, S.K., and Costello, R.M. (1986). Psychoactive substance abuse among medical students. *Am. J. Psychiatry, 143*:187–²191.

41. McAuliffe, W.E., Rohman, M., and Santangelo, S. (1986). Psychoactive drug use among practicing physicians and medical students. *New Engl. J. Med., 315*:805–810.

42. Westermeyer, J. (1988). Substance abuse among medical trainees: Current problems and evolving resources. *Am. J. Drug Alcohol Abuse, 14*:393–404.

43. Conrad, C., Hughes, P., and Baldwin, D.C. (1988). Substance use by fourth-year students at 13 medical schools. *J. Med. Ed., 63*:747–758.

44. Clark, D.C., Gibbons, R.D., and Daugherty, S.R. (1987). Model for quantifying and drug involvement of medical students. *Int. J. Addict., 22*:249–271.

45. Kyriazi, N.C., Schwartz, R.H., Lewis, D.C., and Hoffman, N.G. (1988). Attitudes toward drug use vs. drug use patterns of medical students prior to medical school, *Subst. Abuse, 9*:189–193.

46. Schwartz, R.H., Lewis, D.C., Hoffmann, N.G, and Kyriazi, N. (1990). Drug-use Patterns by Medical Students Before and During Medical School, *Arch. Intern. Med., 150*:883–886.

47. Brewster, J.M. (1986). Prevalence of alcohol and other drug problems among physicians, *J.A.M.A., 255*:1913–1920.

48. DATAGRAM (1984). Substance abuse policies and programs at U.S. medical schools. *J. Med. Ed.*, *63*:759–761.
49. Borenstein, D.B., Cook, K. (1982). Impairment prevention in the training years: A new mental health program at UCLA, *J.A.M.A.*, *247*:2700–2703.
50. Rueben, D.B., Novack, D.H., Wachtel, T.J., and Wartman, S.A. (1984). A comprehensive support system for reducing house staff stress, *Psychosomatics*, *25*:815–820.
51. Siegel, B., and Donnelly, J. (1978). Enriching personal and professional development: The experience of a support group for interns, *J. Med. Educ.*, *53*:908–914.
52. McCrady, B.S. (1989). The distresses or impaired professional: From retribution to rehabilitation, *J. Drug Iss.*, *19*:337–349.
53. Pittman, J.A., and Scott, C.W. (1988). University of Alabama School of Medicine policy on impaired students and faculty with special reference to substance abuse, *Ala. J. Med. Sci.*, *25*:84–90.
54. Vaillant, G.E., Sobowale, N.D., and McArthur, C. (1972). Some psychologic vulnerabilities of physicians, *N. Eng. J. Med.*, *287*:372–375.
55. McCue, J.D. (1982). The effects of stress on physicians and their medical practice, *N. Engl. J. Med.*, *306*:458–463.
56. McCue, J. (1985). The distress of internship: Causes and prevention, *N. Engl. J. Med.*, *312*:449–452.
57. Lewis, D.C. (1986). Doctors and drugs. *New. Engl. J. Med.*, *315*:826–828.
58. Lewis, D.C., Niven, R.G., Czechowicz, D., and Trumble, J.G. (1987). A review of medical education in alcohol and other drug abuse. *J.A.M.A.*, *257*:2945–2948.
59. Lewis, D.C. (1990). Medical Education for Alcohol and other Drug Abuse in the United States, *Can. Med. Assoc. J.*, *143*:1091–1096.

XII

Laboratory Testing for Drugs

44

Laboratory Methodology for Drug and Alcohol Addiction

Karl Verebey
Bureau of Laboratories, New York City Department of Health, New York, New York

I. INTRODUCTION

Drug abuse and addiction is characterized by compulsive drug-seeking behavior with paroxysmal breaks in use and almost certain relapses. A common feature of all drug and alcohol abusers is denial. The patient lies to himself or herself, and to the forbidding outside world to protect the continuity of his obsessive addiction to drugs and/or alcohol. For this reason, physicians dealing with drug and alcohol addicts are seldom, if ever, given voluntarily the diagnostically important information about the patient's addictive habits.

The drug addiction pattern is an important part of the medical history. The attending physician cannot properly design treatment when kept in the dark about the patient's addiction. Depending on the drugs used, symptoms of physical and/or psychiatric illness may be simulated by the presence or the absence of the particular drug(s). The dichotomy of symptoms associated with drug presence or absence is best illustrated with the opioid class of drugs.

While under the influence of an opioid substance, the addict experiences euphoric, anxiolytic sedation, mental clouding, sweating, and constipation. In the absence of the opioid, common withdrawal signs and symptoms appear, characterized by pupillary mydriasis, agitation, anxiety, panic, muscle aches, gooseflesh, rhinorrhea, salivation, and diarrhea [1]. The two different sets of diagnostic symptoms result from the abuse of the same drug, observed at different times, in the presence and absence of an opiod.

Behavior similar or identical to textbook description of psychosis can be induced in predisposed individuals by drugs. For example, phencyclidine (PCP), amphetamines, or cocaine can cause toxic psychosis indistinguishable from paranoid schizophrenia. While drug-induced model psychosis can be produced in anyone given the adequate dose of lysergic acid diethylamide (LSD), PCP, amphetamine, and cocaine. Drug-induced psychosis has a different prognosis and must be treated differently than psychosis related to endogenous organic, anatomical, or neurochemical disorders [2].

Treatment of identified drug abusers would be extremely handicapped if drug abuse testing was not utilized. Therefore, comprehensive drug testing is important for psychiatrists in making precise follow-up evaluations and appropriate treatment of their patients. Thus, the first good reason for laboratory drug testing is to identify objectively drug abusers and the substance they are abusing.

Testing is of great value also after drug addicts are identified. Current treatment strategies are intimately tied to frequently scheduled urinalysis to monitor recovering addicts. Negative results support the success of treatment, whereas positive test results alert the treating physician of relapse. This is the rationale for objective testing as a necessary component of modern treatment of ex–drug addicts.[3]

Public safety may be endangered by intoxicated individuals. Workers in certain fields should not be influenced by psychoactive drugs, especially drugs that cause delusions and impulsive risk-taking behavior. Drug addiction has been identified among, e.g., doctors, nurses, airline pilots, bus drivers, train conductors and engineers, as well as police officers. Drug abuse testing is advantageous to both the drug abuser and his or her environment (relatives and the general public). The abuser gets early identification, early treatment and a chance for early rehabilitation, and the public is saved from the potential dangers of addicts while under the influence of drugs.

Success of compulsory drug abuse testing by decreasing drug abuse has been clearly demonstrated in the military. Prior to testing in 1981, 48% of servicemen used illegal drugs. After 3 years of testing, less than 5% of drug abusers remained in the military [4]. Although critics often attack testing as ineffective, where serious drug testing is in place, the results are clearly decreased drug abuse. Clinically, when relapse is identified by drug testing, early intervention in treatment is implemented.

II. TESTS AVAILABLE

The complexity surrounding drug abuse testing is a result of large numbers of variables. Identification of each individual drug is unique. Detectability depends on the type of drug, size of the dose, frequency of use, the route of administration, the differences in individual drug metabolism and disposition kinetics, the sample collection time, and the sensitivity of the analytical method used to test the sample. All these variables make each test request an individual case, and general rules for all drugs and all situations can not be defined.

Modern analytical toxicology deals with the detection and quantitation of minute amounts of drugs or alcohol in body fluids. This branch of science has grown and expanded in the last few decades after the recognition of widespread drug abuse and addiction in the United States. Qualified drug abuse testing laboratories are now easily accessible to physicians, providing qualitative and quantitative urinalysis results. Laboratory accreditations must be checked by the physicians before ordering tests because poor-quality laboratories still exist. This chapter examines the clinical utility of drug abuse testing.

III. ALCOHOL DISPOSITION AND METHODS OF MEASUREMENTS

Alcohol abuse is a legal version of drug abuse in the United States and most of the world. The addictive chemical substance in all alcoholic beverages is ethanol or ethyl alcohol. Ethanol is present at 3–6% in beer, at 11–13% in wine, and at 22–60% in distilled beverages. Owing to its water solubility, ethanol, after ingestion, is distributed evenly into total body water. Thus, if the amount of ethanol intake and the subject's weight and sex are known, a reasonably accurate estimation of peak blood ethanol level can be calculated. For example, approximately 6×12 oz of beer will result in a 150 mg% blood ethanol level in a 170-lb subject. These calculations are also effected by the adipose tissue mass, hydration, and the state of the stomach as being full or empty. Ethanol is one of the few drugs for which good correlation exists between blood level and central nervous system (CNS) intoxicating effects. However, individual differences in alcohol tolerance do exist, which are inherited and/or induced by chronic sizable alcohol intake. The current legal limit of ethanol concentration in most states for driving is 100 mg/100 ml of blood or 100 mg%. This value is a reasonable reference cut-off point for identifying one fit to drive or being under the influence of alcohol. Although some studies claim significant intoxicating effects in driving skills in driving simulators already at 50 mg% ethanol levels [5].

Ethanol elimination from the body is a linear or zero-order process down to about 20 mg%, at which point it becomes first-order elimination, which is concentration dependent. The average rate of elimination is about 18–20 mg%/h. This value is dependent on the body weight of the subject; larger amounts of ethanol, being eliminated by heavier individuals. Thus, on the average, an intoxicated subject with an ethanol level of 170 mg% must not drive for 4 h before his or her blood ethanol level dips below the legal limit to about 90 mg% (170 mg% − [4 × 20mg%] = 90 mg% [6].

IV. METHODS OF ANALYSIS

Ethanol is analyzed by various methods: enzyme immunoassays, chemical assays, and gas-liquid chromatographic (GC) methods. [7]. The most specific quantitative method is headspace GC. Volatile substances, such as ethanol, are driven out of the aqueous biofluids by heat incubation. Air samples are taken from the sealed test tubes by an airtight syringe and injected into a gas chromatograph for separation and quantitation. This method separates ethanol from other alcohols and possible interferring substances.

If ethanol analysis is performed by a breathalyzer or one of the immunoassays, the results are mostly reliable, but in forensic cases they should be confirmed by GC. Blood is the desired body fluid for ethanol analysis, although saliva and urine can also be used. Since distribution of ethanol is not equivalent in different body fluids, saliva and urine ethanol levels must be multiplied by correction factors to estimate equivalent blood ethanol concentrations.

Alcoholism, just as drug addiction, is hidden by denial. Therefore, when screening for drugs, ethanol analysis should also be ordered. Usually, ethanol measurements must be requested in addition to a drugs of abuse screening because alcohol is not performed routinely by most laboratories.

V. COMPREHENSIVE DRUG SCREEN

A number of different laboratory methods are available for comprehensive drug screening. When the drug-abuse habit of the patient is unknown, physicians request a comprehensive drug screen. Some laboratories usually perform the most inexpensive, insensitive thin-layer chromatography (TLC) test. Results are often negative owing to the low sensitivity of this screening procedure, not because the drug or its metabolite is not present in the sample. By comprehensive drug testing, different laboratories mean different methods of analysis for different sets of drugs, including or excluding alcohol [2]. The important message is that "comprehensive" does not mean "all" drugs and alcohol. If the physician is not familiar with the laboratory procedure for drug testing, he or she loses his or her effectiveness using the laboratory to its full potential.

Urine samples are mostly sent for comprehensive or routine drug screen analysis. Psychiatrists or other physicians assume that this test will detect all abused drugs. The problem is that TLC drug screen detects only high-level drug use of a select number of drugs.

This test is not sensitive enough to detect marijuana, phencyclidine (PCP), LSD, 3,4,methyl-enedioxymethamphetamine (MDA), 3,4-methylenedioxymethamphetamine (MDMA), mescalin and fentanyl, among others (Table 1). Thus, a negative drug screen does not mean that the patient has not used drugs. What it means is that there is no evidence of high-dose abuse of morphine, quinine (a diluent of heroin), methadone, codeine, dextromethorphan, propoxyphene, barbiturates, diphenylhydantoin phenothiazines, cocaine, amphetamines, or phenylpropanolamine. Low-dose drug abuse is not likely to be detected by TLC. Thus, false-negatives are very high for the routine TLC "drug screen" performed by many clinical laboratories. See Table 1 for the time frame of drug detectability by TLC when use is extensive and drugs are not detected by routine TLC.

Table 2 presents an overview of available tests. If for example, the physician suspects marijuana abuse, he must specifically request that a test for marijuana be performed, usually by enzyme immunoassay (EIA) or radioimmunoassay (RIA). In modern laboratories, screening for prescription drugs and drugs of abuse is performed by EIAs, such as the EMIT (enzyme multiplied immunoassay test), or RIA, TDX and ADX or fluorescent polarization immunoassay (FPIA), and a modern version of TLC, such as Toxi Lab, which has improved sensitivity over conventional TLC systems. In exceptional laboratories, drug screening is performed by capillary gas-liquid chromatography (GLC) equipped with a nitrogen phosphorus detector (NPD). In a single analysis, up to 25–40 compounds can be identified. An example is shown in Figure 1. This analytical system is advantageous when there is no clue to the identity of the abused or toxic substance in the sample. GLC-NPD is time consuming, labor intensive, and usually expensive. While the EMIT and RIA tests are significantly cheaper and more practical than the more specific gas chromatography (GC) and GC combined with mass spectrometry (GC/MS).

The EIA and FPIA have technical advantages over other screening techniques, in that no extraction of drugs or metabolites is required. Thus, EIA and FPIA procedures are easily adaptable for high-volume automated screening analysis of drugs. In fact, most good laboratories offer a five- or 10-drug panel with or without alcohol. These tests are usually

Table 1 Drugs Detected and Not Detected by TLC

Detected 24 h or longer after use
1. Amphetamine, methamphetamine, ephedrine, pseudophedrine, phenylpropanolamine, etc.
2. Benzodiazepines: chlordiazepoxide (Librium), Diazepam (Valium), flurazepam (Dalmane), etc.
3. Barbiturates: phenobarbital, secobarbital, pentobarbital, etc.
4. Methadone, propoxyphene.
5. Tricyclic antidepressants: imipramine, desipramine.
Detected for 3–12 h
1. Opiates
2. Cocaine (benzoylecgonine)
3. Pentazocine (Talwin)
Not Detected by TLC
1. Cannabinoids[a]
2. PCP
3. LSD, psylocybin, MDA, MDMA
4. Designer drugs: fentanyl derivatives

[a]Routine TLC does not detect THC. However, special TLC procedures have been developed with sensitivity in 10–20 nq/ml.
Source: Adapted from Ref. 7.

Table 2 Overview of Drug Testing Methods[a]

Screening	Confirmation)
I. TLC (A,D,E), GC (A,C,F), HPLC (A,C,F)	EIA, RIA, FPIA (B,C,E)
II. EIA, RIA, FPIA (B,C,E)	GC, HPLC, OR GC/MS (A,C,F)

Abbreviations: TLC, thin-layer chromatography; GC, gas-liquid chromatography; HPLC, high-pressure liquid chromatography; EIA, enzyme immunoassay; RIA, radioimmunoassay; FPIA, fluorescence polarization immunoassay; *A*, specific; *B*, nonspecific possible interference; *C*, sensitive (ng/ml range); *D*, insensitive (μg/ml range); *E*, inexpensive; *F*, expensive.
[a]Be certain to inquire at the laboratory for the method used and the list of drugs tested. Also, cutoffs are usually set artifically high. Clinically positives are samples with readings above the blank; ask the laboratory to report the presence of even threshold quantities of drugs.

performed by EIA. An example of drug selection of a 10-drug panel plus alcohol is presented in Table 3. Comparative senstivity ranges and cost per sample for the various analysis are shown in Table 4.

VI. ANALYTICAL METHODOLOGY

The choice of methods for the identification of drugs or their metabolites in body fluids depends on the patient's history, physical examination, past history, and available biological samples. Often there is some hint or knowledge about the type of substances used by the subject, which needs to be confirmed. These are the simplest situations for the laboratory because the analyst can compare the suspected drugs present in the sample with known standards by a specific method such as GC or EIA. The method of choice is determined by the knowledge or suspicion of the drug's identity. The biotransformation pathway and pharmacokinetic pattern of excretion influence the length of time the drug or its metabolite is detectable [8].

Most often, the laboratory receives no clue about the suspected substance(s). In this case, a broad-scope drug screening test is required. There are various types of drug screens available, with markedly different panels of drugs, sensitivity, specificity and cost. Analytical methods are described below with specific examples for specific needs.

VII. EXTRACTION

With the exception of some enzyme immunoassays, such as, EIA, FPIA, and RIA techniques, most methods require isolation of drugs from body fluids before they are subjected to instrumental analysis. Drug isolation is accomplished by extraction using appropriate organic solvents at specific hydrogen ion concentrations (or pH) at which drug molecules favor movement from aqueous biofluids into organic solvents. Basic drugs, such as morphine, methadone, and amphetamines are favorably extracted at alkaline pH, whereas acid drugs such as the barbiturates and phenytoin are more soluble in organic solvents at near neutral or slightly acid pH. There is an advantage to the analytical chemist when the abused substance is known; thus, the proper conditions can be selected for isolation. Samples containing unknown substances are extracted at acidic, basic, and neutral conditions hoping to create the most favorable pH for extraction into an organic solvent. Interference by unrelated molecules is minimized by preparing the cleanest possible extract. Biofluids are rank ordered from "clean" to "dirty": saliva, spinal fluid (CSF), serum, urine, and whole blood (hemolyzed). In other words, the least interference is found when using saliva and CSF, whereas urine and hemolyzed whole blood have more background materials. Depending on the distribution of the drug in the body, which in turn is dependent on the drug's physicochemical properties, one or

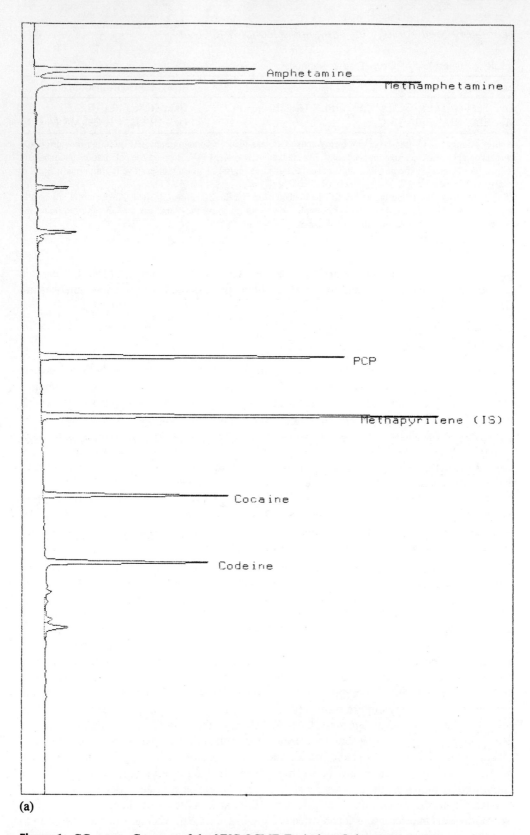

(a)

Figure 1 GC report: Courtesy of the NYC-OCME Toxicology Laboratory

814

```
FOR GC #1, TOM                                              Page  1
LOW TEMPERATURE PROGRAM
Sample Name   :                             Report No :1118.1
Instrument: A3        Calculation: InternalSTD   Quant: HeightUnits
Seq:                     Vial:    0      Result: /DATA/SPEC3008.RES
Run Time    :  18.00 Minutes   Injected on Thu Jan 18, 1990  3:25:09 pm
Run Status: RunStatusOK

Pk#     RT        Height  Code     MG/L       Name
  1    1.989      98980   VV     99107.19    Amphetamine
  2    2.269     161212   VV    161418.9     Methamphetamine
  3    4.636      14046   VB         .03
  4    5.615      16671   PV         .04
  5    8.361     129758   VV    129924.1     PCP
  6    9.666     168932   PV                 Methapyrilene (IS)
  7   11.408      79211   VV     79312.64    Cocaine
  8   12.880      70934   VV     71025.22    Codeine
  9   14.131       3315   VV         .01
 10   14.302       9795   VV         .02

Report Time  : Fri Jan 19, 1990  9:40:04 am

Method       : /DATA/TP3LOTEMP.MTH
Report File  : /DATA/OCME
```

(b)

Figure 1 *Continued*

another biofluid is better suited for analysis. As a rule, urine has 100–1000 times more drug and or metabolite in it than serum. Following extraction and "clean-up" of samples, the extracts are analyzed by various methods differing in sensitivity and specificity.

VIII. Thin-Layer Chromatography

Thin-layer chromatography (TLC) is a technique that is utilized to separate different molecules in a mixture based on their polarity and their chemical interaction with the developing solvents and the thin layer coating. A specific substance given the same physical and chemical conditions will always migrate the same distance from the origin where it is spotted. Thus, if cocaine is present in a mixture, a spot characterized by the cocaine standard will travel to

Table 3 10 Drugs and Alcohol Screen by EIA

Alcohol (ethanol)
Amphetamines (phenethylamines i.e., phenylpropanolamine, ephedrine)
Barbiturates (pento-, amo-, seco-, phenobarbital, etc.)
Benzodiazepines (including chlordiazepoxide (Librium), diazepam (Valium), flurazepam
  (Dalmane), oxazepam (Serax)
Cocaine and/or metabolite (benzoylecgonine)
Methaqualone (Quaalude)
Opiates [morphine, codeine, monoacetyl morphine (heroin metabolite) hydrocodone (Dilaudid) etc.]
Methadone
Phencyclidine (PCP)
Propoxyphene (Darvon)
Cannabinoids (THC metabolite)

Source: Adapted from Ref. 7.

Table 4 Method Sensitivity Ranges and Cost

Detection method	Sensitivity ranges (ng/ml)	Cost/sample range ($)
Chromatography		
TLC	1000–2000	5–10
GLC	10–300	40–50
HPLC	20–300	40–60
GC/MS	5–100	50–100
Immunological assays		
EMIT	20–1000	4–6
RIA	2–20	5–15

the same location on the TLC plate as the cocaine standard. Unfortunately similar molecules, interfering substances in an extract, and various drugs may also travel to approximately the same location. The location of the spot is identified by an Rf number, which is the ratio calculated from the distance traveled by the drug divided by the distance traveled by the solvent front from the origin, where the mixture was originally spotted. TLC is a qualitative method, and it is not very sensitive. Visualization of the spots on TLC is achieved by ultraviolet (UV) or fluorescence lights or by color reactions of the spots after spraying the plates with chemical dyes. Identical molecules are expected to migrate to the same Rf zone and give identical color reactions.

The traditional "toxicology screen" by TLC was primarily designed to detect high-dose and recent drug abuse or intake of toxic levels of drugs. Thin-layer chromatography is an ideal test for emergency room use for unknown drug identification. Drug concentrations in emergency room samples are expected to be high, quick determination of the toxic substance(s) is the primary task, and a single TLC run detects many substances. The TLC toxicology screen is not the method of choice owing to its low sensitivity for the differential diagnosis of drug-induced toxic psychosis, mimicking depression, mania, or schizophrenia. Nor is TLC well suited for the diagnosis of chronic low-dose use of illict drugs. It has been the method used in methadone programs for routine drug screens or tox screens. When TLC is used, false-negatives are the rule rather than the exception. Very often whether a sample is called positive instead of negative depends on the concentration of the drug in the sample and on the sensitivity of the assay. Thin-layer chromatography sensitvity for most drugs is in the low-microgram range (about 2 μg/ml); thus, a negative TLC urine may be positive by methods such as RIA, EIA, FPIA, AND GC/MS, which are sensitive in the low-nanogram range (about 50 ng/ml). Exceptions to insufficient TLC sensitivity are the new TLC methods, such as high-performance TLC (HPTLC), Toxi Lab, and bonded phase adsorption TLC (BPA-TLC). Some of these methods utilize larger volumes of urine (10–15 ml) and sensitive to about 20–100 ng/ml.

A positive TLC result should be confirmed by a scientifically different method, i.e., EIA. Although the color specificity and differential migration makes TLC reliable in the hands of experienced toxicologists, the boredom and labor-intensive nature of TLC makes experienced master-level TLC toxicologists hard to find. Remember that negative results by TLC screen are not always negative by other more sensitive analytical methods [9]. Table 4 shows some of the sensitivity ranges for commonly abused drugs detected by TLC and the more sensitive EIA, RIA, and GC/MS.

Most substances are detected by conventional TLC only when the level of drug in the urine is above 2 μg/ml. This makes cocaine, for example, very difficult to detect by routine

TLC, since the half-life of cocaine is only 1 h in man, the levels of cocaine in body fluids quickly diminish and less than 10% of the cocaine is excreted unchanged in the urine. Marijuana, PCP, LSD, and other important drugs of abuse are not detected at all in conventional TLC systems.

IX. ENZYME IMMUNOASSAY AND RADIOIMMUNOASSAY

The various immunoassays operate on the principle of antigen-antibody interactions. These techniques are commonly used to measure hormones, neurochemicals, and more recently drugs. Antibodies are produced against the drug or drug metabolite of interest by coupling them to large immunoactive molecules and injecting the heptane-bound drug into rabbits or sheep. The animals produce antibodies against the drug, which is used in immunoassays. Immunological methods used for drug detection utilize these antibodies to seek out the drug in unknown biofluids. In the unknown sample, competition exists for available antibody-binding sites between the tagged drug in the test reagent and drug in the unknown sample. The binding ratio determines the presence, absence, or quantity of specific drugs in the unknown sample.

The specificity and sensitivity of the antibodies to drugs are different by different drug assays and manufacturers. Immunoassay can be very specific; however, compounds structurally similar to the drug of interest (their metabolites) often cross react. Thus, in general, specificity of the immunoassays is considered far less than that of GC and GC/MS. Lack of specificity may be an advantage in some cases because interaction of the antibody with both drugs plus metabolites in a sample increases sensitivity in "total" detection of a drug class. In chromatography, single specific molecules are determined. Thus, by GC and GC/MS quantitatively less drug is detected then by immunoassays. For EIA, FPIA, and RIA the sensitivity ranges are between micrograms and picograms per millilter depending on the drug.

Enzyme immunoassay systems are very popular and are commonly used for drug abuse screening because no extraction or centrifugation is required, and the system lends itself to easy automation. Although an EIA screen is more costly than TLC, toxicological screens using EIA are much more sensitive for most drugs and are more likely to detect lower drug concentrations. The physicians or counsellor using EIA screening should inquire as to which drugs are on the screening panel and what are the cutoff values. Often the sensitivity can be lowered by request.

X. GAS CHROMATOGRAPHY AND GAS CHROMATOGRAPHY-MASS SPECTROMETRY

Gas chromatography (GC) is an analytical technique that separates molecules by similar principles as TLC except GC is more sensitive. The sensitivity of GC for most drugs is in the nanogram range, but with special detectors for some compounds, picogram levels can be measured. The TLC plate is replaced by glass or metal tubing (1–2 m long) packed with materials of particular polarity or flexible silica capillary columns 15–30 m long. After extraction and injection, the sample is vaporized by heat at the injection port and carried through the column by a steady flow of gas. The column terminates at a detector, which registers the response to the drugs, which is graphically recorded and quantitated. The response is proportional to the amount of substance present in the sample compared to a known standard. Identical compounds travel through the column at the same speed, since their interaction with the column packing is the same. The time from injection until a response at the recorder is observed, is referred to as the retention time; retention times are often printed above or next to the peaks. Figure 1 shows the capillary gas liquid chromatographic separation of amphetamine, methamphetamine, PCP, methapyrilene (internal standard), cocaine, and codeine. The line, or abcissa, represents time and the ordinate, or peak heights, the quantity of substance present. Identical retention times of substances, run on two different polarity columns, is strong evidence that the substances are identical.

Even stronger evidence than GC can be obtained by the use of GC/MS, which analyzes the drug's migration by GC and fragmentation pattern by a mass spectrometer. Since in various molecules not all bonds are of equal stength, the weak ones are more likely to break under stress. Bombardment of the molecules by an electron beam in the mass detector fragments molecules at the weak bonds. The exact mass of the unfragmented mass molecular ion and the fragments or breakage products is measured by the mass spectrometer. Figure 2 shows the fragmentation pattern of cocaine. The mass molecular ion of cocaine is 303 and two other identifier fragments are 182 and 82 molecular weight fragments. The three identifiers are in a reproducible ratio to one another compared to a known standard. Gas chromatography/ mass spectrometry is referred to as the most reliable, most definitive forensic quality procedure [10]. The breakage of molecules results in unique fragments in specific ratios to one another; thus, the GC/MS method is often called molecular fingerprinting.

The fragmentation pattern of unknowns are compared to standards and checked with a computer library. The library lists the mass molecular ion of the parent compounds, their fragments, and their relative ratios. A perfect match is considered absolute confirmation of a particular drug. The use of GC/MS has been out of the reach of most laboratories in the past because of high cost of equipment, high level of technical expertise needed for operation, and complex sample preparation. However, recent advances in computerization, automated sample preparation, and less expensive analytical technology are placing GC/MS

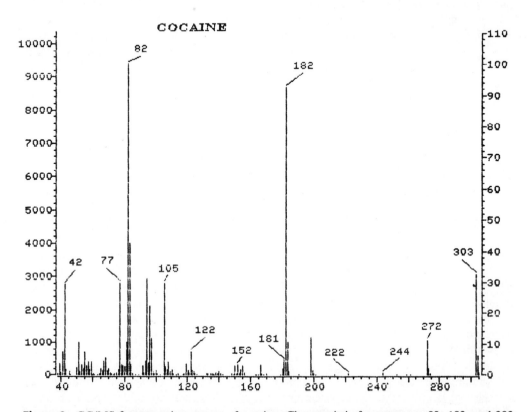

Figure 2 GC/MS fragmentation pattern of cocaine. Characteristic fragments are 82, 182, and 303.

capabilities now within the reach of clinical laboratories. It can also be used quantitatively, which sometimes provides additional information that may help to interpret a clinical syndrome or explain corroborating evidence in forensic cases. Although identification of compounds by GC/MS is considered absolute, this is only true when the instrument is operating in the scanning mode, looking at the full range of fragmentation. When the GC/MS is in the SIM (single ion monitoring) mode, some of the specificity of the MS technique is lost, yet sensitivity for quantitation is increased. The probability is practically impossible of finding interfering substances having the same molecular ions and fragmentation pattern as the drug of interest. Therefore, the chances for error by GC/MS is very little when the instrument is used in the scanning mode and ion ratios of the most characteristic fragments are calculated and compared to known controls.

Gas chromatography for most drugs is about 100–1000 times more sensitive than TLC. It is also more specific, especially when the unknown sample is analyzed on two different columns. Most commonly abused drugs are readily identified by both GC and GC/MS, (e.g., marijuana, cocaine, amphetamines, and opiates). It is also 100–1000 times more sensitive than conventional TLC systems, and when GC/MS is operated in the scanning mode, identification of drugs is considered absolute.

When a routine toxicological screen is ordered, it may be performed by the cheapest (TLC) technique. The physician is often not aware that there are options for more sensitive toxicological methods by either GC, GC/MS, or the practical EIA, FPIA, and RIA techniques. Table 5 shows a comparative sensitivity of the three major methods for a selected group of abused drugs.

XI. THE CHOICE OF BODY FLUIDS AND TIME OF SAMPLE COLLECTION

Some drugs are metabolized extensively and are very quickly excreted, whereas others stay in the body for an extended period of time. Thus, success of detection depends not only on the time of sample collection after the last drug use, but also on the particular drug used and whether the analysis is performed for the drug itself or for its metabolites. In Table 6, the expected time scale of detectability is shown for some commonly abused drugs. [11]

When drug abuse detection is the goal, the following questions should be asked: (1) How long does the particular drug stay in the body, or what is its half-life? (2) How extensively is the drug biotransformed? Thus, should one look for the drug itself or its metabolite(s)? (3) Which body fluid should be analyzed, or what is the major route of excretion? The

Table 5 Sensitivity of Urine Drug Testing Methods for Specific Drugs

Drugs	TLC (ng/ml)	EIA-RIA TDX-EMIT (ng/ml)	GC GC/MS
Amphetamines	2,000	300	25
Barbiturates	2,000	300	50
Benzodiazepines	—	1,000	50
(cocaine) BE	2,000	75–300	20
Marijuana/THC	20	20–100	10
(opiates) (Morphine)	2,000	300	20
PCP	—	25–75	10

[a]Special procedure BPA/TLC not detected by routine TLC.

Table 6 Detectability of Drug Use

Drugs		Half-life (h)	Cutoff (ng/ml)		Detection after Last Use (Days)
			EIA	GC/MS	
Amphetamines		10–15	300	100	1–2
Barbiturates	Short	20–30	300	100	3–5
	Long	48–96	—	—	10–14
Benzodiazepines	Diaz.	20–35	300	—	2–4
	Nordiaz.	50–90	300	100	7–9
Cocaine	C	0.8–1.5	—	—	0.2–0.5
(metabolite)	BE	—	300	50	2–4
Methaqualone		20–60	300	50	7–14
Opiates (codeine, morphine)		2–4	300	100	1–2
Phencyclidine (PCP)		7–16	75	10	2–8
Cannabinoids (THCA)		10–40	20–100	10	Acute 2–8 Chronic 14–42

importance of asking these questions is illustrated by cocaine and methaqualone (Quaalude), which are biotransformed with significant differences.

Cocaine has a half-life of about 1 h in humans. It is rapidly biotransformed into inactive metabolites of benzoylecgonine and ecgoninemethyl ester. Less that 10% of unchanged cocaine and more than 45% of benzoylecgonine is excreted into the urine. Unchanged cocaine is detectable in urine only from 0 to 12 h after use. What does all this suggest to the clinician who wants to know whether or not the patient is taking cocaine? The short half-life indicates that unless use is suspected within hours or the patient is suspected of being under the influence of cocaine, the parent compound is not likely to be found in detectable concentrations in either blood or urine. However, a blood test that includes cocaine and the cocaine metabolite may be reliable for many hours after use to document recent exposure to cocaine. Plasma enzymes continue to metabolize cocaine even after the blood is taken from the body. Therefore, blood samples should be collected into sodium flouride–containing tubes, which inactivates these enzymes (12).

Benzoylecgonine is the major metabolite of cocaine, its half-life is about 6 h and it is excreted in urine at levels of approximately 45% of the dose. It is clear that detection is best accomplished by collecting urine and analyzing it for benzoylecgonine. It has been observed that of those subjects who had enough benzoylecgonine in their urine to be detected, only 2% had enough cocaine present for detection. Thus, 98% of the subjects who were tested for cocaine alone would have been found negative if they were specifically tested for cocaine instead of benzoylecgonine.

A contrasting example is methaqualone (Quaalude). This substance is like cocaine in that it is extremely lipid soluble, but it has a half-life of 20–60 h. Because methaqualone is not biotransformed rapidly, either blood or urine tests are effective for detection of the parent compound itself. Studies showed detection of methaqualone for 21 days in the urine after a single 300-mg oral dose, and in blood for 7 days [13]. Similarly, marijuana metabolites stay very long in the body. Reports indicate that a carboxylic acid metabolite of THC was detectable in a chronic marijuana user's urine 5 weeks after discontinuing marijuana (14). Thus, pharmacokinetic and excretion information are important in deciding what chemical to look for and in which body fluid it is likely to be found.

Which biofluid is best for drug detection analysis? As a rule urine has about 1000 times more drug present in it than serum or plasma. On the other hand, it is often much easier to prepare cleaner extracts from serum than from urine. A cleaner extract greatly reduces background interference, and makes it easier for the chromatographer to interpret and confirm results. Background interference is less important in the immunoassays where no extraction is needed.

Many physicians prefer blood for a drug screen rather than urine because they believe that a drug found in blood is stronger evidence of recent use and better related to brain levels and drug-related behavior than urine drug levels. For example, amphetamine blood levels are directly related to the emergence and persistence of amphetamine-induced psychoses or withdrawal-induced paranoia. Since urine is an ultrafiltrate of plasma, it is also sufficiently accurate for drug and metabolite determination as proof of drug use. However, the collection of urine specimens must be supervised in order to ensure that the person in question is the source of the sample and to guarantee the integrity of the specimen. It is not unusual to receive someone else's urine or highly diluted urine samples when collection of the samples is not supervised or screened by the laboratory for pH, specific gravity, and creatinine. First-morning urine samples are preferred, as they are more concentrated and thus drugs are more readily detected. The decision for using blood or urine should be based on the specific drug's pharmacokinetic and excretion data. As a rule, urine drug levels are higher and should be the biofluid of choice for drug and drug metabolite detection.

XII. INTERPRETATION OF POSITIVE AND NEGATIVE REPORTS

The psychoactivity of most drugs lasts only a few hours after drug ingestion, whereas urinalysis detects many drugs and/or metabolites for days or even weeks. Thus, the presence of drugs (or metabolites) in urine is only the indication of prior exposure, not proof of intoxication or impairment at the time of sample collection. In some cases, quantitative data in blood or urine can corroborate observed behavior or actions of a subject, especially when the levels are so high that it is impossible for the subject to be free of drug effects. Thus, interpretation of drug-induced behavior along with laboratory data belongs to experts of pharmacology, toxicology, and psychiatry.

When one receives drug analysis reports, whether positive or negative, there are certain questions that must be asked about the results: (1) What method was used? (If the lab does not tell you on the report, call and ask.) (2) Did the assay analyze for the drug alone, metabolite only, or both? What is the "cutoff" value for the assay? (Again, call and ask.) (3) Was the sample time close enough to the suspected drug exposure? This information is mostly unavailable, since denial is one of the most typical features of drug abusers. Their use pattern is usually hidden.

First, let us examine positive results. Some scrutiny of the method is needed to determine whether or not a false-positive result is a possibility. Knowledge of the method of determination is helpful. Although TLC is not very sensitive, it is reasonably specific for drugs that have both the parent drug and its metabolite identified on the TLC plate. Also, specific color reactions help to eliminate false-positives for certain drugs. If GLC or GC/MS was the analytical technique, positive results are acceptable with additional assurance.

Use of RIA or EMIT is considered rather sensitive, but chemically similar compounds may readily cross react, with the antibody, registering the "false"-positive results. Cross reactivity depends on the specificity of the antibody used for a particular drug and drug metabolite. Some antibodies are more specific than others. Therefore, each test should be inidividually evaluated for possible false-positive reaction. Positive test results for amphetamines or opiates by immunoassays must be further defined for specific substances to be legally and medically acceptable. Immunoassay results must be confirmed by a chromatographic procedure.

Especially during screening, false-negative results occur easier than false-positives owing to the insensitivity of TLC. Thus, a negative report based on TLC alone is not reliable. Also, if the screening method was RIA or EIA, the cutoff, which separates positives and negatives, may have been set too high. Another possibility for false-negatives is that the sample was taken too long after the last drug exposure. Whatever the case may be, if the suspicion of drug use is strong, repeat testing and inquire at the laboratory for more sensitive drug screening procedures and test for more drugs.

In general, analytical toxicology methods have significantly improved in the past decades and the trend is for further improvement. As technology continues to improve, more drugs and chemicals will be analyzed in biofluids at the nanogram and picogram level. Advancement, however, does not mean that modern methodologies are infallible, nor do they replace the clinician. Theoretically and practically, technical or human error can influence testing results. A solid locally and nationally certified laboratory with the full spectrum of drug abuse tests enables the well-trained clinician to make drug abuse diagnoses that were not possible in the past. With knowledge of the available analytical methods, one can scrutinize the results and be more confident about the validity of the laboratory test results.

XIII. ETHICAL CONSIDERATIONS

The legitimate utilization of drug abuse testing in the clinical setting is indisputable. Denial makes identification of drug abuse difficult; therefore, testing is necessary both in identification and in monitoring treatment outcome. However, drug testing at the workplace and in sports is more controversial. Positive test results may be used in the termination of long-time employees or in the refusal to hire new ones.

Private companies feel that it is their right to establish drug- and alcohol-free workplaces and sport arenas. The opposition feels that it is ill advised to terminate individuals for a single positive test result even when it is confirmed by forensic quality procedures. A testing program is more reasonable which offers a chance for rehabilitation. Probationary periods would provide an opportunity to stop using drugs by entering treatment or self-help programs. Employee Assistance Programs (EAPs) are available in larger companies and governmental organizations which refer employees to drug counseling.

It is important that this new powerful tool, drug testing, is used not as a weapon but judiciously as a means of early detection and prevention of disability. Test results must be interpreted only by individuals who understand drugs of abuse medically and/or pharmacologically. The federal government requires that in their drug testing program the results go directly to Medical Review Officers (MROs) who are trained to interpret such reports. Improper testing in the laboratory or improper interpretation of drug abuse testing data may destroy innocent lives; therefore, it must be prevented.

Federal employees may be tested for drugs of abuse only by locally and nationally certified laboratories. The two most respected forsenic toxicology laboratory regulatory agencies are the National Institute on Drug Abuse (NIDA) and the College of American Pathologists (CAP). Only the most proficient and competent laboratories in the nation are certified by these organizations. The laboratories must pass the most stringent 2-day onsite inspection and frequent proficiency testing programs throughout the year. Owning to the serious consequences of positive test results, employee and pre-employment testing by private companies should also be conducted in certified laboratories.

Is society placed in jeopardy by the drug-related actions of certain drug abusers? How should the test results be used? Who should know the results and under what circumstances?

These are just some of the questions asked by private citizens. The verdict on random testing is not yet decided, but the case for "for cause testing" by the U.S. Supreme Court is on the side of testing. The Court determined that public safety supercedes individual rights to privacy, especially when the person's job in question has significant impact on society. It is predictable that the controversy will continue for some time regarding the civil rights issues and legality of drug abuse testing.

XIV. CONCLUSIONS

As long as illegal drug use is prevalent in our society, drug abuse testing will have an important clinical and forensic role. Testing in the clinical setting will aid the physician treating subjects having psychiatric signs and symptoms secondary to drug abuse, monitoring treatment outcome, and in serious overdose cases. Drug testing in the forensic setting will be utilized for workplace testing and monitoring parolees convicted of drug-related crimes.

Several civil rights concerns must be enforced to protect the innocent. Names of subjects should be known only to the medical office where the sample is collected. Testing must follow strict chain of custody procedures to ensure anonymity and prevent sample mix-up during testing. Some progressive laboratories instituted "bar-code" labeling of samples and related documents to ensure confidentiality, improve accurate reporting, and sample or record tracking.

The reliability of testing procedures is also of foremost importance [15]. Good laboratories instituted internal open, blind, and external quality control systems to assure high quality of testing. Before issuing licenses, governmental agencies require laboratories to adhere to strict standards in personnel qualifications, experience, quality control, quality assurance programs, tight chain of custody procedures, and multiple data review prior to results reporting.

Two nationally recognized agencies are protecting the rights of individual citizens who might be tested and assuring proper procedures in forensic drug testing: the National Institute on Drug Abuse (NIDA's National Laboratory Certification Program) and the College of American Pathologists (CAP's Forensic Toxicology Proficiency Program). In addition, numerous city and state regulatory agencies inspect and license drug testing laboratories. Good laboratories are easily identified by having current certificates of qualification and licenses issued by national and local regulatory agencies.

Conclusively, drug testing has come a long way in accuracy and reliability [16]. Testing started in traditional "wet chemistry" laboratories, using huge sample volumes, crude methodologies, and low sensitivity. Now, auto analyzers perform hundreds of tests on minute sample volumes and measure accurately low-nanogram amounts of analytes. Thus, the insecurity expressed in the popular press about drug abuse testing should not be a concern to anyone using properly certified, licensed laboratories.

ACKNOWLEDGMENTS

The author thanks Dr. Marina Stajic and Michel McGee for their contribution of the illustrations and Debra Verebey for typing the manuscript.

REFERENCES

1. Jaffe J.H., and Martin W.R. (1985). Opioid analgesics and antagonists, *The Pharmacological Basis of Therepeutics*, 7th ed. (A.G. Gilman, L.S. Goodman et al. eds.). Macmillan, New York, pp. 491–531.
2. Gold M.S., Verebey K., and Dackis C.A.(1980). Diagnosis of drug abuse, drug intoxication and withdrawal states. *Fair Oaks Hosp. Psychiatry Lett.* 3(5):23–34.

3. Pottash A.L.C., Gold M.S., and Extein I. (1982). The use of the clinical laboratory, (L.I. Sederer ed.). *Inpatient Psychiatry: Diagosis and Treatment*. Baltimore, Williams Wilkins, pp. 205–221.

4. Willette E. (1986). Drug testing programs, *Urine Testing for Drugs of Abuse*, (R.L. Hawks and N.C. Chiang, eds.). National Institute on Drug Abuse Research Monograph 73. U.S. Government Printing Office, Washington, D.C., pp. 5–12.

5. Perrine M.W. (1974). Alcohol, drugs and driving: Relative priorities for basic and applied research, *Proceedings of the Sixth International Conference on Alcohol. Drugs and Traffic Safety*, (S. Israelstam and Lambert, eds.). Toronto, September 8–13, pp. 107–128.

6. Baselt, R.C., and Cravey, R.H. (eds.) (1989). *Disposition of Toxic Drugs and Chemicals in Man*, 3rd Ed. Yearbook, Chicago.

7. Manno, J.E. (1986). *Interpretation of Urinalysis Results in Urine Testing for Drugs of Abuse*, (R.L. Hawks and N.C. Chiang, eds.) National Institute on Drug Abuse Research Monograph 73. U.S. Government Printing Office, Washington, D.C., pp. 55–61.

8. Chiang, N.C., and Hawks, R.L. (1986): Implicatioans of drug levels in body fluids: Basic concepts, *Urine Testing for Drugs of Abuse*, (R.L. Hawks and N.C. Chiang, eds.). National Institute on Drug Abuse Research Monograph 73. U.S. Government Printing Office, Washington, D.C., pp. 62–83.

9. Verebey, K., Martin, D., and Gold M.S. (1982) Drug abuse: Interpretation of laboratory tests, *Psychiatric Medicine* (W. Hall, ed.). *3*(3):155–167.

10. Hawks, R.L.(1986) *Analytical Methodology in Urine Testing for Drugs of Abuse* (R.L. Hawks and N.C. Chiang, eds.). National Institute on Drug Abuse Research Monograph 73. U.S. Government Printing Office, Washington, D.C., pp 30–42.

11. Wadler, G.I., and Heinline,B. (1989). *Drugs and Athletes, Contemporary Exercise and Sports Medicine*. Davis, Philadelphia, p. 209.

12. Verebey, K. (1987). Cocaine abuse detection by laboratory methods, *Cocaine: A Clinician's Handbook* (A.M. Washton and M.S. Gold, eds.) Guilford Press, New York, London pp. 214–228.

13. Kogan, M.J., Jukofsky, D. Verebey K., et al. (1987). Detection of methaqualone in human urine by radio immunoassay and gas-liquid chromatography after a therapeutic dose. *Clin. Chem.* *24*:1425–1427.

14. Dackis, C.A., Pottash, A.L.C., Annitto, W., et al. (1982). Persistence of urinary marijuana levels after supervised abstinence *Am. J. Psychiatry 139*:1196–1198.

15. Blanke, R.V.(1986). Accuracy in urinalysis, *Urine Testing for Drugs of Abuse*, (R.L. Hawks and N.C. Chiang, eds.). National Institute on Drug Abuse Research Monograph 73. U.S. Government Printing Office, Washington, D.C., pp. 43–53.

16. Frings, G.S., Battaglia, D.J., and White, R.M. (1989). Status of drugs of abuse testing in urine under blind conditions: An AAC study. *Clin. Chem. 35*(5):891–844.

45

Clinical Implications of Federal Regulations on Laboratory Testing for Alcohol and Drugs of Abuse/Addiction

David M. Martin
FirstLab at Horsham Clinic, Ambler, Pennsylvania

Matthew E. Weinstein and Ronald I. Dozoretz
First Hospital Corporation, Norfolk, Virginia

I. INTRODUCTION

Clinical utilization of drug and alcohol abuse/addiction testing has dramatically increased over the last decade, and now promises to become a requirement for employment in the federal and private sectors [1]. Technological variation and lack of standardization within the laboratory industry has created tremendous concern over the accuracy of drug and alcohol abuse/addiction testing [2]. These concerns led to federal regulations detailing the specific technical and administrative aspects of drug abuse testing permissible on federal employees [3]. These regulations not only addressed technical specifics, but also established personnel qualifications and supervisory requirements for reporting positive results, chain of custody documentation procedures, and a detailed set of record-keeping requirements. These regulations have had tremendous beneficial effects leading to greater standardization and consistency within the alcohol and drug abuse testing industry. It has, however, created a entire new set of standards and regulations by which laboratories are allowed to operate and report results. What then should a clinician know and ask a laboratory concerning alcohol and drug abuse/addiction testing? What is the NIDA Drug Screen and NIDA Certification? Can this screen be applied to clinical populations, and how does it compare to a clinically designed drug screen? What is a Chain of Custody Form, when is it necessary, and how can one verify its authenticity? What was the legislative basis for development of these regulations, and who will be required to be tested for drugs as a condition of employment? These and other questions will be addressed with the objective of providing clinicians and Medical Review Officers with a working knowledge of the current regulatory and legislative basis of alcohol and drug testing and its implications from a clinical perspective.

II. OVERVIEW OF FEDERAL REGULATIONS OF LABORATORIES

Federal regulations of clinical laboratories began in 1965 with the signing of the Medicare Act into public law [4]. Under Medicare, the federal government would reimburse medical services for the aged when the providers complied with certain performance standards. Clinical laboratory testing was included in the definition of such medical services and as such, the federal regulation of the laboratory industry began [5].

Clinical laboratories were issued a medicare provider number, an authorization to receive reimbursement under the Act if certain performance, personnel, and efficiency standards were met. Compliance with Medicare standards is required today and for both hospital laboratories and independent laboratories who submit for reimbursement under the Medicare Act or provide services for individuals covered under the Act.

In 1967, the Clinical Laboratory Improvement Act (CLIA) was signed into law [6]. This required clinical laboratories that either solicited or accepted specimens in interstate commerce to be licensed. CLIA licensure standards and administration were separate from the Medicare laboratory program. The Medicare program also had separate standards for hospital-based laboratories and independent laboratories, the latter of which was more stringent. Independent laboratories were defined as those commercial laboratories established outside of hospitals, whereas hospital laboratories by definition were located within a hospital.

In addition to CLIA and the two Medicare programs, various states and cities began enacting their own laboratory regulation and licensure procedures. There are currently 34 states that have individual licensure requirements for laboratories to perform routine clinical tests. In addition, at this writing, nine states and one city, Connecticut, Iowa, Louisiana, Minnesota, Montana, Nebraska, Rhode Island, Utah, Vermont and the city of San Francisco, have enacted laws regulating drug testing [7].

Private agency licensure and proficiency programs for clinical laboratories emerged only in the 1970s, the most notable being the licensure issued by the College of American Pathologists (CAP); its proficiency program and those of the American Association of Clinical Chemistry (AACC) and other discipline-specific organizations soon created a new department within the clinical laboratory; i.e., Proficiency and Quality Control [8]. Hospital or independent laboratories that serviced hospitals also had to comply with standards established by the Joint Commission on Accreditation of Healthcare organizations; i.e., The Joint Commission [9].

Despite the myriad of federal, state, city and private agency regulations to standardize and increase the quality of laboratory testing, the variation was great and in some cases dangerous [10]. This led to a constant stream of media reports on rampant inaccuracies in laboratory services, which spurred the enactment of the Clinical Laboratory Improvement Act of 1988 (CLIA 88) [11]. CLIA 88 is scheduled to go into effect in 1990 and will, for the first time, set a uniform set of federal standards that all clinical laboratories must conform to whether they are independent or hospital based.

Federal regulations by means of CLIA and Medicare coupled with various state, city, and private agency requirements still did not address the complicated issue of drug testing in the workplace. There was no single set of standards that laboratories could be held accountable to in the performance of drug tests. It was not until April 1988 that the Department of Health and Human Services issued mandatory guidelines for laboratories that would be testing for drugs on federal employees [3]. Therefore, only recently has consensus emerged within the laboratory industry and the federal government on how drug testing could technically, administratively, and, therefore, legally be performed. The foundation for these guidelines leading to a legally defensible, technical, and administrative system for drug testing had its origins with the Executive Order for a Drug-Free Federal Workplace and the Drug-Free Workplace Act of 1988.

III. EXECUTIVE ORDER FOR A DRUG FREE FEDERAL WORKPLACE

On September 15, 1986 President Ronald Reagan signed Executive Order 12564 establishing the goal of a drug-free federal workplace [1]. This Executive Order made the 2.8 million civilian employees of the federal government subject to a policy against the use of illegal drugs whether on or off duty. It further orders and authorizes the use of drug testing as a diagnostic tool to identify drug use in certain circumstances and among certain employees. The Executive Order authorized drug testing programs in the following areas:

Federal employees in sensitive positions
Voluntary employee drug testing
Reasonable suspicion
Accident or unsafe practice
Pre-employment

The Executive Order set the stage for drug testing in America. It also charged the Department of Health and Human Services (DHHS) to establish scientific and technical guidelines for drug testing laboratories to be used by the federal government, and to establish standards of certification for laboratories to do such testing for Federal agencies. Two years later, on April 11, 1988, in the *Federal Register*, the Department of Health and Human Services issued mandatory guidelines for federal workplace drug testing programs and charged the National Institute on Drug Abuse (NIDA) for its implementation [3]. For the first time, federal guidelines were issued for laboratories to meet specific criteria in order to perform drug abuse/addiction testing. The laboratory industry struggled throughout 1988 in order to meet these new guidelines which would certify the laboratory to perform drug testing on federal employees, contractors, and grantees. This certification became known in the industry as NIDA Certification.

It, therefore, was the Executive Order that issued the mandate for a drug-free federal workplace and drug testing of individuals in sensitive positions, pre-employment, postaccident, unsafe practices, or on a volunary basis. The Department of Health and Human Services issued the Technical Guidelines for Drug Testing on Federal Employees and, while these events were unfolding, the Omnibus Anti-Drug Abuse Act of 1988 was signed into law on November 18, 1988, by President Reagan. This sweeping legislation on criminal penalties and definition of illegal drug activities had included in Section 4804 a requirement for federal contractors and grantees to maintain a drug-fee workplace, this section is commonly referred to as the Drug-Free Workplace Act of 1988.

IV. DRUG-FREE WORKPLACE ACT OF 1988

Without a question, the 1980s revealed that the United States was indeed at war with an enemy that threatened to invade every citizen both at home and at work. The decade opened with great ethical questions on individual rights under the 4th Amendment preventing unreasonable search and seizure in regard to drug testing. Hundreds of cases and thousands of hours of testimony and deliberation resulted in a sweeping legislation, HR 5210, the Anti-Drug Abuse Act of 1988, which President Reagan signed on November 18, 1988 [12]. The bill became public law 100-690, and it is commonly referred to as the Drug-Free Workplace Act of 1988. (See Appendix)

Interestingly enough, the Drug-Free Workplace Act of 1988 does not include any language or make any mention of drug testing at all. The intent of the bill was to establish the foundation of a drug-free workplace in the areas that the federal government could affect outside the federal government; i.e., the workplaces of federal grantees and contractors. It would affect those grantees and contractors receiving awards of $25,000 or more and require them to meet seven specific requirements:

Drug-Free Workplace Compliance Requirements

1. To publish a statement notifying the employees that the unlawful manufactured distribution, dispensing, possession, or use of a controlled substance is prohibited in the workplace and specifying what actions will be taken against employees for violations of the prohibition.
2. Establish a program to inform employees of the dangers of drug abuse in the workplace and the availability of drug counseling, rehabilitation, and employee assistance programs.
3. Provide all employees working under the contract with a copy of the policy statement.
4. Notify employees in the policy statement that as a condition of continuing employment, the employee will abide by the statement and notify the employer within 5 days if he or she is convicted of any criminal drug offense occurring in the workplace.
5. Notify the contracting officer of an employee conviction within 10 days after the contractor learns of the conviction.
6. Within 30 days of receiving notice of the conviction, impose a sanction on the convicted employee up to and including termination or require the employee to satisfactorily complete an approved drug rehabilitation program.
7. Make a good faith effort to continue to maintain a drug-free workplace by meeting the requirements of the Act.

It was through these seven requirements that employers who were contractees or grantees of the federal government were required to document that their workplaces are drug free. This laid the foundation for further requirements of specific government agencies to begin drug testing and to set down the criteria by which drug testing was to be conducted and reported [13,14].

The Drug-Free Workplace act of 1988 began its implementation subsequent to the Office of Management and Budgets Interim Guidelines to Federal Agencies for Implementing the Drug-Free Workplace Act [15]. This interim guideline was published in January 1989 and was to go into effect on March 18, 1989. These interim guidelines were to coordinate the regulatory development with over 30 federal agencies to ensure uniformed government-wide implementation of the Drug-Free Workplace Act of 1988.

Basically, the requirement for contractors or grantees of federal monies to have a drug-free workplace and to take action to promote a drug-free environment was tucked into the federal acquisition regulation [15]. Now, for the first time a federal contract or grant could be denied on the basis of the applicant not having a drug awareness and antidrug policy statement issued within its company. This covers nearly all federal contractors or grantees, those who fail to comply face suspension of their payments or termination of their contracts, and they can be debarred from future federal contracts or grants up to 5 years. It is estimated that the federal government awarded over $180 billion in contracts, worth more than $25,000, representing over 400,000 individual contracts. There is an additional $100 billion of grants that were awarded in fiscal 1987 that would also fall under the Drug-Free Workplace Act of 1988 [31]. The Drug-Free Workplace Act of 1988 is the legislative basis whereby government contractees and grantees must certify that their workplace is drug free and take actions to maintain it as such.

Although the Drug-Free Workplace Act of 1988 did not require any provisions for drug testing, in anticipation of its implementation and in concert with the Executive Order, the Department of Defense (DOD) and Department of Transportation (DOT), because of the nature of their work, issued guidelines for drug testing [13,14]. This spearheaded mandatory drug testing for nonfederal employees who were either contractors, grantees or regulated by either the Department of Defense or Department of Transportation.

The Department of Defense rule that became effective on October 31, 1988, required the defense contractors must establish and maintain programs for creating a drug-free workplace. A distinguishing aspect of the Defense Department's rule was that it required mandatory drug testing [14]. Employees who would be required to take mandatory drug tests were those employees in sensitive positions. Employers were responsible for determining the extent of criteria for drug testing based on the following factors:

Nature of work being performed
Duties of the employee
Contractors resources
Risks to public health or national security

These rules then went on to allow employers to test under the following conditions: reasonable suspicion, accident, follow-up counseling, or voluntary testing program. The Department of Defense rules did not include random drug testing.

The Department of Transportation regulations for a drug-free workplace affects a wide range of employees who are regulated by the Federal Highway Administration (FHA), Federal Aviation Administration (FAA), Federal Railroad Administration (FRA), Urban Mass Transportation Administration (UMTA), Research and Special Projects Administration, and the U.S. Coast Guard. The Department of Transportation rules not only included drug testing similar to the Department of Defense, but for pre-employment and on a random basis as well. The rule stated that random drug testing was to be administered to all workers so that 50% of the employee population was tested every year. The Department of Transportation published a rigorous seven-part Chain of Custody Form (see Appendix) and defined documentation procedures for collection sites, laboratories, MROs and employers as well [13].

These two departments set the standards for drug testing within the Federal workplace and the private sector companies that fall under the regulations of these departments. Between these two departments, close to 7 million employees became subject to drug testing either as a condition of employment, upon reasonable cause, accident, rehabilitation follow-up, or through random selection. The rules of these departments, coupled with the Drug-Free Workplace Act of 1988 and the Executive Order for a Drug-Free Federal Workplace established the legal and operational basis for drug testing in America.

V. NIDA CERTIFICATION OF LABORATORIES

Certification of laboratories to perform drug testing is administered by the National Institute of Drug Abuse (NIDA) and qualifies laboratories under the U.S. Department of Health and Human Services guidelines to perform testing on federal employees [3]. It is a rigorous three-phase program.

Phase 1. Pre-inspection proficiency testing
Phase 2. On-site inspection
Phase 3. On-going proficiency testing

Prior to qualifying for an inspection from NIDA, an applying laboratory must successfully complete two proficiency samples that are sent to the laboratory. A proficiency sample is a test mix of urine and drugs of known quantities that is blind to the laboratory performing the test. The laboratory must successfully identify the individual compounds with which the sample has been spiked, confirm, and report its findings within a certain tolerance level.

Successful completion of these proficiency samples allow for the laboratory to be inspected on site.

On-site inspection by NIDA-qualified inspectors is a very detailed exercise including another set of proficiency samples to be run on-site during the 2-day inspection. Some of the distinguishing aspects of the inspection versus standard laboratory inspections to meet Medicare, CLIA, state, city, or other agency requirements are as follows:

NIDA Laboratory Characteristics

Rigorous chain of custody procedures for the collection of specimens and handling of specimens during testing and storage.

Specific structural requirements to secure the analytical and accessioning departments. These areas must have floor to ceiling walls and be locked at all times.

Stringent standards for making the entire drug testing laboratory secure, for restricting access to all but authorized personnel, and providing an escort for any others who are authorized to be on the premises.

Precise requirements for quality assurance and performance testing specific to urine analysis for the presence of illegal drugs.

Detailed procedures for the screening and confirmation of drugs indicating their verification and limits of detectability.

Specific educational experience requirements for laboratory personnel to ensue their competence and credibility as experts in forensic urine drug testing.

Once a laboratory has been inspected and issued NIDA Certification, in order to maintain it the laboratory must successfully complete, with 100% accuracy, performance of a continuing proficiency program supplied by NIDA. Should it fail only one part of the proficiency program, licensure is suspended until remedial actions have been put into place.

The laboratory must maintain a very rigorous internal quality control program and subject itself to an external quality control of blind specimens.

NIDA Certification ensures the integrity of the specimen and the technical authenticity of the report throughout the entire analytical process. Other licensing agencies such as various state or city Departments of Health, the College of American Pathologists, Medicare, and the Department of Health and Human Services (CLIA 88) do not address drug testing with such detail. NIDA Certification requires specific performance standards for the analysis of five drugs of abuse, not including alcohol. The five drugs that are included in the certification process and that comprise the NIDA Drug Screen are listed in Table 1.

Table 1 NIDA Drug Screen and Confirmation Guidelines

	Initial test level (ng/ml)	Confirmatory test level (ng/ml)
Marijuana	100	15[a]
Cocaine	300	150[b]
Amphetamines (methamphetamine, amphetamine)	1000	500
Opiates (morphine, codeine)	300[c]	300
Phencyclidine	25	25

[a]Delta-9-tetrahydrocannabinol-9-carboxylic acid.
[b]Benzoylecogonine.
[c]25 ng/ml if using immunoassay specific for morphine.

NIDA Certification requires specific guidelines for the screening and confirmatory levels of each drug or drug class. It also requires specific procedures and associated documentation with the finding of a positive result. Although debated extensively, alcohol was not included in this list as, according to the Executive Order, it is not an illegal drug. Other drugs of abuse such as benzodiazapines, barbiturates, methaqualone, hallucinogens, and other abused drugs were also not included in the guidelines, nor are NIDA Certified Laboratories inspected for the performance of these assays. The first NIDA inspections were carried out in early 1988, and at this writing there are currently 37 laboratories that are certified to perform the NIDA Drug Screen.

A physician acting as a Medical Review Officer (MRO) for an organization would want to ensure that the laboratory performing the drug test is indeed NIDA certified if the employer is required to have testing performed by a NIDA-certified lab. The industries most effected would be those regulated by either the Department of Defense or Department of Transportation. For physicians treating patients clinically either as inpatients or outpatients for alcohol or drug addiction, such certification, and the complexity and expense associated with it, is not required. The NIDA Drug Screen alone owing to its limited constituents and sensitivity is not the best diagnostic or surveillance tool for a clinical patient population.

VI. CLINICAL IMPLICATIONS OF THE NIDA DRUG SCREEN

NIDA Certification of drug testing laboratories was primarily designed to standardize analytical operations and provide a legally defensible basis for implementing federal employee drug testing programs under the Executive Order [16–18]. The consequences of a positive drug test in the workplace and reasons for performing the test are vastly different from those of a clinician in an alcohol or drug rehabilitation program. Because of this, the drugs tested for in a NIDA panel had undergone a different selection process than a clinician would employ in selecting a drug screen to be used diagnostically or as abstinence-assurance device in a rehabilitation program. The NIDA Drug Screen, in testing for only five drugs, may be too narrow in scope to be applied clinically as a relapse prevention or diagnostic tool.

The technological base used in the NIDA Drug Screen was from the early to mid 1980s setting the screening level for drugs much higher (therefore, less sensitive) than it is routinely possible to screen for today. For example, the screening levels for marijuana and cocaine in the NIDA Drug Screen are 100 and 300 ng/ml, respectively. Current technology and manufacturer's recommendation allow marijuana to be detected at 20 ng/ml [21,32], five times the sensitivity in the NIDA Guidelines; and cocaine's metabolite can be safely reported out at 150 ng/ml [19,23], twice the NIDA Guidelines. In the case of amphetamines, the initial screen of 1000 ng/ml is three times what is commonly available to screen for these drugs using standard techniques (22,33). The variation of screening sensitivities was recently reported to result in a greater than 50% rate of false-negative marijuana screens using NIDA Guidelines vs. clinical screening guidelines. The study further documented that the narrow scope of the NIDA Guidelines missed greater than 80% of other commonly abused drugs such as benzodiazepines [39]. These higher levels would result in higher rates of false-negatives within a drug rehabilitation population. This is a dangerous event that does not foster abstinence nor serve as an effective deterrent to continued drug abuse. The reasons for these initial test levels and drug selection are complicated and have their origins in the pioneering work done by the U.S. Navy in the early 1970s [34]. NIDA drug screening guidelines meet the needs within a drug screening program for employment purposes, but may not meet the needs of an individual clinical practitioner.

This is not to say that the NIDA Drug Screen has limited clinical application as a broad screening diagnostic device in the workplace. In that setting, it is extremely appropriate and has laid the foundation for other agencies of the federal government to issue additional regulations. For example, the Department of Transportation (DOT) issued guidelines for the implementation of drug testing using the NIDA Drug Screen [13]. One of the DOT agencies, the Federal Railroad Administration (FRA) issued guidelines that included testing not only for the NIDA Drug Screen drugs but alcohol as well [25].

The NIDA Drug Screen is designed precisely for application in mass screening programs of the general workforce where the likelihood of a positive result triggering legal action is high [16]. It is precisely for this reason that elaborate gas chromatographic mass spectrometry (GC/MS) confirmation procedures and chain of custody documentation are required [18]. Clinically, these issues are less important, expensive and administratively cumbersome. It is important to keep in mind the following points that distinguish the NIDA Drug Screen and clinical drug screens:

NIDA Drug Screen vs Clinical Drug Screens

NIDA drug screening is designed for employment drug testing, not clinical drug testing.
NIDA drug screening has a limited number of drugs tested for: marijuana, cocaine, opiates, amphetamines, and phencyclidine (PCP).
NIDA drug screening positive cutoff values are set higher (therefore, less sensitive) for marijuana, cocaine, and amphetamines than is clinically desirable.
Chain of custody documentation is not required in a clinical environment. If there are legal or professional licensure issues contingent upon the result of a drug test, then a chain of custody is required.
GC/MS confirmation of positive findings is not required in a clinical environment. If there are legal or professional licensure issues contingent upon the result of a drug test, then a chain of custody and GC/MS confirmation is required.
If positive drug test is inconsistent clinically, or the specific drug and concentration would be diagnostically helpful, a GC/MS confirmation can be ordered on the same specimen.

Drug testing has matured rapidly over the last decade since the introduction of commercially available kits for laboratories [36,32]. These new kits employ a wide range of technologies, e.g., radioimmunoassay (RIA), enzyme immunoassay (EIA), and fluorescent polarization immunoassay (FPIA). These techniques have been refined and are at less risk of interference or false-positives than they were upon their introduction [35,37,38].

Because of the technological refinement of these screening assays, GS/MS confirmation is no longer essential in a clinical environemnt [32,38] when contemporary sensitivity and specificity of drug testing is interpreted in light of the prevalence of positive findings in the population [28,29,30].

In a review of 16 studies analyzing 26,941 samples for drugs by various methods, 2833 (10.5%) were found to be positive, and of the positive samples only 47 (1.7%) were not confirmed [38]. These data suggest that in uncontrolled and unstandardized drug testing programs the confirmation of the initial test results is in the area of 98.3%. This high specificity coupled with the prevelence of positives in recovering populations make a confirmatory test routinely unnecessary in clinical populations.

This has several benefits: it increases the speed in which a positive result can be reported, decreases sample size, and overall cost of the procedure. In the cost-containment environment in which the American healthcare market is now in, this approach will not only be rewarded, but it is now essential. It will allow for increased frequency of testing at a lower cost to establish predictable surveillance strategies for relapse prevention. A cost-effective drug screen for clinical application is suggested in Table 2.

Table 2 Clinical and NIDA Drug Screening Guidelines

Drug	Clinical Drug Screen cutoff level (ng/ml)	NIDA Drug Screen cutoff level (ng/ml)
Marijuana	20	100
Cocaine	150	300
Amphetamine	300	1000
Opiates	300	300
PCP	25	25
Benzodiazepines	300	—
Barbituates	300	—
Methaqualone	300	—
Methadone	300	—
Propoxyphene	300	—
Alcohol	20 (mg%)	—
pH	5–8 (units)	—
Specific Gravity	1.005–1.025 (units)	—

The Clinical Drug Screen in Table 2 covers the majority of commonly abused drugs, and is presented with suggested sensitivities that have clinical application along with those required by NIDA for comparison. It is interesting to note that an individual with a 50 ng/ml marijuana reading would be classified as negative using the NIDA Drug Screen, but positive using the Clinical Drug Screen. This has been referred to as administratively negative but chemically positive [38]. The Clinical Drug Screen is designed with administrative cutoff (sensitivity) levels optimized to identify the widest range of chemically positive individuals. The Clinical Drug Screen (Table 2) should employ an antibody-based technology such as RIA, EIA, or FPIA. Quantitation is not required nor desirable owing to the variable nature of the urine compartment, but may be requested on individual patients as the clinical need arises. For example, a consistently positive finding may indicate slow clearance of the drug not continued abuse. Confirmation by GC/MS is not routinely required in a clinical setting that is not litigious. However, its application for specific drug identification and quantitation should be up to the individual clinician's medical judgment and clinical need.

An alternative to using a full Clinical Drug Screen upon every testing event is to narrow to scope, not sensitivity, to the drugs of choice of an individual patient or geographical region. This strategy will provide the constant threat of surveillance while providing the clinician with a flexible program that can be tailored to individual patient needs. For example, a full clinical screen can be ordered upon admission to document an individuals' substance abuse profile. While in treatment the screen can be focused to drug(s) of choice, then expanded if clinically indicated or upon discharge to document abstinence.

Specific gravity and pH are used as tools for the authenticity of the specimen. Extremely low specific gravity can indicate dilution with water; an abnormal pH can indicate adulteration with bleach or vinegar. Additional tests such as chloride and sodium can be added to note adulteration with salt. However, the amount of salt required to alter a test would result in a high specific gravity as well [25]. Temperature-sensitive collection devices and dots can also be used upon collection, as urine temperature will indicate if the specimen is freshly voided [27]. Creatinine has also been used as an indication that the sample is biological and undiluted. Specimens that have creatinine concentrations less than 0.2 gm/L should be viewed suspiciously and be re-collected. Specific gravity, pH, creatinine, temperature, and appearance are all valid indicators of the integrity of the specimen and can be used to verify the authenticity of the specimen.

Federal regulations have had a tremendous impact on increasing the overall performance of alcohol and drug testing laboratories. The most significant effects are the technological refinement of screening assays that no longer require confirmation procedures if applied clinically and the lower sensitivities which administratively expands the detection of chemically positive individuals. Operationally, laboratories have developed standardized internal procedures for ensuring the authenticity of the sample and its integrity throughout the analytical process. These chain of custody procedures are now available to be applied clincially, if needed, to augment the technical findings on a particular specimen or to ensure the specimen's integrity from the point of collection.

VII. CHAIN OF CUSTODY PROCEDURES

The Executive Order, the Drug-Free Workplace Act of 1988, and subsequent NIDA Certification procedures have not only set technical guidelines for the drug testing industry, but have also established acceptance of a Chain of Custody system. The Chain of Custody document follows the specimen from the time it is collected to the point when the report is generated. Anyone who handles the specimen must sign the Chain of Custody Form as either "receiving" or "releasing" the specimen from custody. One could take the Chain of Custody Form and account for any handling of the specimen from the time it was provided up until the time the final report was generated.

In the last half of the 1980s several hundred variations on the Chain of Custody Form have emerged and are being used within the industry. Any drug test that has legal implications should be "chained" with an appropriate Chain of Custody Form. The Department of Transportation (DOT) in its drug testing regulations issued in the *Federal Register* outlined a seven-part form and Chain of Custody tape to be placed over the specimen cap, which is rapidly becoming the standard of the industry (see Appendix B). The DOT form is a seven-part form, a copy for the laboratory (copy No. 1, original), a copy sent by the lab to the Medical Review Officer with the results (copy No. 2), a copy for the Medical Review Officer (copy No. 3), for the donor or employee (copy No. 4), for the collector (copy No. 5), and a copy for the employer (copy No. 6). There is also the provision for a split sample, if required (copy No. 7). The Form is designed so that critical information is conveyed to the laboratory and employer while maintaining confidentiality of the employee's medication history. This is accomplished by having the employee fill in that information on the back of copy No. 4 (donor or employee copy).

Although complicated upon initial review, this form, which is still evolving, satisfies the requirements of confidentiality while providing original copies of nonconfidential information to the employer, lab, collector, and employees. Each laboratory has their own variation on this theme, the form will ultimately reflect the organization's standards it was designed to meet.

It must be noted that a legally defensible Chain of Custody Form does not have to be as comprehensive as the DOT form, but must contain the following key information:

Patient name and signature (code numbers are acceptable)
Collector name and signature
Date of collection
Date and signature of anyone handling the specimen

The specimen itself should be labeled with the employee name, date, and test requested, and should be sealed with a Chain of Custody tape to ensure the sample is not tampered with until its arrival at the laboratory.

Key points to keep in mind when reviewing a Chain of Custody Form are the following:

Chain of Custody Checklist

Check to ensure the *patient name*, date and type of test are properly indicated.
Review *medication history* on form to note if prescription medicines can cause or be responsible for the positive finding.
Scan to ensure that *all areas* are filled in.
Review any *blank spaces* there are in the form.
Ensure the form is *signed by the donor* and the person *collecting* the specimen.
Ensure there is a *signature for each person* who handles the specimen.
If there is any area of the form that is not completed, your first call should be to the laboratory.
   *Review the copy of the form that the laboratory has with the one that you received.
   If any discrepancy exists, the sample should be discarded and a new specimen collected.

The importance of the integrity of the Chain of Custody Form can not be over emphasized. No matter how rigorous the technical aspects of the test were in the laboratory, it is all meaningless unless it can be connected to a complete Chain of Custody Form. Any medical or employment action based on a positive drug test must first have that test backed up with a complete Chain of Custody Form [18]. If any question exists about the integrity of the Form, immediately call the laboratory or personnel department of the organization and have the Form reviewed by the legal department.

In any case that is sure to go to litigation, it is wise to ask for a *Litigation Package* to be prepared by the laboratory. It should include copies of the following:

Drug Testing Litigation Package

Chain of Custody Form
Requisition
Specimen bottle verification sheet
Screening data and worksheet
Screening quality control data
Confirmation data and worksheet
Confirmation quality control data
Proficiency reports for the last year
Letter summarizing the analysis signed by an Analyst and the Director

This will allow for a clinical or employment confrontation with all of the technical and administrative objections already ruled out.

VIII. ALCOHOL AND DRUG TESTING LABORATORY QUESTIONNAIRE

The following is a quick series of questions a clinician or Medical Review Officer can ask to qualify a laboratory and the drug screens they offer:

___ Is the lab NIDA certified? When was certification received?
___ Is the lab Medicare certified?

___ CLIA 88 Licensure? In what areas is the lab licensed?
___ Does the lab have a separate Toxicology Department?
___ Screening method RIA___ EIA___ FPIA___
___ GC/MS confirmation available in house?
___ How long does it take to confirm specific drugs?
___ Is a Chain of Custody Form available?
___ Is the lab familiar with DOT seven-part Chain of Custody Form?
___ What toxicology proficiency does the lab participate in? Are any results less 100% for state, city, or private agency programs?
___ Number of drug screens done per day? (Greater than 50 would be desirable.)

IX. CONCLUSIONS

The impact of federal regulations on clinical laboratories has significantly increased the overall quality of the industry. In no one area has this impact been felt more than in drug testing and its associated technical and administrative guidelines. These regulations have served to improve the consistency and quality of drug testing not only in the workplace, but they have had tremendous beneficial results clinically.

Today clinicians have a powerful array of drug testing tools and strategies to work with that were not available only 10 years ago. Federal regulations on alcohol and drug testing laboratories have forged these devices, equipping modern practitioners with effective diagnostic procedures that can be used cost effectively and as broadly as is clinically indicated.

REFERENCES

1. Executive Order Number 12564 for a Drug-Free Federal Workplace (1986), *Federal Register*, September 15, V. *51* N. 32:889.
2. Hansen, H.J., Candill, S.P., and Boone, J. (1985). Crisis in drug testing: Results of CDC blind study. *J.A.M.A.*, *253*:2382.
3. Department of Health and Human Services (1988). *Mandatory Guidelines for Federal Workplace Drug Testing Programs; Final Guidelines*, Notice, April 11, *Federal Register, 5* 69: part IV.
4. Health Insurance for the Aged Act, the Medicare Act 42 (1965), the United States Code 1395.
5. Medicare's Condition for Coverage of Services of Independent Laboratories, 42 C.F.R., 405.1310.
6. Clinical Laboratories Improvement Act (1967), 42 United States Code 263A.
7. DeCrease, R.P., Lifshitz, M.S., Mazura, A.C., Tilson, J.E., et al. (eds.). *Drug Testing in the Workplace*, 2nd ed. American Society of Clinical Pathologists Press, Chicago, 1989, p. 20.
8. Kenney, M.L. (1987). Quality assurance in changing times: Proposals for reform and research in the clinical laboratory field. *Clin. Chem.*, *33*:328.
9. Joint Commission on Accreditation of Hospitals (1987), *The Accreditation Manual for Hospitals*, Chicago, Illinois JCAH.
10. Van der Graaf, Y. (1987). Screening errors in cervical cytologic screening. *Acta Cytol. 31*(4):434.
11. Clinical Laboratories Improvement Amendments of 1988 (CLIA '88), Public Law #100-578.
12. Drug-Free Workplace Act of 1988, Public Law 100-690.
13. Procedures for Transportation Workplace Drug Testing Programs: Final Rules and Notice of Conference, Part III (1989). *Federal Register*, December 1, 49 CFR, Part 40.
14. Department of Defense Federal Acquisition Regulation Supplement Drug Free Workforce (1988) September 27, 48CFR, Parts 223 and 252.
15. Drug-Free Workplace Requirements: Notice and Final Interim Rules 91989, *Federal Register*, January 31, 54 (N 19): Part II.
16. Susser, P.A. (1985). Legal issues raised by drugs in the workplace. *Labor Law J.*, *42*:54.
17. Bible, J.D. (1986). Screening workers for drugs: The constitutional implications of urine testing in public employment. *Am. Bus. Law J.*, *24*:309.

18. Hoyt, D.W., Finnigan, R.E., Nee, T., Shults, T.F., and Butler, T.J. (1987). Drug testing in the workplace—Are methods legally defensible? *J.A.M.A.*, *258*:504.

19. Poklisa, I.R. (1987), Evaluation of TDx cocaine metabolite assay. *J. Anal. Toxicol.*, *11*:228.

20. Berkabile, D.R., and Meyer, A. False negative rate for EMIT cannabinoids (letter). *J. Anal. Toxicol.*, *13*:63.

21. Frederick, D.L., Green, J., and Fowler, M.W. (1985). Comparison of six cannabinoid metabolite assays. *J. Anal. Toxicol.*, *9*:116.

22. Black, D.L., Goldberg, B.A., and Kaplan, Y.H. (1987). Enzyme immunoassay method for comprehensive drug screening in microsamples of urine. *Clin. Chem.*, *33*:367.

23. Lewis, D.E., Omori, E., Nishio, J., and Schnoll, S.H. (1989). The analysis of cocaine metabolite in urine: A comparison of the TDx FPIA cocaine metabolite assay with gas chromotography-spectrometry (abstract). *Clin. Chem.*, *35*:1186.

24. Colbert, D.L., Gallagher, G., and Mainwaring-Burton, R.W. (1985). Single reagent polarization fluoroimmunoassay for amphetamine in urine. *Clin. Chem.*, *31*:193.

25. Control of Alcohol and Drug Use (1987), 49 CFR, Part 219.

26. Mikkelsen, S.L., and Ash, K.O. (1988), Adulteration causing false negatives in urine drug testing. *Clin. Chem.*, *34*(11):2333.

27. Judson, B.A., Himmelberger, D.U., and Goldstein, A. (1979). Measurement of urine temperature as an alternative to observed urination in a narcotics treatment program. *Am. J. Drug Alcohol Abuse*, *6*:197.

28. Peat, M.A. (1988). Analytical and technical aspects of testing for drug abuse: Confirmatory procedures. *Clin. Chem.*, *34*(3):471.

29. Sunshine, I. (1988). Preliminary tests for drugs of abuse. Clin. Chem., 34:2, 331.

30. Spiehler, U.R., O'Donnell, C.M., and Gokhale, D.U. (1988). Confirmation and certainty in toxicology testing. *Clin. Chem.*, *34*(8):1535.

31. Nogay, B. (1989). *The Drug-Free Workplace Act: The Complete Guide for Federal Contractors and Grantees, Bureau of National Affairs Special Report*, Cat. #14-6075, Washington, D.C.

32. Manufacturers Package Insert (1987). Emit Dau Cannabinoid 20 ng Assay, #3M694 Syva Co., Palo Alto, California.

33. Manufacturers Package Insert (1987). Emit Dau Amphetamine Assay #3M703, Syva Co., Palo Alto, California.

34. Irving, J.(1988). Drug testing in the military: Technical and legal problems. *Clin. Chem.* *34*(3):637.

35. Verebey, K., Mulé, S.J., Alrazi, J., et al. (1986). One hundred EMIT positive cannabinoid urine samples confirmed by BPA/TLC, RIA and GC/MS (letter). *J. Anal. Toxicol.*, *10*:79.

36. Rodgers, R., Crowl, C.T., Einstad, W.M., et al. (1987). Homogenous enzyme immunoassay for cannabionid in urine. *Clin. Chem.*, *24*:95.

37. Duc Vu, T. (1987). Additional results in the validation of the bond elut—THC extraction column—TLC as a confirmation method for emit and RIA positive cannabinoid urines (letter). *J. Anal. Toxicol.*, *11*:83.

38. Kelly, K.L. (1988). The accuracy and reliability of tests for drugs of abuse in urine samples. *Pharmacotherapy*, *8*(5):263.

39. Lakovics, M., Martin, D.M., and Levy, J.M. (1990). *Drug Testing False Negative Rates Using NIDA Criteria* (abstract). American Psychiatric Association 1990 Annual Convention and Scientific Program New Research Abstract 540.

APPENDIX

Excerpts from public law 100-690, referred to as the Drug-Free Workplace Act of 1988

SECTION 4804 OF ANTI-DRUG ABUSE ACT OF 1988

SEC. 5151.   SHORT TITLE.

This subtitle may be cited as the "Drug-Free Workplace Act of 1988".

SEC. 5152. DRUG-FREE WORKPLACE REQUIREMENTS FOR FEDERAL CONTRACTORS.

(a) DRUG-FREE WORKPLACE REQUIREMENT.—

(1) REQUIREMENT FOR PERSONS OTHER THAN INDIVIDUALS.—No person, other than an individual, shall be considered a responsible source, under the meaning of such term as defined in section 4(8) of the Office of Federal Procurement Policy Act (41 U.S.C. 403(8)), for the purposes of being awarded a contract for the procurement of any property or services of a value of $25,000 or more from any Federal agency unless such person has certified to the contracting agency that it will provide a drug-free workplace by—

(A) publishing a statement notifying employees that the unlawful manufacture, distribution, dispensation, possession, or use of a controlled substance is prohibited in the person's workplace and specifying the actions that will be taken against employees for violations of such prohibition;

(B) establishing a drug-free awareness program to inform employees about—

(i) the dangers of drug abuse in the workplace;

(ii) the person's policy of maintaining a drug-free workplace;

(iii) any available drug counseling rehabilitation, and employee assistance programs; and

(iv) the penalties that may be imposed upon employees for drug abuse violations;

(C) making it a requirement that each employee to be engaged in the performance of such contract be given a copy of the statement required by subparagraph (A);

(D) notifying the employee in the statement required by subparagraph (A), that as a condition of employment on such contract, the employee will—

(i) abide by the terms of the statement; and

(ii) notify the employer of any criminal drug statute conviction for a violation occurring in the workplace no later than 5 days after such conviction;

(E) notifying the contracting agency within 10 days after receiving notice under subparagraph (D)(ii) from an employee or otherwise receiving actual notice of such conviction;

(F) imposing a sanction on, or requiring the satisfactory participation in a drug abuse assistance or rehabilitation program by, any employee who is so convicted, as required by section 5154; and

(G) making a good faith effort to continue to maintain a drug-free workplace through implementation of subparagraphs (A), (B), (C), (D), (E), and (F).

(2) REQUIREMENT FOR INDIVIDUALS.—No Federal agency shall enter into a contract with an individual unless such contract includes a certification by the individual that the individual will not engage in the unlawful manufacture, distribution, dispensation, possession, or use of a controlled substance in the performance of the contract.

(b) SUSPENSION, TERMINATION, OR DEBARMENT OF THE CONTRACTOR.—

(1) GROUNDS FOR SUSPENSION, TERMINATION, OR DEBARMENT.—

Each contract awarded by a Federal agency shall be subject to suspension of payments under the contract or termination of the contract, or both, and the contractor thereunder or the individual who entered the contract with the Federal agency, as applicable, shall be subject to suspension or debarment in accordance with the requirements of this section if the head of the agency determines that—

(A) the contractor or individual has made a false certification under subsection (a);

(B) the contractor violates such certification by failing to carry out the requirements of subparagraph (A), (B), (C), (D), (E), or (F) of subsection (a)(1); or

(C) such a number of employees of such contractor have been convicted of violations of criminal drug statutes for violations occurring in the workplace as to indicate that the contractor has failed to make a good faith effort to provide a drug-free workplace as required by subsection (a).

(2) CONDUCT OF SUSPENSION, TERMINATION, AND DEBARMENT PROCEED-INGS.—(A) If a contracting officer determines, in writing, that cause for suspension of payments, termination, or suspension or debarment exists, an appropriate action shall be initiated by a contracting officer of the agency, to be conducted by the agency concerned in accordance with the Federal Acquisition Regulation and applicable agency procedures.

(B) The Federal Acquisition Regulation shall be revised to include rules for conducting suspension and debarment proceedings under this subsection, including rules providing notice, opportunity to respond in writing or in person, and such other procedures as may be necessary to provide a full and fair proceeding to a contractor or individual in such proceeding.

(3) EFFECT OF DEBARMENT.—Upon issuance of any final decision under this subsection requiring debarment of a contractor or individual, such contractor or individual shall be ineligible for award of any contract by any Federal agency, and for participation in any future procurement by any Federal agency, for a period specified in the decision, not to exceed 5 years.

SEC. 5153. DRUG-FREE WORKPLACE REQUIREMENTS FOR FEDERAL GRANT RECIPIENTS.

(a) DRUG-FREE WORKPLACE REQUIREMENT.—

(1) PERSONS OTHER THAN INDIVIDUALS.—No person, other than an individual, shall receive a grant from any Federal agency unless such person has certified to the granting agency that it will provide a drug-free workplace by—

(A) publishing a statement notifying employees that the unlawful manufacture, distribution, dispensation, possession, or use of a controlled substance is prohibited in the grantee's workplace and specifying the actions that will be taken against employees for violations of such prohibition;

(B) establishing a drug-free awareness program to inform employees about—

(i) the dangers of drug abuse in the workplace;

(ii) the grantee's policy of maintaining a drug-free workplace;

(iii) any available drug counseling, rehabilitation, and employee assistance programs; and

(iv) the penalties that may be imposed upon employees for drug abuse violations;

(C) making it a requirement that each employee to be engaged in the performance of such grant be given a copy of the statement required by subparagraph (A);

(D) notifying the employee in the statement required by subparagraph (A), that as a condition of employment in such grant, the employee will—

(i) abide by the terms of the statement; and

(ii) notify the employer of any criminal drug statute conviction for a violation occurring in the workplace no later than 5 days after such conviction;

(E) notifying the granting agency within 10 days after receiving notice of a conviction under subparagraph (D)(ii) from an employee or otherwise receiving actual notice of such conviction;

(F) imposing a sanction on, or requiring the satisfactory participation in a drug abuse assistance or rehabilitation program by, any employee who is so convicted, as required by section 5154; and

(G) making a good faith effort to continue to maintain a drug-free workplace through implementation of subparagraphs (A), (B), (C), (D), (E), and (F).

(2) INDIVIDUALS.—No Federal agency shall make a grant to any individuals unless such individual certifies to the agency as a condition of such grant that the individual will not engage in the unlawful manufacture, distribution, dispensation, possession, or use of a controlled substance in conducting any activity with such grant.

(b) SUSPENSION, TERMINATION, OR DEBARMENT OF THE GRANTEE.—

(1) GROUNDS FOR SUSPENSION, TERMINATION, OR DEBARMENT.—Each grant awarded by a Federal agency shall be subject to suspension of payments under the grant or termination of the grant, or both, and the grantee thereunder shall be subject to suspension or debarment, in accordance with the requirements of this section if the agency head of the granting agency or his official designee determines, in writing, that—

(A) the grantee has made a false certification under subsection (a);

(B) the grantee violates such certification by failing to carry out the requirements of subparagraph (A), (B), (C), (D), (E), (F), or (G) of subsection (a)(1); or

(C) such a number of employees of such grantee have been convicted of violations of criminal drug statutes for violations occurring in the workplace as to indicate that the grantee has failed to make a good faith effort to provide a drug-free workplace as required by subsection (a)(1).

(2) CONDUCT OF SUSPENSION, TERMINATION, AND DEBARMENT PROCEEDINGS.—A suspension of payments, termination, or suspension or debatement proceeding subject to this subsection shall be conducted in accordance with applicable law, including Executive Order 12549 or any superseding Executive order and any regulations promulgated to implement such law or Executive order.

(3) EFFECT OF DEBARMENT.—Upon issuance of any final decision under this subsection requiring debarment of a grantee, such grantee shall be ineligible for award of any grant from any Federal agency and for participation in any future grant from any Federal agency for a period specified in the decision, not to exceed 5years.

SEC. 5154. EMPLOYEE SANCTIONS AND REMEDIES.

A grantee or contractor shall, within 30 days after receiving notice from an employee of a conviction pursuant to section 5152(a)(1)(D)(ii) or 5153(a)(1)(D)(ii)—

(1) take appropriate personnel action against such employee up to and including termination; or

(2) require such employee to satisfactorily participate in a drug abuse assistance or rehabilitation program approved for such purposes by a Federal, State, or local health, law enforcement, or other appropriate agency.

SEC. 5155. WAIVER

(a) IN GENERAL—A termination, suspension of payments, or suspension or debarment under this subtitle may be waived by the head of an agency with respect to a particular contract or grant if—

(1) in the case of a waive with respect to a contract, the head of the agency determines under section 5152(b)(1), after the issuance of a final determination under such section, that suspension of payments, or termination of the contract, or suspension or debarment of the contractor, or refusal to permit a person to be treated as a responsible source for a contract, as the case may be, would severely disrupt the operation of such agency to the detriment of the Federal Government or the general public; or

(2) in the case of a waiver with respect to a grant, the head of the agency determines that suspension of payments, termination of the grant, or suspension or debarment of the grantee would not be in the public interest.

(b) EXCLUSIVE AUTHORITY.—The authority of the head of an agency under this section to waive a termination, suspension, or debarment shall be delegated.

SEC. 5156. REGULATIONS

Not later than 90 days after the date of enactment of this subtitle, the governmentwide regulations governing actions under this subtitle shall be issued pursuant to the Office of Federal Procurement Policy Act (41 U.S.C. 401 et seq.).

SEC. 5157. DEFINITIONS.

For purposes of this subtitle—

(1) ther term "drug-free workplace" means a site for the performance of work done in connection with a specific grant or contract described in section 5152 or 5153 of an entity at which employees of such entity are prohibited from engaging in the unlawful manufacture, distribution, dispensation, possession, or use of a controlled substance in accordance with the requirements of this Act;

(2) the term "employee" means the employee of a grantee or contractor directly engaged in the performance of work pursuant to the provisions of the grant or contract described in section 5152 or 5153;

(3) the term "controlled substance" means a controlled substance in schedules I through V of section 202 of the Controlled Substances Act (21 U.S.C. 812);

(4) the term "conviction" means a finding of guilt (including a plea of nolo contendere) or imposition of sentence, or both, by any judicial body charged with the responsibility to determine violations of the Federal or State criminal drug statutes;

(5) the term "criminal drug statute" means a criminal statute involving manufacture, distribution, dispensation, use, or possession of any controlled substance;

(6) the term "grantee" means the department, division or other unit of a person responsible for the performance under the grant;

(7) the term "contractor" means the department, division, or other unit of a person responsible for the performance under the contract; and

(8) the term "Federal agency" means an agency as that term is defined in section 552(f) of title 5, United States Code.

SEC. 5158. CONSTRUCTION OF SUBTITLE.

Nothing in this subtitle shall be construed to require law enforcement agencies, if the head of the agency determines it would be inappropriate in connection with the agency's undercover operations, to comply with the provisions of this subtitle.

SEC. 5159. REPEAL OF LIMITATION ON USE OF FUNDS.

Section 628 of Public Law 100-440 (relating to restrictions on the use of certain appropriated amounts) is amended—

(1) by striking "(a)" after "Sec. 628."; and

(2) by striking subsection (b).

SEC. 5160. EFFECTIVE DATE.

Sections 5152 and 5153 shall be effective 120 days after the date of the enactment of this subtitle.

Drug Testing Custody and Control Form

EMPLOYEE I.D. No. or SOCIAL SECURITY No.		DATE _____	DONOR'S INITIAL _____
SPECIMEN IDENTIFICATION No. **123456**	PLACE OVER CAP		SIGNATURE OF COLLECTOR

TO BE COMPLETED BY COLLECTOR OR EMPLOYER REPRESENTATIVE

I. EMPLOYER NAME, ADDRESS, AND IDENTIFICATION NUMBER

II. MEDICAL REVIEW OFFICER NAME AND ADDRESS

III. INDICATE WHICH DRUGS SPECIMEN IS TO BE TESTED FOR:
☐ Only THC and Cocaine   ☐ THC, Cocaine, PCP, Opiates, and Amphetamines   ☐ Other *(Specify):*_____

IV. REASON FOR TEST *(Check one)*
☐ Pre-employment   ☐ Random   ☐ Post Accident   ☐ Periodic Medical   ☐ Reasonable Cause   ☐ Other *(Specify):* _____

V. TEMPERATURE OF SPECIMEN
Has been read within 4 minutes   ☐ Yes   ☐ No
TEMPERATURE IS WITHIN RANGE
of 32.5°-37.7°C/90.5°-99.8°F   ☐ Yes   ☐ No—*If NOT, record actual temp:* _____°

TO BE INITIATED BY COLLECTOR AND COMPLETED AS NECESSARY THEREAFTER

VI.

PURPOSE OF CHANGE	RELEASED BY—Signature—Print Name	RECEIVED BY—Signature—Print Name	DATE
Provide Specimen for Testing	— DONOR —		

TO BE COMPLETED BY EMPLOYEE OR APPLICANT PROVIDING SPECIMEN

VII.

SPECIMEN IDENTIFICATION
No.   **123456**

SHIPPING BOX CUSTODY SEAL

FEDERAL REGULATIONS PROHIBIT DISCLOSURE OF THE DONOR'S IDENTITY TO THE LABORATORY.
DONOR SHALL COMPLETE INFORMATION IN SECTION VII (COPY 3) ONLY.

TO BE COMPLETED BY PERSON COLLECTING SPECIMEN *AFTER* DONOR HAS COMPLETED SECTION VII–*(See Copy 3 of Form)*

VIII. COLLECTOR'S NAME—*PRINT (first, middle, last)*   DATE OF COLLECTION

COLLECTION SITE LOCATION

REMARKS CONCERNING COLLECTION: Split sample collected in accordance with applicable Federal requirements. ☐ Yes   ☐ No

I certify that the specimen identified on this form is the specimen presented to me by the donor providing the certification on Copy 3 of this form, that it bears the same identification number as that set forth above, and that it has been collected, labelled and sealed as in accordance with applicable Federal requirements.

SIGNATURE OF COLLECTOR: _____

TO BE COMPLETED BY THE LABORATORY

IX. I certify that the specimen identified by this accession number is the same specimen that bears the identification number set forth above, that the specimen has been examined upon receipt, handled and analyzed in accordance with applicable Federal requirements, and that the results set forth below are for that specimen.   ACCESSION NO.

LABORATORY   ADDRESS

REMARKS:

(PRINT) Certifying Scientist's Name *(Last, First, Middle)*   Signature of Certifying Scientist   Date

THE RESULTS FOR THE ABOVE IDENTIFIED SPECIMEN ARE IN ACCORDANCE WITH THE APPLICABLE SCREENING AND CONFIRMATION CUTOFF LEVELS ESTABLISHED BY THE HHS *MANDATORY GUIDELINES FOR FEDERAL WORKPLACE DRUG TESTING PROGRAMS* (found only on copies one and two):

☐ NEGATIVE

☐ POSITIVE, for the following:
☐ Cannabinoids as Carboxy—THC
☐ Cocaine Metabolites as Benzoylecgonine
☐ Phencyclidine
☐ Opiates
☐ Codeine
☐ Morphine

☐ Amphetamines
☐ amphetamines
☐ methamphetamines

☐ _____

TO BE COMPLETED BY MEDICAL REVIEW OFFICER

X. I have reviewed the laboratory results for the specimen identified by this form in accordance with applicable Federal requirements. My final determination/verification is: *(Check one)* ☐ NEGATIVE   ☐ POSITIVE

SIGNATURE OF MEDICAL REVIEW OFFICER: _____   DATE: _____

COPY 1—ORIGINAL—MUST ACCOMPANY SPECIMEN TO LABORATORY—LABORATORY RETAINS

Drug Testing Custody and Control Form

EMPLOYEE I.D. No. or
SOCIAL SECURITY No.

| | | | | | | | | |

SPECIMEN IDENTIFICATION
No.   123456

TO BE COMPLETED BY COLLECTOR OR EMPLOYER REPRESENTATIVE

I.	EMPLOYER NAME, ADDRESS, AND IDENTIFICATION NUMBER
II.	MEDICAL REVIEW OFFICER NAME AND ADDRESS
III.	INDICATE WHICH DRUGS SPECIMEN IS TO BE TESTED FOR: ☐ Only THC and Cocaine ☐ THC, Cocaine, PCP, Opiates, and Amphetamines ☐ Other *(Specify)*:_____
IV.	REASON FOR TEST *(Check one)* ☐ Pre-employment ☐ Random ☐ Post Accident ☐ Periodic Medical ☐ Reasonable Cause ☐ Other *(Specify)*: _____
V.	TEMPERATURE OF SPECIMEN Has been read within 4 minutes ☐ Yes ☐ No TEMPERATURE IS WITHIN RANGE of 32.5°–37.7°C/90.5°–99.8°F ☐ Yes ☐ No—*If NOT, record actual temp:* _____°

TO BE INITIATED BY COLLECTOR AND COMPLETED AS NECESSARY THEREAFTER

	PURPOSE OF CHANGE	RELEASED BY—Signature—Print Name	RECEIVED BY—Signature—Print Name	DATE
VI.	Provide Specimen for Testing	**— DONOR —**		

TO BE COMPLETED BY EMPLOYEE OR APPLICANT PROVIDING SPECIMEN

VII.	SPECIMEN IDENTIFICATION No. 123456

FEDERAL REGULATIONS PROHIBIT DISCLOSURE OF THE DONOR'S IDENTITY TO THE LABORATORY.
DONOR SHALL COMPLETE INFORMATION IN SECTION VII (COPY 3) ONLY.

TO BE COMPLETED BY PERSON COLLECTING SPECIMEN *AFTER* DONOR HAS COMPLETED SECTION VII–*(See Copy 3 of Form)*

VIII.	COLLECTOR'S NAME—PRINT *(first, middle, last)* DATE OF COLLECTION
	COLLECTION SITE LOCATION
	REMARKS CONCERNING COLLECTION: Split sample collected in accordance with applicable Federal requirements. ☐ Yes ☐ No

I certify that the specimen identified on this form is the specimen presented to me by the donor providing the certification on Copy 3 of this form, that it bears the same identification number as that set forth above, and that it has been collected, labelled and sealed as in accordance with applicable Federal requirements.

SIGNATURE OF COLLECTOR: _____

TO BE COMPLETED BY THE LABORATORY

IX.	I certify that the specimen identified by this accession number is the same specimen that bears the identification number set forth above, that the specimen has been examined upon receipt, handled and analyzed in accordance with applicable Federal requirements, and that the results set forth below are for that specimen. ACCESSION NO.
	LABORATORY ADDRESS
	REMARKS:

(PRINT) Certifying Scientist's Name *(Last, First, Middle)*   Signature of Certifying Scientist   Date

THE RESULTS FOR THE ABOVE IDENTIFIED SPECIMEN ARE IN ACCORDANCE WITH THE APPLICABLE SCREENING AND CONFIRMATION CUTOFF LEVELS ESTABLISHED BY THE HHS *MANDATORY GUIDELINES FOR FEDERAL WORKPLACE DRUG TESTING PROGRAMS* (found only on copies one and two):

☐ NEGATIVE
☐ POSITIVE, for the following:
    ☐ Cannabinoids as Carboxy—THC
    ☐ Cocaine Metabolites as Benzoylecgonine
    ☐ Phencyclidine
    ☐ Opiates
       ☐ Codeine
       ☐ Morphine

☐ Amphetamines
    ☐ amphetamines
    ☐ methamphetamines

☐ _____

TO BE COMPLETED BY MEDICAL REVIEW OFFICER

X.	I have reviewed the laboratory results for the specimen identified by this form in accordance with applicable Federal requirements. My final determination/verification is: *(Check one)* ☐ NEGATIVE ☐ POSITIVE

SIGNATURE OF MEDICAL REVIEW OFFICER: _____   DATE: _____

**COPY 2—2ND ORIGINAL—MUST ACCOMPANY SPECIMEN TO LABORATORY
LAB SENDS TO MRO WITH TEST RESULTS IN SECT. IX**

Drug Testing Custody and Control Form

EMPLOYEE I.D. No. or
SOCIAL SECURITY No.

| | | | | | | |

SPECIMEN IDENTIFICATION
No.   **123456**

TO BE COMPLETED BY COLLECTOR OR EMPLOYER REPRESENTATIVE

I.	EMPLOYER NAME, ADDRESS, AND IDENTIFICATION NUMBER
II.	MEDICAL REVIEW OFFICER NAME AND ADDRESS
III.	INDICATE WHICH DRUGS SPECIMEN IS TO BE TESTED FOR: □ Only THC and Cocaine □ THC, Cocaine, PCP, Opiates, and Amphetamines □ Other *(Specify)*:_____
IV.	REASON FOR TEST *(Check one)* □ Pre-employment □ Random □ Post Accident □ Periodic Medical □ Reasonable Cause □ Other *(Specify)*: _____
V.	TEMPERATURE OF SPECIMEN Has been read within 4 minutes □ Yes □ No TEMPERATURE IS WITHIN RANGE of 32.5°-37.7°C/90.5°-99.8°F □ Yes □ No—*If NOT, record actual temp:* _____ °

TO BE INITIATED BY COLLECTOR AND COMPLETED AS NECESSARY THEREAFTER

VI.	PURPOSE OF CHANGE	RELEASED BY—Signature—Print Name	RECEIVED BY—Signature—Print Name	DATE
	Provide Specimen for Testing	— DONOR —		

TO BE COMPLETED BY EMPLOYEE OR APPLICANT PROVIDING SPECIMEN

VII.	NAME *(Last, First, Middle)*	SPECIMEN IDENTIFICATION No. 123456	DAYTIME PHONE NUMBER	DATE OF BIRTH

DONOR CERTIFICATION: I certify that I provided my urine specimen to the collector; that the specimen bottle was sealed with a tamper-proof seal in my presence; and that the information provided on this form and on the label affixed to the specimen bottle is correct.

SIGNATURE: _____   DATE: _____

Should the results of the laboratory tests for the specimen identified by this form be confirmed positive, the Medical Review Officer will contact you to ask about prescriptions and over-the-counter medications you may have taken. Therefore, you may want to make a list of those medications as a "memory jogger." THIS LIST IS NOT NECESSARY. If you choose to make a list, do so either on a separate piece of paper or on the back of your copy (Copy 4—Donor) of this form—DO NOT LIST ON THE BACK OF ANY OTHER COPY OF THE FORM. TAKE YOUR COPY WITH YOU.

TO BE COMPLETED BY PERSON COLLECTING SPECIMEN *AFTER* DONOR HAS COMPLETED SECTION VII—*(See Copy 3 of Form)*

VIII.	COLLECTOR'S NAME—*PRINT (first, middle, last)*	DATE OF COLLECTION
	COLLECTION SITE LOCATION	
	REMARKS CONCERNING COLLECTION:	Split sample collected in accordance with applicable Federal requirements. □ Yes □ No

I certify that the specimen identified on this form is the specimen presented to me by the donor providing the certification on Copy 3 of this form, that it bears the same identification number as that set forth above, and that it has been collected, labelled and sealed as in accordance with applicable Federal requirements.

SIGNATURE OF COLLECTOR: _____

COPY 3—TO MEDICAL REVIEW OFFICER

Drug Testing Custody and Control Form

EMPLOYEE I.D. No. or SOCIAL SECURITY No.

| , , , , , , , , , |

SPECIMEN IDENTIFICATION
No.   **123456**

TO BE COMPLETED BY COLLECTOR OR EMPLOYER REPRESENTATIVE

I.	EMPLOYER NAME, ADDRESS, AND IDENTIFICATION NUMBER
II.	MEDICAL REVIEW OFFICER NAME AND ADDRESS
III.	INDICATE WHICH DRUGS SPECIMEN IS TO BE TESTED FOR: ☐ Only THC and Cocaine ☐ THC, Cocaine, PCP, Opiates, and Amphetamines ☐ Other *(Specify)*:_____
IV.	REASON FOR TEST *(Check one)* ☐ Pre-employment ☐ Random ☐ Post Accident ☐ Periodic Medical ☐ Reasonable Cause ☐ Other *(Specify)*: _____
V.	TEMPERATURE OF SPECIMEN Has been read within 4 minutes ☐ Yes ☐ No TEMPERATURE IS WITHIN RANGE of 32.5°-37.7°C/90.5°-99.8°F ☐ Yes ☐ No—*If NOT, record actual temp:* _____°

TO BE INITIATED BY COLLECTOR AND COMPLETED AS NECESSARY THEREAFTER

VI.	PURPOSE OF CHANGE	RELEASED BY—Signature—Print Name	RECEIVED BY—Signature—Print Name	DATE
	Provide Specimen for Testing	— DONOR —		

TO BE COMPLETED BY EMPLOYEE OR APPLICANT PROVIDING SPECIMEN

VII.	NAME *(Last, First, Middle)*	SPECIMEN IDENTIFICATION No. 123456	DAYTIME PHONE NUMBER	DATE OF BIRTH

DONOR CERTIFICATION: I certify that I provided my urine specimen to the collector; that the specimen bottle was sealed with a tamper-proof seal in my presence; and that the information provided on this form and on the label affixed to the specimen bottle is correct.

SIGNATURE: _____ DATE: _____

Should the results of the laboratory tests for the specimen identified by this form be confirmed positive, the Medical Review Officer will contact you to ask about prescriptions and over-the-counter medications you may have taken. Therefore, you may want to make a list of those medications as a "memory jogger." THIS LIST IS NOT NECESSARY. If you choose to make a list, do so either on a separate piece of paper or on the back of your copy (Copy 4—Donor) of this form—DO NOT LIST ON THE BACK OF ANY OTHER COPY OF THE FORM. TAKE YOUR COPY WITH YOU.

TO BE COMPLETED BY PERSON COLLECTING SPECIMEN *AFTER* DONOR HAS COMPLETED SECTION VII–*(See Copy 3 of Form)*

VIII.	COLLECTOR'S NAME—PRINT *(first, middle, last)*	DATE OF COLLECTION
	COLLECTION SITE LOCATION	
	REMARKS CONCERNING COLLECTION:	Split sample collected in accordance with applicable Federal requirements. ☐ Yes ☐ No

I certify that the specimen identified on this form is the specimen presented to me by the donor providing the certification on Copy 3 of this form, that it bears the same identification number as that set forth above, and that it has been collected, labelled and sealed as in accordance with applicable Federal requirements.

SIGNATURE OF COLLECTOR: _____

COPY 4—DONOR

BACK-SIDE OF COPY 4—DONOR

LIST PRESCRIPTION DRUGS. *IT IS **NOT** REQUIRED, AND IS FOR **YOUR USE ONLY.***

_____

_____

_____

Drug Testing Custody and Control Form

EMPLOYEE I.D. No. or
SOCIAL SECURITY No.

| | | | | | | | | |

SPECIMEN IDENTIFICATION
No.   **123456**

TO BE COMPLETED BY COLLECTOR OR EMPLOYER REPRESENTATIVE

I.	EMPLOYER NAME, ADDRESS, AND IDENTIFICATION NUMBER
II.	MEDICAL REVIEW OFFICER NAME AND ADDRESS
III.	INDICATE WHICH DRUGS SPECIMEN IS TO BE TESTED FOR: ☐ Only THC and Cocaine ☐ THC, Cocaine, PCP, Opiates, and Amphetamines ☐ Other *(Specify):*_____
IV.	REASON FOR TEST *(Check one)* ☐ Pre-employment ☐ Random ☐ Post Accident ☐ Periodic Medical ☐ Reasonable Cause ☐ Other *(Specify):* _____
V.	TEMPERATURE OF SPECIMEN TEMPERATURE IS WITHIN RANGE Has been read within 4 minutes ☐ Yes ☐ No of 32.5°–37.7°C/90.5°–99.8°F ☐ Yes ☐ No—*If NOT, record actual temp:* _____°

TO BE INITIATED BY COLLECTOR AND COMPLETED AS NECESSARY THEREAFTER

	PURPOSE OF CHANGE	RELEASED BY—Signature—Print Name	RECEIVED BY—Signature—Print Name	DATE
VI.	Provide Specimen for Testing	**— DONOR —**		

TO BE COMPLETED BY EMPLOYEE OR APPLICANT PROVIDING SPECIMEN

VII.	NAME *(Last, First, Middle)* SPECIMEN IDENTIFICATION No. 123456

DONOR CERTIFICATION: I certify that I provided my urine specimen to the collector; that the specimen bottle was sealed with a tamper-proof seal in my presence; and that the information provided on this form and on the label affixed to the specimen bottle is correct.

SIGNATURE: _____   DATE: _____

TO BE COMPLETED BY PERSON COLLECTING SPECIMEN *AFTER* DONOR HAS COMPLETED SECTION VII–*(See Copy 3 of Form)*

VIII.	COLLECTOR'S NAME—*PRINT (first, middle, last)*	DATE OF COLLECTION
	COLLECTION SITE LOCATION	
	REMARKS CONCERNING COLLECTION:	Split sample collected in accordance with applicable Federal requirements. ☐ Yes ☐ No

I certify that the specimen identified on this form is the specimen presented to me by the donor providing the certification on Copy 3 of this form, that it bears the same identification number as that set forth above, and that it has been collected, labelled and sealed as in accordance with applicable Federal requirements.

SIGNATURE OF COLLECTOR: _____

COPY 5—COLLECTOR

Drug Testing Custody and Control Form

EMPLOYEE I.D. No. or
SOCIAL SECURITY No.

| | | | | | | |

SPECIMEN IDENTIFICATION
No.   123456

	TO BE COMPLETED BY COLLECTOR OR EMPLOYER REPRESENTATIVE
I.	EMPLOYER NAME, ADDRESS, AND IDENTIFICATION NUMBER
II.	MEDICAL REVIEW OFFICER NAME AND ADDRESS
III.	INDICATE WHICH DRUGS SPECIMEN IS TO BE TESTED FOR: ☐ Only THC and Cocaine ☐ THC, Cocaine, PCP, Opiates, and Amphetamines ☐ Other *(Specify):*_____
IV.	REASON FOR TEST *(Check one)* ☐ Pre-employment ☐ Random ☐ Post Accident ☐ Periodic Medical ☐ Reasonable Cause ☐ Other *(Specify):* _____
V.	TEMPERATURE OF SPECIMEN Has been read within 4 minutes ☐ Yes ☐ No TEMPERATURE IS WITHIN RANGE of 32.5°–37.7°C/90.5°–99.8°F ☐ Yes ☐ No—*If NOT, record actual temp:* _____ °

TO BE INITIATED BY COLLECTOR AND COMPLETED AS NECESSARY THEREAFTER

VI.	PURPOSE OF CHANGE	RELEASED BY—Signature—Print Name	RECEIVED BY—Signature—Print Name	DATE
	Provide Specimen for Testing	— DONOR —		

TO BE COMPLETED BY EMPLOYEE OR APPLICANT PROVIDING SPECIMEN

VII.	NAME *(Last, First, Middle)*	SPECIMEN IDENTIFICATION No. 123456	

DONOR CERTIFICATION: I certify that I provided my urine specimen to the collector; that the specimen bottle was sealed with a tamper-proof seal in my presence; and that the information provided on this form and on the label affixed to the specimen bottle is correct.

SIGNATURE: _____   DATE: _____

TO BE COMPLETED BY PERSON COLLECTING SPECIMEN *AFTER* DONOR HAS COMPLETED SECTION VII–*(See Copy 3 of Form)*

VIII.	COLLECTOR'S NAME—PRINT *(first, middle, last)*	DATE OF COLLECTION
	COLLECTION SITE LOCATION	
	REMARKS CONCERNING COLLECTION:	Split sample collected in accordance with applicable Federal requirements. ☐ Yes ☐ No

I certify that the specimen identified on this form is the specimen presented to me by the donor providing the certification on Copy 3 of this form, that it bears the same identification number as that set forth above, and that it has been collected, labelled and sealed as in accordance with applicable Federal requirements.

SIGNATURE OF COLLECTOR: _____

COPY 6—EMPLOYER

Drug Testing Custody and Control Form

EMPLOYEE I.D. No. or SOCIAL SECURITY No.

SPECIMEN IDENTIFICATION No. **123456** *-SPLIT*

PLACE OVER CAP

DATE _____

DONOR'S INITIAL _____

_____
SIGNATURE OF COLLECTOR

TO BE COMPLETED BY COLLECTOR OR EMPLOYER REPRESENTATIVE

I.	EMPLOYER NAME, ADDRESS, AND IDENTIFICATION NUMBER
II.	MEDICAL REVIEW OFFICER NAME AND ADDRESS
III.	INDICATE WHICH DRUGS SPECIMEN IS TO BE TESTED FOR: ☐ Only THC and Cocaine ☐ THC, Cocaine, PCP, Opiates, and Amphetamines ☐ Other *(Specify)*:_____
IV.	REASON FOR TEST *(Check one)* ☐ Pre-employment ☐ Random ☐ Post Accident ☐ Periodic Medical ☐ Reasonable Cause ☐ Other *(Specify)*: _____
V.	TEMPERATURE OF SPECIMEN Has been read within 4 minutes ☐ Yes ☐ No TEMPERATURE IS WITHIN RANGE of 32.5°–37.7°C/90.5°–99.8°F ☐ Yes ☐ No—*If NOT, record actual temp:* _____°

TO BE INITIATED BY COLLECTOR AND COMPLETED AS NECESSARY THEREAFTER

VI.	PURPOSE OF CHANGE	RELEASED BY—Signature—Print Name	RECEIVED BY—Signature—Print Name	DATE
	Provide Specimen for Testing	— DONOR —		

TO BE COMPLETED BY EMPLOYEE OR APPLICANT PROVIDING SPECIMEN

VII.	**SPECIMEN IDENTIFICATION** No. **123456** *-SPLIT* **SHIPPING BOX CUSTODY SEAL** FEDERAL REGULATIONS PROHIBIT DISCLOSURE OF THE DONOR'S IDENTITY TO THE LABORATORY. DONOR SHALL COMPLETE INFORMATION IN SECTION VII (COPY 3) ONLY.

TO BE COMPLETED BY PERSON COLLECTING SPECIMEN *AFTER* DONOR HAS COMPLETED SECTION VII–*(See Copy 3 of Form)*

VIII.	COLLECTOR'S NAME—*PRINT (first, middle, last)* DATE OF COLLECTION
	COLLECTION SITE LOCATION
	REMARKS CONCERNING COLLECTION: Split sample collected in accordance with applicable Federal requirements. ☐ Yes ☐ No
	I certify that the specimen identified on this form is the specimen presented to me by the donor providing the certification on Copy 3 of this form, that it bears the same identification number as that set forth above, and that it has been collected, labelled and sealed as in accordance with applicable Federal requirements. SIGNATURE OF COLLECTOR: _____

TO BE COMPLETED BY THE LABORATORY

IX.	I certify that the specimen identified by this accession number is the same specimen that bears the identification number set forth above, that the specimen has been examined upon receipt, handled and analyzed in accordance with applicable Federal requirements, and that the results set forth below are for that specimen. ACCESSION NO.
	LABORATORY ADDRESS
	REMARKS:

_____   _____   _____
(PRINT) Certifying Scientist's Name *(Last, First, Middle)*   Signature of Certifying Scientist   Date

THE RESULTS FOR THE ABOVE IDENTIFIED SPECIMEN ARE IN ACCORDANCE WITH THE APPLICABLE SCREENING AND CONFIRMATION CUTOFF LEVELS ESTABLISHED BY THE HHS *MANDATORY GUIDELINES FOR FEDERAL WORKPLACE DRUG TESTING PROGRAMS* (found only on copies one and two):

☐ NEGATIVE   ☐ POSITIVE, for the following:
   ☐ Cannabinoids as Carboxy—THC   ☐ Amphetamines
   ☐ Cocaine Metabolites as Benzoylecgonine   ☐ amphetamines
   ☐ Phencyclidine   ☐ methamphetamines
   ☐ Opiates
      ☐ Codeine   ☐ _____
      ☐ Morphine

TO BE COMPLETED BY MEDICAL REVIEW OFFICER

X.	I have reviewed the laboratory results for the specimen identified by this form in accordance with applicable Federal requirements. My final determination/verification is: *(Check one)* ☐ NEGATIVE ☐ POSITIVE SIGNATURE OF MEDICAL REVIEW OFFICER: _____ DATE: _____

COPY 7—SPLIT SPECIMEN ORIGINAL—MUST ACCOMPANY SPLIT SPECIMEN
TO LABORATORY—LABORATORY RETAINS

XIII
Family

46

The Family in Drug and Alcohol Addiction

Edward Kaufman
University of California, Irvine, California

Joseph P. Reoux*
University of California, Irvine, Medical Center, Orange, California

I. INTRODUCTION

The importance of family assessment and involvement in the diagnosis and treatment of drug and alcohol addiction cannot be overemphasized. Treatment of some addicted patients may work best when the entire family is available. Family participation is a strongly recommended component of the successful psychotherapy of drug and alcohol addiction [1]. In earlier work, Kaufman [2] has described family therapy as the most promising nonpharmacological intervention for the treatment of drug-dependent individuals and points out that families affect and are greatly affected by drug and alcohol addiction.

This chapter will first review and summarize the current state of knowledge about the family in drug and alcohol addiction. Familial biopsychosocial influences are discussed. Family systems theory is outlined and the family systems of addicted individuals are then examined in detail. Specific methods to involve the family are suggested and the efficacy of family involvement is presented. The chapter concludes with an overview of family treatment approaches and outlines a contemporary approach to family evaluation and treatment with drug- and alcohol-addicted persons.

II. FAMILY INFLUENCES

A. Heredity

Modern research has strongly indicated genetic factors in the disease of alcoholism. Twin studies show a higher concordance rate for alcoholism in monozygotic compared to dizygotic twins. For example, Kaij [3] found that the concordance rate for alcohol abuse in the monozygotic group was 54%, whereas in the dizygotic group it was 24%, a statistically significant difference. Adoption studies have found that children of alcoholics who are adopted away at birth are more likely to develop alcoholism than children of nonalcoholic biological

---

Current affiliation: Indian Health Service, Sitka, Alaska.

parents who are adopted away [4]. Family studies have shown first-degree relatives of alcoholics are more likely to be alcoholic than first-degreee relatives of nonalcoholics [5]. In their review of genetic heritability in the development of alcoholism, Mirin and Weiss [6] state the lifetime prevalence rate of alcoholism in parents and siblings of alcoholics is consistently found to be 30–40%, or three to four times the rate in the general population. Also, they observe about one out of three alcoholics have an alcoholic parent. Individuals may be born with a physical constitution that is more or less susceptible to addiction than other people, and this susceptibility is likely determined by genetics [7,8]. Studies of populations at high risk show children from alcoholic parents respond differently to alcohol than do children of nonalcoholics. The major consistent difference is significantly less intense reaction to alcohol in subjects with a positive family history for alcoholism, including less subjective intoxication, less impaired motor performance postdrinking, less alcohol-related change in cortisol, prolactin, and andrenocorticotropic hormone (ACTH) levels, and differences in certain brain wave measures [9].

Alcoholics with a history of alcoholism in first-degree relatives are found to have earlier onset and greater severity of alcoholism and more alcohol-related problems [10]. Earlier onset is seen in the offspring of two alcoholic parents compared to those of one alcoholic parent [11].

Knowledge in the field of alcoholism is well ahead of studies of other addictive drugs. Little is known about the biological vulnerability and genetic factors in drug addiction other than alcoholism. Pickens and Svikis [12] review the role of genetic influences in drug abuse. They also discuss the interaction of other factors (e.g., cultural, familial, and peer influences) and describe genetic research strategies. As in alcoholism, genetic factors could serve to either protect individuals from developing an addiction or make them more vulnerable.

Evidence suggests that the inheritance patterns may be similar for drug addiction and alcoholism. Cadoret and associates [13] conducted an adoption study of males and females separated from their biological parents at birth and correlated adult diagnoses of drug abuse with biological and environmental factors. They found evidence for two types of genetic factors in drug abuse. The first is drug abuse associated with antisocial behavior, as this study found antisocial behavior in biological relatives results in a higher likelihood of antisocial personality. The second genetic factor is alcohol problems in biological relatives, which correlated strongly with drug abuse in individuals without antisocial personality. Data on nonalcoholic drug use in the biological parents were not available in the adoption agency records, so specificity of transmission could not be determined.

Meller and associates [14] examine the specificity of familial transmission in drug and alcohol addiction. In first-degree relatives of probands who were addicted to drugs only (and not alcohol), 18.5% had a positive history of drug abuse only and 26% of the first-degree relatives abused both drugs and alcohol. Of probands who were addicted to alcohol only, 3% had a first degree family history positive for drug abuse only and a 14% positive history for first-degree relatives who abused both drugs and alcohol. Their results support their hypothesis that a specific transmission occurs. Weiss and associates [15] found a significantly higher rate of alcoholism in the first-degree relatives of alcoholic drug-dependent inpatients compared to the first-degree relatives of nonalcoholic hospitalized drug-dependent inpatients.

The application of family pedigree methods in assessing biological vulnerability to drug addiction is reviewed by Stabenau [16]. He concludes that, as in alcoholism, family pedigree study of drug addiction provides a valuable method for assessing biological vulnerability or risk factors. These studies may suggest personality and biochemical variables and mechanisms of drug-seeking behavior.

B. Family Psychosocial Influence

Investigations into the heredity of alcohol and drug addiction have not proposed that non-biological factors are unimportant. In Cadoret's adoption study [13], environmental factors such as divorce and psychiatric disturbance in adoptive families were also associated with increased drug use. Donovan [17] reviews the present etiological models of alcoholism and emphasizes the multidimensional etiology that involves hereditary, environmental, and psychostructural risk factors. An individual's family is certainly significant to all these risk factors. The popular press literature abounds with works that recognize the family as a factor in the complex etiology of addictive disorders (e.g., see Refs. 18 and 19) and the effects of growing up in a family with an alcoholic member (e.g., see Refs. 20 and 21).

With or without a biopsychosocial predilection for alcohol or drug addiction, use typically begins in adolescence. MacDonald (22) describes the stages of adolescent drug use and the important role of both family and peers. Excessive independence given to adolescents may be related to increased drug use [23], whereas strong parental control tends to be protective [24]. For marijuana, the stronger the family's attitude of disapproval, the less likely the children will use this drug [25]. In an Australian study [26], a significant relationship between perceived family closeness and each of the variables of drinking and drug-taking behavior was found. Perceived helpfulness of the parents appeared to be very important. The results indicate the adolescents want parents to be more interested in them and more involved in their activities.

Swardi's study [27] of 3333 London adolescents showed both family and peers influenced drug taking. When both family and peers used drugs 69% of the adolescents used repeatedly and 79% used at least once. When neither family nor peers took drugs only 3% used repeatedly and 13% reported to ever have tried drugs. When family and peer attitudes were different, peer influence was more important than family attitudes as to whether or not the adolescent took drugs. This study assessed the adolescents' perceived attitudes of the whole family, not only the parents.

Family ethnic and sociocultural differences influence rates of alcohol and drug addiction. Bales [28] analyzed cultural differences in rates of alcoholism and concludes there are three general ways in which culture and social organization can influence rates of alcoholism. The first is the degree to which the culture brings about acute needs for adjustment (inner tension and anxiety) in its members. The second is the group's attitude toward drinking. And third, the degree to which the culture provides substitute relief of inner tension and anxiety is thought to influence the rate of alcoholism.

Ethnicity exerts its influence by affecting family attitudes toward alcohol and drug addiction and by affecting family functioning style [29]. Glassner [30] compares and contrasts Irish American and Jewish American drinking patterns and states each ethnic group in America has its own ways of drinking and control. He outlines the "cultural recipe" in which a culture describes which substances, amounts, and for what reason are proper to use. Cultural recipes help describe the effects of be obtained from the drug and the culturally acceptable circumstances to use it.

In a discussion of sociocultural factors Blum (31) states that relevant research has shown for groups that use alcohol to a significant degree the lowest incidence of alcoholism is associated with the following considerations: early exposure within a strong family or relfgous group that uses diluted small quantities of alcohol, uses alcohol with beverages containing large amounts of nonalcoholic components, and consumption of alcohol with meals (alcohol considered as a food), all of which give low blood alcohol levels. Parents presenting an example of moderate drinking appears to be significant. Other attitudes thought to inhibit destructive drinking patterns include no moral importance attached to alcohol, drinking not viewed as proof of adulthood or virility, social acceptance of abstinence, and social disapproval of excessive drinking or intoxication. Most important Blum concludes, is wide and complete agreement among group members on the rules of drinking.

The groups with the highest reported incidence of alcoholism have been the northern French, Americans (especially Irish Americans), Swedes, Swiss, Poles, and northern Russions. Low-incidence groups include the Italians, some Chinese groups, Orthodox Jews, Greeks, Portuguese, Spanairds, and the southern French [31].

In the United States, high rates of alcoholism appear in Irish Americans [32,33], American Indians [34] and urban blacks and Hispanics. The latter two groups have been understudied but targeted as special populations at risk and in need of study [35]. High rates of alcohol consumption do not necessarily correspond to high rates of alcoholism. For example, Italian Americans traditionally are high consumers but have a low incidence of alcoholism.

Cultural beliefs and traditions help shape a family's and individual's concepts of illness or dysfunction, and may be very different from those of the therapist. Jalali [36] discusses the implications of ethnicity, cultural adjustment, and behavior for working therapeutically with families. The author emphasizes the importance of awareness and understanding of the practice and attitudes of the ethnic group being treated. Furthermore, the generation of immigration, degree of ethnic identification, and expression of traditional values must be considered. Kaufman and Borders [29] delineate familial patterns of interaction and attitudes toward alcohol and drug addiction in several American ethnic groups.

II. FAMILY SYSTEMS

A. Family Systems Theory

Systems theory views the family as an open dynamic system with boundaries, constraints, and subsystems. These interdependent parts are more or less fluid and function together as a basic structural unit or nucleus for the family members to self-organize around. Subsystems consist of individuals, dyads, triads, and more (e.g., parental, sibling, and male subsystems). Affecting one part of the system affects all others, and the system continuously reorganizes and works to reach relative stability. The system is inherently divided horizontally (e.g., siblings) and vertically (different generations). When working with family systems one must consider generations in the upward direction (at least parents and grandparents) as well as the downward (children) [37,38,39].

The family system has certain boundaries (rules defining who can participate in what and how) that range from being inappropriately rigid (disengaged: lack of sufficient connection between individuals) to inappropriately diffuse (enmeshed: lack of sufficient differentiation between individuals). Clear subsystem boundaries encourage proper family functioning and are a useful parameter for evaluation. Subsystems help the family to differentiate its members. The different subsystems contain different hierarchies (levels of power) and different complementary relationships (e.g., a daughter in one subsystem is a sister in another and a mother in still another).

The system must react to change and adapt to stress placed upon it. The system may resist change and has the ability to regulate, balance, and restabilize itself (homeostasis). Systems will show different degrees of flexibility and rigidity when reacting to change and stress. In systems theory causality is seen not as one to one cause and effect, but rather each perturbation affects all component parts, which in turn stimulate a new cycle of perturbation. Important family system constraints include leadership, boundaries (of the family, subsystems, and individuals), and ways of communicating, expressing feelings, and performing family functions. These are also important clinical parameters [37–39].

Drug addiction and alcoholism can be viewed as a symptom of a dysfunctional family system in which the addicted person emerges as the identified patient of the system. The addiction and the associated behaviors evolve within the family and become an integral part of that system, helping to define roles, boundaries, and subsystems. The use of alcohol or drugs becomes a part of the family's sense of equilibrium. Removing the drug use or even addressing it in a new manner significantly stresses the system, and sometimes to intolerable distress, prompting the family to sabotage treatment or drop out. The clinician must be aware of the distress treatment causes, which can intensify alcohol and drug use or elicit an entirely new symptom of family pathology.

Reviewing the history of the family system in alcohol and drug addiction shows that two separate literatures evolved: one for alcoholics and the other for drug addicts. Most studies on families of alcoholics have focused on the male alcoholic in his 40s and his overinvolved spouse [40]. Most studies of drug addicts have focused on youths (in their teens or 20s) and their parents. More recently, on closer examination, it was discovered that frequently these are actually the same family system, but being viewed from different generations. Thus, the most recent focus has been on the three- or four-generational system of the family of addicted individuals regardless of the age of the identified patient or the choice of drug.

B. The Family System in Alcoholism

The Total Family System in Alcoholism

Some family patterns are unique to alcoholism and some are seen in other types of dysfunctional families. Pattison and Kaufman [41] describe four distinct family interactional patterns. The first is the Functional Family System, the family with a practicing alcoholic member. These families have learned to function well and are responsive to external change. A minimum of overt conflict exists and the focus of the family is likely on the alcoholic. Drinking may be more the result of individual personal or social conflicts, and excessive drinking is frequently done away from the home. This type of family system is common in early phases of alcoholism and deteriorates with time.

The second family type is the Neurotic Enmeshed Family System in which the entire family behaves in an "alcoholic" manner, focusing on alcohol. In these families, drinking interrupts normal family tasks and creates conflict, role shifts, and demands for adaptive responses. Physical, emotional, and interpersonal problems due to alcoholism further exacerbate the situation.

A third pattern is the Disintegrated Family System or the separated family. Here progressive biopsychosocial deterioration and family instability leads to a destitute family and an alcoholic alienated from the nuclear family and relatives. This is frequently a later stage of the neurotic enmeshment system. Past history shows adequate family functioning, but at this point the family system has collapsed. These families will not reconstitute during the early treatment phase of the alcoholic. Potential family relationships may be explored and contact initiated where appropriate, but more often substantive work will need to wait for several months of stability to be achieved by the alcoholic.

Last, Pattison and Kaufman [41] described the Absent Family System or the long-term isolated alcoholic. This may be an end-stage deterioration, but more frequently the isolated alcoholic lost the family of origin early in the course of illness. Often such persons have had few if any significant relationships and few life skills. Alcoholics with an absent family system do best in a structured, partially institutionalized social support system [40].

Steinglass [42] uses family systems theory to see family behavior as responsive to two major forces: a morphostatic force (family homeostatic resistance to change and regulatory mechanisms that maintain stability) and a morphogenic force (family reorganization associated with growth, change, or development). In many alcoholic families, alcohol is the central focus and organizing principal around which most family interactions are focused [43], and family stability becomes dependent on alcohol-related phenomena. Acute stability is emphasized, whereas long-term growth is sacrificed. The family's development is distorted by the consequences of alcoholism and the organization of the family around alcohol [42].

In earlier work, Steinglass and associates [44] found that different family behaviors occur in association with active drinking and with sobriety. Alcohol and associated family behaviors offer a temporary solution to perturbations of the family system by conflict or chronic problems. Thus, the family cycles between the sober interactional state (dry) and the intoxicated interactional state (wet).

Steinglass [43] also examined the alcoholic family interactional patterns over periods of months or years. The model suggests the alcoholic family progresses through developmental phases characterized by the drinking status of the alcoholic (wet or dry) and the relative stability of the phase (stable or unstable). The alcoholic family may also be in transition (transitional phase) between phases (unstable or stable wet or dry). These approaches are integrated, and diagrammed schematically by Steinglass [42] with attention being given to family development stage and options which are framed by decisions about alcohol. Steinglass' work has demonstrated when a family is wet, individuals function more independently and disengaged with little coordination between family members. Dry families approach problems together with more unity.

Regardless of the type of family system, alcoholism has a major effect on the family. Alcoholics have extensive problems in their marriages and families [45], including more arguments [46], child and spouse abuse [47,48], and violence [49]. A series of escalating family crises may bring a catastrophic disturbance of the family's system's structure and function. The economic, psychological, emotional, and physical consequences of alcoholism create further conflict and problems that the family system may not know how to respond to in a healthy adaptive manner [41]. Instead, such families tend to exhibit rigid external boundaries [50] with internal interpersonal boundaries that are often diffuse and enmeshed. If family boundaries and rules become organized around alcohol, there is a greater chance alcoholism will be passed on to later generations and the family has a poorer prognosis [51].

Conversely, family problems and conflict serve to evoke, support, and maintain drinking behavior. Conflict between two members of the family system may be displaced onto a third party, issue, or substance such as alcohol [52]. Alcoholism can be a coping mechanism for the alcoholic and the family to deal with dysfunctional patterns and relationships, and in this way be a symptom of pathological family styles, rules, and patterns of alcohol use [51].

Viewed in this manner, alcoholism is both the cause and effect of family dysfunction and problems. Alcohol use and its consequences are dynamically related in a reciprocal manner to the family system and alcohol fills a specific need of the family system in ways that are purposeful, adaptive, and meaningful [53,54].

Early clinical studies of alcoholic families looked at the male alcoholic and his nonalcoholic wife. The stereotype that nonalcoholic spouses chose alcoholics or potential alcoholics as partners to satisfy unconscious needs and then perpetuate alcoholism to gratify these needs does not hold up under empirical research for both women [40,55,56] or men [57,58]. Earlier findings [59] that some wives suffer from psychological or psychosomatic illness upon the husband's recovery has been repeatedly disproven. Psychopathology may not be more prevalent among spouses of alcoholics than spouses of nonalcoholics [60].

As individuals, spouses are certainly impacted by the alcoholic's drinking. They are affected by their partners characteristics as well as by the stressful life events related to drinking. Spouses of alcoholics have more alcohol consumption themselves, more negative life events, fewer social and recreational activities, more depression and medical conditions, more job changes, and less family cohesiveness [61]. When the alcoholic stops drinking, the negative effects upon the spouse diminish [61]. The negative effects upon the spouse do not always worsen when the alcoholic drinks, however. A relationship is found between high alcohol consumption by the alcoholic and higher degree of satisfaction in the spouses of steady drinkers but not binge drinkers [62]. Similarly, symptomatology was reduced in spouses of steady drinkers during times of high alcohol consumption. This demonstrates how alcohol steadies the homeostasis in some family systems.

Frankenstein, Hay, and Nathan [63] showed that alcoholics, while intoxicated spoke more than when sober. The couples they studied increased the numbers of statements indicating approval, agreement, and positive feelings while intoxicated than when sober, especially by the nonalcoholic spouse. The level of statements indicative of criticism and disagreement remained stable.

The extent to which drinking causes problems in family functioning is a significant determining factor of the level of distress in the alcoholic marriage [64]. Factors associated with higher alcohol use correlate with a detrimental impact on the martial relationship, and when alcohol-related problems were statistically controlled, the correlations between consumption and marital satisfaction are greatly reduced or not significant [64].

Examination of marital interactional dynamics, roles, expectations, and patterns, especially as related to alcohol use, show a high incidence of blaming, competition for dominance, responsibility avoidance by alcoholics, and a high incidence of negative affect in alcoholic-spouse interactions. Male alcoholics exceed their spouses, control husbands, and control spouses in the use of responsibility-avoiding messages when communication patterns between couples are examined [65]. Both the alcoholic and his wife are highly competitive and cooperate less than other couples [65]. The alcoholic's wife may appear dominating because she is responsible and direct, but she is unable to control her husband [65]. Paolino and McCrady [66] described how these alcoholic and nonalcoholic spouse "couples blame each other, put each other down, turn each other off, and compete for dominance. They side track each other, do not come up with solutions, and then terminate communication, leading to the alcoholic fleeing the scene to drink."

Chiles and associates [67] compared alcoholic couples with sexual dysfunction to nonalcoholic couples with sexual dysfunction and found no difference in wives dominance as described by either husband or wife. However, alcoholic husbands saw themselves as most submissive, although their wives disagreed. The authors suggest the male alcoholics feel submissive because of their own needs to misperceive the situation.

Male alcoholics tend to present their marriage in an unrealistically favorable manner and report that drinking has not impacted the marriage, whereas the spouse will report considerable marital discord and dissatisfaction [68].

In poorer prognosis alcoholic families, the wives gave and recieved little affection, used few socially desirable adjectives to describe their husbands when sober, and expected their alcoholic husbands to use "hostile-dominance" adjectives or phrases [69]. The marital interactions of alcoholics and their wives were found to be more pathological than nondistressed couples [70]. However, alcoholic couples did not differ significantly from distressed nonalcoholic couples. Both the alcoholic couples and the distressed couples manifested more negative and hostile acts and fewer rational problem-solving statements than the nonalcoholic nondistressed couples [70].

Jacob and associates [71] studied alcoholic families both with the identified patient sober and under the influence of alcohol and compared them to normal families. Interactions between the alcoholic and spouse revealed more negative affect than in the normal family couples. The presence of alcohol increased this type of interaction. This is in contrast to the findings of Frankenstein and associates [63] in which intoxicated alcoholics spoke more and with increased numbers of positive statements than when sober. However, the alcoholics exhibited fewer positive nonverbal communication behavior (e.g., smiling, eye contact, touching) and more negative behavior (e.g., not acknowledging spouses behavior) than their nonalcoholic spouses [63]. Alcoholic fathers showed less leadership, assertiveness, and problem-solving behavior with the spouse and children [71]. Family functioning is affected by how well the alcoholic's nonalcoholic spouse adapts to the pattern of use and the spouse's own level of dysfunction [72].

The Female Alcoholic

Until recently, the alcoholism literature has ignored the specific nature of the female patient. Certain specific aspects of the family of the female alcoholic are consistently different from the family of alcoholic males. Of course, on an individual basis neither all females nor all males are alike and a wide range of variability is seen.

Drinking by women is related to the problems of women in our society in general, such as lack of social power and the external pressure to suppress those aspects of self which do not conform to female sex role stereotypes [73]. When female alcoholics compare themselves to nonalcoholic women, they see themselves as less socially competent and less effective in goal acheivement. Women alcoholics experience more anxiety and feel unworthy and dissatisfied with their purpose in life [74]. Alcoholic women have substantially more depression than do alcoholic men [75].

Alcohol use by the spouse is also an important factor. If both spouses drink addictively, they tend to support each other in continued alcoholism. Women are frequently introduced to alcohol and drugs by men [76], and alcoholic women are more likely to be married to an alcoholic spouse [77]. Women often state that problems in the marriage are the reasons they drink [78]. Alcoholic women have a high divorce rate and they are more frequently left by their spouses than are alcoholic men [79]. Sexual dysfunction in alcoholic women is common [80].

Estep [81] discusses the influence of the family on alcohol and prescription drug use by women. Using interviews and questionnaires, she concludes that those women who sought treatment for their use of both alcohol and depressant drugs, when compared to controls, have companions who drink more heavily and more frequently as well as take prescription depressants more often. These women appear to have been through more marriages and had more abortions, miscarriages, and childbirths. In addition, the women in treatment had higher incidences of arrests, which may create problematic separations from their families. Whether these problems are more a cause or effect of alcohol and drug use was not determined by this study.

Women react with shame and tend to hide their drinking from their families more than men, and their families tend to deny drinking by their maternal figures [77]. Glatt [82] noted that even women who have lost control of their drinking manage to limit their intake with family and friends. Instead, women commonly drink alone during the day at home. Female alcoholics who work may more easily hide alcohol and drug addiction through nonchallenging jobs or excessive absenteeism [83]. Alcoholic women more readily lose their role as wife while holding on to their role as mother, which is the final aspect of social functioning to be lost in alcoholic mothers [79]. Alcoholic mothers are more prone to abuse their children through neglect rather than violently or sexually, however. When they do seek treatment, women experience significantly more problems because of entering treatment (economic, familial, or social) and encounter more opposition to treatment from family and friends than do men [84].

Beyond the nuclear family, the family of origin of female alcoholics has consistently been shown to have high prevalence rates of alcoholism. The finding that female alcoholics are more likely than male alcoholics to have alcoholic parents has been demonstrated by many studies [84], Winokur and Clayton [86] showed that compared to men, alcoholic women had a higher prevalence of alcoholism in their fathers (28 vs 21%), mothers (12 vs 3%), and female siblings (12 vs 3%). Estep [81] found that women who sought treatment for alcohol and prescription depressant problems had parents who more likely drank to excess, more likely to quarrel, and less likely to stay together than the parents of the control group.

An emotionally disruptive family background is a common finding in female alcoholics. Wilsnack [87] noted alcoholic women have a high rate of family disruption, including loss of one or both parents through death, divorce, or separation and alcoholism or psychosis in parents or close relatives. Gomberg [88] found that rates of such disruption are high in both alcoholic men and women, but they are higher in women.

Many female alcoholics perceive that they had cold, severe, bossy, domineering mothers and warmer, gentler, but alcoholic fathers who only when drunk rebelled against their dominant wives [77]. These daughters tended to reject their mothers and felt if the mothers had been more loving, the fathers would have not drank. Not only did these daughters feel that their alcoholic fathers preferred them to their mothers, the daughters gravitated to their fathers for affection and support they felt they did not receive from their mothers. Their lack of positive female role models may have left them with a lack of female identity, making them vulnerable to alcoholism. Strong identification with their fathers also left them increasingly vulnerable to alcoholism as an adult.

Yandow's [89] review of alcoholism in women showed that alcoholism is both the cause and effect of dysfunctional sexuality. Futhermore, she states as many as 75% of women in treatment for alcoholism have a history of sexual abuse, usually starting in childhood and frequently continuing until the time the patient enters treatment. Not addressing the issue of sexual abuse hinders recovery and relapse prevention [90].

In contrast, Glenn and Parsons [91] examined the relationship of gender influences on 27 psychosocial and historical variables in alcoholics with a positive family history for alcoholism, alcoholics with negative family histories, and nonalcoholic controls. They concluded gender is a relatively noninfluential factor in the correlates studied (categorized as family of origin; childhood attention deficit, conduct and learning disorders; psychological variables; peers and family of procreation; and sociocultural - community variables), and that alcoholism and family history of alcoholism are factors having additive effects in a way similar for both men and women.

Children of Alcoholics

Early research on alcoholism neglected the roles and functions of children in the alcoholic family and the consequences of alcoholism on these children. Cork's work [92] helped to focus attention on the children of alcoholics. In their review, El-Guebaly and Offord [93] comment on the lack of well-designed controlled studies in this area and unclear definitions at that time. The review suggest that children of alcoholics are at increased risk for the development of emotional and psychosocial problems. Wilson and Orford [46] discuss the family relationships of their study subjects with the literature in general and found the child's relationship to the nonalcoholic parent and the degree of marital conflict to be important factors influencing the effect of parental alcoholism, which is consistent with the literature reviewed.

More recently, Black and associates [94] studied adult children of alcoholics responses to a questionnaire and found 37% described themselves as alcoholic (compared to 9.5% of controls), more often married alcoholics (20.7 vs 12.9%), and more frequently had alcoholic relatives. These adult children of alcoholics indicated that as children they did not have available interpersonal resources and continued to have interpersonal difficulties in adult life (e.g., problems with trust, dependency, responsibility, expressing feelings). Family disruption (e.g., divorce, death), verbal arguments, physical violence or abuse, and feeling responsible for parental conflict was reported more often in the chilhdoods of adult children of alcoholics than in the control group.

Beletsis and Brown [95] also found adult children of alcoholics to have poor communication skills, difficulty expressing feelings, role and identity confusion, and overresponsibility. They experience problems with trust and intimacy and have emotionally conflicted family relationships. Many alcoholic homes are unstable emotionally with little family unity and family experiences social isolation, parental fighting, spouse abuse, and/or divorce [96,97]. Adult children of alcoholics are at higher risk for divorce, sons are at higher risk for problem drinking, and daughters at increased risk for depression [98].

Giglio and Kaufman [99] review the literature and propose that adult children of alcoholics have certain role behaviors, identity issues, and personality characteristics that relate to childhood family dysfunction as a continuation of psychopathology, an adaptation to childhood roles, or a maladaptive response to trauma. The work of Cermack [100] likens such a childhood to trauma with a reexperiencing of the trauma as adults. The defensive mechanisms and feelings elicited are similar to those seen in posttraumatic stress disorder. While many similarities exist between being raised in an alcoholic home and posttraumatic stress disorder in terms of experiences and responses, differentiating personality traits are being elucidated [101].

Adult children of alcoholics may perceive their family of origin as having rigid coping skills and lacking sufficient adaptability [48]. Childhood opportunities to learn and develop healthier, diverse adaptive behaviors would be limited, and adult children of alcoholics will repeat patterns of drug addiction and patterns of emotional, physical, and sexual abuse across generations [101].

Children of alcoholics who do not develop serious coping problems are distinguished from their peers by more attention from the primary caretaker early in life, absence of prolonged separations, and no additional sibling birth during the first 2 years [102]. Birth order was not examined. Keltner and associates [103] found birth-order effects in children of alcoholics to be significant in that firstborne evidenced less exaggerated psychopathology than later-born siblings.

Wegschieder [104] relates family role to birth order as follows. The eldest is often the family "hero," a compliant overachiever whose function is to provide self-worth to the family system. Inside the hero feels responsible for the family's distress, inadequate, and angry. Frequently the eldest child must function as a responsible parental child and becomes involved intensively with the nonalcoholic parent. The "scapegoat" is typically the second or middle child whose role as troublemaker provides distraction from conflict and focuses the family system. The scapegoat withdraws and often acts out the anger, loneliness, and rejection felt inside in a destructive and irrresponsible manner. The "lost child" functions to offer relief to the family system and withdraws emotionally and physically, not wanting to cause additional problems or demands. Consequently, this child, who is often third born, receives little attention or nurturing, and appears aloof and independent. Inside are feelings of hurt, loneliness, and inadequacy. The youngest child is frequently the family "mascot," who has the role of providing fun and humor for the painful family system. The mascot diverts attention with entertainment. This child remains immature and experiences insecurity, confusion, and loneliness underneath the exterior clowning. Black [105] describes family roles in a similar way. The "responsible one" assumes parental functions and attempts to provide structure and stability for the family system. These children are rewarded for their dependability, organization, and control. The "adjuster role" child detaches and becomes passive or follows an older sibling, underachieving and failing to live up to potential. Third, the "placater" overfunctions on the emotional level and tries to smooth the system over. Like Wegscheider's mascot, the placater tends to underfunction on the functional level.

Rhodes and Blackham [106] looked at these role characteristics in adolescents from alcoholic and nonalcoholic homes. The adolescents from alcoholic homes rated themselves a higher acting-out role and a tendency toward placater and adjuster characteristics, although not to a statistically significant level. No effect of birth order was found.

Bepko [107] describes alcoholic parents as unable to nurture or set limits appropriately, inconsistent with their expectations and messages, and in need of the child's approval. The parent's sense of adequacy is threatened if the child expresses any independent feelings. The children are allowed the roles of parental caretaker, surrogate spouse, or neglected child.

Codependency

The patterns that develop in nonalcoholic family members have been labeled coalcoholism, or more recently codependency. A codependent person is one who has let another person's behavior affect him or her to the point of becoming obsessed with controlling that person's behavior [108]. The codependent passes through an early phase of denial, rationalization, and hopes that the addictive behavior will improve. The codependent feels responsible and directs much attention to taking over responsibility for the addict, enabling the addiction to continue without consequences because of the compulsion to rescue. In the middle phase, hostility, disgust, pity, and protectiveness of the addict are common. In advanced stages, hostility, withdrawal, and suspiciousness become generalized. Finally, feelings of responsibility and a need to control the addict become all encompassing [109].

Cermack [110] states at the core of codependency are denial and an unrealistic relationship to willpower, and he proposes considering codependence as a personality disorder with unique characteristics. The need for a self-help group, such as Alanon, is emphasized to facilitate recovery. Participation in an Alanon program was found to be beneficial to adult children of alcoholics, many of whom reported positive changes in self and improvements in problems [111]. Reported changes in the relationship with the alcoholic were few. The codependent is typically in the prime enabler role [104], repeatedly rescuing the dependent and equates love to being needed by others.

C. Family Systems in Drug Addiction

Much of the literature on family treatment approaches to the addictions focuses on acoholism. However, as Steinglass [42] suggests in his family systems approach to alcoholism, families with other forms of drug addiction have parallels with alcoholism and relevant comments on alcoholic families can be applied to family systems in drug addiction. There is an increasing awareness in the field that many similarities exist between the two types of families. Families with an alcoholic parent frequently produce both drug-addicted and alcoholic children [5,112] and the incidence of drug addiction in alcoholics and alcoholism in addicts is increasing [113], leading to further fusion of the two types of families. Kaufman and Kaufmann [114] describe characteristics of families with an addicted member. They emphasize the drug addict as the symptom carrier of family dysfunction and the addict's role in maintaining family homeostasis. The addict's behavior reinforces a need for the parents to control, yet the addict finds the parenting inadequate. Generational boundaries are diffuse and cross-generational alliances can promote parental divisions and competitions, which in turn allows the addict to provide a displaced focus for parental strife.

Stanton and Todd [115] summarize the distinguishing qualities of family systems of drug-addicted persons from other dysfunctional families. There is a high frequency of multigenerational drug dependency and an extreme incidence of unexpected or untimely deaths, expression of conflict that is direct and primitive, typically a mother who demonstrates symbiotic child-rearing practices which extend into the child's later life, a pseudoindependence through active involvement with a drug-oriented peer group, and pseudoindividuation that maintains family ties through a facade of defiance. A majority of drug addicts maintain close family ties for years [116], and a majority have involvement with their family on a daily (or live with) basis [117]. A large majority (88%) of the families of heroin addicts studied by Kaufman [118] had mothers emotionally enmeshed with their addicted child (mostly sons) to the extent that their happiness or sorrow were totally dependent on the behavior and closeness with these children. Kaufman and Kaufmann [114] found 88% of the mothers of heroin addicts were enmeshed with the addict and 3% disengaged, as rated on videotape observation by experienced clinicians. Forty-three percent of fathers were found to be disengaged, whereas 41% were rated as enmeshed with their addict child. In a study of adolescent drug abusers' families, Friedman and associates [119] found the majority of families categorized themselves as disengaged rather than enmeshed; however, family therapists characterized significantly more of these same families as enmeshed rather than disengaged. Families see themselves differently than the clinicians do.

Cancrini and associates [120] propose a classification of adolescent heroin addicts and their families into four classes. The first is traumatic drug addiction (type A), in which heroin use provides protection from panic and distress in the face of a harmful event (e.g., death, divorce). Typically, these users seek numbness and to mask guilt. Drug addiction from actual neuroses (type B) is characterized by an ongoing active conflict. Family structure is characterized by overinvolvement of one parent, peripheral role of the other parent, weak family subsystem boundaries, polarized "good" and "bad" siblings, and communication with contradictory messages and rapidly escalating conflicts. Transitional drug addiction (type C) families show a tendency to not define relationships and ignore messages from others. The addict's illness is used in a stance of self-sacrifice, and family members tend to manipulate therapists and others to strengthen their own position. There is a high level of mystification within the family and conflicts often are acted out in an inconclusive manner. Sociopathic drug addiction (type D) is characterized by social disadvantages and profoundly disorganized families. Maladaption of these addicts begins early on and is a result of acting out of psychic conflict.

The early literature concerning the family and drug addiction focused on the symbiotic tie between mothers and their drug-addicted sons with absent or uninvolved fathers [121]. In a comparative study of mothers of drug addicts, schizophrenics and normal adolescents, the mothers of the addicts had the highest symbiotic need for the child [122]. Alexander and Dibb [123] studied middle-class families of addicts and noted the presence of a strong father figure who was present and central versus the absent or peripheral fathers in prior studies. All family members tended to perceive the addict as different or flawed, and held the addict in low esteem. The father's position as a strong leader of the family may be a fictional one, with the mother holding the power in the family system [124,125]. Clarifying actual family functioning is difficult because, as demonstrated by studies of social desirability scales of self-reported personal and family functioning, both addicts and their families show a tendency to seek social approval, whereas addicts deny or minimize negative attributes, family members tend to exaggerate positive qualities of themselves and the family [126].

Emmelkamp [127] compared parental rearing practices of drug addicts to control subjects as rated on an inventory for measurement of parental rearing practices. Results show that addicts see their fathers as more rejecting and lacking in emotional warmth, and mothers as more overprotective. Addicts felt more rejected and experienced less emotional warmth from both parents, and rated their parents' rearing behavior as more overprotective than did the control group.

Turner and Saltz [128] examine the literature proposing that an unresolved family grief is responsible for the pathological homeostasis drug addiction provides by pushing the addict toward death in an attempt to resolve grief. They describe the ambivalence and difficulty with separation that both the addict and family experience, and suggest that addiction provides a solution for a family experiencing crisis or system instability related to the child becoming less dependent on the family. They propose families of narcotic addicts are unable to separate because of an incomplete grieving process over interpersonal loss such as emigration [129], parental death or absence [130,131], or loss of an important family member [132].

Spotts and Shontz [133] found that narcotic addicts described psychologically disabled families with one parent absent or overpowering, and the other parent ineffective. Cocaine users described a highly positive overall early family life with warm mothers and strong encouraging fathers. A pattern of success and achievement orientation in the family patterns of cocaine addicts is suspected. The amphetamine-addicted individuals reported strong but manipulative mothers and passive fathers. Barbiturate abusers were felt to be similar to alcoholics and grew up lacking meaningful relationships to either parent [133]. The family characteristics in different types of addictive behavior deserve further investigation.

Anglin and associates [134] reviewed marital relationships found in drug addicts. They point out the available studies often have methodological shortcomings, but in summary the addict is portrayed as a withdrawn, distrusting individual who suffers from low self-esteem and depression, is passive and dependent, and finds it difficult to develop or maintain intimate relationships. These characteristics and drug lifestyle make close relationships unlikely. They also review the stability of interpersonal relationships of addicts that do develop and find that the constraints of heroin addiction do little to promote and maintain enduring intimate relationships, and these relationshipss often end unless they take on a more functional rather than intimate aspect. Addicted women are more likely to live with an addicted man than vice versa, are often introduced to narcotics by men, especially if in an intimate interpersonal relationship with him, and have sexual interest rendered or replaced by drug use and associated activities [134].

In an attempt to explore how narcotic use and its related behaviors interact with couples' relationships, Anglin and associates [134] compared narcotic-addict couples with artificially formed couples (pseudo couples) and observed their use and interactions during the course of methadone maintenance treatment. Pseudocouples were formed for analysis purposes only, and no real relationship existed between assigned partners, so the difference between the experimental and control group was the presence or lack of a real relationship. The concordance for narcotic-using behavior within couples was examined before, during, and after the relationships (real or pseudo) were formed. Strong correlations were found both for narcotic use and abstinence during the relationship when a real relationship existed. Correlation between real relationships and behavior was seen before, during, and after treatment. No correlations of behavior were found before a relationship started or after it ended, nor for pseudocouples.

Relatively few studies have been done on children of drug-addicted parents compared to the literature on the children of alcoholics. It is reasonable to assume both differences and similarities will be found between children of alcoholics and children of drug addicts, but these are not clear at this time. Deren [135] provides an excellent review of the relevant literature. Much of this literature has focused on maternal drug use during pregnancy. Pregnant addicts and their infants are at risk for medical and psychological complications before, during, and after birth, including impaired maternal-infant bonding. Deren's findings show children of addicts may be at risk for developmental disorders or delays. She states the literature on the effects on older children is scanty and results must be considered inconclusive. The results indicate these children may continue to have somatic, intellectual, and behavioral deficits as well as school and socioemotional problems

IV. FAMILY INVOLVEMENT

A. The Intervention

At this point, it should be clear that addictive disorders are multigenerational within families and that considering family biopsychosocial influences is important diagnostically and for full assessment of the patient's addiction. Understanding the many roles drug use and addiction has played in a person's life and the subsequent consequences are helpful in formulating a treatment plan. In addition, family involvement may have significant impact in the patient's recovery as follows.

The family can be instrumental in initiating treatment. Even when the person with alcohol or drug addiction is highly resistant or not participating in treatment, the clinician still may have a highly motivated patient(s); i.e., the family. The technique of the intervention [136], developed for treatment of alcoholism at the Johnson Institute in Minneapolis, Minnesota, but readily adapted for use with all addictions, is especially effective in patients involved with their nuclear families and who are employed.

In this technique, all available family members and the most meaningful support network members such as employer, neighbors, friends, and clergy are coached to confront the addicted person. Ths confrontation is done with deep concern and without hostility. The participants list specific incidents and behaviors consequential to drug use and present them in a nonjudgmental fashion once the intervention meeting is arranged. Family members can be immobilized by their fear and their love, and may find this idea intimidating. They need to be educated about the deadly consequences of their inaction, and they need instruction on how to say, "We love you and because we love you we will not continue to live with you while you abuse alcohol and drugs. If you accept the treatment being offered and continue to work at recovery, we will renew our lifetime commitment to you." The family needs to agree in advance about what treatment is necessary, insist on it in a firm, consistent manner, and follow through with the limits set.

As many family members as possible are included. In addition, involvement of the employer is crucial, and in some cases sufficient of itself to motivate the addicted individual to seek treatment. The employer who clearly makes treatment a precondition for employment, who supports time off for treatment, and agrees to continue support for the patient after initial treatment offers a helpful model for the family and is a valuable ally.

In a nonrandomized study to evaluate the impact of family intervention, Liepman and associates [137] examined the impact on treatment an alcoholic's social network could have. The two groups were differentiated by whether or not a formal intervention by the family with the alcoholic occurred. In the cases in which intervention did occur, 86% entered treatment and a higher rate of continued abstinence was seen in comparison to cases in which the alcoholic's social network received counseling but no formal intervention occurred.

The technique of intervention is very effective, but at times does fail or is not feasible to carry out. Berenson [138] offers a therapeutic strategy for working with spouses of individuals who continue in addictive behavior. The first step is to calm down the family system by clarifying problems, exploring solutions, and teaching coping skills. Second, a support system is mobilized for family members to diffuse emotional intensity. This is effectively done with self-help support groups such as Alanon (discussed later) or other groups that may be more insight oriented. Step three involves giving the spouse three choices: (1) keep doing what you are doing, (2) detach yourself emotionally, or (3) detach yourself physically, When a client does not choose either (2) or (3); it is labeled as choice (1). In choice (2), spouses are helped to live with the alcoholic and accept and not criticize the drinking, and to assume responsibility for their own behavior and reactivity to the drinking. The spouse may move through all three choices in a gradual process toward leaving the relationship.

B. Motivating the Family

If the family needs motivation for treatment, the person who made the initial contact is usually the one who can best get the entire household to come for therapy. The clinician may have to contact reluctant family members directly. If a member claims to no longer be involved with the family, point out that the objectivity he or she could provide would be helpful. If the claim is that too painful of a relationship exists, emphasize the potential relief of pain for that person. Point out the inability to help that patient and family unless they all attend. Most family members will agree to at least an evaluation visit. It then becomes necessary to establish reasons for everyone to continue with treatment.

Stanton and Todd [115] were successful in motivating 70% of families of methadone maintenance patients to come in for an initial interview and to motivate 94% of these to continue. Facilitory principals include delivering a nonblaming message that focuses on helping the patient rather than the family, presenting reasons for family treatment such that to oppose it would be stating explicitly that they want the patient to remain symptomatic.

Weidman [139] describes the following principles and techniques to engage families in treatment. First the decision as to which family members need to be included in treatment is made by the family therapist, not the family. This is done so that critical members are not excluded. The approach for treatment is non judgmental and supportive as parents often feel guilty and responsible. The therapist should join with the family to help conquer the drug problem, and reframe a family member's resistance in positive terms rather than engaging in power struggles (e.g., uninvolvement is reframed as "not wanting to intrude" and the member can then be invited to participate by the rest of the family). With adolescent patients, incorporating the parent's goals for the patient as the treatments goals encourages family participation. Persistence, flexibility, and interest in pursing family involvement are important. Finally, the conviction that family involvement will help needs to be conveyed [139].

C. Efficacy of Family Involvement

The efficacy of family therapy suggested by clinical experience and single case studies is beginning to be demonstrated more rigorously. In his discussion of family treatment for alcohol and drug addiction, Stanton [117] noted only six of 68 studies provided comparative data with other treatment or control groups. Four of six showed family treatment to be superior to other forms of treatment. For example, Hendricks [140] found narcotic addicts receiving 5.5 months of multiple family therapy twice as likely to remain in treatment than addicts who did not respond to multiple family therapy. Of the two studies finding no superiority of family treatment groups, one [141] used therapists new to family therapy and addiction treatment.

Adolescent addicts with multiple family therapy have been shown to have half the recidivism rate than those without [142], and family therapy reduces the number of adolescents who drop out of residential treatment [143]. For residential stays of approximately the same duration, the success rate for treatment increased with family attendance at group therapy [144]. Effect of family treatment was not significant at the extremes of patient duration of stay, however (i.e., < 3 months or > 12 months) [144]. Well-controlled studies of the effectiveness of family-involved treatment are few and limited [145].

Stanton and Todd [115] provided a well-documented controlled study of family therapy of drug addiction. At 1 year followed-up, their family treatment groups were shifted favorably in days free of methadone, illegal opiates, and marijuana compared to the nonfamily treatment group. However, no significant decrease in alcohol use nor increase in work or school productivity was noted. A higher mortality rate (10%) was seen in the nonfamily therapy causes compared to only 2% in those who received family therapy.

McCrady and associates [146] compared the effectiveness on drinking behavior and life satisfaction in three treatment groups: (1) minimal spouse involvement with interventions directed toward the drinker, although the spouse was present, (2) alcohol-focused spouse involvement in which coping skills for alcohol-related situations were emphasized, and (3) alcohol behavioral marital therapy in which the need to modify the marital relationship was also addressed in addiction to alcohol-focused spouse involvement. Results showed better compliance, faster decrease of drinking, and a greater likelihood to stay in treatment and maintain marital satisfaction posttreatment in the subjects receiving alcohol behavioral marital therapy.

Recently the National Institute of Drug Abuse (NIDA) has funded several studies to comprehensively evaluate family therapy's effect and which variables are most significant. Results are eagerly awaited. Although the specifics are not yet known, it is clear that family involvement is important in the treatment of alcohol and drug-addicted individuals. Family involvement enhances the accuracy of assessment, increases the chance of successful intervention, and helps a patient continue motivated in treatment. These factors and the actual changes that can be brought about in a family that is involved in treatment can improve the recovery rates of the alcohol and drug addict.

V. TREATMENT OF FAMILIES

A. Families in Treatment

Families will pass through various phases with differential effects of addiction on the family and different treatment needs at each phase, although few clinical studies have addressed this issue. The initial phase is marked by denial. Family members refuse to accept the fact a problem exists, even though it may be obvious to outsiders. After the denial phase, families tend to overrreact in an enmeshed and chaotic way to drug-related behavior, especially during intoxication and heavy use. There may be marked distress, panic, and anger. Later, a new family homeostasis forms that usually excludes the identified patient. Some families continue enmeshed with the addicted person and are prone to develop severe depression or an addiction themselves. It is expected families will cycle between disengagement and enmeshment. They need maintenance of a long-term positive alliance with treatment professionals so they can return as needed.

The life cycle stage of the family is also a determinant of the type of approach the family needs. The family therapy of an adolescent will be similar regardless of the substance used, whereas treatment of an employed 35-year-old with a family of his or her own will be quite different from the 35-year-old heroin addict still living at home. Individual styles and family systems will have evolved differently over time.

Family therapy that is limited to a dyad (e.g., enmeshed mother and son) is most difficult and some, other person such as a grandparent or ex-spouse must be brought in to faciliate successful family treatment. If no one else is available, a multiple family group can provide surrogate family members to facilitate restructuring of relationships [142]. Therapy limited to an alcoholic and spouse often neglects essential members of the family system such as children or parents of the alcoholic. Family treatment that focuses on addicts and their spouses has been even less effective than with alcoholic couples. This led Stanton and Todd [115] to first work with the addict and the family of origin who must release the addict to the spouse before couples can proceed. When addicts marry, family of origin remains primary and family interactional patterns continue and are expected in the spouse. When the patient has children, parenting skills may need to be taught to the patient and spouse.

Another difficulty frequently encountered is the high numbers of alcohol- and drug-addicted members present in these families. The indentified patient may justifiably feel singled out in a family in which many members have a drug or alcohol problem. Family members may overtly or covertly deny the problem, and powerful confusing mixed messages may be given by family members to the patient and to each other. A person who is not the identified patient may resist participating in family therapy because of the risk of confronting their own addiction. And even if this person does participate, the family may silently agreee to protect him or her from disclosure. Addiction in family members can make diagnosis and treatment of the alcohol- and drug-addicted person difficult, especially when hidden from the health care worker. Multiple family members with addictive disorders should always be considered, and screening all family members for possible alcohol and drug addiction can be helpful.

B. An Overview of Family Treatment Approaches

Six schools of family therapy are briefly summarized. The particular approach used is not as important as the therapist's familiarity in working with and treating the alcoholic or addicted family using a particular treatment method.

Structural Family Therapy

Structural family therapy [38] is a widely practiced form of family therapy used with alcohol- and drug-addicted families. The family system is viewed in terms of boundary clarification, hierarchy of subsystems, flexibility vs rigidity of systems, and the structure of responses to internal and external demands. Symptoms result from family structural imbalance, malfunctioning arrangements (e.g., alliances, splits) and maladaptive reactions to change (e.g., developmental transitions). Techniques may include dyadic confrontations and rearranging seating (reestablish boundaries, hierarchies, alliances) and tasks are given to facilitate goals of treatment.

Strategic Family Therapy

Strategic family therapy [147] sees multiple origins of problems maintained by unsuccessful problem solving, inability to adjust to transitions, and malfuntioning hierarchies with triangulation or coalitions. Techniques such as circular questioning help delineate the family system, and analogical interventions are constructed to encourage a structural shift. Use of paradoxes forces resistant systems to resist by resolving the symptoms, or continue symptomtic, but now under the therapists direction.

Structural-Strategic Therapy

More recently, structural-strategic therapy is a method combined from structural family therapy, which emphasizes restructuring of family systems through interactional change, and strategic family therapy, which views symptoms as homeostatic but maladaptive attempts to regulate family patterns. Techniques of structural-strategic therapists include using tasks, problem solving, emphasis on change outside the session, use of existing family patterns in a positive manner, using paradox (e.g., restraining change and exaggerating roles) and metaphor, and shifting family hierarchies [148,149].

Psychodynamic Family Therapy

Psychodynamic family therapy is not typically used as the sole approach, but the principles can be useful adjuncts for the family therapist who understands the addicted family will require active limit setting and structuring. The therapist uses an understanding of the addiction in context to the historical past of every family member, as well as an understanding of the family's and therapist's emotional reactions to facilitate change in the family system and alleviate the symptoms of family dysfunction. Techniques include interpretation of patterns, overcoming resistance to change, and working through, or repeatedly, issues stemming from the dysfunctional family core conflict.

Systems Family Therapy

Bowen's (39) systems family therapy emphasizes cognitive methods and minimizes use of affect and emotional contact. The focus is on personal differentiation from the family of origin and on analysis of emotional triangles (three-party subsystem, which may include person, issue, or substance of abuse, onto which tension and conflict are displaced). Transgenerational transmission of problems is emphasized. Techniques encourage objectivity and balance between family members, and work to achieve stabilization or detriangulation, individuation, and to increase cognitive functioning and decrease emotional reactivity. A genogram may be constructed to organize information across several generations.

Behavioral Family Therapy

Behavioral family therapy views behavior as a response to a stimulus. The particular behavioral response is maintained by the contingencies and consequences (reinforcement) the behavior (drug use or avoidance) produces, and is also a function of the individuals' prior learning, alternative responses, current state, and genetic constraints. The techniques used help to identify family interactions that trigger and maintain drug use, teaching the family to modify behavior and rearrange contingencies and consequnces, cognitive restructuring, finding alternative behavior, and long-term maintenance planning [150].

C. Multiple Family Groups

Group therapy consisting of multiple families including families of origin, procreation, and couples are extremely useful for treating families of alcoholics and addicts. Separate spouse, adolescent, or children's groups are also helpful. These groups used with individual family therapy can facilitate a shift to new nonaddicted family patterns [151].

The group provides each family system the opportunity to clarify and modify its boundaries and constraints. Feedback from group members outside the individual family challenges family beliefs and defenses, and other families provide role models for alternative behavior. Often families can best identify their own problems by first recognizing similarities with other family systems. Group members provide support and serve as an extended or surrogate family. Bepko [107] states that group members experience relief from being able to identify with others in similar roles. She encourages a technique that is sensitive to family members' sense of pride, encourages self-awareness and responsibility for self, and promotes understanding, flexibility, and adaptability.

D. Alanon

The family is also urged to participate in family self-help groups and this is negotiated as part of the initial treatment agreement. Alanon is a group for members of alcoholic families which arose in the late 1940s as a parallel movement to Alcoholics Anonymous (AA), based on AA's 12 Steps and 12 Traditions. In the mid 1980s other support groups, including Co-Anon (CA), ACA (Adult Children of Alcoholis), and CODA (co-dependents Anonymous), became important factors.

Participation in these self-help groups is a useful adjunct to family therapy. In the short term, they provide the family with the support it needs to set limits and stop enabling the alcoholic or addict to continue in self-destructive behavior. Family members can also benefit from the experience of others and the strength of sharing common problems. The groups also help the families to do something about the addiction problem even if the addict does not, although they are more effective if the alcoholic or addicted member of the family is involved in AA, NA, or CA.

In the long-term, they encourage the families to remain active in treatment and address the addiction as a family problem, since they believe alcohol and drug addiction is a family disease. Family members may profit from the fellowship the groups sponsor, and may be stimulated to explore their own conflicts related to use of drugs and alcohol in the family.

The family group meetings conducted by all of these organizations are similar to AA in their structured format for self-help with a spiritual emphasis. Successful members must accept the disease model of alcoholism and drug addiction, which maintains that the alcoholic or drug addict is not behaving irresponsibly, but has a disease which is totally out of control. Thus, other family members should not take the disease "personally." Members follow three basic principles: (1) a loving detachment from the alcoholic or drug addict, (2) the reestablishment of self-esteem and independence, and (3) reliance on a higher power.

Alanon, Co-Anon, ACA, and CODA have adopted several AA slogans as part of their programs, which embody the self-help philosophy. They include: "First things first," "Easy does it," "Live and let live," "But for the grace of God," and "Just for today." Members are encouraged to recognize themselves in the many similar stories shared by others in the group, and adjust their behavior to the group's operational principles.

New groups such as Cocanon (for the cocaine addict's family), Narconon (narcotics), Alateen (teenagers with alcoholic parent), Parents Anonymous, and Tough Love can also provide support and help. All these groups are extremely helpful in allowing the family to give up their guilty overinvolvement and responsibility for the patient. More insight-oriented groups may exist in some areas that may fill some family members needs not met by 12-Step (Alanon) groups.

VI. A FAMILY-BASED TREATMENT APPROACH

Kaufman [151,152] has described a comprehensive treatment approach to a family treatment approach that will be briefly outlined here. Three phases of treatment are: (1) developing a method for establishing and maintaining a drug-free state, (2) a workable system of family therapy, and (3) family readjustment after the cessation of drug and alcohol addiction.

Family treatment of drug and alcohol addiction begins with an assesment of the extent of use and the difficulties it presents for the patient and family. The presence of the family often facilitates and opens communication between members. In addition, the identified patient may be more honest in front of family who can also provide a more accurate history at times. Some patients may disclose the extent of their drug use only when alone, however. Family patterns of reacivity to drug use is documented.

It is critical to establish a method for detoxification and abstinence so that family therapy can take place effectively. This depends on the severity of the addictive behavior and may involve in or outpatient treatment, medication, self-help groups (e.g., Alcoholics Anonymous), and alternative coping skills. If the pattern is severe (e.g., the patient attends sessions intoxicated), hospitalization may be set as a requirement for continued treatment. Family participation can enhance patient compliance with a method for maintaining abstinence [153].

The second phase involves the development of a workable system of family therapy. Accurate diagnosis is as important in family therapy as it is in individual therapy. Family interactional relationships, conflicts, and communication patterns are examined. Family rules, boundaries, and shifts are explored. Adaptability and conflict-resolution style is also elucidated. Any system of family therapy can work well in alcohol and drug addiction if the typical family system is understood and a method to maintain abstinence (phase 1) is utilized. The treatment techniques will be varied by the family therapist in order to meet the needs of the different individuals and their families. Often it is not the type of drug that demands modifications in technique, rather other variables such as extent of use, ethnicity, stage of life cycle, gender, and stage of disease require a flexible and skillful therapist [151].

Many families will not be ready to accept treatment recommendations or conditions for entering into therapy. The treating or referring clinician must be willing to maintain long-term ties with the family even through multiple treatment failures.

It can be helpful for a therapist to terminate with a family who fails to comply with limits set, or if the identified patient continues to use drugs, as continued family therapy may imply change is occurring when it is not. Working with a family on the requirements for therapy can also help model appropriate limit setting. Families that understand therapy is being terminated in their best interest often return at later time more committed.

The third phase involves the family readjustment after the alcohol and drug use has stopped. The family may enter a "honeymoon" phase in which major conflicts are denied and a superficial harmony based on relief and suppression of negative feelings exists. The family system may readjust to where another family member presents difficulties, the symptom of an underlying family system pathology. The addicted person may feel compelled to return to using in order to stabilize the system at its previous homeostatis and thereby rescuing the new symptom bearer. The family must be worked with for months and often years after the alcohol and drug addiction is first treated if a drug-free state is to continue. All too often, treatment programs include only a short-term intensive family experience and neglect the need for ongoing family treatment and more than temporary impact.

VII. CONCLUSIONS

The family is important for both diagnosis and treatment of alcoholism and drug addiction. As a dynamic, responsive system the family fluctuates around various patterns of relative homeostasis in which alcohol and drug use is a significant component. The family system is seen as a multigenerational interdependent reciprocal interaction between multiple subsystems. The characteristics of some of these relationships are described by means of current literature review and discussion. All clinicians working with addicted patients must be familiar with the importance of family involvement. Frequently the family needs treatment. Treating the family may be the treatment of choice for some addicted individuals, and family treatment improves the chances for recovery in most cases. The clinician must understand what the family is going through, the need and effectiveness of family treatment, and the process of the family's involvement in treatment. Families will go through a readjustment period requiring continued family treatment and resolution of conflicts around past or future drinking that can lead to relapse [153]. Improvement of family functioning is seen in families in which the alcoholic is recovering [72], and studies investigating family life suggests recovered alcoholics attain similar levels of function as nonalcoholic families [154].

REFERENCES

1. Kaufman, E., and Reoux, J. (1988). Guidelines for the successful psychotherapy of substance abusers, *Am. J. Drug Alcohol Abuse, 14*(2):199–209.
2. Kaufman, E. (1986). A workable system of family therapy for drug dependence, *J. Psychoact. Drugs 18*(1):43–50.
3. Kaij, L. (1960). *Studies of the Eitology and Sequels of Abuse of Alcohol*, Lund, Sweden, University of Lund.
4. Goodwin, D.W., Schulsinger, F., Hermansen, Leif, Guze, S.B., and Winokur, G. (1973). Alcohol problems in adoptees raised apart from alcoholic biological parents, *Arch. Gen. Psychiatry, 28*:238–243.
5. Cotton, N.(1979) The familial evidence of alcoholism: A review, *J. Stud. Alcohol., 40*:89–116.
6. Mirin, S., and Weiss, R. (1989). Genetic factors in the development of alcoholism, *Psychiatry Ann., 19*(5):239–242.
7. Schuckit, M.A. (1988). Genetics and the risk for alcoholism, *J.A.M.A. 254*:2614–2617.
8. Schuckitt, M.A., Li, T.K., Clonninger, C.R., and Deitrich, R.A. (1985). The genetics of alcoholism—A summary of the proceedings of a conference convened at the University of California, Davis, *Alcoholism Clin. Exp. Res., 9*(6):475–492.
9. Schuckit, M.A. (1989). The importance of genetic factors in alcoholism, *Drug Abuse Alcohol. Newsletter, XVIII* (1):
10. Penick, E.C., Powell, B.J., Bingham, S.F., Liskow, B.I., Miller, N.S., and Read, M.R. (1987). A comparative study of familial alcoholism, *J. Stud. Alcohol, 48*(2):136–146.
11. Mckenna, T., and Pickens, R. (1981). Alcoholic children of alcoholics, *J. Stud. Alcohol, 42*(11):1021–1029.
12. Pickens, R.W., and Svikis, D.S. (1988). Genetic vulnerability to drug abuse, *N.I.D.A. Res. Monogr. V 89*:1–8.
13. Cadoret, R.J., Troughton, E., O'Gorman, T.W., and Heywood, E. (1986). An adoption study of genetic and environmental factors in drug abuse, *Arch. Gen. Psychiatry, 43*:1131–1136.
14. Meller, W.H., Rinehart, R., Cadoret, R.J., and Troughton, E. (1988). Specific familial transmission in substance abuse, *Int. J. Addict. 23*(10):1029–1039.
15. Weiss, R.D., Mirin, S.M., Griffin, M.L., and Michael, J.L. (1988). A comparison of alcoholic and nonalcoholic drug abusers, *J. Stud. Alcohol, 49*(6):510–515.
16. Stabenau, J.R. (1988). Family pedigree studies of biological vulnerability to drug dependence, *N.I.D.A. Res. Monogr. 89*:25–40.
17. Donovan, J.M. (1986). An etiologic model of alcoholism, *Am. J. Psychiatry, 143*(1):1–11.
18. Bradshaw, J. (1988). *Healing the Shame that Binds You.* Deerfield Beach, Florida, Health Communications.
19. O'Gorman, P., and Oliver-Diaz, P. (1987). *Breaking the Cycle of Addict..* Deerfield Beach, Florida, Health Communications.
20. Woititz, J.G. (1983). *Adult Children of Alcoholics.* Pompano Beach, Florida, Health Communications.
21. Ackerman, R.J., (1983). *Children of Alcoholics*, 2nd ed. New York Simon and Schuster.
22. Macdonald, D.I. (1989). *Drugs, Drinking and Adolescents*, 2nd ed. Chicago, Year Book.
23. Streit, F., Halsted, D.L., and Pascale, P.J. (1974). Differences among youthful users and non users of drugs based on their perceptions of parental behavior. *Int. J. Addict., 9*:749–755.
24. Hunt, D.G. (1974). Parental permissiveness as perceived by the offspring and the degree of marijuana usage among offspring, *Hum. Rel., 27*:267–285.
25. Pendergast, T.J., Jr. (1974). Family characteristics associated with marijuana use among adolescents, *Int. J Addictio., 9*:827–839.
26. Reynolds, I., and Rob, M.I. (1988). The role of family difficulties in adolescent depression, drug-taking and other problem behaviours. *Med. J. Aust., 149*(5):250–256.
27. Swadi, H.S. (1988). Adolescent drug taking: Role of family and peers, *Drug Alcohol Depend., 21*(2):157–160.
28. Bales, R.J. (1946). Cultural differences in rates of alcoholism, *Q. J. Stud. Alcohol., 6*:480–499.

29. Kaufman, E., and Borders, L. (1988). Ethnic family differences in adolescents substance use, *The Family Context of Adolescent Drug Use* (R. Coombs, ed.). New York Haworth Press, pp. 99–120.

30. Glassner, B. (1981). Irish bars and Jewish living rooms: Differences in ethnic drinking habits. *Alcoholism*, 19–20.

31. Blum, K. (1984). *Handbook of Abusable Drugs*. New York, Gardner Press, pp. 276–278.

32. Terry, J., Lolli, G., and Golder, G. (1957). Choice of alcoholic beverage among 531 alcoholics in California, *Q. J. Stud. Alcohol, 18*:417.

33. Lolli, G., Schesler, E., and Golder, G.M. (1960). Choice of alcoholic beverage among 105 alcoholics in New York, *Q. J.Stud. Alcohol, 21*:475.

34. Weibel-Orlando, J.C. (1986/87). Drinking patterns of urban and rural American Indians, *Alcohol Health Res. World*, 8–12.

35. Williams, M. (1985). Special populations, *Alcohol Health Res. World, Spring*:13–14.

36. Jalali, B. (1988). Ethnicity, cultural adjustment, and behavior: Implications for family therapy, *Clinical Guidelines in Cross-Cultural Mental Health* (L. Comas-Diaz, and E.E.H. Griffith, eds.). New York, Wiley, pp.9–32.

37. Kaplan, H.I., Freedman, A.M., and Sadock, B.J. (1985). *Comprehensive Textbook of Psychiatry IV*. Baltimore, Williams & Wilkins, 279–282, 1427–1432.

38. Minuchin, S. (1974). *Families and Family Therapy*. Cambridge, Massachusetts, Harvard University Press.

39. Bowen, M. (1978). *Family Therapy in Clinical Practice*. New York, Jason Aronson.

40. Pattison, E.M., and Kaufmann, E. (1981). Family therapy in the treatment of alcoholism, *Family therapy and Margin Psychopathology* (M.R. Langsley, ed.). New York, Grune & Stratton.

41. Kaufman, E., and Pattison, E.M. (981). Differential methods of family therapy in the treatment of alcoholism, *J. Stud. Alcohol., 42*(11):951–971.

42. Steinglass, P. (1985). Family systems approaches to alcoholism, *J. Subst. Abuse Treatment., 2*:161–167.

43. Steinglass, P. (1980). A life history model of the alcoholic family, *Fam. Proc., 18*:337–354.

44. Steinglass, P., Davis, D.I., and Berenson, D. (1977). Observations of conjointly hospitalized "alcoholic couples" during sobriety and intoxication: Implications for theory and therapy, *Fam. Process, 16*:1–16.

45. O'Farrell, T.J., and Birchler, G.R. (1987). Marital relationships of alcoholic, conflicted, and nonconflicted couples. *J. Marital Fam. Ther., 13*:259–274.

46. Wilson, C., and Orford, J. (1978). Children of alcoholics Report of a preliminary study and comments on the literature, *J. Stud. Alcohol, 39*(1):121–142.

47. Byles, J.A. (1978). Violence, alcohol problems and other problems in disintegrating families, *J. Stud. Alcohol., 39*:551–553.

48. Weatherford, V., and Kaufman, E. (1988). Adult children of alcoholics: Personal and transgenerational patterns. *Proceedings of the American Psychiatric Association 141st Annual Meeting*, Washington,D.C., May 1988.

49. Vanhasselt, V., Morrison, R., and Bellack,A. (195). Alcohol use in wife abusers and their spouses, *Addict. Behav. 10*:127–135.

50. Hindman, M. (1976). Family therapy in alcoholism, *Alcohol Health Res. World, 1*:209.

51. Wolin, S., Bennett, L., and Noonan, D. (1980). Disrupted family rituals: A factor in the intergenerational transmission of alcoholism, *J. Stud. Alcohol. 41*:199–214.

52. Bowen, M. (1974). Alcoholism as viewed through family systems theory and family psychotherapy, *Ann. N.Y. Acad. Sci. 233*:115–122.

53. Davis, D., Berenson, D., Steinglass, P., and Davis, S. (1974). The adaptive consequences of drinking, *Psychiatry, 37*:209–215.

54. Steinglass, P., Winer, S., and Mandelson, J.H. (1971). A systems approach to alcoholism: A model and its clinical application, *Arch. Gen. Psychiatry, 24*:410–408.

55. Edwrds, P., Harvey, C., and Whitehead, P.C. (1973). Wives of alcoholics: A critical review and analysis, *Q. J. Stud. Alcohol, 34*:112–132.

56. Paolino, T.J., Jr., McCrady, B.S., Diamond, S., and Longaburgh,R. (1976). Psychological disturbances in spouses of alcoholics, *Q. J. Stud. Alcohol, 37*:1600–1608.

57. Busch, H., Kormendy, E., and Feverlein, W. (1973). Partners of female alcoholics, *Br. J. Addict. 68*:179–184.
58. Rimmer, J. (1974). Psychiatric illness in husbands of alcoholics, *Q. J. Stud. on Alcohol, 35*:281–283.
59. MacDonald, D. (1956). Mental disorders in wives of alcoholics, *Q. J. Stud. Alcohol, 17*:282–287.
60. Jacob, T., Favorini, A., Meissel, S., and Anderson, C. (1978). The alcoholic's spouse, children and family interactions: Substantive findings and methodological issues, *J. Stud. Alcohol, 39(7)*:1231–1251.
61. Moos, R.H., Finney, J.W., and Gamble, W. (1982). The process of recovery from alcoholism. II. Comparing spouses of alcoholic patients and matched community controls, *J. Stud. on Alcohol, 3(9)*:888–909.
62. Jacob, T., Dunn, N., Leonard, K. (1983). Patterns of alcohol abuse and family stability, *Alcoholism Clin. Exp. Res. 7*:382–385.
63. Frankenstein, W., Hay, W.M., and Nathan, P.E. (1985). Effects of intoxication on alcoholic's marital communictaion and problem solving. *J. Stud. Alcohol, 46(1)*:1–6.
64. Zweben, A. (1986), Problem drinking and marital adjustment, *J. Stud. on Alcohol, 47(2)*:167–172.
65. Gorad, S.L. (1971). Communicational styles and interaction of alcoholics and their wives, *Fam. Process, 10*:475–489.
66. Paolino, T.J., Jr., and McCrady, B.S. (1979). *The Alcoholic Marriage: Alternative Perspectives*, New York, Grune & Stratton.
67. Chiles, J.A., Strauss, F.S. and Benjamin, L.S. (1980). Marital conflict and sexual dysfunction in alcoholic and nonalcoholic couples, *Br. J. Psychiatry, 137*:266–273.
68. Rychtarik, R.G., Tarnowski, K.J., and St. Lawrence, J.S.(1989). Impact of social desirability response sets on the self-report of marital adjustment of alcoholics, *J. Stud. Alcohol, 50(1)*:24–29.
69. Orford, J., Oppenheimer, E., Egert, S., Herrmann, C., and Gutline, J. (1976). The cohesiveness of alcoholism-complicated marriage and its influence on treatment outcome, *Br. J. Psychiatry, 128*:318–319.
70. Bilings, A.G., Kewssler, M., Gomberg, C.A. (1979). Mutual conflict resolution of alcoholic and non-alcoholic couples during drinking and non-drinking sessions, *J. Stud. Alcohol, 40*: 183–195.
71. Jacob, T., Richey, D., Evitkovic, J.F., and Blane, H.T. (1981). Communications styles of alcoholic and nonalcoholic families when drinking and not drinking. *J. Stud. Alcohol, 42*:466–482.
72. Moos, R.H., Moos, B.S. (1984). The process of recovery from alcoholism: III. Comparing functioning in families of alcoholics and matched control families. *J. Stud. Alcohol, 45(2)*:111–118.
73. Sandmaier, M. (1980). *The Invisible Alcoholics: Women and Alcohol Abuse in America*, New York, McGraw-Hill.
74. McLachlan, J.F.C., Walderman, R.L., Birchmore, D.F., and Marsden, L.R. (1979). Self-evaluation, role satisfaction and anxiety in the woman alcoholic, *Int. J. Addict. 14(6)*:609–632.
75. Schuckit, M.A., Pitts, F.N., Reich, T., King, L.T., and Winokur, G. (1969). Two types of alcoholism in women, *Arch. Gen. Psychiatry, 20*:301–306.
76. Reed, B.G. (1985). Drug misuse and dependency in women: The meaning and implications of being considered a special population or minority group, *Int. J. Addict., 20(1)*:13–62.
77. Beckman, J.J. (1975). Woman alcoholics: A review of social and psychological studies. *J. Stud. Alcohol, 36(7)*:797–824.
78. Lindbeck, F.L. (1972). The women alcoholic, *Int. J. Addict., 7(3)*:567–580.
79. Corrigan, E.M. (1980). *Alcoholic Women in Treatment*, New York, Oxford University Press.
80. Forrest, G.C. (1982). *Alcoholism and Human Sexuality*, Springfield, Illinois, Thomas.
81. Estep, R. (1987). The influence of the family on the use of alcohol and prescription depressants by women, *J. Psycoact. Drugs, 19(2)*:171–179.
82. Glatt, M.M. (1982). Reflections on the treatment of alcoholism in women, *Br. J. Alcohol Alcohol. 14(2)*:77–83.
83. Reichman, W. (1983). Affecting attitudes and assumptions about women and alcohol problems, *Alcohol Health Res. World 7(3)*:6–10.
84. Beckman, L.J., and Amaro, H. (1986). Personal and social difficulties faced by women and men entering alcoholism treatment, *J. Stud. Alcohol, 46(2)*:135–145.

85. Beckman, L.J., and Amaro, H. (1984–1985). Patterns of women's use of alcohol treatment agencies, *Alcohol Health Res. World, Winter*:15–25.
86. Winokur, G., and Clayton, P.J. (1968). Family history studies in comparison of male and female alcoholics, *Q. Stud. Alcohol, 29*:885–891.
87. Wilsnack, S.C. (1982). Alcohol abuse and alcoholism in women, *Encyclopedic Handbook of Alcoholism* (E.M. pattison and E. Kaufman, eds.). New York, Gardner Press, pp. 718–735.
88. Gomberg, E.L. (1981). Women, sex roles and alcohol problems, *Profess. Psychol., 12*(1):146–155.
89. Yandow, V. (1989). Alcoholism in women, *Psychiatry Ann.*, 19(5):243–247.
90. Kovach, J. (1986). Incest as a treatment issue for alcoholic women. *Alcoholism Treat. Q., 3*(1):1–15.
91. Glenn, S., and Parsons, O.A. (1989). Alcohol abuse and familial alcoholism: Psychosocial correlates in men and women, *J. Stud. Alcohol, 50*(2):116–127.
92. Cork, M.R. (1969). *The Forgotten Children: A Study of Children with Alcoholic Parents*. Alcoholism and Drug Addiction Research Foundation of Ontario, Toronto.
93. El-Guebaly, N., and Offord, D.R (1977). The offspring of alcoholics: A critical review, *Am. J. Psychiatry, 134*(4):357–365.
94. Black, C., Bucky, S.F., and Wilder-Padilla, S. (1986). The interpersonal and emotional consequences of being an adult child of an alcoholic, *Int. J. Addict. 21*(2):213–231.
95. Beletsis, S., and Brown, S. (1981). A developmental framework for understanding the adult children of alcoholics, *Focus Women J. Addict. Health*, 2:187–203.
96. MacDonald, D.I., and Blume, S.B. (1986). Children of alcoholics. *Am. J. Dis. Child., 140*(8):750–754.
97. Stark, E. (1987). Forgotten victims: Children of alcoholics, *Psychol. Today 21*:58–62.
98. Parker, D.A., and Harford, T.C., (1988). Alcohol related problems, marital disruption and depressive symptoms among adult children of alcohol abusers in the United States, *J. Stud. Alcohol, 49*(4):306–313.
99. Giglio, J., and Kaufman, E. (1989). The relationship between child and adult psychopathology in children of alcoholics, *Int. J. Addict. 25*:263–290.
100. Cermack, T. L. (1985). *A Primer on Adult Children of Alcoholics*. Pompano Beach, Florida, Health Communications.
101. Weatherford, V., Reist, C., Kaufman, E., and Kauffman, C. (1988). Personality patterns of adult children of alcoholics and post traumatic stress disorder. *Proceedings of the American Psyciatric Association 141st Annual Meeting*, Washinton, D.C., May, 1988.
102. Werner, E.E. (1986).Resilient offspring of alcoholics: A longitudinal sutdy from birth to age 18, *J. Stud. Alcohol, 47*(1):34–40.
103. Keltner, N.L., McIntyfe, C.W., and Gee, R. (1986). Birth order effects in second-generation alcoholics, *J. Stud. on Alcohol, 47*(6):495–497.
104. Wegscheider, S. (1981). *Another Chance: Hope & Health for the Alcoholic Family*. Palo Alto, California, Science and Behavior Books.
105. Black, C. (1979). Children of alcoholics, *Alcohol Health Research World., 4*(1):23–27.
106. Rhodes, J., and Blackham, G. (1987). Differences in character roles between adolescents from alcoholic and nonalcoholic homes. *Am. J. Drug Alcohol Abuse, 13*(1–2):145–155.
107. Bepko, C., and Krestan, J.A. (1985). *The Responsibility Trap*. New York, Free Press.
108. Beattie, M. (1987). *Codependent No More*. New York, Harper & Row/Hazelden Foundation.
109. Kaufman, E. (1985). *Substance Abuse and Family Therapy*. Grune & Stratton, pp. 39–40.
110. Cermack, T. (1989). Al-Anon and recovery, *Rec. Dev. Alcohol., 7*:165–182.
111. Cutter, C.G., and Cutter, H.S.(1987). Experience and change in Al-Anon family groups: adult children of alcoholics, *J. stud. Alcohol, 48*(1):29–32.
112. Ziegler-Driscoll, G. (1979). The similarities in families of drug dependents and alcoholics, *Family Therapy of Drug and Alcohol Abuse* (E. Kaufman and P. Kaufman, eds.). New York, Gardner Press, pp. 19–39.
113. Kaufman, E. (1980). Myth and reality in the family patterns and treatment of substance abusers, *Am. J. Alcohol Abuse, 7*(3,4):257–279.

114. Kaufman, E., and Kaufmann, P. (eds.) (1979). Family therapy of substance abusers, *Family therapy of Drug and Alcohol Abuse*, New York, Gardner Press.

115. Stanton, M.D. and Todd, T.C. (1982). *The Family Therapy of Drug abuse and Addiction*, New York, Guilford Press.

116. Noone, R.J., and Reddig, R.L.(1976). Case studies on the family treatment of drug abuse, *Famil. Process, 15*:325-332.

117. Stanton, M.D. (1980). Some overlooked aspects of the family and drug abuse, *Drug Abuse from the Family Perspective* (B.G. Ellis, ed.). National Institute of Drug Abuse, U.S. Department of Health, Education and Welfare, Rockville, Maryland, pp. 1-17.

118. Kaufman, E. (1981). Family structures of narcotic addic ts, *Int. J. Addict. 16*::106-108.

119. Friedman, A.S., Utada, A., and Morrissey, M.R. (1987). Families of adolescent drug abusers are "rigid": Are these families either "disengaged" or "enmeshed," or both? *Fam. Process. 26*(1):131-148.

120. Cancrini, L., Cingolani, S., Compagnoni, F., Costantini, D., and Mazzoni, S. (1988). Juvenile drug addiction: A typology of heroin addicts and their families. *Fam. Process. 27*(3):261-271.

121. Fort, J.P. (1954). Heroin addiction among young men, *Psychiatry, 17*:251-259.

122. Attardo, N. (1965). Psychodynamic factors in the mother-child relationship in adolescent drug addiction: A comparison of mothers of schizophrenics and mothers of normal adolescent sons, *Psychother. Psychosom. 13*:249-255.

123. Alexander, B.K., and Dibb, G.S. (1975). Opiate addicts and their parents, *Fam. Process. 14*:499-514.

124. Schwartzman, J. (1975). The addict, abstinence and the family. *Am. J. Psychiatry, 132*:154-157.

125. Kirschenbaum, M., Leonoff, G., and Maliano, A. (1974). Characteristic patterns in drug abuse families, *Fam. Thera., 1*:43-62.

126. Gibson, D., Wermuth, L., Sorensen, J.L., Menicucci, L., and Bernal, G. (1987). Approval need in self-reports of addicts and family members, *Int. J. Addict. 22*(9):895-903.

127. Emmelkamp, P.M.G., and Heeres, H. (1988). Drug addiction and parental rearing style: A controlled study, *Int. J. Addict., 23*(2):207-216.

128. Turner, F.N., and Saltz, L. (1987). Narcotic addiction and family process: Death wish or countertransference, *J. Subst. Abuse Treat. 4*:29-36.

129. Vaillant, G.E. (1973). A 20-yer follow-up of New York narcotic addicts, *Arch. Gen. Psychiatry, 29*:237-241.

130. Klagsbrun, M., and Davis, D.I. (1977). Substance abuse and family interaction, *Fam. Process, 16*:149-173.

131. Coleman, S.B. (1978). The role of death in the addict family, *J. Marriage Fam. Counsel., 4*: 79-91.

132. Stanton, M.D., Todd, T.C., Heard, D.B., Kurshner, S., Kleiman, J.I., Mowatt, D.T., Riley, P., Scott, S.M., and Van Duesen, J.M. (1978). Heroin addiction as a family phenonmenon: A new conceptual model, *Am. J. Drug Alcohol Abuse, 5*:125-150.

133. Spotts, J.V., and Shontz, F.C. (1980). A life-theme theory of chronic drug abuse. *N.I.D.A. Res. Monogr. 30*:59-70.

134. Anglin, M.D., Kao, C., Harlow, L.L., Peters, K., and Booth, M.W. (1987). Similarity of behavior within addict couples. Part I. Metholodogy and narcotics patterns, *Int. J. Addict, 22*(6):497-524.

135. Deren, S. (1986). Children of Substance Abusers: A Review of the Literature, *J. Subst. Abuse Treat, 3*:77-94.

136. Johnson, V.E. (1980). *I'll Quit Tomorrow*, rev. ed. San Francisco, Harper & Row.

137. Liepman, M.R., Nirenberg, T.D., and Begin, A.M. (1989). Evaluation of a program designed to help family and significant others to motivate resistant alcoholics into recovery. *Am. Drug Alcohol Abuse, 15*(2):209-221.

138. Berenson, D. (1979). The therapist's relationship with couples with an alcoholic member, *Family Therapy of Drug and Alcohol Abuse* (E. Kaufman and P. Kaufmann, eds.). New York, Gardner Press, pp. 233-242.

139. Weidman, A.A. (1985). Engaging the families of substance abusing adolescents in family therapy, *J. Subst. Abuse Treat. 2*:97-105.

140. Hendricks, W.J. (1971). Use of multifamily counseling groups in treatment of male narcotic addicts, *Int. J. Group Therapy, 22*:34–90.

141. Ziegler-Driscoll, G. (1977). Family research study at Eagleville Hospital and Rehabilitation Center, *Fam. Process, 61*:175–189.

142. Kaufman, E., and Kaufmann, P. (1977). Multiple family therapy: A new direction in the treatment of drug abusers, *Am. J. Drug Alcohol Abuse, 4*:467–478.

143. Weidman, A. (1987). Family therapy and reductions in treatment dropout in a residential therapeutic community for chemically dependent adolescents, *J. Subst. Abuse Treatment., 4*(1):21–28.

144. Clerici, M., Garini, R., Capitanio, C., Zardi, L., Carta, I., and Gori, E. (1988). Involvement of families in group therapy of heroin addicts, *Drug Alcohol Depend., 21*(3):213–216.

145. McCrady, B. (1989). Outcomes of family-involved alcoholism treatment, *Rec. Dev. Alcohol., 7*:165–182.

146. McCrady, B.S., Noel, N.E., Abrams, D.B., Stout, R.L., Nelson, H.F., and Hay, W.M. (1986). Comparative effectiveness of three types of spouse involvement in outpatient behavioral alcoholism treatment. *J. Stud. Alcohol, 47*(6):459–467.

147. Haley, J. (1977). *Problem Solving Therapy*, San Francisco, Jossey Bass.

148. Madanes, C. (1981). *Strategic Family Therapy/Cloe Madanes*. San Francisco, Jossey-Bass.

149. Stanton,M. (1981). An integrated structural/strategic approach to family therapy, *J. Marital Fam. Ther., 7*:427–429.

150. Noel, N.E., McCrady, B.S. (1984). Behavioral Treatment of an alcohol abuser with the spouse present, *Power to Change: Family Case Studies in the Treatment of Alcoholism* (E. Kaufman, ed.). New York, Gardner Press, pp. 23–78..

151. Kaufman, E. (1985). *Substance Abuse and Family Therapy*. Orlando, Florida, Grune Stratton.

152. Kaufman, E. (1989). Family therapy in substance abuse treatment, *American Psychiatric Association: Treatment of Psychiatric Disorders*: A Task Force Report of the American Psychiatric Association, Washington, D.C., pp. 1397–1416.

153. O'Farrell, T.J., and Bayog, R.D. (1986). Antabuse contracts for married alcoholics and their spouses: A method to maintain antabuse ingestion and decrease conflict about drinking, *J. Subst. Abuse Treat., 3*:1–8.

154. Callan, V.J., and Jackson, D. (1986). Children of alcoholic fathers and recovered alcoholic fathers: Personal and family functioning, *J. Stud. Alcohol. 47*(2):180–182.

47

Coaddiction: Treatment of the Family Member

David J. Nyman and James Cocores
Fair Oaks Hospital, Summit, New Jersey

I. INTRODUCTION

During the past 25 years, significant strides have been made in the treatment of alcohol and drug addiction. Minnesota model treatment programs [1] have gained increasing recognition as the treatment of choice for addiction and are now readily available throughout the country. Today, physicians and other health care providers have a wide variety of alternatives, such as detoxification, inpatient rehabilitation, and comprehensive outpatient services, available to them when they are formulating an appropriate course of treatment for their alcohol and drug-addicted patients. However, the conceptualization and treatment of the psychological reaction of family members living with an active addiction have not made similar advancements. Scant attention has been paid to the family member's experience, and in turn the affect that these same individuals have, if untreated, on the long-term recovery of the addicted patient. Less than a handful of papers have been published on the topic and the amount of empirical research conducted has been even more limited.

In general, the psychological and behavioral disturbances exhibited by family members that are a direct result of regular interaction with an addict have been labeled *codependency* or *coaddiction* [2]. While these terms are often used interchangeably, we have chosen to employ the latter term throughout this chapter because it more clearly denotes the family member's experience as an outgrowth of the addictive process. Schaef [3] traces the development of the coaddiction concept to the initial recognition in the late 1970s that family members often exhibit a specific set of behavioral responses that allow an addiction to continue unabated and within a family system that has insidiously become organized around the addiction. While described more fully below, this constellation, referred to as enabling, is the inadvertent effort by coaddicts to protect their alcohol- and drug-addicted loved one from the deleterious consequences that inevitably develop from chemical use.

This realization that an enabling system develops and supports an evolving addiction was the field's initial attempt to examine the psychic and behavioral responses of family members and their role in the natural course of addiction. Drug and alcohol addiction treatment centers began designing family programs that were intended to begin dismantling the enabling system. Today, these programs usually consist of a weekly education hour, concerning addiction and coaddiction, and a multifamily group therapy. Almost all treatment centers offer these programs, which have become essential components of effective alcohol and drug addiction treatment programs.

While the identification of enabling was an important first step in studying the role of family members in addiction and recovery, the application of this concept has had limited utility. In one sense, it has been a recapitulation of the experience that coaddict's have within the family system: they are important only to the extent that they are relevant to the addicts well-being. While this is obviously important, and a good part of this chapter examines this aspect of coaddiction, this focus inadvertently reinforces a secondary role for the family member. Attention stays on the addict and the coaddict remains peripheral.

II. THE ADDICTIVE ENVIRONMENT

Family members live in a chaotic and disruptive environment that is bred by addiction. To fully comprehend this experience, one needs to appreciate the nature of addictive illness [4] and the kind of personality it shapes [5]. The compulsion to locate, use, and conceal alcohol and drug use frequently forces a change in the addict's characterological style to include a strongly defensive posture that helps create the chaos that envelops family members [6]. Addicts must build an insulated world that prevents them from examining their own use and experiencing its consequences. Their entire world view and personality style becomes organized around this goal. Central to this defensive system, and perhaps the most difficult aspect of addiction for family members to accommodate, is the addict's use of denial that is designed to obfuscate the alcohol and drug use. This denial can reach psychotic-like proportions, and a family member who is continuously confronted with this can, at best, become highly frustrated and stressed, and, at worst, begin to question their own perceptions and memory. The authors have interviewed numerous coaddicts who were convinced they had significant cognitive impairments because their observations and memories of alcohol and drug-related incidents were widely discrepant with their addicted family members.

In addition to denial and further battering coaddicts is the tendency for their addicted family member to use externalizing defense. Addicts will frequently project responsibility for their use onto others ("If you were a better wife, I wouldn't have to drink"), allowing them to avoid examination of their addicted behavior and justify the chemical use ("I drink because of stress"). The coaddict often accepts these accusations and rationalizations because of his or her ignorance about the nature of the addictive process (as discussed below) and adherence to the traditional societal view that dysfunctional families or marriages drive individuals into addiction. Frequently, the addicted individual capitalizes on this mistaken belief with a further and a more pronounced use of projection and rationalization. The result is that many family members feel even more responsible for the addiction and this guilt fuels the enabling behaviors so detrimental to recovery. A cycle is created in which the addict's uncontrolled and outwardly focused behavior reinforces a family member's guilt and sense of responsibility, which only compels him or her to continue enabling and maintain the protective environment in which the addiction flourishes.

Coaddiction frequently leads to significant psychiatric disturbances. In an attempt to identify the kind of disorders most typically developed, Cocores [7] interviewed 50 parents and 50 spouses of alcohol- and drug-addicted patients consecutively admitted to the Outpatient Recovery Centers of Fair Oaks Hospital, Summit, New Jersey. He found that each one, at a minimum, met the diagnostic criteria for adjustment disorder. Many also met criteria for more severe disorders, such as dysythmic disorder (parents and spouses, 32 and 67%, respectively), and generalized anxiety disorder (10 and 12%, respectively). In a separate investigation, Cocores and his colleagues also found that spouses of addicted individuals reported significant sexual dysfunction on a comprehensive survey of such behavior [8]. While not systematically examined, ancedotal evidence in both these studies suggested that the anxiety, depression, and other psychiatric symptoms reported by the coaddicts were secondary to the onset of their family member's addiction.

III. THE COADDICTION SYNDROME

Several attempts have been made to identify the major characteristics of the coaddiction syndrome [3,7,9,10]. Based upon a review of this limited literature, and the authors' own clinical experience, the following represents the most frequently observed psychic and behavioral responses of family members who live in an addictive family system.

A. Enabling

Frequently begun out of genuine concern, the budding enabler's desire is to simply protect a fellow family member from problematic circumstances (e.g. lending money because the addicted individual expended available funds on purchasing cocaine, making excuses to an employer for a family member "ill" with a hangover). Initially, the enabling act can be construed as a healthy support for another member of the family whose predicament requires providing guidance, protection, or encouragement. As noted previously, this inadvertently prevents the developing addict from experiencing the natural consequences of alcohol and drug use. Denial is supported rather than responsible behavior. The addict is assisted by the enabler to avoid the environmental consequences that might propel him or her to recognize the impact of his or her alcohol and drug use. The illusion of control can continue. Unless enabling behaviors are checked, the natural downward progression of addiction will continue unabated because the addict is left insulated and protected from the consequences of his or her behavior.

The initial basis for enabling, providing assistance to a family member in difficulty, and thus maintaining a cohesive unit in the face of external threats, is deeply rooted in the societal norm for the family. Frequently, when enabling behaviors are identified in treatment, the coaddict argues that not protecting the addict is a betrayal of the family. In addition, just as alcohol and drug use becomes an autonomous function for the addict and his or her behavior becomes increasingly stereotyped, so do the actions of the enabling coaddict. Loss of voluntary control over enabling acts are often seen. Statements such as "I don't know that I do it until after it's done" are frequently voiced by family members. Of all the coaddict characteristics noted in affected family members, enabling behavior is often the most resistant to intervention.

B. Ignorance

The addictive process contradicts much of the layperson's understanding of behavior and its causes. Addiction is neither voluntary nor willful, and despite the individual's best efforts, concious attempts at control are not effective. This inability to curb alcohol and drug addiction despite the pleadings of others is very difficult for family members to understand. They naturally conclude that their addicted loved one cares less for them than they do for alcohol and drugs. It frequently leaves them feeling angered and abandoned, further contributing to their sense of failure and stress. This ignorance about addiction is usually at the heart of the coaddiction experience. Many family members, like most individuals, are not knowledgeable about addiction. They make inaccurate assumptions concerning their addicted loved ones' motivations for continued alcohol and drug use, and attribute malevolant intent to that individual that usually does not exist. Most of the other coaddict characteristics grow and fester within this bed of ignorance.

C. Denial

As in addiciton, denial is one of the hallmarks of coaddiction. For some, the denial serves to avoid the reality of the addiction. It is not uncommon for these family members to collude with their family member in a joint attempt to ward off any awareness that an addiction is present. In the following case example, the coaddict's denial is sufficiently intact as to withstand considerable data contrary to her perception.

> Michael, age 24, presents for an addiction assessment at the request of his lawyer. He had been charged with is second DWI (driving while intoxicated) in the past 2 years. As is routine procecure, the intake counselor requested that a family member accompany Michael to the evaluation and he brought his mother. She is Edith, aged 52, mother for four children, Michael being her second oldest. Her husband, Michael's father, died of cirrhosis of the liver 4 years ago and Michael's older brother has been arrested several times in alcohol-related incidents. During the interview, Michael denies any significant alcohol or drug problem. He states that he drinks socially and that it was only by chance that the two times he was stopped by the police he was intoxicated. He does state that his life is stressed and sometimes he has a drink on his way home after work with his coworkers. When interviewed, Edith supports her son's report. She states that he does have a stressful job and while he does drink a lot to unwind, he usually knows how to control his intake. She strongly feels he does not have a problem, stating he is a "good son" and in any event "boys will be boys." She asks several times during the interview as to when they can leave because they both have errands to run that afternoon.

Recognition that an addiction has taken hold in their family is actively resisted by some coaddicts because it allows them to successfully avoid the guilt and/or painful reality that a family member has a problem. In the example above, Edith's denial may have served to prevent her from associating Michael's behavior with her husband's alcohol-related death and recognizing that the family has another addicted member.

For others, the denial is not of the addiction, but of their own coaddiction. They can readily recognize that an addiction has affected their family member. Frequently, they are the force that drives the addict into treatment. However, it is their own pain that they cannot acknowledge.

> Barbara, aged 33, accompanied her husband Tom, aged 35, to the evaluation. They have been married for 7 years, and during the past 3, Tom's cocaine use has escalated dramatically. He has frequently not been at home. The family's finances are in a shambles, and his job in jeopardy. However, during the evaluation Tom is unable to recognize any of the consequences of his cocaine use and refuses to participate in treatment. During the interview, several indications are present that Barbara is suffering significantly from Tom's addiction. She is very tearful, reporting sleep disturbances and having recently left her job so that "I could have more time to be a better wife and help Tom stop using cocaine." The assessment counselor explores with Barbara these behaviors and informs her that they are frequently characteristic of the coaddiction syndrome. However, stating that "I'm really O.K., and if I went to the treatment center for myself, Tom will probably use because I won't be there watching him."

Barbara's denial keeps her trapped within the addicton system and enables her husband to continue his use of cocaine.

D. Irrational Reliance on Control

Despite contradictory evidence, addicts continue to cling to the belief that their alcohol and drug use can be contained through willpower. Maintaining adherence to this inaccurate perception helps them remain locked into the addictive cycle. Coaddicts operate in a similar manner with the same result. They are often relentless in their attempts to control their addicted family members and cannot recognize that their efforts will be fruitless. They regularly sacrifice time and energy toward this goal, despite experiencing repeated frustration and failure. Resigning from a job or relocating a residence so as to be more available to monitor an addict's behavior is not uncommon. Family members sometimes seek treatment with the stated intent of learning how to more effectively control their addict's behavior. When the predictable failure in this task is realized, rather than acknowledge that the addiction cannot be controlled through their efforts, they frequently re-double their efforts and simply compound their own sense of failure and importance.

E. Poor Self-Image

Regardless of the coaddict's self-esteem prior to the onset of the addiction, many suffer an impaired self-image after it develops. Family members are routinely bombared with the denial, attacks, and irritability that frequently comprise the addictive personality style. Many internalize these onslaughts and this, within the context of their ignorance about addiction, renders the coaddict feeling worthless and guilt ridden. Moreover, as the addict sinks lower into the addiction, he or she will escalate the attempt to focus responsibility for the chemical use on the family member, who by this time will readily accept the additional responsibility.

F. Stress-Related Illness

Many coaddicts somatasize and have stress-related illnesses such as ulcers, colitis, and migraine headaches [7,11]. In Cocores' [7] sample, a high incidence of physical complaints for parents and spouses were reported 45% and 52%, respectively. Internalizing responsibility for the family's difficulties, and the resultant stress, seems to be a commonly observed characteristic of coaddicts.

These traits tend to be the hallmarks of the coaddiction syndrome; they represent the kinds of feelings and behaviors that most individuals who have an ongoing familial relationship with an addict develop. However one should not infer that all family members have each of these hallmarks. Some may have none, but most have at least several to at least some degree. Each coaddict usually develops their own constellation of coaddiction symptoms as a function of their respective characteriological style, family background, or type of relationship with the addicted individual.

Much of the limited scientific literature available has been devoted to examining the utility of the coaddiction concept and whether it represents a formal condition that requires treatment. As with other evolving descriptive or diagnostic categories (i.e., borderline conditions in the late 1970s), coaddiction has had multiple conceptualizations and descriptions.

This diffusion in clarity has, in part, been a function of the arena in which the concept has been developed. After enabling was identified, several books appeared, written mostly for the public, that painted coaddiction in very broad strokes [3,9,10]. While these works, judging by their sales, touched a chord inside many people, they inadvertently created confusion in the professional world because they were not written with sufficient specificity with respect to the diagnosis and treatment of coaddiction. The result was to create confusion among professionals concerning the definition of coaddiction. For example, Mulry [12] strongly endorses the coaddiction concept as a "companion illness classically occurring in persons who are (or have been) in close relationships with chemically dependent persons," and one that is frequently seen by family physicians. He sees coaddiction as a major contribution to the field's understanding of the addictive system and frequently underidentified. However, Asher and Brussert [13] argue against the medicalization of the experience, and find that coaddiction is simply a social construction consistent with the traditional passive female role. In addition, Gierymski and Williams [14] assert that coaddiction behaviors are frequently not observed among family members and see coaddiction as having little specificity in conceptualizing the generic experience of family members. They also see little support from their anecdotal observations and the several quazi-experimental studies they review to warrant the recognition of coaddiction as a useful concept. Nevertheless, they do conclude that "wives (and possibly other members) in families containing an alcoholic, as a group, are likely to suffer more emotional problems then do spouses of nonalcoholics." They also concede that family groups and Al-Anon participation is essential to the treatment of addiction.

This struggle over coaddiction is, in part, a result of the fact that no single set of clinical phenomenon has been examined, and that much of the work has not been scholarly in characteristic. Numerous investigators indicate that many family members experience adverse emotional consequences secondary to an addiction in the family (7,13,15). However, as noted above, the concept of coaddiction has become somewhat blurred because of poorly conceived attempts to universalize the experience among almost all family members. Gierymski and Williams [14] are not incorrect when asserting that the concept has been applied without consideration to specific criteria.

III. COADDICTIVE PERSONALITY DISORDER

Cermak [11], in an outstanding contribution to the field, attempted to clarify the confusing connotation of coaddiction. He argued that it can best be conceptualized as a personality disorder with its own enduring characterological style that frequently predisposes an individual to emeshment with an alcohol and drug-addicted individual. Cermak proposed specific criteria for his codependent personality (he employed the codependent term rather than the coaddict). They were as follows:

1. Continued investment of self-esteem in the ability to control oneself and others in the face of serious adverse consequences.
2. Assumption of responsibility for meeting other's needs to the exclusion of acknowledging one's own.
3. Anxiety and boundry distortions around intimacy and separation.
4. Emeshment in relationships with personally chemically dependent, other codependent, and/or impulse behaviors.
5. Three or more of the following:
    (a) Excessive reliance and denial
    (b) Construction of emotions (with or without dramatic outburts).
    (c) Depression
    (d) Hypervigilant
    (e) Compulsions
    (f) Anxiety
    (g) Substance abuse
    (h) Has been (or is) the victim of received physical or severe abuse.

    (i)   Stress-related medical illnesses.

    (j)   Has remained in a primary relationship with an active substance abuser for at least 2 years without seeking outside help.

In these criteria, Cermak [11] has taken the hallmarks of coaddiction and made them more pronounced, fixed, and rigid. In addition, as presented in criterian B and C, there is a significant focus on identity and boundry disturbances within the individual that occur when he or she is interacting with the addict. Such an individual experiences the loss of self in the service of satisfying the needs, real or imaginary, of the addict. The ability to acknowledge or differientiate one's own needs from those of the addict is limited and therefore, the coaddict takes on the addict's needs as his or her own. When there is a threat to this symbiotic relationship, the coaddict becomes anxious and "fears the loss of the false self he or she has created for that relationship" [11]. For this reason, coaddicts, as discussed below, are the most capable of sabotaging their addict's treatment.

The coaddiction personality disorder is a major contribution to our understanding of the family member's experience in an additive family system. It allows us to develop a continuum of coaddiction that is somewhat analogous to that of depression in current psychiatric nosology. Depression arising out of a specific environmental circumstance and not disabling, but disruptive to effective interpersonal functioning, is diagnosed as an adjustment disorder with depressive features. Individuals with a depression that causes major dysfunction and includes vegetative signs and symptoms is diagnosed as a major depression. One is short-lived and a function of an individual's adjustment to environmental circumstances; the other is more severe and frequently not necessarily a function of situational occurrences. The two disorders may also coexist in the same patient.

Applying this concept of tying the diagnosis to the severity of the disturbance and having one denoting a condition that is purely a situational disturbance to coaddiction allows us to develop two different coaddictions. One is a reactive coaddiction, or alternately, reactive codependence* and denotes an individual who, as a function of living with an addicted family member, develops a situational disturbance. This classification is similar to an adjustment disorder with mixed emotional features, but has more specificity concerning the experience of the addictive system. The second is coaddiction personality disorder and denotes a long-standing characterological style that lends itself to establishing and maintaining destructive relationships with alcohol- or drug-addicted individuals.

Almost inevitably, an individual who presents for treatment with coaddictive personality disorder has an overlay of reactive coaddiction that is driving them into treatment. The reactive coaddiction must be treated first, similar to an addiction treatment in which the addiction must be arrested before a coexisting or preexisting psychological disturbance can be addressed [16]. However, the reverse is not true. There are many instances when a family member does not have the more severe and long-standing coaddict disorder. They have been swept up in the additive process and develop the disorder of reactive coaddiction. Of course, many individuals have traits of the characterological style, but do not qualify for the diagnosis [11].

In our experience, many individuals with coaddict disorders are adult children of alcoholics (ACOA's), and their behavior is an extension of the style they learned as a child. While outside the scope of this chapter, individuals raised in alcoholic homes have several conflicts that lend themselves to the development of coaddict disorder. Such individuals tend to have

---

*The authors wish to thank Carl Ryder for suggesting the use of this term.

boundary distortions and frequently develop enmeshed interpersonal relationships with abusive individuals who can recapitulate their early childhood experiences.

IV. TREATMENT CONSIDERATIONS

Treatment is essential for coaddiction. As reviewed here, the coaddiction disorders tend to be highly disruptive and cause significant physical and psychiatric disturbances. However, as discussed throughout this chapter, the utility of providing such care extends beyond the need of the coaddict to that of ensuring proper treatment of the alcohol- and drug-addicted patient. Untreated coaddicts, especially those with sever reactive coaddiction or coaddictive personality disorder, may undermine the addiction treatment. Coaddiction insidiously influences the perceptions, attitudes, and motivations of family members. Their cognitive and affective functioning becomes organized around the addict, especially those with coaddictive personality disorder. When the addict enters treatment, the world of this individual becomes severely threatened and anxiety ensues. The role in which the family member was accustomed becomes irrelevant and significant change is necessary. The false self that is created by the coaddict for the addict is no longer supported by the addictive system and the family member frequently feels empty and without purpose. As a result, untreated coaddicts frequently try to coerce their addicted family members to withdraw from treatment or join with them is a collusion against it. Rationalizations such as family obligations, childcare, or conflicting employment schedules are frequently heard as justification for the addict's withdrawal from treatment; it is not uncommon to observe instances in which the addict reports that a family member (untreated) is covertly pressuring him or her to withdraw from treatment or to not attend Alcoholics Anonymous or Narcotics Anonymous (AA/NA) meetings.

Treatment of the family member also significantly enhances the therapeutic leverage [17] of the clinical staff when managing resistance in the addict. Through treatment, the coaddict can become educated about the disease concept, addictive defenses, and the almost predictable flight that addicted patients make from treatment. An alliance can grow between the staff and the coaddict, and when the addict's resistance emerges, the staff and coaddict can act in unison to maintain a firm stance about the need for the addict's continued treatment. This joint effort is frequently effective in containing avoidance behaviors in the addicted patient. However, if the coaddict is not treated, the potential alliance is much more limited, and the necessary therapeutic leverage is frequently not available to effectively challenge the addict's resistance.

In addition to the family member's own need for treatment and its positive impact on the addict's rehabilitation, coaddiction treatment, especially when conducted in conjunction with the addict's treatment, can be essential in preventing the strain that relationships often suffer during early recovery. Separation and divorce are not an uncommon outcome when one spouse is successfully treated for an addiction but the other is not for coaddiction. Joint treatment allows both to begin their recovery simultaneously and with increased empathy for the other's condition. The result is typically an increased cohesion for the family unit, without the previous emeshment and/or antagonism coloring the relationship.

This development is usually critical for successful treatment. If the cohesion does not emerge, it is often predictive of poor outcome. In one of the only empirial studies conducted to date concerning the quality of marital interactions and addiction treatment outcome, Orford's group found that marital cohesion was predictive of 12-month treatment outcome: alcoholic patients in cohesive marriages were significantly more likely than those in noncohesive ones to have a good treatment outcome [18].

VII. ASSESSMENT AND MOTIVATION

At the Outpatient Recovery Centers of Fair Oaks Hospital, Summit, New Jersey, our experience has been that addicted patients who have a coaddict participate in treatment have a better outcome than those treated alone. All individuals seeking services for alcohol and drug addiction are requested to bring a family member to the initial evaluation. At that interview, the assessment counselor interviews both individuals jointly and independently. As denial is a hallmark of addiction, it is necessary to have a family member counter the distortions and omissions of the addicted individual concerning the extent of his or her alcohol and drug use. Unless the family member is in collusion with the addict, his or her input is critical to gaining an accurate picture of the presenting problem. The counselor also assesses the family member for coaddiction. If present, treatment is recommended regardless of whether the addicted individual agrees to treatment. Often, health care providers assessing alcohol and drug abuse will interview family members, but only as part of the addiction assessment and as such are unable to identify codependency in family members.

Coaddicts who seek treatment independently of their addicted family member are typically motivated and become excellent patients. While they often have significant cases of reactive coaddiction and/or coaddictive personality disorder, recognition that they require their own treatment is highly useful and allows the treatment to progress rapidly.

Coaddicts who enter treatment on a collateral basis with an addict are often much more resistant to treatment. With these individuals, motivating them to accept treatment is a major task. The style used to motivate family members for treatment is a function of the nature of the coaddict's denial. For those who do have an awareness of their own psychic distress, motivational techniques do not significantly vary from those used for any form of psychotherapy. During the assessment, the counselor offers a rationale for the treatment and attempts to instill hope in its efficacy. For those with a denial that prevents them from recognizing the deletertous effects that their family members use has had on them, the counselor can "play into" the coaddiction by focusing not on the family member but on the addict. They are accurately told that their addict needs their assistance and such participation will increase the individual's chance for successful recovery. When conducting an initial interview with the family member, the clinician should not limit his or her examination to coaddiction. Addiction can coexist with other disorders [16], and the same holds true for coaddiction. In addition, coaddiction itself may lead to major psychiatric illness, such as clinical depression, and it should be identified and monitored. If such illness does not remit with coaddiction treatment, psychotropic medication should be considered.

VIII. TREATMENT MODALITIES

Many coaddicts seeking treatment at our facility have previously undergone a course of individual psychotherapy. However, these treatments have often been unsuccessful because, in part, the therapists lacked a cohesive understanding of coaddiction. The interventions employed were not designed to integrate and organize the patient's chaotic behaviors around the codependency dynamic. However, even when such a coaddiction theme was cultivated, individual psychotherapy was still often unsuccessful. Family members often enter treatment in acute crisis and a weekly individual psychotherapy does not provide sufficient structure, intensity, or support to maintain them. In addition, the same kind of denial and avoidant defenses that impede the efficacy of individual treatment for addiction operate similarly to limit its effectiveness for coaddiction. We have found that a treatment emphasizing group therapy, especially with frequent sessions, is highly effective. The group setting provides the support and sense of universality [18] that allows the coaddict to identify with, and be supported by, his/her peers. Only then is the coaddict in a position to accept feedback about denial, enabling, and other coaddictive behaviors. One of the goals for the coaddiction therapist is to help create a cohesive group in which the social norm is adherence to a non-coaddictive lifestyle. Through the use of group process, confrontation, experiential learning, and role modeling by senior group members for junior ones, coaddictive behaviors can then be regularly identified and altered.

Yalom's [19] model of interpersonal group therapy is an excellent one for developing a cohesive group and activating coaddictive behaviors. Typically, the same style that patients exhibit within their addictive system are recapitulated in the treatment group. Group members will protect one another from self-examination and painful affective states. Identification, elucidation, and the working through of this recapitulation of the addict–coaddict relationship is critical to a successful treatment of a family member.

Our treatment programs also require active participation in self-help groups, such as Al-Anon [20]. These groups help the coaddictive patient become inculcated with the behaviors and values of a non-coaddictive lifestyle and also provides a larger group on which the patient can rely upon for support, structure, and guidance during times of particular crisis and after treatment has been completed. The group at times is devoted to addressing the patient's resistance of such participation. When explored, these resistances are frequently rooted in the codependent's denial, either of the addiction or their own psychic distress, or an inner sense of humiliation and shame for being part of an addictive family system.

We also present didactic material to complement the group therapy. Educational films and lectures provide patients with basic information about coaddiction, addiction, and recovery [21]. This can help rectify the patient's frequent lack of knowledge about the addictive system which, as discussed previously, contributes to the development of coaddiction.

We provide two coaddiction treatment programs. The first is a 24-week program consisting of a weekly educational hour followed by a discussion and then a group therapy. The purpose of this program is to help patients identify and modify coaddictive behaviors, gain basic information about addiction and coaddiction, and begin participation in Al-Anon. Referrals made to this program are generally of individuals with mild forms of coaddiction, particularly reactive coaddiction.

Family members with more severe reactive coaddiction, or coaddictive personality disorder are generally referred to our second program, a comprehensisve year-long treatment that includes intensive group and individual counseling. During an initial 6 weeks (primary care), patients participate in three group treatment sessions each week and after a 4-week transition period, they then join the weekly aftercare program for the remainder of 1 calendar year. Throughout this treatment, individual counseling is provided on a regular basis and is generally focused on supporting participation in the group. If indicated, individual psychotherapy can be provided independently of the program for patients that require this additional care.

A unique feature of this program, and critical to its success, is how the program interfaces with the evening addiction treatment program that is described elsewhere in this text. Throughout primary and aftercare, coaddict patients participate in joint groups with their alcohol- and drug-addicted family members. Those addicts and coaddicts who enter treatment alone are typically able to make significant gains despite the absence of their family member, principally through surrogate work and participation in the group process. All addicts and coaddicts are assigned to a treatment team consisting of an addiction counselor and a coaddiction counselor. Each independently conducts their respective group therapies and coleads joint groups. These sessions offer an opportunity for both addict and coaddict to gain empathy for the other's experience. Both individuals have often taken a hostile or distant stance in the relationship. An appreciation for how the addiction has affected the other family member has not developed. In these joint groups, the rage or distance from the other individual typically emerges and can be worked through with the support and encouragement of the peers. At the same time, appropriate boundries between addict and coaddict can be drawn and the responsibilities of both identified. The group is also an excellent opportunity for the dismantling of the enabling system. Such behaviors and how they are elicited by addicted family members can be easily elucidated in the group process or brought into it from external addict-coaddict interactions.

> Jeff, an alcoholic, and Pam, a coaddict, have been married 9 years and had been in primary care treatment for 6 weeks. Jeff had been secretly drinking throughout this time and with the knowledge of Pam. Only as they were about to begin transitioning to aftercare did Pam confide in her coaddiction group about her husband's drinking. Pam explained that her silence throughout treatment was a function of her guilt about betraying her husband and fear of his verbal retribution. With the support of her peers, Pam confronted her husband with this information in the joint group. Jeff became enraged and started to verbally abuse his wife. However, with the direction and support of the cotherapists and peers, Pam and Jeff were able to identify their addictive and codependent behaviors and how they interacted to maintain the addictive family system.

This conflict and its resolution became a turning point in treatment for both patients. During the group, each graphically portrayed their contribution to the on-going conflict. The result was an increased understanding of the other's experience; the addict feeling compelled to use and angry at his wife for not supporting it, and the coaddict feeling guilty and believing that continued enabling was her only alternative as a loyal wife.

IX. CONCLUSIONS

Coaddiction is a significant psychic and behavioral disturbance that has traditionally gone undetected by those health care professionals providing treatment for alcohol and drug addiction. Most family members of addicted individuals exhibit characteristics of the syndrome to at least some degree. These characteristics include enabling, ignorance about the nature of addiction, denial, irrational reliance on control, poor self-image, and stress-related illness. Some personality-disordered coaddicts are predisposed to developing relationships with active addicts because of their own childhood experiences, which is often in a previous addictive system.

Treatment of the coaddiction is essential not only because of its inherent value to the family member, but of its importance to the alcohol- and drug-addicted patient's rehabilitation. Through treatment, the enabling system can be dismantled, boundries clarified, self-esteem enhanced, and the potential sabotaging of the addict's treatment by a coaddict threatened by changes in the addictive system prevented. Treatment for the coaddicted patient is most effective when it is conducted in a group format and supplemented by didactic presentations and the patient's participation in the self-help community.

ACKNOWLEDGMENTS

The author's wish to acknowledge Lisa DeSarno Herrejon and Patricia Recchia DeSarno for their effort and assistance toward completing this chapter.

REFERENCES

1. Anderson, D.J. *Perspectives On Treatment*, Hazeldon, Center City, Minnesota, 1986.
2. Cocores, J.A. New treatment for coaddiction disorder. *Psychiatr. Times*, May 13–15 (1988).
3. Schaef, A. *Co-dependence Misunderstood-Mistreated, Harper & Row*, San Francisco, 1986.
4. Miller, N.S., Klahr, A.L., Sweeney, D.R., Sweeney, K., and Cocores, J.A. The diagnosis of alcohol dependence in cocaine dependence. *Am. J. Psychiatry*, (1988).
5. Cocores, J.A., and Gold, M.S. *Recognition*. Crisis intervention treatment with cocaine abusers, *Crisis Intervention handbook*, A.R. Roberts (ed.). Wadsworth, Pacific Grove, California, 1990.
6. Wallace, J. Working with the preferred defense structure of the recovering alcoholic, *Practical Approached to Alcoholism Psychotherapy* (S. Zimberg, J. Wallace, and S.B. Blum, (eds.) Plenum Press, New York, 1978.
7. Cocores, J.A. Co-addiction: A silent epidemic. *Psychiat. Lett.*, 5(2):5–8 (1987).
8. Cocores, J.A., Gold, M.S. Sexual function in co-dependents. *Hum. Sexual.*, February 26 (1989).
9. Beattie, M. *Codependent No More*, Harper & Row, San Francisco, 1987.
10. Mellody, P. Miller, A.W., and Miller, J.K. *Facing Codependency*, Harper & Row, San Francisco, 1989.
11. Cermak, T.L. *Diagnosing and Treating Co-Dependence*, Johnson Institute Books, Minnesota, 1986.
12. Mulry, J.T. Codependency: A family addiction. *Am. Fam. Pract.*, 35(4):215–219 (1987).
13. Asher, R., and Brissett, D. Codependency: A view from women married to alcoholics, *Int. J. Addict.*, 23(4):331–350 (1987).
14. Gierymski, T., and Williams, T: Codependency. *J. Psychoactive Drugs*, 18(1)7–12 (1986).
15. Steinglass, P. The impact of alcoholism on the family: Relationship between degree of alcoholism and psychiatric symptomatology. *J. Stud. Alcohol*, 42(3):288–303 (1981).
16. Cocores, J.A. Treatment of the dually diagnosed adult drug user, *Dual Diagnosis Patients* (M.S. Gold and A.E. Slaby, (eds.). Marcel Dekker, New York, 1990.
17. Zimberg, S. Psychiatric office treatment of alcoholism, *Practical Approaches To Alcoholism Psychotherapy*, S. Zimberg, J. Wallace, and S.B. Blum, (eds.). Plenum Press, New York, 1978.
18. Orford, J. Oppenheimer, E., Egert, S., Hensman, C., and Guthrie, S. The cohesiveness of alcoholism complicated marriages and its influence on treatment outcome. *Br. J. Psychiatry*, 128:318–39 (1976).
19. Yalom, I.D.: *The Theory and Practice of Group Psychotherapy*, Basic Books, New York, 1985.
20. *First Steps*, Al-Anon Family Group Headquarters, Inc., New York, 1986.
21. Cocores, J.A. *The 800 Cocaine Book of Drug and Alcohol Recovery*, Villard Books, New York, 1990.

XIV
Special Topics

48

Drug and Alcohol Addiction and AIDS

Nathan M. Kravis, Carol J. Weiss, and Samuel W. Perry
Cornell University Medical College, New York, New York

I. INTRODUCTION

A. HIV Transmission and Epidemiology

Intravenous drug users (IVDUs) and their sexual partners and children constitute the fastest growing subpopulations of the human immunodeficiency virus (HIV) epidemic. There can no longer be any doubt (as there once was in the mid-1980s) that HIV is transmitted heterosexually. Unprotected vaginal or anal intercourse with an IVDU has become an increasingly prominent vector of HIV transmission. It is estimated that 80% of male IVDUs have their primary sexual relationship with women who are non-IVDUs [1]. This means that in New York City alone there are approximately 120,000 current or former male IVDUs who are presently heterosexually involved with non-IVDU women [2]. As the rate (but not the number) of newly diagnosed cases of AIDS among gay and bisexual men peaks and begins to decline in the 1990s, IVDUs and their sexual partners will constitute an increasingly large percentage of the people who become infected with HIV and are newly diagnosed with acquired immune deficiency syndrome (AIDS).

The HIV seroprevalence rate varies among different geographical populations of IVDUs. In a review of 92 studies of seroprevalence rates among IVDUs across the country, Hahn et al. found a range from 0 to 65%, with the highest rates in the Northeastern part of the United States and Puerto Rico [3]. The reasons for this wide range are not completely clear, but it presumably reflects differing patterns of drug-using behaviors. "Shooting galleries," for example, are primarily (though not exclusively) a Northeast phenomenon. Since drug injection paraphernalia is commonly rented or shared in shooting galleries—practices that promote HIV transmission—it is not surprising to find their presence positively correlating with high seroprevalence among IVDUs. The greater tendency among black and Hispanic IVDUs to share "works" and to frequent shooting galleries may partially explain their higher rates of HIV infection compared to white IVDUs in the same region.

In 1988, 10,747 cases of IVDU-associated AIDS (i.e., AIDS in IVDUs, their sex partners, and in children born to women who were IVDUs or partners of IVDUs) were reported to the Centers for Disease Control (CDC) by the 50 states, the District of Columbia, and U.S. territories [4]. These cases represent about a third of the 32,311 AIDS cases reported to the CDC in 1988. Male heterosexual IVDUs represented over half and male homosexual/bisexual IVDUs approximately one-fifth of all IVDU-associated AIDS. As noted in a 1989 CDC report, "IVDU-associated AIDS accounts for most AIDS cases in heterosexual men, women, and children" [4].

B. Cocaine and the HIV Epidemic

Cocaine use increases HIV transmission by increasing the frequency of injection and needle sharing, and by increasing the frequency and likelihood of practicing unsafe sex.

The impaired judgment associated with drug intoxication and withdrawal contributes to HIV transmission because it effects needle sharing, needle cleaning, and sexual behavior. It is unclear what proportion of IVDU-associated AIDS is due to sexual transmission as opposed to needle sharing. Nevertheless, studies confirm that common sense would predict: Drug and alcohol use is associated with failure to practice safer sex, even in individuals who are well informed about the risks of HIV transmission and know what to do to reduce those risks during sexual activity [5,6].

All drugs of abuse are disinhibiting and may promote unsafe sexual practices. Because it is short acting, cheap, and widely available, cocaine, especially in its purified, smokable, and highly addictive form, "crack," is often implicated in unsafe sex. Heavy cocaine and crack users are apt to experience surges of hypersexuality characterized by prolonged periods of intense sexual arousal and promiscuity. Needless to say, during these hypersexual binges, condom use, let alone judicious and discriminating selection of sexual partners, is rarely a consideration. Prostitution, which has always been associated with drug addiction, is an all-too-frequent outcome of crack addiction. Although figures are unavailable, it is well known that women in crack houses often end up trading sex for drugs. These are hardly circumstances conducive to controlling an epidemic caused largely by sexual transmission.

Needle sharing is a devastatingly "efficient" mode of HIV transmission. In a 1986–1987 study of IVDUs in San Francisco, roughly half of the subjects acknowledged "using drugs in a shooting gallery where they did not know who had previously used the needle and syringe" [7]. It appears that educational efforts have been more effective in encouraging IVDUs to clean their syringes with bleach than in decreasing their sharing of needles [8,9]. Given the socioeconomic factors involved in obtaining clean needles, it may be more feasible for a needle user to clean needles rather than stop sharing altogether [10]. Here too, because of its shorter half-life and greater frequency of injection, cocaine plays a subversive role. Those who share a needle with only one partner are more readily persuaded to cease needle sharing altogether, whereas those who share needles with multiple partners are more likely to be cocaine users and less likely to respond to interventions aimed at decreasing needle sharing [8].

Indeed, cocaine plays a particularly pernicious role in the burgeoning HIV epidemic among current and former IVDUs and their sexual partners. Intravenous and intranasal cocaine use is not uncommon among heroin addicts, both before and during methadone maintenance treatment. In the previously cited study of San Francisco IVDUs by Chaisson et al. [7], almost one-third of the cocaine-using subjects either initiated or accelerated cocaine injection during long-term methadone maintenance treatment. Because of the relatively short-lived "high" associated with its use, intravenous cocaine addicts inject more frequently than heroin users—sometimes more than 10 times a day. They are also more likely to withdraw blood into the syringe to mix with the drug [7], a practice known as "booting." Booting may enhance HIV transmission by increasing the likelihood of exposure to contaminated blood.

Ominously, most heroin addicts prefer injectable cocaine over crack [11]. Cocaine injection alone is associated with a higher risk of HIV infection than either injecting cocaine mixed with heroin ("speedballing") or alternating injection of cocaine and heroin. In brief, all drug use that includes cocaine injection in one way or another is associated with a much higher risk of HIV infection than heroin injection alone [7].

II. MEDICAL ASPECTS OF DRUG AND ALCOHOL ADDICTION AND AIDS

A. Drug Addiction and Immune Functioning

Drugs of abuse have long been implicated as contributing to endocrinological and immunological disturbances [12], though it has been difficult to distinguish specific drug effects from other factors such as poor nutritional status, lack of adequate clothing and shelter, and previous illness.

The hepatotoxic and neurotoxic effects of alcohol are well known. Although it is accepted that alcohol has an adverse effect on the immune system, neither the extent of this effect nor the mechanism(s) have been clearly elucidated. Alcohol abuse in humans significantly decreases the weight of peripheral lymphoid organs; the spleen and thymus. Circulating leukocytes are also diminished. Both humoral immune mechanisms and cell-mediated immunity are impaired by alcohol consumption, contributing to the alcoholic's well-recognized increased susceptibility to infectious agents [13].

Tetrahydrocannabinol may have marked suppressive effects on various components of the immune system, both cellular and humoral. Cannabinoids at nontoxic doses can depress the in vitro functional activity of T and B lymphocytes as well as macrophages. Cannabinoids have the ability to serve as cofactors in altering the immune status of the host, conferring increased susceptibility to retroviral infection [14].

It has also been well established that opiate addicts have a variety of endocrine disturbances, most importantly involving the hypothalamic-pituitary-gonadal axis [12,15]. Opiate addicts have been shown to have depressed levels of total T cells [16]. More recent studies demonstrate specific deficiencies in immune function (natural killer cell activity) among parenteral drug abusers that improve with methadone maintenance [17].

The effect of cocaine on the immune system cannot be characterized as solely enhancing or depressing [16]. Cocaine hydrochloride added to cultures of human peripheral blood lymphocytes suppresses some immune functions, while enhancing others [18]. Investigators are presently pursuing the possibility that cocaine "may have direct immunologic effects that bear either on the transmissibility from persons infected with HIV-1 or on an individual's risk of acquisition given exposure" [11].

It has been long known that IVDUs have higher rates of tuberculosis (TB), bacterial pneumonia, bacterial endocarditis, and sexually transmitted diseases (STDs) than the non-drug-using population. Since the advent of HIV infection and AIDS, however, these problems have been compounded.

B. Bacterial Pneumonia and Tuberculosis

The medical ramifications of HIV infection extend far beyond opportunistic infections by nonpathogenic organisms. Current and former IVDUs without AIDS who are HIV-positive have a fivefold increase in risk over seronegative IVDUs for serious bacterial pneumonias owing most often to either *Streptococcus pneumoniae* or *Haemophilus influenzae* infections, indicating a possible role for pneumococcal vaccines in the medical management of seropositive IVDUs [19]. The seropositives experience a higher mortality rate from these pneumonias than the seronegatives [19,20].

Increased TB morbidity has been known to be associated with AIDS since 1987 [21]. In a prospective study of 520 IVDUs in a methadone maintenance program, Selwyn et al. showed that HIV- seropositive IVDUs have a significantly higher risk of active TB over seronegatives, presumably owing to greater susceptibility to reactivation of latent tuberculous infection [22]. This finding implies a need to consider linking prophylaxis with anti-TB agents such as isoniazid with daily methadone doses for PPD-positive clients who also test positive for the presence of the HIV antibody [22,23].

C. STDs and Other Infectious Diseases

The resurgence of syphilis that has accompanied the HIV epidemic has received attention in the medical [24–26] and lay [27] press. Here, too, cocaine is implicated, particularly in its role in driving the promiscuity and prostitution known to take place in crack houses. The concomitant rise in incidence of chancroid, particularly in minority men and women, has been less heralded [28]. Most experts believe that syphilis, chancroid, and herpes—STDs that cause genital ulcers—increase the efficiency of HIV transmission by providing a portal of entry for the virus at the site of the lesion.

Recent evidence suggests that in addiction to these associations between HIV infection and other infectious diseases, IVDUs may, independent of HIV serological status, be at greater risk for infection with human T-cell leukemia viruses, especially HTLV-II [29]. Needle sharing is the presumed mode of contagion. Like HIV-I, HTLV-I, HTLV-II, and HIV-II are thought to be associated with long latency periods. The laboratory technology for detecting subtypes of HTLV infection is too new to indicate what hematological, immunological, or neurological complications asymptomatic carriers of HTLV-II infection will develop.

D. Pregnancy and Reproductive Health

Although habitual heroin injection can adversely affect reproduction [12,30], female IVDUs are relatively fertile. The overwhelming majority of female IVDUs are black or Hispanic. Compared to their white age-matched counterparts, they have more babies and fewer abortions, and probably use contraceptives less frequently and/or less effectively [31,32]. Furthermore, HIV seropositivity in female IVDUs does not appear to be associated with a decreased pregnancy rate, nor does asymptomatic HIV infection adversely affect pregnancy outcome [33]. Taken together, these factors emphasize the high risk for perinatal HIV transmission posed by female IVDUs.

III. NEUROPSYCHIATRIC ASPECTS OF DRUG AND ALCOHOL ADDICTION AND AIDS

A. Diagnosis

Facing the stress of HIV testing and receiving the diagnosis of HIV infection may lead to transient, reactive psychiatric symptoms that include depression, anxiety, and preoccupation with physical symptoms [35,35]. Major depression may occur in both early and late stages of HIV infection.

Neurological and psychiatric abnormalities may be among the first symptoms of HIV infection [36,37]. Many of the neuropsychiatric manifestations of AIDS are directly attributable to the presence of HIV in the central nervous system (CNS) and are not simply epiphenomena.

Physical weakness or dementia may obscure or confound a depressive episode; both of these conditions may also occur simultaneously. Suicidal ideation is common among HIV-infected individuals, and patients with AIDS have increased rates of suicide [35,38,39]. Opiates and cocaine are frequently used by drug users to treat the psychological and physical distress associated with AIDS-related depression and dementia.

The most common organic mental disorders in patients with HIV infection are delirium, dementia, and organic mood syndrome. AIDS dementia complex (ADC) is the most common CNS complication of HIV infection [40]. HIV-1 infects the CNS early in the infectious process and may be sequestered in the cerebrospinal fluid, remaining latent for several years. AIDS dementia complex usually manifests itself after patients develop major opportunistic infections, though some patients present with this syndrome prior to developing major systemic complications. Only a small number of patients develop dementia when they are otherwise medically well, but the majority eventually become afflicted with ADC [41]. In one study, 10% of HIV-infected individuals sought medical attention for cognitive disturbances, and 40% had symptoms of cognitive impairment before AIDS was diagnosed [41]. Over two-thirds of AIDS patients autopsied have evidence of neurological involvement [41].

HIV-1 affects the central and peripheral nervous system with relative sparing of the cortex. The principal neuropathological abnormalities are in the subcortical structures, notably the central white matter, deep gray structures (including the basal ganglia and thalamus), and the brain stem. Therefore, ADC is a subcortical dementia. Other subcortical dementias are the dementias associated with Huntington's disease, progressive supranuclear palsy, and Parkinson's disease. These dementias are marked by psychomotor slowing, decreased mental flexibility, and decreased spontaneity. By contrast, a cortical dementia such as Alzheimer's disease includes aphasia, apraxia, abnormalities of cortical sensation, and disorientation.

AIDS dementia complex is particularly noted to produce cognitive slowing and deficits in recent memory and attention. The degree of cognitive impairment that is present when ADC is diagnosed varies among patients. Approximately 10% of asymptomatic HIV seropositives have slight to moderate cognitive impairment [41]. Early signs include poor concentration, slowed processing, impaired initiation, and forgetfulness. Global dementia is seen in later stages.

In addition to these cognitive deficits, motoric and behavioral impairments are also seen as part of ADC. The early motor disturbances include clumsiness, incoordination, ataxia, poor balance, abnormal reflexes, and weakness. As symptoms progress, paraparesis and incontinence may develop. Behavioral disturbances range from withdrawal and apathy to hallucinations and other psychotic symptoms. Mutism occurs in the terminal stage.

The diagnosis of ADC must be distinguished from treatable neurological complications of AIDS such as cerebral toxoplasmosis, primary CNS lymphoma, and cryptococcal meningitis. Peripheral neuropathies and vacuolar myelopathy are also common neurological complications of AIDS and may occur concurrently with ADC.

Delirium may appear in persons with HIV infection at any point in their illness, though it is more common at times of systemic illness. Drug withdrawal and drug intoxication significantly contribute to the development of delirium in all patients, especially those with HIV infection. Organic mood syndromes also may occur at any point in the course of HIV infection and are also importantly affected by drug use.

B. Treatment

In treating the neuropsychiatric manifestations and complications of HIV infection, it must be remembered that the drug-abusing patient continues to battle his addictive disorder while struggling with the ravages of HIV. Clinicians must be aware of the sensitivity of HIV-spectrum patients to the side effects of psychotropic medications while at the same time providing symptomatic relief. They should avoid the relatively common error of undermedicating the drug abuser in pain for fear of causing or abetting further addiction [42].

Mild insomnia or anxiety usually does not require medication. Patients should be encouraged to discuss these matters in psychotherapy or in individual or group counseling/support meetings before resorting to medication. When medications are prescribed, dependency-producing medications like the benzodiazepines should be avoided. Instead, sedating medications such as diphenhydramine (Benadryl), chloral hydrate, sedating antidepressants such as trazodone, or even clonidine, may be used. More debilitating anxiety or the disruptive agitation associated with delirium and dementia may need to be managed with neuroleptics if these sedating medications fail, although neuroleptic use in HIV-infected patients is known to cause unusually frequent and severe dystonias and neuroleptic malignant syndrome [45].

Depression can be treated with tricyclic antidepressants. Monoamine oxidase inhibitors (MAOIs) should be avoided in the drug abuser because of their interaction with alcohol, opiates, and cocaine. Psychostimulants have been recommended for the treatment of depression and dementia in AIDS [46], though their use has not been studied in drug abusers with AIDS. However, psychostimulants have been known to precipitate cocaine craving in drug abusers [47], and may do so during their medical illness as well; therefore, they should be used cautiously, if at all, in anyone with a history of cocaine use.

Azidothymidine (AZT) has been reported to improve neurological symptoms in some AIDS patients [48]. It appears to slow progression of symptoms of dementia, and, in some cases, improve cognition.

IV. PSYCHOSOCIAL ASPECTS OF DRUG AND ALCOHOL ADDICTION AND AIDS

The most prominent psychological traits of many drug abusers and alcoholics—their low frustration tolerance, difficulty tolerating intense affect, and tendency to use denial—render them extremely ineffective in coping with the demands of a contagious, chronic, and fatal condition such as HIV infection. HIV infection poses formidable challenges to such a personality organization. Facing the daily fear, uncertainty, anxiety, anger, and depression that accompany HIV infection requires considerable emotional fortitude and psychological health. The alcohol or drug addict, lacking an adequate repertoire of coping skills, naturally turns to familiar, albeit destructive, behavior.

HIV testing and counseling of drug addicts is complicated by numerous factors related to the varying ego strengths and weaknesses and the diverse lifestyles of this heterogeneous group. The powerful pull of denial may prevent some addicts from ever obtaining testing. Pretest counseling calls on the patient to imagine his or her response to a positive or negative test result; this is problematic for those addicts who have difficulty envisioning a future as near as a few hours away. For some, notification may not be possible because of homelessness or transience.

Response to notification is quite variable among drug addicts; systematic studies in this area are few [38]. Both health care providers and patients often harbor the belief that seropositive notification will have a salutory effect on drug use. This may occur transiently, but rarely in an enduring fashion unless drug rehabilitation measures are initiated. Regarding the effects of notification on parenteral drug use and HIV transmission, Cox et al. [49] found an association between seropositive notification and decreased needle use, and Casadonte et al. [50] found that notified seropositive IVDUs showed significantly greater risk reduction than notified seronegative IVDUs—but not a greater reduction than in serologically untested subjects. Conversely, Marlink et al. [51] reported higher rates of drug relapse with needle injection in seropositive than in seronegative or untested subjects at 3 months follow-up, but no significant differences between the three groups at the 9- and 12-month assessments.

Anxiety, shame, rage, and denial may precipitate drug binges or medical noncompliance. Relapse has been seen in former drug addicts who have done well for many years, typically in the context of self-medication for illness-related symptoms such as depression and fatigue. Loss of social and occupational supports and organic brain disorder may also result in relapse into drug use.

For some addicts, cognitive and developmental deficits may better explain their behavior. Many come from backgrounds of social and intellectual impoverishment. They may be unable to project themselves into the future and imagine themselves attaining goals or realizing aspirations. In this setting, the notion of future risk may be meaningless; the future itself is either unimagined or foreseen with despair. "Tomorrow" is an abstraction. An impoverished drug user weighs the hopelessness and futility of his environment against the pleasure of intoxication.

Intellectual deficits account for some noncompliance with preferred medical interventions. It is often hard for some addicts to understand the difference between a treatable infection and AIDS; some may therefore refuse antibiotics that may return them to relative health. Similarly, many have difficulty grasping the difference between HIV infection and AIDS; hence, the role of AZT or pentamidine prophylaxis may be obscured.

V. CULTURAL AND SOCIOECONOMIC ASPECTS OF DRUG AND ALCOHOL ADDICTION AND AIDS

The urban poor comprise the vast majority of parenteral drug users. This is a disenfranchised class with poor family and social supports, both of which are important and lacking in the battle against a chronic, fatal illness. These are often people with little to live for or few resources to support the struggle their survival will entail. This group also lacks the social power or political clout to organize themselves and compete for scarce funding and other state-administered resources [52].

This population's relationship with the medical community also places them at a disadvantage. Often they do not use health care services in a structured way and do not follow through with recommended treatments or diagnostic procedures. Alternative belief systems, such as spiritism in Hispanic cultures, as well as cognitive difficulty negotiating a path through labyrinthine medical facilities and hospital bureaucracies may contribute to inconsistent use or avoidance of medical services.

The disruptive behavior sometimes seen among drug abusers in hospitals and clinics should be viewed in light of the street culture from which many of them come. These are often people who are rarely sedentary except when intoxicated. In the street, they are constantly on the move, making deals, and subject to few rules. The structure of the hospital is foreign and foreboding to them. The alien hospital milieu combined with the addict's intolerance of anxiety and boredom, and his or her vulnerability to irritablity or agitation on the basis of delirium or withdrawal explains why some drug addicts can be exasperating patients.

Inner city drug-using cultures have certain deeply rooted mores that are *not* changing rapidly, despite AIDS. In the predominantly male-dominated Hispanic cultures, it is generally not accepted for men to use condoms and women are expected to bear their men children regardless of circumstances, which often include youth, poverty, and disease. Women who advocate the use of condoms or not bearing a child owing to HIV infection may be subject to beatings or abandonment by their mates.

For female drug addicts, many of whom feel deviant and stigmatized [53], bearing a child may be their only hope at being "normal" and accepted by society or by their man.

Pregnant seropositive addicts weigh this hope against the 30–40% risk of bearing an infected child. Many choose to accept that risk.

The practice of sharing needles is also reinforced by strong social forces that are not easily altered [54,55]. The user's first injection experience is usually at the hand of, and with the equipment of, a veteran IVDU. Intimate friendships and sexual relationships are often entwined with needle sharing. Drug use in group settings commonly entails sharing of equipment or drugs. Not to share is considered an affront, or, more recently, an unspoken accusation that your drug partner is infected with HIV [10].

VI. DRUG ADDICTION AND AIDS: SPECIFIC INTERVENTIONS

Behavioral change in the IVDU is not effectively achieved through educational efforts alone. Concrete, practical, and long-term interventions are needed. Street outreach programs and storefront centers for education, counseling, and medical care are important ways of reaching this population. Tangible inducements need to be provided, such as food or food stamps, clothes, toys, or assistance with shelter or with managing social service bureaucracies.

Drug abuse rehabilitation services, particularly methadone maintenance treatment programs (MMTPs), remain the most promising conduit for changing behavior [56–60]. Methadone maintenance treatment programs offer a number of practical advantages for initiating and maintaining behavior change, above and beyond the narcotic blockade that prevents injection of opiates. These programs provide frequent and long-term therapeutic contacts. Clients can be regularly exposed to AIDS prevention education each time they come to the clinic to receive their medication. Even when clients do not totally recover, they sustain a relationship with care providers that may influence their behavior in small ways that would otherwise not have been possible; this leaves the door open for future change.

Traditional addiction treatment programs have typically shunned the use of pharmacotherapy in the management of anxiety or mild depression; behavioral interventions, counseling, and group support have been preferred. Only recently has the use of major tranquilizers or antidepressants become accepted within these treatment programs. Sedative-hypnotics and benzodiazepines are still avoided. The current challenge facing addiction treatment programs is learning when—and which—pharmacological interventions are indicated in the management of the seropositive patient.

The seropositive drug-addicted patient in addiction treatment who is still relatively medically healthy should continue to be taught that not all psychological symptoms get medicated; for example, he or she might receive antidepressants for depression, but not benzodiazepines for irritability or chronic insomnia. When such patients are in the medical hospital where the available resources and general milieu do not permit the inculcation of the principles of addiction treatment, more expedient prescribing practices may be necessary. Even in the hospital, however, medications that are not easily abused or sold on the street are preferable. In the later stages of AIDS, if the patient is infirmed or no longer able to benefit from addiction treatment, or has little ability to obtain illicit drugs, more liberal prescribing practices are sensible and humane. In sum, the clinician will need to consider the patient's current position in the projected course of HIV-spectrum illness as well as the circumstances of treatment in determining the appropriate treatment approach.

Patients need to be helped to cope with the news of seropositivity and the subsequent stresses attendant to the illness without resorting to drug abuse. Their nihilism, hopelessness, fear, rage, and anxiety may be tempered with the knowledge that the course of their illness will likely be accelerated by further illicit drug use.

Often the clinician can provide invaluable assistance by helping the seropositive patient involve his or her family in his or her care. Many of these patients feel rejected by their families, ashamed of their behavior, or believe their families are too impaired (usually with alcohol or drug addiction) to be helpful. Assisting the patient in telling the family can lead to rapprochement and additional support.

VII. Problems and Future Prospects

At the end of nearly a decade of AIDS—an initial decade of shock and devastation as well as productive (if belated) response—the path leading into the 1990s is studded with hopeful prospects and obstacles yet to be surmounted.

A. Problems

Given its invidious role in promoting high-risk behavior, the lack of specific, pharmacological treatment for cocaine addiction and the relative unavailability of comprehensive drug-free cocaine addiction treatment to the urban poor deserves a place at the top of the list of unresolved dilemmas in the struggle against AIDS.

The hidden nature of asymptomatic HIV infection has wrought havoc and tragedy in the lives of many. Thousands of women who are already infected have no idea that they have even been exposed to HIV. A substantial fraction—probably between one-third and one-half—of women who give birth to HIV-seropositive babies will report no self-identified risk factors [61]. Clearly this points to a continued and massive need for educational efforts tailored expressly for sexually active women.

It would certainly be naive to expect counseling and education to translate neatly, directly, or linearly into behavior change. Success in reaching high-risk groups with information about AIDS and HIV transmission has not been matched by success in getting these groups to actually modify practices that place them at risk [62]. This is so regardless of the target population or targetted high-risk behavior. For instance, it is uncertain how knowledge of HIV seropositivity and risk of perinatal transmission affects the decision-making process in infected women who are grappling with whether to continue or electively terminate pregnancy [63]. Nevertheless, drug addiction rehabilitiation, counseling, and supportive follow-up remain our only viable clinical interventions for this group, and the demand for these services will undoubtedly rise as HIV antibody testing of pregnant women becomes more widespread, resulting in greater numbers of identified seropositives.

The long latency or incubation period of HIV is both a blessing and a curse. While promising longer life and greater opportunity for timely medical intervention among identified seropositives, the typically lengthy period of asymptomatic HIV infection (10 years or longer) complicates detection and risk reduction. A risk (such as that posed by HIV infection) that lacks immediate consequences is surely more likely to be ignored by most IVDUs than the relentless threat of withdrawal. In the IVDU's day-to-day struggle to survive, the need to obtain the next "fix" reigns paramount; the possibility of acquiring or transmitting a virus whose effects will probably not be felt for several years is, by comparison, a pale abstraction.

B. Prospects

On the other hand, there are indications that IVDUs are neither impervious to educational compaigns nor disinterested in implementing safer injection practices. A robust if not altogether welcome sign of this is the increased demand for and illicit marketing of sterile needles and syringes by drug dealers [64]. In addition, there is some evidence of risk reduction among certain subpopulations of IVDUs, apparently in response to interventions such as methadone treatment programs, HIV antibody testing and counseling programs, and a host of community-based efforts to distribute AIDS information as well as bleach, condoms, and clean syringes.

For example, the HIV-seroprevalence rate among New York City IVDUs appears to have stabilized in recent years. While this does not mean that there are no new HIV infections in this group, it does imply that the rate of new infections is being counterbalanced by other factors. Des Jarlais et al. report a seroprevalence rate stabilized between 55 and 60% among IVDUs in the borough of Manhattan from 1984 through 1987 [65]. They suggest that successful treatment of IVDUs and risk-reduction measures adopted by IVDUs are the constructive factors contributing to this apparent seroprevalence rate stabilization, along with negative factors such as death or serious illness eliminating seropositives from the pool of active IVDUs and the entry into the pool of new, as yet uninfected IVDUs.

The partial success of chemoprophylaxis with zidovudine—also known as azidothymidine (AZT)—in asymptomatic seropositives as well as its proven value in treating early manifestations of AIDS has provided new impetus for widespread HIV antibody testing of individuals at risk. Though its bone marrow toxicity poses a serious limitation, timely treatment with AZT can substantially prolong survival from HIV infection. With the growing recognition among at-risk individuals that knowledge of HIV antibody status can in some cases enhance the quality and duration of life, the demand for testing, and hence the concomitant need for competent pre- and posttest counseling, will increase.

Although the development of an AIDS vaccine still appears distant, the prospects for new and better medications to bolster the fledgling pharmacological armamentarium against HIV infection and the many debilitating opportunistic infections of AIDS are encouraging. Dideoxyinosine (DDI) is a promising new antiviral agent that acts like AZT only with substantially less hematopoietic toxicity [66]. Medications approved by the U.S. Food and Drug Administration (FDA) in 1989 for use against selected opportunistic infections of AIDS include ganciclovir for cytomegalovirus (CMV) retinitis and aerosolized pentamidine for *Pneumocystis carinii* pneumonia prophylaxis. The FDA has also granted investigational new drug for treatment (IND) status to recombinant human erythropoietin for treatment of AIDS-related anemia [66].

Pending further basic science research and pharmacological breakthroughs, a great deal of psychosocial and public health research still needs to be done. The unresolved question of the possible utility and efficacy of distributing free sterile needles to IVDUs is a case in point. It is also an example of a matter that can only be rationally decided by empirical study getting bogged down in politics and ideological debate [67]. Helping addicts inject drugs safely should not be disparaged as antithetical to the goals of drug addiction treatment, even though these typically include helping addicts curtail or eliminate drug injection. It may well be that promoting safer injection practices among IVDUs complements rather than contradicts the aim of decreasing drug injection in a necessarily multifaceted AIDS prevention effort [68].

VIII. CONCLUSIONS

As a group, IVDUs are now the major vector of heterosexual and perinatal HIV transmission in the United States and Europe [68]. This makes it incumbent upon all clinicians involved in combating the HIV epidemic to cultivate some expertise in drug abuse. Attitudinal changes on the part of many clinicians unaccustomed to treating drug addicts may also be in order, hand-in-hand with increased knowledge. It is important for them to be aware of the heterogeneity of the IVDU population, which encompasses people with a wide variety of attitudes about health and treatment as well as a range of socioeconomic and cultural backgrounds. It may also be useful for clinicians to be taught to view alcoholism and drug addiction as chronic medical illnesses on the model of diabetes mellitus or congestive heart failure. A better understanding of the chronicity of drug addiction might mitigate some of the countertransference hazards of treating people who are prone to relapse despite our best efforts.

Likewise, for all clinicians who specialize in treating drug addicts, knowledge of AIDS and HIV is essential, as is committment to making HIV risk reduction a high-priority treatment goal. Drug addiction services need to become more multifaceted to meet the current complex situation. Parochialism among alcoholism services, self-help groups, drug-free treatment programs, MMTPs, and general psychiatric facilities is ultimately a disservice to patients with the dual problems of drug addiction and HIV-spectrum illness. Methadone programs will need to develop services to treat their growing number of multiple-drug addicts and psychiatrically impaired addicts, and drug-free programs will need to recognize the use of pharmacological agents [69]. Antabuse, naltrexone, and antidepressants may all facilitate abstinence [70,71].

The HIV epidemic has highlighted the need for an integration of medical and drug addiction services. Drug treatment programs should receive funding to have medical services on site and medical facilities should have on-site addiction treatment services. Without such an integration of services, the medically ill drug addict will not be able to obtain optimal care.

Clinicians must be backed by societal efforts, including attempts by local politicians and community leaders to resolve the conflicts engendered by community resistance to establishing drug rehabilitation programs in residential neighborhoods. Despite some encouraging evidence that the interventions at our disposal can be efficacious, their limited availability and underutilization have precluded dramatic results. For example, during the first year of its operation (1987–1988), 92% (635) of the 688 IVDUs who were offered HIV antibody testing and counseling at Boston City Hospital's Project TRUST accepted the testing, and nearly 80% of the 635 who received the testing returned for their test results and counseling [72]. These relatively high voluntary testing and return rates suggest that IVDUs can be recruited for and interested in HIV antibody testing and counseling, and therefore are generally within reach of deliverable AIDS prevention measures. Yet apart from this one project, only 473 of the estimated 14,000 IVDUs in the Boston metropolitan area received HIV antibody testing and counseling at anonymous testing sites and sexually transmitted disease (STD) clinics in 1988 [72].

Clearly, the clinical, scientific, social, and pedagogic challenges posed by the HIV epidemic are enormous. Yet these challenges, daunting as they are, need not occasion hopelessness or despair. Analogous to a medical crisis in the life of an individual, the AIDS crisis should be viewed as presenting our society with a window of therapeutic opportunity—an opportunity, in part, to rethink our response to drug addiction.

ACKNOWLEDGMENT

Supported by NIMH grants #MH42277 and #ES87008.

REFERENCES

1. Friedman, S.R., Des Jarlais, D.C., and Sotheran, J.L. (1986). AIDS health education for intravenous drug users. *Health Ed. Q. 13*:383–393.
2. Women and AIDS Resource Network. *Women and AIDS: The Silent Epidemic*. New York, 1988.
3. Hahn, R.A., Onorato, I.M., Jones, S., and Dougherty, J. (1989). Prevalence of HIV infection among intravenous drug users in the United States. *J.A.M.A. 261*:2677–2684.
4. Centers for Disease Control. (1989). Acquired immunodeficiency syndrome associated with intravenous drug use—United States. *M.M.W.R. 38*:165–170.
5. Stall, R., McKusick, L., Wiley, J., et al. (1986). Alcohol and drug use during sexual activity and compliance with safe sex guidelines for AIDS: the AIDS Behavioral Research Project. *Health Ed. Q. 13*:359–371.
6. Goldsmith, M.F. (1988). Sex tied to drugs = STD spread. *J.A.M.A. 260*:2009.

7. Chaisson, R.E., Bacchetti, P., Osmond, D., Brodie, B., Sande, M.A., and Moss, A.R. (1989). Cocaine use and HIV infection in intravenous drug users in San Francisco. *J.A.M.A.* *261*:561–565.

8. Sorensen, J.L., Guydish, J., Costantini, M., and Batki, S.L. (1989). Changes in needle sharing and syringe cleaning among San Francisco drug abusers (letter). *N. Engl. J. Med.* *320*:807.

9. Chaisson, R.E., Osmond, D., Moss, A.R., Feldman, H.W., and Bernacki, P. (1987). HIV, bleach, and needle sharing (letter). *Lancet 1*:1430.

10. Magura, S. Grossman, J.I., Lipton, D.S., Siddiqi, Q., Shapiro, J., Marion, I., and Amann, K.R. (1989). Determinants of needle sharing among intravenous drug users. *Am. J. Public Health* *79*:459–462.

11. Weiss, S.J. (1989). Links between cocaine and retroviral infection. *J.A.M.A.* *261*:607–609.

12. Kreek, M.J. Multiple drug abuse partners and medical consequences, *Psychopharmacology: The Third Generation of Progress*. (H.V. Meltzer, ed.). New York, Raven Press, 1987.

13. Jerrells, T.R., Marietta, C.A., Bone, G., Weight, F.F., and Eckardt, M.J. Ethanol-associated immunosuppression, in *Psychological, Neuropsychiatric, and Substance Abuse Aspects of AIDS*. (T.P. Bridge, A.F. Mirsky, and F.K. Goodwin, eds.). New York, Raven Press, 1988.

14. Friedman, H., Klein, T., Specter, S., Pross, S., Newton, C., Blanchard, D.K., and Widen, R. Drugs of abuse and virus susceptibility, *Psychological, Neuropsychiatric, and Substance Abuse Aspects of AIDS*. (T.P. Bridge, A.F. Mirsky, and F.K. Goodwin, eds.). New York, Raven Press, 1988.

15. Cushman, P. Some endocrine and immunological observations in heroin and methadone maintained opioid addicts, *The Social and Medical Aspects of Drug Abuse* (G. Serban, ed.). New York, Spectrum, 1984.

16. Donahoe, R.M., and Falek, A. Neuroimmunomodulation by opiates and other drugs of abuse: Relationship to HIV infection and AIDS, *Psychological, Neuropsychiatric, and Substance Abuse Aspects of AIDS*. (T.P. Bridge, A.F. Mirsky, and F.K. Goodwin, eds.). New York, Raven Press, 1988.

17. Novick, D.M., Ochshorn, M., Ghali, V., Croxson, T.S., Chiorazzi, N., and Kreek, M.J. (1988). Natural killer activity and lymphocyte subsets in parenteral heroin abusers and long term methadone maintenance patients. *Clin. Res. 36*:798A.

18. Klein, T.W., Newton, C.A., and Friedman, H. Suppression of human and mouse lymphocyte proliferation by cocaine, *Psychological, Neuropsychiatric, and Substance Abuse Aspects of AIDS* (T.P. Bridge, A.F. Mirsky, and F.K. Goodwin, eds.). New York, Raven Press, 1988.

19. Selwyn, P.A., Feingold, A.R., Hartel, D., Schoenbaum, E.E., Alderman, M.H., and Klein, R.S., Freidland G.H. (1988). Increased risk of bacterial pneumonia in HIV-infected intravenous drug users without AIDS. *AIDS 2*:267–272.

20. Centers for Disease Control (1988). Increase in pneumonia mortality among young adults and the HIV epidemic—New York City, United States. *M.M.W.R. 37*:593–596.

21. Centers for Disease Control (1987). Tuberculosis and acquired immunodeficiency syndrome—New York City. *M.M.W.R. 36*:785–795.

22. Selwyn, P.A. Hartel, D., Lewis, V.A., Schoenbaum, E.E., Vermund, S.H., Klein, R.S., Walker, A.T., and Friedland, G.H. (1989). A prospective study of the risk of tuberculosis among intravenous drug users with human immunodeficiency virus infection. *N. Engl. J. Med.* *320*:545–550.

23. Braun, M.M., Truman, B., DiFerdinando, G., and Morse, D. (1989). Drug abuse, HIV infection, and tuberculosis (letter). *J.A.M.A. 262*:616.

24. Centers for Disease Control (1988). Continuing increase in infectious syphilis—United States. *M.M.W.R. 37*:35–38.

25. Centers for Disease Control (1988). Relationship of syphilis to drug use and prostitution—Connecticut and Philadelphia, Pennsylvania. *M.M.W.R. 37*:755–758,764.

26. Centers for Disease Control (1989). Update: heterosexual transmission of acquired immunodeficiency syndrome and human immunodeficiency virus infection—United States. *M.M.W.R. 38*:423–434.

27. Kerr, P. (August 20, 1989). Crack and resurgence of syphilis spreading AIDS among the poor. *The New York Times*, pp. 1,36.

28. Landesman, S.H., Minkoff, H.L., and Willoughby, A. (1989). HIV disease in reproductive age women: a problem of the present. *J.A.M.A. 261*:1326–1327.

29. Lee, H., Swanson, P., Shorty, V.S., Zack, J.A., Rosenblatt, J.D., and Chen, I.S.Y. (1989). High rate of HTLV-II infection in seropositive IV drug users in New Orleans. *Science 244*:471–475.

30. Finnegan, L.P. (1985). The effects of maternal opiate abuse on the newborn. *Fed. Proc. 44*:2314–2317.

31. Brown, L.S., Mitchell, J.L., DeVore, S.L., and Primm, B.J. (1989). Female intravenous drug users and perinatal HIV transmission (letter). *N. Engl. J. Med. 320*:1493–1494.

32. Ralph, N., and Spigner, C. (1986). Contraceptive practices among female heroin addicts. *Am. J. Public Health 76*:1016–1017.

33. Selwyn, P.A., Schoenbaum, E.E., Davenny, K., Robertson, V.J., Feingold, A.R., Shulman, J.F., Mayers, M.M., and Klein, R.S. Friedland, G.H., and Rogers, M.F. (1989). Prospective study of human immunodeficiency virus infection and prgenancy outcomes in intravenous drug users. *J.A.M.A. 261*:1289–1294.

34. Tross, S., and Hirsch, D.A. (1988). Psychological distress and neuropsychological complications of HIV and AIDS. *Am. Psychol. 43*:929–934.

35. Jacobsen, P.B., Perry, S.W., and Hirsch, D. (1990). Behavioral and psychological responses to HIV antibody testing. *J. Consult. Clin. Psychol. 58*:31–37.

36. Perry, S., Belsky-Barr, D., Barr, W., and Jacobsberg, L. (1989). Neuropsychological function in physically asymptomatic HIV seropositive men. *J. Neuropsychiatry 1*:296–302.

37. Marotta, R., and Perry, S. (1989). Early neuropsychological dysfunction caused by human immunodeficiency virus. *J. Neuropsychiatry 1*:225–235.

38. Perry, S., Jacobsberg, L., and Fishman, B. (1990). Suicidal ideation and HIV testing. *J.A.M.A. 263*:679–682.

39. Marzuk, P.M., Tierney, H., Tardiff, K., Gross, E.M., Morgan, E.B., Hsu, M.A., and Mann, J.J. (1988). Increased risk of suicide in persons with AIDS. *J.A.M.A. 259*:1333–1337.

40. Price, R.W., Brew, B., Sidtis, J., Rosenblum, M., Scheck, A.C., and Cleary, P. (1988). The brain in AIDS: Central nervous system HIV-1 infection and AIDS dementia complex. *Science 239*:586–592.

41. Tross, S., Price, R.W., Navia, B., Thaler, H.J. et al. (1988). Neuropsychological characterization of the AIDS dementia complex. *AIDS 2*:81–88.

42. Perry, S. (1985). Irrational attitudes towards addicts and narcotics. *Bull. NY Acad. Med. 61*:706–727.

43. Edelstein, H., and Knight, R.T. (1987). Severe parkinsonism in two AIDS patients taking prochlorperazine. *Lancet 2*:341.

44. Breitbart, W., Marotta, R.F., and Call, P. (1988). AIDS and neuroleptic malignant syndrome. *Lancet 2*:1488–1489.

45. Swenson, J.R., Erman, M., Labell, J, et al. (1989). Extrapyramidal reactions: Neuropsychiatric effects in patients with AIDS. *Gen. Hosp. Psychiatry 11*:248–253.

46. Holmes, V.F., Fernandez, F., Levy, J. K. (1989). Psychostimulant response in AIDS–related complex patients. *J. Clin. Psychiatry 50*:5–8.

47. Gawin, F., Rirdan, C., and Kleber, H.: Methylphenidate treatment of cocaine abusers without attention deficit disorder: A negative report. *Am. J. Drug Alcohol Abuse 11*:193–197.

48. Schmitt, F.A., Bigley, J.W., McKinnis, R., Logue, P.E., Evans, R.W., Drucker, J.L., and the AZT Collaborative Working Group (1988). Neuropsychological outcome of zidovudine (AZT) treatment of patients with AIDS and AIDS-related complex. *N. Engl. J. Med. 319*:1573–1578.

49. Cox, C. Selwyn, P., et al. (1986). Psychological and behavioral consequences of HTLV/LAV antibody testing and notification among intravenous drug users in a methadone program in New York. *Second International Conference on AIDS*, Paris.

50. Casadonte, P.P., Des Jarlais, D.C., et al. (1988). Psychological and behavioral impact of learning HIV test results in IV drug users. *Fourth International Conference on AIDS*, Stockholm.

51. Marlink, R.G., Foss, B., et al. (1987). High rate of HTLV/LAV exposure in IVDAs from a small sized city and the failure of specialized methadone maintenance to prevent further drug use. *Third International Conference on AIDS*, Washington, D.C.

52. Friedman, S.R., Des Jarlais, D.C., Lotheran, J.L., Garber, J. Cohen, H., and Smith, D. (1987). AIDS and self-organization among intravenous drug users. *Int. J. Addict. 22*:201–219.

53. Sandmaier, M. *The Invisibile Alcoholics*. New York, McGraw-Hill, 1980.

54. Des Jarlais, D.C., Friedman, S.R., and Strug, D. AIDS and needle sharing within the IV-drug use subculture, in *The Social Dimensions of AIDS: Method and Theory*. (D.A. Feldman and T.M. Johnson, eds.). New York, Praeger, 1986.

55. National Research Council. *AIDS, Sexual Behavior, and Intravenous Drug Use* (C.F. Turner, H.G. Miller, and L.E. Moses, eds.). Washington, D.C., National Academy Press, 1989.

56. Cooper, J.R. (1989). Methadone treatment and acquired immunodeficiency syndrome. *J.A.M.A.* 262:1664–1668.

57. Dole, V.P. (1988). Implications of methadone maintenance for theories of narcotic addiction. *J.A.M.A. 260*:3025–3029.

58. Dole, V.P. (1989). Methadone treatment and the acquired immunodeficiency syndrome epidemic. *J.A.M.A. 262*:1681–1682.

59. Ball, J.C. Lange, W.R., Myers, C.P., and Friedman, S.R. (1988). Reducing the risk of AIDS through methadone maintenance treatment. *J. Health Social Behav. 29*:214–226.

60. Magura, S., Grossman, J.I., Lipton, D.S., Amann, K.R., Koger, J. (1989). Correlates of participation in AIDS education and HIV antibody testing by methadone patients. *Public Health Rep. 104*:224–231.

61. Landesman, S., Minkoff, H., Holman, S., McCalla, S., and Sijin, O. (1987). Serosurvey of human immunodeficiency virus infection in parturients: Implications for human immunodeficiency virus testing programs of pregnant women. *J.A.M.A. 258*:2701–2703.

62. Fineberg, H.V. (1988). Education to prevent AIDS: prospects and obstacles. *Science 239*:592–596.

63. Selwyn, P.A., Carter, R.J., Schoenbaum, E.E., Robertson, V.J., Klein, R.S., and Rogers, M.F. (1989). Knowledge of HIV antibody status and decisions to continue or terminate pregnancy among intravenous drug users. *J.A.M.A. 261*:3567–3571.

64. Des Jarlais, D.C., Friedman, S.R., and Hopkins, W. (1985). Risk reduction for the acquired immunodeficiency syndrome among intravenous drug users. *Ann. Internal Med. 103*:755–759.

65. Des Jarlais, D.C., Friedman, S.R., Novick, D.M., Sotheran, J.L., Thomas, P., Yancovitz, S.R., Mildvan, D., Weber, J., Kreek, M.J., Maslansky, R., Bartelme, S., Spira, T., and Marmor, M. (1989). HIV-1 infection among intravenous drug users in Manhattan, New York City, from 1977 through 1987. *J.A.M.A. 261*:1008–1012.

66. Goldsmith, M.F.(1989). AIDS drug development, availability intensify. *J.A.M.A. 262*:452–453.

67. Marriott, M. (June 7, 1989). Drug needle exchange is gaining but still under fire. *The New York Times*, pp. B1,B5.

68. Des Jarlais, D.C., and Friedman, S.R. (1989). AIDS and IV drug use. *Science 245*:578.

69. Gordis, E. (1988). Methadone maintenance and patients in alcoholism treatment. *Alcohol Alert 1*:1–4.

70. Millman, R.B. (1988). Evaluation and management of cocaine abusers. *J. Clin. Psychiatry 49*:27–33.

71. Kosten, T.R., and Kleber, H.D.(1984). Strategies to improve compliance with narcotic antagonists. *Am. J. Drug Alcohol Abuse 10*:257.

72. Centers for Disease Control (1989). Counseling and testing intravenous drug users for HIV infection—Boston. *M.M.W.R. 38*:489–496.

49

Protracted Abstinence

Anne Geller
Smithers Alcohol Treatment Center, New York, New York

I. INTRODUCTION

It is a common observation that following cessation of drug use patients remain symptomatic long after the acute withdrawal syndrome has passed. In those who maintain abstinence, symptom intensity and frequency usually wane over a time course which can be weeks or years. Relapses also occur with the greatest frequency during the first 3–6 months of abstinence and thereafter decline. It is reasonable to assume that one of the factors in early relapses might be the abnormal physiological and psychological state of the newly abstinent person. There are, however, a number of possible causes for symptoms in early abstinence which must be distinguished if rational therapy is to be pursued. These include the manifestations of endorgan damage, the recrudescence or unmasking of symptoms which were suppressed by the drug, the presence of an unrelated complicating disorder, the psychological effects of the patient's emerging awareness of painful consequences of his or her drug use, the disruption caused by the radical change in habits as well as a true protracted abstinence syndrome.

A basic conceptual model for drugs producing tolerance and dependence is that some functions which are altered in the presence of the drug react to cessation of drug intake by a shift in the opposite direction, the severity of the shift being a measure of severity of dependence. This shift is often accompanied by an overshoot or rebound, the abstinence syndrome, and is a manifestation of changes in the central nervous system (CNS) brought about by repetitive contact with the drug. The protracted abstinence syndrome is thought to be a continuing manifestation of the same process at a reduced intensity. In some cases, the persistent alteration in central nervous system function may be latent not manifesting itself directly but only when provoked, for example, by reexposure of the drug.

The long duration of withdrawal symptoms was studied initially among heroin users. Himmelsbach [1] in 1942 reported the persistence of an increased cold pressor response following withdrawal in abstinent heroin addicts. In 1968, Martin and Jasinski [2] found abnormalities lasting for at least 6 months into abstinence. These included miosis, hyperthermia,

tachycardia, increased catecholamine excretion, and decreased respiratory response to CO^2.
Insomnia, persisting for 6 weeks, was reported by Kay in 1975 [3]. In alcoholics Kissin et
al. [4] noted that abstinent patients displayed autonomic irregularities such as reduced cold
pressor response and parasympathetic over activity as well as abnormalities in psychomotor
performance and in endocrine and respiratory functions. Similar, though less marked, deficits
were found in a group of alcoholics abstinent from 2–10 years. Sleep patterns and sleep architecture were also abnormal long into sobriety in some studies.

In a series of animal experiments in the 1970s [5–7], chronic alcohol intake was shown
to produce measurable central nervous system changes which persisted long after alcohol
was withdrawn. These changes were in the form of neural hyperexcitability which could be
revealed by reexposure to alcohol. These changes in neural excitability were not uniform
throughout the brain, but were most marked in the reticular formation, hippocampus, and
frontal and parietal cortices [7]. In mice previously exposed to narcotic drugs, Brase [8] and
his associates unmasked residual abnormalities long into abstinence by a priming injection
of morphine followed by naloxone. Following induced alcohol dependence, rats abstinent
for 6 months showed abnormal locomotor and rapid eye movement (REM) sleep patterns
[6] after a challenge dose of alcohol. The time limits of this model have not been tested.
In humans, alterations in saccadic eye movement velocity have been shown to be correlated
with changes in activity of the benzodiazepine–gamma aminobutyric acid (GABA) receptor
complex. Alcoholic subjects abstinent for more than 4 weeks showed increased sensitivity
to diazepam as measured by subjective feelings of sedation as well as objectively by decreased saccadic eye movements [9].

About one-half of newly abstinent alcoholics [10] show evidence of persistently increased
central noradrenergic transmission measured by metabolites 3-methoxy-4-hydroxy-phenyl-
glycol (MHPG) in cerebrospinal fluid. This correlates clinically with a syndrome of irritability
and grandiosity. Fall of MHPG over several weeks of abstinence also parallels a decline in
CNS hyperexcitability as measured by auditory-evoked potentials [11].

Detoxified alcoholics may also show nonsuppression in the dexamethasone suppression
tests as well as blunted thyrotropin response to thyrotropin-releasing hormone [12].

There have been clinical descriptions of symptoms persisting into abstinence and waning with time for alcohol, benzodiazepines, opiates, and stimulants. In practice it is not always
easy to distinguish symptoms due to protracted withdrawal from those due to the other causes
mentioned before. The dysphoria in opiate abstinence, anxiety in benzodiazepine abstinence,
and cognitive impairment in alcohol abstinence for example, have many possible etiologies.
Indeed, this is particularly true for alcohol, where the drug can cause neuronal damage both
directly and as a consequence of nutritional deficiencies. The cognitive impairment so common in early abstinence from alcohol provides an illustration of the complexity of analysis.
It could be a preexisting condition, it could be due to a direct neurotoxic effect of alcohol,
it could be secondary to hepatic damage, or to impaired absorption of thiamine. It could be
a consequence of CNS hyperexcitability. Most probably the deficts which are noted are the
total of several factors acting in a similar direction. With awareness of this complexity, we
will turn to some of the clinical descriptions of abstinence.

II. PSYCHIATRIC SYMPTOMATOLOGY

A high proportion of alcoholic patients have shown persistent symptoms of anxiety and depression [13] during the first 3–6 months of abstinence, in the absence of clear comorbid
psychopathology. A Swedish study [14], unfortunately limited to the first 90 days of abstinence
from alcohol, described fatigability, reduced sleep, reduced sexual interest, apparent sadness
and hostility. Symptoms which might be a consequnce of CNS hyperexcitability such as

inner tension pains, reduced sleep and fatigability improved over the 90 days. A number of biochemical measures were also studied. Of interest, platelet monoamine oxidase (MAO) activity remained low during the entire observation period. The highest values were found in the early recovery phase, suggesting a temporary increase in MAO during acute withdrawal against a generally low background. Transaminases were normal in patients with more than 10 days of abstinence, whereas gamma-glutamyltranspeptidase (GGTP) and high-density lipoprotein (HDL) cholesterol remained high for up to 60 days. Polyunsaturated fatty acids in blood lipids only slowly increased toward normal, a finding which may be related to function of synaptic membranes.

In an extensive survey of abstinent alcoholics, DeSoto [15,16] investigated psychiatric symptomatology over a 10-year period in a cross-sectional sample from Alcoholics Anonymous (AA) studied initially in 1982–1983 and again 4 years later. Using the SCL-90-R which provides an overall measure of severity of symptomatology (the global severity index), DeSoto divided his 312 subjects into five groups depending on length of abstinence. Figure 1 shows his finding of declining severity over a 10-year period. Initial scores for the less than 6 months abstinent group are close to the clinical range (i.e., a severity only obtained by about 2.5% of the population). The 10-year group approximates what might be expected from a general population sample. Items which might be related to CNS hyperexcitability (trouble falling asleep, restless disturbed sleep) start out high but normalize fairly quickly; that is, over a 1- to 2- rather than a 10-year time frame. Items which might be related to permanent CNS damage (e.g., trouble remembering things, mind going blank) were the only ones which, though improving, remained above population norms after 10 years of abstinence.

Although there were considerable differences among subjects at any time period, the scores are not accounted for by just a few highly symptomatic individuals. From a clinical point of view, it is important to note that in the first 6 months of abstinence, approximately 40% of the sample scored within the clinical range on dimensions of depression, interpersonal sensitivity, anxiety, and obsessive-compulsive symptoms. This last group is also clearly tapping functions related to cognitive impairment rather than obsessional behavior per se.

III. SLEEP DISTURBANCES

Sleep disruption and sleep fragmentation, as opposed to simple decreased sleep time, have been shown to result in daytime sleepiness and decreased performance on a variety of tasks

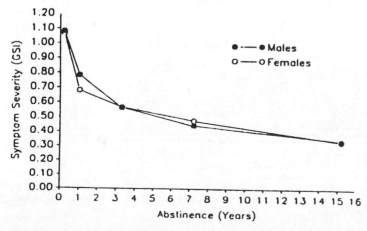

Figure 1 Severity of symptoms (mean scores on the Global Severity Index of the Brief Symptom Inventory) for subjects grouped by sex and length of abstinence. (From Ref. 16, used with permission.)

[17]. Complaints of restless, disturbed sleep are common in early abstinence from alcohol, opiates, benzodiazepines, and stimulants and are most likely a component of the protracted abstinence syndrome. Sleep has been studied in sober alcoholics with a general finding of decreased slow-wave sleep, more arousals, and frequent changes in sleep stage [18–20]. In a study by Snyder and Karacan [21], they failed to confirm slow-wave sleep loss in alcoholics abstinent 3 weeks, but did not find decreased total sleep time, increased latency to sleep, and markedly less sleep efficiency with frequent changes in sleep stages. It is not known for how long the general quality of sleep remains impaired. In one, rather limited study, recovery occurred only after 1–4 years of sobriety [18]. In a study of sleep in opioid abstinence, changes persisted for 3 months, but longer time periods were not examined. The sleep disruptions in early abstinence may well be in part responsible for some of the cognitive disturbances, particularly difficulties with concentration as well as some of the mood changes, irritability, and lability seen during this period.

IV. SYMPTOM REEMERGENCE

In studying both acute and protracted abstinence from benzodiazepines, the confounding problem of symptom reemergence has to be examined [22]. Nonetheless, it is clear that there is a withdrawal reaction after long-term therapeutic use of benzodiazepines [23], and some of these withdrawal symptoms, e.g., tinnitus, involuntary movements, and perceptual changes are new and distinguishable from the symptoms of anxiety for which the drug was originally prescribed.

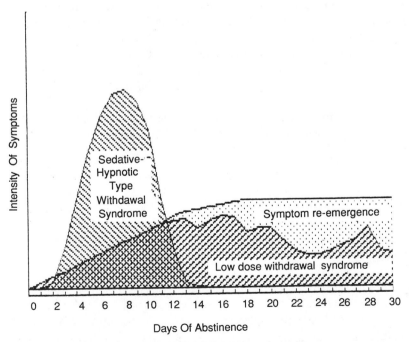

Figure 2 Comparison of relative intensity and time course of enzodiazepine withdrawal syndromes. (From Ref. 22, used with permission.)

V. PROTRACTED WITHDRAWAL

While many clinical investigators have estimated the duration of withdrawal symptoms as from 4–6 weeks, there are reports of protracted withdrawal lasting for 6 months to 1 year [24,25]. Symptoms include hypersensitivity to sensory stimuli, paresthesias, perceptual distortions, muscle pains, twitching, tremors, headache, and sleep disturbances as well as anxiety symptoms such as tension, irritability, lack of energy, impaired concentration, derealization, and depersonalization. Busto [26] described three cases of persistent tinnitus lasting up to 1 year of abstinence in patients withdrawing from therapeutic doses of diazepam. None of the patients had had tinnitus prior to withdrawal. Duration of benzodiazepine use appears to be more important than dose [23] in determining the severity of acute benzodiazepine withdrawal symptoms, though no studies have been done as yet on the protracted withdrawal. Clinical experience suggests that discontinuation of the triazolobenzodiazepines (triazolam, alprazolam) may result in particularly persistent symptoms. Prolonged use of benzodiazepines has been shown to result in poor performance on tasks of visual spatial ability and sustained attention [27]. The extent to which these impairments persist in abstinence and influence symptomatology is not yet known.

There have been systematic investigation of protracted abstinence symptoms with stimulants. Chronic administration of amphetamine and methamphetamine depletes the stores of serotonin and dopamine in rat brains [28,29], and these changes may be long lasting or permanent. Administration of amphetamines or cocaine causes a significant decrease in tyrosine hydroxylase which lasts for more than 3 months [30].

A. Anhedonia and Anergia

Clinically, cases of long-lasting anhedonia and anergia have been described with amphetamine abstinence [31], and an intermittent course of recurrent periods of depression and anergia has been charted in the first 12 weeks of abstinence from cocaine [32].

B. CNS Changes

In monkeys smoking the equivalent of three marijuana cigarettes a day for 3 months, Heath [33] reported changes in activity recorded from septal electrodes which persisted for many months after discontinuation of the drug. More recently, ventricular enlargements in frontal and caudate areas were found in monkeys given daily tetrahydrocannabinol (THC) for 5 years [34]. In humans, abrupt discontinuation of marijuana is followed by irritability, restlessness, nervousness, and insomnia which lasts accurately for 4–5 days [35], but which has been reported clinically to persist for many months in a low-grade form.

It is clear that the CNS changes that occur in response to the chronic use of certain drugs can be long lasting and may even in some cases be permanent if neurotransmitter function is sufficiently disrupted. Protracted abstinence symptoms as a consequence of these changes may then in fact become manifestations of endorgan damage. It is important to recognize that the outside time limits of some of these phenomena have not been explored. This is particularly of interest when considering the latent abnormalities which can be revealed by reintroduction of the drug in an abstinent subject. Do the abnormalities which underlie the symptoms of protracted withdrawal completely disappear with the passage of time, or is the reactivity of the CNS permanently changed so that reintroduction of the drug results in an abnormal response for the rest of the lifetime?

C. Conditioned Responses

Another interesting question is the relationship between the protracted withdrawal syndrome and conditioned responses. Wikler's [36] observation in the 1940s that former opiate addicts exhibited measurable signs of withdrawal when returning to the environment where they had used drugs has been confirmed by conditioned withdrawal responses elicited by the odor of peppermint alone, after methadone maintained subjects had been repeatedly exposed to pairings of peppermint odor with naloxone injections [37].

D. Withdrawal Signs Associated with Drug-Using Cues

Videotapes of drug-related scenes induced tachycardia and decreased skin temperature (withdrawal signs) in detoxified opiate addicts accompanied by reports of craving. Craving has also been produced in cocaine addicts by exposure to drug-using cues. Do conditioned withdrawal responses summate with protracted abstinence symptoms to produce intense craving in early abstinence, thus setting the stage for relapse? Marlatt [38] has described the abstinence violation effect, the tendency for an abstinent addict to go on a drug binge after a single exposure to the drug, as being largely due to psychological factors such as a change in one's cognitive set from abstainer to user. How much of this is, in fact, related to the production of withdrawal-like symptoms because of latent CNS abnormalities which can be activated by reexposure to the drug?

VI. PHARMACOTHERAPY AND THE PROTRACTED ABSTINENCE SYNDROME

One of the core problems of drug treatment is that of the high frequency of relapse in early abstinence. Considering its importance, surprisingly little research has been done on the protracted abstinence syndrome since the 1970s. Research on the CNS changes associated with protracted abstinence is particularly necessary to determine whether the syndrome can be modified by pharmacotherapy in a way which reduces the risk of relapse. Pharmacotherapy could be directed at any of the components of the protracted withdrawal syndrome, either on the basis of specific symptoms or more directly on the neurotransmitter changes which underly the symptoms. Dole and Nyswander [39], on the basis of what they believed to be persistent changes in cell function brought about by chronic exposure to heroin, proposed that the dismal relapse rate among addicts might be due to protracted abstinence, or a continuing unpleasant state of low-grade withdrawal which could be immediately reversed or normalized by an opioid drug such as methadone. Dole's more recent formulation [40] is that

> the narcotic receptor ligand acts as a modulator adjusting the intensity of suffering and the body's hormonal response to stress. In non tolerant patients, the reactions to tissue damage and related stresses are modulated by the natural ligand, the opioid peptides; while pain can be abolished therapeutically for a limited time by a dose of narcotic drug. However, repeated injections of narcotic lead to down regulation of the modulating system and possibly also to suppression of endogenous ligands. The receptors become insensitive to narcotic drugs and to their natural ligands. A new stability is achieved if methadone is given in an adequate daily dose, but at the price of continued dependence on the medication.

Thus, a fundamental question of long-term users of narcotics is whether the modulating systems can return to normal function after termination of narcotic input. Substitution of long-acting methadone for heroin has been an effective treatment for many heroin addicts, eliminating the symptoms of protracted withdrawal and permitting stability and improved function. Even with vast improvements in all areas of life, however, it has proved to be extremely difficult for patients to endure the protracted abstinence from methadone withdrawal without relapsing to opiate use again. The partial agonist buprenorphine appears to produce only mild withdrawal and may emerge as a better substitution drug than methadone. Using less problematic, same class, long-acting drugs to eliminate the protracted abstinence syndrome and decrease relapse has not been successful with sedative-hypnotics and stimulants, with the possible exception of nicotine chewing gum.

Kissin [41] proposed the use of chlordizepoxide to help alcoholics cope with protracted withdrawal symptoms. However, the action of sedative-hypnotics at receptor sites is not analogous to that of opiates and there is no equivalent receptor blockade. Furthermore, cognitive deficits are a feature of sedative-hypnotic use and will summate with those already present in the early abstinent alcoholic. Clinicians are generally agreed that benzodiazepines do not have a place in the treatment of alcoholism beyond that of acute withdrawal [42].

Methylphenidate was proposed as a substitution treatment for cocaine addicts but has been unsuccessful due to abuse of methylphenidate itself or relapse to cocaine abuse. Clearly some drug class substitution is not a universal solution to the problems of protracted abstinence. Other approaches have been proposed but are in the experimental or conceptual stage.

The dysphoria and drug craving during abstinence from cocaine is thought to be related to dopamine depletion. The precursor tyrosine and the agonist bromocriptine have been tried with minimal success. The antidepressant desipramine has had somewhat more positive results [43], though the early tricyclic jitterness syndrome may actually exacerbate craving in some patients [44]. The role of calcium channel blocking drugs [45] in ameliorating the symptoms of protracted withdrawal in alcoholics is interesting but remains hypothetical at present.

VII. CONCLUSIONS

Protracted abstinence syndromes are poorly understood but enormously important consequences of drug dependence and may explain why highly motivated patients inexplicably relapse in early abstinence in spite of otherwise good prognostic indicators. An elaboration of the cellular mechanisms for these phenomena may lead to the development of appropriate pharmacological interventions. Meanwhile an appreciation on the part of health care professionals of the genuine distress being experienced by the newly abstinent addict and an appropriate education of the patient can do much to mitigate the consequences.

REFERENCES

1. Himmelsbach, C.K. Clinical studies of drug addiction. *Arch. Int. Med. 69*:766–772 (1942).
2. Martin, W.R., Jasinski, D.R., Sapira, J.D., Flanary, H.G., Kelly, O.A., Thompson, A.K., and Logan, C.R. The respiratory effects of morphine during a cycle of dependence. *J. Pharm. Exp. Ther. 162*:182–89 (1968).
3. Kay, D.C. Human sleep and EEG through a cycle of methadone dependence. *Electroencephalogr. Clin. Neurophysiol. 38*:35–43 (1975).
4. Kissin, B., Schenker, V., and Schenker, A. The acute effects of ethyl alcohol and chlorpromazine of certain physiological functions in alcoholics. *Q. J. Stud. Alcohol 20*:481–93 (1959).
5. Begleiter, H., and Porjesz, B. Persistence of brain hyperexcitability following chronic alcohol exposure in rats. *Adv. Exp. Med. Biol. 85B*:209–222 (1977).
6. Gitlow, S.E., Dziedzic, S.W., and Dziedzic, L.M. Tolerance of ethanol after prolonged abstinence. *Adv. Exp. Med. Biol. 85A*:511–591 (1977).
7. Begleiter, H., Denoble, V., and Porjesz, B. Protracted brain dysfunction after alcohol withdrawal in monkeys. *Biological Effects of Alcohol* (H. Begleiter, ed.) New York, Plenum Press, 1980, pp. 231–249.

8. Brase, D.A., Iwamoto, E.T., and Loh, H.H. Re-initiation of sensitivity to naloxone by a single narcotic injection in post addict mice. *J. Pharmacol Exp. Ther. 197*:317–325 (1976).

9. Weingartner, M.V., Adinoff, B., and Linnoila, M. Effects of diazepam on human saccadic eye velocity antagonized by RO 15-1788 and increased sensitivity in chronic alcoholics. *Soc. Neurosci. Abstr. 12*:663 (1986).

10. Borg, S., Kvande, H., and Sedvall, G. Central norepinephrine metabolism during alcohol intoxication in addicts and healthy volunteers. *Science 213*:1135–37 (1981).

11. Begleiter, H., and Porjesz, B. Persistence of a subacute withdrawal system following ethanol intake. *Drug Alcohol Depend. 4*:353–7 (1979).

12. Khan, A., Ciranlo, D.A., and Nelson, W.H. Dexamethasone suppression test in recently detoxified alcoholics. *J. Clin. Psychopharm. 4*:94–97 (1984).

13. Brown, S.A., and Schuckit, M.A. Changes in depression among abstinent alcoholics *J. Stud. Alcohol 49*:412–417 (1988).

14. Alling, C., Balldin, J., Bokstrom, K., Gottfries, C.G., Karlsson, I., and Langstrom, G. Studies on duration of a late recovery period after chronic abuse of ethanol. *Acta. Psychiatr. Scand. 66*:384–397 (1982).

15. DeSoto, C.B., O'Donnell, W.E., Alfred, L.J., and Lopes, C.E. Symptomatology in alcholics at various stages of abstinence. *Alcoholism Clin. Exp. Res. 9*:505–512 (1985).

16. Desoto, C.B., O'Donnell, W.E., and DeSoto, J.L. Long term recovery in alcoholics *Alcoholism Clin. Exp. Res. 13*:693–697 (1989).

17. Bonnet, M.H. Effects of sleep disruption on sleep, performance and mood. *Sleep 8*:11–19 (1985).

18. Wagman, A.M.I., and Allen, R.P. Effects of alcohol ingestion and abstinence on slow wave sleep of alcoholics, *Alcohol Intoxication and Withdrawal, Experimental Studies II* (Gross, ed.). New York, Plenum, 1975, pp. 453–466.

19. Adamson, J., and Burdick, J.A. Sleep of dry alcoholics. *Arch Gen Psychiatry 28*:146–149 (1973).

20. Zarcone, V.P., Cohen, M., and Hoddes, E. WAIS, MMPI and sleep variables in abstinent alcoholics, *Alcohol Intoxication and Withdrawal, Experimental Studies II* (Gross, ed.). New York, Plenum, 1975, pp. 431–451.

21. Synder, S., and Karacan, I. Sleep patterns of sober chronic alcoholics. *Neuropsychobiology 13*:97–100 (1985).

22. Smith, D.E., and Wesson, D.R. Benzodiazepine dependency syndromes. *J Psychoactive Drugs 15*:85–89 (1983).

23. Noyes, R., Garvey, M.J., Cook, B.L., and Perry, P.J. Benzodiazepine withdrawal: A review of the evidence. *J. Clin Psychiatry 49*:382–389 (1988).

24. Ashton, H. Benzodiazepine withdrawal: An unfinished story. *Br. Med. J. 288*:1135–1140 (1984).

25. Higgit, A.C., Lader, M.H., and Fonagy, P. Clinical management of benzodiazepine dependence. *Br. Med. J. 291*:688–790 (1985).

26. Busto, V., Fornazzari, L., and Naranjo, C.A. Protracted tinnitus after discontinuation of long term therapeutic use of benzodiazepines. *J. Clin. Psychopharm 8*:359–362 (1988).

27. Golombok, S., Moodley, P., and Lader, M. Cognitive impairment in long term benzodiazepine users. *Psychol Med. 18*:365–374 (1988).

28. Ricaurte, G.A., Schuster, C.R., and Seiden, I.S. Long term effects of repeated methylamphetamine administration on dopamine and serotonin neurons in the rat brain. *Brain Res. 193*:153–163 (1980).

29. Ricaurte, G.A., Bryan, D., Strauss, L., Seiden, L.S., and Schuster, C.R. Hallucinogenic amphetamine selectively destroys brain serotonin nerve terminals. *Science 229*:986–988 (1985).

30. Trulson, M.E., Babb, S., Joe, J.C., and Raese, J..D. Chronic cocaine administration depletes tyrosine hydroxylase immunoreactivity in rat brain nigral striatal systems. *Exp. Neurol 94*:744–756 (1986).

31. Elinwood, E.H. The epidemiology of stimulant use, *Drug Use: Epidemiology and Sociological Approaches* (F. Josephson and E. Carroll, eds.). Washington, D.C., Hemisphere, 174, pp. 303–309.

32. Gawin, F.H., and Kleber, H.D. Abstinence sysptomatology and psychiatric diagnoses in cocaine abusers. *Arch. Gen. Psychiatry 43*:107–113 (1986).

33. Heath, R.A., Fitzjarrell, A.T., Garey, R.E., and Myers, W.A. Chronic marijuana smoking: Its effects on function and structure of the primate brain, *Marijuana: Biological Effects* (G.C. Hahas and W.D.M. Patton, eds.) Oxford, England, Plenum, 1979.

34. McGraham, J.P., Dublin, A.B., and Sassenrath, E. Long term Δ9 tetra-hydrocannabinol treatment: Computed tomography of the brains of rhesus monkeys. *Am. J. Dis. Child. 138*:1109–1112 (1984).

35. Jones, R.T. Cannabis and health. *Am. Rev. Med. 34*:247–258 (1983).

36. Wikler, A. Recent progress in research on the neurophysiological basis of morphine addiction. *Am. J. Psychiatry 105*:328–338 (1948).

37. O'Brien, P.O., Childress, A.R., McLellan, A.T., Ehrman, R., and Ternes, J.W. Types of conditioning found in drug dependent humans, *Learning Factors in Substance Abuse* (B.A. Ray, ed.). National Institute on Drug Abuse Research Monograph No. 84, U.S. Government Printing Office, Washington, D.C., 1988, pp. 44–61.

38. Marlatt, G.A., and Gordon, J.R. *Relapse Prevention.* New York Guilford Press, 1985.

39. Dole, V.P., and Nyswander, M.E. Methadone maintenance and its implication for theories of narcotic addiction, *The Addictive State* (A. Wikler, ed.) Baltimore, Williams & Wilkins, 1969, pp. 359–366.

40. Dole, V.P. Implications of methadone maintenance for theories of narcotics addiction. *J.A.M.A. 260*:3025–3029 (1988).

41. Kissin, B. The use of psychoactive drugs in the long term treatment of alcoholic. *Am N.Y. Acad. Sci. 252*:385–395 (1975).

42. Meyer, R.E. Prospects for a rational pharmacotherapy of alcoholism. *J. Clin Psychiatry 50*:403–412 (1989).

43. Garwin, F.H., Kleber, H.D., Byck, R., et al: Desipramine facilitation of initial cocaine abstinence. *Arch. Gen. Psychiatry 46*:117–121 (1989).

44. Weiss, R.D. Relapse to cocaine abuse after initiating desipramine treatment *J.A.M.A. 260*:2545–2546 (1988).

45. Little, H.J., Dolin, S., and Halsey, M.J. Calcium channel antagonists decrease ethanol withdrawal syndrome. *Life Sci. 39*:2059–2065 (1986).

50

Protracted Withdrawal Syndromes from Benzodiazepines

Heather Ashton
The University of Newcastle upon Tyne, Newcastle upon Tyne, England

I. INTRODUCTION

Drug withdrawal syndromes, in general, tend to consist of mirror images of the drugs' initial effects. Thus, abrupt withdrawal from chronic usage of beta-adrenoceptor antagonists such as propranolol may give rise to tachycardia and palpitations; abrupt withdrawal from antihypertensive doses of clonidine may be followed by hypertension, anxiety, and other signs of increased sympathetic activity. Brenzodiazepines are no exception: On sudden cessation after chronic use, anticonvulsant effects may be replaced by epileptic seizures, muscle relaxation by increased muscle tension, hypnotic effects by insomnia or nightmares, and anxiolytic effects by increased anxiety. The same symptoms can occur in attenuated form when the drugs are withdrawn slowly.

However, all these symptoms are not inevitable in any individual patient. The particular features of the withdrawal syndrome, their time of onset, duration, and severity are greatly modified by many other factors. Such factors include pharmacokinetic variables, dosage and duration of drug use, rate of withdrawal, the presence or absence of the original disorder (such as anxiety) for which the drug was prescribed, personality characteristics, physical makeup and susceptibility, and the use of concomitant treatments. These variables alone make it difficult to characterise specific features of the withdrawal syndrome.

This difficulty is compounded by the fact that, as long-term medication, benzodiazepnines have mainly been prescribed for anxiety and insomnia, disorders which themselves include most features of the drug withdrawal syndrome. When such patients undergo reduction of benzodiazepine dosage, especially slow reduction, how can one specify which emergent symptoms are "true," drug-related withdrawal symptoms, which are "pseudowithdrawal" symptoms (Tyrer et al., 1983), which represent a return of the original anxiety state, and which are the natural reactions of an anxious personality undergoing the stress of withdrawal? In circumstances such as these, the benzodiazepine withdrawal syndrome becomes largely a matter of definition.

Nevertheless, the existence of a benzodiazepine withdrawal reaction, from both high and low (therapeutic) doses of benzodiazepines, is no longer in dispute, and many attempts have been made to define and measure it and to estimate its incidence and duration.

II. DEFINITIONS AND MEASUREMENTS

Symptoms occurring during benzodiazepine withdrawal have been described by many authors (Ashton, 1984, 1987; Busto et al., 1986, Hallstrom and Lader, 1981; Murphy et al., 1984; Owen and Tyrer, Petursson and Lader, 1981a, 1981b, Smith and Wesson, 1983, Tyrer et al., 1981, 1983; Winokur et al., 1980 among others). Commonly described symptoms are shown in Figure 1. None of these symptoms are specific to benzodiazepine withdrawal: They include all the psychological and somatic symptoms of anxiety, although certain symptom clusters are characteristic. Petursson and Lader (1981a, 1981b) and Owen and Tyrer (1983) emphasized the appearance of new symptoms, not experienced before withdrawal and un-common in anxiety states. These new symptoms include hypersensitivity to sensory stimuli (sound, light, touch, taste, and smell) and perceptual distortions (e.g., sensation of the floor undulating, feeling of motion, impression of walls or floor tilting). There also appears to be a higher incidence than usually seen in anxiety of depersonalization, derealization, paresthesias, and extreme dysphoria, an amalgam of anxiety, depression, nausea, malaise, and depersonalization (Petursson and Lader, 1981). Visual hallucinations, distortion of body image, psychotic reactions, formication, muscle fasiculation and twitching (occasionally resembling myoclonus), and considerable loss of weight are also described during ben-zodiazepine withdrawal and are unusual in anxiety states.

Smith and Wesson (1983) and Ashton (1984) drew attention to the characteristic fluctua-tion of symptoms which may wax and wane without obvious psychological provocation. Smith and Wesson (1983) suggest that this wavelike symptomatology is an important marker to distinguish the low-dose benzodiazepine withdrawal syndrome from symptom reemergence. However, since symptoms may fluctuate in the course of the day or over periods of days or weeks, accurate recording is difficult.

Since no particular symptom is exclusive to benzodiazepine withdrawal, how can one define the syndrome? Tyrer et al (1981, 1983) have attempted various methods in placebo-controlled studies:

1. The appearance of two or more new symptoms during the withdrawal period. New symp-toms in one study included perceptual disturbances, sensory hypersensitivity, and fear of imminent death (Tyrer et al., 1981); and also psychotic symptoms, depression and dysphoria, muscle twitching, and abnormal sensations of movement in another (Tyrer et al., 1983). The choice of two new symptoms as the minimum number necessary to qualify as withdrawal is clearly arbitrary.
2. An increase in self-rated symptoms (Comprehensive Psychiatric Rating Scale) to greater than 50% of baseline levels, followed by a return to lower values. Symptom resolution is clearly an important feature in differentiating between symptoms due to withdrawal and symptom reemergence, emergence, or overinterpretation. As Smith and Wesson (1983, p. 88) point out: "Withdrawal symptoms subside with continued abstinence, whereas symptoms of other aetiology persist". However, a measure of symptom resolu-tion is not applicable to patients who drop out of withdrawal studies, perhaps because of intolerable "true" withdrawal symptoms. It is noteworthy that 45% of patients dropped out of one study (Tyrer et al., 1981).

	0	1	2	3

PSYCHIC

- Drowsiness/fatigue
- Excitability (jumpiness, restlessness)
- Unreality
- Poor memory/concentration
- Perceptual distortion
- Hallucinations
- Obsessions
- Agoraphobia/phobias
- Panic attacks
- Depression
- Paranoid thoughts
- Rage/aggression/irritability
- Craving

SOMATIC

- Headache
- Pain (limbs, back, neck)
- Pain (teeth, jaw)
- Tingling, numbness, altered sensation (limbs, face, trunk)
- Stiffness (limbs, back, jaw)
- Weakness ("jelly legs")
- Tremor
- Muscles twitches
- Ataxia
- Dizziness/lightheadiness
- Blurred/double vision
- Tinnitus
- Speech difficulty
- Hypersensitivity (light, sound, taste, smell)
- Insomnia/nightmares
- Fits
- Nausea/vomiting
- Abdominal pain
- Diarrhoea/constipation
- Appetite/weight change
- Dry mouth
- Metallic taste
- Difficulty in swallowing

- Flushing/sweating
- Palpitations
- Overbreathing

- Thirst
- Frequency/polyuria, pain on micturition
- Incontinence
- Menorrhagia, PMT
- Mammary pain/swelling

- Skin rash/itching
- Stuffy nose/sinusitis
- Influenza-like symptoms
- Sore Eyes
- Other Symptoms (specify)

Figure 1 Withdrawal Symptom Rating Scale. 0 = none, 1 = mild, 2 = moderate, 3 = severe.

917

3. A combination of methods 1 and 2 so that a withdrawal reaction is defined as the appearance of new symptoms that resolved before the end of the study (20 and 14 weeks after the end of withdrawal; Tyrer et al, 1983). More recently, Tyrer et al. (1989) have produced a questionnaire of symptoms that are relatively specific to benzodiazepine withdrawal in that they mainly occur during periods of drug withdrawal and return toward baseline levels after withdrawal.
4. Pseudowithdrawal symptoms were defined as symptoms occurring when patients thought they were reducing drug intake but their drug consumption and blood concentrations of benzodiazepines were unchanged.

Such definitions, derived from double-blind, placebo-controlled studies, have been extremely helpful in the recognition of benzodiazepine dependence, especially low-dose dependence. However, they are of necessity arbitrary and can only be approximate, since the appearance or severity of any particular symptom or symptom cluster may actually represent a variable combination of true withdrawal, pseudowithdrawal, and reemergence of anxiety, and the same patients liable to pseudowithdrawal reactions are also likely to be most vulnerable to true withdrawal effects.

Furthermore, definitions based on differences from prewithdrawal symptoms do not take into account the possibility that, owing to the development of tolerance, withdrawal symptoms may already be present while patients are still taking benzodiazepines. Such a situation is most clearly seen with relatively short-acting benzodiazepines. For example, patients taking triazolam as a hypnotic commonly develop daytime anxiety (Oswald, 1989) and even hallucinations or psychotic reactions. These are almost certainly withdrawal effects, since they are immediately relieved by taking the drug, but eventually disappear after the drug is stopped (Ashton, 1987). Similarly, with lorazepam and alprazolam (Hermann et al., 1987) patients often develop increasing anxiety and panic as well as craving between doses (Ashton, 1984). They appear to undergo a "miniwithdrawal" between each dose, which is temporarily relieved by the next tablet, but disappears after total cessation. An analogous condition is seen with alcohol: Alcoholics commonly complain of tremor and insomnia, symptoms which are temporarily relieved by alcohol, but which only disappear after a period of abstinence. Even with long-acting benzodiazepine such as diazepam, there is usually a history in long-term users of steadily increasing anxiety, with the development over the years of new symptoms such as agoraphobia, often with perceptual distortions and depersonalization, despite continued usage of these supposedly anxiolytic drugs. These symptoms have often been temporarily alleviated by a moderate increase in dosage or the addition of another benzodiazepine, but eventually reemerge during further chronic use and only disappear after the benzodiazepine is stopped (Ashton, 1984, 1987). Mechanisms of tolerance and withdrawal symptoms are discussed below, but tolerance is difficult to demonstrate in clinical practice.

Because of these many immeasurable factors, it is doubtful whether the boundaries of a "true" benzodiazepine withdrawal syndrome can ever be clearly demarcated.

III. INCIDENCE

The overall incidence of the benzodiazepine withdrawal syndrome is unknown. As with cigarette smokers (Ashton and Stepney, 1982), there may be a large, uncounted population who quit regular benzodiazepine usage after months or years without ever coming to medical attention. Tyrer (in press) notes that it is surprising how many patients in ordinary practice have no difficulties whatsoever in reducing their benzodiazepine dosage, and the incidence of a benzodiazepine withdrawal syndrome in general practice appears to be around 30% (Tyrer, in press; Tyrer, 1989; Tyrer et al., 1981, 1983). On the other hand, in selected patients referred for specialist treatment, the incidence may be 100% (Ashton, 1987; Lader and Ola-jide, 1987; Petursson and Lader, 1981a). It is also worth noting that withdrawal syndromes in the form of rebound insomnia (Kales et al., 1978) or more general symptoms can occur in experimental subjects and in nonanxious patients prescribed benzodiazepines for sports injuries (Lader, 1988). In addition, a benzodiazepine withdrawal syndrome has been described in neonates whose mothers took "therapeutic" doses of benzodiazepines during pregnancy (Rementeria and Bhatt, 1977).

Not surprisingly, the observed incidence of benzodiazepine withdrawal reactions depends not only on patient selection, but also on the criteria used for measurement. In the study of Tyrer et al. (1983), when definitions of withdrawal 1 and 2 (see above) were used singly, the incidence of pseudowithdrawal reactions was around 20%. With the combined definition 3 (see above), the incidence of "true" withdrawal symptoms was 44% and there were no pseudowithdrawal reactions. This incidence of course only applies to those consenting to take part in the study and managing to finish it. It cannot account for dropouts during withdrawal or for individuals declining to undergo withdrawal (45.5% of eligible patients in the study of Tyrer et al., 1981). Thus, the incidence of benzodiazepine withdrawal, like its diagnosis, becomes largely a matter of definition.

IV. DURATION

The identification of the benzodiazepine withdrawal syndrome is difficult enough; its duration is even more difficult to delineate. Most estimates suggest a duration of approximately 5–28 days, with a peak in severity around 2 weeks postwithdrawal, after which most symptoms return to prewithdrawal levels (Busto et al., 1986; Murphy et al., 1984; Owen and Tyrer, 1983; Petursson and Lader, 1981a, 1981b; Tyrer et al. 1981, 1983).

To a large extent, the apparent duration of withdrawal depends upon how long the patients are followed up, and several authors have drawn attention to the prolonged nature of postwithdrawal symptoms in some cases. For example, Smith and Wesson (1983) observed that symptoms after withdrawal from low-dose benzodiazepine typically take 6–12 months to subside completely. Prolonged symptoms include anxiety, insomnia, paresthesias, altered sensation, muscle spasms, and psychosis. Ashton (1984, 1987) reported a similar protracted time course. Tyrer (in press) refers to a postwithdrawal syndrome in the 6 months after withdrawal. Hallstrom and Lader (1981) found the Hamilton Anxiety Score still raised above baseline levels 30 days after withdrawal from low-dose benzodiazepines, but it had returned to baseline levels by follow-up several months later when successfully withdrawn patients "had resumed their normal life" (Hallstrom and Lader, 1981 p. 237). Olajide and Lader (1984) suggested that depression may be an integral part of the benzodiazepine withdrawal syndrome and may last several months after withdrawal in susceptible individuals; this phenomenon was also observed by Ashton (1987). Busto et al. (1988) described two cases in whom severe tinnitus first appeared during benzodiazepine withdrawal and persisted for 6 and 12 months after discontinuation before finally diminishing or disappearing. In one of these cases, the tinnitus was immediately alleviated by diazepmam in a double-blind placebo-controlled trial conducted over 1 week, 6 months after withdrawal; after a further 6 months of abstinence, the tinnitus had become tolerable.

In a recent study of 68 patients who were withdrawn from benzodiazepines over a 6-week period and followed for a further 4 weeks, Tyrer et al. (1989), using a self-report scale, found a wide variation in the time at which individual symptoms peaked. Mean scores for some symptoms (depression; dizziness, paresthesia, feelings of unreality) peaked early, whereas mean scores for others (nausea, memory impairment, faintness, touch sensitivity, and motor impairment) were maximal 8 weeks after the start of withdrawal. Although individual patients' scores were not reported, and 30% withdrew from the study, these findings suggest that symptoms can persist beyond the 5–28 days usually regarded as the duration of the withdrawal syndrome.

Ashton et al., (1989) used the rating scale shown in Figure 1 to record the symptoms of patients undergoing diazepam withdrawal under double-blind placebo-controlled conditions. Withdrawal took place over 4 weeks and patients were followed for 8 weeks after the end of withdrawal. Half the patients received placebo and the other half buspirone before, during, and for 4 weeks after withdrawal. Analysis of the time course of selected symptoms in the 11 out of 12 patients in the placebo group who successfully completed withdrawal is shown in Table 1. Eight weeks after the end of withdrawal, mean scores for headache, dizziness, depression, tinnitus, paresthesias and motor symptoms remained higher than prewithdrawal scores; other symptoms had declined although few had disappeared. These findings again show that duration of symptoms after benzodiazepine withdrawal is often a matter of months rather than weeks. Different symptoms persisted in the Tyrer et al. (1989) and Ashton et al. (1989) studies, which differed also in size of sample, patient selection, and rate of withdrawal. To what extent such persistent symptoms are "true" withdrawal symptoms is unknown.

A further problem in assessing the duration of the withdrawal syndrome is the interpretation of the baseline (prewithdrawal) symptoms and anxiety scores. Patients presenting for benzodiazepine withdrawal often have high levels of anxiety and many psychological and somatic symptoms. Figures 2 and 3 show Hospital Anxiety Depression (anxiety) (Zigmond and Snaith, 1983) and symptom rating scores for 12 patients on benzodiazepines compared with the scores of 18 healthy university students approaching their examinations. Both groups took placebo tablets and were followed for 20 weeks. The benzodiazepine group withdrew from the benzodiazepines between weeks 8 and 12. It is clear that the patients had considerably higher scores than the normal subjects on both scales, even at the beginning of the study while they were still taking benzodiazepines.

Certainly in these patients the benzodiazepines were not effectively controlling anxiety and, as argued above, it is possible that at least some of the presenting symptoms were due to "withdrawal" symptoms even in the presence of the drug, as a result of the development of drug tolerance. Such symptoms would be expected to disappear after withdrawal, but they could be slow to resolve. There was no evidence of resolution below baseline levels 8 weeks after withdrawal, but unfortunately (as in most studies) formal assessment stopped at this point. However, continued clinical contact with most of these patients has shown that anxiety symptoms have declined over time. This slow improvement bears out the observations quoted above (Ashton, 1984, 1987; Busto et al., 1988; Hallstrom and Laber, 1981; Olajide and Lader, 1984; Smith and Wesson, 1983) that symptoms improve gradually for many months after withdrawal and some patients are able to resume normal lives after years of incapacity before withdrawal.

Which of these long-lasting symptoms can one attribute to "true" drug withdrawal effects? Is it possible to pinpoint a time at which the benzodiazepine withdrawal syndrome ends and to say with certainty that any residual symptoms must be due to other factors? The problem is similar to that of designating which effects of a bout of influenza or infectious mononucleosis can be attributed to the specific virus. Do such effects include only those of the viral toxemia? Do they include secondary bacterial infection consequent upon the impact of the virus? Do they include the period of postviral lethargy and depression which, like benzodiazepine withdrawal syndromes, tend to recur to wavelike fashion for several months? Once again, the benzodiazepine withdrawal syndrome appears to slip through the fingers and one is led back to a question of definition. Probably a clear definition of duration is

Table 1 Scores for Selected Symptoms Before, During, and After Diazepam Withdrawal (n = 11; mean total scores on Withdrawal Symptoms Rating Scale shown in Fig. 1)

Symptom	Score at start of 4-wk withdrawal period	Maximum score	(Weeks after start of withdrawal)	Score 8 wks after end of withdrawal
Declining symptoms (postwithdrawal score equal or less than prewithdrawal)				
insomnia/nightmares	8	14	(1)	8
nausea/vomiting	6	8	(5)	4
perceptual distortion	0	5	(2–6)	0
excitability/restlessness	14	18	(5)	14
sensory hypersensitivity[a]	9	13	(4)	6
poor memory/concentration	7	12	(5)	6
Persisting symptoms (postwithdrawal score greater than prewithdrawal)				
anxiety[b]	9.09	11.9	(5)	11.75
depression[b]	7	9	(4–8)	9
tinnitus	5	10	(2–3)	9
headache	10	18	(2)	13
dizziness	5	19	(6)	8
paresthesia[c]	8	14	(6)	12
motor symptoms[d]	24	46	(5)	35

[a]Sensory hypersensitivity: to light, sound, taste, smell.
[b]Hospital Anxiety Depression scores.
[c]Paresthesia: tingling, numbness, altered sensitivity in limbs, face, trunk.
[d]Motor symptoms: total score for stiffness, weakness, tremor, muscle twitches, ataxia.

ANXIETY

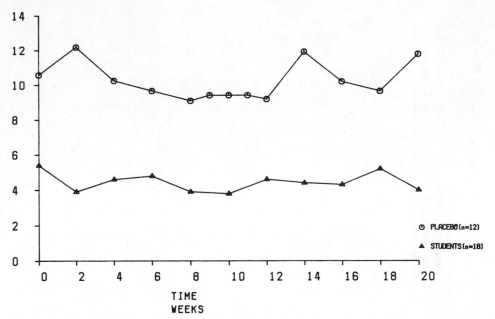

Figure 2 Hospital Anxiety Depression (HAD) Scale scores for anxiety over 20 weeks in 18 healthy students and 12 patients taking diazepam (7.5 mg SD 4.6 daily). Patients and students took placebo tablets until week 20. Patients withdrew from diazepam during weeks 8–12. One patient dropped out after 12 weeks for domestic reasons.

SYMPTOM SCORE

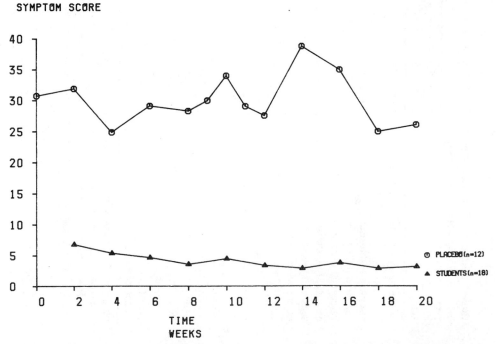

Figure 3 Withdrawal symptoms scores over 20 weeks in 18 healthy students and 12 patients taking diazepam (7.5 mg SD 4.6 daily). Patients and procedures as in Figure 2. Withdrawal Symptom Rating Scale shown in Fig. 1.

impossible because drug-induced perturbations of central neurotransmission merge imperceptibly into the background of individual, genetically determined and learned, patterns of brain activity.

V. PROTRACTED SYMPTOMS AFTER BENZODIAZEPINE WITHDRAWAL

All the problems of definition discussed above are multiplied in any attempt to describe protracted benzodiazepine withdrawal syndromes. Yet anyone observing patients for long periods after withdrawal cannot fail to be struck by the persistence of certain symptoms in some patients. These may not be "true" benzodiazepine withdrawal symptoms; nevertheless, they are possibly related to benzodiazepine use and often present a clinical problem. Listed below are examples of some protracted symptoms which from personal observations and other reports appear to be relatively common after benzodiazepine withdrawal. Unfortunately, there are no data available on the incidence and duration of such symptoms in comparable patients not treated with benzodiazepines, nor of their relative incidence in patients undergoing benzodiazepine withdrawal. Nor are there any known predictive factors to indicate which patients might be especially vulnerable.

A. Anxiety

As discussed above, anxiety may persist for many months after benzodiazepine withdrawal, yet slowly decline below prewithdrawal levels after 1–2 years (Ashton, 1987). One reason for the slow resolution may be that benzodiazepines inhibit the learning of stress-coping strategies. Such effects have been demonstrated in animals and man (Gray,1987). Consequently there is a long period after benzodiazepine withdrawal when patients have a decreased ability to cope with stressful situations (Ashton, 1989; Murphy and Tyrer, 1988; Owen and Tyrer, 1983). Recovery may require many months of learning new strategies of stress control to replace the years of stress coping by means of exogenous drugs.

Hence, persisting anxiety after benzodiazepine withdrawal does not necessarily imply the reemergence of an anxiety state existing before benzodiazepine treatment; it may represent the uncovering of a type of learning deficiency induced by long-term benzodiazepine use. People who take benzodiazepines tend to have high ratings for trait anxiety (Ashton and Golding, 1989; Golding and Cornish, 1987; Golding et al., 1983) which may confer a particular vulnerability to the stress of withdrawal. Nevertheless, even without formal treatment, protracted anxiety symptoms, including agoraphobia and panic, many gradually resolve after benzodiazepine withdrawal (Ashton, 1987), although the process may be hastened by behavioral treatments.

B. Depression

Depression can be caused or aggravated by chronic benzodiazepine use (Lader and Petursson, 1981), yet it also appears to be a feature of the withdrawal syndrome (Olajide and Lader, 1984). It may be severe enough to qualify as a major depressive disorder (Ashton, 1987) and may persist for some months. Olajide and Lader (1984) suggest that the mechanisms for postwithdrawal depression may be central serotonin depletion, but there is no direct evidence for this. Clinically, the depression is no different from depressive illness in general, and it responds to antidepressant drugs. It is not clear whether protracted depressive symptoms are more common in patients with a previous history of depression or whether it recurs in subsequent years after withdrawal.

C. Tinnitus

Tinnitus is a common symptom of benzodiazepine withdrawal and may initially result from the characteristic general hypersensitivity to sensory stimuli. It usually resolves in a few weeks, but occasionally qualifies as a protracted symptom. Busto et al. (1988) describe two cases in which tinnitus persisted for 6 and 12 months after withdrawal and mention a third patient who was unable to withdraw from benzodiazepines because of severe tinnitus at each attempt. Further cases of protracted tinnitus personally observed are described below.

Case 1

Female aged 54. Duration of benzodiazepine usage: 8 years. Withdrawn slowly from oxazepam, 45 mg daily, in 1986. Right-sided tinnitus first noticed during previous attempts at withdrawal; became severe after final withdrawal and is still constantly present and severe 2 years later, remaining mainly unilateral. No abnormality detected on skull x-ray, CAT scan, EEG, and ENT examination, apart from slight bilateral (symmetrical) high-tone deafness. Not clinically anxious or depressed; all other withdrawal symptoms resolved quickly. Taking no medication.

Case 2

Female aged 62. Duration of benzodiazepine usage: 18 years. Withdrawn slowly from diazepam, 15 mg daily, in 1988. Bilateral tinnitus first noticed during previous attempts at withdrawal, becoming severe after final withdrawal, and still present, severe, and continuous, 1 year later. ENT investigations: moderate bilateral high-tone deafness; wears hearing aid. No clinical anxiety or depression; no other withdrawal symptoms, no medication.

Case 3

Female aged 58. Duration of benzodiazepine usage: 20 years. Withdrew from diazepam, 20 mg daily, over 4 weeks in 1988. Developed acute psychotic reaction which resolved in 1 week. First noticed left-sided tinnitus 1 month after withdrawal. Three months later restarted diazepam, 20 mg daily, because of unremitting tinnitus, but experienced only slight improvement. Second withdrawal over 1 year, 1988–1989. Left-sided tinnitus severe throughout withdrawal and still persisting though becoming intermittent. ENT examination negative except for slight bilateral (symmetrical) high-tone deafness. Medication: mianserin 30 mg daily, started after onset of tinnitus; carbamazepine recently added with no effect on tinnitus.

Case 4

Female aged 70. Duration of benzodiazepine usage: 20 years. First noticed tinnitus, mainly right sided, on withdrawal from flurazepam, 30 mg daily in 1985. Tinnitus continuous ever since, not relieved by a course of diazepam. ENT examination normal. Drugs: no psychotropics, inhalers for asthma.

Tinnitus is fairly common in the general population and the apparent relation to benzodiazepine use may be incidental, but these cases raise the suspicion that benzodiazepines may occasionally cause permanent or only slowly reversible brain damage. Such damage may not be detectable on CAT scans; one study (Lader et al., 1984) suggested a mild degree of cortical shrinkage in chronic benzodiazepine users, but this finding was not confirmed in a later study (Perera et al., 1987). Two of the above patients also complained of unilateral headaches.

D. Paresthesias

Paresthesia, in the form of tingling, "pins and needles," or numbness of the extremities or circumoral region, are another common symptom of benzodiazepine withdrawal. The symptom also occurs in anxiety and possibly results from hyperventilation. Benzodiazepines depress the sensitivity of the respiratory center to carbon dioxide (Gilmartin et al., 1988), and it is possible that the respiratory center becomes hypersensitive during withdrawal, triggering hyperventilation. Resolution of paresthesia usually occurs within a few weeks of withdrawal. Occasionally, however, patients complain of numbness or of a burning sensation affecting the fingers, feet, and legs, which may be protracted for months or years. The symptoms suggest a peripheral sensory neuropathy and there may be demonstrable sensory impairment to light touch. Two patients summarized below typify several similar cases personally observed at a benzodiazepine withdrawal clinic.

Case 1

Female aged 56. Duration of benzodiazepine usage: 15 years. Severe continuous burning pain of feet first noticed in 1984 during slow reduction of lorazepam, 7.5–1.5 mg daily. Changed to diazepam and slowly withdrawn over 1 year, 1987–1988. Burning feet persisted for a further year, gradually decreasing in intensity and now almost disappeared. No abnormal signs; good peripheral pulses. Medication; promethazine, 50 mg nocte since 1988.

Case 2

Female aged 67. Duration of benzodiazepine usage: 12 years. First noticed severe burning pain in feet and legs in 1981 during reduction of medazepam, 15–5 mg daily. Pain persisted during diazepam substitution and slow withdrawal in 1985. 1986: still severe burning pain in legs not relieved by chlordiazepoxide. 1989: pain still present. Neurological examination, nerve conduction studies, serum folate, and B_{12} levels normal; peripheral pulses present and normal.

Formication is also common during benzodiazepine withdrawal and many patients temporarily complain of a feeling of insects crawling on the skin or of lice or nits in the hair. Occasionally more bizarre sensations are reported, such as a feeling of slime or water running over the body, a sense of inner vibration, or a feeling of "trembling inside," and these symptoms may be protracted. Such symptoms may be variants of the burning sensations described above or may possibly be psychotic, but have a temporal relationship to benzodiazepine withdrawal.

E. Motor Symptoms

Increased muscle tension, hyperreflexia, tremor, fasiculation, and muscle jerking are common features of benzodiazepine withdrawal but usually resolve within weeks. Occasionally, muscle jerking persists for a year or more after withdrawal, and the clinical picture may suggest myoclonus, tics, or exaggerated startle reactions. Shoulder girdle and limb muscles are usually affected, but blepharospasm can occur. Some patients complain of violent jerking of the whole body at the onset of sleep, which may occur 20 or more times a night. The restless legs syndrome may also be protracted. Some of these symptoms may result from increased peripheral sympathetic tone, since they are often improved by propranolol. Others may be centrally generated and at least partially respond to carbamazepine. Blepharospasm can be controlled by local injection of botulinum toxin at 3-month intervals. Protracted motor symptoms such as these raise the possibility that benzodiazepines are capable of causing long-term hyperexcitability of motoneurons or central motor pathways.

F. Gastrointestinal Symptoms

Gastrointestinal symptoms are extremely common during chronic benzodiazepine use and in withdrawal. Many chronic benzodiazepine users have been investigated by gastroenterologists and found to have irritable bowel syndrome (Ashton, 1987). Gastrointestinal symptoms may be aggravated by hyperventilation (Lum, 1987), and may disappear completely after benzodiazepine withdrawal, even in patients who have had irritable bowel syndrome for years. Nevertheless, there remains a sizable core of patients who complain of food intolerance and gaseous abdominal distension which first appears during withdrawal and is protracted for many months. Tests for specific food allergies almost always prove negative, and the condition is unresponsive to conventional treatment. Patients often turn to alternative or "fringe" medication, undergo various forms of diet, and become convinced that they have intestinal candidiasis or damage to the immune system. None of these claims have scientific support, although Lum (1987) reports that hyperventilation provokes histamine release and that the incidence of food intolerance and pseudoallergic reactions is high in chronic hyperventilators. The effect of benzodiazepine withdrawal on gastrointestinal function and on corticosteroid and immune responses (known to be affected by stress) perhaps merits further attention.

VI. BRAIN MECHANISMS OF BENZODIAZEPINE WITHDRAWAL SYMPTOMS

The primary effect of benzodiazepines is enhancement of gamma-aminobutyric acid (GABA) activity on postsynaptic $GABA_A$ receptors in the brain. The effect results from an interaction with specific benzodiazepine binding sites on the GABA-receptor complex (Mohler and Okada, 1977; Squires and Braestrup, 1977), which increases the affinity of the receptors for GABA (Costa, 1981). The GABA neurons consist of small interneurons forming local circuits which exert a powerful influence on the excitability of other neurons passing through their spatial domain (Bloom, 1985). Such local GABA circuits are widely distributed throughout the brain, including the reticular formation, limbic system structures, and cerebal and cerebellar cortices (Young and Kuhar, 1980). Gamma-aminobutyric acid is a universal inhibitor of nervous activity and also inhibits the release of excitatory neurotransmitters (Benton and Rick, 1976). Thus, the actions of benzodiazepines include not only enhancement of GABA activity at many brain sites, but also decreased release of acetylcholine, norepinephrine, dopamine, and serotonin (Haefely et al., 1981). The clinical effects of benzodiazepines probably result from a combination of these primary and secondary effects at critical sites. For example, the anxiolytic effects may be due to decreased serotonergic and noradrenergic activity in septohippocampal pathways (Gray, 1981). Thus, benzodiazepine's actions are by no means confined to a particular neurotransmitter or brain pathway.

Any chronically used drug gradually engenders a series of homeostatic responses which tend to restore normal function despite the presence of the drug. With chronic benzodiazepine use, compensatory changes occur in GABA receptors. Such changes consist of decreased sensitivity of these receptors to GABA, probably as a result of alterations in affinity state and decreased density (Cowan and Nutt, 1982; Nutt, 1986). In addition, there are changes in the secondary systems controlled by GABA, so that the output of excitatory neurotransmitters tends to be restored, and/or the sensitivity of their receptors increases. The whole complex of primary and secondary changes eventually results in benzodiazepine tolerance.

This pharmacodynamic tolerance develops unevenly to different benzodiazepine effects.

For example, tolerance appears more rapidly to hypnotic and anticonvulsant than to anxiolytic effects (Sepinwall and Cook, 1979). Tolerance to different effects may also vary between individuals, possibly due to variations in intrinsic GABA activity in different parts of the brain, which are in turn reflected in personality characteristics and susceptibility to stress. Tolerance is never complete and probably never reaches a perfect equilibrium in all brain systems, which may be one reason for the high morbidity among chronic benzodiazepine users (Ashton, 1987). Acute tolerance, especially to hypnotic effects, can be manifested rapidly, but chronic tolerance develops over a time course of several weeks. Once established, chronic tolerance can last for months or even years after cessation of some central nervous system depressants such as alcohol (Cicero, 1978) and probably also benzodiazepines.

The development of pharmacodynamic tolerance sets the scene for the withdrawal syndrome. Cessation of the drug exposes all the adaptations which have accrued to counteract its presence, releasing a rebound of unopposed activity involving many neurotransmitters and their receptors and many brain systems. Clinically this state is manifested as the withdrawal syndrome, consisting of effects which are largely the opposite of those originally induced by the drug. The distribution, duration, and severity of symptoms depend on the particular systems which have undergone adaptive modulations and the degree of the adaptive changes induced as well as on the rate of drug withdrawal. Some authors distinguish between rebound and withdrawal effects, but the mechanism is the same for both (Lader, 1988). Acute withdrawal effects are reversed by an appropriate dose of the drug which restores the status quo.

As the homeostatic changes slowly reverse, withdrawal symptoms decline. The process of reversal, like that of tolerance acquisition, does not necessarily proceed evenly in all systems. The variable time of emergence and duration of individual symptoms during benzodiazepine withdrawal noted by Tyrer (1989) and Ashton et al. (1989) (see Table 1) may reflect this uneven course. The perturbations of brain function induced by benzodiazepines are exceedingly complex, and it is not surprising that withdrawal symptoms are many and variable. Different symptoms may reflect disturbance of the balance between different neurotransmitter systems as suggested by Ashton (1984), and are likely to show large interindividual differences depending on personal characteristics and susceptibilities. As discussed above, it is difficult to set a definite time limit on the reversal of tolerance, and therefore the end of the withdrawal syndrome. In general, tolerance declines over a matter of weeks, but in some cases it may endure for a year or more (Cicero, 1978). Delayed or slow reversal of tolerance may account for some protracted withdrawal symptoms.

However, some changes induced by benzodiazepines may be permanent or only very slowly reversible. Since benzodiazepines apparently inhibit learning, especially of stress-coping strategies (Gray, 1987), cessation after many years of use may expose a learning deficit, especially in the ability to cope with stress. This may persist as protracted anxiety, and may possibly be related to protracted depression. Anxiety symptoms are likely to endure until a new learning has induced the appropriate synaptic changes which probably involve modification of endogenous GABA activity.

VII. CONCLUSIONS

Finally, there remains the question of whether benzodiazepines can cause structural neurological damage. Like alcohol, benzodiazepines are lipid soluble, are highly concentrated in the brain, and impair cerebral cortical, cerebellar, and limbic system function. It is possible that use over many years could cause physical changes such as cortical shrinkage, which may be only partially reversible. Such changes have been demonstrated by computed tomographic (CAT) scan studies in young alcoholics (Lee et al., 1979; British Medical Journal,

1981), although not conclusively in chronic benzodiazepine users (Lader et al., 1984; Perera et al., 1987). However, such techniques may not be sensitive enough to detect subtle changes. Nor are standard tests of intellectual function sensitive enough to detect minor degrees of cognitive impairment which may persist after withdrawal in some long-term users. It remains possible that some protracted benzodiazepine withdrawal symptoms (including tinnitus and other neurological and psychological symptoms) could result from physicochemical neuronal damage. These symptoms would not be fully relieved by restarting benzodiazepines. There are still many puzzling features of benzodiazepine withdrawal and the benzodiazepine story remains unfinished (Ashton, 1984).

REFERENCES

Ashton, H. (1984). Benzodiazepine withdrawal: An unfinished story. *Br. Med. J., 288*:1135–1140.

Ashton, H. (1987). Benzodiazepine withdrawal: Outcome in 50 patients. *Br. J.Addict.82*:665–671.

Ashton, H.(1989). Risks of dependence on benzodiazepine drugs: A major problem of long-term treatment. *Br. Med. J., 298*:103–104.

Ashton, H., and Golding, J.F. (1989). Tranquillisers: Prevalence, predictors and possible consequences. Data from a large United Kingdom Survey. *Br. J. Addict., 84*:541–546.

Ashton, H., and Stepney, R. (1982). *Smoking: Psychology and Pharmacology.* London, Tavistock.

Ashton, H., Rawlins, M.D., and Tyrer, S.P. (1989). A double blind placebo controlled study of buspirone in diazepam withdrawal in chronic benzodiazepine users. *Br. J. Addict., 157*:232–238.

Benton, D., and Rick, J.T. (1976). The effect of increased brain GABA produced by amino-oxyacetic acid on arousal in rats. *Psychopharmacology, 49*:85–89.

Bloom, F.E. (1985). Neurohumoral transmission in the central nervous system, *The Pharmacological Basis of Therapeutics.* (A.G. Gilman, L.S. Goodman, T.W. Rall, and F. Murad, eds.). New York, Macmillan, pp. 236–259.

British Medical Journal (1981). Minor brain damage and alcoholism. *Br. Med. J., 2*:455–456.

Busto, U., Fornazzari, L., and Naranjo, C.A. (1988). Protracted tinnitus after discontinuation of long-term therapeutic use of benzodiazepines. *J. Clin. Psychopharmacol., 8*:359–362.

Busto, U., Sellers, E.M., Naranjo, C.A., Cappell, H.P., Sanchez, C.M., and Sykora, K. (1986). Withdrawal reaction after long-term therapeutic use of benzodiazepines. *N. Engl. J. Med. 315*:654–659.

Cicero, T.J. (1978). Tolerance to and physical dependence on alcohol: behavioural and neurobiological mechanisms, *Brain and Pituitary Peptides.* Munich, Ferring Symposium 1979, pp. 1603–1617.

Costa, E. (1981). The role of gamma-aminobutyric acid in the action of 1,4 benzodiazepines, *Towards Understanding Receptors.* (J.W. Lamble, ed.). Elsevier/North Holland, Amsterdam, pp. 176–183.

Cowen, P.J., and Nutt, D.J. (1982). Abstinence symptoms after withdrawal from tranquillising drugs: Is there a common neurochemical mechanism? *Lancet, 2*:360–362.

Gray, J. A. (1981). Anxiety as a paradigm case of emotion. *Br. Med. Bull. 37*:193–197.

Gray, J.A. (1987). The neuropsychology of emotion and personality, *Cognitive Neurochemistry*, (S.M. Stahl, S.D. Iverson, and E.C. Goodman, eds.). Oxford, England, Oxford University Press, pp. 171–190.

Haefely, W., Pieri, L., Pole, P., and Schaffer, R. (1981). General pharmacology and neuropharmacology of benzodiazepine derivatives, *Handbook of Experimental Pharmacology* Vol. 55, II (H. Hoffmeister and G. Stille, eds.). Berlin, Springer-Verlag, pp. 13–262.

Hallstrom, C., and Lader, M. (1981). Benzodiazepine withdrawal phenomena. *Int. Pharmacopsychiatry, 16*:235–44.

Hermann, J. B., Brotman, A.W., and Rosenbaum, J.F. (1987). Rebound anxiety in panic disorder patients treated with shorter-acting benzodiazepines. *J. Clin. Psychiatry, 48* (Suppl. 10):22–28.

Gilmartin, J.J., Corris, P.A., Stone, T.N., Veale, D., and Gibson, G.J. (1988). Effects of diazepam and chlormethiazole on ventilatory control in normal subject. *Br. J. Clin. Pharmacol., 25*:766–770.

Golding, J.F., and Cornish, A.M. (1987). Personality and life-style in medical students: Psychopharmacological aspects. *Psychol. Health, 1*:287–301.

Golding, J.F., Harper, T., and Brent-Smith, H. (1983). Personality, drinking and drug-taking correlates of cigarette smoking. *Person. Individ Diff.*, 4:703–706.

Kales, A., Scharf, M.B., and Kales, J.D. (1978). Rebound insomnia: A new clinical syndrome. *Science*, 201:1039–1041.

Lader, M. (1988). The psychopharmacology of addiction—benzodiazepine tolerance and dependence, *The Psychopharmacology of Addiction* (M. Lader, ed.). Oxford, England, Oxford University Press, pp. 1–14.

Lader, M.H., and Olajide, D.(1987). A comparison of buspirone and placebo in relieving benzodiazepine withdrawal symptoms. *J. Clin. Psychopharmacol.*, 7:11–15.

Lader, M.H., and Petursson, H. (1981). Benzodiazepine derivatives - side effects and dangers. *Biol. Psychiatry, 16*:1195–1212.

Lader, M.H., and Petursson, R.H. (1984). Computed axial brain tomography in long-term benzodiazepine users. *Psychol. Med., 14*:203–206.

Lee, K., Moller, L., Hardt, F., Haubek, A., and Jenson, E. (1979). Alcohol-induced brain damage and liver damage in young males. *Lancet, 2*:759–761.

Lum, L.C. (1987). Hyperventilation syndromes in medicine and psychiatry: A review. *J. R. Soc. Med., 80*:229–231.

Mohler, H., and Okada, T.(1977). Benzodiazepine receptors: Demonstration in the central nervous system. *Science, 198*:849–851.

Murphy, S.M., and Tyrer, P. (1988). The essence of benzodiazepine dependence, *The Psychopharmacology of Addiction* (M. Lader, ed.). Oxford, England, Oxford University Press, pp. 157–167.

Murphy, S.M., Owen, R.T., and Tyrer, P.J. (1984). Withdrawal symptoms after six week's treatment with diazepam. *Lancet, 2*:1389.

Nutt, D. (1986). Benzodiazepine dependence in the clinic: Reason for anxiety? *Trends Pharmacol. Sci., 7*:457–460.

Olijade, D., and Lader, M. (1984). Depression following withdrawal from long-term benzodiazepine use: A report of four cases. *Psychol. Med., 14*:937–940.

Oswald, I.(1989). Triazolam syndrome 10 years on. *Lancet, 1*:451–452.

Owen, R.T., and Tyrer, P. (1983). Benzodiazepine dependence: A review of the evidence. *Drugs, 25*:385–398.

Perera, K.M.H., Powell, T., and Jenner, F.A. (1987) Computerised axial tomographic studies following long-term use of benzodiazepines. *Psychol. Med., 17*:775–777.

Petursson, H., and Lader, M.H.(1981a). Withdrawal from long-term benzodiazepine treatment. *Br. Med. J., 283*:634–635.

Petursson, H., and Lader, M.H. (1981b). Benzodiazepine dependence. *Br. J. Addict., 76*:133–145.

Rementeria, J.L., and Bhatt, K. (1977). Withdrawal symptoms in neonates from intrauterine exposure to diazepam. *J. Paediatr., 90*:123–125.

Sepinwall, J., and Cook, L. (1979). Mechanisms of action of the benzodiazepines: Behavioural aspects. *Fed. Proc. 39*:3024–3031.

Smith, D.E., and Wesson, D.R. (1983). Benzodiazepine dependency syndromes. *J. Psychoact. Drugs, 15*:85–95.

Squires, R.F., and Braestrup, C. (1977). Benzodiazepine receptors in the rat brain. *Nature, 266*:732–734.

Tyrer, P., Murphy, S., and Riley, P. (1989). The benzodiazepine withdrawal symptom questionnaire. *J. Affect. Disord., 19*:53–61.

Tyrer, P., Owen, R., and Dawling, S. (1983). Gradual withdrawal of diazepam after long-term therapy. *Lancet, 1*:1402–1406.

Tyrer, P., Rutherford, D., and Huggett, T. (1981). Benzodiazepine withdrawal symptoms and propranolol. *Lancet, 1*:520–522.

Winokur, A., Rickels, K., Greenblatt, D.J., Snyder, P.J., and Schatz, N.J. (1980). Withdrawal reaction from long-term low dosage administration of diazepam. *Arch. Gen. Psychiatry, 37*:101–105.

Young, W.S., and Kuhar, M.J. (1980). Radiohistochemical localisation of benzodiazepine receptors in rat brain. *J. Pharmacol. Ex. Ther., 212*:337–346.

Zigmond, A.S., and Snaith, R.P. (1983). The hospital anxiety and depression (HAD) scale. *Acta Psychiatr. Scand., 6*:361–370.

51

Countertransference Issues in the Treatment of Drug and Alcohol Addiction

John E. Imhof
North Shore University Hospital–Cornell University Medical College, Manhasset, New York

I. INTRODUCTION

Since the 1933 publication of Rado's *The Psychoanalysis of Pharmacothymia* [1], a vast amount of psychiatric literature has explored the issue of drug and alcohol addiction from several perspectives: etiological, demographical, sociological, criminological, and psychological causation. In addition, significant attention continues to focus upon the myriad of diagnostic, treatment, and rehabilitation approaches in drug and alcohol addiction. For example, Lettieri, Sayers, and Pearson [2] have detailed 43 separate and distinct theories of drug abuse, just one indicator of the disparities inherent in treatment of drug and alcohol addiction. Yet in the majority of all surveyed articles, chapters and books on addiction, little if any attention is given to that one factor which often determines whether or not treatment will succeed: the attitudes and feelings of the treatment provider towards the drug- and alcohol-addicted patient. In major reviews of addiction treatment and research studies, (3–6), the role of the provider as being influential in treatment outcome is generally not acknowledged. However the addiction treatment provider may possess such a significant amount of negative feelings or attitudes towards the addicted patient that any hope for objective and effective diagnosis, treatment, and rehabilitation becomes diminished, if not completely eliminated.

Case Vignette

By the time Harry R. was referred to the company's Employee Counseling Services, he had been late for work several times, had caused one major accident that resulted in serious injury to himself and another worker, and had initiated several shouting matches with his co-workers and supervisors. Since beginning with the printing firm in 1974, Harry had, with the exception of occasional Monday morning latenesses, an exemplary work record until 4 months ago, when the accident occurred. He stated he "forgot" to get a safety lock switch on one of the presses, which suddenly started up when Harry and co-worker began to change the printing fluids. Harry and the other worker sustained third-degree burns on their hands and wrists. At the time, Harry's supervisor noted he smelled alcohol on Harry's breath, to which Harry responded with several expletives and threats of physical confrontation.

Rather than initiate more stringent disciplinary measures, the supervisor recommended that Harry speak to the firm's counseling psychologist, primarily because of Harry's many years of service, and the fact he was most usually "just a great guy." Th supervisor proceeded to arrange a meeting on Monday morning at 9:30 A.M. with Dr. B. That recommendation was forwarded by a note which was attached to Harry's time card just prior to his leaving work on a Friday afternoon.

On Monday morning Harry arrived 10 min late at the consultation, and he was visibly upset and annoyed. He appeared somewhat disheveled and unkempt. He sat down, lit a cigarette, and refused to put it out in spite of Dr. B.'s reminding him of the No Smoking sign. Dr. B. decided she would pursue the interview in spite of the smoking, and asked questions such as, "Why do you think you're here, Harry?", and "Your supervisor thinks you have a drinking problem—do you agree"? Harry quickly became agitated, verbally abusive, and questioned whose decision it was that he be referred for "mental help." He expressed his outrage that he was singled out, saying that "plenty of guys around here screw up a hell of a lot more than I do, and they sure as hell drink more than I do." Then, in a quick reversal of tactics, Harry began to question the youthful-looking Dr. B.'s credentials and experience. He became seductive and rather obnoxious, sensing he had the upper hand in the confrontation.

The longer Harry was in the room, the angrier Dr. B. became. She felt flushed, increasingly agitated, and, for a moment, feared she may be in some physical danger. Without making any further attempts to engage Harry, she abruptly stood up and ended the meeting by saying, "I don't think we can help you. Unless, you get to work on time, stop abusing people, and stop your drinking, you're probably going to lose your job in a very short time." Perhaps taken aback by Dr. B.'s sudden candor, Harry stood up calmly, said, "Go to hell, sweetheart," and walked out. Almost prophetically, Harry came in late the following morning, reeked of alcohol on his breath, and was summarily fired.

In discussing this incident later with a supervisor, Dr. B. recounted, "You want to know how I felt? Plain and simple, I wanted to kill him on the spot! He was abusive, obnoxious, chauvanistic, hostile, and certainly not interested in my helping him." She also commented on her strong sense of guilt in having such negative feelings toward an individual who obviously had serious emotional problems. Nonetheless, Dr. B. was unable to determine any manner in which she could have handled the situation differently, thereby possibly resulting in a more satisfactory outcome.

It should be noted at the onset that the concept of countertransference itself is one that continues to undergo a continuing dialogue regarding its very usefulness in the therapeutic relationship. Slakter [7] notes that, "Clearly, no agreement exists as to the meaning of countertransference. Just as each individual countertransference experience is unique, so we seem to have many unique approaches in conceptualizing the phenomenon." [p. 200].

However, for the purposes of further understanding the interactive processes of providing evaluation, diagnosis, and treatment to the addicted individual, *countertransference* shall be conceptualized as the total emotion reaction of the treatment provider to the patient, with consideration of the entire range of conscious, preconscious, and unconscious attitudes, beliefs, and feelings in the provider. The treatment provider, or therapist, is considered to be any individual charged with the responsibility of providing drug and alcohol treatment services. Such a category would include physicians, psychologists, clinical social workers, clinical nurse specialists, and former drug- or alcohol-addicted individuals, commonly referred to as ex-addict counselors or recovery specialists.

In addition to the presence of countertransference within the one-to-one treatment relationship, this chapter shall also address other forms of countertransference, including institutional and societal countertransference, the origins of which may be found in the history of our nation's legislative efforts in attempting to reduce and eliminate drug addiction and alcoholism.

II. LITERATURE REVIEW

Upon a careful review of more than 60 years of psychiatric literature that addresses the treatment of drug and alcohol addiction, one may easily realize that the current negative attitudes toward drug and alcohol patients in large part stems from the manner in which most of the addiction treatment pioneers themselves viewed their subjects. When we learn that many of the most skilled and talented clinicians found little hope for improvement in their subject populations, it is not difficult to draw from them an essentially pessimistic view regarding the prognosis of treating drug and alcohol patients.

In 1929, Simmel [8] indicated that because of murderous impulses and the need for self-punishment, the treatment of the drug addict carries several risks, especially the heightened possibility of the patient's suicide. After 30 years of investigation into treating drug-addicted patients, Rado (1) concluded that the "prognosis of drug addiction is quite unfavorable." [p. 34] Fenichel [9] urged against the treatment of addicts in any location other than an institutional setting, in particular because of the tendency of the drug addict to act out while in treatment. Meerlo [10] cautioned against drug addicts who attempt to bribe therapists with passive, compliant, and limited drug-free behavior while waiting for the first perceived error by the therapist as justification for falling back to a pattern of using drugs.

In 1948, when Ausubel [11] wrote that "drug addiction constitutes more than a rare and isolated phenomenon of behavioral maladjustment (which psychiatrists and other medical men approach with disinterest, dread and despair..." [p. 219], his parenthetical comment was the first literature reference that acknowledged the actual personal, subjective reaction that could be induced in addiction treatment providers by drug-addicted patients. Ten years later, Ausubel [12] expounded on his views of the treatment relationship:

> ...Yet despite the need for establishment of rapport and positive transference the physician only too frequently, even in the best institutions, openly displays a cynical, unrealistic and hostile attitude towards the addict: he is indifferent to the latter's genuine complaints, assumes in advance that he is a liar, and maintains that it is a waste of effort and money to attempt a cure. Such an attitude must be deplored as...contributing toward the resentment and lack of personality reintegration that helps pave the way for relapse. In the case of the voluntary patient, it leads to his immediate discharge. [p. 61]

In writing of the countertransferential difficulties in the treatment of alcoholism, Selzer [13] noted that "...when hostility enters the picture as part of the defensive armor, not of the patient, but of the therapist, and is directed against the patient, the changes for establishment of a positive therapeutic relationship are markedly diminished. If anything, this situation will intensify the patient's difficulties and make recovery more unlikely." [p. 301] Selzer [13] further states that such countertransference "often perpetuates the drinking pattern" [p. 305]. Furthermore, the "hostility may be expressed on an overt or conscious manner, or may operate so that both patient and therapist are unconscious of its presence" [p. 305]. In this regard, Kaufman [14] suggests that relabeling countertransference as "therapist codependency, or enabling" may be a useful concept in assisting clinicians to more effectively grapple with their feelings toward drug and alcohol addicted patients.

In an article concerning reaction formation as a countertransference phenomenon in the treatment of alcoholism, Moore [15] postulates:

> because of renounced infantile cravings, the therapist is angered by the constant seeking of indulgence by the alcoholic patient. He may express this directly by rejection of the patient. Because the therapist is often made anxious by any awareness of anger at his patients, he may defend himself by establishing a reaction formation in the form of an overly indulgent and permissive attitude.... This attitude is destructive of the patient's chance of recovery as it impairs his reality testing and encourages denial of the severity of the drinking problem. Thus, the therapist's unconscious hostility ultimately finds its mark. [p. 485]

In an expansive review and summary of the major psychoanalytic contributions to the understanding of the etiology and treatment of drug addiction, Rosenfeld [16] acknowledges that "only a few of the authors mentioned in the review have discussed the technical difficulties which arise in the treatment of both alcoholics and drug addicts." [p. 242]

Wurmser [17] has written that "drug abuse is the nemesis to haunt psychiatry itself. The enormousness of emotional problems dwarfs our skills, more than our knowledge; we understand far more than we can actually influence...." [p. 406] How might treatment providers feel about dealing with a group of patients who are thought to dwarf the skills of experienced clinicians?

Merry [18] noted that owing to both personality disorders and the tension and urgency frequently associated with (heroin) addiction, physicians often have to contend with noncomformist behavior such as lateness, bad manners, and bad tempers. To deal with this situation, Merry calls for a "tolerant and sympathetic staff." [p. 206] In exploring the management of the drug-addicted patient in treatment, Rosenfeld [16] states that the "drug addict is a particularly difficult patient to manage because the analyst has not only to deal with a psychologically determined state but is confronted with the combination of a mental state and the intoxication and confusion caused by drugs." [p. 128]

Davidson [19] is one of the few authors that explores the impact of the patient's psychological defense structure on the therapist, and the manner in which this interaction is managed on a clinical level. In writing of the transference and countertransference phenomena regarding the treatment of methadone maintenance patients, Davidson notes that often extreme affects of methadone patients present enormous problems for staff. "Expressions of strong hostility, anger and blamefulness in patients arouse equally powerful emotions in staff, whose most common response is to retaliate—overtly or covertly, against the patient." [pp. 121-122]

Case Vignette

The psychiatric attending was rudely awakened by the 3 A.M. call from the emergency room resident, whose voice belied a sence of both anger and confusion: "Dr. L., I'm sorry to call you at this time, but we have a problem here. About 2 hours ago, the police ambulance brought in a junkie—a real dirtbag if I ever saw one. This guy is filthy, cursing everyone in the E.R. and plainly refusing to cooperate. The police say they received an anonymous phone call and were directed to Sunset Park, where they found him unconscious on one of the benches. His breathing was labored, but he awoke in the ambulance and has been in and out of consciousness since then. He has fresh needle marks on his left arm, but won't tell us anything about what he took, or how much. The medical people pumped his stomach and say he's out of danger. His girlfriend arrived an hour ago and according to her, this guy has tried to kill himself a couple of times. I think I could convince him he should be admitted, but we've only got one bed left, and I know Dr. J. has an admission scheduled later this morning. Frankly, I'd like to get this bum the hell out of here. I think he'll be nothing but trouble upstairs. Remember that last junkie we had about 3 months ago—took a swing at the security guard and nearly started a riot on the unit? Anyway, the medical people insist he has to be admitted, and I don't want them telling us what to do. I figured I should call you, because I'm not sure what to do here."

III. THE DRUG- AND ALCOHOL-ADDICT PATIENT: PSYCHIATRIC IMPLICATIONS

Recognition and management of countertransference phenomena are especially relevant in the treatment of drug- and alcohol-addicted patients. Such patients, already labeled in society as addicts, junkies, garbageheads, dopefiends, rummies, boozers, and drunks, may often find themselves in the care of therapists who, while well intentioned, find themselves experiencing a formidable and often unwanted array of feelings, reactions, and attitudes toward their patients. It is essential to emphasize that such reactions are not at all uncommon in working with drug- and alcohol-addicted patients, but rather reflect the necessity of further understanding the emotional status of the addicted patient.

The drug- and/or alcohol-addicted patient arrives for treatment in a state of psychological and physiological decompensation. As with any individual who experiences a major destabilizing and stressful crisis, he or she is desperate for immediate relief. The drug- and alcohol-addicted individual is often terror stricken, anxiety ridden, depressed, demanding, and often communicates these and other needs in a pleading, if not pathetic manner. The clinical composite illustrates significant ego regression, with demonstrable states of fragmentation, depersonalization, and, most commonly, an immobilizing depression. The addicted patient is no longer able to utilize, exploit, or manipulate the environment. He or she is concurrently dependent upon the external world for survival, yet terrified of this dependency because of his or her basic mistrust and rage [20].

Furthermore, the drug-addicted patient abuses himself or herself in a most vengeful and ultimately masochistic manner. In this regard, Stolorow [21] notes that

> by actively producing his own failure and defeat and actively provoking humiliation, abuse and punishment, the masochistic character experiences the illusion of magical control and triumphant power over his object world....Such illusions of magical control enable the masochist to deny his narcissistic vulnerability by retaining his fantasies of infantile omnipotence. [p. 445]

For the drug- and alcohol-addicted patient, the attendant psychological and physiological pain is enormous, and the drug(s) serve as the analgesic. In effect, the patient asks, "What can you offer me that is better than heroin [or whatever the drug of choice]?" Considering the patient's extensive drug use, lifestyle, social milieu, and the years of "drug rewards" prior to the onset of deterioration, it is indeed a difficult question to answer. Also to be considered is the physical effect that the drug provides. One patient told his therapist that a shot of heroin made him feel as if he were experiencing a 3-hour continuous orgasm, and wanted to know what the therapist had to offer in its place. The therapist replied, "Hard work, emotional struggles, painful remembrances and, for a time, incredible frustration." The patient laughed and asked which choice the therapist would select.

As noted by Hirsch, Imhof, and Terenzi [20], a fundamental operational definition of drug and alcohol addicted individuals is that

...they are psychiatric patients with varying degrees of psychopathology, and that the drug use is symptomatic of the basic, underlying pathological state. The absence of this conceptual view in the continuing development, refinement and application of...treatment modalities would perpetuate the historical status of the drug abuser: a nonpsychiatric patient, a sociomedical outcast viewed as untreatable and unmanageable. It has not been uncommon that these patients have been shunned by mental health professionals and agencies, not only as a result of professional abdication but perhaps more often by the therapist's subjective feelings of ineffectiveness and impotence. [p. 25]

Further understanding toward treatment of drug- and alcohol-addicted patients may be obtained by clarification of their diagnostic categories. Many authors [5,15,17,20] have stated their impression that drug- and alcohol-addicted patients most appropriately fall into the diagnostic categories of borderline and narcissistic personality disorders. When we understand that two of the primary defenses of these categories are splitting and projective identification, further light is shed upon the treatment challenge posed by these patients.

In writing of the therapeutic significance of splitting and projective identification, Grotstein [22] notes that

Powerful feelings are more than not expressed by giving another person the experience of how one feels...All human beings seem to have the need to be relieved of the burden of unknown, unknowable feelings by being able to express them, literally as well as figuratively into the flesh, so to speak, of the other so that this other peson can know how one feels. We are each projections and ultimately wish the other to know the experience we cannot communicate or unburden ourselves, or until we have been convinced that the other understands. We cannot be convinced that they understand until we are convinced that they now contain the experience. [pp. 201–202]

Masterson [23] provides further illustration of this concept when he writes that

...the borderline patient projects so much and is so provocative and manipulative, particularly in the beginning of therapy, that he can place a great emotional stress on the therapist. Unless the therapist can understand both what the patient is doing and how it is affecting his own emotions, he will be unable to deal with it therapeutically. It is important to keep in mind that the patient is a professional at provocation and manipulation while the therapist is an amateur at the use of these mechanisms. [p. 105]

So in addition to considering the clinical challenges of borderline and narcissistic patients with their attendant intense transference manifestations, the diagnostic label of drug addicted or alcoholic is now further imposed on the clinical picture. Accordingly, one can now begin to understand that the therapeutic challenges awaiting treatment providers working with drug- and alcohol-addicted patients are at least profound.

Case Vignette

Mary C. is a 29-year-old woman who sought professional help when she realized she had become addicted to the Xanax (alprazolam) that her physician had been prescribing for the past 2 years. She had complained of nervousness, agitation, and difficulty sleeping. Her physician, an internist, considered Mary to be a "whiner" and "complainer," and once even commented that "you shouldn't get so hysterical about everything." He diagnosed Mary as having a generalized anxiety disorder, prescribed 0.25 mg of Xanax three times daily, and mildly recommended she contact a psychotherapist to help her with her day-to-day problems in living. During her subsequent intake evaluation at the Island Metropolitan Drug Treatment Center, Mary commented on the initial physical relief she experienced with Xanax, which led her to indefinitely postpone any further thoughts about beginning therapy.

About 6 months prior to her drug program application, Mary noticed that her agitation and nervousness were increasing. She had difficulty sleeping and experienced complications in a number of her interpersonal relationships. She broke up with her fiancé, and was constantly quarreling with her parents and sisters. Her internist suggested she increase the Xanax dosage to 0.50 mg three times a day. While this provided relief for about 2 weeks, her anxiety symptoms returned in full force. She asked her physician for an even higher dosage and, when he refused, stormed out of his office and made an appointment with another physician whom she knew would more freely prescribe the Xanax. A few weeks prior to her calling the drug program, she was taking between 8 and 10 Xanax a day and, for the first time, began experiencing a severe and immobilizing depression.

During her intake, the counselor wrote that the "patient speaks in a rapid and anxious manner, is somewhat argumentative and demanding, though there is a likeable quality about her." She was diagnosed as being dependent on the benzodiazepines, while her anxiety symptoms were viewed as iatrogenically induced, as well as secondary to a major depressive disorder. Mary denied any suicidal ideation, though she was deemed at risk because of the recent suicides of her aunt and first cousin, both to whom she felt close.

It was the Center's recommendation that Mary be admitted to the inpatient unit for detoxification from the Xanax, to be followed by outpatient individual and group therapy upon discharge. While Mary accepted the recommendation for therapy, she refused hospitalization and stated she would detoxify herself, cutting back a few pills each day. Five days later Mary had a seizure and was brought to the emergency room. She was diagnosed as having withdrawal symptoms resulting from abrupt cessation of the benzodiazepines (she stopped all medication within 3 days) and was admitted to the inpatient unit. The unit staff found her to be a difficult and demanding patient, and she insisted on signing out against medical advice following 3 days of hospitalization. After failing to convince her to remain in the hospital to complete the detoxification, the resident physician, feeling totally exasperated and angry, finally told Mary, "Look, do whatever the hell you want. Just don't think you're going to get back in here so easy if things don't work out. You can't expect to get everything you want when you want it."

Mary was discharged from the hospital. Three days later she attempted suicide, ingesting 30 Xanax with several glasses of wine. She was found unconscious by her mother, rushed to the hospital, and admitted to the Intensive Care Unit, where she remained for 3 days until she regained consciousness.

In subsequent discussions with his supervisor following Mary's readmission to the inpatient psychiatric unit, the resident stated how unsympathetic and angry he still felt toward Mary, and expressed surprise at her suicide attempt. "I never saw that at all. I figured she was too feisty and assertive to consider hurting herself. I was in fact happy to discharge her, and I feel somewhat depressed about having her as my patient again."

IV. THE THERAPEUTIC ENCOUNTER

Unless the treatment provider has an awareness of the antitherapeutic implications of unrecognized and/or unmanaged countertransference, continuing and effective treatment with the drug-addicted and alcoholic patient will probably be short lived. As Krystal and Raskin [24] note regarding the treatment of drug addiction: "With these patients the problems of countertransference are especially difficult because of the agression they include. Because patients are very demanding, expressing insatiable, endless oral fantasies, the analyst has to deal with their fears of being devoured or destroyed, and often becomes concerned with giving too much or too little with them. [pp. 103–104]

Cohen, White, and Schoolar [25] have written that the therapist:

> must be ready to assume a position which allows him to empathize with the drug abuser's feeling of isolation and impotence. Therapy will of necessity involve a ...long term commitment. Not only is this inherent in severe identity problems but there will be many resistances to involvement combined with acting out, designed at some point to test the genuineness and stability of concern exhibited by the therapist. In some respects, the challenge to the mental health treatment community seems almost overwhelming. How does one move unflinchingly into an arena where he is made to feel unwanted, incompetent and even malevolent? [p. 358]

While the presenting symptomatology of the drug-addicted and alcoholic patient may vary from neurotic to overtly psychotic, so too may the countertransference reactions of therapists vary in marked degrees—at times overt and transparent, at other times subtle and not so easily detected. Table 1 is a list of various presenting defenses and transference manifestations of drug-addicted and alcoholic patients, along with those corresponding countertransference reactions that may be evoked in the therapist. Such a list is by no means intended to be complete, but rather to serve as an illustration of some possible interactive combinations to which clinicians should be attuned.

V. FURTHER SOURCES OF COUNTERTRANSFERENCE REACTIONS

In addition to the interactive combinations presented in Table 1, there are additional factors inherent in drug and alcohol treatment that, unless recognized and addressed, may very well lead to inappropriately managed countertransferential reactions to drug and alcohol patients.

A. Staff Burnout

Mental health professionals understand the concept of the burnout syndrome, yet perhaps might be unfamiliar with the countertransferential implications of the syndrome. Pines and Maslach [26] have defined burnout as "a syndrome of a negative self-concept, negative job attitudes, and a loss of concern and feeling for clients." [p. 233] Imhof, Hirsch, and Terenzi [27] note that

> The clinical picture [of a staff member exhibiting burnout symptoms] generally centers around a withdrawal mechanism—a self-protecting, narcissistic distancing which manifests itself as indifference, tiredness, boredom, and in general, a separation from the therapeutic environment. Such burnout features are not uncommon when considering the consistent and intense demands that the [drug and alcohol addicted] patient makes, and the recidivistic and chronically relapsing manifestations of the addictive disorders. [p. 28]

Unless the clinician strives to consistently remain aware of his or her physical and emotional well-being, the potential for burnout is heightened when working with demanding treatment populations. And as noted by Patrick [28],

> There comes a time, therefore, when the clinician must attend to the issue of self-preservation: the nurture, care, stimulation and preservation of one's person as a valuable resource. Without such attention to the self, the clinician working in the substance abuse treatment field cannot attain professional or personal achievement and satisfaction of goals. ...If the clinician is sincerely committed to the helping role, it is incongruent to neglect self-help. [p. 85]

Table 1   A Sampling of Patient Defenses and Transference Manifestations and Various
Countertransference Reactions by Treatment Staff

Patient	Therapist/Counselor
1. The patient as victim—"Poor me—I'm helpless," or "Everyone is against me", or "Why does everything happen to me"	Anger at the helplessness Feeling the need to rescue and save the patient Becoming an advice giver Experiencing sadistic feelings toward the masochistic element of patient's transference Identify with the helplessness; i.e., "I know just how you feel—it happens to me too" "You and me against the world"
2. Overt anger and hostility by patient toward therapist and other treatment staff	Emotional withdrawal from patient's anger Becoming frightened for one's safety Meet anger with greater anger Discharge patient for inappropriate behavior Passive-aggressive behavior toward anger; i.e., appearing to listen, then making changes with regard to patient's appointment time, date of session, frequency, lateness, etc.
3. The perfect patient—does everything right: on time, verbal, drug free—seeming appropriate in all aspects	Becoming complacent and bored Experiencing a sense of great therapeutic effectiveness, if not grandiosity
4. The perfect patient acts out: misses appointments, overdoses, gets arrested, etc.	Therapist becomes enraged Feelings of inadequacy, incompetence; shattering of illusion of the effective therapist Depressive reaction, as a defense against rage Impulsive acting out by the therapist; i.e., discharge patient Provoke patient to leave therapy
5. The patient intellectualizes behavior and experiences; no apparent contact with emotions and feelings	Therapist resorts to interpreting Attacks the primary defense of intellectualization, telling patient she or he is using his or her head, not heart Anger at patient for not conforming to role of the "good" patient who should talk about feelings Therapist becomes complacent with intellectualizing, as it avoids necessity of addressing underling emotions
6. Provocative and obnoxious toward therapist: belittling, devaluing, confronting	Anger at patient Emotional withdrawal; cowering under attack Seek to discharge patient as uncooperative, and/or "unsuitable for outpatient therapy"
7. Patient insists on knowing personal information about therapist prior to self-revelations	Reveal personal information to soothe patient Silence Anger at feeling intruded upon

(continued)

Table 1   *Continued*

Patient	Therapist/Counselor
8. Cannot maintain ground rules of session. Wants to eat and drink during therapy; several phone calls throughout the week; a scattered, often chaotic patient	Therapist permits eating and drinking in session Anger at phone calls, and feeling intruded upon Warns patient about discharge if calls don't cease Changes patient's appointment time, or cancels sessions
9. Insists that she or her cannot be helped; wants to constantly leave therapy unless results are seen quickly	Feels pressure and sense of being manipulated Anger at patient Feelings of helplessness and ineptitude Recommends discharge

B. Acquired Immune Deficiency Syndrome (AIDS)

Given the now well-established relationship between intravenous drug use and human immune virus (HIV) infection, substance abuse treatment clinicians are compelled to explore the countertransferential implications of working with AIDS patients as well as those patients whose prior drug-taking and/or sexual history may have exposed them to the AIDS virus. It has not been uncommon for even experienced treatment professionals to specifically state that under no circumstances will they work with a patient who has been diagnosed as having AIDS. Faltz and Madover [29] identify the specific countertransference issues for clinicians working with AIDS patients: "fear of the unknown, fear of contagion, fear of death and dying, fear of homosexuality, denial of helplessness, overidentification with the patient, anger, and the need for professional omnipotence." [pp. 28–29] Treating a patient who is both HIV–infected and has history of drug addiction may indeed present a difficult challenge to the clinician, in that there exists two treatment issues whose existence has been subject to stereotypical categorization: drug addiction and AIDS.

C. Counselors With Former Drug and Alcohol Use Histories

A substantial number of therapeutic communities, methadone maintenance programs and inpatient rehabilitation centers today have a particularly distinctive and historical personnel requirement that stands alone in the mental health treatment field today. Specifically, having prior drug and alcohol use experience (and of course successfully becoming drug free) is often considered a prerequisite for counselor positions, and such prior drug-using experience is viewed as equally important as one's formal clinical training. Alternately referred to as ex-addicts, addiction specialists, rehab counselors, or recovery specialists, the formerly addicted drug/alcohol user-turned-clinician presents special considerations regarding awareness of countertransferential issues. In this regard, Imhof, Hirsch, and Terenzi [27] note that

> The drug patient may serve as a constant and perhaps uncomfortable reminder of the therapist's past....the therapist who is a former compulsive drug abuser might inadvertantly seek to utilize the identical therapeutic framework with the patient that the therapist himself experienced, and currently views as being responsible for his own successful

rehabilitation. In such cases, a "what worked for me will work for you" attitude may result in unreasonable therapeutic expectations, often leading to premature treatment termination. [p. 29]

Furthermore, utilizing one's own personal experiences as a basis for treating others obviously neglects psychological and physiological individuality. And readers are furthermore advised to consider the countertransferential implications for an area of mental health treatment (i.e., drug and alcohol addiction) that places similar emphasis on personal drug experience in relation to clinical training. In many drug and alcohol programs today, and unlike any other area of mental health treatment, having had the illness is a requirement for treating the illness.

D. Therapist's Family History

Given the epidemic nature of drug and alcohol addiction in the United States today, and the specific intergenerational nature of alcoholism, there is substantial likelihood that at least one member of most therapists' families has experienced a problem with drugs or alcohol. Accordingly, it is imperative that each therapist understand the extent of drug and or alcohol use in his or her family, and how that may affect the manner in which the therapist approaches treatment of individuals and other families with addicted members. In particular, it is essential for the clinician to be aware of identification issues that may be aroused when treating patients who bear resemblances to member(s) of the therapist's own family who have been or are currently involved with drugs and/or alcohol.

E. Societal Influences on the Therapist

Drug and alcohol treatment personnel are members of society and, as such, are vulnerable to the same antidrug stereotypes to which everyone else is subjected. Societal countertransference is especially prominent given the recurrent wars on drugs in which our country has engaged since President Kennedy's White House Conference on Drug Abuse in 1962 [30]. Little sympathy or understanding can be found today for those who willingly and knowingly sell, deal, or ingest drugs, and the proliferation of drug wars has contributed to our national consciousness of fighting the "enemies", i.e., those associated with all the illicit channels of drug addiction.

It should be noted that the origins of the current anti-drug sentiment today may be traced to the early part of the twentieth century. While few of the moral sanctions evidenced today could be found in 1900, the Harrison Narcotics Act of 1914, which limited the manufacture, volume, and distribution of narcotics, also initiated an anti-drug user sentiment that continues to the present day. Within a relatively brief period of time (from 1900 to 1914), addicted law-abiding citizens suddenly found themselves branded as criminal and had to pay very high prices for what became, as a result of the legislation, black market drugs [31].

Because of society's general anti–drug user sentiment, it is not uncommon for drug-addicted individuals to withhold knowledge of their drug use from both family members and employers for fear of being ostracized and, in the work-related areas, fired. While provision of health insurance for alcohol rehabilitation programs has continued to deemotionalize the acknowledgment of a drinking problem, there still exists today great fear of openly stating that one has a drug problem. This societal countertransference perpetuates the notion of a drug-addicted person as a social outcast; a sociological and criminological phenomenon rather than an individual in need of medical and psychiatric intervention.

F. Institutional Countertransference

Case Vignette

Evelyn Kramer, the intake social worker for Island Metro's Drug Program, was quite unprepared for the experience of meeting William, a 34-year-old white, homosexual intravenous drug user, who was diagnosed as having AIDS 3 years ago. Accompanied by his lover, and two aunts, William had, at 3 A.M. that morning, flamboyantly presented to Island Metropolitan Hospital's Emergency Room insisting he was addicted to Valium (diazepam), Darvocet (propoxyphene and acetaminophene), and Seconal (secobarbital) and, in dramatic gestures, demanding immediate inpatient hospitalization in order to detoxify from the drugs. His reason for wanting admission to Island Metro was primarily related to the fact that his AIDS doctors were on the staff at Island, and he reasonably expected he would receive greater coordination of care if he were admitted there. William's personality is usually brittle and provocative, and he was no less provocative the morning he sought admission. Alternately demanding his rights as a patient, and accusing the doctors of not wanting to admit him because he had AIDS, William angrily confronted the psychiatric resident with a threat that, unless he were admitted "within the hour," he would "bite someone and give them AIDS."

The psychiatry resident, Dr. Andrea Martin, found herself feeling both panic and rage. Her first impulse was to call Security, which she did immediately, and then contacted the medical resident. Dr. Martin felt it essential to first assess William's medical status prior to proceeding with a mental status examination as part of his inpatient evaluation. With a Security guard now present in the consultation room, William was no less belligerent with the medical resident, Dr. Richard Smith, with whom William now started to flirt, and wondered aloud, so all in the Emergency Room could here, if Dr. Smith himself was homosexual. In an attempt to set limits with the patient, Dr. Smith informed William that he would refuse to proceed with the examination unless William refrained from his now obnoxious behavior. Dr. Smith suspected, as was later confirmed by toxicology, that William was indeed stoned.

While Dr. Smith was conducting his medical evaluation, Dr. Martin had also contacted the chief resident in psychiatry, to inquire whether or not, since the psychiatric unit was at full census, a consideration should be made to go over-census. In learning of the circumstances of the case, the chief resident decided he would not consent to admitting the patient and would instead recommend a referral to the county hospital. That recommendation was supported by the medical resident, who stated that, despite William's stoned condition and his insistence on being addicted to three substances, a referral should be made to the County hospital, since "all the beds at Metro are full."

Upon hearing he would not be admitted to the hospital of his choice, William suddenly began crying and pleading for help, stating he was out of drugs and would start withdrawal soon. Dr. Martin insisted that the county hospital would attend to his medical and psychiatric needs, but that he could always pursue other treatment choices at Island Metro's Drug Treatment Center. At that point, William put on his clothes and, without another word, bolted from the Emergency Room.

When Evelyn arrived for work at 9 A.M., William was seated in the Intake Unit, having announced he was referred from the Emergency Room, where he was told the drug program would find him a bed in a hospital "other than the county hospital." True to his style, William continued to act in a provocative and confronting manner, at which point Evelyn immediately stated, "Listen, unless you just talk to me in a respectful manner, you can go and sit in the waiting room for another two hours." Her tone and demeanor apparently motivated William to address his presenting problem without the usual attendant drama, and Evelyn proceeded with an intake evaluation.

She determined that William did indeed require inpatient detoxification, though he again insisted on being hospitalized at Island Metro, so he could be near his AIDS doctors. He expressed a willingness to be placed on a waiting list, and overall began comporting himself in a manner quite different as had been evidenced in the Emergency Room. Evelyn arranged for an evaluation with Dr. Judd, the program's staff psychiatrist, who supported the intake counselor's findings and himself began to make a number of phone calls to investigate why William had not originally been admitted to Island Metro earlier that morning.

Drug treatment professionals are familiar with both institutional and milieu countertransference, wherein the negative feelings in society toward drug- and alcohol-addicted patients are reflected in unwritten, informal policies that seek to limit, if not in fact bar, certain types of patients from being admitted to hospitals, or certain units within hospitals. For example, while there exists greater acceptance and understanding of the drug-addicted patient as having psychiatric problems, inpatient treatment services for addicted patients are usually found in discrete settings, apart from the inpatient psychiatric and medical units of most hospitals. Commonly referred to as rehabilitation centers, these programs cater exclusively to the drug and alcohol population, who often are unable to obtain the services they need in a general hospital setting.

VI. RECOMMENDATIONS

In order to assist clinicians in recognizing and managing a wide range of possible countertransferential reactions, the following recommendations are provided for review and discussion. While these recommendations may be considered for all individuals treating drug- and alcohol-addicted patients, they may have greater relevance and applicability for those individuals in therapist and counseling roles.

A. The Therapist's Own Therapy

It has been the writer's experience that the most critical factor in ensuring that negative countertransference factors are minimized is whether or not the therapist has had a successful personal therapy experience. It is very difficult, if not impossible, to provide for another what has not been provided for oneself.

It should be clarified that, for the purposes of this discussion, a successful therapy experience is defined as one in which the individual has had an opportunity to understand, to accept, and, when indicated, to appropriately modify his or her conscious and unconscious impulses, motivations, and behaviors to enhance intrapsychic and interpersonal functioning. This includes the capacity to be in touch with one's own thoughts and feelings as they relate to the self, and to relationships with others. The well-analyzed therapist has the capacity for empathy without overidentification, compassion without pity, listening without judging, and reflecting without imposing one's own values and opinions. Given the complexities inherent in the treatment of drug-dependent individuals, it is postulated that only through examining, with another, the process of one's own emotional development, can the therapist most effectively recognize, tolerate, and understand the range of countertransferential and attitudinal considerations that may arise in the treatment of not only drug and alcohol addicted patients, but other patients as well.

B. Clinical Supervision

The second critical factor in assisting the therapist to recognize countertransferential factors that can be damaging to treatment is individual clinical supervision. Without the opportunity to have a well-qualified professional objectively reflect on the process of therapy sessions, the therapist may not recognize feelings within him or herself that may contaminate interventions and adversely affect the course of treatment. Maintaining the availability of clinical supervision is a responsibility not only to the patient, but also to the therapist himself or herself, and the profession which he or she represents. In addition to individual supervision, group supervision and peer supervision provide rich opportunities for the therapist to continuously review his or her work with patients and receive feedback. A particularly significant advantage of group supervision is that the therapist has the opportunity to hear about other treatment situations and how they are managed.

C. Clinical Training

It is incumbent upon the substance abuse treatment clinician to have a knowledge of and attunement to the dynamics of a wide range of pathological and nonpathological verbalizations. Therefore, the third factor relating to the effective management of countertransference is the quality of one's training. As noted earlier, drug and alcohol patients can often induce chaotic, turbulent, and hateful feelings in the treatment provider. Unless the provider clinically understands the diagnostic picture of the patient and the manifestations of a particular diagnostic category, the therapist may find himself/herself unable to separate from and manage the feelings he or she is experiencing from the patient.

In addition to the clinical training programs that are germane to individual professional categories, i.e., psychiatry, psychology, clinical social work, and nursing, it is essential that the clinician have some grounding in both the drugs of abuse, and the particular physiological and psychological manifestations presented by those drugs.

D. Continuing Education

It is this writer's position that deciding to work with a particular clinical population strongly suggests that the clinician continue to keep abreast of latest developments in his or her field of practice. Attending continuing education seminars, workshops, lectures, training institutes, graduate programs, grand rounds, and specialized conferences are but a few of the continuing education options available to substance abuse treatment personnel.

E. Exacting Personnel Standards

Given the large numbers of former drug- and alcohol-addicted individuals who are currently working in the field of addiction treatment, it is imperative that treatment agencies place particular emphasis on the personnel standards for employment, especially those for former substance abusers. This may be accomplished through a vigorous interview process that, in particular with regard to interviewing former drug users, develops inquiries into (1) the reasons for the applicant seeking employment in the substance abuse field (2) the length of time the individual has been drug and/or alcohol free, (3) the individual's capacity for flexibility in developing treatment plans and in providing counseling and therapy services, (4) expounding on the individual's philosophy of the causative factors related to drug and alcohol addiction, and (5) determining the applicant's awareness of countertransference. Such standards are viewed as essential given the demanding nature of providing drug treatment services and the high recidivism rates associated with drug abuse.

F. Drug and Alcohol Addiction Criteria

The majority of medical school, psychology, social work, and nursing programs allocate an insufficient amount of time to addressing the myriad of treatment issues in drug and alcohol addiction. It is postulated that specific courses that address treatment situations in difficult populations, including drug and alcohol addiction, would substantially enhance the clinician's ability to more objectively treat those patients who are presented with drug and alcohol problems. Furthermore, such courses would optimally provide opportunities for studies to explore their own personal attitudes toward drug and alcohol use, both their own and that of others.

VII. CONCLUSIONS

It has been my clinical impression through the years that countertransference is not a necessarily popular topic. This holds true not only as it pertains to the treatment of addictive disorders, but to psychotherapy in general. A number of clinical presentations I have attended seem to endlessly detail the clinical composite of the patient, and how that patient was treated, without a word mentioned as the the subjective experience of the treatment provider as a partner in the outcome. It is far easier to review the pathology of our patients rather than our own. Perhaps the Ecclesiastes proverb, "In much wisdom is much grief; and he that increaseth knowledge increaseth sorrow," speaks to the hesitancy of many therapists to avoid or neglect recognition of their subjective experience of the patient. Therapists and counselors seek to help people get better, and the notion of countertransference generally implies that we, the therapists, have to first get better before the patient can improve.

This chapter has explored the countertransferential and attitudinal implications regarding the diagnosis, treatment, and rehabilitation of drug- and alcohol-addicted patients. While exploration and analysis of one's own participation in the treatment relationship is not necessarily an easy undertaking, it is only through examining our own thoughts, feelings, and attitudes toward our patients that we may be able to provide the most objective and effective care that each individual seeking treatment is entitled to receive. The author hopes these comments may serve as a springboard for further critical review and discussion of this essential component in the treatment of drug and alcohol addiction.

REFERENCES

1. Rado, S. (1933). The psychoanalysis of pharmacothymia. *Psychoanalyt. Q.*, 2:1–23.
2. Lettieri, D., Sayers, M., and Pearson, H.W. (eds.) (1980). *Theories on Drug Abuse*. National Institute on Drug Abuse Research Monograph No. 30. Washington, D.C., Government Printing Office.
3. Austin, G.A., Macari, M.A., and Lettieri, D.J. (1979). *Guide to the Drug Research Literature*. National Institute on Drug Abuse Research Series No. 27. Washington, D.C., Government Printing Office.
4. Anderson, W.H., O'Malley, J.E., and Lazare, A. (1972). Failure of outpatient treatment of drug abuse: II. Amphetamines, barbiturates, hallucinogens. *Am.J.Psychother.*, 128:122–125.
5. Renner, J.A., and Rubin, M.S.(1973). Engaging heroin addicts in treatment. *Am. J. Psychiary*, 130:976–980.
6. Simpson, D.D., and Savage, L.J. (1980). Drug abuse treatment readmissions and outcomes. *Arch. Gen. Psychiatry*, 37:896–901.
7. Slakter, E.(1987). *Countertransferences*. New York. Jason Aronson.
8. Simmel, E. (1929). Psycho-analytic treatment in a sanitarium. *Int.J. Psychoanaly.*, 10:70–89.
9. Fenichel, O. (1945). *The Psychoanalytic Theory of Neurosis*. New York, Norton.
10. Meerloo, J.A.M. (1952). Artificial ecstasy: A study of the psychosomatic aspects of drug addiction. *J. Nerv. Ment. Dis.*, 155:246–266.
11. Ausubel, D.P. (1948). The psychopathology and treatment of drug addiction in relation to the mental hygiene movement. *Psychiatr. Q.*, 22:219–250.

12. Ausubel, D.P. (1958). *Drug Addiction: Physiological, Psychological and Sociological Aspects*. New York, Random House.
13. Selzer, M.L. (1957). Hostility as a barrier to therapy in alcoholism. *Psychiatr. Q.*, *31*:301–305.
14. Kaufman, E. (1989). The psychotherapy of dually diagnosed patients. *J. Subst. Abuse Treat.*, *6*(1):9–18.
15. Moore, R.A.(1961). Reaction formation as a countetransference phenomenon in the treatment of alcoholism. *Q. J. Stud. Alcohol.*, *22*:481–486.
16. Rosenfeld, H.A. (1964). *Psychotic States*. New York, International Universities Press.
17. Wurmser, L. (1972). Drug abuse: Nemesis of psychiatry. *Am. Scholar, 41*:393–407.
18. Merry, J. (1967). Outpatient treatment of heroin addiction. *Lancet, 1*:205–206.
19. Davidson, V. (1977). Transference phenomena in the treatment of addictive illness: Love and hate in methadone maintenance, *Psychodynamics of Drug Dependence* National Institute on Drug Abuse Research Monograph No. 12). (J.D. Blaine and D.A. Julius, eds.) Washington, D.C., Government Printing Office.
20. Hirsch, R., Imhof, J.E., Terenzi, R.E., and Fried M. (1980). The drug treatment and education center: An overview. *North Shore Univ. Hosp. Clin. J., 3*:8–16.
21. Stolorow, R. (1975). The narcissistic function of masochism (and sadism). *Int. J. Psychoanal. 56*:441–448.
22. Grotstein, J. (1981). *Splitting and Projective Indentification*. New York, Jason Aronson.
23. Masterson, J.F. (1976). *Psychotherapy of the Borderline Adult*. New York, Brunner/Mazel.
24. Krystal, H. (1977). Self and object representation in alcoholism and other drug-dependence: Implications for therapy, National Institute on Drug Abuse, *Psychodynamics of Drug Dependence* National Institute on Drug Abuse Research Monograph No. 12). (J.D. Blaine and D.A. Julius, eds.). Washington, D.C.: Government Printing Office.
25. Cohen, C.P., White, E.H., and Schoolar, J. (1971). Interpersonal patterns of personality for drug abusing patients and their therapeutic implications. *Arch. Gen.Psychiatry, 24*:353–358.
26. Pines, A., and Maslach, C. (1978). Characteristics of staff burnout in mental health settings. *Hosp. Commun. Psychiatry, 29*(4):233–237.
27. Imhof, J.E., Hirsch, R., and Terenzi, R.E. (1984). Countertransferential and attitudinal considerations in the treatment of drug abuse and addiction. *J. Subst. Abuse Treat. 1*:21–30.
28. Patrick, P.K.S. (1984). Self-preservation: A non-negotiable requirement for the substance abuse clinician. *J. Subst. Abuse Treatment, 1*:85.
29. Faltz, B.G., and Madover, S. (1988). Treatment of substance abuse in patients with HIV infection. *AIDS Subst. Abuse*, Hayworth Press.
30. Proceedings, White House Conference on Narcotic and Drug Abuse. (1962). Washington, D.C., U.S. Government Printing Office.
31. Imhof, J., and Terenzi, R. (1990). Substance Abuse in America: An overview, *Community Psychology* (M.S. Gibbs, J.R.L. Lachenmeyer, J. Segal, eds.). Gardner Press, New Jersey.

52

Drug and Alcohol Use and Addiction Among Physicians

Gregory B. Collins
Cleveland Clinic Foundation, Cleveland, Ohio

I. INTRODUCTION

The physician who has become impaired from drugs or alcohol poses a dilemma for the profession and for society. The obligation to help the physician is keenly felt by the profession, whose numbers are dedicated to assisting others, including their own colleagues. Since the physician's impairment may jeopardize the well-being of patients, however, there is also a strong obligation for the profession to protect the public. Accomplishing both of these laudable objectives is not necessarily an easy matter: The physician's stress, training, access to drugs, and professional stature predispose to the use of drugs and may undermine the treatment process; concerns for protection of the public raise difficult questions about confidentiality, workplace reentry, monitoring, probation, or even license suspension, all of which may deter the physician from obtaining treatment.

Even the extent to which physicians have problems with drugs or alcohol is a matter of controversy. In an extensive review of the literature on physician drug and alcohol abuse, Brewster [1] states that "The principal conclusion to be drawn...is that no one really knows how many practicing physicians are having problems with alcohol and other drugs." She goes on to state that while several studies seem to suggest that problems with drugs other than alcohol are unusually prevalent among physicians, "on closer examination the studies are seen to be inadequate to support firm conclusions." She concludes that "the survey data suggest that the overall prevalence of problems with alcohol and other drugs among physicians may not be different from that found among the general population." Finally, she notes that "Conclusive studies on the occurrence of drug problems among physicians have yet to be done." She cautions against extreme statements about the prevalence of drug dependence among physicians until such studies have been carried out [1].

On the other hand, substance abuse is frequently present in disciplinary cases involving physicians. Gualtieri et al. [2] described the formation of the California Diversionary Program for Impaired Physicians, which originated a legislatively mandated merger between the Board of Medical Quality Assurance (BMQA) and the California Medical Association

(CMA) in 1980. As a result, involuntary and voluntary impaired physician referrals were made to the Impaired Physician Program and were "diverted" from disciplinary action. Following the formation of the Impaired Physician Program in California, drug abuse was the most common referring complaint (38%), followed by alcohol abuse (29%), alcohol and drug abuse (17%), mental illness and substance abuse (8%), mental illness (6%), and physical disorder and substance abuse (1%). An analysis of type of medical practice in this cohort reflected that general or family medicine practitioners were the most frequently referred group (20%), followed by those in anesthesiology (14%), internal medicine (13%), obstetrics/gynecology (10%), emergency medicine (7%), psychiatry (7%), and others [2].

In recent years, however, the profession has seen very encouraging progress in dealing with the problem of impaired physicians. There is a far better appreciation of the risk of chemical dependency for physicians generally, and especially for high-risk practice patterns such as general practice or anesthesia. A better understanding has emerged regarding the development of chemical dependency among physicians, a process which often begins well before entry into professional school. There has also been an explosion of interest in the impaired physician, interest which has been spurred by the American Medical Association, International Doctors in Alcoholics Anonymous (IDAA), and the American Society of Addiction Medicine (ASAM). The Peer Assistance Movement, borrowing principles from the Employee Assistance Movement, has developed an extensive network of Impaired Physician Committees in state medical societies, and has fostered an advocacy-based, constructive-coercion approach to obtaining treatment for physicians. At present, the outlook is bright for impaired physicians. Specific treatment is widely available, and there is a strong emphasis on professional reentry under therapeutic supervision, with the assistance of peer assistance programs. The outcomes are good in the large majority of cases. Clearly, the physician can be helped—and the public can be protected—by a humane, but firm, continuing program which incorporates elements of both treatment and monitoring.

II. PHYSICIANS IN TRAINING

Impaired physicians who have been asked when their problems first began, almost universally state that their medical school days provided the "right" mixture of stress, insufficient social life, and lack of support to allow for development of destructive, dysfunctional coping mechanisms which eventually lead to impairment [3]. In Clark's questionnaire study of 120 medical students, 63% of the alcohol abusers had a history of abuse that predated their admission to medical school [4]. Alcohol abusers were not more anxious or depressed than their peers, but were more likely to have a family history of alcoholism than peers. In Clark's study, excessive drinking had no measurable impact on academic performance in the first 2 years of medical school. Alcohol abuse was associated with better grades in the first year and a strong tendency toward better National Board of Medical Examiners Part 1 scores at the end of the student's year in medical school. Alcohol abuse also had no discernable impact on clerkship performance in the third and fourth year. The author concludes that this finding contradicts those of most studies of high school and college students which have reported that alcohol abuse was associated with poorer grades. Clark also notes that many students, particularly those motivated to excel, feared being stigmatized or penalized in their career progress for admitting to any psychological problems or for using psychotherapy. Hard-drinking students or physicians may be prone to discount warnings about the hazards of alcohol abuse because of their demonstrated competence and success. Clark also found that 11% of the class under study met clinical research criteria for drug abuse (e.g., habituation, tolerance, withdrawal symptoms, and drug-related arrests), during the course of medical school. There was no significant relationship between alcohol abuse and drug abuse in this student sample

[4]. Widespread recreational drug use, especially cocaine use, by medical students suggests that these groups do not believe that such use places them at risk [5].

Baldwin, using a questionnaire on a large, nationally representative sample of senior medical students (n=2047), found that, in general, medical students used much less of mood-altering substances than comparable groups of young people in the population, with the exception of alcohol and tranquilizers [6]. The findings of the study also supported the notion that the use of such substances usually begins well before medical school and frequently as early as grade or high school. Few of the medical students felt they needed help for substance abuse (1.6%), and indeed only nine students out of 2023 admitted to being currently dependent on any substance other than tobacco. For lifetime ever use, the most common drug reported was alcohol, with 98.1% reporting lifetime ever use, followed by marijuana, with 66.2% reporting lifetime ever use. Cocaine was the third most frequently used substance, with 32.5% reporting lifetime ever use. Tranquilizers were used by 19.5% over their lifetime. Amphetamines appear to have lost some favor with 22.6% reporting some lifetime ever use [6].

McAuliffe et al. found that drug-use surveys of nonclinical samples of young physicians and premedical, medical, and nursing students in New England indicate that between 56 and 70% have used marijuana, and that some of them (15–21%) now have progressed to recreational experimentation with higher-risk drugs, especially cocaine [7]. The authors found that the use of amphetamines for studying and staying awake appears to have declined in prevalence. Approximately 40% of the young physicians in this sample also treated themselves with one or more psychoactive drugs, mostly opiates (27%), tranquilizers (17%), and sedatives (8%). Most subjects reported using the drugs only a few times, and future health care professionals consistently had slightly lower drug-use rates than many other graduate and college students [7].

McAuliffe, et al. reported on risk factors of drug impairment in random samples in physicians and medical students [8]. In a questionnaire study of 500 physicians and 504 medical students, background characteristics that were likely to be risk factors of impairment included drug access, a family history of substance abuse, and a lack of substance abuse education. These authors found 22% of physicians and 27% of medical students had family histories of substance abuse. Symptoms of life stress were frequently reported, including chronic fatigue, family burdens, marital or love-life difficulties, and personal neglect. Physicians and medical students reported especially high amounts of job and school stress. The most frequently experienced types of job or school stress in the physician and medical student samples were the interference of work with family or social life, inability to relax at the end of a day's work, frustation over paperwork, the possibility of mistakes that could cause harm to patients, and having a workload that cannot be finished in a day. Eighteen percent of the physicians and 25% of the students reported ever having a serious emotional problem. Twice as many of the students (15%) as practitioners (7%) currently had such problems. The most important historical correlates for both medical student and physician drug use were sensation seeking, life stress, and a family history of drug dependence, whereas for physicians, family history was somewhat less important, and chronic pain was more important [8].

Conard, et al. in a national survey of substance use and abuse among resident physicians, found that the stage of education at which initial drug use occurs for the great majority of young physicians was at the high school and college level for tobacco, alcohol, marijuana, cocaine amphetamines, lysergic acid diethylamide (LSD), other psychedelics, and heroin [9]. The authors suggest that medical school and residency were not breeding grounds for spread of these substances. Of particular concern were the high rates of first use for tranquilizers and opiates during medical school and residency. It was noted that medical students had a higher rate of use of tranquilizers and opiates than a national age-matched cohort. The data on reasons for use suggested three major profiles of drug use in the resident population. For recreation, residents chose alcohol, marijuana, cocaine, and psychedelics. To improve performance and maintain alertness, they used tobacco and amphetamines. The third major pattern was self-treatment or treatment under another physician's supervision, for which tranquilizers, opiates, and barbiturates were used. Only a quarter of the respondents knew of a clear policy and/or educational program on alcohol and drug abuse in their workplace, but 20% indicated they had colleagues they considered impaired by alcohol or drugs. The findings suggested to the authors the need for postgraduate institutions to address the issues of drug-abuse policy, education, and prevention among physicians in training. The data were noted to reaffirm the importance of the recently introduced federal policy requiring residents assistance programs (RAPs) to be in place for the award of federal funds [9].

III. THE IMPAIRED PHYSICIAN

In our experience, the diagnosis of addiction in physicians is difficult because of the well-entrenched denial system, the sophistication (from training and experience) employed in avoiding detection, and the ability of physicians to find plausible rationalizations for their use of drugs. Nonetheless, family consequences are generally the first indicator of drug-abuse problems. As the spouse becomes aware of the physician's "eating the mail" (ingesting samples), self-prescribing, or using family members' supposed ailments to obtain drugs for self-use, concern gives way to arguments and fights over the drug use. Eventually, more profound mistrust, anger, and alienation set in, and separation and/or divorce may occur. Personality changes and ethical deterioration may be the next step, with gross changes of behavior and attitude being evident, especially regarding outbursts of anger, irritability, paranoia, or inappropriate behavior sexually or financially. Legal problems, such as charges of driving while intoxicated, domestic violence, tax evasion, or personal bankruptcy may occur, but the most frequent legal problem is related to prescribing irregularities. Oddly, physical deterioration often occurs before occupational impairent. The classic physical stigmata of alcoholism may of course become evident, but also, with physicians, the stigmata of chronic long-term medication abuse are often present. These stigmata include septic, necrotic skin lesions and hardened, fibrotic, boardlike fibrositic changes of muscular tissue from self-injection. Finally, job performance deterioration in the form of chronic latenesses or long, unexplained absences from work begin to set in. Patients and staff note alcohol on the breath, slurred speech and other evidences of intoxication, inappropriate remarks and behavior toward patients and staff, being asleep or unarousable on call, unanswered and unreturned phone calls, record-keeping deterioration, practice errors, and often, coverups by staff and family.

In our experience, physician misuse of drugs through the route of self-prescribing often begins with a legitimate reason for the drug use. Commonly seen examples are depression, kidney stones, irritable bowel syndrome, chronic headache, and neck or back spasms. A physician soon finds that the medication works well to relieve physical and psychological discomfort and contiues its use. The physician gradually takes over the responsibility for diagnosis and treatment of his or her own ailment, and begins the process of self-prescribing, often with the excuse that self-treatment is more "convenient" and takes less time away from practice and patients. This pattern of self-prescribing is maintained with the rationale that "I need it to function in spite of my ailment." Finally, the addicted physician comes to feel that the ailment will be unbearable without constant and chronic-self-medicating.

A 1987 study by Talbott et al. examined 1000 physicians referred to the Medical Association of Georgia Impaired Physician Program (IPP) [10]. Of this physician cohort, 920 (92%) had a primary diagnosis of drug dependence, 59 (5.9%) had a psychiatric diagnosis with or without drug dependence, and 21 (2.1%) had no evidence of either disorder. The mean age of the group was 45.3 years and was becoming progressively younger over time. Male physicians were over represented in this study as 96.1% of the group were male, compared to 86.6% of all U.S. physicians being male. Of those with the diagnosis of chemical dependency, alcohol was the most commonly used drug, followed by meperidine hydrochloride and diazepam. While 28% reported abuse of a single drug, younger physicians more frequently used multiple drugs. The authors noted a trend toward cocaine abuse, which was seen in two of every seven physicians presented for evaluation in 1986; parenteral substance abuse also seemed to be on the increase, being seen in 38.8% of the study sample. The authors concluded that anesthesia and family or general practice specialties were significantly over-represented in the impaired group. The authors also reported that the anesthesiologists tended to be younger and that family and general practitioners tended to be older. The family and general practitioners were more likely to be solo practitioners in rural areas and appeared to abuse alcohol, suffering severe physical sequelae [10].

In an analysis of health care professionals referred to the Medical Association of Georgia (MAG) program, physicians, pharmacists, and dentists were compared with nurses in evaluations of substance abuse characteristics. The results of this study reflect that pharmacists and nurses appear more likely to be polydrug addicted and are less likely to be exclusively alcohol abusing. Simultaneous use of two or more drugs was common in these groups. Over half reported addiction to four or more drugs. Nurses frequently reported abusing narcotics and often chose parenteral routes of administration. Physicians, and particularly pharmacists, frequently abused many different classes of drugs. Pharmacists were more likely than any other professional groups to abuse stimulants. Sedative abuse and narcotic abuse were frequently seen in the pharmacist group also. Alcohol also appeared to be the drug most frequently abused by each group, and there was no significant difference between groups with respect to cocaine abuse. Most of the health professionals in the study reported obtaining the substances they abused from the workplace or from another health professional peer [11].

The issue of concomitant psychopathology in addicted physicians is addressed in a recent study. In this study of 50 physicians treated in the alcoholism recovery program of the Menninger Clinic, psychopathology ranged from overt schizophrenia to no demonstrable psychiatric syndrome other than addiction. Physicians experiencing addiction problems before age 40 were more likely to exhibit serious psychopathology in the borderline range, whereas physicians older than 40 years were more likely to exhibit organic brain impairment and depression. In 72% of these cases, important negative childhood factors were implicated. The authors noted that in all physician-patients younger than 40 years, significant parental deprivation was evident. In this group, drug abuse escalated rapidly and was unabated once it started. In the group older than 40 years, 36% showed evidence of significant parental deprivation. The authors also noted a possible contribution of stress from adjustment problems secondary to moving from a lower-class background to a higher one. Four percent of the physician-patients were found to have psychotic functioning. Severe borderline personality organization, characterized by impulsiveness, unstable and intense interpersonal relationships, affective instability, and identity disturbance, was reported in 32%. "Higher-level" personality traits, characterized by obsessive-compulsive and hysterical patterns of functioning, were found in 36%. They conclude that the earlier an addiction problem develops in the physician's career, the more likely it is to be associated with serious psychopathology [12].

In a report on a physician mortality project, conducted jointly by the American Medical Association and the American Psychiatric Association, a preliminary profile of the physicians that took their own lives showed that they more often made prior suicide attempts, verbalized suicidal intentions, self-prescribed psychoactive drugs, and suffered financial losses [13]. When compared to a control group of nonsuicide deceased physicians, the greatest difference between the suicide and nonsuicide physicians lay in their use of drugs and alcohol. More than one-third (34%) of the physicians who committed suicide were believed to have had a drug problem at some time in their lives. The corresponding figure for those in the nonsuicide control group was one-seventh (14%). More than half of those in the suicide group had prescribed a psychoactive drug for themselves, whereas only one-fifth (22%) of those in the control group had done so. Although frequency of drinking did not vary between the two groups, those who commited suicide were reported to have had more social problems caused by drinking than those who died by other causes. Frequently noted were interference with work, interference with social life, drinking to the point of unconsciousness, alcohol-related blackouts, and intoxication. Each of these problems was more prevalent in the last 2 years of life for physicians who committed suicide. The report suggests, among other things, that the AMA auxiliary consider offering educational programs for spouses to help detect early signs of excessive stress, alcohol and other drug abuse, and major depression [13].

Physicians dependent on mind- and mood-altering chemicals have difficulty acknowledging their illness or seeking treatment without encouragement, according to Harris [14]. The author notes that it is usually not until progressive behavioral deterioration becomes obvious to family or colleagues that the individual seeks assistance. Even then, through misjudgments related either to the toxic effect caused by any of these various drugs or to addiction to those drugs, many physicians continue their alcohol and drug addiction. Such physicians often will either leave or curtail practice rather than seek help. Harris also lists the following characteristics that may be recognized by persons referring impaired physicians for treatment [14]:

Disruptions in family life
The development of legal problems
Neglectful of practice routines
Social isolation
Driving while intoxicated
Intoxication while attending social functions
Noticeable odor of alcohol at the work site
Making hospital rounds at unusual times
Canceling office appointments without obvious conflict of time
Giving unusual or dangerous orders over the telephone, particularly from home during
    the evening or night
Disruptive behavior at meetings, or failure to complete committee assignments
Forgetting social appointments
Holding telephone conversations with slurred speech or tangential conversation
Dressing sloppily or in a noticeably different style

Talbott et al. [10] conclude that

The following factors play a role in development of impairment in physicians: 1) genetic predisposition and environmental exposure, 2) stress and poor coping skills, 3) lack of education regarding the various kinds of impairment that effect a physician's ability to practice medicine with reasonable skill and safety to patients, 4) the absence of effective prevention and control strategies, 5) drug availability in the context of a permissive professional and social environment, and 6) denial.

They also conclude that the most effective means of prevention appears to be early detection and treatment [10].

Accidental death from drugs is a serious risk for health professionals. Talbott and Wright [15] note that

...a major threat to the health of the patient/professional even in the early stages is the risk of severe or lethal drug effect. Scrupulous in the handling of these agents and their patients, the physician or nurse will take excessive doses of medicine and endure toxic reactions which shock those who later care for them. Many die from overdose, idiosyncracy and drug sensitivity in the early stages of abuse, before the late signs and symptoms of addiction become maniest.

Risk factors cited by Talbott and Wright for physicians include the following: availability, ignorance, uniqueness, occupational stress, and the medical marriage [15]. Availability may be a particular problem in anesthesia or in small general practice settings. Ignorance of all aspects of the disease concept may arise from the fact that physicians tend to treat the sickest, most hopeless members of the chemically dependent population. This limited sample may produce a skewed and unnecessarily negative view of the disease of addiction and the prospects for recovery. Talbott and Wright [15] note that uniqueness is a problem for physicians since

> the natural tendency for upper class individuals to regard themselves as "special" is made more severe for professionals as they progress through a series of ever more difficult educational and occupational examinations. When this is combined with the common use of denial in those who must deal with daily human suffering, the result is the often amazing sense of invulnerability seen in professionals and documented in the very high private aviation accident rate for physicians. Most programs aimed at intervention attempt to bring the professional recovering from chemical dependency into contact with those at risk, to attempt to break through this denial.

Talbott and Wright also comment on the destructive role of occupational stress, primarily from overwork. They also note that "it can become a catchall defense against all kinds of emotional or situational pain." These authors also report that the marriages of medical professionals do not seem to be especially durable, nor do they seem to be viewed as sources of strength by each of the partners. Why this should be is not clear, but "flight into work," dysfunctional communication, divorce, behavioral disorder, and sexual dysfunction are common in the professional marriage [15].

IV. IMPAIRED FEMALE PHYSICIANS

Until recently, women comprised only a small percentage of practicing physicians. With their increasing numbers, however, attention has come to be focused on their own problems of impairment, particularly those regarding drug and alcohol dependency. In a survey of 100 women in medicine (95 physicians and five students) in Alcoholics Anonymous (AA) with at least 1 year of sobriety, Bissell and Skorina threw some light on this long-neglected subject [16]. In their cohort, relationship difficulties appeared to be extremely common. Thirty-four of the physicians and all of the five students had never been married. In the remainder, marital instability was common. Only 13 physicians were still in the first marriage. Fifty-three percent were certain that at least one parent was alcoholic. Interestingly, of the 80 physicians who knew their class standing in medical school graduation, 50% had been in the upper third of the class, 34% in the middle third, and 16% in the lower third. Three subjects ranked first in their class, two ranked number two, and a total of 16 said they were in the upper tenth. Many belonged to the honor society, Alpha Omega Alpha, and many more had received a variety of awards, prizes, and scholarships. The only training speciality that appeared overrepresented was psychiatry [16].

These female subjects reported a high incidence of addiction to drugs other than alcohol, with 40% reporting addiction to alcohol only. A total of 15 subjects had been sued for professional liability—three of them twice, another three times, and one "seven or eight times." Thirty-two of the female physicians reported having attempted suicide, as did two medical students, which the authors note was twice as frequent as suicide among male counterparts. Those subjects who reported a history of addiction to stronger narcotics were much more likely to report suicide attempts than were those addicted to alcohol alone [16].

The small percentage (4%) of women physicians referred to the large Georgia Impaired Physician's Program (IPP), has been noted by Martin and Talbott [17]. These authors noted that the female impaired physicians in the Georgia program appeared to be high achievers in medicine. The authors identified numerous psychological issues which may be active in cases of female physician impairment. They note that female physicians may experience more stress than male physicians, and that female physicians seem to come to the Program with "fewer coping skills, less self-esteem and less ability to withstand the stresses involved in the IPP treatment milieu than the men do. They have fewer ways to gain ego strength during treatment due to lack of role models and lack of interaction with 'true peers' in residential living." The authors note that these women physicians often reported having experienced sexual, physical, and emotional abuse as children, for the most part perpetrated by members of their own family or known members of their community. Often such women have cultivated the skill of hiding their true feelings to protect themselves from further violence. When such women stay in treatment, their

> pain, loneliness, and fear are all likely to surface with self-disclosure. These feelings are often accompanied by a sense of range at having been used and rejected by either parents or others they looked to for love and nurturing as children. They also express rage at being considered by society as more deviant in their chemical dependence than men, with the stigma associated with it, and deviant in their attempts to achieve and be accepted in a male dominated profession.

It seems that a lack of trust for people both within medicine and outside it is a major stumbling block for recovery in women physicians. Psychodynamic differences between impaired female and male professionals are also noted.

> Men in recovery talk about needing to get rid of their big egos, to look outside themselves to achieve their proper focus for their lives, and to be sensitive to the feelings of others. Women for the most part, express a sense of fragmented egos, of having looked after others and having looked to others in the past for their definition of themselves. For men the task of recovery may be giving up the desire for complete power over their own lives and the lives of those around them. For women, it may be accepting responsibility for their lives and using appropriately the power they do have.

The authors note that women physicians, like nonphysician drug-dependent women, face issues of abandonment and isolation far more often than their male counterparts. Those who do not return to intact support networks must often rely heavily on the treatment center staff to help them [17].

C. Anesthesia: A Special Risk

The special risk of anesthesiologists for chemical dependency has been noted previously [2,10]. In a survey of 289 anesthesia training programs (with a response rate of 85.5%), 184 of these programs had at least one suspected incident of drug dependence during the period 1970–1980. These programs reported a total of 334 confirmed cases of substance dependency, including a substantial number of instructors. Meperidine and fentanyl were the most frequently mentioned drugs in this study. Significantly, 30 of these anesthesiologists died of drug overdose. The majority of the impaired anesthesiologists were referred for psychiatric care, with few in need of actual detoxification. A detailed follow-up was available on only

40% of the total, and only 71 persons were offered to return to their original employment. The authors conclude that chemical impairment may be more common than usually thought in anesthesia, perhaps because of drug availability [18].

Gallegos et al. reported that 11.9% of the 1225 physicians seen by the Medical Association of Georgia Impaired Physician Program between July, 1975 and September, 1987 were anesthesiologists [19]. Gualtieri, in the California Diversionary Program Study, found 14% of physicians referred to be anesthesiologists [2]. Since only 4% of U.S. physicians are anesthesiologists [20], anesthesiologists appear to be heavily overrepresented in the population of chemically dependent physicians. In the Georgia study [19], the authors compared the impaired anesthesiologists (IAs) with all U.S. anesthesiologists and all U.S. physicians and noted the following findings: the IAs were younger than the other two groups; women, blacks, and other minority groups were significantly underrepesented among the IAs; residents and fellows (physicians who have completed their residencies and are taking further training) appear to be significantly overrepresented in this study sample; and IAs were more frequently unemployed (as a direct result of chemical dependence) or retired than physicians in the other two groups. This study also found that the IAs were significantly more likely to be poly-drug-addicted than other impaired physicians, and that narcotic addiction, especially with fentanyl and morphine, was more prevalent than in the larger group of impaired physicians. Although meperidine (Demerol) was frequently abused by both groups, non-IA controls more frequently used the drug orally, whereas the IAs were more likely to abuse it parenterally. Impaired anesthesiologists were more likely to abuse narcotics (most often obtained in the work setting) and to abuse these drugs intravenously. They were also more likely to have been confronted about drug use at work and had been reported for having abused drugs at work. Significantly, the authors report that 85% of the IAs who are residents reported that one of the reasons they were attracted to anesthesiology was drug access. These authors noted additional explanations for the apparently excessive prevalence of drug dependence among anesthesiologists as including the following: anesthesologists more frequently abuse potent drugs that cause them to become addicted very quickly; drug handling and access for anesthesiologists is greater than for any other specialty; many of the drugs used in anesthesiology require only small amounts for their full therapeutic effects; and diverting small amounts of such drugs without getting caught is easy. The authors additionally note that drug testing for high-potency drugs of the fentanyl class is difficult and not routinely obtained, even with routine blood or urine screening. While these authors have found that most of these individuals are able to successfully return to the field of anesthesiology and maintain solid recovery, our experience is that the decision to return to the high-risk environment of anesthesiology is a highly individual one and must be evaluated carefully by the treatment team as well as by the supervising institution. The authors have also noted occurrences of "closed-mindedness among professional peers" when considering reentry for addicted anesthesiologists [19]. In our experience, careful monitoring and insistence on a thorough, comprehensive, high-quality recovery program, with vigorous activity in the addicted physician's self-help network will generally lead to a favorable result.

One response to the anesthesia risk problem is suggested by Adler et al., who developed and reported a system to better control the accountability of narcotics and other potentially addictive drugs [21]. Their system consisted of a three-phase approach: (1) an individual anesthesia cart/narcotics box, (2) computer analysis of drug usage, and (3) an anesthesia drug audit. A standard stock issue of drugs is maintained by each resident. Drugs are issued daily to those residents administering anesthesia. Each drug transaction is recorded by the resident according to the patient's name, hospital number, type and length of surgical procedure, type and amount of drug use, and the amount of each drug discarded. A weekly computer-generated report shows individual usage trends for each drug and the summary of "high" users for that period. The compuer does not "flag" an individual as a drug abuser, but monitors trends and controls substance usage. Those residents having a significant alteration in their drug usage pattern that is not explained legitimately are comprehensively audited [21].

Talbott et al. recommend tight controls over narcotics in anesthesia departments, and comment that tight controls appear to be well established in urban large medical centers rather than in smaller hospital settings [10]. The authors note "We also know from our investigations that many anesthesia residents who have presented for treatment in the MAG's IPP report drug availability, or access, as a major reason for choosing that field of practice." The authors go on to state that "prevention for this speciality may need to come at the level of resident selection and the education of medical students and residents about the disease [10].

In our experience, a comprehensive approach to the high risk-problem in anesthesia is warranted. This would include additional attention to resident selection issues and motivation for this particular specialty. As training is initiated, ongoing emphasis on vigilance and prevention/avoidance should be maintained, with frequent medical education presentations on this subject. "Double signouts" of medications should be initiated and drug usage should be carefully audited. The high level of awareness and sensitivity on the part of instructors and supervisors for incipient problems in trainees should be maintained. Nonthreatening help should be offered and reinforced by hospital administration. Reentry into the field should be encouraged wherever prudent and feasible. All in all, a nonpejorative, nondiscriminatory attitude should be taken toward drug dependency problems as an occupational hazard, generating a response which is both objective and humanitarian. Although patient protection must remain the highest priority, many anesthesiologists will be able to return successfully to practice in this specialty, and should be helped to do so, under appropriate monitoring and supervision.

V. TREATMENT OF ADDICTED PHYSICIANS

In our experience, the drug involved physician is a difficult patient to treat. His or her emotional makeup, training, and experience reinforce denial and the myth of invulnerability. The impairment may be well hidden behind a superficial appearance of success and intelligence. Physicians are products of a training regimen that reinforces self-reliance and self-discipline; often physicians have difficulty giving up work and practice responsibilities to assume a patient role. Their long experience as authority figures makes it difficult for them to listen, accept the diagnosis or treatment recommendations, and conform to treatment requirements. In the earlier stages, there is little accountability to others. The family, often dependent on the physician's income or prestige, may be reluctant to "blow the whistle." The unique status of the physician, and the history of good service to the community may mean that the physician is literally "killed with kindness" by the community which reacts in protective (enabling) role rather than a coercive one. Confidentiality fears may be extreme as the physician fears that "everybody will know; my patients will go to other physicians; no other doctors will refer me patients in the future." These fears have seldom been found to be valid in our experience, as generally the community and peer physicians are delighted that the physician is taking measures to get help. Like other executive or VIP patients, physicians can be intimidating when confronted. The tendency to pull rank or status, or to try to blunt the constructive coercion process by intimidation or threats of retaliation are extremely common. Finally, the physician may "flee into health" with firm resolutions and promises to be good. These tactics indicate continued inability to accept the need for help and monitoring and are far less desirable than an attitude of doing whatever is recommended to get well.

Treatment of addicted physicians is often a turbulent and problematic affair. Johnson noted that the treatment process was often stormy, with drug use occurring at times in the hospital, attempts at exploitation and manipulation, angry and hostile outbursts, and periods of hopelessness and despair [12]. The authors note that it is the physician who proceeds through treatment with the expectation that a "cure" will be accomplished by others while he or she remains uninvolved, or expects that he or she can accomplish his own recovery without others, presents the greatest dilemma because he or she continues to isolate himself or herself from others. Dealing with these resistances of denial and isolation has been frequently met with an angry response from the physician-patient [12].

Comprehensive, long-term alcohol and drug treatment appears to work best for physicians. One such comprehensive approach is described by Herrington et al. in the De Paul Hospital (Milwaukee) Program [22]. There, the 33 physicians in their cohort remained in the inpatient program for an average of 30 days, where treatment was provided by a multidisciplinary team. Treatment modalities included individual and group counseling, psychotherapy, orientation sessions regarding Alcoholics Anonymous (AA) and Narcotics Anonymous (NA), occupational-recreational therapy sessions, and the involvement of family members in the treatment process. On completion of this phase of the recovery program, physician-patients were referred to a 2-year, intensively monitored outpatient phase, a fundamental aspect of which was the provision of unpredictably random urine screening tests, often weekly or more. Continuing AA and NA participation was strongly encouraged, including attendance at local meetings of the Milwaukee Doctors in AA. Spouse participants were also engaged in continuing follow-up treatment, including Al-Anon meetings and specialized Milwaukee Physician's Spouses Al-Anon Group. Individual therapy, family psychotherapy, or both, with a psychiatrist or psychologist familiar with the dynamics and treatment of drug abuse disorders, was also recommended during this outpatient phase. The third phase, assisting the participant in resuming his or her professional practice, was accomplished through a cooperative effort among treatment personnel, state and local medical and dental societies, and hospital medical staffs. The authors note that resumption of professional activities may be gradual or partial, full or complete, depending on stipulations or limitations imposed by the licensing body and by treatment progress. Quarterly progress reports are sent to the appropriate monitoring or regulatory body [22].

Talbott and Martin describe 14 keys to a successful treatment program for impaired physicians [23]. These keys, as they describe them, are as follows:

1. The strength and virtues of having an impaired physician program headed by the State Medical Society, with the promise of advocacy for physicians if they sign contractual agreements to undergo treatment and maintain recovery;
2. Acceptance of alcoholism and drug addiction as a psychosocial, biogenetic disease;
3. Utilization of a 72-hour triage for comprehensive assessment;
4. True peer-group therapy to overcome the sense of omnipotence, uniqueness, and professional immunity to loss of control found in impaired physicians;
5. Two-year program, including an intensively monitored and structured aftercare component;
6. AA-oriented treatment program, including, but not limited to, involvement in IDAA (International Doctors in Alcoholics Anonymous);
7. Family involvement;
8. Mirror image therapy in which impaired physicians, independent of their own specialty, work (under supervision) as alcohol and drug counselor-trainees, seeing themselves reflected in their own patients;
9. The use of medical students;
10. A 4-week outpatient program specially designed for impaired health care professionals living in recovery houses;

11. Caduceus outpatient recovery residences—peer group apartments or houses in which recovering professionals remain for 3 months;
12. The Caduceus Club, a quasi-scientific club which acts as a bridge into the self-help groups;
13. A formal plan for spiritual development;
14. A quality control function supplied by a Data and Statistics Division of the Impaired Physicians Program.

The authors note that these keys to treatment are structured to counter several features unique to impaired physicians. In particular, they note the lack of understanding of the disease concept of alcoholism and drug addiction in the physician population, the easy access to mood-altering drugs, and a tendency to diagnose and treat themselves for pain, stress, depression, and other conditions. The massive denial of vulnerability is seen to cause extreme isolation, facilitated by a conspiracy of silence by peers, friends, family, and patients. These physicians progessively isolate and "depeopleize" their world so that they are left with a sparse life-support network and an extremely limited repertoire of nondrug coping skills for dealing with issues of living. The program emphasizes rebuilding of a healthy support network to maintain wellness and to acquire habits of healthy living [23].

Family therapy is unquestionably an important aspect of the treatment process for the impaired physician. Talbott and Martin [23] note that "family therapy has proved to be absolutely essential to recovery. In our experience, the single most important factor contributing to the relapse of the impaired physician is the family that remains ill. For a family member, compulsive preoccupation with the alcoholic, isolating oneself from other members of the family and the community, experiencing fear over losing control of the addict and over what might happen in spite of all one can do, are a few of the symptoms of this parallel condition, producing shame, fear, and anger. These feelings are repressed and an uncommon tolerance to pain is exhibited instead [23]. These authors have developed a 3-day Family Workshop which is held each month at the treatment center. This Workshop includes spouses or significant others, adult children, as well as adolescents and young children, and is designed to help the whole family increase its knowledge, sharpen its perception, and enhance its acceptance of chemical dependence as a family disorder, according to the authors [23]. In our experience, treatment begins with an *evaluation* by a chemical dependency professional. A professional with specialized training, certification, and/or extensive experience in the treatment of impaired physicians is advisable. Evaluation may be done under circumstances of high or low motivation; the outcome will not be dependent on the level of motivation at the time of the initial contact. As a result of the evaluation, which may and should include information from the family and coworkers or supervisors, treatment recommendations are made and the formal treatment process begins. Invariably, abstinence from all mood-altering and potentially addictive drugs is required, including abstinence from alcohol. Often it is best to proscribe the use of any medication without the expressed approval of the treatment program. Strong emphasis is placed on developing a drug-free lifestyle, avoiding the former pattern of using substances for "good" reasons, which have often arisen from subjective physical or emotional complaints.

Inpatient treatment is most frequently recommended for physicians for a variety of reasons. Typically the high level of initial resistance presented by physicians requires intensive supportive psychotherapy to overcome. Issues of stigma, powerlessness, surrender, "disease concept", and the need for help and full compliance require heavy emphasis on education and attitude change. Because physicians, like other executives or professionals, have a great deal to lose with a relapse, intensive efforts are often made at the outset to "do it right the first time" and to prevent a catastrophic occurrence later. Concerns about liability, professional reputation, and credibility also favor an inpatient treatment solution, as the physician or hospital may be under pressure to demonstrate the everything possible is being done to correct the situation and prevent a recurrence. Because of the often well-entrenched denial system of the patient and family, a "total immersion" approach involving an inpatient stay in an intensive milieu is frequently essential. In our experience, a 28-day inpatient stay is adequate intensive treatment for about 50% of the physicians. For the other 50%, a transitional phase of residential treatment in a specialized residential treatment facility may give the newly sober physician additional time to practice recovery skills, attitude change, AA involvement, and drug-free living, with group support and freedom from family and occupational pressures.

Attendance at 12 Step–based self-help meetings is a major support for all phases of the program, and is strongly encouraged as a lifetime commitment. These self-help groups may include Alcoholics Anonymous, Narcotics Anonymous, International Doctors in Alcholics Anonymous, specialized hospital-sponsored self-help groups [24], and Caduceus Clubs. These clubs, now scattered across the United States, are specially designed as transitional support groups for the special needs of drug-involved physicians, and are based on the 12-Step program initiated by Alcoholics Anonymous.

For alcoholic physicians, especially those under age 55, disulfiram (Antabuse) is a very useful adjunct in the treatment process, and probably accounts for a 15% increase in favorable outcomes in our hands. The use of disulfiram serves as a psychological reminder and a deterrent to the physician, but also provides reassurance to family members, hospital administrators, licensing bodies, and courts that the physician is doing everything possible to avoid relapse.

For drug-involved physicians, frequent urine monitoring for unauthorized substances is essential. In our experience, twice weekly urine checks, with supervised collections, will suffice initially for 3–6 months. If abstinence is maintained during that period, a random urine collection schedule can be substituted. Occasional testing for nonroutine drugs of abuse, such as drugs in the fentanyl class for anesthesiologists, is definitely indicated. Also, occasional body surface checks are indicated, especially in cases of previous use by injection. We strongly encourage voluntary self-referral to State Medical Association Impaired Physicians' Committee for specialized peer support, and, when risk is high or when motivation is marginal, we often encourage self-referral (by the impaired physician) to the state licensing body to introduce greater accountability. Periodic reporting, done on a quarterly basis, ensures compliance, and acts as an ongoing reminder for the physician to satisfy program requirements.

Special considerations may require attention in the treatment of women physicians. Bissell and Skorina note that treatment options for women physicians may be somewhat limited, since many impaired physician committees even now are comprised exclusively of men, and that posttreatment support groups for physicians are also composed largely of men [16]. The authors report that the issue of whether to put women physicians in with male physician counterparts or to put them in with all-women's groups, with nurses for example, is a confounding one. With the advantage of hindsight, most of the women physician-patients felt that treatment experiences with other women were more valuable to them than were those with men. The authors cautioned against conflicts of interest, real or apparent, on the part of those who force a colleague into treatment, and suggest that the one recommending a particular treatment must not be in the position of profiting financially or in terms of status by one decision rather than another. The authors conclude by suggesting that "when a women physician is involved, it may be particularly important to be alert to the danger of denial or more judgmental attitudes based on unacknowledged gender stereotypes and attitudes" [16].

In our experience, drug-involved residents and medical students present special problems. Students and trainees have significant drug exposure and experience in undergraduate and graduate school [4,6,9]. Addiction may be well established by the time residency training begins. Institutions themselves contribute to the problems of drug-involved trainees by lacking clear, consistent institutional policies for such issues. As a result, staff attitudes vary widely with respect to treatment or discipline. The institution (and its staff) may have legitimate concerns about liability or possible harm to patients as well as about "consistency" of training or discipline. Leaves of absence for drug dependency treatment may present real difficulties for an institution which must provide medical services to patients and which relies heavily on residents for this care. Cross-coverage by resident peers may be thin or nonexistent, and can generate resentment. Resident benefits for salary continuatioin and treatment expense may be inadequate. Finally, the resident is, in reality, a "job applicant in the medical industry" and issues of confidentiality, mandatory reporting, stigma, and even discrimination may cause the trainee to delay the process of getting much-needed help.

In response to the problem of drug and alcohol abuse or addiction in physician trainees or residents, hospitals are beginning to use preemployment urine toxicology screening tests. In one such program, a group of 164 house staff were tested, with the result that 100% were found to be negative for drugs [25]. The Cleveland Clinic Foundation and other medical training institutions are now using preemployment drug screening on all employees, including physicians, both trainees and staff. While such a preemployment drug-screening program is not foolproof, Lewy reports at least some benefit [25].

> Because prospective house staff receive adverse notification, routine pre-employment drug testing is not an accurate indicator of recent drug use. However, drug testing does provide a clear message that drug use by house staff is not condoned. Inclusion of drug testing provides an opportunity to discuss issues of substance abuse and to inform house staff of available treatment resources.

The author concludes that if carefully planned and implemented, a policy of preemployment drug testing for physicians may be "a useful adjunct to the broader approach to managing drug use among physicians" [25].

VI. THE PHYSICIAN PEER ASSISTANCE MOVEMENT

The peer assistance movement for impaired health care professionals has been gaining momentum steadily. Peterson, in a review of this subject, notes that the success achieved by intervention programs in the workplace—occupational alcoholism programs and employee assistance programs (EAPs)—have inspired these peer assistance programs for impaired professionals [26]. This EAP format has provided a basic prototype that could be modified to meet the needs of the impaired health care professional. Many of these peer assistance programs rely on intervention techniques worked out and described by Johnson [27] and also use a form of benevolent coercion. Peterson points out that these intervention techniques can be applied in industry, in a family setting, and in dealing with the impaired professional [26]. Because of the denial which is an integral part of the alcoholic syndrome, outside intervention has proven to be an effective means of interrupting the disease process at an earlier time. Since the effects of alcoholism can be more readily measured and observed in a work setting, and since the threat of job loss is a powerful motivator for alcoholics to seek help, intervention programs in the workplace have been gaining an acceptance as effective modalities. These intervention programs appear well suited to the task of overcoming the denial and rationalization that is so much a part of the alcoholic syndrome [26]. A helpful intervention, especially when done by recovering professional peers, fosters identification with the recovery process, minimizes resistance and antagonism, and "models" a new, sober way of life for the suffering alcoholic physician.

The principles upon which these interventions are based are exemplified by those adopted by the Subcommittee on Physician Effectiveness of the Ohio State Medical Association's Committee on Mental Health [28]. They are: (1) We should be motivated by humanitarian concerns for the public and the impaired physician. (2) We should recognize that alcoholism, drug abuse, and mental illness among physicians are often ignored or untreated. (3) We should recognize that alcoholism, drug addiction, and mental illness are treatable conditions—and that treatment and rehabilitation personnel skilled in these areas have a good success record. (4) We should encourage all impaired physicians to seek help and cooperate in treatment at the eariest possible time in order for them to retain or regain full effectiveness to practice. (5) We should employ constructive coercion if a physician refuses all offers for assistance at a time when his impairment poses a threat to reasonable delivery of medical care. (6) We should employ involuntary coercion where all efforts fail—and the physician's impairment threatens the public or physician's health. The Ohio Subcommittee notes that "as practitioners of the healing arts, physicians more than any other professional group should be prepared to help troubled colleagues [28].

Similar objectives are noted in the Disabled Doctors Plan for Georgia, which is based on two major premises, according to Talbott et al. [29]: (1) The disabled physician, for psychological reasons, is usually unable to reach out for help, no matter how perilous his situation becomes. (2) Fellow-physicians who would help the disabled physician must take the initiative, being careful to use a sincerely compassionate, nonjudgmental, nonpunitive approach, and such an approach must be made under the aegis of the State Medical Association. The goals of this plan are: first, to identify physicians who are disabled by reason of their addiction to, or abuse of, drugs, including alcohol; and, second, the plan is intended to persuade as many of these physicians as possible to seek treatment voluntarily.

During this process, it is intended to protect their dignity, preserve their anonymity, and spare them embarrassment to the fullest extent possible. It is also intended to give compassionate assistance not only to the disabled doctor, but also to his or her family from the time of identification until the time that the doctor's professional activities are restored. A third major purpose of the Georgia plan is to provide a considerate, practical, and effective means of dealing with those doctors whose disability has been verified, but who either continue to deny their illness or else have refused to complete a course of treatment. It is the intention of the Georgia plan not only to protect the recalcitrant disabled doctor himself, but also to protect his family, his patients, and his whole medical community against the irresponsible behavior which is characteristic of addiction [29].

Talbott et al. in describing the model Medical Association of Georgia (MAG) Disabled Doctor's Plan, note that two specialized and essentially independent committees of the State Medical Association jointly carry full responsibility for the plan [29]. A Physician's Consultant Committee (PCC) has the primary role of advocate for the disabled physician. This committee carries out a statewide program of eduction about the nature of addictions and the services offered by the committee; establishes identification of disabled physicians; creates a trusting relationship with the disabled physician and his or her family; motivates the disabled physician to seek and complete effective treatment; acts as an advocate of the disabled physician in his or her troubled personal and professional relationships; helps to develop with the disabled physician a realistic plan of rehabilitation and reentry into medical pracice; provides moral support and practical aid to the disabled physician and his or her family during the rehabilitation process; and relates to and is responsive to requests from the other committee. This other committee, identified as the Professional Conduct and Medical Ethics Committee (PCMEC), refers complaints of addiction and drug abuse to the PCC for validation in the hope of promoting motivation for voluntary treatment; requires the PCC to determine the status of any physician who has begun treatment; and makes recommendations to the State Medical Board regarding any disabled physician when a majority of the PCMEC membership agrees that the reasonable efforts of the PCC have failed to produce the desired rehabilitation. Talbott et al. also emphasized that strong attempts are made to encourage voluntary entry into treatment for the impaired physician. If these motivational efforts fail, however, coercive or disciplinary action can be taken by the PCMEC [29].

Peterson lists the typical elements of the peer assistance process which functions first as a referral resource [26]. At the state level, a hotline is usually available to take requests for assistance and to offer advice. At the local level, a team of three or four committee members often functions in an intervention capacity. Members who act as intervenors usually undergo special training as part of the intervention team and support group. These members conduct fact finding, help to document the fact that a problem does exist, and if so, they meet with the impaired individual and attempt to motivate the impaired practitioner to accept help and proceed toward treatment and rehabilitation. Committee members also provide ongoing support during the recovery process [26].

Harris also notes that the most caring and constructive act from any potential referral source is early referral to the helping agency [14]. The almost universal reaction of physicians in recovery from chemical dependence is gratitude for intercession, regardless of how much they resisted diagnosis and treatment during their illness [14].Steindler suggests that more women may have to join the ranks of organized medicine to counter the present massive over-representation of males in local impaired physician committees, since "those persons in need of help are also more likely to come forward if they perceive that the 'change agent' is not overwhelmingly unrepresentative of their sex" [30].

VII. OUTCOMES

Using these general guidelines, outcomes for physicians are generally favorable. Morse et al., reporting on 73 physicians compared to 185 middle-class patients treated for alcoholism of drug addiction, found that the prognosis was more favorable for physicians [31]. When the groups were selected for study on the basis of completion of inpatient treatment, availability at time of contact, and not having died, 83% of physicians and 62% of the general group were noted to have favorable outcomes. The authors ascribe close monitoring, in part, for the better prognosis for physians. Although this study focused on abstinence, and did not measure other outcomes, such as work adjustment or social stability, the likelihood of correlation between these parameters and sobriety is evident. The authors also noted a lack of correlation between severity of addiction (as measured by adverse professional consequences and times previously treated) and treatment outcome. Physicians with multiple previous admissions and with severe professional difficulties recovered as favorably as did those with lesser problems in this study. Morse et al. [31] offered the following reasons why physicians seemed to recover at higher rates than nonphysicians: Most physicians were forced to begin their rehabilitation under a probationary reporting system overseen by others. Urine checking was commonly done, and involvement in impaired physician programs was frequent. The authors felt that this structured monitoring system is "therapeutic in itself and may force longer periods of abstinence from drugs and alcohol, during which time other rehabilitation efforts can become effective and the behavioral effects of addiction can moderate."

Kliner et al. analyzed 1-year follow-up data on addicted physicians and found that they generally have a favorable prognosis [32]. Most of the 67 patients studied reported improvements. One year after discharge from treatment, three-fourths of the physicians studied had been abstinent for 1 year, and most reported improvement in five other areas—drug use, general physical health, self-image, professional performance, and personal adjustment.

Favorable outcomes for addicted physicians have also been reported by Shore in describing the experience of the Oregon Board of Medical Examiners over an 8-year period [33]. Of the 63 addicted or impaired physicians who had been on probation with the Oregon Board, 75% were rated as stable and improved. In this group, the physicians had been on formal probation for an average of 6 years. The physician cohort included both drug-addicted (78%) and psychiatrically ill physicians (22%). At follow-up there had been two suicides, and two deaths in five physicians for whom the status was unknown. Overall improvement was seen in 75% of the subjects. The author noted a dramatic difference in the improvement rates (96%) for those subjects who had received urine monitoring for drug addiction compared with subjects who had no urine monitoring (64%), and who had been treated before there had been a strict requirement for a urine-monitoring program [33].

In this cohort of Oregon physicians, practitioners of family medicine represented 35% of the impaired physicians, compared with 21% of family practitioners among all of Oregon's MDs in 1980. Ten percent of the impaired physicians were psychiatrists, compared with 6% psychiatrists among all Oregon physicians. The author also noted that several of the impaired physicians sought employment in the state hospitals as part of their rehabilitation and were subsequently identified with psychiatry as a field of practice. These physicians were all successfully rehabilitated and had stable and reliable job performance. The author notes that the positive outcome associated with contingency contracting, urine monitoring, and a medically oriented addiction treatment philosophy in both voluntary and required programs is encouraging. The author also states that relapses were not statistically associated with a poorer prognosis, noting there was not a significant correlation between relapse and the long-term outcome rating. After 6 years, 57% of the subjects with alcohol dependence and 44% of those with other drug dependence had a history of relapse. Subjects with a history of relapse had a lower improvement rate (71 vs 91%), which was not statistically significant in this study [33].

Coexisting psychopathology may influence outcome. Johnson noted that physician patients with psychoses or features of borderline psychopathology were doing less well than others at outcome. The authors noted that one common denominator for successful outcome seemed to be the extent that the physician-patient was able to internalize important elements of the treatment experience [12].

Herrington et al., using a comprehensive approach, noted that 40 physicians entered the program, with 33 completing treatment [22]. Thirty-one have returned to full practice and 22 have experienced no relapse. The authors conclude that drug-abusing physicians have a generally favorable prognosis for rehabilitation, in terms of both resumption of a medical career, and maintenance of an alcohol- and drug-free lifestyle. These authors report a favorable outcome in 82.5% of physician-patients treated [22].

VIII. LEGAL ISSUES

Angres and Busch [34], in a review of legal matters surrounding the impaired physician, note that

> the ability of the physician, like any other individual, to obtain medical help and rehabilitation for his or her disease is a right. The ability to receive rehabilitation and then to have reentry into the medical profession is a privilege. In order for such rehabilitation and reentry to occur appropriately for the well-being of patients, certain guidelines that are specific to physicians must be utilized in treatment and aftercare monitoring.

Because the treating physician may have a dual (and conflicting) responsibility, the authors describe the problem of "agency" on the part of the treating physician; that is "is the treating physician an agent of the patient solely, or automatically also an agent of society for monitoring other physicians?" Also, the issue of mandatory reporting is a thorny one. Angres and Busch define the problem presented by the conflict between the mandatory reporting requirements of many "sick doctor" statutes and the duty to maintain doctor-patient confidentiality, especially when the physician enters treatment voluntarily. The authors note that some states allow breaches of doctor-patient confidentiality when patients are assessed as dangerous to self or others, whereas some states do not allow these breaches. The authors also note that "court decisions in malpractice cases indicate that physicians and hospital staff who know or should have known of compromised patient care from the practice of an impaired physician can and often will be held liable for any harm that may arise [34]. There are instances in which physicians have been fined or assessed civil penalties for failure to report another physician's drug induced impairment [35]. Angres and Busch [34] note that hospitals have a legal responsibility to monitor the competence of physicians given staff privileges under the legal doctrine of *respondeat superior*, which holds the employer responsible for acts committed by an employee in that setting. The authors note that the "threat of reporting" can be used to encourage the physician to voluntarily self-refer to the local or state voluntary impaired physician program, but if the physician refuses, involuntary referral to the licensing board may be required [34].

Finally, Angres and Busch comment about the role of coercion in the physician's entry into treatment, nothing that "most will come into treatment as a result of some degree of coercion," whether from a disciplinary body, employer, family member, or other influence. The authors additionally note that "the greatest degree of coercion really comes from the disease process" through its financial and interpersonal consequences. While the initial response to the coercive consequences of the disease may be anger and resentment, the treatment process generally involves progression to a healthier appreciation of recovery as a gift [34], or is replaced by an "attitude of gratitude" for the perserverence and help of the many "agents of change" involved in the physician's recovery process.

Thanks to the Impaired Physician Movement, spearheaded largely by the International Doctors and Alcoholics Anonymous (IDAA), there has been a tremendous increase in our understanding and awareness of the unique risks of physicians in their exposure to drugs and alcohol. While the profession has done much to respond to the needs of the drug-involved physician once identified as such, a much more vigorous effort at prevention still needs to be undertaken. This prevention effort should educate and train physicians for a different attitude toward drug use by themselves and their family members. This new (and more cautious) attitude should recognize that mood-altering drugs are inherently dangerous, and that they and the their places of storage or distribution should be regarded with caution and respect. It should recognize that peer pressure to use alcohol, recreational drugs, or medications operates on everyone, and that there needs to be reinforcement and approval for abstemious and drug-free socialization and recreation by physicians. This new physician wellness attitude should recognize that a life that is drastically out of balance because of chronic overwork or stress is an unhealthy and risky condition, which does not justify the use of substances for coping. Finally, the physician needs to accept responsibility for much of the "stress" that he or she perceives. Our own achievement orientation, drive to excel, and exaggerated sense of responsibility and importance may lead to the view that we as physicians are helpless victims of awesome and uncontrollable stresses, the only solution for which is drug comfort and refuge. Perhaps as physicians, we need to begin to cultivate a life that is not only "dedicated," but is also balanced and healthy in mind, body and spirit.

REFERENCES

1. Brewster, J.M. Prevalence of alcohol and other drug problems among physicians. *J.A.M.A.* 255(14):1913–1920 (1986).
2. Gualtieri, A.C., Cosentino, J.P., and Becker, J.S.. The California experience with a diversion program for impaired physicians. *J.A.M.A.* 249(2):226–229 (1983).
3. Scharrer, A.J. A dangerous mix: Alcohol, drugs and medical students. *Ill. Med. J.* 169(4):224 (1986).
4. Clark, D.C. Alcohol and drug use and mood disorders among medical students: Implications for physician impairment. *Q.R.B.* 14(2):50–54 (1988).
5. McAuliffe, W.E., Weschler, H., Rohman, M., Soboroff, S.H., Fishman, P., Toth, D., and Friedman, R. Psychoactive drug use by young and future physicians. *J Health Soc. Behav.* 25(1):34–54 (1984).
6. Baldwin, D.C., Conard, S., Hughes, P., Achenbach, K.E., and Sheehan, D.V. Substance use and abuse among senior medical students in 23 medical schools. *Ann. Conf. Resident Med. Ed.* 27:262–267 (1988).
7. McAuliffe, W.E., Rohman, M., Fishman, P., Friedman, R., Wechsler, H., Soboroff, S.H., and Toth, D. Psychoactive drug use by young and future physicians. *J. Health Soc. Behav.* 25:34–54 (1984).
8. McAuliffe, W.E., Santangelo, S., Magnuson, E., Sobol, A., Rohman, M., and Weissman, J. Risk factors of drug impairment in random samples of physicians and medical students. *Int. J. Addict.* 22(9):825–841 (1987).
9. Conard, S.E., Hughes, P., Baldwin, D., Achenbach, K., and Sheehan, D. Substance use and the resident physician: A national study. *Ann. Conf. Resident Med. Ed.* 27:256–261 (1988).
10. Talbott, G.D., Gallegos, K.V., Wilson, P.O., and Porter, T.L. The Medical Association of Georgia's Impaired Physicians Program. Review of the first 1000 physicians: Analysis of specialty. *J.A.M.A.* 257(2):2927–2930 (1987).
11. Gallegos, K.V., Veit, F.W., Wilson, P.O., Porter, T., and Talbott, G.D. Substance abuse among health professionals. *Md. Med.J.* 37(3):191–197 (1988).
12. Johnson, R.P., and Connelly, J.C. Addicted physicians: A closer look. *J.A.M.A.* 245, (3):253–258 (1981).
13. Council on Scientific Affairs: Results and Implications of the AMA—APA physician mortality project, stage II *J.A.M.A.* 257(21):2949–2953 (1987).
14. Harris, B.A. Not enough is enough. The physician who is dependent on alcohol and other drugs. *N. Y. S. J. Med.* 86(1):2–3 (1986).
15. Talbott, G.D., and Wright, C. Chemical dependency in health care professionals. *Occup. Med. S. Art Rev.* 2(N 3):581–591.
16. Bissell, L., and Skorina, J.K. One hundred alcoholic women in medicine. An interview study. *J.A.M.A.* 257(21):2939–2944 (1987).
17. Martin, C.A. and Talbott, G.D. Special issues for female impaired physicians. *J.M.A.G.* 75(8):483–488 (1986).
18. Ward, C.F., Ward, C.G., and Saidman, L.J. Drug abuse in anesthesia training programs. *J.A.M.A.* 250(7):922–925 (1983).
19. Gallegos, K.V., Browne, C.H., Veit, F.W., and Talbott, G.D. Addiction in anesthesiologists: Drug access and patterns of substance abuse. *Q.R.B.* 14(4):116–122 (1988).
20. Roback, G., et al. *Physician Characteristics and Distribution in the U.S.* Chicago, American Medical Association, 1986.
21. Adler, G.R, Potts, F.E., Kirby, R.R., LoPalo, and Hilyard, G.R. Narcotics control in anesthesia training. *J.A.M.A.* 253(21):3133–3141 (1985).
22. Herrington, R.E., Benzer, D.G., Jacobson, G.R., and Hawkins, M.K. Treating substance-use disorders among physicians *J.A.M.A.* 247(16):2253–2257 (1982).
23. Talbott, G.D., and Martin, C.A. Treating impaired physicians: fourteen keys to success. *Va. Med.,* 113(2):95–99 (1986).

24. Collins, G.B., Janesz, J.W., Thrope, J.B., and Manzeo, J. Hospital-sponsored chemical dependency self-help groups. *Hosp. Commun. Psychiatry 36*(12):1315–1317 (1985).

25. Lewy, R. Preemployment drug testing of housestaff physicians (letter). *N.Y. St. J. Med.* 553–554 (1988).

26. Peterson, R.L. Reaching the impaired practitioner: The peer assistance network. *J. Mich. Dent. Assoc. 70*(6):265–269 (1988).

27. Johnson, V.E. *I'll Quit Tomorrow*, 2nd ed. New York, Harper & Row, 1980.

28. New Help for Disabled Physicians. Ohio St. Med. J. 641–643 (1975).

29. Talbott, G.D., Holderfield, H., Shoemaker, K.E. and Atkins, E.C. The disabled doctors plan for Georgia. *J. Med. Assoc. Ga.* 71–76 (1976).

30. Steindler, E.M. Alcoholic women in medicine: still homeless. *J.A.M.A. 257*(21):2954–2955 (1987).

31. Morse, R.M., Martin, M.A., Swenson, W.M., and Niven, R.G. Prognosis of physicians treated for alcoholism and drug dependence. *J.A.M.A. 251*(6):743–746 (1984).

32. Kliner, D.J., Spicer, J., and Barnett, P. Treatment outcome of alcoholic physicians. *J. Stud. Alcohol 41*(11):1217–1219 (1980).

33. Shore, J.H. The Oregon experience with impaired physicians on probation. *J.A.M.A. 257*(21):2931–2934 (1987).

34. Angres, D.H., and Busch, K.A. The chemically dependent physician: Clinical and legal considerations, *New Direct. Ment. Health Serv.* San Francisco, Jossey-Bass, 1989, No. 41.

35. Kalstrom, J. Chemically dependent physicians: Colleagues now pay for looking the other way. *Kansas Med.* 69–70, 72–73.

53

Gambling Problems in Alcoholics and Drug Addicts

Sheila B. Blume
South Oaks Hospital, Amityville, New York

> A tremendous exhilaration swelled within me. A wild shout burst from my lips. People turned and stared at me, but I rushed to join the winning line that formed in front of the cashier's window. I walked toward my parked car. My step was light and I felt as one who had been reborn...Like a man under dope, I was carried far beyond the realm of reality. For a time I knew a happiness I had never known before. I could do no wrong. The money poured in. But the time came when my luck changed.
>
> Anonymous [1]

I. INTRODUCTION

There are many parallels between mankind's use of alcohol and other mood-altering drugs and participation in various forms of gambling. Both kinds of activities are thought to predate recorded history. Both alcohol use and games of chance are mentioned in the Bible as well as in the great traditional literary masterpieces of both Eastern and Western cultures. In the case of alcohol use, approximately two-thirds of the adult population of the United States report that they drink at least once a year [2]. The proportion of American adults who gamble to some extent was very similar in the 1970s, reported at about 60–65% [3]. However, as a result of the spread of state lotteries and other forms of legal gambling, the proportion of the population who gamble has increased through the 1980s to 80% or above [4]. It is interesting that this increase has occurred at the same time that American's alcohol use, as measured by per capita consumption, has shown a slow but stead decline [2].

Much like drinking, gambling is a widely accepted, socially approved form of recreation. Like drinking and drug taking, wherever gambling has been widespread, governments have found it necessary to develop legal controls on its availability, access by minors, quality, auspices, management, and other aspects of the industry and market. These controls have been designed in part to protect the public from unscrupulous entrepreneurs. However, they are also based on society's perception that both psychoactive substance use and gambling can lead to serious social and personal problems. Whereas for most drinkers and gamblers the activity is a pleasant, if not very profitable, recreation, for a significant minority these activities become the focus of a life-threatening disease.

Societies have experimented with a multiplicity of prohibition and legalization policies toward the various psychoactive drugs and gambling. At present, the pendulum in the United States is swinging toward increasing social acceptance of gambling, with legalization of lotteries, casinos, bingo games, on- and off-track betting, and sports betting. The states are looking to lotteries as a relatively painless way of raising revenue. Governments have tended to run these state-sponsored games as bottom-line business enterprises, concerned with attracting the greatest number of players and encouraging each to bet as much as possible [5]. This intense public promotion of gambling by state governments is distinctly different from state involvement in alcoholic beverage marketing. In the so-called "monopoly" states (states in which only state-run stores sell alcohol for off-premise consumption), beverages are sold as a public convenience, but drinking is neither encouraged nor is it promoted by massive advertising campaigns. The State promotions of lotteries, with their promises of attaining wealth without work and their glorification of the excitement of gambling, undoubtedly recruit many new gamblers into wagering of all kinds. By glorifying lottery winners while never mentioning the much larger population of losers, these promotional campaigns are basically dishonest. They also help to maintain societal denial of the importance of gambling problems. Although several states (notably Iowa and Massachusetts) have passed legislation devoting a small proportion of their lottery profit to support prevention and treatment programs, most states and the federal government offer little if any assistance. One group trying to reverse this trend is the National Council on Problem Gambling in New York. The Council has approximately 15 state council affiliates, either in operation or currently being organized. These councils are struggling to increase public awareness and to develop resources to combat gambling problems.

II. PATHOLOGICAL GAMBLING AS A DISEASE

Pathological gambling, a disorder first listed by the American Psychiatric Association (APA) in the third edition its *Diagnostic and Statistical Manual of Mental Disorders* (DSM-III) in 1980 (6), has been known to mankind for centuries. Famous people afflicted with this disease have abounded in history. One example was the famous Jewish scholar and musician, Rabbi Leon Modena, who lived in Venice during the late sixteenth and early seventeenth centuries [7]. Another was the great Russian novelist Fyodor Dostoyevsky, who wrote his novella *The Gambler* in 1866 as a desperate measure to rescue his finances [8].

In 1928, Sigmund Freud wrote about Dostoyevsky's gambling in his essay *Dostoyevsky and Parricide*. Freud hypothesized that guilt relating to Dostoyevsky's father's violent death bore a fundamental relationship to the writer's later gambling addiction [9]. Both before and after Freud's contribution, a number of other psychoanalysts took an interest in studying and treating compulsive gamblers. The most notable of these was Edmund Bergler, whose psychoanalytic study of more than 60 "neurotics addicted to gambling" led him to hypothesize an overwhelming unconscious need to lose as one of several important aspects of the compulsive gambler's psychopathology [10]. The various psychodynamic theories of this disorder, reviewed in depth by Rosenthal [11], make fascinating reading.

During the past few decades, an alternative conception of pathological gambling has been developed (e.g., see Refs. 12 and 13). This model looks at pathological gambling as an addictive disorder; as an addiction to being "in action." Being in action describes an aroused state experienced while betting, characterized by intense excitement and a feeling of power and hopeful anticipation. Although the 1987 revision of DSM-III (DSM-III-R) continues to categorize pathological gambling as a Disorder of Impulse Control Not Otherwise Classified, its diagnostic criteria have been revised to a form almost exactly parallel to the revised criteria for Psychoactive Substance Dependence [14]. The current DSM-III-R diagnostic criteria require evidence of maladaptive gambling behavior as indicated by a minimum of four of nine behaviors:

1. Frequent preoccupation with gambling or with obtaining money to gamble
2. Frequent gambling of larger amounts of money or over a longer period of time than intended
3. A need to increase the size or frequency of bets to achieve the desired excitement
4. Restlessness or irritability if unable to gamble
5. Repeated loss of money by gambling and returning another day to win back losses ("chasing")
6. Repeated efforts to reduce or stop gambling
7. Frequent gambling when expected to meet social or occupational obligations
8. Sacrifice of some important social, occupational, or recreational activity in order to gamble
9. Continuation of gambling despite inability to pay mounting debts, or despite other significant social, occupational, or legal problems that the person knows to be exacerbated by gambling

The core of this conception is the loss of control of gambling, as evidenced by the need to bet more money more often to get the desired effect (tolerance), preoccupation with gambling, the increased importance of gambling in the subject's life to the exclusion of other, previously valued activities, and interference in the individual's functioning. In these respects pathological gambling is very like other addictions. In addition, a central feature of pathological gambling is the "chase" or "chasing losses" [15]. This involves making larger and more risky bets in an attempt to win back money already lost. When a pathological gambler begins to chase losses, a phenomenon also referred to as "going on tilt" [16], losses characteristically accelerate, as described below.

III. EPIDEMIOLOGY OF PATHOLOGICAL GAMBLING

A. Adults

A variety of methods have been employed to estimate the prevalence of compulsive or pathological gambling in the general public. Among adults, rates of between 1.5 and 3.0% have been found (17–20). Most recently, Volberg and Steadman, using the South Oaks Gambling Screen (SOGS) in a telephone-poll model, found that in New York, 1.4% of adults scored in the probable pathological gambling range and an additional 2.8% reported some gambling-related problems [18]. A later study by the same authors in the states of New Jersey and Maryland found comparable results [19].

B. Adolescents

Less is known about the epidemiology of this disorder among adolescents. Lesieur and Klein surveyed 892 eleventh and twelfth grade students in four New Jersey high schools (three public, one parochial) [21]. Using an extensive questionnaire covering many aspects of gambling behavior and gambling-related problems, they found that 91% of the students had gambled at some time in their lives, and 86% had done so in the past 12 months. Thirty-two percent gambled at least weekly, with playing cards for money, casino gambling, sports betting, and lotteries the most popular forms of wagering. With Probable Pathological Gambling defined as three or more DSM-III criteria [6], 5.7% of the students (2% of the girls and 9.5% of the boys) fell into this group. Rates of gambling problems also correlated with lower grades in school and heavy gambling by parents.

In an interview reported in the *Journal of the American Medical Association*, Lesieur points out that every year 200,000 teenagers are refused admission to New Jersey casinos and another 35,000 are evicted from casino floors [22]. In the high school study quoted above, in which all of the subjects were underage, 46% claimed to have gambled in casinos and 3% reported doing so once a week or more [21]. Most adults who reach treatment report that they began to gamble as teenagers or preteens, and many date their preoccupation and problems with gambling to that period. Thus, a serious concern about gambling in U.S. adolescents seems to be justified.

C. Risk Factors

Although the etiology of pathological gambling is unknown, risk factors have been identified through both epidemiological and clinical studies. Volberg and Steadman found overrepresentation of males, nonwhites, and less educated adults among those with gambling problems in the general public [17,18]. In addition, in New York, but neither in New Jersey nor in Maryland, they found gambling problems overrepresented among people under age 30 and among those with incomes of $25,000 or less [17]. It is notable that men outnumbered women 2 to 1 in all of their surveys, whereas both clinical and Gamblers Anonymous (GA) population studies have yielded sex ratios closer to 9 to 1 of males to females [17,23]. Clinical population studies have also characteristically yielded an overrepresentation of educated professional men, especially lawyers and financiers. I believe this disparity between general population and clinical population findings is a function of the very inadequate state of our present casefinding and treatment systems. At present, only late-stage, heavily indebted individuals are recognized as having gambling problems—and often only after they have been caught embezzling or in some other illegal activity uncharacteristic of their general way of living. Those who do not have access to large amounts of cash or credit, and whose losses take place in a context of lower sums are seldom referred to treatment or Gamblers Anonymous at present. Thus, women, the less educated, and those of lower income are not reaching treatment in proportion to their representation among problem gamblers in the community.

A series of risk factors were identified in the South Oaks study of compulsive gambling among 458 adult inpatients who entered treatment for alcohol and drug addiction [24]. They include the following:

Being male (25% had gambling problems compared to 6% of the female patients)
Having a father whom the patient believed was a compulsive gambler (62% had gambling problems)
Reporting a mother who was a heavy gambler (30% had gambling problems)
Reporting heavy gambling by a sibling (40% had gambling problems)
Reporting an alcoholic father (28% had gambling problems)
Gambling as a teenager, taking part in a wider variety of forms of gambling, and placing larger bets

All of the above were found to be correlated with rates of gambling problems higher than the overall rate of 19%.

A similar study of 100 youthful multidrug-addicted inpatients at South Oaks Hospital (mean age: 17 years) revealed many of the same risk factors (25):

Being male (30% had gambling problems compared to 21% of the females)

Having a parent whom the patient reported had a gambling problem (50% had gambling problems compared to 28% of the group as a whole)
Starting gambling at an earlier age.

IV. PHENOMENOLOGY OF PATHOLOGICAL GAMBLING

A. Pathophysiology

Little is known about the pathophysiology of pathological gambling. Roy and his associates
have studied a wide variety of neurotransmitters and their metabolites in the body fluids of
male pathological gamblers as compared to normal subjects [26]. Their findings focus on
the noradrenergic system, with increased levels of centrally produced 3-methoxy-4-hydroxy-
phenylglycol (MHPG) in the cerebrospinal fluid and of norepinephrine itself in the urine during
the early period of withdrawal from gambling. This same group of researchers subsequently
analyzed their data to correlate biochemical findings with personality ratings [27]. They found
that scores on the extraversion scale of the Eysenck Personality Questionnaire correlated
significantly with both cerebrospinal fluid and plasma MHPG as well as with levels of
norepinephrine metabolites in the urine. Although the significance of these correlations has
yet to be fully understood, the findings point to a relationship between personality
characteristics and noradrenergic functioning in pathological gamblers.

   Still other studies have looked at elecroencephalographic (EEG) patterns in pathological
gamblers in comparison to normal controls [28,29]. The researchers identified patterns of
decreased hemispheric differentiation between right and left sides of the brain in response
to a simple task in pathological gamblers, similar to patterns found in patients with attention
deficit disorders. As a follow-up to these findings, Carlton and is colleagues administered
questionnaires to male pathological gamblers and matched controls assessing their childhood
behaviors [30]. The gamblers rated themselves consistently higher in traits associated with
attention deficit disorder.

   Furthermore, in a study of beta endorphins in pathological gamblers, Blaszczynski and
his colleagues found lower baseline levels of these endorphins in horse-race addicts than in
poker-machine addicts or controls [31]. Evidence of deficits in the endorphin system could
support a theory linking pathological gambling with other addictive disorders through a final
common brain pathway. However, such formulations must await further research and a better understanding of central addictive mechanisms.

B. Clinical Features

The clinical features of pathological gambling have been described by Custer (23,32–34).
Custer has differentiated three phases of the disease: the winning phase, the losing phase,
and the desperation phase. These phases are not uniform for all cases. Women, for example,
usually begin gambling later in life than men and often do not experience a winning phase.
They are more likely to report using gambling as a means of escape from a chronic and overwhelming life problem for which they have no other coping mechanism (e.g., an alcoholic
or abusive husband).

Winning Phase

The winning phase sometimes begins with a "big win" (an amount equal to or greater than
half the subject's annual income), which creates a feeling of extreme elation and an immediate
strong interest in gambling. Dostoyevsky's novella includes a character who becomes absorbed in roulette through this means. For most pathological gamblers, however, the winning phase is a result of careful attention to handicapping horses, studying sports team records,

etc. The individual becomes absorbed in gambling and becomes a skillful gambler. Although the gambler both wins and loses during this phase, he or she tends to recall and talk about the wins and deny the losses. This leads to an occasional or frequent inability to account for money claimed to be won. The gambler's self-esteem becomes increasingly dependent on being both smarter than the average person and favored by Lady Luck, and able therefore to achieve wealth, power, and status without hard labor. During this phase the size and frequency of betting increases, but indebtedness is not a major problem, since the gambler continues to work and wins frequently enough to support his or her need to stay "in action." This period is also characterized by an increasing psychological dependence on being in action as a remedy for dysphoric states such as boredom, resentment, and anxiety as well as a source of pleasure and self-esteem.

Losing Phase

The losing phase often begins with the kind of chance loss experienced by anyone who gambles. To pathological gamblers, however, losses represent severe injuries to their self-esteem. Therefore, instead of cutting back, they begin to chase losses, staking more and more in an effort to recoup money already lost. This kind of betting accelerates losses. There are often ups and downs, compared by families to an "emotional roller coaster" and by clinicians to alternating depressive and hypomanic periods. However, the general trend is toward increasing debt and deterioration of social, vocational, and interpersonal functioning. Family possessions, savings, and legitimate sources of borrowing are exhausted.

Desperation Phase

Pathological gamblers who have reached the desperation phase may engage in behaviors inconsistent with their previous moral standards, such as lying, embezzling, and forgery. These behaviors are justified by the gambler as temporary expedients until the next big win. Financial crises lead to the plea for a "bailout" (a large loan or gift meant to relieve immediate financial pressure), usually in return for a promise to give up gambling entirely. The bailout, however, like detoxification for a heroin addict who is only interested in decreasing his dosage, simply leads to more of the same. Like the opiate addict, the gambler has experienced an impairment of control of gambling. Like the addict, the gambler's craving is stimulated either by dysphoric states or by exposure to others engaging in the behavior. For both, abstinence is the appropriate treatment goal.

Most pathological gamblers who enter treatment or Gamblers Anonymous (GA) do so in the desperation phase. Major depression is common (76% in one VA inpatient study [35] and 72% in a study of GA members [36]. Bipolar disorder, hypomanic states, panic disorder, and agoraphobia have also been reported. Suicide attempts are common, with rates of 17–24% reported in surveys of GA members and higher rates in treatment populations.

C. Sex Differences

Sex differences between male and female pathological gamblers have been described by Lesieur [37] and Lesieur and Blume [38]. Lesieur studied 50 female members of GA, and found that their illness had begun at a later age than is characteristic for men. For more than half, gambling was a form of escapism from the beginning. As a group, they showed less indebtedness and illegal activity than men. They had high rates of other addictive and psychiatric diagnoses. Fully 58% had undergone psychotherapy before reaching GA. However, only four of these women were referred to GA by their psychotherapists. In many cases, they had not discussed their gambling with the therapist. When they had, the gambling was often considered unimportant. Their eventual entry into GA was mostly by self-referral and on the advice of family members [37]. As has been pointed out above, women are currently grossly undeserved in the GA and treatment systems. Thus, it is not clear whether these women's patterns are characteristic for female pathological gamblers in general.

D. Relationship to Crime

Another important aspect of pathological gambling is its relationship to crime [39,40]. The most common crimes involve appropriating money with which to gamble, and therefore include embezzelment, forgery, larceny, and working in illegal gambling operations (bookmaking, numbers running etc.). Violent crime is less common but not unknown. Women's patterns are similar but they report less criminal activity in general. Although many inmates of jails and prisons are there because of gambling problems, few correctional institutions have developed screening or rehabilitation programs.

V. RELATIONSHIP TO ALCOHOLISM AND ADDICTION

A major 1986 study of 458 adult inpatients at South Oaks Hospital in Amityville, New York, elucidated the relationships between pathological gambling and other addictive disorders (24). The patients, hospitalized for alcoholism and other drug addictions, were studied by means of questionnaires, direct interviews, and interviews with family members. Gambling was very common in this population. Eighty-nine percent had gambled at some time and 72% had done so in the previous year. Drinking and drug taking often accompanied gambling (44% used alcohol or drugs some, most, or all of the time they gambled). Conversely 34% said they gambled some of the time and 5% most or all of the time they drank or took drugs. For the group as a whole, 9% satisfied a lifetime DSM-III diagnosis of pathological gambling, whereas an additional 10% satisfied some criteria but fell short of the full diagnosis. These patients were considered problem gamblers. Risk factors for gambling problems are listed above, in Section III. Patients who suffered from alcoholism alone had lower rates of pathological gambling than those with combined addictions or drug addiction alone. The rates for alcoholism alone were 5% pathological and 10% problem gamblers; other drug addiction alone, 18% pathological and 11% problem gamblers; and dual addiction, 12% pathological and 10% problem gamblers. Those in treatment for drug addiction alone were chiefly cocaine and heroin addicts.

A similar study was subsequently carried out among younger inpatients in another of the addiction treatment units at South Oaks Hospital [25]. This survey of 100 multidrug addicts in an inpatient therapeutic comunity was reported by Lesieur and Heineman in 1988. In this group, with an average age of 17 years (contrasted with an average age of 37 years for the adults), the researchers found a prevalence of gambling problems even greater than the adult study. Overall, 14% were diagnosed as pathological gamblers and an additional 14% were categorized as problem gamblers. Risk factors are summarized above in Section III. Only 16% of the patients said they had never gambled. Over half had played cards for money and bet on sports, and about 15% gambled on each of these activities once a week or more. The results point up the common occurrence of pathological and problem gambling among youthful addicts.

Gambling by these patients puts them at risk for relapse into alcohol and/or drug use, as well as at risk for switching addictions (substituting the "high" derived from the action of gambling for that previously obtained from alcohol or drugs). The findings of these studies led the South Oaks Hospital to rethink its policies for its addiction units. The units now make an effort to educate patients and families about gambling, and to prevent gambling problems in all patients treated for addiction (see Sect. VIII).

VI. IDENTIFICATION OF PATHOLOGICAL GAMBLING IN ALCOHOLICS AND ADDICTS

Since few pathological gamblers consider their gambling a problem until they reach the desperation phase, patients presenting themselves for alcoholism or addiction treatment do not spontaneously discuss their gambling histories. The denial associated with pathological gambling is very similar to that encountered in other addictive disorders. Questions like Are you a compulsive gambler?, or Do you have gambling problems?, are likely to be met with denial. The need for a valid, reliable screening tool for use in this group inspired the development of the South Oaks Gambling Screen (SOGS) (Figs. 1 and 2) [41]. The SOGS can be given as a paper and pencil test or a structured interview. Not all of the 16 questions count toward the total score, although all of them yield information important for prevention and treatment planning. The maximum SOGS score is 20. A score of 5 or more correlates well with a DSM-III and DSM-III-R diagnosis of Pathological Gambling. A score of 1–4 indicates some history of gambling problems with presumed risk for future problems as well. The SOGS can be obtained by writing the author at South Oaks Hospital, 400 Sunrise Highway, Amityville, New York 11701.

Patients identified by the SOGS should be carefully assessed to establish a diagnosis. An article by Glen presents an excellent guide to patient assessment [42]. Information obtained from family members may also be helpful, although family members are often unaware of the full extent of the patient's gambling activity.

VII. TREATMENT OF PATHOLOGICAL GAMBLING IN ALCOHOLICS AND ADDICTS

A variety of inpatient and outpatient treatment models have evolved over the past few years [43]. Some of these models treat compulsive gamblers separately from other patients, whereas others, employing an addictions model, treat them in a special track within an addiction treatment program [44,45]. The alcoholic or other drug addict who is found to have a problem with gambling can be best treated for both addictions at the same time.

The techniques used in gambling treatment involve the same psychoeducation, individual, group and family therapy, and self-help approaches used in other addiction treatment. Attention must be paid to overcoming the denial of both patient and family, and the development of motivation for abstinence.

Because the patient initially sought treatment for alcohol or drug addiction, it is often necessary to explore the relationship between the patient's alcohol and/or drug use and gambling in detail. It is also important for the patient to discover the similarities in patterns of dependence on the high of being in action and on the drug-induced feeling of euphoria or relief.

Financial problems require special attention in the treatment of pathological gambling. Gradual repayment of debts is preferred to a family bailout or declaring bankruptcy. The gradual return of a sense of pride through repaying those injured through the patient's illness is as helpful in this diseasse as it is in other addictions. At South Oaks we have found psychodrama a useful therapeutic tool in the treatment of the multiply addicted [46], as it has been in alcoholism treatment [47]. Attendance at Gamblers Anonymous is also an integral part of treatment.

Long-term follow up through outpatient counseling and Gamblers Anonymous are critical to recovery. As in other addictions, a great deal of harm is done to family members, who need help as well [48–50]. Heineman compared 39 wives of pathological gamblers with an equal number of wive of alcoholics [51]. She found that gambler's wives had several types of problems rarely seen in the alcoholics' families. These included threatening phone calls

SOUTH OAKS GAMBLING SCREEN

Name_____ Date_____

1. Please indicate which of the following types of gambling you have done in
    your lifetime. For each type, mark one answer: "not at all," "less than
    once a week," or "once a week or more."

	not at all	less than once a week	once a week or more	
a.	___	___	___	play cards for money
b.	___	___	___	bet on horses, dogs or other animals (at OTB, the track or with a bookie)
c.	___	___	___	bet on sports (parlay cards, with bookie, or at Jai Alai)
d.	___	___	___	played dice games (including craps, over and under or other dice games) or money
e.	___	___	___	went to casino (legal or otherwise)
f.	___	___	___	played the numbers or bet on lotteries
g.	___	___	___	played bingo
h.	___	___	___	played the stock and/or commodities market
i.	___	___	___	played slot machines, poker machines or other gambling machines
j.	___	___	___	bowled, shot pool, played golf or some other game of skill for money

2. What is the largest amount of money you have ever gambled with on any one day?

    ___never have gambled   ___more than $100 up to $1000

    ___$1 or less   ___more than $1000 up to $10,000

    ___more than $1 up to $10   ___more than $10,000

    ___more than $10 up to $100

3. Do (did) your parents have a gambling problem?

    ___both my father and mother gamble(d) too much

    ___my father gambles (or gambled) too much

    ___my mother gambles (or gambled) too much

    ___neither one gambles too much

4. When you gamble, how often do you go back another day to win back money you lost?

    ___never

    ___some of the time (less than half the time I lose)

    ___most of the time I lose

    ___every time I lose

Figure 1 South Oaks Gambling Screen. South Oaks Foundation. Copyright (1986) printed with permission.

from creditors, loans for which the wives had cosigned, prolonged financial problems, and a shortage of self-help groups. Finally, the wives of recovering pathological gamblers complained of loneliness because their husbands were often working at two or three jobs and spending their few spare hours at GA meetings and aftercare. Both psychotherapy (preferably in groups) and Gamanon are of great help to these family members.

5. Have you ever claimed to be winning money gambling but weren't really? In fact, you lost?

   ___never (or never gamble)

   ___yes, less than half the time I lost

   ___yes, most of the time

6. Do you feel you have ever had a problem with gambling?

   ___no

   ___yes, in the past but not now

   ___yes

7. Did you ever gamble more than you intended to?......................... ___ ___
                                                        yes no

8. Have people criticized your gambling?................................. ___ ___
                                                        yes no

9. Have you ever felt guilty about the way you gamble or what happens when you gamble?... ___ ___
                                                        yes no

10. Have you ever felt like you would like to stop gambling but didn't think you could?.. ___ ___
                                                        yes no

11. Have you ever hidden betting slips, lottery tickets, gambling money, or other signs of gambling from your spouse, children or other important people in your life?.................................... ___ ___
                                                        yes no

12. Have you ever argued with people you live with over how you handle money? ___ ___
                                                        yes no

13. (If you answered yes to question 12): Have money arguments ever centered on your gambling?... ___ ___
                                                        yes no

14. Have you ever borrowed from someone and not paid them back as a result of your gambling?.. ___ ___
                                                        yes no

15. Have you ever lost time from work (or school) due to gambling?......... ___ ___
                                                        yes no

16. If you borrowed money to gamble or to pay gambling debts, who or where did you borrow from? (check "yes" or "no" for each)

                                                                                     no   yes

a. from household money...( ) ( )

b. from your spouse...( ) ( )

c. from other relatives or in-laws...( ) ( )

d. from banks, loan companies or credit unions.............................( ) ( )

e. from credit cards...( ) ( )

f. from loan sharks ("Shylocks")...( ) ( )

g. you cashed in stocks, bonds or other securities.........................( ) ( )

h. you sold personal or family property....................................( ) ( )

i. you borrowed on your checking account (passed bad checks)...............( ) ( )

j. you have (had) a credit line with a bookie.............................( ) ( )

k. you have (had) a credit line with a casino.............................( ) ( )

Figure 1 *(continued)*.

Few studies have traced pathological gamblers after treatment. Taber and his colleagues followed 57 of 66 male patients 6 months after they completed the inpatient phase of treatment at a Veterans Administration Hospital unit [52]. In 80% of the cases, collateral interviews with family members, GA sponsors, close friends, or counselors were also held. Fifty-six percent of the expatients contacted had remained abstinent for the full 6 months. Sixty-seven

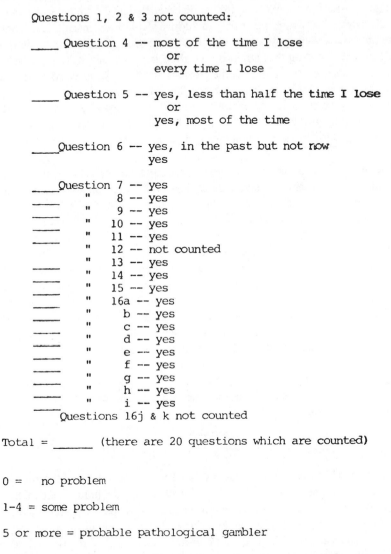

Scores on the SOGS are determined by adding up the number of questions which show an "at risk" response:

Questions 1, 2 & 3 not counted:

_____ Question 4 -- most of the time I lose
                    or
                    every time I lose

_____ Question 5 -- yes, less than half the time I lose
                    or
                    yes, most of the time

_____ Question 6 -- yes, in the past but not now
                    yes

_____ Question 7 -- yes
_____   "   8 -- yes
_____   "   9 -- yes
_____   "   10 -- yes
_____   "   11 -- yes
         "   12 -- not counted
         "   13 -- yes
_____   "   14 -- yes
_____   "   15 -- yes
_____   "   16a -- yes
_____   "   b -- yes
_____   "   c -- yes
_____   "   d -- yes
_____   "   e -- yes
_____   "   f -- yes
_____   "   g -- yes
_____   "   h -- yes
_____   "   i -- yes
         Questions 16j & k not counted

Total = _____ (there are 20 questions which are counted)

0 =   no problem

1-4 = some problem

5 or more = probable pathological gambler

Figure 2 South Oaks Gambling Screen Score Sheet. South Oaks Foundation. Copyright (1986) printed with permission.

percent were abstinent at contact and had been so for at least a month. There were significant gains in all areas of functioning and decreases in both subjective distress and behavioral disturbance.

Politzer and his collagues studied the cost-effectiveness of treatment for pathological gambling at the Johns Hopkins program in Maryland [53]. They concluded that the overall societal benefit-to-cost ratio was in excess of 20:1.

VIII. PREVENTION OF GAMBLING PROBLEMS IN ALCOHOLICS AND DRUG ADDICTS

An important part of most alcoholism and addiction rehabilitation programs is the education of the patient and family about the nature of addictive disease. Patients are taught that they must abstain from all drugs of addictive potential, including alcohol and marijuana. They are further instructed to advise their physicians and dentists about their risk for addiction so that any analgesic or sedative drug that might be required is prescribed with great care. This education is not complete, however, unless the patients and families are also educated about pathological gambling and informed that they may be at increased risk of developing this disorder. Patients with a positive family history, those who have gambled heavily, and those who have been especially attracted to the feeling of being in action require special attention. They should be helped to review their attitudes and gambling behavior, and to develop abstinence strategies.

In a residential setting, it is also important to review the kinds of recreational activities offered to patients. Alcoholics and addicts have a great deal of difficulty in structuring free time when they stop their alcohol and drug use. The recreational activities in which they participate while inpatients are often their first "clean and sober" activities in years. It is, therefore, important to avoid inadvertently socializing these patients into forms of recreation normally acompanied by gambling in the outside world. Games of cards, billiards, and dice games are common in addiction treatment facilities. Even though house rules in most facilities do not allow gambling, "unofficial" bets are often made. Some units even sponsor bingo games. A safer policy encourages physical fitness activities as well as hobbies or games that are not customarily related to gambling. A combination of educational and recreational approaches will provide the most effective preventiion possible at our present stage of knowledge.

The final segment in the prevention design involves family education and intervention. We must never assume that the significant others in the treatment of our addicted patients are themselves free of addictive disease. Some have alcohol, drug, and gambling problems themselves. Others, as offspring or spouses of addicted people, need psychotherapeutic help in finding a rewarding way of life.

IX. CONCLUSIONS

The study of pathological gambling, the development of a treatment network and the education of the public about this disease are at a level of development not unlike that of the alcoholism field in the 1950s. Public and professional interest are low, public policy makers have yet to face the nature and extent of societal gambling problems, and only the most severely and acutely ill patients reach treatment (if they do not commit suicide or land in prison first).

The current popularity of gambling legalization and its role as a quick fix for public budget deficits makes it easy to predict that our society will see more pathological gambling problems before we see less. That is, the problem will have to get significantly worse before public attention leads to widespread and effective prevention and treatment efforts. In the meantime, it is important that research into the causes and mechanisms of this disease continue, and that professional and citizen groups continue to agitate for attention. Those of us who are interested in the treatment of alcoholics and other drug addicts, however, can do much more. We can learn to identify and treat this illness in our patients, and to prevent its development in our patients and their families. That is our own special challenge.

REFERENCES

1. Gamblers Anonymous (1984). *Sharing recovery through gamblers anonymous*, Gamblers Anonymous Publishing, Los Angeles, California.
2. U.S. Department of Health and Human Services (1987). *Sixth Special Report to the U.S. Congress on Alcohol and Health*, National Institute of Alcohol Abuse and Alcoholism, Washington, D.C.
3. Commission on the Review of the National Policy Toward Gambling (1976). Gambling in America, U.S. Government Printing Office, Washington, D.C.
4. Lesieur, H.R., Personal communication, December 1989.
5. Clotfelter, C.T., and Cook, P. (1989). *Taking Lotteries Seriously*. Institute of Policy Sciences and Public Affairs, Duke University, Chapel Hill, North Carolina.
6. American Psychiatric Association (1980). *Diagnostic and Statistical Manual of Mental Disorders*, 3rd ed. Washington, D.C.
7. Hertzberg, L. (1985). Leon Modena, Renaissance rabbi: 1571–1648, *Harvard Mag.*, Sept–Oct., pp. 41–43.
8. Dostoyevsky, F. (1966). *The Gambler/Bobok/A Nasty Story* (translated by J. Coulson). Penguin Books, New York (See translator's Introduction, pp. 7–16.)
9. Freud, S. (1928). Dostoyevsky and parricide, *Collected Papers*, Vol. III. Hogarth Press, London.
10. Bergler E. (1957). *The Psychology of Gambling*. Bernard Hanison, London.
11. Rosenthal, R.J. (1987). The psychodynamics of pathological gambling: A review of the literature, *The Handbook of Pathological Gambling* (T. Galski, ed.). Thomas, Springfield, Illinois.
12. Orford, J. (1985). *Excessive Appetites: A Psychological View of Addictions*, Wiley, Chichester, New York.
13. Blume, S.B. (1988). Compulsive gambling and the medical model, *J. Gambl. Behav. 3*:237–247.
14. American Psychiatric Association (1987). *Diagnostic and Statistical Manual of Mental Disorders*, 3rd Ed., *Revised*. Washington, D.C.
15. Lesieur, H.R. (1984). *The Chase: Career of the Compulsive Gambler*. Schenkman, Cambridge, Massachusetts.
16. Browne, B.R. (1989). Going on tilt, *J. Gambl. Behav., 5*:3–21.
17. Culleton, R., and Lang, M. (1985). *The Prevalence Rate of Pathological Gambling in the Delaware Valley in 1984*. Forum for Policy Research and Public Service, Rutgers University, Piscataway, New Jersey.
18. Volberg, R.A., and Steadman, H.J. (1988). Refining prevalence estimates of pathological gambling, *Am. J. Psychiatry, 4*:502–505.
19. Volberg, R.A., and Steadman, H.J. (1989). Prevalence estimates of pathological gambling in New Jersey and Maryland, *Am. J. Psychiatry, 146*:1618–1619.
20. Transition Planning Associates (1985). *A Survey of Pathological Gamblers in the State of Ohio*, (Available from Ohio Lottery Commission.)
21. Lesieur, H.R. and Klein, R., (1987). Pathological gambling among high school students,, *Addict. Behav. 12*:129–155.
22. Breo, D.L., (1989). In treating the pathological gambler, MDs must overcome the attitude "why bother?" *J.A.M.A., 262*:2599–2606.
23. Custer, R. L. (1984). Profile of the pathological gambler, *J. Clin. Psychiatry, 45*:35–38.
24. Lesieur, H.R., Blume, S.B., and Zoppa, R.M., (1986). Alcoholism, drug abuse and gambling, *Alcoholism Clin. Exp. Res.*, 10 (1):33–38.
25. Lesieur, H.R., and Heineman, M., (1988). Pathological gambling among youthful multiple substance abusers in a therapeutic community, *Br. J. Addict., 83*:765–771.
26. Roy, A., Adinoff, B., Roehrick, L., Lamparski, D., Custer, R., Lorenz, V., Barbaccia, M., Guidotti, A., Costa, E., and Linnoila, M., (1988). Pathological gambling: a psychobiological study, *Arch. Gen. Psychiatry, 45*:369–373.
27. Roy, A., DeJong, J., and Linnoila, M. (1989). Extraversion in pathological gamblers, correlates with indices of norodrenergic function, *Arch. Gen. Psychiatry, 46*:679–681.
28. Carlton, P., and Goldstein, L., (1987). Physiological determinants of pathological gambling, *A Handbook of Pathological Gambling*, (T. Galski, ed.). Thomas, Springfield, Illinois.

29. Goldstein, L., Manowitz, P., Nora, R., Swartzburg, M., and Carlton, P.L., (1985). Differential EEG activation and pathological gambling, *Biol. Psychiatry, 20*:1232–1234.

30. Carlton, P.L., Manowitz, P., McBride, H., Nora, R., Swartzburg, M., and Goldstein, L., (1987). Attention deficit disorder and pathological gambling. *J. Clin. Psychiatry, 48*:487–488.

31. Blaszczynski, A.P., Winter, S.W., and McConaghy, N. (1986). Plasma endorphin levels in pathological gambling, *J. Gambl. Behav., 2*:3–14.

32. Custer, R.L., and Milt, H. (1985). *When Luck Runs Out*, Facts on File, New York.

33. Custer, R.L. (1987). The diagnosis and scope of pathological gambling, (T. Galski, ed.). *The Handbook of Pathological Gambling*, Thomas, Springfield, Illinois.

34. Custer, R.L., (1986). An overview of compulsive gambling, *Addiction in the Jewish Community* (S.J. Levy, and S.B. Blume eds.). Federation of Jewish Philanthropies, New York.

35. McCormick, R.A., Russo, A.M., Ramirez, L.F., and Taber, J.I., (1984). Affective disorders among pathological gamblers seeking treatment, *Am. J. Psychiatry, 141*:215–218.

36. Linden, R.D. (1986). Pathological gambling and major affective disorder: Preliminary findings, *J. Clin. Psychiatry, 47*:201–203.

37. Lesieur, H.R. (1988). The female pathological gambler, *Gambling Research: Proceedigns of the Seventh International Conference on Gambling and Risk Taking*, (W.R. Eadington, ed.). University of Nevada, Reno.

38. Lesieur, H.R., and Blume, S.B. (in press). When lady luck loses: Women and compulsive gambling, *Feminist Perspectives on Treating Addictions* (N. Van Den Bergh, ed.). Spring, New York.

39. Lesieur, H.R. (1987). Gambling, pathological gambling and crime, *The Handbook of Pathological Gambling* (T. Galski, ed.). Thomas, Springfield, Illinois.

40. Lesieur, H.R. (1989). *Female Pathological Gamblers and Crime Paper presented at the American Society of Criminology*, Reno, Nevada, Nov. 9, 1989.

41. Lesieur, H.R., and Blume, S.B., (1987). The south oaks gambling screen (SOGS): A new instrument for the identification of pathological gamblers, *Am. J. Psychiatry, 144*(9):1184–1188.

42. Glen, A.M. (1985). Diagnosing the pathological gambler, *J. Gambl. Behav., 1*:17–22.

43. Taber, J.I., and McCormick, R.A., (1987). The pathological gambler in treatment, The Handbook of Pathological Gambling, (T. Galski, ed.). Thomas, Springfield, Illinois

44. Blume, S.B. (1986). Treatment for compulsive gambling: An overview, *Addictions in the Jewish Community* (S.J. Levy and S.B. Blume, eds.). New York Federation of Jewish Philanthropies.

45. Blume, S.B. (1986). Treatment for the addictions: Alcoholism, drug dependence and compulsive gambling in a psychiatric setting, *J. Subst. Abuse Treat., 3*:131–133.

46. Blume, S.B. (1989). Treatment for the addictions in a psychiatric setting, *Br. J. Addict. 84*:727–729.

47. Blume, S.B. (1985). Psychodrama and the treatment of alcoholism, *Practical Approaches to Alcoholism Psychotherapy* S. Zimberg, J. Wallace, and S.B. Blume (eds.). 2nd ed., Plenum Press, New York.

48. Gaudia, R. (1986). The challenge of the compulsive gambling family, *Addictions in the Jewish Community*, (S.J. Levy, and S.B. Blume eds.). Federaton of Jewish Philanthropies, New York.

49. Lorenz, V.C., and Yaffee, R.A. (1989). Pathologial gamblers and their spouses: Problems in interaction, *J. Gambl. Behav., 2*:113–126.

50. Lesieur, H.R., and Rothschild, J. (1989). Children of gamblers anonymous members, *J. Gambl. Behav., 5*:269–281.

51. Heineman, M. (1987). A comparison: the treatment of wives of alcoholics with wives of compulsive gamblers, *J. Gambl. Behav., 3*:27–40.

52. Taber, J.I., McCormick, R.A., Russo, A.M., Adkins, B.J., and Ramirez, L.F., (1987). Follow-up of pathological gamblers after treatment, *Am. J. Psychiatry, 144*:757–761.

53. Politzer, R.M., Morrow, J.S., and Leavey, S.B. (1985). Report on the cost-benefit/effeciveness of treatment at the Johns Hopkins center for pathological gambling, *J. Gambl. Behav., 1*:131–142.

54

A Multidisciplinary Team Approach to the Treatment of Drug and Alcohol Addiction

Gregory B. Collins, Kathleen Weiss, Dennis Cozzens, Jan Thrope, Margaret Kotz, and Joseph W. Janesz
Cleveland Clinic Foundation, Cleveland, Ohio

I. INTRODUCTION

At first glance, it would seem that the founders of Alcholics Anonymous (AA), "Dr. Bob" Smith and "Bill" Wilson, did not rely on multidisciplinary team to find their own sobriety and launch the fellowship of AA. Nonetheless, if one studies the roots of the AA movement, it is clear that the multidisciplinary approach was one of the main strengths of the movement as it gathered in the knowledge of physicians, psychiatrists, clergy, nurses, and recovering individuals all working together to help the alcoholic attain the elusive goal of lasting sobriety [1]. This early "multidisciplinary" approach in AA has evolved into a highly specialized, but nonetheless multidisciplinary, methodology widely used in drug dependency treatment programs. With assistance from many disciplines, the drug-dependent person is first detoxified and then is restored to physical, emotional, and spiritual health. The effective accomplishment of this broad restorative goal requires the input of people with different skills—a true multidisciplinary group. It would seem obvious that such a group would need to work together in a harmonious fashion in order to accomplish its goal of total recovery of the drug-dependent person. Nonetheless, the very diversity of the backgrounds and experiences of the team members in many ways works against this harmonious interaction, often resulting in rivalry, resentment, and even therapeutic sabotage. Since the alcoholic can easily divide and conquer, splitting staff and playing on biases and rivalries to remain entrenched in the addictive cycle, staff coordination and teamwork must be achieved and maintained to facilitate the process of change and recovery.

II. THE NEED FOR A MUTLIDISCIPLINARY TEAM APPROACH

As Ruth Fox, M.D., Medical Director of the National Council on Alcoholism, has noted, "Treatment of the alcoholic, to be successful, must be mutlidisciplinary [2]. One of the primary reasons is the many diverse types of knowledge and skill that a treatment professional would need to possess in order to treat cases of drug dependency independently and alone.

Drug dependency is a physical, emotional, social, and spiritual disease, and the skills needed to treat all aspects of this disease process are of such breadth that it is all but impossible for one person to treat the whole person adequately. Brotman, in an attempt to enumerate the disciplines required for the treatment of alcoholism, states, "While only time and extensive research will yield the clue to the optimum composition of such a team, I would suggest that it might include the disciplines of medicine, psychiatry, nursing, social case work, community organization and research. Thus the team would incorporate a broad array of skills addressed to the major areas of functioning in the patient's life" [3]. Addiction is often a life-threatening disease. Medical treatment is often the necessary first priority, and thus the skills needed would include a medical understanding of all the possible physical consequences of the disease, including withdrawal syndromes and types of organ pathology. These medical skills would also include the ability to intervene both diagnostically and therapeutically so as to arrest the progress of these physical consequences. The prevention and treatment of the alcohol withdrawal syndrome, seizures, neuropathies, malnutrition, hepatitis, and severe anemia are frequent necessities, for example.

The emotional and cognitive consequences of the disease are no less important, since the "alcoholic thinking" reinforces the disease process through denial, minimization, and rationalization. As Fox notes, "Most patients are not motivated to stop drinking, since alcohol has given rewards they are unwilling to give up [4]. Most patients refuse to face their alcoholism for many years, using the defense mechanisms of denial, rationalization, regression, and projection of blame onto the person closest to them. When finally confronted with the threat of divorce, loss of employment, or loss of health and prestige, they may agree to undergo therapy [2]. Intervention at this level requires skills in individual and group therapy and requires the ability to change or influence the attitudes and behaviors of patients. Since brain damage is a frequent concomitant of substance abuse, assessment skills are needed using psychological testing and other forms of psychiatric/psychological evaluation. The psychosocial component of the chemical dependency disease process also requires special skills. Social stabilization and restructuring are very important, as the patient who has a severely damaged social support system will be at a great disadvantage in developing a new, recovery-oriented support system after leaving the treatment center. For example, the alcoholic salesman who has to contend with client entertainment may require intensive counseling in nondrinking social skills or may need vocational change. Likewise, the alcoholic who lives in close proximity to a bar may need social service help in moving to protect sobriety. Lastly, but certainly not of least importance, are the spiritual skills required to treat the disease process. These spiritual skills involve the treatment team in endorsing the AA 12-Step Program which would emphasize certain aspects of healthy spirituality and deemphasize pathological aspects of spirituality. This spiritual approach to the disease process places a strong emphasis on examination of spiritual deficits and needs while promoting a process of spiritual revitalization. These widely divergent skills needed to treat the many facets of the addictive disease process illustrate why it is so important for the patient to be treated, not by one individual, but by a team in order to assure the best chance of recovery.

From the staff point of view, it is important that there is a team approach to drug dependency problems, as these patients are often complex, and potential pitfalls are numerous. If a physician is attempting to treat a drug-dependent patient independently, there may be difficulty and danger in "enabling" the patient by providing continued prescriptions of the drug of abuse or a substitute drug. Endless demands and manipulations for chemicals can sabotage well-intentioned physicians unless the emotional-cognitive or "thinking part" of the disease process is altered at the same time. O'Connor and Morgan have also noted that "many patients exhibit a great deal of pathological manipulation" [5]. To treat this symptom, the maintenance of lines of communication between many part-time personnel of various disciplines must be maintained. Coordination and supervision of the treatment team constitutes a major activity of the clinic administrator and psychiatric consultant. Also, the issue of counter-transference (feelings or reactions of the therapist toward the patient) may help or hinder the treatment of these difficult patients. Many times, if treated in a one-to-one setting, the therapist may "act out" personal issues with the patient, especially since many professionals in this field have had personal experience with some type of drug dependency process, either through their own addictions or through addictions in the spouse or family of origin. These past experiences, if not modulated through a team approach, can introduce therapeutic "blind spots" and distortions and might make one-to-one treatment very difficult and much less successful. For example, the therapist may begin to act out repressed anger at the drug-dependent family members of long ago through inappropriate irritability with the patient. Or, the therapist may be enabling of the patient's addiction, perhaps by "rescuing" or rationalizing relapses, and may not be aware of this. Therefore, it is important that a team of people be available to support each other in reality testing and in evaluating their own behaviors. This personal emotional energy can be very useful in the treatment of drug-dependent patients if it is recognized for what it is, and if it is then channeled appropriately. It is clear that it is much easier to manipulate a person working in solitary fashion, than to manipulate a group of therapists working in unison.

A team approach to drug dependency treatment is also important in that treating these patients on an individual basis can be very time consuming, demanding, and emotionally exhausting. The high frequency of "burnout" for professionals treating these patients is well known. Not being able to share with team members the inevitable feelings of frustration, anger, and confusion can contribute to a more rapid rate of burnout. It is important that the team itself function as a supportive, reality-oriented group, allowing an individual team member to be redirected in a gentle, nonthreatening way, should involvement with a patient become unhealthy or dysfunctional. Without this group interaction, an individual therapist could continue with a formulation for treatment that would either ignore or exaggerate aspects of the patient's personality and/or dysfunction to the detriment of recovery. These errors are less likely when there are other professionals involved in the patient's care who also feel a responsibility for the patient's progress and treatment.

Team size is important, as the team needs to work with maximum efficiency and effectiveness. Team size should be relatively small to allow for cohesiveness and some closeness. Spratley recommends a team of six to eight therapists to be the most effective [6]. A high level of trust and respect should exist among the team members, so that their work can be shared openly and in a safe environment. It is also essential that communication between team members be honest and empathic. Too large a team makes close support and trust difficult, and could lead to splitting within the team. Too small a team can lead to enabling of each other, lack of perspective, or to a situation in which new ideas and attitudes are not tolerated. A mature team, as described by Spratley, has six Cs: clarity, congruence of purpose, competence, confidence, continuity, and caring attitudes [6].

The next question is what kind of team, and how should the team be composed? The team could be focused in many ways.

1. There could be a medically based team in which the focus would be to attain physical health for the patient. This would be done through medications (such as for detoxification), laboratory procedures, bed rest, and a focus on the patient's medical condition. The team would consist of physician, possibly an internist, gastroenterologist, pulmonary specialist, and a nursing staff. In the past, drug dependency (especially alcoholism) was treated this way, once the patient became sick enough to be admitted to the hospital for physical illness as a result of his alcoholism.

2.   Another type of focus team would be a psychiatrically based one, the goal of which would be to help the patient achieve emotional health. This is commonly done through individual, group, or family therapy from an analytic, cognitive, or Gestalt approach, or any combination of the above. Additional tools of the psychiatrically based team approach to drug dependency are the use of psychiatric medications and hospitalization.

3.   Another example of a team approach would be a socially based one which would have the focus of helping the patient to achieve social health. This could be achieved through recreational, occupational, and social-adjustment therapy that would be focused primarily upon the patient being more socially appropriate.

4.   A final example of a team approach would be a 12 Step–based team, which would have the goal of leading to spiritual health for the patient. The tools used in this team are the 12 Steps and 12 Traditions of Alcoholics Anonymous [7], the AA *Big Book* [8], and the AA slogans, prayers, and meetings. These allow the patient to become spiritually healthy, hopefully promoting sobriety by developing a new spiritual way of life.

While all of the above teams offer valid and reasonable approaches to a drug dependency problem, none of these can stand alone as adequate treatment in giving patients the best chance of attaining and maintaining sobriety and recovery. It is important then to see that just a team approach is inadequate if a team is described as any two people working toward a patient's well-being. The team must be multidisciplinary also to be truly effective. For example, a true multidisciplinary team would not consist solely of an internist, gastroenterologist, and pulmonary specialist, as those disciplines are not broad enough to treat the whole patient. Also, a team which would include only a social worker, counselor, and therapist would not be adequate, in that the patient's medical and spiritual needs would not be addressed adequately. A multidisciplinary approach should be one that would include many different disciplines and should not be based from one point of view, perspective, or philosophy.

This multidisciplinary team approach might not be as critical in the treatment of other types of illnesses. In other words, patients can be (and are) treated very appropriately for many psychiatric problems in individual therapy, such as in psychoanalysis or cognitive therapy. A multidisciplinary team is not essential in certain disorders, and in some may be contraindicated, as in the analysis of certain neuroses. In order for patients to work through neurotic concerns, such as depression or phobias, it may not be essential that a multidisciplinary team be present to treat them. In many such cases, a group therapy situation would be appropriate, but this does not mean that there would be a multidisciplinary team treating that patient or that group. In therapy groups, usually only one or two therapists are present, and they are commonly from the same discipline or very close disciplines; i.e., psychology and social work. Also, when treating medical problems, such as hypertension, there is not so pressing a need for a team approach, let alone a multidisciplinary team. Purely socially based problems may not need a multidisciplinary team approach, as the patient generally needs guidance and direction as to more appropriate handling of his or her affairs in society. The program of Alcoholics Anonymous is a fellowship which promotes a new, sober, spiritual way of life. Since anyone can live by or advocate these principles, the AA Program is not in itself discipline bound; rather it is the organizing philosophy around which the disciplines unite. A true multidisciplinary team approach is far broader and more inclusive than a narrower, discipline-based team approach.

Also implied in the term multidisciplinary team, is the sense that all disciplines are of great value in the treatment process. There is recognition and consensus that an important contribution is made by each discipline in the treatment of the drug-dependent patient, and, therefore, all disciplines are necessary in treating these complex patients. For example, a drug-dependent patient who is medically stabilized and doing well emotionally is in danger of relapse if his or her social situation is chaotic and dangerous to him. A patient who is emotionally and socially well adjusted by the end of the treatment, but who has no real understanding of the value of being spiritually healthy, may have a difficult time maintaining sobriety during stressful periods.

Since the goal of treatment is to allow the patient his or her best chance for recovery, a multidisciplinary team will afford the best opportunity as the contribution of each member of the team will be different because of specific training. In all cases, physical health, or at least a stable physical condition, is an essential aspect of recovery, necessitating the skills of physicians and nurses. Additionally, a psychiatrist will see subtleties of the patient's emotional state that may need specific treatment that others might miss. Likewise, a social worker may see "slippery areas" in the patient's social network that a psychiatrist might not be attuned to. A psychologist will be able to identify nuances in the patient's cognitive functioning that might not otherwise be discovered. The 12 Step component [7], provided by counselors and AA volunteers, also is essential after discharge, since the patient cannot take the treatment team home. The 12 Steps and peer support are essential in continually reinforcing the changes in attitude and perspective for the maintenance of stable, "quality sobriety." A true multidisciplinary team approach to treatment allows the widest possible range of modalities in helping the person to restore health physically, emotionally, cognitively, socially, and spiritually.

III. THE TEAM APPROACH: THEORY AND PRACTICE

According to Francis and Young, "The team approach is a distinctive style of working aimed at harnessing the collective talent and energy of people [9]. While many of the same characteristics necessary for an effective group are also necessary for an effective team, the notion of *team* adds a dimension to the word group. A team develops a distinctive spirit to accomplish its task. Let us now explore the factors influencing the effectiveness, maturity, and functioning of a team.

A team is a collection of two or more individuals who *must* coordinate with each other in order to get a job done. The group becomes a team when there is a task which requires that the group members must interact and influence each other in order to accomplish that task. There is no best way to organize a team to create the elusive quality necessary for the team to complete its task. However, the recognition that the team is larger, greater, and more able to complete its task than any individual in the team could complete the task single handedly is a primary assumption. The team is more than the composite of individual members. It has an emotional component and a task component that can best be realized in its wholeness.

The emotional and task components rely on some basic assumptions. These assumptions depend on the culture of the organization where the team completes its task. In general, the assumptions reflect the values, norms, philosophy, rules, climate, and system of organization within which the team functions. In our drug dependency treatment milieu, these values, norms and philosophies include the 12 Steps of Alcoholics Anonymous [7], the Four Absolutes of the Oxford Group Movement (purity, honesty, unselfishness, and love), plus three other absolutes added pragmatically (self-discipline, humility, and gratitude). Beyond these unifying virtues or principles is the tacit assumption that team members will *live* by these principles and not merely mouth the words, and will, in their individual ways, be living "powers of example" for role modeling of healthy attitudes and behaviors. "Walking the walk, not just talking the talk" is a highly valued group norm. In our experience, it is not necessary that staff members be recovering individuals themselves. Rather, the ability to live by the principles, and the ability to empathize and lead others to a better life are issues which supersede personal recovery experience. Additional group norms may extend to dress (casual or "professional"), language (use of profanity by patients or staff), or attitude (competition vs cooperation). The establishment of these norms is by no means an easy or natural aspect of team evolution. The varied backgrounds and experiences of typical drug dependency team members yield a diversity of opinions on these subjects which can lead to rivalry. The fine balance between a fractious diversity and a "working consensus" around group norms is an elusive and fragile thing. In our milieu, the operating consensus around the disease concept of drug dependency, and the philosophical unity around the Steps and Absolutes offer a solid conceptual framework that all team members can comfortably "buy into," buffering differences and interpersonal frictions.

Even within this framework of philosphical unity, the team must exist in a larger system. The larger system, for example, a hospital, social service network, or even a self-help fellowship, must be understood in order to define the team context as well as emotional and task contributions. Since all the systems are fluid, dynamic, and interactive, the team must be able to respond to the demands and norms of the larger system in which it exists; it cannot merely look inside itself for validation, as self-serving myopia and complacency will soon result. Finally, how the team accomplishes its task requires set procedures and patterns of communication within the team and within the larger system.

Rubin has described a model of organizational development in terms of the organization's goals, roles, procedures, and interpersonal relationships [10]. While many other variables and models are significant in our interdisciplinary team situation, it has been useful for us to employ this particular organizational development model to examine and enhance our own team functioning. As Rubin states, "The effective coordination of a team's resources rests, in part, on the ability to specify the goals or objectives one is trying to achieve [10]. A useful scheme for analyzing team functioning is to simply ask the questions: What is this team trying to do? What are its tasks? For the team to function well, the members need to know why it is that they are working together. The primary goal of the team may be to provide outstanding patient care. This goal may be defined by the larger system, such as a hospital, and while there may be general agreement about this goal and principle, consensus may not be so easily reached about specifics. For example, team may not be well defined, especially with regard to who is in and who is out. Quality may not be defined either. Quality goals such as abstinence from mood-altering drugs, patient satisfaction, high productivity, program solvency, and "caring" may be, to a degree, mutually exclusive. The extent to which component members of the team prioritize these valued goals and the way they go about attaining them constitutes the dynamic web of tension which exists in the organizational team. This goal-setting step can be accomplished by fiat (this is what we're going to do and this is how we're going to do it), or by a consensus-based approach, utilizing discussion, deliberation, debate, and finally, decision making. In our drug dependency treatment center, the attainment of abstinence and the development of a new way of life in accordance with the philosophy of Alcoholics Anonymous are generally agreed-upon philosophical goals for our patients.

A working assumption about our goal is that all of the team members are willing to operationalize and "own" a part of that goal. Not only has the larger system mandated that the functional team will contribute to the goal, but each team member vigorously supports the goal and actually is unwilling to settle for less responsibility or completeness in its achievement. Team members who do not buy into or adequately prioritize the goal are soon out of step with group norms and introduce disharmony and friction into the smooth flow of the organizational conponents. Leadership (and peers) must recognize these distances, and address them in a way that reestablishes cohesion and unity rather than in a way which fosters further alienation and antagonism. Generally, we have found that such corrective actions are best handled in one-to-one encounters with team leaders. The goal of these corrective actions is always the reestablishment of a spirit of inclusion, commitment, excellence, and ownership.

Without these vital and healthy team attitudes, the elusive goal of lasting sobriety in the context of a new, AA-oriented way of life will founder on the rocks of divisiveness and competition. In our center, we frequently remind ourselves that each team member fully shares in the ownership and responsibility for providing high-quality, sobriety-oriented patient care. Thus, an exciting sense of meaningful participation and team spirit permeates the team task.

IV. ROLES

In order to achieve the goal or to complete the task assigned to the team, members assume a variety of roles. The problem of clarifying the goal of the group is not nearly as difficult or complicated as the problems relate to role. Each team member enters the team with multiple expectations about who should be doing what, and about how each member "should" behave. According to Rubin and Beckhard [11], there exist questions about role ambiguity, role conflict, and role overload in any group. There will be less uncertainty for team members if there is role clarity and specific agreement with external role expectations. Job descriptions assist with some of the role clarification, but can only partially delinate the operational issues involved in accomplishing the team task. External group membership held by individual team members, i.e., reference groups, can also assist with clarification of role and contribution to task; however, "reference group loyalties can create significant problems for an individual in terms of his behavior as a member of the team [8]. Richard Hall's summary of the characteristics of a professional mentality defines some of the role expectations imposed by professional reference groups [12]. Feelings of autonomy which support the professional's right to make decisions and control work may be in conflict with the decision-making process of the team. Membership in professional organizations (or self-help groups) may reinforce values, beliefs, and identities within the profession (or group) to develop a "colleague-consciousness," influencing standards of practice that may be unknown or unacceptable in the interdisciplinary team. One profession's belief in its indispensable and beneficial qualities to public service may inadvertently devalue the contributions of another discipline on the same team. Self-regulation may be interpreted as colleague control and lack of open communication within the work team. Finally, the amount of dedication the practitioner has to the profession may blind him or her to the contributions made by other team members [9]. One can easily extrapolate the complexity of establishing roles within an interdisciplinary team of professionals when one considers the sheer number of individuals representing different disciplines in an inpatient treatment setting.

To illustrate, in a drug dependency treatment setting, the overinvestment of staff members in discipline-bound, "reference-group-thinking" can easily emerge. In the case of physician (including psychiatrist) team members, a sense of physician leadership and ultimate physician responsibility can render the doctor heedless to the valued and appropriate inputs of other team members, as the physician reserves the right to make all diagnostic and treatment decisions. The nurse, on the other hand, may feel entitled to exert excessive influence out of a sense of proprietary overinvolvement, noting that "No one spends as much time with the patient as I do, as I know best." The social worker may overvalue a focus on social manipulation of the social support network to facilitate recovery or perhaps overvalue a particular therapeutic modality, such as transactional analysis or Gestalt therapy, to the detriment of other inputs. Recovered personnel and AA volunteers tend to overvalue their experience in "having been there," and often have strong feelings that only they can "break through denial" and give the patient guidance in a way that he or she will accept. All of these reference-group perspectives are devaluing and demeaning to other members of the team, even if inadvertently so, and must be muted somewhat and blended so that the component parts work together to produce an enhanced team work-driven result. In our program, we frequently refer to a "links in the chain" approach, which emphasizes both individual strength but also the interdependence of each link in producing the result. Other programs refer to "quilts" or fabrics of interwoven threads, blending individual contributions into a unified whole. Once again, the team has to find a balance point, in this case, between the energy and structure provided by discipline-bound training and the potential divisiveness and authoritarianism that it engenders.

Compounding the problems inherent in the integration of numbers of discipline-bound personnel is the issue of degree of membership. Francis and Young [9] suggest three levels of membership:

1. Core team members whose contributions are necessary over an extended period, and significant reorganization would be necessary should they withdraw.
2. Supportive team members whose contributions aid the team to do its work effectively, to ease, support and provide assistance, raw materials, or information. They do not greatly assist tasks to be performed or spark creative effort.
3. Temporary team members whose contributions are specific and timebound.

This level of membership configuration adds yet another degree of complexity to the interplay of the team components. Most of the drug dependency treatment programs we know have been organized around a core team member or two. Such a person(s) often provides the philosophical leadership, vision, and goal clarity needed to unify the team. Because of this leadership, the core member or members may have a high public profile and may account for attracting a sizable proportion of the patients to the center. Such individuals can be from many disciplines and the drug dependency field has seen outstanding core members who are physicians, nurses, social workers, psychiatrists, and psychologists. These core members have also included both recovering addicts and nonaddicted individuals as well. Indeed core membership may convey influence and status in a real or. presumed way which may also inadvertently devalue the important contributions of supportive and temporary members. The dynamic tension that is created between these components can produce friction or erupt into overt rebellious hostility.

Finally, the role each individual plays on the team is constantly changing. Certain team members may exhibit group task roles that are clearly relevant to the team's fulfillment of its tasks. This same individual, at other times, may function in a group maintenance role to contribute to the team's optimal working order, enhancing its positive climate, and promoting good internal communication and relationships. At still other times, the same person's unconscious reliance on self-oriented or discipline-bound roles may block group satisfaction, limit productivity, or disorganize team synergy. In a drug dependency program, for example, a physician core member might provide essential medical tasks and might strongly influence the program in other ways, deciding who gets treated, for how long, and in what way. On the other hand, the same physician could exert excessive discipline-bound influence which might devalue the role of nurses, social workers, or counselors by insisting that he or she, rather than the group process, knows best in all cases and at all times.

Finally, leadership roles may (and should) shift with the specific task or problem at hand. Organizing an annual alumni reunion for example, may be an important task which binds patients emotionally to the philosophy of the treatment program, but the organizing of such an activity would probably best be left to an individual with the time, motivation, and skills to ensure a successful outcome. Such a leadership designation might have little to do with discipline of origin, or with core membership status. Rather the nature of the task itself and the skills that are required for its successful completion strongly influence the leadership needed.

In summary, then, the effective interdisciplinary team incorporates a dynamic, interactive, fluid pattern of interrelating to achieve internal and external goals important for the completion of its task. The team must move from an amorphous state of nondefinition of role to one that incorporates a certain amount of role clarity, without inflaming role-based rivalries and "turf battles." The team must also function within the philosophical framework in which the input of all members is valued and important, balancing the strong influence of core members, whereas at the same time fostering participation and ownership by supportive and temporary team members as well. All these issues must be dealt with smoothly and imperceptibily in order for critical internal goals to be achieved, i.e., fostering the recovery of the drug dependent patient, whereas at the same time addressing external pressures as well. These external pressures may come from governmental funding agencies, hospital administrations, insurance companies, professional reference groups, and even recovered volunteers; each of these groups may have its own agenda for who should be doing what and how it should be done. The team must address itself to the needs and wants of these constituencies, and must negotiate an acceptable *modus operandi* with these external influences on its functioning. The complexity of these interactions is truly astounding and must often, of necessity, give way before task-driven initiatives. Who is best suited for the job by skill, experience, and interest is a decision the group must resolve by its deliberative, decision-making process. The team must then support the decision and enthusiastically buy into its implementation with their expertise and energy.

V. PROCEDURES

Accomplishing this interplay of people, roles, and goals is a highly complex organizational task which is best achieved by developing and adhering to effective team work-oriented procedures. The procedural aspects of team function and development deal with the process aspect of the work group. While the goal of the team answers the question "what" and the roles answer the question "who," the procedures need to identify "how." A team must be able to make decisions about the task it has been assigned. Yet, the entire team need not make all decisions as a group. Questions about who makes what decisions and how the decisions are made, implemented, and evaluated require serious procedural effort. Teams can choose how to decide from a full range of possibilities, including total unanimity, consensus, majority rule, authority rule, or default. Any form of decision making may be appropriate in certain circumstances, but who defines those circumstances, and what permission is required from team members may give rise to other procedural issues. What time frame, how much information, and who provides information about areas of decisions add still other dimensions to the decision-making procedure. Finally, questions about how the decisions are implemented, what sort of acceptance or "buy-in" is expected from the team, and who validates the decision-making process and the outcomes may need to be determined.

The effective flow of communication is essential to all the procedural aspects of team play. Some of the rules governing information flow are found in the decision-making procedures. In fact, some of the same questions need to be raised when discussing communication or decision making, e.g., who, when, how, how often, why, and where. Similarly, many styles of communication patterns may be employed: hierarchical, round-robin (everyone speaks), authoritarian (power speaks), informational, and educational, to name a few. Each form is appropriate in given situations, however.

Factors influencing team communication patterns need to be addressed frequently. Active participation must be encouraged for all members. Time must be allotted for the free exchange of ideas and feelings. Openness to new ideas and divergent opinions encourages active participation and values the contributions made by each member. The notion of dialogue in both directions of the heirarchy and across interdisciplinary lines promotes the sense of team spirit and ownership of goals.

Open communication also assists with the procedural aspects involved in conflict management. Francis and Young note that "as the team develops, it becomes necessary to sort out personal relationships of power and influence [9]. Conflict is inevitable, but can lead to a higher level of team functioning when carefully managed. Often, team change institutes conflict, so that some of the same tools used to manage change can manage conflict. Identifying the problem and the needs, generating possible outcomes, negotiating differences with a "win-win" vision, treating the problem and not the team member, keeping the mission goal clearly fixed, and finally, reviewing our progress, has been a process that works for our team.

Leadership issues may strongly influence procedures of decision making, conflict management, and communication flow. In a team of professional interdisciplinary members, hierarchies within the larger system can obscure team hierarchies. Yet, when the larger system supports interdisciplinary team efforts, empowerment of all team members is possible, and leadership roles can fluctuate drive by need or demand. The traits of successful leaders can be shared, modeled, employed, encouraged, and expanded to the team membership. The willingness of the leader to be a risk taker, decision maker and supporter of team members, establishes and models team norms. Style of leadership on the team also determines communication patterns, atmosphere, structure, and expectations. Bennis notes that when leaders are effective, four themes of empowerment are evident: "People feel significant, learning and competency matter, people are a part of a community [team], and work is exciting [13].

Finally, process issues lead to the development of norms, the unwritten rules governing behaviors, Norms are simply the way things are done by a certain team. Norms are often the unspoken guidelines for socialization into systems. Their existence is most felt when violated. Like feelings, norms are neither good or bad—they just are. Their appropriateness should be measured by their usefulness to the team in completing its assigned task. In our experience, these norms pertain to just about every circumstance of team interaction. Our team norms affect where people sit at a conference table, their style of clothing, who speaks first (and last), and the use of "therapeutic language" (AA, psychiatric, "street," or a mix, for example). Other issues such as uniforms, punctuality, degrees on name tags, and even argument styles fall into the category of team norms, all of which must be negotiated and resolved.

In summary, the process of developing procedures parallels the formation of the team. Different stages of team development promote different procedural and practice patterns. All processes of the team are fluid, dynamic, and interactive.

VI. INTERPERSONAL RELATIONS

The evolution of a team follows patterns that are similar to the formation of any group. Certain stages of development can be predicted. The interpersonal relationships within the team mirror those of any process-oriented task group.

When the team first forms, people tend to seek their own place in the team in relationships to other team members. There is a gradual growth of personal exchange of values, styles, attitudes, and readiness, as each group member brings his or her own uniqueness to the whole. The team task begins to be accomplished and interpersonal relationships begin to develop. However, each member also contaminates this team's process with attitudes and training accrued through prior living and learning.

It then becomes necessary for the team to deal with conflict. This is an expected developmental stage for any team to experience. Alliances, internal and external role expectations, hidden agendas, and struggles for power/influence/control need to be resolved in ways that will promote the accomplishment of the team task. Conflict management with positive resolutions assist the team in its developmental journey. Failure to deal effectively with conflict impedes the team in its task and stunts further growth or success within the team. How disagreements are handled very much influences the ongoing work of the team, not only through the modeling of successful problem solving to team members, but also by developing healthy work norms.

In the drug dependency treatment setting, conflict and interpersonal tension are an expected and inevitable consequence of the multidisciplinary nature of the team. The varied backgrounds and personal experiences of the individuals lead to a collision of ideas and priorities which, when overlaid with role-related personal issues, becomes a major obstacle to the team's accomplishing of its task. Perhaps fundamental to conflict resolution in a drug dependency treatment setting, is the recognition that the patient's sobriety is the top priority. How that goal can best be achieved is an issue which can be argued ardently from every side, but ultimately it is the patient who wins from this discourse, and the entire staff can derive satisfaction from that knowledge. In acting conscientiously toward the goal of helping the patient attain sobriety, self-serving, competitive tendencies can be set aside without much loss of face and without a sense of losing the therapeutic argument. This fervent discourse, especially in treatment planning sessions, should not be viewed as an argument but rather as an energized dialogue in which everybody puts forth maximum effort. Usually, in our experience, when this happens a consensus gradually or rapidly emerges, which sweeps all before it. The consensus is powerful and palpable and is generally not to be denied even by authoritarian core members. Hearing and heeding this consensus is analogous to searching for the group conscience of AA, an AA tradition which recognizes that the collective wisdom of the group is generally superior to that of any one individual [7]. The enactment of this tradition in a professional team setting generally works well and can serve as a role model to the patient in heeding this group conscience very carefully in the AA program. Even so, at times the energy level and intensity of dialogue among team members can become so passionate that conflicts escalate beyond the comfort zone. At those times, deferring final resolution of the problem to another time, seeking new information, or smoothing ruffled feathers by verbal or physical expressions of friendly concern may be needed. Carrying a grudge or getting even are behaviors which work counter to the spirit of unity and compromise which must be part of any organizational team's functioning.

A meaningful and fulfilling work experience has been characterized by Ruch and Goodman as having four components: knowledge, care, respect, and responsibility [14]. Creating work norms around these areas assists the team members with their tasks. Members of the team want to know what is happening with their work in relation to the team and the larger system. They want to know that their contribution is important, valued, respected, and necessary to the mission of the team. Norms must be established about responsibility and accountability both to team members and to the larger system. Even to what extent the team spirit empowers the team needs to be developed as a norm. Do team members believe that collectively the team works better than the sum of its parts?

As members gain the freedom to participate fully in the team, team maturity occurs and performance of its task improves. Interpersonal relationships, often informal, are based on positive regard, mutual respect, and trust. Rigid roles become much less important. Complimentarity and reciprocity of respect provide the interactive "lubrication" for smooth team functioning. The team gains strength, identity, and success within the larger system as a result. Teams are dynamic systems that require change for maintenance. Each change offers the opportunity for chaos or growth. The process of team growth and development provides an ongoing challenge to all team members.

Our experiences at interdisciplinary teamwork are not unlike those of Ottenberg at The

Eagleville Hospital and Rehabilitation Center [15]. As Ottenberg remarked,

> When one gathers together a staff of physicians, psychiatrists, psychologists, nurses, social workers, recovered alcoholics as counselors, and assorted rehabilitation workers, one has assembled a group of highly trained and skilled professionals, each of whom has vague and uneasy feelings about the competence and intensions of the others.

Ottenberg commented that conflicts frequently arose around the issue of focusing on "alcoholism" per se, or taking a whole-patient viewpoint in addressing recovery problems. Another problem Ottenberg observed was the disease of alcoholism itself [15].

> Ubiquitous as discarded beer cans and obvious as a rum nose, yet it lacked any generally accepted and validated method of treatment. Out of necessity we designed our own therapeutic program. One portion was oriented along lines of conventional group therapy, with emphasis on insight, psychogeneis, and social interplay in the group situation. The other major thrust was a broad-band behavior-therapy approach.

Ottenberg also commented on the problems inherent in changing well-entrenched alcoholic or addictive psychopathology with long ingrained characteristics of isolation and manipulativeness, all to be changed within a short period of time in the hospital setting. A breakthrough for Ottenberg's team seemingly came about after a training visit to the Daytop Village Program in New York [15].

> We were surprised by the aggressive, even assaultive, attacks on the psychological defenses of the residents in some of the therapeutic encounters. We recognize the same hardened mechanisms of self-deception and denial that had been thwarting our efforts. The uninhibited hammering away seemed to have no ill effects when carried out in the therapeutic setting within a community based on mutual concern and respect for just treatment...human beings are less fragile and more redeemable than we had thought.

Staff exposure to a marathon training session led to the incorporation of "minithons" at the Eagleville Hospital where

> the staff gathered at about 7 in the evening and have continued in session until 5 or 6 in the morning. These extended meetings offered an opportunity to relate to one another at a level of honesty and candor that is far different from the usual hospital staff meeting. Of course, expressing feelings, even when it does go on all night, does not necessarily solve problems; but it does define them and bring them into the open where we can commit ourselves to do something about them, to the benefit of staff, patients, and the entire community [15].

These marathoms were extended to patients as well, with the result that "the intense involvement that goes with marathons gives off an aura of excitement and vitality that tends to diffuse among patients and staff. Even visitors sense a charge in the atmosphere, and many, within a few hours, begin to feel 'turned on'" [15]. Ottenberg observed that these therapeutic techniques produced "a positive effect on the therapist, the patients and the whole community," he also noted the washing away of "false lines of demarcation between staff and patients, and between disciplines [15].

The gradual process of program maturation has been described by Costello et al. [16] as follows:

> Ongoing in-service training over the past three and one-half years has proven both extremely frustrating and heartening. As the problem grows in stability, the character of the ongoing staff training has developed from painful confrontations between non-AA'ers and AA'ers, or between professionals and non-professionals, to healthy effective and intellectual interchanges. Staff attrition has accounted for the elimination of

individuals with rigid ideological positions and has left a core of fairly flexible individuals who are capable of honest give-and-take about sensitive issues without personal regression or program sabotage. New staff have been recruited by a procedure more sensitive to problems and issues regarding the melding of ideologies into a team identification.

Shared decision-making appears to be a byproduct of program maturation. "Decision-making power is shared by staff members so that the AA influence does not dominate the counselor-patient relationship, and so that the professional staff does not try to mold the counseling staff into miniprofessionals' who would be shackled by a model they do not fully understand or accept [16].

It is perhaps not an accident that a multidisciplinary team approach with active participation has been fostered in the Alcohol and Drug Recovery Center (ADRC) at the Cleveland Clinic Foundation, since participatory and democratic processes have long been fostered at our institution. As Srivastva and Cooperrider have noted [17],

Consensus about the primary task of organizing went beyond the economizing functional one (to make profits or fulfill a market demand) and centered around a broader, open-ended psychosocial one. The efficiency logic of instrumental rationality was by no means inoperable or rejected; it was simply circumscribed by the professionals' practical concern for the ongoing development of an active, responsive, and cooperative social system in an organization committed to a democratic/participatory process.

This sense of participatory and democratic involvement by all the practitioners has fostered a strong sense of purpose and unity among staff members; indeed, a recent book on the history of the Clinic is revealingly titled *To Act as a Unit: The History of the Cleveland Clinic Foundation* [18].

VII. PRACTICAL APPLICATION

In actual practice, the ideal of a smoothly functioning team of interrelated but distinctly different disciplines is a difficult state to achieve and sustain. Our own experience at the Cleveland Clinic Foundation Alcohol and Drug Recovery Center (ADRC) would certainly support that view, since the fine tuning of the milieu and staff occupies a tremendous amount of the time and energy of our six "core" managers. Our interdisciplinary team consists of three full-time psychiatrists (one of whom is the Head of the Section), a program manager (master's level psychologist), a head nurse (master's degree with psychiatric and drug dependency experience), and a master's level program coordinator/counselor supervisor, 15 additional registered nurses (five of whom are master's prepared), seven counselors (five of whom are master's prepared), four clerical pesonnel, one research coordinator, and one full-time housekeeper. These people run a 20-bed inpatient unit with a 28-day inpatient program combining detoxification and rehabilitation psychotherapy, in addition of a sizeable outpatient practice.

Because of its location in the Cleveland Clinic Foundation, an institution well-known for its medical and surgical capabilities, a sizable number of our patients have had or do have life-threatening degress of organ damage from drug abuse. In addition, although we do not operate a dual diagnosis unit per se, approximately 70% of our patients are sufficiently psychosocially impaired to warrant the designation of dual diagnosis. Outpatients are served in an evaluation clinic and aftercare counseling clinics. The approach is eclectic with a strong emphasis on AA plus family therapy and psychosocial rehabilitation. Urine testing and disulfiram (Antabuse) are frequently used, and nonaddictive psychotropic medications are used for those dual diagnosis patients in whom functioning or sobriety would be impaired without pharmacotherapy. An outcome study from this program, published in 1983, found 78.4% of drug-involved patients and 65.1% of alcohol-involved patients had returned to a high level of sobriety and psychosocial functioning [19]. Staff has published on the development of hospital sponsored self-help groups [20] and recruiting, retaining [21], and involving AA volunteers [22]. Research activities have centered on alcoholic family members of bulimics [23], presurgical evaluation of alcoholics for organ transplantation [24], and the biochemical aspects of alcoholism [25]. Our approach is truly eclectic, multidisciplinary, and emphasizes teamwork in a healthy, vibrant staff milieu. Active participation by all staff members is vigorously encouraged. Everyone can justly feel that his or her contribution is an important part of the overall effort of rehabilitating the whole person. Although each physician heads a "team" (two inpatient and one outpatient/consult), case managers (nurses or counselors) strongly influence treatment decisions. A consensus approach is employed in arriving at treatment plans, and this consensus is forged and modified daily at morning chart rounds conference and at a weekly treatment planning meeting with all team members present (including those from the second shift).

It is at the weekly treatment planning sessions that the really difficult decisons about patient management are developed. The case managers present background information, progress, and treatment, and a proposed plan of action. Usually active debate follows and additional suggestions are laid on the table. A consensus gradually emerges and becomes, by group endorsement, the treatment plan. The case manager usually implements the plan with physician input and authorization. At times, the debate about the treatment plan becomes heated; since we actively foster "ownership" by everyone, sometimes this can go a bit too far. Debate can be impassioned and overlaid with an attitude of "I must win or else." Usually the group conscience prevails, however, and heated tempers cool off, generally within 24 h. Sometimes this cooling-off process must be facilitated by another team member to step in to provide some perspective, reassurance, support, and reintegration. With this process operating smoothing, staff members can take some risk with their clinical judgments knowing that the group will carefully correct them if this is needed. A degree of creativity—hard to achieve in the tradition-bound drug dependency field—can be allowed to flourish with the group conscience providing the safety net.

A sense of ownership and participation is actively fostered by seemingly endless celebrations of the individual's presence in the milieu. Birthday parties, showers, transition parties, Friday parties, honorary breakfasts, and even commemorative parties for no particular reason seem to abound to celebrate and commemorate the importance of everyone's participation. Numerous attractive plaques dot the wall commemorating present, past, and deceased staff members. The sense of special people belonging to a special team is constantly reinforced.

The sense of specialness is communicated to patients as well. Treatment plans are individualized and take into account strengths, weaknesses, and psychosocial realities in building a long-term sobriety program. There is great attention to detail altering old (alcoholic or addictive) ways of doing things. There is constant attention to putting one's best foot forward, with emphasis on good grooming, manners, language, attitude, and conduct. Old strengths and talents, long buried by addictive neglect, are strongly encouraged and allowed to flourish anew. Often the person rediscovers him or herself as an attractive and competent individual without the distorting influences of drugs. This sense of personal specialness is reinforced by encouraging some reverence for the rebirth process as a unique, remarkable, and almost mystical experience. Patients often feel physically, emotionally, and spiritually transformed by the process. This transformation is hopefully sustained by progression to the aftercare phase of the program with its emphasis on outpatient group support in the hospital and in the community. Twelve-Step work is encouraged after discharge, as "alumni" (with stable sobriety) take newcomers to community AA meetings. An annual reunion brings hundreds of alumni and their family members together with the staff for a huge celebration. The reinforcing potential of this event is tremendous. Many patients look to these reunions as milestones in recovery, often "staying sober for the next one." These celebrations, volunteer activities, and hospital-based self-help groups give our patients a sense of specialness and pride in their recovery. The patients quickly become an all-important part of the team instead of the "product."

Decision-making is often the true test of teamwork in a multidisciplinary setting, and our setting is no exception. Our group has grappled with who decides and how to decide inumerable times. A Steering Committee has evolved as our major decision-making and policy-implementing body. Members of his committee include three psychiatrists, the head nurse, the program manager, and the counselor supervisor. These six members operate on an open, sharing, consensus basis in decision making and policy implementation. Seating is varied. No one sits at the head of the table. The task of writing minutes is rotated. Status and role-related prerogatives are deemphasized in what is an informal yet earnest dialogue. Members bring lunch and the meeting always starts late. The informality and casualness of the meeting offset the seriousness and built-in tensions when strong personalities with strong reference group loyalties get together. Members have learned to set these loyalties aside and to become more interactive, interdependent, and less authoritarian. An observer would notice a high degree of trust, commitment, and enthusiasm from all the participants. This level of interactive trust does not happen by accident, rather it is the end result of years of struggling, readjusting, negotiating, clarifying, and talking. Individual members start out programmed for conflict with their reference group loyalties, past experiences, and individual agendas at the ready. Only gradually are these diminished with disclosure, negotiation, and compromise. A fine balance point is sought in which members retain their individuality but are not blinded or motivated solely by that. Note unlike the Eagleville experience [15], we soon discovered our need for minimarathon steering committee meetings—3- to 4-h hour quarterly sessions where things are thrashed out or gone over in more detail. The meeting agenda can be sharply or loosely defined, and can be set by anyone present. These minimarathon meetings allow individuals time to talk in depth about their points of view, often referencing their own opinions based on past experience. Personal priorities and strong feelings, which may be well hidden on a day-to-day basis, have time to come forth and are evaluated in a caring atmosphere. The group process is always supportive. No one goes away mad. Rather, most often the participants feel electrified and uplifted by the experience and have the glow of realization that the end result of the deliberation was better by far than the thinking of any one individual present.

VIII. SELF-HELP GROUPS IN THE TREATMENT TEAM

The involvement of the self-help groups' philosophies and members is both crucial and complicated at the same time. Alcoholics Anonymous (AA) is an independent "fellowship" whose principles, articulated largely in the form of 12 Steps and 12 Traditions [7], has provided the philosophical structure for many other self-help groups today, including Narcotics Anonymous, Cocaine Anomymous, Sex Anomymous, and many others. Since its founding by two alcoholics in 1935, AA has provided a philosophy which provides the foundation for many treatment programs. Furthermore, treatment programs may rely heavily or even exclusively on self-help group members to fill their staff position. Typically, patients receive strong, comprehensive orientation to the principles of AA and are given vigorous encouragement to join and become active in the fellowship as a means of sustaining sobriety. Many then return to the treatment center as AA volunteers, providing additional helping resources to patients and families in the center [22].

Outcome research and clinical experience has proven that meaningful relationships between professionals and self-help groups are extremely valuable. "Research on treatment outcomes among alcoholics increasingly finds that participation in AA improves chances for successful rehabilitation [26]. In addition "several mental health agencies and alcoholism programs have demonstrated that volunteers can make important contributions [22]. Featherman and Welling found that volunteers can be successfully integrated into a community health center [27]. Van Meulebrouck and Fikany established a training program to teach volunteers to work with alcoholics [28]. Slaughter and Torno involved "senior" alcoholic patients as patient-counselors for newly hospitalized alcoholics [29], and Covner concluded that volunteers can be successful, under supervision, in counseling alcoholics [30].

The role that AA assumes is both philosophical and organizational. A new patient in a treatment program can be inspired by a recovering volunteer who can expose him or her to the philosophy and methodology of learning to live sober one day at a time. Hospitalized patients can actually see others who have recovered from the illness of alcoholism and who have rebuilt their shattered lives and restored themselves to health and sanity. The patients have an opportunity to "tell it like it is" to others who have suffered similarly, and patients who hesitate to discuss their situations with professionals often confide in other alcoholics [21]. The AA philosophical approach encompasses mental, emotional, and spiritual aspects, and the volunteers who embody these principles act as positive peer supports and credible role models. Functionally, AA structures patients' rehabilitation through the 12 Steps and 12 Traditions [7] and outlines how to "work the program." Through anecdotal experiences and a "what will work for me will work for you" approach, therapeutic changes occur [21]. The AA program "directly alters the individual's narcissistic, grandiose perceptions of the self and assists in the development of a more mature, less egoistic self-concept [31]. An AA-based recovery program is a spiritual, cognitive, and behavioral way of life that enhances a personal and interpersonal sense of well-being while promoting a value system based on honesty and humility.

However, several pitfalls can occur between treatment professionals and members of AA, primarily involving conflict and rivalry. "Historically one of the major impediments to the development of partnerships is the natural antithesis between the philosophies of self-help and professional health care. This antithesis [notes Emerick]is especially strong in these times of increasing specialization and professionalism [32].

Emerick continues that "self-help groups are extremely conscious of the potential for co-optation by professionals and are apt to consider professional partnerships as professional attempts to redirect traditional self-help goals, such as independence and empowerment, into more typical professional-client relationships [32]. Boundary disputes and ideological differences may also create conflict. The roles and responsibilities of the AA member and the professional differ significantly. For example, the helping professional is bound by federally mandated confidentiality laws and operates by a legally regulated medical approach. An AA member, however, although respectful of anonymity, is not necessarily governed by as many guidelines when he or she interacts with the newly recovered patient. He or she may feel comfortable breaching anonymity when it is within the fellowship, or if it is intended to help a patient. Thus, in this way and in many others, professionals and AAs operate under different guidelines. At times when the two groups vigorously disagree, rivalry rather than cooperation ensues. A study done by Kurtz indicated that "cooperation between professionals and AA members involves frequent interaction, congruent ideas about treatment, and appropriate linking strategies [26]. The most cooperative centers interacted often with AA because half of the staff belonged to AA or Al-Anon, and they were linked to the AA community by accepted practices, such as by employing volunteers from AA [26]. Appropriate linking activities reduce the threat of co-optation [26]. One program which successfully bridged the gap was the Friendship Room project at the Cleveland Metropolitan General Hospital. This program provided AA volunteers to do consultations in the emergency room and at the hospital bedside every evening throughout the year. The project was sponsored by 14 AA groups, which adopted 1 or 2 nights per month in the hospital [22].

Indeed, integration of self-help group members into the treatment team is not always, in our experience, easily accomplished or maintained. Staff members who are involved in self-help groups themselves may realize that their dual involvements may evoke conflicting loyalties and may have a difficult time separating appropriate behaviors for each circumstance. For many years, it was felt that AA members could not even serve as paid staff in an alcohol treatment setting because of possible violations of AA traditions, especially those regarding receiving money for AA work, anonymity, and nonaffiliation. More significantly, the problems inherent in adapting a self-help group approach to a professional setting may be difficult. For example, the AA injunction "let go and let God" may be a reasonable guideline in a self-help group, but in a hospital setting with an expectation of care, such an approach might not be appropriate. Those "two-hatters" (staff members in self-help groups) who are too narrowly focused or rigid will find it difficult or impossible to accommodate to the realities of a professional setting with its red tape, bureaucracy, paper work, accountability, and team work emphasis. On the other hand, other two-hatters will adapt sucessfully and find the treatment setting to be an opportunity to help others when they are most receptive, even if compromises must be made with external constaints [33].

Many of the same problems with reference group loyalty in professionals impact on the integration of self-help group members as volunteers or staff. While the achievement of sobriety would be a generally accepted goal, the question of what is the best way to get there might be fraught with dissention. The decision of whether the team takes a whole-person or narrower alcoholic approach, or the degree to which AA attendance must be insisted upon, are examples of potentially controversial subjects. The necessity for team members to buy into group norms is somewhat at odds with the AA tradition of cooperation but not affiliation, and there may be a need on the part of the AA to hold back a bit of the self to assure that he or she has not been coopted by the professionals. The issue of degree of membership is also a compounding problem. Are the AA members core members? [9] Or are they supportive or even temporary members? Often there is a wide discrepancy between the staff or administrative view and that of the AA volunteers or staff.

The resolution for such obstacles to teamwork lies, of course, in communication, negotiation, and compromise. A clear understanding of AA philosophy and tradition is of great help to the self-help members (who may not have studied the original traditions carefully) and to professional/administrative staff (who need to understand the sensitivities and needs of self-help group members). Special programs for recruiting and retaining the special skills of recovering Alcoholic Anonymous volunteers have worked well in hospital settings [21]. Integration into a professional team does in fact require special skills; namely, the ability to be flexible and to adapt to the needs, circumstances, and norms of the team. Not everyone has these skills, and recruitment and selection processes must be undertaken with this limitation in mind. Specialized orientation and training, with clearly defined norms and expectations, may also be of great help. Using a nonprofessional staff intermediary may help promote acceptance of accountability by AA volunteers. Such an intermediary may be a hospital alcohol services committee, a volunteer coordinator, or even a neutral administrator. Such an arrangement avoids the tension generated by AA members feeling accountable to professional staff, and when corrections have to be made, there will be much less bitterness between the AA volunteers and the professionals [21].

IX. CONCLUSIONS

A multidisciplinary team approach to the treatment of drug dependency is a concept which goes well beyond the mere presence of different disciplines. The illness itself requires specialized inputs from medicine, psychiatry, psychology, social work, nursing, self-help programs, and many more. None of these disciplines can carry the whole weight of rehabilitating the recovering patient. All must work together to accomplish this task. Yet the *way* in which they work together is critically important as well. Team members must overcome their natural reference group loyalties and competitive biases from past training and experience to work together in a cooperative fashion to facilitate the process of recovery. It is only by setting limits on individual ownership and entitlement that real team work can emerge. Such individuality if left unchecked, is destructive to team morale and functioning in the long run. Ultimately, the group process or the group conscience (as the AAs put it), will show that its wisdom is superior to that of any one individual.

REFERENCES

1. *Alcoholics Anonymous Comes of Age.* Alcoholics Anonymous Publishing, Inc., 1957.
2. Fox, R. A multidisciplinary approach to the treatment of alcoholism. *Int. J. Psychiatry 5*(1):34–44 (1968).
3. Brotman, R. Total treatment. *Int. J. Psychiatry, 5*(1):45–46 (1968).
4. Fox, R. Psychiatric aspects of alcoholism. *Am. J. Psychother. 19*:408–416 (1965).
5. O'Connor, W.J. and Morgan, D.W. Multidisciplinary treatment of alcoholism: A consultation program for team coordination. *Q. J. Stud. Alcohol, 29*(4):903–908 (1968).
6. Spratley, T.A. The practical business of treatment—1. A multidisciplinary and team approach. *Br. J. Addict., 84*(3): 259–266 (1989).
7. Twelve Steps and Twelve Traditions. Alcoholics Anonymous World Services, Inc., New York, 1953.
8. *Alcoholics Anonymous*, 3rd ed. Alcoholics Anonymous World Services, Inc., New York, 1976.
9. Francis D., and Young, D. *Improving Work Groups: A Practical Manual for Team Building.* University Associates, San Diego, 1979.
10. Rubin, I.M., Fry, R.E. and Plovnick, M.S. *Managing Human Resources in Health Care Organizations: An Applied Approach.* Reston, Virginia, Reston, 1978.
11. Rubin, I.M., and Beckard, R. Factors influencing the effectiveness of health teams. *Milbank Q. July*:317–335 (1972).
12. Hall, R. Professionalization and bureaucratization. *Am. Sociol. Rev. 33*:92–104 (1968).
13. Bennis, W. The four competencies of leadership. *Train. Dev. J. August*: 16–19 (1984).
14. Ruch, R.S. and Goodman, R. *Image at the Top: Crisis and Renaissance of Corporate Leadership.* New York, Free Press, 1983.
15. Ottenberg, D.J. The Eagleville Interdisciplinary Rehabilitation Program for Alcoholics: Lessons after two years. *Q. J. Stud. Alcohol, 30*(2):449–452 (1969).
16. Costello, R.M., Giffen, M.B., Schneider, S.L., Edgington, P.W., and Manders, K.R. Comprehensive alcohol treatment planning, implementation, and evaluation. *Int. J. Addict. 11*(4):553–570 (1976).
17. Srivastva, S. and Cooperrider, D.L. The emergence of an egalitarian organization. *Hum. Relat. 39*(8):683–724 (1968).
18. Hartwell, S. *To Act as a Unit: the Story of the Cleveland Clinic Foundation*, 1985.
19. Collins, G.B., Janesz, J.W., Byerly-Thrope, J., Forsythe, S.B., and Messina, M.J. The Cleveland Clinic Alcohol Rehabilitation Program: A treatment outcome study. *Cleve. Clin. Q. 52*:245–251 (1985).
20. Collins, G.B., Janesz, J.W., Byerly-Thrope, J., Manzeo, J. Hospital-sponsored chemical dependency self-help groups. *Hosp. Commun. Psychiatry, Dec.*:1315–1317 (1985).
21. Collins, G.B., Barth, J., and Zrimec, G.L. Recruiting and retaining volunteers in a hospital alcoholism program. *Hosp. Commun. Psychiatry,32*(2).130–132 (1981).

22. Collins, G.B. and Barth, J. Using the resources of AA in treating alcoholics in a general hospital. *Hosp. Commun. Psychiatry, 30*(7):480–482 (1979).

23. Collins, G.B., Kotz, M., Messina, M., and Ferguson, T. Alcoholism in the families of bulimic anorexics. *Cleve. Clin. Q. 52*:65–67 (1985).

24. Kotz, M., Collins, G.B., Stagno, S., Currie, K., and Zuti, R. Chemical dependency: A transplant issue. *Alcoholism Clin. Exp. Res.*, (1988).

25. Collins, G.B., Zuti, R., Brosnihan, K.B., Messina, M., Kotz, M., and Gupta, M. *Neurohormonal Response to Acute Ethanol Intake in Alcoholics*. The Endocrine Society, 69th Annual Meeting, 1987, p. 153.

26. Kurtz, L.F. Cooperation and rivalry between helping professions and members of AA. *Health Social Work, 10*(2):104–112 (1985).

27. Featherman, R.E., and Welling, M. Using volunteers in a community mental health center. *Hosp. Commun. Psychiatry, 22*:113–114 (1971).

28. Van Meulebrouck, M. and Fikany, E.O. Training program teaches volunteers to work with alcoholics. *Hosp. Commun. Psychiatry, 24*:10 (1973).

29. Slaughter, L.D., and Torno, K. Hospitalized alcoholic patients: IV. The role of patient-counselors. *Hosp. Commun. Psychiatry, 19*:209–210 (1968).

30. Covner, B.J. Screening volunteer alcoholism counselors. *Q. J. Stud. Alcohol, 30*:420–425 (1969).

31. Mack, J.E. Alcoholism, AA, and the governance of the self, *Dynamic Approaches to the Understanding and Treatment of Alcoholism* H. Bean and N. E. Zinberg eds.). New York, Free Press, 1981, pp. 128–162.

32. Emerick, R.E., Self-help groups for former patients: Relations with mental health professionals. *Hosp. Commun. Psychiatry, 41*(4): (1990).

33. *A.A. Guidelines for Members Employed in the Alcoholism Field*. From General Service Office Box 459, New York, N.Y., 10017.

XV
Emergencies

55

Drug and Alcohol Emergencies

Andrew E. Slaby
Fair Oaks Hospital, Summit, New Jersey; The Regent Hospital, and
New York University, New York, New York

Steven D. Martin
Parkview Episcopal Medical Center, Pueblo, Colorado

I. INTRODUCTION

Drug and alcohol addiction may be the primary reason for a person presenting as a psychiatric emergency, or it may accompany another psychiatric disorder obfuscating the clinical diagnosis and complicating both acute management and aftercare. The term *dual diagnosis* is used when substance abuse coexists with another psychiatric disorder. Practically speaking, there are many instances of triple, quadruple, or even more diagnoses given the reality that the abuse of one substance is often accompanied by abuse of another, and by the fact that substance abuse leads to a myriad of medical, surgical, and psychiatric problems cocaine users, for instance, often use drugs such as alcohol, barbituates, heroin, or marihuana to calm them after the stimulant "high." Intravenous heroin use may lead to cotton emboli to the lungs, hepatitis, and the acquired immune deficiency syndrome (AIDS); the latter may present as depression, phobias, panic, delirium, or dementia [1,2].

A good history and physical examination alerts clinicians to many drug emergencies, but a drug screen is needed to assure that a chemically induced psychiatric disorder is not inadvertently mistaken to be functional [3]. Symptomatic psychoses, such as those seen with phencyclidine, dextroamphetamine, and cocaine, perfectly simulate paranoid psychoses. Ideas of reference and delusions of persecution are seen with a clear sensorium.

All substance-abusing patients should be evaluated for and continued to be suspect of suicidial and homocidal ideation and risk. In one study of all admissions to an emergency department [4], it was found that 20% of those presenting to medicine and surgery and 15% to psychiatry were alcohol related. Of those admissions related to alcohol, 90% had social problems, 50% reported depression, and 25% had made a recent suicide attempt. A study of those voluntarily seeking acute care for drug and alcohol abuse indicated an overrepresentation of women, more recent onset of abuse, and a greater incidence of suicide attempts than those coerced into treatment by the courts or police [5]. Self-destructive, or other types of destructive behaviors, may be conscious or unconscious or owing to the perceptual distortions due to drug intake.

II. ALCOHOL-RELATED EMERGENCIES

The neurology and epidemiology of alcohol use disorders has always been confounded by coexistence of both psychiatric and medical disorders. The *(Diagnostic and Statistical Manual of Mental Disorders*, 3rd ed, revised, American Psychiatric Association) Washington, D.C., 1987 DSM-III-R presents the best classification to date, and serves as a guide to diagnosis as well as to direct diagnostic–specific interventions. Occult medical and surgical disorders should always be entertained. Delirium tremens may be accompanied by congestive heart failure secondary to an alcoholic cardiomyopathy and the Wernicke-Korsakoff syndrome owing to thiamine deficiency. A patient who is "stone drunk" may also be bleeding internally owing to a ruptured splen and be confused on account of an evolving subdural hematoma.

A. Alcoholic Amnestic Disorder

The alcoholic amnestic disorder (Korsakoff's syndrome) develops insidiously or acutely following an episode of delirium tremens. Differential diagnosis includes the hallucinatory dilirium associated with alcohol withdrawal. Tremors and seizures, however, are not seen with the alcohol amnestic disorder. Korsakoff's syndrome is not limited to alcoholics. Confabulation and polyneuritis is also seen in some pregnant women [1,2]. Men are more often affected than women. Prolonged alcohol use and poor dietary intake is usual.

The disorder is rare before the age of 35. Peripheral nerve damage ranges from minimum to severe. Thiamine deficiency is responsible for the core feature: short-term memory disturbance without impairment of immediate memory. The sensorium remains clear. A patient has a normal digit span, but cannot remember three objects after 20 min. This rare condition has become even more rare through prophylactic use of 50—100 mgm of thiamine and high-potency vitamin B complex preparations whenever alcoholics are seen. Prolonged alcohol use leads to malabsorption even if dietary intake is sufficient.

The irreversible memory changes that follow Wernicke's encephalopathy may be arrested by early aggressive use of thiamine.

B. Alcohol Hallucinosis

Alcohol hallucinosis is a rare disorder characterized by the development of hallucinations, usually auditory but sometimes visual, 1 or 2 weeks after cessation of a period of drinking of sufficient duration to engender dependence. The illness spares no sex or age, but it is generally seen in men between the ages of 30 and 40, and persists for weeks to years without remission. Friends or relatives may be needed to corroborate drinking history (e.g., with housewives and executives). A family history or schizophrenia is a risk factor. The sensorium remain clear and the patient is oriented. Voices may be threatening or accusatory (particularly of sexual indiscretions). Command or imperative hallucinations increase risk of suicide or homicide. Patients are often angry, fearful and litigious.

Differential diagnosis includes schizophrenia, hyperthyroidism, affective illness, and stimulant and phencyclidine (PCP) use. Hospitalization with physical restraints is necessary if a patient is violent. Sedation with a benzodiazepine (e.g. chlordiazepoxide [Librium], 20–100 mg or lorazepam [Ativan], 0.5–2 mg) or a neuroleptic (e.g., 5–10 mg of haloperidol [Haldol] or thiothixene [Navane] may be needed acutely followed by evaluation for long-acting neuroleptics such as depot Haldol or fluphenazine (Prolixin). Patients should be kept oriented and night light used. Sleep and appropriate dieting and vitamin intake must be provided. Prevention for self-destructive and other destructive behaviors is required until patients' symptoms spontaneously remit or psychopharmacotherapy is adequate.

C. Alcohol Idiosyncratic Intoxication

Some individuals behave acutely intoxicated after taking only small amounts of alcohol with serum levels less than 10–30%. Disinhibited and sometimes assaultive behavior occurs suddenly and lasts a few minutes to 24 h or more if untreated. There is amnesia for the episode after it occurs.

The onset of this disorder is generally in adolescence or the 20s. The etiology was once felt to be due to epileptic discharges evoked by alcohol use. Individuals are usually out of contact with others when aggressive and impulsive action occurs. Temporal lobe spikes are found in the electroencephalograms of a small number of those affected. In some instances, there is a history of encephalitis or trauma. Use of sedative-hypnotics, tranquillizers, fatigue, and debilitating medical illness contribute. Loss of tolerance may be temporary or permanent [2].

Untreated, episodes usually abate in a long sleep with amnesia on awakening. Benzodiazepines may be required to control assaultive behavior with protection provided for the patient and others. Physical retraints may be needed until medication is effective.

Although much is written about this phenomenon, its existence as a discrete diagnostic entity is still a matter of controversy.

D. Alcohol Intoxication

All patients who present acutely intoxicated with alcohol should be suspected of other drug ingestion and medical problems. Reaction time is slowed at 5–150 mg%. A patient acts intoxicated at 150–300 mg%. Above this problems with respiration and severe neurological complications appear. Respiratory depression and coma leading to toxic death are an extreme risk at 400–500 mg%. Serum alcohol levels in the toxic range require supportive care, gastric lavage, thiamine, and glucose [6]. If a patient has been taking Antabuse (disulfiram), intravenous ascorbic acid and monitoring of the blood pressure are usually required. Severe alcohol intoxication may be accmpanied by head injury, internal bleeding, communication problems, other drug abuse problems (corroborated by serum drug screen), and acid-base imbalance [7,8].

High alcohol levels do not preclude life-threatening medical problems. Intubation and intravenous fluids may be required until the diagnosis is clear [6,8]. Thaimine is given in all instances [9]. Restraints and benzodiazepines are required for aggressive behavior. Intravenous fluids (D50W), vitamins, and monitoring of vital signs are required if a patient is to be withdrawn from alcohol [9]. If a history of seizures exists, Dilantin (phenytoin) or Tegretal (cambamazapine) is added to the regimen [10]. In addition to a serum drug and alcohol screen, a CBC, SMA—22 and skull films are required [11] with careful attention to the anion gap [12]. The serum glucose level must be drawn before D50W is provided.

Alcohol coma, which usually sets in at serum alcohol levels of 400–500 mg% is characterized by subnormal body temperature, decreased respiratory rate, weakened pulse, stertorous breathing, decreased or absent reflexes, pale or cyanotic skin, contraction or dilation of the pupils, and incontinence or retention of urine. Serum levels of 600–800 mg% are usually fatal.

In most instances of alcohol intoxication and coma, friends or family are available to provide history of use. Sometimes a person has been challenged at such events as a fraternity party or groom's party to drink a large amount of alcohol (e.g., a quart of vodka) in a brief period of time. In such cases, there is a real threat of death from respiratory depression owing to the achievement of very high serum levels when the ability of the liver to metabolize the alcohol is taxed to a maximum. Alcohol is usually metabolized at the rate of 1 oz liquor. Symptoms generally appear as levels rise rather than when they are falling, and are present as long as 12 h after drinking. Fractures, sunburn, frostbite, subdural hematomas, automobile crashes, drowning, airplane accidents, and household and industrial accidents have been associated with drinking. More than a quarter of suicides and one-half of murders occur when a person has been drinking. Rape, incest, and spouse abuse have also been associated with drinking. Intoxicated individuals misuse prescription drugs as well as recreational drugs, further complicating the picture [1,2].

The first task in the management of alcohol intoxication is identification and treatment of medical conditions such as diabetes, acidosis, hepatic failure, AIDS, gastrointestinal bleeding, hypoglycemia, seizures, or meningitis which may be accompanying the condition. Use of sedatives, even benzodiazepines, is minimized to prevent obfuscation of the emergence or the presence of an evolving medical condition. Physical restraints and a room free of distractions is needed. Mildly intoxicated individuals sometimes respond to coffee and support. Death when it occurs is normally due to aspiration of vomitus or respiratory depression.

E. Alcohol Withdrawal Delirium

Alcohol withdrawal delirium (delirium tremens, DTs) generally occurs within 3–4 days (but may as early as 2 and as late as 10 days) after cessation or reduction of heavy alcohol use of some duration. Symptoms of alcohol withdrawal are identical to those of withdrawal of other central nervouse system depressants such as phenobarbitol, methaqualone (Quaaludes), benzodiazepines, and meprobamate [13]. Withdrawal symptoms are dose dependent. The greater the amount of alcohol ingested or the greater the addictive effects of similar acting CNS depressants taken, the greater the withdrawal symptoms. Reduction of heavy intake to 50% can cause withdrawal symptoms while drinking [14] at a lower dose. Increased CNS and hepatic tolerance due to increase liver metabolism and cross tolerance with other sedatives is found in many chronic users. The cross tolerance with barbituates has led some [15] to suggest the use of phenobarbitol for withdrawal in patients who have a probability of seizures on withdrawal.

Delirium, once it commences, may last hours to days. The mortality rate today due to complications such as hyperthermia and circulatory collapse remains as high as 15% in treated cases [16] and even greater (25–50%) in those untreated. The clinical presentation is often complicated by concurrent substance intoxication or withdrawal, the Wernicke-Korsakoff syndrome, infections, dehydration with electrolyte inbalance, hyperthermia, vascular collapse, cirrhosis, meningitis, malnutrition, cerebral lacerations, anemia, and gastritis with hematemesis. Computed tomographic (CT) scans, lumbar puncture, and skull films are recommended to identify epidural or subdural hematomas due to falls, muggings, or seizures while intoxicated or withdrawing. Concurrent physical illness predisposes a user to withdrawal delirium. Only about 5% of individuals treated for alcohol withdrawal actually develop delirium [2].

Seizures may be the first manifestation of withdrawal [13]. Alcohol use both lowers the seizure threshold directly in the CNS as well as increases the risk of seizures as the serum alcohol level falls [17,18]. The risk of seizures is increased when a patient is a chronic alcohol user [19]. Seizures tend to occur 13–48 h after cessation of alcohol use [19]. Typically, they are generalized motor seizures. In 65% of the cases there are multiple motor seizures, with 3% experiencing status epilepticus [14]. Seizures may be due to hyperventillation with decreased pCO_2 and an increased pH and decreased magnesium, or due to a direct effect on the brain. Posttraumatic seizures and meningitis are ruled out by CT scan, lumbar puncture, and skull films.

Other early symptoms of DTs are nightmares, anxiety attacks, paranoia, agitation, illusions, disorientation, vacillating levels of consciousness, tactile hallucinations, increasing psychosis, coarse tremor, speech disturbance, and tachycardia. A hyperalert agitated state is a particularly ominous sign. Patients typically have dilated pupils, are diaphorectic, restless, have elevated blood pressure, and exhibit dry lips and a coated tongue. Their heart rate is accelerated. Early in the course of alcohol withdrawal there is decreased sleep time with increased latency, increased awakening, increased REM (rapid eye movement) time, and decreased stage 4 sleep. The hallucinosis in untreated DTs can last 1–6 days. Auditory hallucinations are not as frequent as visual and tactile hallucinations. Duration of tremulousness is dependent on prewithdrawal daily alcohol use [14]. Disorientation, vacillating levels of consciousness, and short-term memory deficit characterize the cognitive changes. The time course and rapidity of onset distinguishes it from dementia. Age, brain damage, and addiction are predisposing factors [20].

Patients with impending or acute DTs are placed in a well-lit room. All procedures (e.g., restraints or blood drawing) should be explained to reduce fear. An available family member or significant other may help to calm the patient. Delirious patients should be placed to allow observation for complications (e.g., seizures and aspiration) without disturbing other patients. Mechanical restraints serve to protect patients from harming themselves or others.

Maintenance of fluid and electrolyte intake is imperative. As much as 6L of fluids may be needed, with at least 1500 ml normal saline to counter lost through profuse perspiration and agitation. Serum electrolytes, BUN, and hemotocrit are monitored to guide treatment.

Benzodiazepines are drugs of choice for alcohol withdrawal. Ativan (lorazepam) is particularly good because it can be given intramuscularly, has a short half-life, and is not metabolized by the liver. Valium (diazapam) and Librium (chlordiazepoxide) are also used, but their longer half-life and poor absorption makes them not suitable for intramuscular use. Paraldehyde, which is effective orally and rectally [14], is less commonly used because of its excretion through the lungs and the danger of nerve damage and sterile abscesses when given intramuscularly in the buttock. Chloral hydrate and alcohol itself are used in rare instances. Alcohol potentiates the sedation of other tranquillizing drugs. Management of withdrawal from more than one drug is dependent on the class of the drug. If a patient is withdrawing from alcohol and a barbituate, phenobarbitol may be used for both. Benzodiazepines are used to cover alcohol cessation prior to withdrawal for opiates in the dually addicted. When a patient has used both a sedative and an opiate, the sedative is withdrawn first.

Sedation should be liberally provided to the patient with DTs to prevent exhaustion, reduce agitation, make the patient more comfortable, and produce sleep and rest. Physicians should be aware of the danger of oversedation. Sedation may mask symptoms of an epidural or subdural hematoma. Risk is minimized if the physician reassesses the situation before each dose of medication is ordered and writes a new order at the time. The risk is greatest when intramuscular medication is provided.

The temperature is monitored with vigilence for emergence of a superimposed infection such as pneumonitis. Cooling blankets, sponge baths, and aspirin are used to keep the temperature down in the absence of infection. Appropriate antibiosis is provided for infection. Thiamine (50–200 mg intramuscularly followed by 100 mg p.o. orally b.i.d.), and multivitamins are provided to prevent progression of Wernicke's disease and other vitamin deficiency disorders. During the height of withdrawal, the pulse, blood pressure, and temperature are recorded at half-hour intervals to minimize the occurrence of delirium, circulatory collapse, and hyperthermia. Ice packs and cooling mattresses are used for hyperthermia; fluid replacement, vasopressors, and even whole blood, if required, are used to combat shock.

Grand mal, nonfocal seizures occur [19] with 3% of patients progressing to status epilepticus. Phenobarbital and phenytoin are of little value, but are both effective prophylaxis once seizures have stopped. Diazepam is used for status epilepticus. Seizures tend to recur unless a sufficient serum level of benzodiazepines is maintained because of their short half-life. The airway is controlled and precaution is taken to prevent harm when seizures occur. Seizures may be symptomatic of a traumatic bleed, mengingitis, or hypoglycemia and require assessment by skull films, CT scan, lumbar picture, and serum chemistries. Glucose is administered if the blood sugar is low [22].

All drugs used to manage alcohol withdrawal have limitations. Benzodiazepines are not always effective in severe cases. Paraldehyde is addicting, and sudden death has been reported following its use. Barbituates comparably addict and produce paradoxical excitement. Phenothiazine lower the seizure threshold and are hepatotoxic [2].

Alcohol withdrawal is a medical emergency. Once delirium tremens appears or is suspected, a patient must be hospitalized, and delirium and attendant medical problems (e.g., gastritis, cirrhosis) addressed. The mortality rate of DTs is still given at 15% [14].

F. Alcohol Jealousy

Unfortunately, patients with alcohol jealousy are less likely to be seen in emergency settings than victims of their projections and delusions. Friends and relatives of the patients are usually required to corroborate the diagnosis. The patients, usually with a long history of alcohol use, are angry, suspicious, and distrustful. The jealousy can lead to assaults, homicide, self-destructive behavior, and suicide. Affected patients accuse their wives or lovers of illicit sexual affairs with friends, strangers, children, and relatives. Wives are accused of insatiable sexual appetites. The patient finds "semen stains" on sheets, suspects showing or changing of clothes to be preparation to meet a lover, and perceive the wife or lover as being more "cold." Obviously, the ideas of reference and accusations lead to a partner's withdrawal and fear. There is often an absence of mature heterosexual relationships. The jealousy can occur in both alcohol and nonalcoholic states. Some believe the paranoia is precipitated by alcohol in individuals with a predisposition to paranoid schizophrenia and other disturbances associated with paranoia.

The prognosis is guarded. Acute administration of neuroleptics reduces symptoms, but a patient will discontinue medication because of the fear he is being controlled, leading to reemergence of delusions and violent behavior. Long-acting haloperidol and fluphenazine offer some relief.

G. Alcohol Nonpsychiatric Emergencies

There are a number of other disorders associated with chronic alcohol use that complicate the diagnosis of psychiatric illness or appear independently requiring immediate attention [21,22]. Alcohol has a direct toxic effect on the heart. Cardiomyopathy leads to low-output congestive heart failure with dyspnea and anxiety or frank aggitation, which may be misconstrued as being due to alcoholic intoxication. Sedation of someone in heart failure can lead to death by obfuscating increasing distress. Tachydysrhythmias occur but most do not require treatment [22]. Alcohol reduces alveolar macrophage activity with an increased risk of asphyxiation pneumonia, one of the causes of death with delirium tremens.

The use of alcohol is a risk factor for a number of cancers, including oral and esophageal tumors. Persistent vomiting can result in Mallory-Weiss tears and Boerhaave's syndrome. Hematemasis when it occurs may be due to gastritis, thrombocytopenia, varicosities, esophagitis, Mallory-Weiss tears, and platlet disorders with prolonged clotting times. One of the most common early problems of chronic alcohol use is fatty liver, which is usually asymptomatic. Harbingers of frank alcoholic hepatitis include elevated liver function tests, right upper quadrant pain, jaundice, leukocytosis, fever, and increased prothrombin time. Cirrhosis leads to portal hypertension, ascites, and varicosities. While all liver disease may be accompanied by neurasthenia and depressed mood, hepatic failure leads to encephnalopathy and psychosis. Impaired absorption occurs in the intestine. Acute pancreatis is seen with excessive prolonged intake [22].

Coma may be due to alcohol alone, mixed alcohol and drug use, hypoglycemia, sepsis, Wernicke's syndrome, postictal confusion, subdural hematomas, head trauma, hemorrhagic shock from gastrointestinal bleed or pancreatis, hyperthermia, hepatic encephalopathy, alcohol or lactic acidosis, and methanol or isopropyl alcohol ingestion. Computed tomographic scan and appropriate laboratory studies, including spinal tap, are indicated in instances of coma. Symmetrical neuropathies occur with sensorimotor impairment. The Wernicke-Korsakoff syndrome is characterized by ocular palsies, apathy, retrograde and anterograde amnesia, ataxia, confabulation, and nystagmus, and is treated with thiamine.

Chronic subclinical myopathy occurs [22] as well as acute rhabdomyloysis associated with myoglobinuria and muscle cramps, weakness, and tenderness. Cerebellar degeneration is a correlate of chronic alcohol use. Anemia of chronic disease occurs as well as iron deficiency anemia due to chronic blood loss. Hemolytic syndromes have also been reported, all of which may present as depression or fatigue. Impaired immunological response results in increase risk of infections and cancer. There is decreased leukocyte mobilization and decreased phagocytic activity with decreased serum bacterocidal activity and defective chemotaxis [22]. Streptococcal pneumonia, spontaneous pneumonites, and fever result.

Endocrine changes that are associated with changes in mood, cognition, and behavior include hypoglycemia, hyperurecemia, hypertriglyceridemia, and electrolyte imbalances with alterations in phosphate, magnesium, and calcium levels. Alcoholic ketosis results in a large anion gap. Twenty to 30% of patients with bipolar and unipolar affective disorders, antisocial personalities, and schizophrenia are heavy users of alcohol [2].

III. NON–ALCOHOL-RELATED DRUG EMERGENCIES

One of the paramount problems associated with drug abuse is the need to ascertain whether one is confronting drug abuse coupled with major or minor nondrug abuse disorders or confronting the myriad manifestations of polydrug abuse. Alcohol use frequently accompanies the use of cocaine. Cocaine and other stimulant ("upper") use is associated with sedative ("downer") use. Recreational drugs such as the glue used for sniffing can lead to brain damage, further complicating the picture. Cocaine causes cardiac arrythemias and myocardial infarction that may present as anxiety and panic. Judgment is decreased, which may lead to indiscriminate sexual ventures that may result in AIDS, syphilis, and assaults that may cause brain damage. Finally, major psychiatric disorders (e.g., bipolar illness) and minor (e.g., panic disorder) may drive a person to use drugs to self-medicate and to impaired judgment that results in drug use.

A. Amantadine Intoxication

Hallucinations, delirium, disorientation, and delusions are seen with abuse of the antiparkinson drug amantadine. The insidious onset of sensory changes makes recreational interest in this drug limited. Visual hallucinations associated with the use of the drug alert clinicians to the chemical basis of the symptoms. Abuse is rare but when it does occur it is often seen (as with use of other antiparkinson drugs) in patients prescribed the drug for an associated psychiatric disorder. Symptoms abate with cessation of use [2].

B. Amphetamine Intoxication and Withdrawal

Oral and intravenous use of amphetamines ("crank," "bennies," "speed," "ice", "crystal meth", "uppers") and other stimulants lead to intoxication, delirium and delusion, and in some instances violent outburts, including assaults and homicides [23–26]. Increased violence with amphetamine use (as with PCP and "crack") is attributed to the paranoid thinking, panic, emotional liability and lowered impulse control that occurs with use [24]. Abrupt cessation of amphetamine use leads to depression and in some instances suicide [2,13]. Chronic anhedonia, anergy, and stimulant craving may exist for an extended period of time due to neurotoxicity [27,28]. Vascular changes including hypertension and fibroid necrosis of the media and interna of the vessels has been reported [29,30]. Amphetamines and other stimulants are the only drugs that produce a psychosis in a clear sensorium that is indistinguishable from paranoid disorder or paranoid schizophrenia of psychogenic origin. In one study, 12 of 14 subjects given intravenous methamphetamine developed an acute psychosis [31].

Individuals presenting with psychological and behavioral manifestations of delusion with use are said to be intoxicated. Chronic use with or without increase in dosage can lead to paranoia. Fragmented thinking, dysattention, difficulty in goal-directed behavior, and confusion within 24 h of use is referred to as delirium. Symptoms of psychosis are common when the dose exceeds 90–100 mg of dextroamphetamine a day, although as little as a single dose can precipitate a panic state in someone predisposed. Paranoia tends to fluctuate with amount of drug taken. A myriad of other psychological symptoms occur with acute intoxication: impaired judgment, disinhibition, stereotype, activation, hypersexuality, and impulsivity [28], hallucinations in a clear sensorium, and a less profound thought disorder than with schizophrenia [32]. Physiological symptoms occurring concommitently are those of sympathetic arousal: increased blood pressure and heart rate, hyperthermia, increased respiratory rate and pupillary size, and tremor. In the extreme, there is a pseudocatatonic picture [30].

The clinical picture of a sympathomimetic psychosis is produced by cocaine and a number of amphetaminelike drugs. These include, in addition to amphetamines themselves, dextroamphetamine, metamphetamine, and substances differing from substituted phenylethyamine that have amphetaminelike actions such as methylphenidate and a variety of diet pills. Intoxication usually begins within 24 h of intake. A prolonged high or moderate dose use is required for the development of a delusional state. Intravenous use leads to almost immediate symptom development. When delusional symptoms develop after a single dose, one should think of an underlying paranoid disorder or paranoid schizophrenia. Use of other drugs such as sedatives, hallucinogens, and "designer" drugs may complicate the clinical picture and complicate management of withdrawal, especially with CNS depressant use cessation and delirium tremens with its risk of mortality. Heroin in combination with cocaine or amphetamines is called a "speedball" or "croak." Some people use heroin alone to bring themselves "down."

The clinical presentation of cocaine and amphetamine intoxication is indentical. The distinguishing feature is that symptoms due to cocaine are transient unless there is other psychopathology. Symptoms due to amphetamines can persist long beyond the time of use. All drug toxic states represent an interaction of a patient's premorbid psychological and physical condition, the environment in which the substance is taken, the dose and duration of drug intake, and the quantity and kind of other drugs taken. Symptoms of amphetamine intoxication and delirium (with dysattention and vacillating levels of consciousness) generally abate within 6 h of cessation of use. The delusional disorder may last as long as a year, but it is generally gone within a week. Attention is usually maintained and delusions are the principal symptom. Serum and urine screens for amphetamines and other drugs corroborate the diagnosis.

Untreated amphetamine psychosis subsides in 2–3 days after cessation of use it the abuser does not suicide. Visual hallucinations tend to persist for 24–48 h; delusions last for a week or 10 days. Delusions in an attenuated form may continue for as long as year. Users generally "crash," sleeping as long as 18–20 h per day for 2–3 days and experience a depression that can reach suicidal proportions and endure for weeks, requiring antidepressants or electroshock therapy if the magnitude and acute intensity of suicidal behavior dictates. More apathy, fatigue, and flattening of affect is seen than with endogenous depression. Acutely, restraints and sedation may be required if the patient acts out violently. A quiet room, reassurance, and efforts to keep the patient calm coupled with 2–5 mg t.i.d. of haloperidol or thiothixine is usually sufficient to manage even the most delusional patients [12,13,16,32,33]. Frequently, no medication or a benzodiazepine such as diazepam [11] is sufficient. If a patient has ingested significant amounts of drugs with antiecholinergic effect in addition to the stimulant, diazepam or lorazepam is used instead of an antipsychotic. With severe intoxication (accompanied by hyperthermia, seizures, hypertension, and tachycardia), anticonvulsants, cooling with a cooling blanket or ice packs, gastric lavage, intravenous fluids, and antihypertensive medication are required on a medical unit [30].

Withdrawal symptoms generally commence with 3 days of cessation of use of amphetamines, with a peak within 2–4 days. A paranoid confusional psychosis with the same features as seen with intoxication may appear, although the more usual picture is that of depression or irritability that lasts weeks to months, sometimes necessitating the use of antidepressants or electroconvulsive therapy (ECT). Psychiatric symptoms require neuroleptics if they are particularly distressing such as 2–5 mg b.i.d. or t.i.d. of haloperidol or thiothixene, or 2–4 mg b.i.d. or t.i.d of perphenazine or fluphenazine. The changes in mood, thought and behavior are due to alterations in dopamine metabolism. Suicide is a major concern, necessitating precautionary measures involving hospitalization if necessary. Antidepressants are gradually decreased over days as symptoms remit. Antidepressants may be required for months if depression is severe.

There is no need to taper the amphetamine dose. It may be discontinued abruptly. Patients should be allowed to sleep. Fatigue, apathy, and hypersomnia are characteristic of sympathomimetic withdrawal. If there is a history of chronic drug abuse, Narcotics Anonymous (NA), Cocaine Anonymous (CA), or Alcoholics Anonymous (AA) are the treatments of choice in addition to whatever inpatient or outpatient medical and/or psychiatric treatment is required. In instances of dual diagnosis (e.g., amphetamine addiction and anorexia nervosa), diagnostic- specific treatment is indicated. Periodic urine screens are necessary for repeated abusers. Even when sympathomimetic substances are prescribed for attention deficit hyperactivity disorder, narcolepsy, and enhancement of antidepressant therapy, withdrawal symptoms may be seen on cessation of use.

C. Angel's Trumpet Intoxication

Patura savvealens (Angel's trumpet), a poisonous plant that grows wild in Southeastern and Gulf states, can be eaten or brewed in tea to produce a central nervous system anticholinergic syndrome of appeal to halllucinogen users. Scopolamine (hyoscine) and, to a lesser degree, atropine and hyosyamine produce the toxic state. Those who have inadvertently ingested the derivatives of the plant or sought it for its hallucinogenic properties experience strong symptoms of an anticholinergic psychosis: widened pulse pressure; dry, hot, and flushed skin; confusion; visual hallucination; agitation; dysmnesia; clouding of the sensorium; and in the extreme conditions, paralysis and death. The skin is flushed because of dilation of the cutaneous vessels. Fever is due to inhibition of sweating and to the hyperthermic response. Scopolamine, in addition, increases the basal metabolic rate.

Supportive measures and protection from harm to self and others is provided where needed, coupled with gastric lavage and physostigmine (1–4 mg intramuscularly) in extreme cases to reverse the effects of alkaloids. Antipsychotics are not given because their own anticholinergic properties enhance rather than diminish symptoms. Alpha-blocking activity can precipitate cardiovascular collapse and death [2].

D. Anticholinergic Intoxication

Signs and symptoms of an atropine psychosis are a result of the parasympathetic blockade seen with ingestion of hyoscine, stramonium, thorn apple pods, hyosyamine, jimsom weed, belladonna, scopolamine, and henbane taken recreationally, medicinally, or inadvertently. Scopolamine is found in some antitussives. Over-the-counter sedatives, eye-drop preparations, antispasmotics, and nonprescription asthma preparations may contain atropine and scopolamine, and in the last mentioned, belladonna and stramonium [2]. Tricyclics, neuroleptics, benztropine (Cogentin), antihistamines, and hypnotics such as glutethimide have anticholinergic properties. Symptoms occur with intranasal use and with a few eye drops (especially in the very young and very old). Laboratories do not tend to screen for anticholinergics unless specifically requested to do so. The rapid rate of excretion requires immediate sampling of serum and urine. Belladonna alkaloids are rapidly absorbed from the gastrointestinal tract and distributed throughout the body, with most being excreted in the urine within 12 h of ingestion. Untreated symptoms tend to abate in 24 h. Xerostoma and dryness of other mucus membranes, hoarseness, increased thirst, restlessness, disorientation, dry hot skin, rapid weak pulse, hyperthermia, and widely dilated inactive pupils are seen. There is difficulty urinating, dysphagia, burning of the eyes and throat and stangury. Visual hallucinations without perceptual distortion and double vision is experienced. Dysattention, dysmnesia, loquaciousness, flushed skin, and body-image distortion also occur. Blood pressure is normal or decreased. Scopolamine intoxication differs from atropine toxicity by presence of a slow pulse, the presence of the Babinski sign, lack of skin flushing, and lethargy and somnolence due to central nervous depression rather than excitement.

Patients scopolomine intoxication are provided water, moistening of the mucus membranes (including use of artifical tears if needed), and catherization if necessary. Gastric lavage is performed after oral ingestion. Mild stimulation with caffeine or amphetamine counters scopolomine-induced CNS depression. Artificial respiration is required if breathing is failing or inadequate. Methacholine and pilocarpine relieve peripheral symptoms. Coma and anticholenergic delirium are reversed by the anticholinesterase physostigmine. There are reports of asystole with the use of physostigmine, so its use should be restricted to extreme cases of need. Unlike neostigmine, this drug crosses the blood-brain barrier, thereby reversing both peripheral and central blockade. One to 3 mg of physostigmine intramuscularly or intravenously reverses CNS toxicity by inhibiting the destructive action of cholinesterase, prolonging and exaggerating the action of acetycholine. Physostigmine is completely broken down in the body within 1.5–2.0 h, requiring an additional 0.5–2 mg i.m. or i.v. at that time if symptoms persist. Minor tranquilizers such as alprazolam (Xanax) (1–4 mg) and lorazepam (Ativan) (1–4 mg) are prescribed for agitation if there is no chronic pulmonary disease. Neuroleptics enhance the symptoms because of their anticholinergic properties [1,2].

E. Barbiturate Intoxication and Withdrawal Disorders

Hypnotics, barbiturates, benzodiazepines, and similar acting drugs can cause serious behavioral disturbances when taken in excess (and even at therapeutic and subtherapeutic doses in some individuals) and upon abrupt withdrawal after prolonged use at moderate to large doses [1,2]. Sedative-hypnotics include chloral hydrate, paraldehyde, meprobamate, methyprylon, glutathimide, methaqualone, and ethchlorvynol. The short-acting barbiturates are the most frequently abused and include secobarbital, amobarbital, and pentobarbital. Phenobarbital addiction is rare. Benzodiazepines include alprazolam, chorazepam, chlordiazepoxide, diazepam, flurazepam, oxazepam, and triazepam. Prolonged usage of benzodiazepines is required to produce the sedative withdrawal syndrome. Severe overdose and withdrawal is always a medical emergency [1,2,34,35].

It is difficult to get a good history of sedative-hypnotic abuse. Individuals with a well-cultivated social demeanor can overtly or unconsciously be quite deceptive about their drug use, with the result that the sudden emergence of psychosis at the time of hospitalization for traumatic injury may be the first evidence of a sedative-hypnotic, alcohol, or combined sedative-hypnotic/alcohol problem. Untreated, withdrawal can be fatal and is indistinguishable from delirium tremens of alcohol withdrawal. Urine and serum screens confirm the diagnosis.

The absorption, metabolism, and distribution rates of the various barbiturates, benzodiazepines, and sedative-hypnotics vary, but the signs and symptoms of intoxication and withdrawal are comparable. Duration of use, individual susceptibility, and particular drug used determine the duration of withdrawal and the severity of symptoms. Pentobarbital and secobarbital users of 400 mg or less for 3–12 months are unlikely to experience withdrawal. Users of 600 mg/day for 3–4 weeks may experience minor withdrawal symptoms: tremor, weakness, anxiety, nausea, vomiting, and involuntary twitching. Similar symptoms will be seen upon cessation of the use of greater than 60 mg/day of diazepam [36]. Abrupt withdrawal of 800 mg or more of pentobarbital or secobarbital leads, in addition, to life-threatening delirium and grand mal seizures [37,38]. Other symptoms of withdrawal include sleep disturbance, malaise, dysattention, depression, hallucinations, confusion, formication, and headaches. Reflexes are hyperactive, and the heart rate is increased. The patient is hyperpyrexic and sweats. The blood pressure is elevated, but the patient experiences postural hypotension, blepharospasm, coarse tremor of the tongue and eyelids, and psychomotor agitation or excitement is also seen. Delusions generally commence with 1 week of cessation of use [39].

Essential symptoms seen with hypnotic/sedative/benzodiazepine withdrawal are similar to those of alcohol withdrawal with the exception that coarse tremor is more common with alcohol withdrawal. Similarly, intoxication symptoms resemble those of alcohol intoxication. Paradoxical disinhibition is seen, particularly in the elderly, who may also present with psychotic symptoms when intoxicated [21]. In spite of the fact that tolerance develops to the sedative-hypnotic effects of barbiturates, the lethal dose is not *significantly* increased, so that acute intoxication can be superimposed on chronic intoxication [37]. When alcohol and barbituate intoxication occur concurrently, as is often the case, it is difficult if not impossible to determine which symptoms are due to alcohol and which are due to barbiturates or similar acting drugs. Although disinhibition is seen early, inhibition occurs as the quantity of the drug taken increases.

Intentional overdose and inadvertent overdose with these drugs occurs. Sedative-hypnotics, barbiturates, and benzodiazepines are commonly taken by depressed people in suicide gestures and attempts. The usual time this occurs is late afternoon [40]. Drug paroxysm is a particular risk in older people. In such cases, a person forgets he or she has taken a dose and persists until a near lethal or lethal dose is achieved. Characteristics of overdose include respiratory depression, hypotension, isoelectric EEG, flaccid coma of varying depths, gastrointestinal paralysis, vesicles and bullae on the skin, hyperthermia, lack of pupillary response, and pneumonia [41,42]. Death results from respiratory depression. Glutethimide coma is comparable to that of barbiturates with the exception that it is longer with variations in depth owing to the accumulation of the active metabolite [43], and there is less respiratory depression. The pupils are widely dilated, and there is an increase in frequency of hypotension [39]. Administration of naloxine or another opioid antagonist [44,45] parenthetically distinguishes severe barbituate intoxication with depression from opioid intoxication. Opioid antagonists do not impact intoxication of other drugs [1,2].

When a patient presents loquacious and ataxic with slurred speech, irritability, labile mood, feeling in a dreamlike state, and uninhibited sexual and agressive behavior, barbituate of a similar acting drug intoxication should be suspected. Serum and urine screens coupled with the history and the use of the barbiturate tolerance test [46] allow one to estimate the amount taken and to determine what is required for withdrawal. The process of withdrawal once commenced is slow and usually involves a short-acting barbiturate to allow better control over the half-life. Phenobarbital, when it is used [47], is chosen because its longer duration of action produces less fluctuation in barbiturate levels, producing protection against withdrawal symptoms. It does not produce the highs seen with shorter-acting barbiturates.

If one is using phenobarbital for withdrawal after the daily dose is estimated using a shorter-acting drug [36,38], the amount of phenobarbital to be administered is calculated substituting 30 mg of phenobarbital for each 100 mg of the short-acting barbituate. Withdrawal begins after 2 days on this dose. If there has been an overestimation of the amount to be taken, slurred speech, ataxia, and other signs of toxicity appear. If withdrawal symptoms emerge, 200 mg of pentobarbital is given and the amount of phenobarbital increased. Upon stabilization, the dose is reduced by 30 mg daily as long as there are no remarkable withdrawal symptoms. The dose is given in four divided amounts to allow more careful monitoring of withdrawal symptoms. When there is no sign of withdrawal, one of the four doses may be omitted.

Flexibility is greater with the use of short-acting drugs like secobarbital or pentobarbital whose action is limited to about 4 hs. Again, the initial dose is estimated by the history and the barbiturate tolerance test. Consideration must be given to other drugs used with mixed addictions. For instance, 100 mg of pentobarbital is equivalent for withdrawal purposes to 3– 4 oz of spirits. Comparably, 400 mg of meprobamate is equivalent to 100 mg of pentobarbital. The daily dose is administered in four amounts, with omission of one of the doses if intoxication occurs. If withdrawal symptoms emerge, 100–200 mg of pentobarbital may be given until intoxication occurs. The dose is then reduced by 100 mg until there is evidence of withdrawal. The bedtime dosage is the last to be eliminated. The danger of severe medical complications with withdrawal (e.g., status epilepticus) requires inpatient treatment for withdrawal. After the process is completed, psychotherapy to elicit the reasons for drug addiction and a drug rehabilitation program are necessary to prevent readdiction.

Major overdose in suicide attempts requires admission to a medical intensive care unit where supportive measures are coupled with efforts to prevent further drug absorption through gastric emptying and the use of activated charcoal. Elimination is enhanced through alkalization of the urine [42] and diuretics [41]. Hypothermia is treated with external and internal warming [42]. Chest x-rays are required to detect an evolving pneumonia.

F. Benzodiazepine Withdrawal and Intoxication

Withdrawal and intoxication symptoms have been well-documented with the use of both short- and long-acting benzodiazepines, as mentioned in the previous sections. Symptoms appear even when these drugs have been administered at therapeutic doses for a long period of time. Symptoms of withdrawal are relieved with reintroduction of the drug that was abruptly discontinued [1,2]. Symptoms persist for days or weeks and even months after withdrawal because of slow elimination of active metabolites. Long-acting benzodiazepines such as flurazepam (half-life 47–100 h) and diazepam (half-life 26–96 h) are eliminated over a week or more, whereas short-acting benzodiazepines such as oxazepam (half-life 7–20 h) and lorazepam (half-life 10–20 h) are rapidly eliminated over 2 days. The rapid decline in plasma levels of drugs such as alprazalam and the other short-acting benzodiazepines leads to greater severity in symptoms upon cessation of use.

Withdrawal is milder with benzodiazepines with half-lives greater than 36 h, which appear to have a built-in tapering mechanism. Rebound insomnia is common with as little as a single dose of a short-acting benzodiazepine over a short period of time. Discontinuation of longer-acting benzodiazepines used for sleep is not associated with worsening of sleep duration. Symptoms of withdrawal of benzodiazepines increase and then decrease after withdrawal. If symptoms persist, and in fact worsen, underlying affective illness or an anxiety disorder should be suspected [1,2].

G. Caffeine Intoxication

Caffeine intoxication (caffeinism) is characterized by actue or chronic anxiety, insomnia, restlessness, palpitations, tachycardia, tachypnea, diuresis, diarrhea, irritability, nausea, and epigastric pain. Extrasystoles and other cardiac arrhythmias, muscle twitching, and hyperesthesia are also seen. Ringing in the ears has been reported, and sometimes flushing of the skin occurs. Caffeinism is in the differential diagnosis of anxiety disorders, mania, delirium, and depression. In addition to coffee, substances containing caffeine such as various over-the-counter analgesics, stimulants, cold preparations, and prescription drugs as well as tea and cola drinks contribute to symptom formation. As little as one cup of brewed coffee may cause the reaction. Ironically, some depressed people with sleep problems drink coffee in the middle of the night, enhancing the sleep problems and furthering the development of an anxiety component of the primary affective illness. A single cup of brewed coffee contains 100–150 mg of caffeine. Doses in excess of 1000 mg (seven to 10 cups of coffee) result in muscle twitching, cardiac arhythmias, and psychomotor excitement. Increased amounts leads to tinnitis. In the extreme (10 gm or more), grand mal seizures and death from respiratory failure may occur. The absence of sleep improvement with the administration of adequate antidepressant may be due to the use of coffee in the mid-afternoon or evening [1,2].

Management of caffeine intoxication entails cessation or reduction in the intake of coffee and other caffeine-containing compounds. This may be difficult because of withdrawal symptoms such as fatigue, irritability, dysphoria, inability to work effectively, headache, nervousness, and depression. Benzodiazepines may be needed to treat an acute episode of anxiety. Symptoms pass within 24–48 h of cessation of the use of caffeine-containing substances.

H. Cannabis Intoxication

Cannabis (marijuana) in all its forms (thetrahydrocannabinal [THC] and hashish) is usually smoked, but it may be taken in pill form as pure THC or eaten in brownies and other preparations. Proffered under a number of appellations (e.g., "MJ", "pot," "grass," "dope," "bhang", "Mary Jane," "reefer"), the use of cannabis varies from experimentation a few times to chronic daily use for years. Some users report being drugged daily from age 9 or 10 through their 20s! Obviously, heavy drug use during the developmental stages can lead to a distortion of the personality, which in the extreme become relatively enduring personality disorders such as borderline personality and narcissistic character disorders. Symptoms relate to set (expectations as to what should happen), setting (a conventional setting as opposed to a disco with incense, strobe lights, dry ice, and heavy metal music), personality (e.g., obsessive-compulsive vs histrionic), and dose (hashish soaked in opiate vs "grass" that is literally mostly grass). Most marijuana smokers, like alcohol users, are occasional users with only mild to moderate reactions that are either pleasurable or not sufficiently disabling to cause the need for medical assistance. There is no physiological dependence and, therefore, in the strictest sense of the word, addiction does not occur. There are no withdrawal symptoms.

Symptoms characteristic of cannabis intoxication include disinhibition, euphoria, silliness with laughter, a sensation of flowing of time, increased appetite, suggestibility, lightheadedness, impaired judgment, a sensation of floating, and enhanced sensuality. Distressing symptoms in those predisposed include derealization, depersonalization, paranoia, free-floating and panic anxiety, incoherence, dysmnesia, disorientation, altered reality testing, fears of dying, illusion, depression, and suicidal thoughts. Rarely a person feels he or she is going crazy and experiences hallucinations and delusions. The pupils are not changed in size, but the conjunctivae are injected. The mouth is dry and tachycardia may occur. Intoxication occurs immediately after smoking, which, of course, is also the case with crack or pencylidine (PCP). The latter may be surreptiously sold as marijuana to introduce the unsuspecting to a new more powerful and addicting drug. Symptoms peak in 0.5 h and disappear nearly entirely within 3 h if no more is taken. Oral use leads to a slower and lower peak level with symptoms of duration of about 6 h. The sweet smell of cannabis may be on the patient's clothing. Presentation in the emergency room may follow such trauma as industrial, automobile, motorcycle, or airplane accidents due to impairment of concentration and judgment from the drug [1,2].

Clinicians must use serum screens to distinguish cannabis symptoms from those of cocaine derivatives, stimulants, alcohol, and hallucinogens. If the premorbid personality was stable and drug screens show only cannabis derivatives and no concurrent physical illness is present, symptoms may be attributed to marijuana intoxication. In other instances in which a person is chronically psychotic or undergoing a schizophrenic deterioration, the drug may have been taken to help organize the internal chaos, to seek insight, or to be accepted by a deviant drug-impaired subculture. If there is a family history of psychiatric illness, marijuana may be the sufficient stress to evoke a latent psychiatric disorder.

Suicidal or homicidal precautions must be instituted if evaluation proves the need. Concurrent psychiatric and medical disorders must be identified and documented. Most patients can be "talked down" from a cannabis high in a supportive safe atmosphere with or without addition of benzodiazepines (e.g., alprazolam, lorazepan) to reduce panic. Psychiatric symptoms require a neuroleptic such as haloperidol or thiothixine, 5–10 mg. These drugs are discontinued as soon as it appears they are no longer needed (usually in 1 or 2 days). A person should be seen in follow-up to ascertain whether the symptoms of cannabis intoxication have fully remitted. If symptoms continue, another process is suggested if no further drug use has occurred. Flashbacks occur less frequently with cannabis than with hallucinogens, but are treated similarly (i.e., benzodiazepines for anxiety; neuroleptics for psychotic symptoms).

I. Clonidine Withdrawal

The emergence of psychiatric symptoms has been reported upon withdrawal of the imidazoline antihypertensive clonidine hydrochloride [1,2], used alone or in combination with naltrexone hydrochloride to suppress the signs and symptoms of opiate withdrawal, when it has been prescribed as an antipsychotic for manic and schizophrenic patients, or when it has been abruptly discontinued when prescribed for hypertension. Frank violence has been seen when clonidine has been withdrawn from psychiatric patients. Anxiety and irritability are more common symptoms. The mechanism for induction of psychiatric symptoms is unclear.

Gradual withdrawal of clonidine minimizes violence and anxiety. Neuroleptics are used acutely if needed, but the symptoms of clonidine withdrawal abate with time. Safety precautions are required if a patient is violent.

J. Cocaine Intoxication and Withdrawal

Cocaine is a drug associated with a myriad of psychiatric medical and surgical problems. The good news is the fact that this once fashionable drug of those in the "fast lane," intellectuals, artists, politicians, and the power elite has lost its popularity as those who passively or actively once supported its use has either experienced addiction themselves, or have seen their friends or family members become addicted and even die. The bad news is that never before in history have so many young people been involved with the production, distribution, and use of a cocaine derivative. Crack houses and crack wars blight our cities and are a source of millions of dollars in revenue for enterprising, but ruthless entrepreneurs, who capitalize on the fact that the unsuspecting use of this potent agent leads to addiction, robbery, assaults, suicide, and homicide.

Crack is inexpensive and readily available. Smoked alone or mixed with marijuana, it impacts in seconds to minutes. The immediate sensation is described by many as a constant orgasm. Many experienced users when asked whether they prefer sex or cocaine respond: "Doctor, you are very naive. Sex lasts seconds, cocaine highs can last hours." Indeed, they can. Afterward, however, comes the crash with or without the ravages of psychiatric and medical complications. Crack is so addicting because the high is so great and the crash so severe. Users will sometimes do literally anything to avoid crashing. Adolescents murder. Lawyers, doctors, and stockbrokers sell wives' and lovers' jewelry. Adolescents sell grand-parents' rare silver. And young men and women sell themselves as hetero- and homosexual prostitutes.

Cocaine is generally sold as crystalline flakes or powder ("snow") or as a gummy residue ("bazoka"). The usual route of use is intranasally ("snorting") or smoking ("free-basing" or "roach"). Once popular, intradermal use ("skin popping") has diminished in frequency owing to the ascent of smoking as the favored mode of use, and to the fact it is associated with necrotic skin lesions. Application of cocaine to the mucous membrane of the mouth is known as "freezing." The arm veins or the internal jugular (accessed in the "pocket" above the clavicle) are the most common areas of intravascular administration. Cocaine is also taken in the eye, the rectum, and the vagina. It is placed inside the penis to delay ejaculation by inhibition of sensation. Prolonged nasal use results in perforation of the nasal septum. In some instances, a white powdery substance is found in the nose.

Valsalva maneuvers [49] (e.g., at stool) after smoking can lead to alveolar rupture [50]. Pneumothorax and reduction in the carbon monoxide diffusion capacity are also seen [48,51–55]. Over time, the entire nasal septal (bony and cartilagenous structures) necroses. A saddle nose deformity and osteolytic sinusitis appears [56,57]. In addition to snorting, the use of sympathomimetic nasal sprays to combat rebound nasal congestion contributes to the symptom picture. Tracheobronchial rupture results in subcutaneous emphysema, pneumomediastinum, and pneumocardium [50,56,58].

Cocaine intoxication resembles amphetamine and other sympathomimetic intoxication states. As with all drug states, clinical presentation represents an interaction of the patient's personality, genetic endowment, the enviornment in which the drug is taken, concurrent psychiatric and medical illnesses (including, in this instance, those caused by cocaine use), dose of cocaine, route of administration, and kind and quantity of other drugs taken [2].

Onset is more rapid than with amphetamines. If snorted, the symptoms cocaine intoxica-tion begin within minutes and are usually gone within hours. Effects may be brief or last hours if cocaine is taken intravenously. Depression, fatigue, anxiety, irritability, and tremulousness appear within 1 h of cessation of cocaine use. Heroin and cocaine taken together is referred to as a "speedball."

Euphoria is the most common affectual response to cocaine followed by hypomania, dysphoria, and paranoia with overtly violent behavior, including homicide. Formication (tactile hallucinations of insects crawling under the skin) may lead to excavations of the skin with bleeding and infection [59,60]. This sensation is referred to as "cocaine bugs." Other symptoms of a cocaine psychosis [61] include sleep disturbance, loose associations, delusions and ideas of reference, auditory and visual hallucinations ("snow lights" resembling migraine headaches), anorexia, impaired judgment, and confusion. There is a feeling of immunity to fatigue and great muscle power. The pupils are dilated and the patient, diaphorectic. The skin is pale, the temperature and blood pressure are elevated, and the patient appears haggard and tremulous. The intake of large doses of cocaine over a brief period of time leads to seizures and death from hyperthermia, cardiac arrhythmias, or respiratory paralysis.

Myocardial infarctions and sudden death have been reported to be associated with cocaine use in young people without a history of arteriosclerotic vascular disease by angiography or at autopsy [48,62]. Ischemia without infarction leads to chest pain and arrhythmias [55,63,64]. The sympathomimetic action of cocaine upon the heart is believed to be responsible for these arrhythmias, which include sinus tachycardias and ventricular tachycardia, fibrillation, and asystoyle [63]. Cocaine-induced systolic hypertension causes rupture of the ascending aorta [63,65]. Cocaine-induced heart attacks are both due to the direct action of a sympathomimetic substance on the heart causing electrical arrythmias as well as by spasm leading to thrombosis in infarction. Both events can occur in the very young without any underlying heart disease [63,65,66–74]. Intravenous use of cocaine can lead to pulmonary edema [75]. Subarachnoid hemorrhage has been reported with only snorting cocaine [29,76,77]. Those with berry aneurysms and arteriovenus malformations are at particular risk [63,78].

Since the use of cocaine is greatest among the young, a number of obstetrical and gynecological problems have been reported in young women users in addition to whatever impact cocaine has on the developing fetus. Abruptio placentae occurs with large retroplacental clots secondary to acute hypertension [63] and increased risk of spontaneous abortion [79–81]. In addition, perinatal cerebral infarction has been seen in an infant delivered of a mother intoxicated with cocaine [80]. In this instance, the child's urine was also positive for the drug.

Cocaine is seldom taken orally, but when it is it has been reported as being as effective as nasal cocaine, although onset of action may be longer [63]. The danger of oral ingestion of cocaine is ischemia with subsequent infarction of the bowel or gangrene due to alpha-adenergic stimulation and vasoconstriction [82]. Massive oral overdose of cocaine occurs with "body packing" (i.e., transportation of cocaine by swallowing packet of the drug often fashioned with a condom). When the packet ruptures, massive amounts of the drug are absorbed. The individual may seize [71]. The symptoms of intoxication occur, and include tachycardia, diaphoresis, agitation, hypertension, delirium, and hallucinations [83]. Ultimately, the patient dies of cardiopulmonary arrest and cardiac arrhythmias [84,85]. Extreme hyperthermia is also seen, and this is attributed to resetting of the hypothalamic heat center and to vasoconstriction [86]. Most of the packets (usually composed of cellophane and latex) used to smuggle cocaine pass uneventually [87].

Other complications seen with cocaine addiction include fungal cerebritis due to a diminished immune response (seen more with intravenous users) [63], hyperglycemia, interference with antihypertensives, hepatitis septicemia, acquired immune deficiency syndrome (AIDS), wound botulism, and bruxism [54].

Cocaine intoxication is usually self-limited to 24 h. There are no major withdrawal symptoms, but there is some depression and craving. During the immediate hours and days pursuant to cessation, depression and irritability are great with a concurrent intense desire to recommence drug use. This may be even greater if the individual was using the medication to self-medicate an affective disorder [1]. In addition in predisposed individuals, a psychosis (e.g., schizophrenia) may be precipitated that may require extended evaluation and management, particularly if symptoms are recurrent and chronic care necessitated. Neuroleptics such as haloperidol and thiothixine will mollify psychotic symptoms both due to cocaine intoxication as well as to schizophrenia. Antipsychotics with strong anticholinergic properties will tend to lower the blood pressure. Neuroleptics interestingly reduce paranoia without impacting on experienced euphoria [27]. If an anticholinergic drug has been taken with the cocaine, a benzodiazepine should be given (e.g., 0.5–4.0 mg of lorazepam) for psychomotor excitement. Most antipsychotics have anticholinergic properties.

Ingestion of large doses of cocaine results in chest pain, syncope, tremulousness, delirium, and seizures with a temporal lobe discharge pattern. Death results from respiratory paralysis or cardiac arrythmias. Treatment is supportive. Diazepam is given for seizures as anticonvulsants are not effective [63].

Intravenous barbiturates can enhance respiratory depression and, therefore, are somewhat dangerous to give in cocaine intoxication. Hyperthermia can be a severe problem and requires cooling with cooling blankets, ice and other measures [88–91]. Chlorpromazine also appears to help [57,86,88,92]. Intravenous fluids and respiratory support are also required. Laboratory studies are required to indentify concurrent and evolving medical problems as well as concurrent drug use. Naloxone (Narcon) should be provided immediately after blood have been drawn for studies to reverse opiate toxicity [13]. Breathing must be monitored and assistance provided when indicated [11] because heroin and other substances are often taken to temper the cocaine high. The use of propranolol in the treatment of acute cocaine intoxication is controversial [93,94]. While the heart rate is decreased, blood pressure may increase due to imposed alpha stimulation with beta blocking [95]. Labetalol has been used for both alpha and beta blocking. Calcium channel blockers appear to be an antidote to the cardiac effects of cocaine intoxication [96].

K. Hallucinogenic Intoxication and Flashbacks

In addition to the drugs already mentioned in dedicated sections (e.g., anticholhergic drugs), a number of drugs are taken specifically for their perceptual changing action. These drugs, the hallucinogens, include lysergic acid diethylamide (LSD), mescaline, psilocybin (mushrooms), peyote (cactus buttons), dimethyltryptamine (DMT), phencyclidine (PCP) [2,5] and dimethoxy-4-ethyl-amphetamine (STP). Typical alterations in mood and sensation include intense panic, intensification of colors, paranoia, intense loneliness, depersonalization and derealization, visual illusions, synesthesias, paresthesias, and depression at times to suicidal proportions. The pupils are frequently dilated with LSD. Time-limited recurrences of these symptoms days or months after hallucinogen use are referred to as "flashbacks." These generally only last minutes. When longer they can be quite frightening, and they can be confused with the micropsychotic episodes of borderline personalities. The etiology of flashbacks is a subject of controversy. These occur after one or several uses of the drug.

Support alone will suffice if symptom intensity is not such as to require medication or protection from self-destructive or other destructive behavior. In most instances, if pharmacotherapy is required, anxiolytics are appropriate, as it is panic associated with perceptual distortions that is disabling, not the actual changes themselves. If, for instance, someone is intoxicated with alcohol, he or she sleeps it off and generally awakens with a "hangover" and some modicum of remorse. They do not, however, require medication save perhaps aspirins for headache, nor do they require psychiatric help unless they are alcohol dependent of self-medicating a mood or anxiety disorder. Patients in continued treatment should be monitored for recurrence of drug use if new psychiatric symptoms emerge or chronic ones do not abate. If the same person voluntarily takes or has been "slipped" a hallucinogen, and the people about him or her begin melting into the floor, that person would panic and require a drug such as lorazepam (Ativan) or alprazolam (Xanax) if they could not be talked down. A Southwestern United States Native American on the other hand who uses cactus buttons (peyote) or mushrooms (psilocyin) in a religious ceremony does not respond negatively to the alterations in perception and mood. The changes are expected and familiar [1,2].

If the symptoms of hallucinogen intoxication or flashback achieve psychotic proportions, a neuroleptic may be required. The danger to using such is twofold. The anticholinergic properties may act synergistically to enhance hallucinogen intensity. Secondly, the atropinlike properties may act to increase the risk of a cardiac arrhthymia or blood pressure problems. Drugs are mixed and a hallucinogen may be taken coupled with a more potent agent such as "croack" (a sandwich of crack and heroin), requiring special vigilence for cardiovascular and respiratory problems [12,97–98]. Naloxone is required for opiate intoxication [11]. Uncomplicated flashbacks are self-limited, lasting only minutes to (rarely) hours. After treatment, the patient is advised to avoid all further hallucinogenic use, including that of marijuana. If flashbacks persist and/or intensify in severity or frequency, evaluation for other pathology such as schizophrenia should be undertaken, and if found to be present, treated [1,2,16,32].

L. Meperidine Toxicity

Meperidine (Demerol) addiction tends to be limited to health professionals, pharmacists, and those with ready access to a supply. Street sale is limited by supply. Agitation and confusion occur with elevated serum levels, which occur if the amount is increased or clearance reduced as in the case of impaired renal clearance as evinced by elevated serum creatinine levels, Dysphoria, shakiness, visual disturbances, disorientation, tremors, hallucinations, and myoclonus have been reported. If a patient prescribed the drug becomes toxic and analgesia necessary, an agent of equal potency such as morphine or methadone is prescribed. If the drug is abused, management is comparable to that of methadone or heroin withdrawal. Meperidine, like amphetamines and cocaine, can cause seizure at higher doses. This is the opposite of alcohol and barbiturates, which cause seizures on withdrawal [99].

M. Nitrous Oxide Intoxication

Laughing gas (nitrous oxide) is used to induce mild euphoria and light-headedness. Dentists have access to it as an anesthetic agent. Adolescents get it from aerosol cans of whipped cream (hence the term "whipped"). Hold the can erect and pressing the release can give five to six hits [2]. The effect is mild. Duration of symptoms are time limited.

N. Nutmeg Intoxication

The aromatic evergreen, *Myristica fragrans*, is the source of one of the oldest spices in use: nutmeg., Myristicine, a psychoactive substance, is found in both the seed coat and oil of the seeds. Taken directly or mixed with food, the spice purchased in the spice department of a grocery store is a source of an inexpensive high. Inadvertent use of inappropriate proportions of nutmeg in preparations of pies has led to visual hallucination, agitation, severe headaches, flushing, palpitations, and numbness in the extremities. Temporal and spatial perception is also reported impaired. Although symptoms are time limited, death due to fatty degeneration of the liver has been reported.

O. Opiate Intoxication and Withdrawal

Heroin, methadone, and meperidine cause similar intoxication and withdrawal symptoms. The first mentioned is associated with a panoply of physical complications due to the illegality of its trafficking and irresponsibility of those who produce and supply it. In some instances, it may be cut with a lethal substance to enhance a high, reduce cost, or eliminate an undesirable user. Taken in usual amounts, euphoria, drowsiness, and apathy are experienced. Respiratory and heart rate are decreased, face flushed, blood pressure increased, and pupils constricted (they dilate as a person withdraws). Memory, judgment, and attention are impaired. Constipation occurs and is sometimes associated with nausea. Analgesia is common. Body temperature is decreased, speech slurred, and psychomotor retardation appears. In the extreme, opiate overdose leads to pulmonary edema, coma, and death. In the instance of meperidine, psychosis, muscle twitching, and seizures are seen. Meperidine does not cause miosis [100]. In addition to narcotics, pulmonary edema may be the initial presentation of methaqualone, acetylsalicylic acid (ASA) and meprobamate intoxication [101–109].

A single dose of intravenous or subcutaneous morphine peaks within 20 min to 1 h and is diminished within 4–6 h accompanied by a down and craving for more. Tolerance develops to the euphoria, sedation, analgesia, and respiratory depression, but not to the miosis and decreased bowel activity over time [110]. This creates problems after successful withdrawal if opiate abuse recurs. The naive user may take the dose that was sufficient to maintain euphoria without respiratory problems just prior to withdrawal and die with respiratory depression because he or she is no longer tolerant of such high doses. Multiple addiction to opiates barbiturates, and alcohol or concurrent hallucinogen use creates problems of intoxication, withdrawal, and management [11].

Codeine and glutethimide in combination (referred to as "hit," "loads," "doors and fours" [109]) provide an extended "heroin" high. Coma, convulsions, trauma, and peripheral neuropathies are reported with concurrent codeine/glutethimide use [112].

Medical problems abound with heroin abuse. Infections are common. Abcesses, pneumonia, subacute bacterial endocarditis, tuberculosis, venereal disease, viral and serum hepatitis, and AIDS have been reported. Polymicrobial infections are common with intravenous drug use. Septic emboli and mycotic aneurysms develop [29]. Septic emboli occur secondary to endocarditis, but embolizations of filters [29] and broken needles to the lungs are also seen [113–115]. Mycotic emboli lead to vascular rupture with resultant stroke [29]. Computerized tomography demonstrates cerebral abscesses and jugular venous thrombosis [116,117]. Needle emboli result when over-the-counter insulin syringes are used which bend, break, and fragment easily [114].

Traumatic pneumothorax is a complication that occurs when intravenous users elect a central approach to the internal jugular vein [118]. This is referred to as "the pocket shot." In some instance, the carotid arthery itself is inadvertently punctured [116], and cerebral infarction follows. Both focal lesions and lesions secondary to cardiopulmonary arrest occur [29].

The signs and symptoms of opiate intoxication are reversed by the intravenous administration of a narcotic antagonist if irreversible cerebral anoxia has not occurred. Narcotic antagonists include naloxone (Narcan) nalorphine, and levallorphan. Because of the short half-life of Narcan, symptoms of overdose may reappear, requiring further attention [9,12,98,102,108,110]. When a packet of heroin has been swallowed in an effort to avoid prosecution for smuggling, ipecacuanha (ipecac) may be required to induce vomiting [107]. Clonidine may be used with naltraxone for rapid detoxification [119,120].

Vital signs are supported and intravenous fluid and other specific measures provided as complications and drugs concommitantly taken dictate [121–123]. An airway must be provided with support for both breathing and blood pressure. Pulmonary edema is a medical emergency and must be treated accordingly [9,12,16,103,108,110]. Evidence of trauma must be sought and managed. Fifty percent of deaths with opiates are due to overdose, 25% are due to trauma, and the remainder to infection [110]. Traumatic pneumothorax requires treatment with either needle aspiration or chest tube [118].

Tetanus shots should be provided and systematic review for common infections in this group—hepatitis B, AIDS, septicemia, endocarditis, osteomyclitis, arthritis, syphilis, malaria, and tuberculosis [101,110]. Specific treatment is required for the management of other substances that may be present in the body. Severe hypocalcemia is associated with chronic glutethimide addiction [124]. Gluthethimide, rarely used in medical practice these days, is associated with sudden apneic spells, especially with manipulation of the oropharnyx [109].

When withdrawing a person from opiates, similar problems arise regarding questions of amount of drug taken, number of drugs taken, medical/surgical complications, and associated medical and psychiatric illnesses that are not directly related to opiate use or withdrawal. Alcohol, cocaine, amphetamines, methadone, meperidine, salicylates, gluthethamine, and propoxyphene (Darvon) may be present [125]. The patient may sequester opiates or other drugs to take if the withdrawal is intolerable. Opiate withdrawal may commence owing to a lack of supply or to an inability to obtain a source, following administration of an opiate agonist, or voluntarily. It rarely occurs after opiate administration for pain.

Withdrawal symptoms usually commence within 6–8 h following the last dose of morphine or heroin and peak in 2–3 days. They have run their course in 7–10 days. Meperidine withdrawal is more time limited. Withdrawal commences within hours, peaks at 8–12 hours, and has run its course in 4–5 days. Methadone withdrawal may take 24 h to occur and continue for as long as 10–14 days. Death is rare. If it occurs, a medical problem such as coronary heart disease exists. History and serum and urine assay are required to identify drugs used. Patients tend to be anxious, irritable, depressed, and aggressive. They feel nauseous with decreased appetite, weakness, malaise, joint pains, and hot and cold flashes. Diarrhea, rhinnorhea, ejaculation, vomiting, and perspiration are seen. They yawn, cry, and are restless sometimes with frank tremor. The pupils are dilated (the opposite of opiate intoxication) and fixed with piloerection. Muscles twitch and blood pressure, heart rate, and respiratory rate are increased [2].

Cross tolerance with a number of opiates allows withdrawal with methadone, a long-acting synthetic opiate, over 1 or 2 weeks. Sufficient amount of methadone is provided to control symptoms. Time is allowed for gradual reduction in physical dependence. Detoxification from heroin lasts about 1 week. Insomnia, joint pains, gastrointestinal symptoms, sweating, and other symptoms appear if withdrawal is more rapid. Signs and symptoms of withdrawal are monitored daily. In most instances, 10 mg of methadone b.i.d. or q.i.d. is sufficient to keep symptoms at bay. After giving the dose for 2 days, the dose is cut by 5–10 mg daily. For instance, 20 mg is given for the first 2 days, 15 mg on the third day, 10 mg on the fourth day, and so on. In no instance should the rate of withdrawal be greater than 20% of the daily dose above 20 mg of methadone per day. Higher doses, greater number of doses, and a longer period of withdrawal is required when opiate tolerance and severity of withdrawal symptoms is increased by inflammatory or febrile illness. Clonidine is also used for withdrawal [16,100,105,120]. The side effects of clonidine include dry mouth, lethargy, and hypotension [119]. A protracted abstinence syndrome has been reported that lasts as long as 4–6 months [13].

Seizures are not usual with opiate withdrawal unless mixed addiction is present with a drug such as alcohol or a barbiturate [126–128]. Serum and urine screens will provide evidence of this. Neuroleptics are not required unless a patient is psychotic in addition to being addicted. If vomiting is not managed by the clonidine or methadone withdrawal schedule, trimethobenzamide (Tigan) or hydroxyzine (Vistaril) can be given. A patient may be concomittently toxic with salicylates or acetaminophen because of the source of codeine [109,112]. If a patient is coaddicted to alchol and barbiturates, withdrawal from these substances in the best of circumstances should precede heroin withdrawal. Phenobarbital would cover both alcohol and sedative-hypnotic withdrawal. For alcohol and heroin withdrawal, a patient may be provided methadone and phenobarbital with a decrease of the two together. The same is true for sedative-hypnotic and heroin withdrawal [126].

Narcotic-addicted mothers in the third trimester of pregnancy should be maintained on methadone because of the risk of fetal death secondary to the intrauterine abstinence syndrome and decreased birth weight [9,103].

P. Phencyclidine Intoxication

Phencyclidine (PCP) is one of the drugs that can create a paranoid psychosis in a clear sensorium. A number of brutal deaths have been associated with this drug's use (ironically marketed under the appelation "angel dust") as there have been with crack. Prior to 1978, the drug was available as Sernylan, a veterinary anesthetic with sympathomimetic properties. Ketamine is a structurally related anesthetic. Phencylidine is a white crystalline solid, easily manufactured in a kitchen laboratory. The fact that it may be snorted, smoked, injected intravenously, or swallowed allows it to be made available for sale as cocaine alone or as a dilutent. It is also marketed as marihuana, mescaline, LSD, amphetamine, and psilocybin. Serum assays reveals the presence of PCP. The clinical picture seen with phencyclidine is less dependent on the users' personalities than with other hallucinogens. Onset of symptoms is rapid. Symptoms resemble schizophrenia and are quite disabling. Patients are agitated, assaultive, anxious, and disoriented. Homicide and suicide attempts may occur. Thoughts are distorted and the patient is tangential, circumstantial, and disoriented. Paranoia and ideas of reference are common. Auditory, visual, and tactile hallucinations appear with or without paresthesias or analgesias. There is a disassociation of somatic sensation. The blood pressure is elevated and the pupils are constricted or of normal size. Diaphoresis, vomiting, tachycardia, hyperpyrexia, hypersalivation, and clouding of the sensorium are also seen. The patient is ataxic and rigid. Myoclonus and psychomotor excitement appear. Deep tendon reflexes are increased. Horizontal and vertical nystagmus, decreased position sense, hyperacusis, tachypnea, and muscle spasticity are found on physical examination. Phencylidine intoxication is always considered serious until proven otherwise [1,2,32].

While symptoms in mild instances pass rapidly with cessation of use, enduring or more severe symptoms require continuing evaluation and diagnostic-specific management. A person may have used other recreational drugs or have coexistant psychiatric or physical illness. In the former case, a primary psychiatric disorder may have led to abuse of the drug. Ammonium chloride, cranberry juice, or ascorbic acid taken orally or by nasogastric tube enhance excretion of PCP by acidifying the urine [16]. Benzodiazepines and neuroleptics are both used for the management of PCP intoxication. Benzodiazepines such as diazepam (Valium) sedate without anticholinergic effects, which may contribute to arrhythimias or problems with blood pressure, but inhibit excretion of the drug despite acidification of the urine. Neuroleptics such as thiothixine (Navane) and haloperiodol (Haldol), on the other hand, sedate the patient but may contribute to cardiovascular problems. Neuroleptics are frequently used with careful monitoring of the heart rate and blood pressure when rapid remission of symptoms is desired to obviate need for hospitalization [1,2,11,16,97,98]. This minimizes the dangers of orthostatic hypotensive crises.

Young children, the elderly, those with concurrent medial illness, and those who have taken intentionally or unintentionally large doses of the drug may develop status epilepticus, adrenergic crises, lethargy, hypertensive encephalopathy, or coma, and in some instances die if they are not provided emergency medical measures to support vital functions [1,2,29]. Opisthotonus in such instances precedes seizures [32]. Phentolamine is used for acute hypertension. Instrumentation is avoided where possible. Muscles are massaged and diazepam, 10–30 mg provided. Patients must always be provided with protection from harming themselves and others, even in instances of severe overdose. The half-life in overdoses in 1–3 days. Accentuation of laryngeal and pharyngeal reflexes with marked increase in secretions requires careful suctioning from the corners of the mouth. Propranolol, 40–80 mg, is suggested to protect patients from adrenergic crises. Ipecac is contraindicated in cases of PCP intoxication because of the risk of convulsions. Sponging and cooling blankets are required to dissipate heat and obviate hyperthermic crises. Intubation and deep suctioning is avoided save when absolutely necessary in coma. Large cannula intravenous infusion should be instituted in coma with ascorbic acid in solution. Bladder catherization may be necessary to relieve PCP-induced urinary retention. Anticonvulsants may be required to manage seizures. Cholinergics are avoided because bronchial secretions are already in excess. As a patient regains consciousness in cases of coma, voice contact is made and extended evaluation of suicide risk and coexistant psychopathology undertaken. Examining clinicians should always be aware of the occult effects of trauma due to attendant anesthesia and analgesia. Urinary PCP levels are not of use in the prediction of either hypotensive episodes or violence [2].

Q. Psychotropic Drug Withdrawal

Patients who experiment with recreational drugs as well as many who do not may abruptly discontinue neuroleptics, thymoleptics, and benzodiazepines and experience a panoply of symptoms, such as anxiety, agitation, malaise, tremor, irritability, myalgia, insomnia, abdominal pain, dizziness, chills, and fatigue. Moodiness, worsening of depression, coryza, chills, diarrhea, vomiting, delirium, perspiration, and nausea also have been reported. Twenty-one to 55% of those who suddenly stop antidepressants experience withdrawal, presumably due to central cholinergic overdrive [112]. Appropriate instructions for management is particularly important when antidepressants must be discontinued in instances of allergic reactions. Withdrawal symptoms are greater with neuroleptics with strong autonomic properties and when they are discontinued with antiparkinson agents. In the later instances, akathisia may appear with severe discomfort to the patient. Sinus tachycardia with frequent extrasystoles associated with bligeminy is reported with cessation of imipramine, suggesting the drug may have masked cardiac instability or that rebound arrhythmias occur [2]. Withdrawal from alprazalam may last months. Changes in the electroencephalogram are seen with withdrawal.

Gradual reduction in dose over 2–4 weeks generally prevents symptoms. Antidepressant withdrawal has been successfully treated with anticholinergics (i.e., atropine) [2].

R. Steroid Abuse and Intoxication

Steroids are abused by athletes and patients with eating disorders. In addition, toxic symptoms are seen in patients prescribed the drugs for diagnostic-specific purposes such as in Addison's disease and neoplastic illness. Mania, delirium, schizophreniform symptoms, depression, and dementiform symptoms have been reported. Dosage is correlated with the risk of the development of symptoms, but the duration, severity, onset, or type of symptoms is not impacted on by dosage, or duration of treatment or use of the steroid. Females are more prone to the development of symptoms than males. Depression, euphoria, and psychosis are the most frequent symptoms reported. Antipsychotic medication can relieve symptoms without necessarily decreasing the dose if continued steroid use is recommended to alleviate a patient's symptoms. Symptoms nearly always abate the discontinuation of the use of steroids. Symptoms emerge during an increase or decrease of the dose as well as at a steady dose. If symptoms emerge while increasing the dose, decrease the amount given and more slowly increase the dose to the desired amount. If they emerge during decrease of the drug, withdraw it more slowly.

S. Solvent Intoxication

Glue, dyes, cleaning fluid, paint thinner, toluene, finger nail polish remover (acetone), and other solvents or their derivatives are a source of "cheap highs." Use of these modes of escape are both correlated with psychopathology in the user (usually children and adolescents) and with the development of enduring neuropsychological impairment. Initial excitement is followed by depression, disorientation, and confusion. Generalized muscle weakness may appear with or without cardiac arrythmias and increase serum creatine phosphokinase levels. Patients have gastrointestinal discomfort and ataxia. Supportive and symptomatic care is provided [97]. Unless permanent brain damage has occurred, symptoms remit with cessation of use [11].

T. Volatile Nitrate Intoxication

Light-headedness and fluctuating levels of consciousness, dysattention, and disorientation have been reported with the use of volatile nitrate ("popper") use. Amyl nitrate has been used for the relief of angina for over a century, and it is sold in small thin glass capsules covered by webbing, so they may be crushed and used by those suffering angina pain. Other sources are butyl nitrate and isobutyl nitrate. Nitrates are sold in "head" shops and novelty shops and through mail order houses under the name of Rush, Aroma of Man, Heart-On, Gas Bullet, Toilet Water, and Poppers. These drugs have been sought to create abandonment in sex, dancing, and art. The specific symptom picture is related to the setting the drug is used in, personality of the user, amount of drug taken, concurrent physical and psychiatric illness, and expectations of the user.

Physical signs of use include tachycardia, flushing, decreased blood pressure, weakness, syncope, ataxia, and tachycardia. Pulsating headaches are experienced. Inverted T waves and depressed ST segments are seen transiently on the EKG. Symptoms generally pass rapidly with cessation of use [97].

REFERENCES

1. Slaby, A.E. Other psychiatric emergencies, *Comprehensive Textbook of Psychiatry/V*, Vol. Two, 5th ed. (H.I. Kaplan and B.J. Sadock, eds.). Baltimore, Williams & Wilkins, 1989.
2. Slaby, A.E., Lieb, J., and Tancredi, L.R. *The Handbook of Psychiatric Emergencies*, (3rd ed.) New York, Medical Examination, 1986.
3. Kellerman, A.L., Fihn, S.D., LoGarto, J.P., and Copass, M.K. Impact of drug screening in suspected overdose. *Am. Emerg. Med., 16*:1206–1216 (1987).
4. Mendelson, E.F. Alcohol-related psychiatric emergencies: Their characteristics and care at a walk-in clinic. *Br. J. Psychiatry, 150*:121–124 (1987).
5. Kontaxaleis, V., Markids, M., Vaslamatzia, G., and Christodoulou, G.N. Substance abusers seeking emergency psychiatric care: Motivation to treatment. *Drug Alcohol Depend., 16*:185–189 (1985).
6. Olson, E., McEhrue, J., and Greenbaum, D.M. Alcohol and miscellaneous agents. *Heart Lung, 12*(2):127–130 (1983).
7. Gibb, K. Serum alcohol levels, toxicology screens and use of the breath alcohol analyzer. *Am. Emerg. Med., 15*(3)349–353 (1986).
8. Olson, E., McEhrue, J., and Greenbaum, D.M. Recognition, general considerations and techniques in the management of drug intoxication. *Heart Lung*, 12(2):110–114 (1983).
9. Chapel, J.L.: Emergency room treatment of the drug-abusing patient. *Am. J. Psychiatry, 130*:257–259 (1973).
10. Sellers, E.M., and Kalant, H. Alcohol intoxication and withdrawal. *N. Engl. J.Med., 294*(14):757–762 (1976).
11. Felter, R., Izsak, E., and Laurence, H.S. Emergency department management of the intoxicated adolescent. *Pediatr. Clin. North Am., 34*:399–421 (1987).
12. Greenblatt, D.J. and Shader, R.J. Drug abuse and the emergency room physician. *Am. J. Psychiatry, 131*:559–562 (1974).
13. Czechowicz, D. *Detoxification Treatment Manual*. USUA&AS, National Institute of Drug Abuse, Washington, D.C. (U.S. Government Printing Office.)

14. Thompson, W.Z. Management of alcohol withdrawal syndromes. *Arch. Intern. Med., 138*:278–283 (1978).

15. Isbell, H., Fraser, H.F., Wiler, A., Belleville, R.E., and Eisenman, A.J. An experimental study of etiology of "rum fits" and delirium tremens. *Q. J. Stud. Alcohol, 16*:1–33 (1955).

16. Dubin, W.R., Weiss, K.J., and Dorn, J.M. Pharmacotherapy of psychiatric emergencies. *J. Clin. Psychopharmacol., 6*(4):210–222 (1986).

17. No, S.K.E., Hauser, W.A., Brust, J.C.M., and Susser, R. Alcohol consumption and withdrawal in new-onset seizures. *N. Engl. J. Med. 319*(11):666–673 (1988).

18. Simon, R.D. Alcohol and seizures. *N. Engl. J. Med., 319*(11):715–716 (1988).

19. Wilbur, R., and Kulitz, F.A. Anticonvulsant drugs in alcohol withdrawal: Use of pheytoin, primadone, carbamazepine, valproic acid and the sedative anticonvulsants. *Am. J. Hosp. Pharm., 138*:1138–1143 (1981).

20. DeVaul, R.A., and Jervey, F.L. Delirium: A selected medical emergency. *A.F.P., 24*(6):52–157 (1981).

21. Tarain-Petrone, C. Psychiatric emergencies, *Emergency Medicine for the Primary Care Physician* (J.E. Hocuh, ed.). Philadelphia, Saunders, 1986.

22. McMichen, D.B. Alchol-related disease, *Emergency Medicine* (P. Rosen, eds.). St. Louis, Mosby, 1983.

23. Allen, R.P., Sater, D., and Cori, L. Effects of psychostimulants on aggression. *J. Nerv Ment. Dis., 160*:138–145 (1975).

24. Ellinwood, E. Assault and homicide associated with amphetamine abuse. *Am. J. Psychiatry, 127*(9):1170–1175 (1971).

25. Ellinwood, E. Amphetamine psychosis: Individuals, settings and sequences. *Current Concepts on Amphetamine Abuse* (E. Ellinwood and S. Cohen, eds.). Rockville, Maryland, National Institute of Mental Health, 1972.

26. Greenbaum, D.M. Clinical aspects of drug intoxication: The St. Vincent's Hospital Symposium–Part 1. *Heart Lung*, (1983).

27. Gawin, F.H. Neuroleptic reduction of cocaine-induced paranoia but not euphoria. *Psychopharmacology, 90*:142–143 (1986).

28. Gawin, F.H. and Ellinwood, E.H.: Cocaine and other stimulants: actions, abuse and treatment. *N. Engl. J. Med., 318*(18):1173–1182 (1988).

29. Caplan, L.R., Hier, D.B., and Banks, G: Current concepts of cerebrovascular disease: Stroke and drug abuse. *Stroke, 13*:869–872 (1982).

30. McMullen, M.J. Stimulants, *Emergency Medicine: Concepts & Clinical Practice*, P. Rosen, F.J. Baker,G.R. Braen, R.H. Daily, and R.E. Levy (Eds.) St. Louis, Mosby,1983.

31. Bell, D.S. The experimental reproduction of amphetamine psychosis. *Arch. Gen. Psychiatry 29*:35–37 (1973).

32. DiSclatarri, A., Hall, R.C.W., and Gardner, E.R. Drug-induced psychosis: Emergency diagnosis and management. *Psychosomatics, 22*(10):845–855 (1981).

33. Angrist, B., Lee, H.K., and Gershon, S. The antagonism of amphetamine-induced symptomotology by neuroleptics. *Am. J. Psychiatry, 131*(F):817–819 (1974).

34. Allgulander, C. History and current status of sedative hypnotic drug use and abuse. *Acta Psychiatr. Scand., 73*:465–478 (1986).

35. Fauman, B.J., and Fauman, M.D. Recognition and management of drug abuse emergencies. *Comp. Ther. 4*:38–43 (1978).

36. Perry, P.J., and Alexander, B. Sedative/hypnotic dependence: Patient stabilization tolerance testing and withdrawal. *Drug Intell. Clin. Pharm., 20*:532–537 (1986).

37. Jaffe, J.H. Drug addiction and drug abuse, Goodman and Gilman's *The Pharmacological Basis of Therapeutics* (A.G. Gilman, L.S. Goodman, and W. Roll, eds.).

38. Janeceh, E., Kapur, B.M., and Divany, P. Oral phenobarbital loading: A safe method of babiturate and nonbarbiturate hypnosedative withdrawal. *Canad. Med. Assoc. J., 137*:410–412 (1987).

39. Maher, J.F., Schrainer, G.E., and Westervelt, F.B. Acute glutethimide intoxication. *Am. J. Med., 33*:70–82 (1982).

40. Morris, R.W. Circadian and circannual rhythms of emergency room drug-overdose admissions. *Adv. Chronobiol.* 451–457 (1987).

41. Lankin, D.L., and Baltarowich, L.L. Sedative-hypnotics, *Emergency Medicine: Concepts and Clinical Practice*. (P. Rosen, F.J. Baker, G.R. Braen, R.H. Daily, and R.C. Levy eds.). St. Louis, Mosby, 1983.

42. Gay, N.E., and Tresznewsky, O. Barbiturates and a potpourri of other sedatives, hypnotics and tranquilizers. *Heart Lung, 12*(2):122–127 (1983).

43. Hausen, A.R., Kennedy, K.A., Ambre, J.J., and Fisher, L.O. Glutethimide poisoning: A metabolite contributes to morbidity and mortality. *N. Engl. J. Med., 292*(5):250–252 (1975).

44. Ward, J.T. Endotrachial drug therapy. *Am. J. Emerg. Med., 1*:71–82 (1983).

45. Taudberg, D. Endotracheal nalozone. *Am. J. Emerg. Med., 3*:366–367 (1983).

46. Shader, R.I., Caine, E.D., and Meyer, R.E. Treatment of dependence on barbiturates and sedative-hypnotics, *Manual of Psychiatric Therapeutics* (R. Shader, ed.) Boston, Little Brown, 1975.

47. Smith, D.E., and Wesson, D.R. Phenobarbital techique for treatment of barbiturate dependence. *Arch. Gen. Psychiatry, 24*:56–60 (1971).

48. Cregler, L.L., and Mark, H. Medical complications of cocaine abuse. *N. Engl. J. Med., 315*(23):1495–1500 (1986).

49. Shesser, R., Davis, C., and Edelstein, S. Pneumomediastium and pneumothorax after inhaling alkaloidol cocaine. *Ann. Emerg. Med., 10*::213–215 (1981).

50. Awesty, D.J., Stanley, R.B., and Crochalt, D.M. Pneumonediastinum and cervical emphysema from inhalation of "free base" cocaine: Report of three cases. *Otolarygol. Head Neck Surg, 94*:372–374 (1986).

51. Weis, R.D., Goldenheim, P.D., Mirin, S.M., Hales, C.A., and Mendelson, J.H. Pulmonary dysfunction in cocaine smokers. *Am. J. Psychiatry, 138*(8):110–112 (1981).

52. Van Dyke, C., and Byck, R. Cocaine, *Sci. Am., 246*(3):128–141 (1982).

53. Itkonem, J., Schnoll, S., and Glassroth, J. Pulmonary dysfunction in 'free base' cocaine users. *Arch. Intern. Med, 144*:2195–2197 (1984).

54. Cohen, S. Cocaine: Acute medical and psychiatric complications. *Psychiatry Ann. 14*(10):747–749 (1984).

55. Coleman, D.L., Ross, T.F., and Naughton, J.Z. Myocardial ischemia and infarction related to recreational cocaine use. *West. J. Med., 136*:444–446 (1982).

56. Schweitzer, V.G. Osteolytic sinusitis and pneumomediastinum deceptive otolaryngologic complications of cocaine abuse. *Laryngoscope, 96*:206–210 (1986).

57. Gay, G.R. Clinical management of acute and chronic cocaine poisoning. *Ann. Emerg. Med., 11*:562–572 (1982).

58. Morris, J.B., and Shuck, J.M. Pneumomediastinun in a young male cocaine user. *Ann. Emerg. Med., 14*(2):194–196 (1985).

59. Magnan, E., and Saury, T. Trois cas de cocainisme chronique. *Cr. Soc. Biol. (Paris) 1*:60–63 (1889).

60. Post, R.M. Cocaine psychoses. A continuum model. *Am. J. Psychiatry, 132*:225–231 (1975).

61. Lesho, L.M., Fischman, M.W., Javaid, J.I., and Davis, J.M. Iatrogenic cocaine psychosis. *N. Engl. J. Med. 307*:1153 (1982).

62. Kossawsky, W.A., and Lyon, A.F. Cocaine and acute mycoardial infarction, probable correlation. *Chest, 86*:729–731 (1984).

63. Cregler, L.L., and Mark, H. Cardiovascular danger of cocaine abuse. *Am. J. Cardiol., 57*:1185–1186 (1986).

64. Cregler, L.L., and Mark, H. Relation of acute myocardial infarction to cocaine abuse. *Am. J. Cardiol. 56*:784 (1983).

65. Benchimal, A., Bartal, H. and Desser, K.B. Accelerated ventricular rhythum & cocaine abuse. *Am. Intern. Med., 8*:519–520 (1978).

66. Vincent, G.M., Anderson, J.L., and Marshall, H.W. Coronary spasm producing cornary thrombosis and myocardial infarction. *N. Engl. J.Med. 309*(4):220–223 (1983).

67. Pasternack, P.F., Calvin, S.B. and Bauman, F.G. Cocaine-induced angina pectoris and acute myocardial infarction in patients younger than 40 years. *Ann. J. Cardiol., 55*:847 (1985).

68. Weiss, R.D., Goldenheim, P.D., Mirin, S.M., Hales, C.A., and Mendelson, J.H. Pulmonary dysfunction in cocaine smokers. *Am.J. Psychiatry., 138*(8):110–112 (1981).

69. Schachue, J.S., Roberts, B.H., and Thompson, P.D. Coronary artery spasm and mycoardial infarction associated with cocaine use. *N. Engl. J.Med., 310*(25):1665–1666 (1984).

70. Simpson, R.W., and Edwards, W.D. Pathogenesis of cocaine-induced ischemic heart disease. *Arch. Pathol. Lab. Med., 10*:213–215 (1981).

71. Bethinger, J. Cocaine intoxication: massive oral overdose. *Ann. Emerg. Med., 9*:429–430 (1980).

72. Nanji, A.A., and Filipanlio, J.D. Esystole and ventricular fibrillation associated with cocaine intoxication. *Chest, 85*:132–133 (1984).

73. Guinn, M.M., Bedford, L.J.A., and Wilson, M.C. Antagonism of intravenous cocaine lethality in nonhuman primates. *Clin. Toxicol, 16*:499–508 (1980).

74. Isner, J.M., Estee, N.A.M., et al. Acute cardiac events related to cocaine abuse. *N. Engl. J. Med., 315* (23):1438–1443 (1986).

75. Allred, R.J., and Ewer, S. Fatal pulmonary edema following intravenous "free base" cocaine use. *Ann. Emerg. Med., 10*(8)441–442 (1981).

76. Lichtenfeld, P.J., Rubin, D.B., and Feldman, R.S. Sabarachnoid hemorrhage precipitated cocaine snorting. *Arch. Neurol., 41*:223–224 (1984).

77. Schwartz, K., and Cohen, J.A. Subarachnoid hemorrhage precipitated by cocasine snorting. *Arch. Neurol, 41*:2050, 1984.

78. Westle, C.V., and Wright, R.K. Death caused by recreational cocaine ris. *J.A.M.A. 241*:2519–2522 (1979).

79. Archer, D., Sachs, B.P., Tracey, K.J., and Wise, W.E. Abruptio placentae associated with cocaine use. *Am. J. Obstet. Gynecol, 146*(2):220–221 (1983).

80. Chasnoff, I.J., Bassey, M.E., Savach, R., and Stack, C.M. Perinatal cerebral infraction and maternal cocaine use. *Pediatrics, 108*(3):456–459 (1986).

81. Chasnoff, I.J., Burn, W.J., Schnol, S.H., and Burns, K.A. Cocaine use in pregnancy. *N. Engl. J. Med., 313*(11):666–669 (1985).

82. Nalbandian, H., Sheth, W., Dietruch, R., and Georgion, J. Intestinal ischemia caused by cocaine ingestion; report of two cases. *Surgery, 97*(3):374–376 (1985).

83. Fishbain, D.A., and Wetli, C.V. Cocaine intoxication, delirium and death in a body packer. *Ann. Emerg. Med., 10*:531–532 (1981).

84. Jonsson, S., O'Meara, M., and Young, J.B. Acute cocaine poisoning-importance of treating seizures and acidosis. *Am. J. Med., 75*:1061–1064 (1983).

85. McCarron, M.M., and Wood, J.D. The cocaine body packer syndrome. *J.A.M.A., 250*(11):1417–1420 (1983).

86. Menashe, P.I., and Gottlieb, J.E. Hyperthermia, rhabdomyolysis and myoglobinuric renal failure attribute to recreational use of cocaine. *South. Med. J. 81*(3):379–380 (1988).

87. Caruana, D.S., Weinbach, B., Ery, D., and Gardner, L.B. Cocaine-packet ingestion diagnosis, management and natural history. *Ann. Intern. Med., 100*:73–74 (1984).

88. Catravas, J.D., Waters, F.W., Walz, M.A., and Davis, W.M. Acute cocaine intoxication in the conscious dog: Pathophysiologic profile of acute lethality, *Arch. Int. Pharmacodyn. Ther., 235*:328–340 (1978).

89. Catravas, J.D., Waters, F.W., Walz, M.A., and Davis, W.M. Acute cocaine intoxication in the conscious dog: studies in the mechanism of lethality. *J. Pharmacol. Exp. Ther. 217*(2):350–356 (1981).

90. Roberts, J.R., Quattrucci, E., and Howland, M.A. Severe hyperthermia secondary to intravenous drug abuse. *Am. J.Emerg. Med., 2*:373 (1984).

91. Gold, M.S., Ehrenkranz, J.R.L., Jonas, J.M., and Dackis, C.A. Treatment of acute cocaine toxicity, *Soc. Neurosci. Abst. (Toronto), 14*:1 (1988).

92. Olson, K.A., Benowitz, N.L., and Pentel, P. Management of cocaine poisoning. *Ann. Emerg. Med., 12*:655–656 (1983).

93. Catravas, J.D., Waters, I.W., and Davis, W.M. Antidotes for cocaine poisoning. *N. Engl. J. med., 295*:1238 (1977).

94. Catravas, J.D., Waters, I.W., Waltz, M.A., and Davs, W.M. Antidotes for cocaine poisoning. *N. Engl. J. Med., 297*:1238 (1977).

95. Ramiska, E., and Sacchetti, A.D.Propranolol-induced hypertension in treatment of cocaine intoxication. *Ann. Emerg. Med., 14*:1112–1113 (1985).

96. Nahas, G., Tronve, R., Demus, J.F., and von Stibon, M. A calcium-channel blocker as antidote to the cardiac effects of cocaine intoxication. *N. Engl. J. Med., 313*(8):519–520 (1988).

97. McGuigan, M.A. Toxicology of drug abuse. *Emerg. Med. Clin. North Am., 2*(1):87–101 (1984).

98. Ellison, J.M., and Jacobs, D. Emergency psychopharmacology: A review and update. *Ann. Emerg. Med., 15*:962–968 (1986).

99. Goehing, M.G., Thirman, M.J. Neurotoxicity of meperidine. *Ann. Emerg. Med., 14*:1007–1009 (1985).

100. Allen, T. Narcotics, *Emergency Medicine: Concepts and Clinical Practice.* (P. Rosen, F.S. Baker, G.R. Braeh, R.H. Daily, and R.C. Levy. eds.) St. Louis, Mosby, 1983.

101. Dunlop, M.G., and Steedman, D.J. Opiod intravenous drug abuse and the accident and emergency department. *Arch. Emerg. Med., 2*:23–77 (1985).

102. Dole, V.P., Foldes, F.F., Trigg, H., Robinson, J.W., and Blatman, S. Methadone poisoning. *N. Y. State J. Med.,* 541–543 (1971).

103. Connaughton, J.F., Reeser, D., Schut, J., and Finnegan, L.P. Perinatal addiction: outcome and management. *Ann. J. Obstet. Gynecol., 129*(6):679–686 (1977).

104. Chappel, J.W. Treatment of morphine-type dependence. *J.A.M.A., 221*:1516 (1972).

105. Freitas, P.M. Narcotic withdrawal in the emergency department. *Ann. J Emerg. Med., 11*:562–572 (1982).

105. Hawlem, J.A., and Mathewson, H.S. Emergency control of convulsions. *J. Am. Assoc. Nurse Anesth.* 47:182–186 (1979).

107. Robins, J.B., and Rae, P.W. Recovery of ingested heroin packets. *Arch. Emerg. Med.* 3:125–127 (1983).

108. Mofenson, H.C., and Caraccio, T.R. Toxidromes. *Compr. Ther., 11*(2):46–52 (1985).

109. Chartier, D.M. Glutethimide and codeine overdose. *J.E.N., 9*:307–309 (1983).

110. Gold, F.L., Bresnitz, E., and Weisman, R. Opiods, and opiates. *Heart Lung, 12*(2):114–122 (1983).

111. Ellinwood, E.H. Amphetamine psychosis: description of individuals and process. *J. Nerv. Ment. Dis., 144*:273–283 (1967).

112. Khajawall, A.M., Sramek, J.J., and Simpson, G.M. "Loads" alert. *Est. Jr. Med., 137*(2):166–168 (1982).

113. Galdun, J.P., Paris, P.M., Weiss, L.D., and Heller, M.B. Central embolization of needle fragments. A complication of intravenous drug abuse. *Am. J. Emerg. Med.* 5(5):379–382 (1987).

114. Horattas, M.C., and Moorman, D.W. Cardiopulmonary needle embolization: A complication of central venous drug abuse. *Am. J. Emerg. Med., 6*(1):27–30 (1988).

115. Greenbaum, D.M., and Marschell, K.E. The adult respiratory disease syndrome. *N.Y. Med.,* 2:27–35 (1980).

116. Lewis, L.W., Jr., Grona, N., and Elliott, J.P. Complications of attempted central venous injection performed by drug abusers. *Chest, 78*:613–617 (1980).

117. Merha, G.L., Colley, D.P., and Clark, R.A. Computed tomographic demonstration of cervical abscesses and juglar vein thrombosis. *Arch.Otolaryngal., 107*:313–315 (1981).

118. Wisdom, K., Kovak, R.M., Richardson, H.H., Martin, G.V., Obaid, F.N., and Tomlanovich, MC., Alternate therapy for traumatic pneunrothorax in "pocket shooters." *Ann. Emerg. Med., 15*:428–432 (1986).

119. Gossop, M. Clonidine and the treatment of the opiate withdrawal syndrome. *Drug Alcohol Depend., 21*:253–259 (1988).

120. Gold, M.S. Pottash, A.C., and Extein, I. Clonidine in acute opiate withdrawal. *N. Engl. J. Med., 302*:1421–1422 (1980).

121. Barth, C.W., Bray, M., Roberts, W.C. Rupture of the ascending aorta during cocaine intoxication. *Am. J. Cardiol., 57*:496 (1986).

123. Gay, G.R., Loper, K.A. Control of cocaine-induced hypertension with Labetalol. *Anesth. Anaolog., 67*:91 (1988).

124. Ober, K.P., Dennessy, J.F., and Hellman, R.M. Severe hypocalcemia associated with chronic gluthethimide addiction. *Am. J.Psychiatry,*

125. Mihleman, R.E., and Weth, C.V. Death caused by recreational cocaine use. *J.A.M.A., 252*(14):1889–1893 (1984).

126. Novick, D.M. Major medical problems and detoxification treatment of parental drug-abusing alcholics. *Adv. Alchol Subst. Abuse 3*(4):87–105 (1984).

127. Sampliner, R., and Iber, F.L. Diphenyhydantoin control of alcohol withdrawal seizures. *J.A.M.A., 230*(10):1430–1432 (1979).

128. Victor, M., and Adams, R.D. The effect of alcohol on the nervous system. *Res. Publ. Assoc. Res. Ment. Dis., 32*:526–673 (1953).

XVI
Prevention

56

Children and Adolescents and Drug and Alcohol Abuse and Addiction: Review of Prevention Strategies

Karol L. Kumpfer
University of Utah, Salt Lake City, Utah

I. IMPORTANCE OF SUBSTANCE ABUSE PREVENTION

A. Medical and Social/Economic Costs

The contribution of chemical dependency to health care costs is unknown, but it has been estimated to range from 14% to over 50% (Harwood et al., 1984). Because of antibiotics and other advances in modern medicine, styles of living rather than infectious diseases are the major causes of death in young people today (MacDonald, 1984). Hence, as medical research increasingly demonstrates the importance of healthy lifestyles to the prevention of disease and mortality, more physicians are becoming concerned about the impact of alcohol, tobacco, and other drugs on their patients in terms of both mortality and morbidity. Adolescent alcohol and drug abuse can quickly destroy the health benefits of years of careful pediatric and parental care.

Alcohol and other drugs have been linked with problems associated with acute use (e.g., auto accidents, fires, injuries), chronic use (e.g., cirrhosis, ulcers, cancers, malnutrition), and a behavioral pattern of chronic use called dependency. Associated with use of drugs and alcohol is a significant increase in the death rate of 15- to 24-year-olds. Alcohol is associated with more than 50% of the reported cases of the three major causes of death for youth—accidents, homicides, and suicides. Alcohol and tobacco greatly increase a youth's risk for a broad range of health problems, including cardiovascular disease and cancer. Cigarette smokers have a life expectancy 7 years shorter than nonsmokers. Recent studies have linked marijuana use to chronic cough, emphysema, and lung cancer (Tashkin and Cohen, 1981), endocrine problems such as decreased testosterone and gynecosmastia (Copeland et al., 1980, Harmon and Aliapoulis, 1972), immune system suppression (Munson and Fehr, 1982),

This chapter is based on a paper presented at the American Academy of Child and Adolescent Psychiatry's (AACAP) 1989 Annual Conference in New York City, based on material developed for the Project Prevention Initiative of the AACAP.

ophthalmological problems (Hepler et al., 1972), and alterations in blood pressure and tachycardia (Tennant, 1982).

According to estimates from the Research Triangle Institute on the economic and social costs of alcohol and drug abuse (Harwood et al., 1984), the economic costs of chemical dependency equalled about $850 per person in America in 1986. This is $100 more than the $754 per capita cost ($499 for alcohol abuse and $255 for drug abuse) in 1983 (Harwood et al., 1984). The total drain on our economy is staggering and estimated to be over $200 billion in 1986 because of accidents, crime, health care costs, fires, and lost productivity due to alcholism and drug abuse. The lifetime cost of a single drug abuser is estimated at $85,000 in lost productivity and direct economic burden on the welfare system. These costs do not include the tangible emotional suffering and negative impact on health, welfare, and productivity of family and friends caused by substance abusers. In addition, these costs estimates appear to greatly underestimate the impact of alcohol and drug abuse on our escalating national health care costs, since the Research Triangle Institute's report only attributed 1.9% or $4.3 billion of the total health care cost ($223.8 billion in 1980) to drug- or alcohol-related illnesses and trauma.

B. Health/Wellness Concepts

As styles of living become more prominent in the causes of today's diseases and health care costs continue to soar, health are providers are rethinking their role. They are more interested in preventing accidents and diseases by improved health and consumer education. Prevention as a health care concept is increasingly stressed in health curriculums at universities, and is promoted and supported by state governors, legislators, and health departments.

According to a survey of states by the National Association of State Alcohol and Drug Abuse Directors (NASADAD), in fiscal year 1984, about 13% (or $173.8 million) of the total allocations for alcohol and drug abuse services (over $1.3 billion) was spent on prevention services (Butynski, Record, and Yates, 1985). This equal 77¢ per person spent on prevention. States estimated that nearly 6.7 million persons received prevention services in over 6200 prevention programs. One-third of all persons served were youth in prevention programs in the schools. The other two-thirds were primarily adults served through public media campaigns.

C. Conclusion

The increases in prevention funding in the last few years is a godsend, and has revised substance abuse and health care providers' concepts about alcohol and drug abuse. More people consider substance abuse to be preventable, though the question of how is still to be answered. We are finding it more difficult to stop many youth from engaging in peer-supported drinking and drug use than educational programs alone can handle. We are discovering that the majority of youth who end up in treatment programs have sustance-abusing parents and that chemical dependency runs in families. Still, there are many questions which are left unanswered. Such as how to find the most developmentally appropriate and effective programs for reaching youth in schools? What are the best prevention strategies for children of chemically dependent parents and other high-risk groups? How can improved behavioral change technologies be used in prevention programming?

II. RISK AND PROTECTIVE FACTORS

Prevention programs must be based on etiological information which specified the likely causes and correlates of alcohol and drug abuse. Because childhood prevention programs, lacking longitudinal findings, are rarely able to test effectiveness, it is important to develop theoretical etiological models against which to measure theoretically specified changes. If one considers the prior etiological research can be placed on a continuum from investigations of correlates to causes, most empirical findings to date have largely clustered on the "correlate" end of the scale. These studies, while helpful, do not inform prevention specialists of how to design their programs as well as empirical studies of the causes of chemical dependency. Researchers reporting their findings have frequently had to stop short of attributing causality to any given factor or combination of factors because of the lack of an explicit articulation of the theoretical bases for the causal relationships. In addition, it is exceedingly difficult to determine causality in applied research when lacking experimental controls. Causality also implies that a temporal relationship has been established, with causal variables preceding or precipitating the onset of the chemical dependency. Interpretation of causal sequencing of events involves the application of repeated measures of the same cohorts over a period of time. Hence, both theoretical models and longitudinal studies are needed to help determine causality.

Unfortunately, the majority of prior prevention programs in the field of substance abuse have not been guided by empirical data, but by intuitive notions about the causes of chemical dependency. Prevention program designers must not assume that certain environmental or family variables cause substance abuse, or that substance-abusing youth or their families have certain deficits which prevention specialists must rush out to correct.

One striking example of prevention programming poorly grounded in etiological research involved the use of family communication training for prevention of delinquency. During the 1970s, a number of deliquency specialists developed family-based prevention programs aimed at teaching appropriate family communication patterns. In his dissertation, Parsons (1972) observed that families of delinquents behaved as if they had already taken family communication courses (e.g., they did not interrupt, they took turns, etc.), whereas the communication patterns of normal families resembled utter chaos.

Designers of substance abuse prevention programs must understand the essential and real differences between abusing and nonabusing families and also which factors are most predictive of adolescent drug abuse. Intuition and educated guesses are undependable guides.

III. EFFICACY AND TYPES OF DRUG AND ALCOHOL ABUSE AND ADDICTION PREVENTION PROGRAMS

A. The Public Health Services (PHS) Model of Prevention

This model, which consists of a triad of host, agent, and environment factors, provides a method for categorizing the many different types of prevention activities for drug dependency. Approaches which attempt to influence the attitudes and normative behaviors of society in relation to alcohol and drugs (such as advertising and the portrayal of alcohol and drugs in the mass media) fall on the AGENT-ENVIRONMENT axis. Prevention approaches which work to decrease one's motivation to use alcohol and drugs are placed along the HOST-AGENT axis (i.e., decreasing accessibility, increasing age, taxes, and price). Most prevention approaches typically considered prevention by the general public lie along the ENVIRONMENT-HOST axis. The etiological factors influencing youth's drug and alcohol abuse can be organized as a continuum of influence from the most distal—national, state, and local community; to intermediate influence with coworkers, peers, friends, role models, and teachers; to most proximal or close influences in family of origin and immediate family or spouse (Kumpfer and DeMarsh, 1984). Drug and alcohol dependency programs can also be categorized along this traditional prevention axis by the primary site of influence they are attempting to chance—community, school, or family.

Some prevention programs have several simultaneous sites of influence. For instance, national medial countercampaigns (primarily classified as a distal approach impacting national norms) could have broad influence across the entire ENVIRONMENT-HOST continuum. Likewise, server training and education on liability (Peters, 1985; Saltz, 1985) impact servers at several points on this continuum (i.e., in local lounges, taverns, and restaurants; public events, business socials, fraternities/sororities; and friends or family members who regularly use alcohol or drugs to entertain). In addition, school-based programs which seek to involve the parents and siblings through family homework assignments and televised smoking cessation programs (Flay et al., 1982, 1983b, 1983c) or volunteer efforts will impact more sites of influence.

Prevention approaches can also be dichotomized into those which attempt to modify or remove the causes of chemical dependency versus those which attempt to buffer the consequences. Some researchers and practitioners in alcoholism attempt to prevent the adverse consequences of drug and alcohol abuse and addiction by creating a low-risk environment through technological and social engineering. They attempt to find better ways to decrease the approximately 100,000 deaths and hundreds of thousands of injuries caused by encounters between drinkers and high-risk environments. Advocates of this approach (Beauchamp, 1976; Ryan, 1972, Wittman, 1985) point out that current prevention policy often places the onus for drug abuse problems solely on the individual, despite scientific information clearly implicating the environment. Environmental risk reduction strategies have been quite successful in the public health prevention field. Removal of lead from paint to protect babies from lead poisoning and control of air pollution are examples of cost-effective reduction strategies. In the alcohol field, recommended measures to mitigate drunk-driving accidents include mandatory seat belt and air bag laws (Wagenaar, 1985, personal communication), ignition starter control devices which require skills needed to drive safely, increasing the penalties and enforcement for driving while intoxicated (DWI) and driving under the influence (DUI) laws, increasing liability and education of servers (Saltz, 1985), and Students Against Drunk Driving (SADD) contracts for parents to drive teenagers home who have been using alcohol or drugs.

Other environmental risk reduction policies include public intoxication legislation which attempts to remove public drunks from parks and abandoned buildings to safe, supervised settings like walk-in and detoxification centers. Other consequences of drug and alcohol dependency, such as increased family violence, child neglect and abuse, decreased worker productivity, and increased crime, accidents, and fires are addressed in prevention programs such as employee assistance programs for early indentification and intervention, crime prevention programs, and family violence and neglect prevention programs. Many of these prevention programs are not the primary activity of drug abuse agencies, but of other social service or juvenile justice agencies.

Etiological research (see Kumpfer, 1987 for a complete review of biological and environmental risk factors) supports the proposition that some children are more vulnerable to becoming substance abusers because of biological and psychosocial risk factors. The degree and type of inherited biochemical and neuropsychological vulnerability will differ for each child. In addition, the extent and type of psychosocial damage sustained by the child raised in a household with a drug- or alcohol- dependent or dysfunctional parent will also vary. This author believes that for these reasons and cost effectiveness, prevention programs should be primarily targeted to high-risk populations. These programs should be flexible and tailored to the specific needs of the participants.

An ideal strategy for developing tailored prevention interventions would be to start with an extensive biological and psychosocial risk assessment (see DuPont, 1988 for several suggested lists of risk factors). One could then create specific prevention interventions designed for each risk factor. At first glance, this would appear to be very costly and involve agencies and specialities not generally directly associated with the prevention of drug dependency (pediatricians, child psychiatrists and other child development specialists, special educators, juvenile justice specialists). However, a number of research studies have found that the most effective prevention programs are generally those that are most intensive (Kumpfer, 1987; Moskowitz, 1986) and tailored to the specific needs of high-risk populations.

Some prevention specialists (Hawkins et al., 1987) believe that prevention efforts should target high-risk neighborhoods, schools, or communities rather than high-risk individuals because of the concern for labeling individuals as high risk, or involving youth and families in interventions that they do not need if they turn out to be "false-positives." This would be one possible solution to getting as many high-risk children into a program without specifically labeling them as high risk. Currently, the prevention field provides prevention services to many false-positives in general school or public programs; namely all school children and the general population in expensive, obtrusive, and overly simplistic prevention programs that so far have occasionally been found to increase alcohol and drug use (Hansen, 1988). Involving children and families in the general population in interventions they do not need and that may have negative effects, is closely, ineffective, and potentially unethical.

Some health professionals may well be afraid to provide needed early intervention and prevention services to a child who has an identified problem (abused or neglected children, emotionally or behaviorally disturbed children, learning-disordered children, depressed or suicidal children, to name a few) because of some nebulous concern for "labeling." (Introductory psychology classes often discussed the Rosenthal "expectancy" Effect, though this research has never been replicated.) If this ill-founded fear of labeling is not countered, these children will be denied, in many cases, empirically proven beneficial services. The child or the parents need not be told the child is at high risk for drug or alcohol abuse.

The new prevention programs created with Office of Substance Abuse Prevention (OSAP) funding will taret high-risk or vulnerable children and youth, but in general they do not label these children or youth. Youth are selected for these special services because they are members of high-risk groups of youth, such as children of abusers, children living in public housing or high-density housing, children already manifesting problems (behavioral, academic, or emotional) and gateway drug users. These high-risk child demonstration programs are generally advertised to the teachers, community members, and parents as extra services that will help children in any of these groups to be happier, better adjusted, more skillful, and more successful in life.

To date, many drug and alcohol abuse prevention programs have focused on providing education in schools. These educational approaches are designed to provide information to the general student body. They are a good beginning, but it should be obvious from the prior review of risk factors that more intensive interventions are needed to impact high-risk youth. The next secton will review the type of prevention programs that have been implemented and evaluated. In general, adequate evaluations of these programs are very rare and makes a critical review difficult.

IV. MAJOR DRUG AND ALCOHOL ABUSE PREVENTION CENTERED APPROACHES

Within the Public Health System (PHS) model of prevention, three major approaches have been promoted by the federal government and the states—namely, school-based prevention interventions, community-based prevention interventions, and family-focused prevention interventions. All three of these major approaches are reviewed in depth in Ezekoye, Kumpfer, and Bukoski, 1986. Each of these approaches are reviewed below. In addition to these three approaches, two more recent approaches to prevention are reviewed in this chapter—comprehensive, multiple-component prevention programs that attempt to improve school or community environment or climate, and environmental public policy approaches that often rely on legislation and pertain primarily to alcohol.

A. School-based Prevention Interventions

One-third of all prevention programs are conducted in the schools. School-based programs are the primary method for accessing youths for the prevention of alcohol and drug abuse. Many readers may remember the lessons on tobacco, drugs, and alcohol which they received in their school health classes, Today's programs are much improved and do not rely on scare tactic methods promoted by Harry J. Anslinger, and the Bureau of Narcotics, because they were shown to be counter productive or ineffective (Bukoski, 1979; Wepner, 1979). One study demonstrated that knowledge retention in students is better in a low fear versus high fear appeal, and better with a credible communicator (Williams, Ward, and Gray, 1985).

As the "back to basics" educational revolution grows, this route of easy access to a large number of youth is declining (Adler & Raphael, 1983). The percentage of high school sensors reporting having received any drug education information in schools has declined from 79% in 1976 to 68% in 1982—a surprising result given the increase in funding for prevention in recent years. Of these students, only 20% reported receiving a special course on drug abuse, with 59% of these students reporting that the course was valuable (Johnston et al., 1985).

A wide variety of school-based programs are being implemented and tested in our nation. These approaches have been categorized by Bukoski (1986) into five domains: incognitive, affective/interpersonal, behavioral, environmental and therapeutic. Each of these will be discussed briefly, but under the headings of cognitive, affective, alternative, behavioral, community, and family-focused programs.

Knowledge About Alcohol and Drugs—Cognitive Programs

Programs influencing the cognitive domain focus on increasing the students' knowledge about (1) pharmacological effects of alcohol and drugs, (2) health and social causes and consequences of abuse, (3) school and community attitudes and norms and legal sanctions, and (4) general health education. These programs often consist of films and didactic instruction by classroom teachers or health educators. Occasionally, law enforcement officials or physicians are asked to present to the classes health consequences or legal realities. Reality-oriented assemblies presented by exaddicts and drug paraphenalia displays have been found to be ineffective, but are occasionally still used. A teacher who passes around a joint to a class should not be surprised to get two back. These educational programs are generally effective in increasing students' knowledge about alcohol and drugs, but whether they have any impact on decreasing or delaying the onset of alcohol or drug use is not known because most educational programs do not include evaluation of behavioral objectives (Moskowitz, 1983).

Issues to be faced by proponents of these programs are:

1. The knowledge/attitudes/intentions/behavior theory: The primary theory of change underlying these programs, which assumes that a change in knowledge will affect a change in attitudes, intentions to use, and eventually behavioral use, has never been empirically demonstrated. A number of studies have provided little empirical support for this theory (Goodstadt, 1981; Wallack and Barrows, 1981). Some researchers have been able to demonstrate knowledge retention without changes in attitudes, intentions, or behavior (Moskowitz et al., 1984; Schaps et al., 1982; and Williams et al., 1985), whereas other researchers have been able to demonstrate attitude changes, but no change in intentions or behavior (Schlegal and Norris, 1980). In addition, some researchers have found changes

in intentions and opposite changes in behavior (Kumpfer & DeMarsch, 1986). In our study, we found youth in one condition (the Family Skills Training groups), who significantly increased their intentions to use drugs (like their drug-using parents), but those who were users significantly decreased their use. A number of studies found that intentions to use drugs accounted for little of the variance in subsequent use after controlling for prior use (Bentler and Speckart, 1979; Huba et al., 1981).

2. Decreased exposure to educational programs by high risk youth: Many high-risk children, including children of alcohol or drug abusers, do not regularly attend school and are likely to "skip out" on an alcohol or drug lecture or film. In addition, these are the children who drop out of school earlier and are lost to the pretest or follow-up evaluation of outcomes owing to frequent moves of the family.

3. Quality control is very difficult when teachers, students, or trainers with many different attitudes toward alcohol and drug use are implementing the programs. Process evaluations are rarely conducted to determine whether the trainers are implementing the program as specified.

4. Weak Programs: Most of these programs are not intensive or enduring enough to have much impact unless their goals are very simple. One study has found that longer programming may not be necessary if the goals are to increase knowledge and the curriculum simply presents the facts. Schlegal, Manske, and Page (1984) found that students exposed to a 3-session "fact"'s curriculum had lower alcohol consumption at posttest and 6-month follow-up than students who had the facts sessions plus four more sessions of values clarification and decision-making skills.

5. Some educational programs are ineffective because they are not developmentally or culturally appropriate. Prevention programs should be designed to match the cognitive level of the child and fit with the child's cultural and ethnic traditions.

Despite the fact that few of these knowledge-oriented prevention programs have had measurable impacts on reduced alcohol or drug abuse, some researchers are still supportive of this approach and say that more research is needed on this approach. It is the author's opinion that providing information about the short-term negative consequences of alcohol or drug abuse may help to deter low-risk youth from experimentation with these drugs. This effect will help to reduce stress on a number of families that worry that their children will become drug abusers. Knowledge about the highly addictive qualities of some drugs (i.e., "crack" or "designer" drugs) may be more important, since even low-risk youth could become addicted to these drugs through occasional use.

It is the author's opinion that educational programs could also be used to help high-risk youth understand the behavior of adults; namely, their parents, grandparents, relatives, or friends when they drink too much. Low-risk children can also be taught to be supportive and helpful to children less fortunate than themselves who are living in homes with drug- or alchol-addicted dependent parents. Teachers could be trained to recognize the signs of a child of drug- or alcohol-addicted parents and could then refer the child for help or provide extra understanding and support for the child when at school (Ackerman, 1983).

Affective and Interpersonal Education Programs

Affective and interpersonal prevention activities indirectly hope to prevent drug abuse by increasing the child's self-concept, understanding of feelings and interpersonal relationships, and awareness of the communication and decision-making processes. A wide variety of programs are grouped under this approach. Some programs involve youth in discussion groups or peer counseling sessions about feelings, decision making, problem solving, communications, or values clarification. Occasionally, professional consultation is provided on an individual or group basis.

Evaluations have found little support for the effectiveness of this approach in decreasing adolescents' intentions to use or not use drugs as well as changing attitudes or delaying the onset of use (Huba et al., 1980; Goodstadt, 1980; Goodstadt and Sheppard, 1983; Moskowitz et al., 1982, 1984). The Napa Project, which was based primarily on this model, demonstrated no effects on seventh-grade males or eighth grade males or females. The only positive effect on use was found for alcohol and marijuana, but not cigarettes among seventh-grade girls at posttest and not at a 1-year follow-up (Moskowitz et al., 1984; Schaps et al., 1982). Another program that combined values decision making with social competency skills training in a 12-session program found a positive effect on tobacco use at posttest, but a negative effect on alchol use and no effect on marijuana use (Gersick, Grady and Snow, 1985). Johnson and his associates (1985) report negative effects on alcohol and marijuana by a decision-making and social competency curriculum compared to their social influences, peer-resistance training program. It is not clear, however, that both programs were implemented with the same degree of enthusiasm.

These studies show conflicting results on different substances, but overall these affective education programs have not been demonstrated to be very effective given limited programming funding and time. It is the author's belief that the goals of these programs are laudable, but they are to far removed from the goal of reduced drug abuse. More intensive programming for high-risk youth who are actually found to be deficient in these skills may be more productive.

Alternative Programs

This type of approach to prevention is based on the theoretical assumption that providing youth with "alternative highs" or skill- and competency-building activities will reduce sustance abuse. Schaps and his associates (1981) found in a review of 122 prevention evaluation studies only 12 dealt with alternative programming. The effectiveness of this approach was equivocal. Five of the programs had positive outcomes, but seven reported no program impact. Stein and associates (1984) found that the Channel One nationwide program, in which many high-risk youth were involved in community recreation and business projects, failed to prevent the short-term increase in frequency of drunkenness and use of some drugs expected developmentally in high-risk youth. However, it is possible that these programs were actually effective in reducing high-risk youth's use of alcohol and drugs, and that this result would have been shown if the participating youth had been compared to similar high-risk youth in control groups. When evaluating prevention programs with youth already manifesting behavior and drug problems, one needs to remember that these "in trouble" youth often have a rapidly escalating base rate of problem behaviors and that a decrease in this rapid increase of drug use is progress. However, in alternative programs that bring a number of gateway drug-using youth together, one must also consider the contagion effect. An experimental evaluation of three of the Channel One sites showed slight positive findings for improved democratic problem solving and participation in alternatives, but increased use of inhalants, hallucinogens, and alcohol (Hu et al., 1982).

An important discovery by Swisher and Hu (1983) that helps to explain some of the contradictory findings for this approach is that *some alternative activities promote decreased use and others promote increased use* depending on the social environment and people associated with each type of activity. Activities such as those involving entertainment, sports, social, extracurricular, and vocational activities are associated with increased use of alcohol or drugs, whereas activities such as academic activities, religious activities, and active hobbies are associated with decreased use.

Murray and Perry (1985) are in the process of evaluating an alternatives program that is based on the functional relevance of drugs for youth at different ages. They have found that transition marking and social acceptance are important functions of alcohol and drugs among younger youth, whereas stress reduction appears more important among older youth. All of the youth used alcohol and drugs to enhance personal energy, for recreation, and relief from boredom or loneliness. They are evaluating their school-based program, called Amazing Alternatives, which helps youth to identify health-enhancing alternative activities for each function served for them by substance use.

Behavioral Prevention Programs

These programs attempt to behaviorally train students to resist peer pressures to use tobacco, alcohol, and marijauna through social learning, reciprocal determinism, and efficacy theory (Bandura, 1977, 1986). The currently popular social competency approaches to prevention include three different strategies: (1) the social influences approach as found in social inoculation and peer resistance social skills training strategies promoted initially by Evans and his Houston associates (1978, 1981); (2) modeling or training health-promoting behaviors; and (3) the broader life/social skills approaches promoted by Botvin and Eng (1980, 1982).

Social influences prevention programs have been well supported fiscally, and have been researched by a large number of well-known prevention specialists, e.g., McAlister and his Stanford associates (1979, 1980), Perry and her Minnesota associates (1980a, 1980b; 1983a, 1983b), Tell and associates in Oslo (1984), Vatiainen and associates in North Karelia, Finland (1983), Schinke, Gilchrist, and their Seattle associates (1983, 1986), Pentz and her Tennessee or USC associates (1982, 1983), Johnson and his Minnesota or USC associates (1984, 1985), Flay and his Waterloo or USC associates (1982, 1983a, 1983b, 1983c; 1985), Fisher and his associates in Australia (1983), Dielman and his Michigan group (1984a, 1984b), and Biglan, Severson, and colleagues in Oregon (1985) to name a few.

These programs appear to have some effectiveness in delaying onset of tobacco use in junior high school students, though Moskowitz (1986) points out that the "pattern of effects is inconsistent across studies even of the same program. Some studies find reductions in new smoking; others find reductions in experimental or more regular smoking." The reason for the delayed onset is unknown because of the large number of mediating variables in these programs. Some researchers have speculated that if real changes are occurring in these programs that the changes may be due to reinforcement of existing school norms not to use tobacco (Kumpfer, Moskowitz, and Klitzner, 1986), or recent changes in the social climate not to smoke cirgarettes or the informal social control climate (Moskowitz, 1983; Perry et al., 1980; Polich et al., 1984, Rodin, 1985). Botvin and McAlister (1982) report that student interviews revealed a positive change in the entire social atmosphere regarding smoking following their life skills antismoking intervention.

Because of increased awareness of the health risks of tobacco due to the antismoking campaign beginning with the 1964 U.S. Surgeon General's Report, many American citizens have chosen to decrease their use of health-compromising, mild stimulants, such as tobacco. This may not have been as difficult to change as for other drugs because there are more acceptable mild stimulants available—caffeine, sugar, and zanthene—that can serve a similar function. In fact, the caffeinated soft drink market has increased significantly in recent years and sugar and chocolate consumptions are very high. Hence, antismoking "Say No" programs did not have to address the basic functions of nicotine. Brauch (1980) and Murray and Perry (1985) have stressed that we need to understand the different psychosocial functions played by alcohol and other drugs before effective prevention programs can be designed for these substances. This author believes that we also need to understand the biological functions that alcohol and drugs play in designing the best replacement strategy.

There is growing concern among prevention researchers and practitioners about the high percentage of prevention research funding supporting this single prevention approach when there is little empirical data to support its effectiveness (Bell and Battjes, 1985). A preliminary evaluation of the application of this approach to alcohol and marijuana prevention in the USC Project Smart suggests disappointing outcomes as this program did not prevent any significant number of children from using alcohol or marijuana (Johnson et al., 1985). Recently, prevention practitioners and researchers expressed concern about the real as opposed to statistical effectiveness of these programs even with antismoking applicatiaons. For instance, because of the high attrition (25–64%) in these school-based programs, the often cited 50% reduction in youth who begin use can mean very few youth when percentages are translated to actual members. Hence, because of their high cost and intrusiveness into the daily academic schedule of schools, these programs do not at this time appear to be cost effective. The highest-risk youth are often missing from schools and do not receive the benefits of the continuity of these school-based programs. Also, these programs rarely report what happens to high-risk youth who are already users or any youth who are already using tobacco, alcohol, or drugs. It is entirely possible that these programs are having a negative impact in increasing alcohol, tobacco, or drug use in youth who have already tried them.

In a review of this prevention approach, Flay (1987) concludes:

> Overall, the findings from the most rigorous studies to date suggest that the social influences approach to smoking prevention can be effective some of the time. However, this conclusion seems somewhat fragile, given the considerable differences between studies in the patterns of reported results. Also, at least two plausible alternative interpretations of the reported effects remain—namely, sensitizing effects of the pretest testing (or screening), and the Hawthorne Effect, since many control group schools receive no special program.

In addition, Moskowitz (1986) points out that "the effect sizes and significance levels reported in these studies are biased and cannot be trusted as the statistical analyses were not conducted on the units assigned to conditions, schools or classrooms, but rather on students (Biglan and Ary, 1985; Cook, 1985; Moskowitz; 1983)." So it appears that even the "fourth-generation studies" suffer from major methodological weaknesses and claimed positive effects of the "Say No" skills training programs need to be closer evaluated.

This author does not believe that such a simplistic approach can be very effective with high-risk youth who by this point in their development will have multiple reasons to "say yes" to drugs and alcohol. These programs do not address the main reasons that vulnerable youth use drugs. A nuber of researchers have also suggested that the peer pressure notion as the primary determinant of substance abuse is overly simplistic (Moskowitz, 1983; Eiser and van der Pligt, 1985; Sheppard et al., 1985). A young student representative of the "Say No Clubs" recently explained at a Chicago conference that "peer pressure is more like Adidas. If you are the only one without them, you want them." This doesn't sound much like the type of peer pressure promoted by the social inoculation program providers or researchers, which present a picture of drug-using youth who are badgering a nonusing youth to "just try it, you'll like it." A recent research study by Shope and Dielman (1985) found that most fifth and sixth grade students alrady had sufficient refusal skills (or "saying no") skills before the program, and that a four-session social skills training curriculum did not decrease their alcohol consumption

School Climate Change Approaches

Several prominant drug-abuse theorists hae recognized the importance of the social environment in drug abuse prevention. Hawkins and Weis (1985) developed the social development model that hypothesizes that youth who bond to their school are less vulnerable to the influence of negative peers. School bonding, which they define as committment, attachment, and belief, is determined by opportunities for successful involvement in school activities and positive peer groups. Many schools today are not designed to be conducive to involvement by high-risk students. Some schools actively attempt to eliminate high-risk students from their activities and even from the school by expulsion. Gottfredson (1986) has found in studies of several hundred schools that students bond more readily in a positive social environment that discourages the use of drugs and alcohol without jeopardizing opportunities for involvement and recognition by using and high-risk students. Bascially, we need to create "kinder and gentler schools," just as President Bush had called us to create a "kinder and gentler nation".

Gottfredson (1986) evaluated a comprehensive, multicomponent program aimed to improve school climate and make faculty, staff, and students more cohesive and supportive of each other. This program organizes all school prevention activities through a School Prevention Coordinator and several planning and implementation teams—a student team, a faculty team, a parent team, a business/school partnership team, and a "high-risk students" team, consisting primarily of counselors and vice principals responsible for high-risk students. Each team plans prevention activities guided by the school data and the basic philosophy of developing programs that improve school pride and climate, increase school involvement and bonding, and improve academic performance. The plans are coordinated by a core executive team made up of the leaders of each team. This program was evaluated and found effective in reducing alcohol and drug use in junior and senior high school students and in increasing school academic performance.

Kumpfer and her associates (1989) are currently evaluating an adaptation of the Project PATHE for high-risk students, called Project HI PATHE. In Project HI PATHE a broad variety of prevention programs were implemented and tested. All of the programs were designed to increase the involvement of high-risk and low socioeconomic students. Examples of projects implemented include cooperative learning, life skills courses, teen talk lines run cooperatively by counselors and trained students, peer counseling and peer leadership programs, alternative sports and hobby activities, faculty retreats to improve faculty morale and bonding, school pride days, new student welcome projects, entering class support activities, treatment aftercare support groups, after-school tutoring to improve academic achievement, in school suspension programs, alcohol and drug presentation's and musicals involving high-risk students, and student-producted teen guides to the local community and businesses. The results of the first year of operations indicate positive reductions in use in the high-intensity school as compared to the low-intensity control schools.

B. Community- Based Prevention Interventions

Public Media

This approach to prevention is one of the major methods for providing prevention for adults. The primary techniques used are mass media or public awareness campaigns. A coordinated media campaign could involve one or all of the following: radio, television, newspaper, magazine, billboard, and poster consumer awareness adertisements; special face-to-face presentations in workshops, classes, conferences, campaigns; and supporting publications such as pamphlets, books, films, video tapes, and direct-mail flyers. This prevention strategy is one of the earliest used in this country. The goal of this approach is generally to provide increased information about the health consequences of alcohol and drug abuse or use. Unfortunately, evaluations of these public-awareness programs, particularly those that employed scare tactics, have not been encouraging (Blum, Blum, and Garfield, 1976). More research suggests that information-only programs can be more effective if they communicate in a straightforward way the adverse effects of drugs, use credible communicators, target behavioral changes needed to support nonuse, and influence the recipients' perceptions about the acceptability of use/addiction (Durrell and Bukoski, 1983; Polich et al., 1984).

A primary weakness of these early information-only prevention programs was that they assumed a knowledge (attitude) behavior model. A considerable body of research suggests that increased knowledge has little effect on attitudes, and changes in attitudes seldom lead to behavior changes (McGuire, 1969). In fact, the more common scenario is that change in behavior lead to changes in attitudes. Fishbein (1973) and other social psychologists have discovered that attitude change can influence behavior change if two conditions are satisfied: (1) that attitude is specifically about the behavior to be measured, and (2) other social and environmental factors support the attitude-behavior change relationship (Ostram, 1969; Rockeach and Kliejunas, 1972; Wicker, 1971).

The conclusion concerning media campaigns is that they do provide needed information and through a slow process do affect the community's social norms in the long run when combined with other community prevention strategies. In addition, the public demand for credible information about alcohol and drugs is increasing and should be satisfied by accurate and scientifically credible messages.

Parent Groups

Increasingly, prevention planners are advocating efforts to create a community climate of nondrug use (Durrell and Bukoski, 1983). The current involvement of parents' groups in promoting community substance abuse prevention of both drugs and alcohol is significant. These parental groups generally focus on one or more of three goals: (1) changes in the home to counter prodrug messages. (2) changes in the youth's social environment, and (3) community-awareness campaigns. Actually, because of the spontaneous nature of these parent groups, little is known about the actual activities of these parent groups and their effectiveness. The National Institute of Drug Abuse (NIDA) has funded a descriptive study of these national parent groups in hope of better understanding their impact (Klitzner, 1984). A national examples of the usefulness of parent groups in macroapproaches to prevention are Chemical People, the Cottage Program International's Family Friendship Circles, and the National Federation of Parents for Drug Free Youth. The focus on these macrocommunity prevention efforts is on creating a climate in which children are getting "don't do drugs" messages from respected adults and peers in schools, media, and the community at large.

Community Groups

Over the years, a number of public service clubs, church groups, corporations, and private nonprofit organizations have helped in the fight against alcohol and drug abuse. Civic groups such as the Junior League, the Lion's Club, Service Clubs of America, and the Rotary have sponsored their own alcohol and drug prevention programs or worked with state and local officials to enhance the effectiveness of a state or national campaign. A number of businesses have volunteered to sponsor high-risk youth in the Channel One Programs.

C. Family-Focused Prevention Interventions

Importance of the Family in Drug and Alcohol and Addiction Abuse Prevention

Prevention specialists are beginning to recognize the valuable resource that parents and families are for increasing the effectiveness of drug and alcohol abuse and addiction prevention programs for youth. The author's recent research with children of drug- and alcohol-abusing parents (DeMarsch and Kumpfer, 1986; Kumpfer and DeMarsch, 1986a) supports the fact that the family is highly involved in the genesis and maintenance of drug and alcohol abuse and addiction and can be very influential in the alleviation of risk factors in children.

Prevention Programs for Children of Drug- and Alcohol Addicted Parents

These results suggest cost-effect, family-based prevention interventions must be developed to prevent drug and alcohol abuse and addiction in children of alcohol and drug abusers or addictions. Few family-focused drug and alcohol abuse prevention programs have been developed for high-risk children, despite the fact that the application of parent training and family skills training programs to other problems in children have been highly effective (Dinkmeyer and McKay, 1976; Forehand and McMahon, 1981; Gordon, 1970; Guerney, 1964; L'Abate, 1977; Miller, 1975; Patterson et al., 1975). One reason for this effectiveness is that parents can be trained to be effective change agents and their effect will be enduring and powerful. In the last 10 years, the NIDA has supported several family-focused prevention programs, namely, the author's Strengthening Families Program (DeMarsh and Kumpfer, 1986; Kumpfer and DeMarsh, 1986a) for children of drug and addicts in treatment, Alvy's Confident Parenting Program (1985) for parents of black youth, and Szapocznik's Family Effectiveness Training (1983, 1986, 1987) for parents of high-risk Hispanic adolescents.

The Kumpfer and DeMarsh Strengthening Families Program.   Once the characteristic differences between drug- and nondrug-addicted families and children were supported by empirical findings, the author developed and tested three different types of family oriented prevention program—a parent training program, a children's social skills training program, and a family skills training program—to determine their effectiveness in reducing the children's risk factors. Preliminary analyses of the pre- and posttest data suggest that all three programs were successful in reducing the risk factors in the children, though each program's effect depended on its intended goals. Hence, the behavioral parent training program was successful in reducing the children's problem behaviors and improving the parent's ability to discipline the children; the family skills training program improved the family relationships and some of the children's problem behaviors; and the children's social skills program improved the children's social skills. Only in the complete Strengthening Families Program that combines all three interventions was alcohol and drug use actually decreased in the older children. A proposed longitudinal study is needed to determine in the long run which of these changes will be most successful in preventing alcohol and drug abuse in the younger children. Another important finding of this research is that regardless of the parents' dysfuntionality, most parents can be coached and assisted in developing more effective parenting styles that will affect risk factors in their children.

Parent training program results.   Following exposure to the Parent Training Program parents report having less problems handling school-aged children, and demonstrated increased knowledge of child behavior management principles. This increased knowledge and improved parent discipline effectiveness had direct impact on the behavior of the children, who were reported to scream less, have fewer temper tantrums, get angry less, have improvements in their home behaviors, and display fewer problems than other children their own age. Further, the children were reported by their parents to be happier, and to like school better, and also to have shown an increase in their outside activities. The children reported a significant decrease in intention to smoke and to drink, but not to use drugs.

Family skills training program.   This program combined three different phases—a filial play therapy phase in which parents are taught to enjoy the child, called Child's Game; a family communications training phase; and an effective discipline training phase called Parent's Game. Preliminary outcome effectiveness evaluations indicate improvements in three theorectically specified areas that are thought to influence a child's "risk status": (1) family functioning, (2) children's behavior problems, and (3) children's expressiveness.

Family function seemed to improve on several dimensions following participation in the Family Skills Training program, including increased family communication of problems, improved relations among siblings, improved ability to think of family-oriented activities, clarity of family rules, and more social contacts by parents.

Likewise, improvements in children's behavior problems were found. Parents reported their children behaved less impulsively, were more well-behaved at home, and had fewer problem behaviors in general. Also, children self-reported improved relations with peers.

The Family Skills Training component of the Strenghtening Families Program curriculum also appears to have impacted the extent to which children are able to express themselves within the family context—both verbally and otherwise. Children were found to ask for more help with their homework, to talk to people more when they feed sad, to seek more attention from parents, and to cry more. Similar to the Parent Training Program, the children reported at posttest significant decreases in their intentions to use tobacco and alcohol, but not drugs.

Obviously, the author believes that this approach has considerable promise for reducing drug and alcohol abuse in high-risk youth. The positive effects of a parent training program, a family skills training program, and a children's social skills training program need to be tested for durability in a follow-up study and the program effectiveness with other high-risk populations (minorities, conduct-disordered children) needs to be tested.

Family Therapy

A number of clinicians are using family therapy as a prevention or early intervention strategy for high-risk children and youth. Klein et al., (1977) discovered that Functional Family Therapy is an effective prevention strategy for younger siblings of delinquents was a major breakthrough in this area. Hence, to the degree that family therapy reduces risk factors for nonusers or nondrug-dependent members of the family (the spouse and the children), it is a prevention strategy. Unfortunately, many public and private funding sources for drug and alcohol abuse prohibit payment for anyone but the abuser.

Family therapy can take many forms. Gallant et al. (1970) have experimented with the use of multiple-couple groups. Steinglass (1975) briefly employed the free use of alcohol (while being videotaped) in the initial assessment stages of an experimental inpatient program at National Institute of Alcohol Abuse and Alcoholism's (NIAAA) Laboratory for Alcohol Research to help the staff and couples better understand the role that alcohol played in the family dynamics. In Utah, the Teen Alcohol and Drug Schools have employed multiple family therapy principles successfully for years. One unique feature of this program is that the children and parents are switched for initial communication exercises. It often appears for people to practice new skills with different parents and children.

To work successfully with drug- and alcohol-addicted families, the therapist or trainer needs to have a thorough understanding of the dynamics and typical developmental stages of these families (see Kaufman, 1980; Steinglass, 1980). The pioneering work of Wegscheider (1981) and Ackerman (1983) in family therapy with alcoholics has promoted understanding in this filed. Since recruitment is often a problem, Szapocznik and his associates (1984) have experimented with one-person family therapy and found it effective. In addition, Szapocznik has developed culturally relevant family therapy for Hispanic families of Cuban descent. Maldanado and his associates have successfully used their family model as an early intervention strategy for Hispanic (Spanish and Mexican descent) first-offender youth, and as a prevention strategy for siblings (Courtney, 1984; Kumpfer et al., 1985).

Family Self-Help Groups

Self-help groups, such as Al-Anon for spouses of alcholics and Alafam for families of alcoholics, are increasing in popularity. Over 5000 Alafam groups exist throughout the world, making them the single largest prevention program involving families of alcohol-dependent persons. These groups closely parallel Alcoholics Anonymous meetings. According to Ablon (1974), they teach the basic lesson that alcoholism is a disease, and three basic principles: loving detachment from the alcoholic, reestablishment of their own self-esteem and independence, and reliance on a "higher power." Through shared experiences, the groups teach that many families have the same problems, and that they are not alone. Some treatment clinics for alcohol dependency also involve spouses (para-alcoholics) or families in groups. One of the authors (Kumpfer, 1975) specializes in prevention groups for wives of alcohol-dependent men using a specially structured curriculum. Through increased understanding, these spouses and families are not only increasing the probability that the alcoholic will achieve and maintain sobriety, but they are decreasing their own risk of becoming alcoholics. (For further information on para-alcoholics and co-alcoholics, see Greenleaf, 1981).

D. Multicomponent Prevention Programs

All of the above prevention approaches involve a single strategy. More recently, prevention programmers and planners have become excited about the possible interactive and enhancing potential of sustained, integrated, multicomponent community programs or campaigns. School-based programs are limited in their influence on youth because the majority of an adolescent's time is spent outside of school (at home, watching TV, in the community, etc.). In addition, the highest-risk youth are the least likely to be at school, and also significant onset of drug and alcohol abuse occurs after high school graduation. Hence, an optimal prevention program would incorporate mass media, community organization, and families as well as schools.

Evaluation

Evaluations of multicomponent prevention programs have been encouraging and suggest that by combining a number of programs a synergistic effect may increase the effectiveness of all components. Flay and his associates (1983b, 1983c) combined a school and media smoking prevention program with written homework assignments to be completed with parents. The junior high school youth in this program were only half as likely to start smoking during the 2 months between pre- and posttests. Significant secondary effects were observed in parents involved in the program, with 35% quitting smoking and 69% attempting to cut back or quit. This research did not test the individual components; hence, it was not possible to determine the efficacy of the multicomponent approach.

Bien and Bry (1980) did employ a dismantling design to improve academic performance (one of the covariants of substance abuse). They found that only the seventh graders with all three components (teacher conferences, student goal-setting groups, and home notes or calls to parents) had significant improvements in grades and attendance over a nonintervention group. This research tends to support the increased effectiveness hypothesis of the multicomponent prevention strategy; however, it is possible that the most important component is the family involvement added last.

Health Promotion Program

Additional support for the multicomponent community prevention approach can be gleaned from the heart disease prevention and health promotion community programs: the Oslo Study (Holmes et al., 1982), the Stanford Three Community Study (Maccoby, 1976; Solomon, 1982), and the North Karelia Project (McAlister, et al., 1980, 1982). The Stanford Three Community Study demonstrated that the combination of in-home or group prevention sessions with public media significantly reduced the risk of heart disease, increased knowledge (Meyer et al., 1980), and decreased smoking and number of hypertensives (Farquhar et al., 1981) when comparing intervention to no intervention control communities. Intermediate results were found for the media-only communities at 1- and 3-year follow-ups. Likewise, the intensive community prevention programming in the North Karelia, Finland Project suggests that multicomponent programs may have synergistic effects. A higher percentage of persons in North Karelia who viewed the nationally televised smoking cessation programs had ceased smoking over persons in unorganized communities.

A number of new community heart disease prevention programs are currently underway in the United Sates: the Stanford Five Cities Study (Farquhar, 1978), the Minnesota Heart Health program (Leupker et al., 1982), the Pawtucket Heart Health Program (Elder et al., 1982), and the Lycoming Community Health Improvement Program (Felix, 1983). These community programs seek to be more integral to the communities by involving key community leaders and fewer outsiders to run programs. Unfortunately, none of these prevention programs include an evaluation design which can demonstrate the relative effectiveness of the individual program components.

Several community-based drug prevention programs have been developed in San Francisco (Wallack and Barrows, 1981), Charlotte, North Carolina (Kim, 1981, 1982), Ventura, California (NIDA, 1982a), and Seattle, Washington (Resnik, 1982). According to Johnson (NIDA, 1982b), it is "not clear that any meaningful evaluation of these projects will be forthcoming."

E. Environmental Prevention Approaches

Some prevention approaches, particularly in the prevention of alcoholism, alcohol abuse, and alcohol problems (drunk driving, accidents, illness), are concerned with community environmental changes as mentioned earlier for informal and formal social controls. For instance, specialists in the alcohol field have advocated numerous environmental and regulatory approaches to prevent alcohol-related problems. Recommended measures include regulating the content of alcoholic beverage advertising (Mosher and Wallack, 1981), increasing the accuracy of portrayals of the consequences of alcohol use in the mass media (Wallack, in press), increasing counteradverting via industry funding (Wallack, 1984), increasing excise taxes and price (Mosher, 1982; Grossman, Coate and Arluck, 1984), and decreasing availability by (1) increasing the minimum age for legal purchase (Vingilis and DeGenova, 1984; Wagenaar, 1981, Williams and Lillis, 1985), (2) reducing the number of outlets selling alcoholic beverages for off-premise consumption (Hooper, 1983; MacDonald and Whitehead, 1983), (3) eliminating alcholic beverage sales from several stations, and (4) restricting sales at public events (Wittman, 1985).

Moskowitz (1986) has recently completed a review of these community environmental prevention approaches. Conclusions in this field are hindered by the lack of experimental designs, comparable control groups, lack of data on mediating variables, and the absence of process or implementation data (Judd and Kenny, 1981); however, at this time it would appear that some public policy changes can have modest impact in reducing alcohol problems. Moskowitz (1986) states that: "A substantial body of well-designed research indicates that increasing the minimum legal drinking age to 21 is an effective means of reducing alcohol-related automobile crashes, injuries and fatalities among the affected age group." Wagenaar (1983) estimates that 20% of all alcohol-related crashes and 13% of all fatal crashes involving young drivers can be prevented (Arnold, 1985).

The effectiveness of increased cost of alcohol on decreased use is unknown because of the substantial overlap of differences in community values or informal social controls with the amount of excise tax on alcohol. It does appear that if increased taxes are added to liquor, then youth and adults will switch to lower cost beer. Beer is now very similar in price to soft drinks because from 1967 to 1983 the price of alcoholic beverages increased only half as much as nonalcoholic beverages (Cook, 1984).

The effectiveness of drinking-driving laws appears to have short-term effectiveness depending on the enforcement of the laws and the degree of media coverage concerning the crackdown. This policy approach is more costly to implement than the prior mentioned policy approaches of increased minimum age and increased taxation. The increased taxation approach as an additional benefit in the general state funds raised through this policy can be earmarked, as some states have done, for drug and alcohol abuse treatment and prevention programs.

Another secondary or tertiary prevention strategy designed to reduce alcohol problems and drunk driving is server intervention (Mosher, 1983). O'Donnell (1985) estimates that about half of all alcohol-impaired drivers are driving to or from licensed on-premise establishments. Server intervention involves developing new policies and training managers and servers to refuse service to intoxicated customers and to increase profits by promoting food and nonalcoholic drinks. There are two evaluation studies of server interventions currently in progress, but no result to date (Saltz, 1985).

Most of these formal control prevention strategies are only appropriate for the prevention of abuse of a legal substance like alcohol. They are less applicable to the drug abuse prevention field except for over-the-counter and prescription drugs. Also, because these environmental and regulatory approaches tend to legislate personal choice, they often face public and private resistance (Bell and Levy, 1984) and raise ethical and moral questions (Roffman, 1982).

V. PUBLIC POLICY ISSUES

Alcohol and drug abuse, dependency, and problems are a significant drain on the health and economic wellbeing of this nation. Despite the significant drop in use of alcohol and drugs by youth in this nation since 1981, a substantial percentage of adults are using drugs. The commitment in this country to the prevention of substance abuse has been limited to verbal commitments rather than financial commitments. Despite the fact that in 1986 drug and alcohol abuse cost each person in this country about $850 (economic cost estimated from lost productivity, treatment costs, societal costs in accidents, fires), only the equivalent of 77¢ per person was spent on abuse prevention.

Public concern appeared to change dramatically last fall and the U.S. Congress authorized several billion dollars for the prevention of alcohol and drug abuse. Unfortunately most of this money will be spent on supply reduction techniques that have demonstrated little effect on actual use patterns. According to Lloyd Johnston (in press), 200 times more funding is going toward supply reduction as compared to demand-reduction strategies of prevention. The Rand Corporation Report on Strategies for Controlling Adolescent Drug Use (Polich et al., 1984) details why the use of supply-reduction interventions are ineffective in decreasing drug use and probably have pushed youth into harder drugs.

In addition, a very small amount of the new funding will be target to high-risk children and youth as advocated in this paper. Only about $24 million of the total amount will be used to fund demonstration/evaluation projects for comprehensive prevention and treatment, targeted prevention projects, and early intervention projects for high-risk youth. The creation of the new Office of Substance Abuse Prevention (OSAP), which will administer these new targeted prevention projects, is a step in the right direction. Hopefully, many new and innovative programs will be created and evaluated for dissemination by this funding.

VI. COST-BENEFIT OF PREVENTION PROGRAMS

Cost-effectiveness or cost-benefit analyses of current drug and alcohol abuse prevention approaches need to be conducted as advocated by the American Academy of Child and Adolescent Psychiatry's prevention project. Currently, it is very difficult to determine cost effectiveness because effectiveness for many prevention approaches are not well established. However, gross estimates are possible and should be used in advance of establishing a prevention program to determine whether the project is worthwhile. Little is published on the costs of programs from which to estimate cost effectiveness. In 1977, the NIDA published some information that could be used to determine gross estimates of cost effectiveness. Their general estimates, at that time, were that in order to be cost effective information or media campaigns needed to affect 0.15% of the participants, education programs needed to affect 6.25% of the participants, alternative programs needed to affect 8.53% of the participants, and intervention programs needed to affect 4.48% of the participants.

Research evaluations rarely ever publish their effectiveness rates and compare them to the costs of continued use of alcohol or drugs or unexpected benefits. The 1986 estimated yearly cost to society of a dysfunctional drug user is about $8000, whereas it was about $6200 in 1982. Hence, this figure on estimated cost of dysfunctional use needs to be indexed each year. Cost-effectiveness evaluations are obviously the best indicator of whether the program was really the most cost-effective because outcomes are compared across several programs with the same type of participants. However, cost-benefit analyses are possible with programs that have only one experimental group and one randomly assigned control group. In addition, this type of analysis has the added advantage of allowing the evalutor to add other spin-off or unexpected benefits to society. For example, the author has conducted a cost-benefit analysis of an alternative, job skills–building prevention program for high-risk youth. This program proved to be cost beneficial only when the value of the youth's community home-building projects were entered into the equation.

Cost-effective programs are likely to be those that include the following elements: community volunteers working with youth in community settings, strategies that target high-risk youth, messages that stress healthy lifestyles and focus on short-term health consequences, and integrated programs with enduring, coordinated, and pervasive strategies that address many of the environmental domains addressed in this chapter.

VII. RECOMMENDED DIRECTIONS

In a presentation to the American Academy of Child Psychiatry in 1985, the author discussed several promising directions for the prevention of substance abuse (Kumpfer, 1985). The most important points are summarized below:

1. Prevention interventions need to be tailored to the intended audience, including age, race, culture, gender, and life circumstances.
2. Prevention interventions need to be based on the best known etiological factors contributing to or protecting a youth from substance abuse.
3. More etiological research is needed that longitudinally track high-risk youth from childhood into the drug-using adolescent and early adult stages of their lives.
4. Increased prevention effectiveness research is needed for a broad range of different prevention interventions, rather than the current strategy of putting most funding into education-based approaches using one major strategy—"Say No" skills training.
5. Cost effectiveness and cost-benefit analyses (even if very crude) should be conducted to determine in general whether a particular prevention strategy is likely to be worthwhile

to develop. This type of analysis may help prevention designers to consider ways to cut costs and increase benefits.

6. Preferred prevention strategies are those that coordinate local community involvement, include messages that stress healthy lifestyles, target high-risk youth, and are enduring, naturalistic prevention programs.

VIII. CONCLUSIONS

There are no simple solutions in the fight against alcohol and drug abuse, which due to long term, complex causes that to begin early in life. Early childhood risk factors put some children on a different developmental path than most children that terminates in drug and alcohol abuse and other problem behaviors. Health care providers need to use their professional training and knowledge to attempt to help these children by early intervention and referral efforts.

REFERENCES

Ablon, J. (1974). Al-Anon family groups: Impetus for change through the presentation of alternatives. *Am. J. Psychother., 28*(1):30.

Ackerman, R. (1983). *Children of Alcoholics*. Holmes Beach, Learning Publications.

Adler, R., & Raphael, B. (1983). Children of alcoholics *Aust. N. Z. J. Psychiatry, 17*:3–8.

Alvy, K.T. (1985). *Parenting Programs for Black Parents*. Paper presented at the Primary Prevention of Psychopathology Conference (Families in transition: Primary prevention programs that work), sponsored by the National Institute of Mental Health, University of Vermont, Burlington.

Arnold, R. (1985). *Effect of Raising the Legal Drinking Age on Driver Involvement in Fatal Crashes: The Experience of Thirteen States*. (Department of Transportation Report No. HS 806 902). Washington, DC: National Highway Traffic Safety Administration.

Bandura, A. (1977). *Social Learning Theory*. Englewood Hills, New Jersey, Prentice-Hall.

Bandura, A (1986). *Social Foundations of Thought and Action: A Socialcognitive Theory*. Englewood Cliffs, New Jersey, Prentice-Hall.

Beauchamp, D. (1976). Exploring new ethics for public Health: Developing a fair alcohol policy. *J. Health Polit. Policy Law 1*:338–354.

Bell, C., and Battjes, R. (1985). *Prevention Research: Deterring Drug Abuse Among Children and Adolescents*. Washington, D.C., National Institute on Drug Abuse Research Monograph.

Bell, C.S., and Levy, S.M. (1984). Public policy and smoking prevention: Implications for research, *Behavioral Health*, (J.D. Malarazzo et al., eds.). New York, Wiley, pp. 775–785.

Bentler, P., and Speckart, G. (1979). Models of attitudes—behavior relations. *Psychol. Rev. 86*:452–464.

Bien, N.Z., and Bry, B.H. (1980). An experimentally designed comparison of four intensities of school-based prevention programs for adolescents with adjustment problems. *J. Commun. Psychol. 8*:110–116.

Biglan, A., and Ary, D. (1985). Methodological issues in research on smoking prevention. In C. Bell and R. Battjes (Eds.), *Prevention Research: Deterring Drug Abuse Among Children and Adolescents* (C. Bell and R. Battjes, eds.), U.S. Department of Health and Human Services Publication No. ADM 85-1334. Rockville, Maryland, National Institute on Drug Abuse, pp. 170–195.

Biglan, A., Severson, H.H., Ary, D. V., Faller, C., Thompson, R., Nautel, C., Lichtenstein, E. and Weissman, W.W. (1985). *Refusal Skills Training and the Prevention of Adolescent Cigarette Smoking*.

Blum, R., Blum, E., and Garfield, E. (1976). *Drug Education: Results and Recommendations*. Lexington, Massachusetts, Lexington Books.

Botvin, G.J., and Eng, A. (1980). A comprehensive school-based smoking prevention program. *J. School Health, 50*:209–213.

Botvin, G., and McAlister, A. (1982). Cigarette smoking among children and adolescents: Causes and prevention, *Annual Review of Disease Prevention* (C. Arnold, ed.). New York, Springer.

Braucht G. (1980). Psychosocial research on teenage drinking: Past and future, *Drugs and the Youth Culture*. (F. Scarpitti and S. Batesman, eds.). Beverly Hills, California, Sage Press.

Bukoski, W. (1979). *Drug Abuse Prevention Evaluation: A Meta-Evaluation Process*. Paper presented at the Annual Meeting of the American Public Health Association, New York.

Bukoski, W.J. (1986). School-based substance abuse prevention: A review of program research. *J. Child. Contemp. Soc.*.

Butynski, W., Record, N., and Yates, J. (1985). *State Resources and Services Related to Alcohol and Drug Abuse Problems: An Analysis of State Alcohol and Drug Abuse Profile Data—FY 1984*. Developed in part under contract No. ADMS 271-84-7314. Washington, D.C., National Association of State Alcohol and Drug Abuse Directors, Inc.

Cook, T. (1985). Priorities in research in smoking prevention, *Prevention Research: Deterring drug abuse among children and adolescents* U.S. Department of Health and Human Services Publication No. ADM 85-1334.) Rockville, Maryland, National Institute on Drug Abuse, pp.196-220.

Cook, P., and Tauchen, G. (1984). The effect of minimum drinking age legislation on youthful auto fatalities, 1970-1977, *J. Legal Stud. 13*:169-190.

Copeland, K.C., Underwood, L.E., and VanWyk, J.J. (1980). Marijuana smoking and pubertal arrest. *N. Engl. J. Med., 96*:1079-1080.

Courtney, R.J. (1984). *Functional Family Therapy Intervention for Hispanic Juvenile Offenders and Their Parents*. Project consultation on the Institute for Human Resources Development Prevention Program. Salt Lake City, Utah State Division of Alcoholism and Drugs.

DeMarsh, J., and Kumpfer, K.L. (1986). Family-oriented interventions for the prevention of chemical dependency in children and adolescents. *Childhood and Chemical Abuse: Prevention and Intervention* (S. Ezekaye, K. Kumpfer, and W. Bukoski, eds.). New York, Haworth Press.

Dielman, T.E., Horvath, W.J., Leach, S.L., and Lorenger, A.L. (1984a). *Peer Pressure in Recruitment to Smoking*. Final report to NIDA, University of Michigan.

Dielman, T.E., Leach, S.L., Lyons, A.C., Lorenger, A.T., Klos, D.M. and Horvath, W.J. (1984b). Resisting pressures to smoke: Fifteen-month follow-up results of an elementary school based smoking prevention project. *Int. J. Health Ed.*

Dinkmeyer, D., and McKay, G.D. (1976). *Systematic Training for Effective Parenting*. Circle Pines, Minnesota, American Guidance Service.

DuPont, R.I. (1988). *Stopping Drug Abuse Before It Starts: The Future of Drug Abuse Prevention*. A Report of a Committee of the Institute for Behavior and Health, Inc., Rockville, Maryland.

Durrell, J., and Bukoski, W. (1983). *The Prevention of Substance Abuse: State-of-the-Art*. (Unpublished paper).

Eiser, R., and van der Pligt, J. (1985). *Attitudinal and Social Factors in Adolescent Smoking: In Search of Peer Group Influence*. Exeter, England, Department of Psychology, University of Exeter.

Elder, J.P., Artz, L.M., Carleton, R.A., Kinsley, P.M., Peterson, G.S., Rosenberg, P.E., and Snow, R.C.K. (1982). *Establishing Cost-Efficient Member-Owned Heart Health Programs in Organizational Settings*. Paper presented at the annual convention of the Society of Behavioral Medicine Baltimore, Maryland.

Evans, R.I., Rozelle, R.M., Mittelmark, M., Hansen, W.B., Bane, A., and Havis, J. (1978). Deterring the onset of smoking in children: Knowledge of immediate physiological effects and coping with peer pressure, media pressure, and parent modeling. *J. Appl. Soc. Psychol. 8*(2):126-135.

Evans, R.I., Rozelle, R.M., Maxwell, S.E., Raines, B.E., Dill, C.A., Guthrie, T.J., Henderson, A.H. and Hill, P. C. (1981). Social Modeling films to deter smoking in adolescents: Results of a three-year field investigation. *J. Appl. Psychol. 66*:399-414.

Ezekoye, S., Kumpfer, K., and Bukowski, W. (1986). *Childhood and Chemical Abuse*: Prevention and Intervention. New York, Haworth Press.

Farquahar, J.W. (1978). The community-based model of life style intervention trials. *Am. J. of Epidemiol. 108*(2):103-111.

Farquahar, J.W., Magnus, P.F., and Maccoby, N. (1981). The role of public information and education in cigarette smoking controls. *Canad. J. Public Health, 72*(6):412-420.

Felix, M.R.J. (1983). *The Pennsylvania County Health Improvement Program* (CHIP). Unpublished project description.

Fishbein, M. (1973). Introduction: The prediction of behaviors from attitudinal variables, *Advances in Communication Research* (C.D. Mortensen and K.K. Sereno, eds), New York, Harper & Row.

Fisher, D.A. Armstrong, B.K., and de Klerk, N.H. (1983) *A Randomized-Controlled Trial of Education for Prevention of Smoking in 12-Year-Old Children*. Presented at 5th World Conference on Smoking and Health, Winnipeg, Canada.

Flay, B. (1987). Psychosocial approaches to smoking prevention: A review of the findings. *Health Psychol.*

Flay, B.R., Johnson, C.A., Hansen, W.B., Ulene, A. Grossman, L.M., Alvarez, L., Sobel, D.F., Hochstein, G., and Sobel, J.L. (1982). Evaluation of a mass media enhanced smoking prevention and cessation program, *Experimental Research in Televised Instruction*, (Vol V.) (J.P. Baggaley and P. Tanega, eds.). Montreal, Concordia University Press.

Flay, B.R., D'Avernas, J.R., Best, J.A., Kersell, M.W., and Ryan, K.B. (1983a). Cigarette smoking: Why young people do it and ways of preventing it, *Pediatric and Adolescent Behavioral Medicine* (P. McGrath and P. Firestone, eds.) New York, Springer-Verlag.

Flay, B.R., Hansen, W.B., Johnson, C.A. and Sobel, J.L. (1983b). *Involvement of Children in Motivating Smoking Parents to Quit Smoking with a Television Program*. Paper presented at the 5th World Conference on Smoking and Health, Winnipeg, Canada, July, and the 91st Annual Convention of the American Psychological Association, Anaheim, California.

Flay, B.R., Johnson, C.A., Hansen, W.B., Grossman, L.M., Sobel, J.L., and Collins, L.M. (1983c, October). *Evaluation of a School-Based, Family-Oriented, Television-Enhanced Smoking Prevention and Cessation Program: The Importance of Implementation Evaluation*. Presented at the Joint Meeting of Evaluation Network and the Evaluation Research Society, Chicago.

Flay B.R., Ryan, K.B., Best, J.A., Brown, K.S., Kersell, M. W., d'Avernas, J. R. and Zanna, M.P. (1985). Are social psychological smoking prevention programs effective? The Waterloo Study. *J. Behav. Med.*, 8(1):37–59.

Forehand, R.L., and McMahon, R.J. (1981). *Helping the Noncompliant Child. A Clinician's Guide to Parent Training*. New York, The Gilford Press.

Gallant, D.M., Rich, A., Bey, E., and Terranova, L. (1970). Group psychotherapy with married couples: A successful technique in New Orleans alcoholism cliic patients. *J. La. State Med. Soc.*, 122:41.

Gersick, K., Grady, K., and Snow, D. (1985). *Social-Cognitive Skill Development with Sixth Graders and Its Initial Impact on Substance Use*. Unpublished manuscript. New Haven, Connecticut, Yale University, Department of Psychiatry.

Goodstadt, M. (1980). Drug Education: A turn on or a turnoff. *J. Drug Ed.*, 10:89–99.

Goodstadt, M. (1981). Planning and evaluation of alcohol educaton programmes. *J. Alcohol Drug Ed.*, 26:1–10.

Goodstadt, M., and Sheppard, M. (1983). Three approaches to alcohol education. *J. Stud. Alcohol*, 44(1):362–380.

Gordon, T. (1970). *Parent Effectiveness Training*. New York, Wyden.

Gottfredson, D.C. (1986). An empirical test of school-based environmental and individual interventions to reduce the risk of delinquent behavior. *Criminology*, 24(4):705–730.

Greenleaf, J. (1981). *Co-Alcohoic, Para-Alcoholic*. Los Angeles, Greenleaf Associates.

Grossman, M., Coate, D., and Arluck, G. (1984). *Price Sensitivity of Alcoholic Beverages in the United States*. Unpublished manuscript. New York, National Bureau of Economic Research.

Guerney, B.G., Jr. (1964). Filial therapy: Description and rationale. *J. Consult. Psychol.*, 28(4):304–310.

Hansen, W.B. (1988). *Theory and Implementation of the Social Influence Model of Primary Prevention*. Paper presented at the National Prevention Network and NASADAD Prevention Research Conference, Kansas City.

Harmon, J., and Aliapouluis, M.A. (1972). Gynecomastia in marijuana users., *N. Engl. J. Med.*, 287:936.

Harwood, H.J., Napolitano, D.M., Kristiansen, P.L., and Collins, J.J. (1984). *Economic Costs to Society of Alcohol and Drug Abuse and Mental Illness: 1980* Contract No. ADM 283-83-002. Research Triangle Park, North Carolina, Research Triangle Institute.

Hawkins, J.D., and Weis, J.G. (1985). The social development model: An integrated approach to delinquency prevention. *J. Primary Prevention.* 6(2):79.

Hawkins, J.D., Catalano, R.F., Jones, G., and Fine, D. (1987). Delinquency prevention through parent training: Results and issues from work in progress, *From Children to Citizens, Vol. 3: Families, Schools, and Delinquncy Prevention* (J.Q. Wilson and G.C. Loury, eds.). New York, Springer-Verlag, pp. 186–206.

Hepler, R.S., Frank, I.M., and Ungerleider, J.T. (1972). Pupillary constriction after marijuana smoking. *Am. J. Ophthalmol. 74*:1185–1190.

Holme, E.I., Helgeland, A., Hjermann, I., and Leren, P. (1982). Socio-economic status as a coronary risk factor: The Oslo study. *Acta Med Scand., 660* (Suppl.):146–151.

Hooper, F. (1983). *The Relationship Between Alcohol Control Policies and Cirrhosis Mortality in the United States Countries*. Paper presented at the annual conference of American Public Health Association in Dallas, Utah.

Hu, T., Swisher, J., McDonnell, N., and Stein, J. (1982). *Cost-Effectiveness Evaluation: A Drug Abuse Prevention Alternatives Program*. Research report for the Prevention Branch of the National Institute on Drug Abuse. Grant No. E07 DAO2464-02.

Huba, G.J., Wingard, J.A., and Bentler, P.M. (1980). Longitudinal analysis of the role of peer support, adult models, and peer subcultures in beginning adolescent substance use: An application of setwise canonical correlation methods. *Multivar. Behav. Res. 15*:259–279.

Huba, G.J., Wingard, J., and Bentler, P. (1981). Intentions to use drugs among adolescents: A longitudinal analysis. *Int. J. Addict. 16*:331–339.

Johnston, L.D., O'Malley, P., and Bachman, J.G. (1985). *Use of Licit and Illicit Drugs by America's High School Students, 1975–1984*. (U.S. Department of Health and Human Services Publication No. ADM 85-1395). Washington, D.C., U.S. Government Printing Office.

Johnson, C.A., Hansen, W.B., Collins, L.M., and Grahan, J.W. (1984). *Final Report: The High School Anti-Smoking Project*. (Report to National Institute on Drug Abuse). University of Southern California.

Johnson, C.A., Hansen, W.B., Flay, B.R., Graham, J., and Sobel, J. (1985). *Prevention of Multiple Substance Abuse in Youth*. Paper presented at National Prevention Network Conference, Nashville, Tennessee.

Judd, C., and Kenny, D. (1981). *Estimating the Effects of Social Interventions*. Cambridge, England, Cambridge University Press.

Kaufman, M. (1980). Myth and reality in the family patterns and treatment of substance abusers. *Am. J. Drug Alcohol Abuse, 7*(3&4):257–279.

Kim, S. (1981). *An Evaluation of Ombudsman Primary Prevention Program on Student Drug Abuse*. Charlotte, North Carolina, Charlotte Drug Education Center.

Kim, S. (1982). Feeder area approach: An impact evaluation of a prevention project on student drug abuse. *Int. J. Adict., 17*(2):305–313.

Klein, N.C., Alexander, J.F., and Parsons, B.V. (1977). Impact of family systems intervention on recidivism and sibling delinquency: A model of primary prevention and program evaluation. *J. Consult. Clin. Psychol., 45*:469–474.

Klitzner, M. (1984). *Descriptive Study of National Parent Groups*. A grant submitted to the National Institute on Drug Abuse. Pacific Institute for Research and Evaluation.

Klitzner, M., and Schoenberg, S.K. (1988). Concerns Regarding the indirect assessment for drug abuse among adolescents. *Dev. Behav. Pediatr., 9*(1):

Kumpfer, K.L. (1975). *TBO: Therapy by Objectives. A New Clinical Program for Promoting Change*. Symposium on new psychotherapy techniques for women, Rocky Mountain Psychological Association, Salt Lake City, Utah.

Kumpfer, K.L. (1985). *Prevention Approaches to Adolescent Substance Use/Abuse*. Paper presented at the American Academy of Child Psychiatry Institute on Substance Abuse and Adolescence, San Antonio, Texas.

Kumpfer, K.L. (1987). Special populations: Etiology and prevention of vulnerability to chemical dependency in children of substance abusers. *Youth at High Risk for Substance Abuse*. (Brown, B.S, and A.R. Mills, eds.). National Institute on Drug Abuse Technical Review, No. 65, 1-99, Rockville, Maryland.

Kumpfer, K.L., and DeMarsh, J. (1984, February). *Prevention Services to Children of Substance-Abusing Parents: Project Rationale, Description and Research Plan.* Technical report submitted to National Institute on Drug Abuse, Rockville, Maryland.

Kumpfer, K.L., and DeMarsh, J. (1985). Genetic and family environmental influences on children of drug abusers *J. Child. Contemp. Soc.*, (3/4):

Kumpfer, K.L., and DeMarsh, J.P. (1986a). *Prevention Strategies for Children of Drug-Abusing Parents.* (Unpublished). Social Research Institute, University of Utah, Salt Lake City.

Kumpfer, K.L., and DeMarsh, J. (1986b). Family oriented interventions for the prevention of chemical dependency in children and adolescents, *Chlildren and Chemical abuse: Prevention and Early Intervention* (S. Ezekoye, K. Kumpfer, and W. Bukoski, eds.). New York, Harworth Press.

Kumpfer, K., Moskowitz, J., and Klitzner, M. (1986). Future issues and promising directions in the prevention of chemical dependency. *J. Child. Contemp.Soc.*.

Kumpfer, K.L., Alvarado, R., Turner, C., and Bosich, M. (1989). *Reducing Drug Abuse Through School Climate Improvements: The Final Report on Project: HIPATHE.* Department of Education, Washington, D.C.

L'Abate, L. (1977). *Enrichment: Structued Interventions with Couples, Families, and Groups.* Washington, D.C., University Press of America.

Leupker, R.V., Blackburn, H., Mittelmark, M., Jacobs, D.R., and Cline, F.G. (1982). *A Community Research and Demonstration Project on the Prevention of Cardiovascular Diseases: The Minnesota Health-Health Program.* Paper presented at the Ninth World Congress of Cardiology, Moscow.

Maccoby, N. (1976). The Stanford heart disease prevention program, *Consumer behavior in the Marketplace* (I.M. Newman, ed.). Symposium proceedings. Nebraska, Nebraska Center for Health Education, pp. 31–44.

MacDonald, D.I. (1984). *Drugs, Drinking and Adolescents.* Chicago, Year Book.

MacDonald, S., and Whitehead, P. (1983). Availability of outlets and consumption of alcoholic beverages. *J. Drug Iss.*, (Fall):477–486.

McAlister, A., Perry, C., and Maccoby, N. (1979). Adolescent smoking: Onset and prevention. *Pediatrics, 63*:650–658.

McAlister, A., Puska, P., Koskela, K., Pallonen, V., and Maccoby, N. (1980). Mass communication and community organization for public health education. *Am. Psychol. 35*(4):375–379.

McAlister, A.L., Puska, P., Salonen, J.T., Tuomilehot, J., and Koskelia, A. (1982). Theory and action for health promotion: Illustratons from the North Karelia project. *Am. J. Public Health, 72*(1):43–50.

McGuire, W.J. (1969). The nature of attitudes and attitude change, *The Handbook of Social Psychology*, 2nd ed. (G. Linzey and E. Aronson, eds.). Reading, Massachusetts, Addison-Wesley.

Meyer, A.J., Nash, J.D., McAllister, A.L., Maccoby, N., and Farquhar, J.W. (1980). Skills training in cardiovascular health education campaign. *J. Consult. Clin. Psychol.*, *48*(2):129–142.

Miller, W. (1975). *Systematic Parent Training: Procedures, Cases and Issues.* Champaign, Research Press.

Mosher, J.F. (1982). Federal tax law and public health policy: The case of alcohol-related tax expenditures. *J. Public Health Pol.*, *3*(3):260–283.

Mosher, J. (1983). Server intervention: A new approach for preventing drinking driving. *Accid. Anal. Prevent.*, *5*:483–497.

Mosher, J.F., and Wallack, L.M. (1981). Government regulation of alcohol advertising: Protecting industry profits versus promoting the public health. *J. Public Health Pol.*, *2*(4):333–353.

Moskowitz, J.M. (1983). Preventing adolescent substance abuse through drug education, *Preventing Adolescent Drug Abuse: Intervention Strategies* (T.J. Glynn, C.G. Leukefld, and J. P. Ludford, eds.). Rockville, Maryland, National Institute on Drug Abuse Research Monograph 47 (ADM) 83-1280, pp. 233–249.

Moskowitz, J. (1986). *The Primary Prevention of Alcohol Problems: A Critical Review of the Research Literature.* Monograph of Prevention Research Center, Berkely, California, 94704, pp. 1–63.

Moskowitz, J., Malvin, J., and Schaeffer, G. (1984). The effects of drug education at follow-up. *J. Alcohol Drug Ed.*, *30*:45–49.

Moskowitz, J., Schaps, E., and Malvin, E. (1982). A process and outcome evaluation of a Magic Circle primary prevention program. *Eval. Rev.*, *6*:775–788.

Moskowitz, J., Malvin, J., Schaeffer, G., and Schaps, E. (1984). An experimental evaluation of drug education course. *J. Drug Ed., 14*:9–22.

Munson, A.E., and Fehr, K.P. (1982). Immunological effects of cannabis, Cannabis and Health Hazards: Proceedings Consequences of Cannabis Use. Toronto, Addiction Research Foundation, p. 257.

Murray, D.M., and Perry, C.L. (1985). The prevention of adolescent drug abuse: Implications of etiological, developmental, behavioral, and environmental models, *Etiology of Drug Abuse Implications for Prevention* (C.L. Jones and R.J. Battjes, eds.). National Institute on Drug Abuse Research Monograph 56, U.S. Department of Health and Human Services Publication No. ADM 85–1335. Washington, D.C., U.S. Government Printing Office, pp. 236–256.

National Institute of Drug Abuse (1982a). A chronology of growth: How the parent movement evolved. *Prev. Resources, 6*(1):11–12.

National Institute of Drug Abuse (1982b). Networking: Allies in prevention/parents and youth. *Prev. Resources, 6*(2):4-6.

O'Donnell, M. (1985). Research on drinking locations of alcohol impaired drivers: Implications for prevention policies. *J. Public Health Pol., 6*:510–525.

Ostram, T.M. (1969). The relationship between the affective, attitudinal, and social correlates of drug use. *Int. J. Addict., 15*:869–881.

Parsons, B.V. (1972). "*Family Crisis Intervention; Therapy Outcome Study.*" Unpublished doctoral dissertation, Salt Lake City, University of Utah.

Patterson, G.E., Reed, J.B., Jones, R.R., and Conger, R.E. (1975). *A Social Learning Approach to Family Intervention*. Eugene, Oregon Castalia.

Pentz, M.A. (1982). *Social Skills Training: A Preventive Intervention for Drug Use in Adolescents.* Paper presented at American Psychological Association, Meeting, Washington, D.C.

Pentz, M.A. (1983). Prevention of adolescent substance abuse through social skill development. *Preventing Adolescent Drug Abuse: Intervention Strategies* (T.J. Glynn, C.G. Leukefeld and J.P.Ludford, eds.). (National Institute on Drug Abuse Research Monograph 47, U.S. Department of Health and Human Services Publication No. ADM 83-1280. Washington, D.C., U.S. Government Printing Office.

Perry, C., Killen, J., Slinkard, L.A. and McAlister, A.L. (1980a). Peer teaching and smoking prevention among junior high students. *Adolescence, 9*(58):277–281.

Perry, C., Killen, J., Telch, M., Slinkard, L.A., and Danaher, B.G. (1980b). Modifying smoking behavior of teenagers: A school-based intervention. *Am. J. Public Health, 70*(7):722–725.

Perry, C.L., Murray, D.M., Pechaceck, T.F., and Pirie, P.L. (1983a). Community-based smoking prevention: The Minnesota Heart Health Program, Unpublished. University of Minnesota.

Perry, C.L., Telch, M.J., Killen, J., Dass, R., and Maccoby, N. (1983b). High school smoking prevention: The relative efficacy of varied treatments and instructions. *Adolescence, 18*(71):

Petchers, M.K., Singer, M.I., Angelotta, J.W. and Chow, J. (1988). Revalidation and expansion of an adolescent substance abuse screening measure. *Dev. Behav. Pediatr., 9*:

Peters,J. (1985). Director, Intermission, Ltd., 56 Main Street, Northampton Massachusetts 01060.

Polich, J.M., Ellickson, P.L., Reuter, P. and Kahan, J.P. (1984). *Strategies for Controlling Adolescent Drug Use*. Santa Monica, California, Rand.

Resnick, H.S. (1982). *It Starts with People—II. Drug Abusze Prevention Programs for the 1980s.* Unpublished. Lafayette, California, Pyramid.

Rodin, J. (1985). The application of social psychology. *The Handbook of Social Psychology*, Vol. II (G. Lindzey and E. Aronson, eds., New York, Random House, pp. 805–882.

Rockeach, M., and Kliejunas, P. (1972). Behavior as a function of attitude-toward-object and attitude-toward-situation. *J. Person. Soc. Psychology, 22*:194–201.

Roffman, R.A. (1982). *Marijuana as Medicine*. Seattle, Madrona. Rousch, G.C., Thompason, B.A., and Berberian, R.M. (1980). Psychoactive medicinal and non-medicinal drug use among high school students. *Pediatrics, 66*:709–715.

Ryan, W. (1972). *Blaming the Victim*. New York, Vintage Press.

Saltz, R. (1985). Prevention Research Center, Server Intervention Project, 2532 Durant Avenue, Berkeley, California 94704.

Schaps, E., DiBartolo, R., Moskowitz, J., Palley, C., and Churgin, S. (1981). Primary prevention evaluation research: A review of 127 impact studies. *J. Drug Iss., 11*:17–43.

Schaps, E., Moskowitz, J., Condon, J., and Malvin, J. (1982) Process and outcome evaluation of a drug education course. *J. Drug Ed., 12*:353–364.

Schinke, S.P., and Gilchrist, L.D. (1983a). Preventing cigarette smoking with youth. *J. Primary Prevent.*,

Schinke, S.P., and Gilchrist, L.D. (1983b). Primary prevention of tobacco smoking. *J. of School Health, 53*(7):416–419.

Schinke, S.P., and Gilchrist, L.D. (1986). Preventing cigarette smoking with youth. *J. Primary Prevent.*

Schlegal, R., and Norris, J. (1980). Effects of attitude change on behavior for highly involving issues: The case of marijuana smoking. *Addict. Behav., 5*:113–124.

Schlegal, R., Manske, S., and Page, A. (1984). A guided decision making program for elementary school students: A field experiment in alcohol education, *Prevention of Alcohol Abuse* (P. Miller and T. Nirenberg, eds.). New York, Plenum Press.

Sheppard, M., Wright, D., and Goodstadt, M. (1985). Peer pressure and drug use—Exploding the myth. *Adolescence, 20*:949–958.

Shope, J., and Dielman, T. (1985). *An Elementary School-Based Peer Resistance Program of Prevention Adolescent Alcohol Misuse.* Paper presented at Illinois Alcoholism and Drug Dependence Association Annual Conference Workshop. Ann Arbor, Michigan, University of Michigan.

Solomon, D.S. (1982). Health campaigns on television. *Television and Behavior: Ten Years of Scientific Progress and Implications for the Eighties*, Vol. 2 (D. Pearl, I. Bouthilet and J. Lazar, eds.). Technical Reviews, Washington, D.C., National Institute of Mental Health, pp. 308–321.

Sowder, B., and Burt, M. (1978a). *Children of Addicts and Nonaddicts: A Comparative Investigation in Five Urban Sites.* Report to NIDA. Bethesda, Maryland, Burt Associates.

Stein, J.A., Swisher, J.D., Hu, T., and McDonnell, N. (1984). Cost-effectiveness evaluation of a Channel One program. *J. Drug Ed.,14*:251–269.

Steinglass, P. (1975). Family therapy in alcoholism, *Treatment and Rehabilitation of the Chronic Alcoholic* (B. Kissin and H. Begleiter, eds.). New York, Plenum Press, pp. 259–299.

Steinglass, P. (1980). The alcoholic family at home: Patterns of interaction in dry, wet and transitional stages of alcoholism. *Arch. Gen. Psychiatry, 24*:401–408.

Swisher, J.D., and Hu, T.W. (1983). Alternatives to drug abuse: Some are and some are not, *Preventing Adolescent Drug Abuse: Intervention Strategies* (T.J.Glynn, C.G. Leukefeld, and P. Ludford, eds.). (National Institute on Drug Abuse Research Monograph 47, U.S. Department of Health and Human Services Publication No. ADM 83-1280. Washington, D.C., U.S. Government Printing Office, pp. 141–153.

Szapocznik, J. (1983). *Family Effectiveness Training.* Unpublished final report. University of Miami Family Guidance Center.

Szapocznik, J. (1986). Executive Summary: The NIAAA - WHO Collaborating Center Designation Meeting. In the *Proceedings of the NIAAA - WHO Collaborating Center Designation Meeting and Alcohol Research Seminar.* Rockville, Maryland.

Szapocznik, J., et al. (1984). One person therapy. Tarter, R.E., Alterman, A.I., and Edwards, K.L. (1985). Vulnerability to alcoholism in men: A behavior-genetic perspective. *J. Stud. Alcohol., 46*:329–356.

Szapocznik, J. Perez-Vidal, A., Hervis, O., and Brickman, A.L. (1987). Innovations in family therapy: Strategies for overcoming resistance to treatment. *Handbook of Brief Psychotherapies* (R.A. Wells and V.J. Giannetti, eds.). New York, Plenum Press.

Tashkin, D.L., and Cohen, S. (1981). *Marijuana Smoking and Its Effects on the Lungs.* Rockville, Maryland, American Council for Drug Education.

Tell, G.S., Klepp, K.I., Vellar, O.D. and McAlister, A. (1984). Preventing the onset of cigarette smoking in Norwegian adolescents: The Oslo youth study. *Prevent. Med.* 13:256–275.

Tennant, F.S., Jr. (1982). Clinical toxicology of cannabis use. Cannabis and health hazards: *Proceedings of the ARF/WHO Scientific Meeting on Adverse Health and Behavioral Consequences of Cannabis Use.* Toronto, Addiction Research Foundation, p. 69.

Vatiainen, E., Pallonen, U., McAlister, A., Koskela, K., and Puska, P. (1983). Effect of two years of educational intervention in adolescent smoking (The North Karelia Youth Project). *Bull. W.H.O., 61*(3):529–532.

Vingilis, E.R., and DeGenova, K. (1984). Youth and the forbidden fruit: Experiences with changes in legal drinking age in North America. *J. Crim. Just., 12*:161–172.

Wagenaar, A.C. (1981). Effects of an increase in the legal minimum drinking age. *J. Public Health Pol.* 2(3):206–223.

Wagenaar, A.C. (1982). Aggregate beer and wine consumption: Effects of changes in the minimum legal drinking age and a mandatory beverage container deposit law in Michigan. *J. Stud. Alcohol.,* 43(5):469–487.

Wagenaar, A.C. (1983). *Alcohol, Young Drivers and Traffic Accidents; Effects of Minimum Age Laws.* Lexington, Massachusets, Lexington Books.

Wallack, L. M. (1984). *The Prevention of Alcohol-Related Problems: Recommendations for Public Policy Initiatives.* Berkely, California, Prevention Research Center.

Wallack, L. (in press). Mass media, youth and the prevention of substance abuse: Towards an integrated approach. *J. of Child. Contemp. Soc.*

Wallack, L.J., and Barrows, D.C. (1981). *Preventing Alcohol Problems in California: Evaluation of the Three Years "Winner Program."* California Department of Alcohol and Drug Programs. Contract A-0345-8. Berkeley, Social Research Group.

Wegscheider, S. (1981). *Another Chance: Hope and Help for the Alcoholic Family.* Palo Alto, California, Science and Behavior Books.

Wepner, S. (1979). Which way drug educaton? *J. Drug Ed.,* 9:93–103.

Wicker, A.W. (1971). An examination of the "other variables" explanation of attitude-behavior inconsistency. *J. Pes. Soc. Psychol.,* 19:18–30.

Williams, T.P. and Lillis, R.P. (1985, April 18–21). *Changes in Alcohol Consumption by Eighteen Year Olds Following an Increase in New York State's Purchase Age to Nineteen.* Paper presented at the National Council on Alcholism, National Alcoholism Forum, Washington, D.C.

Williams, R., Ward, D., and Gray, L. (1985). The persistence of experimentally induced cognitive change: A neglected dimension in the assessment of drug prevention programs. *J. Drug Ed.,* 15:33–42.

Wittman, F. D. (1985). *Reducing Environmental Risk of Alcohol Problems.* Berkely, California, Prevention Research Center.

SELECTED READING

Battjes, R.J. and Jones, C.L. (1985). Implications of etiological for preventive interventions and future research, *Etiology of Drug Abuse: Implications for Prevention*, (C.L. Jones and R.J. Battjes, eds.). National Institute on Drug Abuse Research Monograph 56, U.S. Department of Health and Human Services Publication No. ADM 85-1335, pp.269–276. Washington, D.C., U.S. Government Printing Office.

This NIDA publication reviews the most important etiological research on causes of drug abuse and the implications for prevention programs. Many of the most important theories of drug abuse as well as developmental research are covered. This publication is free from the NIDA Clearinghouse.

Bell, C., and Battjes, R. (1985). *Prevention Research: Deterring Drug Abuse Among Children and Adolescents.* U.S. Department of Health and Human Services Publication No. ADM 895-1334, Rockville, Maryland. National Institute on Drug Abuse Research Monograph, Number 63, GPO Stock #017-024-01263-7.

This NIDA RAUS: Research Analysis and Utilization System Research Monograph is another excellent source of information on prevention programs that have been evaluated by researchers.

Bukoski, W.J. (1985). School-based substance abuse prevention: A review of program research. *J. Child. Contemp. Soc.,* 18(1/2):95–117.

Recent reviews of school-based substance abuse prevention research indicate that a variety of prevention activities have been implemented in schools throughout the country. This review classifies prevention programs into one of five educational domains: cognitive, affective/interpersonal, behavioral, environmental, and therapeutic. Research findings for each domain are discussed. This chapter can also be found in the Ezekoye, Kumpfer, and Bukoski (1986).

DeMarsh, J., and Kumpfer, K.L. (1986). Family-oriented interventions for the prevention of chemical dependency in children and adolescents, *Childhood and Chemical Abuse: Prevention and Intervention* (S. Ezekoye and W. Bukoski, eds.). New York, Haworth Press.

Researchers and clinicians are beginning to recognize the valuable resource that parents and families are for increasing the effectiveness of substance abuse prevention programs for youth and adolescents. This article reviews family-oriented interventions and discusses outcome effectiveness data when available.

DuPont, R.L. (1989). *Stopping Alcohol and Other Drug Use Before It Starts: The Future of Prevention.* A report of a Committee of the Institute for Behavior and Health, Inc. Published by the Office of Substance Abuse Prevention and available from the Alcohol and Drug Abuse Clearinghouse.

The report covers the shape and current state of the alcohol-and drug-use epidemic, what prevention program have been tried and work, identification of youths at high risk, and the next steps needed. This report also includes several drafts of risk assessment instruments.

Ezekoye, S., Kumpfer, K., and Bukoski, W. (1986). *Childhood and Chemical Abuse: Prevention and Intervention.* New York, Haworth Press.

This book covers the etiology of drug abuse and prevention and intervention strategies. Many of the best-known researchers in drug and alcohol abuse prevention (Hawkins, Catalon, Wallack, Johnson, Hansen, Pentz, Moskowitz, Klitzner, Kumpfer, DeMarsh, and Bukoski) contributed reviews of the literature in their area for this book. Ezekoye contributed a multicultural model and Beschner discussed treatment approaches.

Goodstadt, M. (1980). Drug Education: A turn on or a turnoff. *J. Drug Ed., 10*:89–99.

A critical review of the early approaches to school-based prevention.

Gottfredson, D.C., and Gottfredson, G.D. (1986). *The School Action Effectiveness Study: Final Report.* Center for Social Organization of Schools. Baltimore, The Johns Hopkins University.

The final report of the Project PATHE, which is a comprehensive coordinated approach to improving school climate as an approach to reducing drug and alcohol abuse.

Hawkins, J.D., Lishner, D., and Catalano, R.F. (1985). Childhood predictors and the prevention of adolescent substance abuse, *Etiology of Drug Abuse: Implications for Prevention* (C.L. Jones and R.J. Battjes, eds.). (National Institute on Drug Abuse Research Monograph 56, U.S. Department of Health and Human Services Publication No. ADM 85-1335, pp. 75–126). Washington, D.C., U.S. Government Printing Office.

A very complete review of risk factors for substance abuse and the implications for prevention approaches. This article make a strong plea for prevention approaches to be based on risk factors.

Johnston, L.D., O'Malley, P.M. and Bachman,J.G. (1986). *Drug Use Among American High School Students, College Students, and Other Young Adults: National Trends Through 1985.* University of Michigan, Institute for Social Research, National Institute on Drug Abuse publication.

Presents the results of the high school senior survey conducted annually in the United States. This particular monograph covers a review of the prior years and analyzes trends. Since this monograph is published annually by the National Institute on Drug Abuse, a more recent issue may be available from the NIDA Clearinghouse.

Kumpfer, K.L. and DeMarsh, J. (1986). Family environmental and genetic influences on children's future chemical dependency, *Children and Chemical Abuse: Prevention and Early Intervention.* (S. Ezekoye, K. Kumpfer, and W. Bukoski, eds.). New York Haworth Press.

Reviews possible genetic and environmental factors which contribute to future drug and alcohol dependency in children of alcohol and drug abusers Studies on genetic vulnerability and biological markers of alcoholism and drug abuse are reviewed. Research on the characteristics of drug- and alcohol-abusing families are discussed. The article concludes with recommendations concerning the need for more family-focused prevention interventions for children of drug and alcohol abusers.

Kumpfer, K., Moskowitz, J., and Klitzner, M. (1986). Future issues and promising directions in the prevention of chemical dependency. *J. of Child. Contemp. Soc. 18*(1/2):249–278.

This article reviews environmental and public policy approaches to prevention. Then it covers a scheme for conceptualizing the various approaches to prevention in relation to the Public Health Services prevention model. The article concludes with speculations about the future of prevention, based on possible positive and negative changes in society and drug-use patterns. Finally, recommendations are made for the most promising programs.

Kumpfer, K.L. (1987). Special populations: Etiology and prevention of vulnerability to chemical dependency in children of substance abusers, *Youth at High Risk for Substance Abuse* National Institute on Drug Abuse Monographs, U.S. Department of Health and Human Services Publication No. (ADM)87-1537, Rockville, Maryland, pp. 1–73.

A very thorough, well-organized review chapter, which covers the research findings on biological and environmental risk and protective factors for substance abuse in children of alcohol and drug ab users. This review is much more comprehensive than the earlier Kumpfer and DeMarsh (1986) article on this topic. This book should also be available from the NIDA clearinghouse.

Swisher, J.D., and Hu, T.W. (1983). Alternatives to drug abuse: Some are and some are not, *Preventing Adolescent Drug Abuse: Intervention Strategies* (T.J. Glynn, C.G. Leukefeld, and J.P. Ludford, eds.). National Institute on Drug Abuse Research Monograph 47, U.S. Department of Health and Human Services Publication No. ADM 83-1280. Washington, D.C., U.S. Government Printing Office, pp. 141–153.

Reviews the research on alternative approaches to prevention of substance abuse and concludes that alternative approaches that are related to or involve persons known to use or abuse alcohol or drug abuse are likely to increase use in youth. On the other hand, alternative approaches that involve persons who do not use drug or alcohol are likely to reduce use in youth.

XVII
Interventions

57

Interventions for Recovery in Drug and Alcohol Addiction

David J. Mersy
St. Paul–Ramsey Medical Center/Ramsey Clinic, St. Paul, Minnesota

I. INTRODUCTION

Drug and alcohol addiction is one of the most frequently occurring problems in medical practice. In spite of this, drug and alcohol addiction often goes undiagnosed [1]. Part of the problem is that the physician may not have delved deeply enough into the problem to be able to make the diagnosis. Several studies, however, have indicated that there is a hesitancy on the part of the physician to make the diagnosis because he or she lacks confidence as how to proceed once the diagnosis is made [2,3]. Many physicians have never received training in the skills necessary to diagnose and manage drug and alcohol addiction problems. If a systematic approach to the patient is used, many of these obstacles can be overcome. This chapter will discuss techniques for confirming the diagnosis of drug and alcohol addiction once it is suspected, ways to confront the patient, and ways to intervene (including formal intervention).

II. FIRMING UP THE DIAGNOSIS

It is absolutely essential that the physician have as much information and "ammunition" as possible before confronting the patient with possible drug or alcohol addiction. In this section, we will discuss how to obtain information from the patient (including screening tests), information from the family and others, information from the clinical examination, and information from the laboratory.

A. Information from the Patient

One may be suspicious that a patient seen in the office or hospital is addicted to drugs or alcohol based on a variety of factors, including: (1) problems in the person's home life or relationships, (2) problems at work, and (3) problems with his or her health (such as elevated blood pressure or gastritis of unknown etiology).

Drug or alcohol addiction will usually affect a person's relationships first. Thus, the person who complains of marital discord or difficulties with children should raise the physician's suspicions. Frequently those closest to the drug- or alcohol- dependent person will begin to manifest many of the same defense mechanisms as the drug- or alcohol-addicted person. The next major area which becomes affected is the person's physical health. The type of physical deterioration will be determined by the stage of the illness as well as by the drug used and the amounts. Early on mild tremor and slightly elevated blood pressure may occur. Later on in the illness cirrhosis in the alcoholic as well as the serious mental problems of the abuser of stimulant drugs are seen. The final major area which becomes affected is job performance or occupational status. This is often late in the course of alcohol and drug addiction, since the person will try to preserve his or her job as long as possible. The early signs of impaired work performance can be manifested by tardiness and a decreasing level of performance as well as the "Monday-Friday flu syndrome."

Relying on the patient's history of the amount of alcohol or other drugs consumed is frought with difficulty [4]. This is largely because of the denial which is a universal symptom of drug and alcohol addiction [5]. Denial is defined as the inability to accept and deal with the reality of the emotional distress that alcohol/drug abuse is causing. Many physicians have difficulty grasping that this not a conscious effort on the part of the patient. The person knows there is a problem but at the same time is not able to let himself or herself appreciate the damaging effects of his or her drug or alcohol use. The significance of denial in a drug- or alcohol-addicted person cannot be overemphasized. Later in this chapter, we will discuss the various ways that the denial can be broken through and the person helped to get into a recovery program.

While the patient's history of the amount of use is not usually reliable, the physician can get some indication from the patient's response when asked about drug or alcohol use. The person for whom drugs and alcohol is not really a problem is going to be forthright and honest when discussing these issues. The person who looks uncomfortable or gets defensive may be minimizing the possible role of drugs or alcohol in his or her life.

Other helpful suggestions from the medical history are a history of driving while intoxicated (DWI) or blackouts. While receiving one DWI does not label a person as alcoholic, having two or more DWIs is very suggestive of the condition [6]. Blackouts are characteristic of drug and alcohol addiction. During a blackout the person has a memory loss of his or her behavior. This is to be contrasted with passing out, which is a total loss of consciousness that sometimes occurs with very heavy drinking. The drug- or alcohol-dependent person may behave entirely normally during the blackout. It is only later when some aspect of their behavior is pointed out to them and they cannot remember any of it that they realize they have memory loss for the time period. This can be very frightening for the person experiencing a blackout and is a hallmark of drug and alcohol addiction.

Because of the unreliability of patient reports about the amount and effects of alcohol or drug use, several screening tests have been developed. These screening tests vary from extremely simple questions that the physician can ask in the course of the examination to more elaborate questionnaires which the patient must fill out. For the busy practitioner, the simpler screening tests are the most useful.

One of the simplest things that the physician can do is to ask the patient the following two questions: (1) Have you ever had a drinking problem? (2) When was your last drink? (With a positive response being drinking within the preceding 24 h.) A positive response to either or both questions carries a sensitivity of 91.5% and a negative response to both questions holds a negative predictive value of 98% [7].

A slightly more elaborate set of questions, but a very useful one, is the CAGE questionnaire [8]. The CAGE questions are: (1) Have you ever felt you should *Cut* down on your drinking? (2) Have people *annoyed* you by criticizing drinking? (3) Have you ever felt bad or *guilty* about your drinking? (4) Have you ever had a drink first thing in the morning to steady your nerves or to get rid of a hangover (*eye-opener*). Before the CAGE questions are asked, it must first be determined whether the person drinks or uses drugs or not. These questions can be asked by the physician in the course of a general history. A positive answer to two or more of the items is highly suggestive for alcohol problems. The CAGE questionnaire can be used for screening for drug problems other than alcohol by substituting the name of the drug for alcohol.

Another screening test that can be used for the diagnosis of alcoholism is the Michigan Alcoholism Screening Test (MAST) [9]. The MAST questions are depicted in Table 1 with the value listed for each positive response. The scoring for the MAST is as follows: A score of 3 points or less is considered nonalcoholic. A score of 4 points is considered to be suggestive of alcoholism, and a scored of 5 or more is consistent with the diagnosis of alcoholism.

The MAST has been shortened to a 13 question version called the SMAST (Table 2). It has been shown to be as effective as the MAST and to have greater than 90% sensitivity [10]. One benefit of the SMAST is that it can be given to either the patient or the spouse.

B. Information from Family and Others

Because the person with a drug or alcohol addiction problem is often in denial (which makes getting an accurate drinking or chemical use history quite difficult), family members can be a good source of accurate information. Family members can provide good information because drug or alcohol addiction in its early stages affects relationships before work or physicial health. Thus, family members will be well aware of problems and will usually connect them to the drug or alcohol use. Obtaining permission to speak to the family can be a delicate situation. One simple method is to simply say to the patient that you wish to speak with the spouse and/or other family member. You can point out that this should not be a problem if "as you say there really is not a problem with your use of drugs or alcohol." One problem which must be recognized, however, is that often family members will be affected almost as much by the disease process as the patient and there may be a certain amount of denial or enabling behavior on the part of the family members. This enabling behavior can be manifest by protecting the patient from the consequences of his or her chemical use.

In the absence of close family members, friends can also be a good source of information. A similar sort of permission must be obtained. Getting information from employers can present two problems. The first problem is that performance in the workplace is affected relatively late in the course of the disease, and the second is that the drug- or alcohol-dependent person is likely to want to protect his or her job at all costs, and he or she may be even more reluctant to give you permission to contact the employer than the family member.

C. Clinical Examination

The physicial examination can be helpful in confirming the diagnosis of drug or alcohol addiction. Physical findings are most commonly seen in more advanced forms of the disease when the diagnosis may be quite evident. It is helpful to know that trauma and gastrointestinal disease tend to occur earlier in the course of alcohol dependency than neurological disease or cirrhosis of the liver.

The examination may show epigastric tenderness. Moderate to severe antral gastritis has been found in 46% of alcohol abusers [11]. If the liver is enlarged, of course, this is quite suggestive of alcoholic liver disease in the person who consumes alcohol.

Unfortunately there is much overlap of clinical manifestations of the various liver disorders which precludes differentiation on clinical grounds with any degree of accuracy [12]. If the

Table 1 Michigan Alcoholism Screening Test

		YES	NO
0.	Do you enjoy a drink now and then? If answer is yes, then continue with the following questions.		
1.	Do you feel you are a normal drinker? (by normal we mean you drink less than or as much as most other people.)	——	(2)
2.	Have you ever awakened the morning after some drinking the night before and found that you could not remember a part of the evening?	(2)	——
3.	Does your wife, husband, or parent or other near relative ever worry or complain about your drinking?	(1)	——
4.	Can you stop drinking without a struggle after one or two drinks?	——	(2)
5.	Do you ever feel guilty about your drinking?	(1)	——
6.	Do friends or relatives think you are a normal drinker?	——	(2)
7.	Are you able to stop drinking when you want to?	——	(2)
8.	Have you ever attended a meeting of Alcoholics Anonymous (AA) for yourself?	(5)	——
9.	Have you gotten into physical fights when drinking?	(1)	——
10.	Has your drinking ever created problems between you and your wife, husband, a parent or other near relative?	(2)	——
11.	Has your wife, husband (or other family member) ever gone to anyone for help about your drinking?	(2)	——
12.	Have you ever lost friends because of your drinking?	(2)	——
13.	Have you ever gotten into trouble at work or school because of your drinking?	(2)	——
14.	Have you ever lost a job because of drinking?	(2)	——
15.	Have you ever neglected your obligations, your family or your work for two or more days in a row because you were drinking?	(2)	——
16.	Do you drink before noon fairly often?	(1)	——
17.	Have you ever been told you have liver trouble? Cirrhosis?	(2)	——
18.*	After heavy drinking have you ever had delirium tremens (DT s) or severe shaking or heard voices or seen things that really weren't there?	(2)	——
19.	Have you ever gone to anyone for help about your drinking?	(5)	——
20.	Have you ever been in a hospital because of drinking?	(5)	——
21.	Have you ever been a patient in a psychiatric hospital or on a psychiatric ward of a general hospital where drinking was part of the problem that resulted in hospitalization?	(2)	——
22.	Have you ever been seen at a psychiatric or mental health clinic or gone to any doctor, social worker or counselor for help with any emotional problem where drinking was part of the problem?	(2)	——
23.	Have you ever been arrested for drunk driving, driving while intoxicated or driving under the influence of alcoholic beverages? (If yes, how many times? ____)	(2)	——
24.	Have you ever been arrested or taken into custody, even for a few hours, because of other drunk behavior? (If yes, how many times? ____)	(2)	——

*5 points for bona fide delirium tremens
2 points for each arrest

person has been abusing alcohol and is physically dependent upon it, and it has been some time since the last use, the clinical examination may show some signs of early withdrawal. These mild withdrawal reactions will manifest as tremor, anxiety, and hyperreflexia.

Trauma and accidents are another indication of potential drug or alcohol addiction, and you should ask about traumatic incidents and look for scars. One survey reported that 36% of regular drinkers had reported at least two accidental injuries in the preceding year compared with an accident rate of only 8% in nondrinkers [13].

Table 2 Short Michigan Alcoholism Screening Test (SMAST)

1. Do you feel you are a normal drinker? (By normal we mean you drink less than or as much as most other people? (No)
2. Does your wife, husband, a parent or other near relative ever worry or complain about your drinking? (Yes)
3. Do you ever feel guilty about your drinking? (Yes)
4. Do friends or relatives think you are a normal drinker? (No)
5. Are you able to stop drinking when you want to? (No)
6. Have you ever attended a meeting of Alcoholics Anonymous? (Yes)
7. Has drinking ever created problems between you and your wife, husband, a parent or other near relative? (Yes)
8. Have you ever gotten into trouble at work because of your drinking? (Yes)
9. Have you ever neglected your obligations, your family or your work for two or more days in a row because you were drinking? (Yes)
10. Have you ever gone to anyone for help about your drinking? (Yes)
11. Have you ever been in a hospital because of drinking? (Yes)
12. Have you ever been arrested for drunken driving, driving while intoxicated or driving under the influence of alcoholic beverages? (Yes)
13. Have you ever been arrested, even for a few hours, because of other drunken behavior? (Yes)

Answers related to a diagnosis of alcholism are shown in parenthesis after each question. Three or more of these answers indicate a diagnosis of alcoholism; two such answers indicate the possibility of alcoholism; fewer than two answers indicate that alcoholism is not likely.

Questionnaire reprinted with permission from *Journal of Studies on Alcohol* 1975;*36*:124. Copyright by Journal of Studies on Alcohol, Inc., Rutgers Center of Alcohol Studies, New Brunswick, NJ 08903.

Elevated blood pressure can be a red flag to lead you to suspect alcoholism. Klatsky and associates [14] surveyed 84,000 persons and reported that the prevalence of hypertension was 11.2% in individuals ingesting six or more drinks per day compared with 4.6% in nondrinkers.

For drugs other than alcohol, the findings are less common, but the following can be helpful: The person using marijuana will lack ambition and will have injected conjunctivae. Heavy cocaine snorters may have a perforated nasal septum or simply unilateral nasal inflammation. They may also have a hyperactive appearance. This can be true of any person using stimulants. Red flags for cocaine abuse are any atypical acute symptoms reflecting vascular compromise in a person less than 40 years of age. This would include cerebral vascular accidents, aneurysms, transient ischemic attacks, or myocardial infarcts and angina. Another tipoff to cocaine use and abuse is rapidly remitting psychiatric symptoms such as panic anxiety attacks, transient paranoid psychosis, or acute depression.

D. Laboratory Tests

Although many laboratory tests have been used to confirm drug or alcohol abuse, no laboratory test is specific for this purpose. Laboratory tests should only be used in conjunction with the previously described techniques to help confirm the diagnosis. The most useful laboratory tests are the use of the mean corpuscular volume (MCV) and gamma-glutamyltransferase (GGT) for helping to confirm alcohol problems and the urine toxicological screen for other drugs of abuse.

The serum GGT level has been used as an early indicator of alcohol consumption and has been shown to be raised in about three-fourths of alcoholic patients who had no evidence of hepatomegaly or other clinical signs of liver disease [15,16]. A number of studies have indicated that an increased MCV indicates heavy alcohol consumption. In a study of 8000 employees of a large insurance company, Unger and Johnson [17] found that 3% had macrocytosis (MCV more than 96 for men and 100 for women). A large proportion (65%) of the individuals with a high MCV were considered to be consuming excessive amounts of alcohol. Several attempts have been made to combine these two tests (as well as others) to increase their usefulness. One such study [18] found significant correlations between daily alcohol intake and corresponding GGT and MCV values. They found the GGT to be superior to the MCV, but when both are elevated it is very suggestive of alcohol abuse. It should also be noted that these parameters worsen over time with continued alcohol use. Thus, a GGT which is abnormal and higher than a value obtained some months or a year or two prior can be used as hard data to get the patient to look at their alcohol use.

For drugs other than alcohol, the urine toxicological screen can be quite helpful. These screens are now readily available. They can be particularly useful if a physician suspects that a patient's problems may be due to drug or alcohol problems and has met with severe forms of denial. Some drugs such as marijuana stay in the urine for long periods of time, whereas others, such as cocaine, can be detected for much shorter periods.

III. INFORMAL PHYSICIAN INTERVENTIONS

Once the physician is quite suspicious that the patient is addicted to drugs or alcohol, he or she needs to decide the best method to present this to the patient. Informal physician intervention is one aspect of giving information to the patient on a continuum from sharing of information to formal intervention (which will be discussed in Sect. IV). When we speak of informal physician intervention and formal intervention we are speaking of situations in which there is strong or definite evidence of drug or alcohol addiction. In cases in which there is not yet a definite drug or alcohol addiction problem, education alone of the patient is very important. The Canadian and British literature emphasize this approach even for persons with more severe alcohol or drug problems [19]. It is my belief that when there is a drug- or alcohol-addiction problem then informal physician intervention or perhaps formal intervention is necessary. When the problem is one of early problematic use, then education and counseling alone can be somewhat effective in getting the person to cut down their use.

A. Simple Physician or Family Interventions

These are the type of encounters in which physicians or family members can intervene with a person who may have a problem with drugs or alcohol. They will be discussed first before we describe the specific examples of physician intervention and formal intervention.

Feedback About Behavior

A person affected by the drug or alcohol use of a close associate or family member can let the person known exactly how the person appears when using drugs or alcohol. For example, a physician might say to a colleague, "John, I have always liked and respected you, but last night at the hospital staff party you had been drinking and obviously slurred your words and made inappropriate comments to my new associate. You also stumbled when you walked back to your car. I am concerned for you and wish you would look at your drinking."

Description of Feelings

A person can describe to someone with a possible drug- and alcohol-addiction problem how they feel about his or her behavior while under the influence. This could take the form of being embarassed, angry, hurt, or frightened around the drug or alcohol use. For example, using the same situation as above, the physician could say, "Last night at the staff party after you had four or five drinks and made inappropriate remarks to my young colleague, I felt embarassed and angry."

Stop Enabling

Enabling refers to the kinds of behavior of those around the person with a drug- or alcohol-addiction problem to protect him or her from experiencing the harmful consequences of the drug or alcohol abuse. For example, enabling behavior on the part of the spouse of the physician described above would be to call his clinic the morning after the staff party and report that he is ill and unable to come to work. Dropping the enabling behavior would be simply to do nothing at all and allow her husband to experience the consequences of not showing up at work.

Offer the Person Help

It might be possible to offer a person with a drug or alcohol problem help with an evaluation or treatment. For example, in the example quoted above, the physician could say to his colleague, "This isn't the first time that I have seen you have difficulty with your behavior after having some drinks at a party. I am concerned about you. I know of a group of physicians who have gotten together to help other physicians with problems like this. Here is the name of Dr. Smith and his phone number."

Independent Actions by Family Members

Family members can intervene in an indirect way by starting to do something for themselves. A good example is a spouse who becomes concerned about drug or alcohol abuse in her husband and begins to attend Al-Anon meetings. This will often cause enough change in her and the family system that the drug- and alcohol-addicted person will eventually be guided and directed into a recovery problem.

B. Specific Physician Interventions

Physician Intervention with Minimal Denial

The physician who wants to discuss a patient's possible drug and alcohol addiction has two tasks: (1) The physician must present the evidence that makes him or her feel that the drug- or alcohol-addiction problem may exist. (2) A discussion must be held with the patient about the disease concept of drug and alcohol addiction. This makes it easier for the patient to accept help because it implies that factors other than personal irresponsibility are at work. In our society, there are still times when drug or alcohol addiction is viewed as a moral problem and the physician discussing the disease concept with the patient removes that stumbling block. The patient also needs to know that drug and alcohol addiction is a treatable disease and that recovery is indeed possible. It is important to be as caring and nonjudgmental as possible in presenting the diagnosis (or suspicions) and recommendations.

In the person with minimal denial, a simple review of the hard data and your recommendation that he or she obtain further help may be sufficient. In this situation, it is not usual that the denial has always been minimal but the several types of hard evidence such as DWIs and now the physician talking to the patient have finally broken through the wall of denial.

The following case example will illustrate this situation:

John Smith is a 38-year-old blue-collar worker who comes to the physician's office for a general physical examination, which was prompted by vomiting up a small amount of bright red blood 3 days prior. His wife insisted that he come in. His history is remarkable for a family history of alcoholism in his father, who has been sober and in Alcoholics Anonymous (AA) for 5 years. The patient admits to several beers each day after work and sometimes more on weekends. His first marriage ended in divorce 3 years ago, and on close questioning he admits to some marital conflict and that his wife is concerned about his drinking. He had a DWI 2 years ago and was advised to stop drinking at that time, but declined treatment saying he could do it on his own. His physical examination is normal except for mildly elevated blood pressure and epigastric tenderness. His MCV and GGT are both elevated. His stool guaiac is negative. When confronted with the abnormal physical findings and advised to get a formal evaluation the patient agrees.

This is a good example of a decreased amount of denial because of the patient's DWI and the fact that he was not able to quit drinking on his own. The physician's presentation of hard data in the form of elevated MCV and GGT finished breaking through the denial because the patient was obviously quite concerned about his alcohol use. In this type of case, it is very important that the physician have his or her referral sources lined up so that the patient can be sent directly to a drug and alcohol addiction counselor or treatment facility for evaluation. It is also important to note that the physician has not labeled the patient as drug or alcohol addicted, but has merely suggested that alcohol might be a problem and has suggested a more formal evaluation.

If the patient does not have insurance and cannot afford inpatient or outpatient treatment, or the community lacks treatment resources, you can refer the patient to AA, which has chapters in almost every community in this country. In many larger communities, AA Intergroup (a central referral resource) is listed in the local telephone directory. AA Intergroup will provide, at no cost, the names and telephone numbers of several recovering alcoholics or drug addicts who are willing to talk about their personal experiences in recovery and to accompany the patient to an AA meeting. Also, if a physician knows of recovering alcoholics or drug addicts who are in his or her practice who are active in AA, they can ask them if their names and telephone numbers may be given to other patients. Those with a good recovery program are almost always willing to do this and can be a tremendous help in dealing with drug- or alcohol-dependent patients.

Physician Intervention with Major Denial

Many drug and alcohol addicted patients are in major or complete denial [20]. The patient in major denial will insist there is no problem and will not accept the diagnosis. If the patient can be persuaded to seek a second opinion, he or she should immediately be referred to a drug and alcohol addiction counselor or a physician with special interest and expertise in drug and alcohol addiction. Often, this "expert" can convince the patient of the need for further evaluation and help.

Like most alcoholics and drug addicts, patients in major denial may claim that they can quit using at any time, and therefore do not have a problem. In this event, an attempt should be made to negotiate a contract that either limits the amount of drug or alcohol use or calls for total abstinence. (It is usually more difficult to limit use than to abstain.) The patient must agree beforehand to obtain help if he or she is unable to abstain or limit use. If possible, the family and/or employer should be made aware of the contract and convinced to agree to an alternative plan (which usually stipulates that the patient will go to treatment) if the patient is unable to comply with the terms of the contract.

Using the same case example as before, the patient in major denial will probably become quite angry at the physician when informed about the elevated MCV and GGT. It might take considerable effort on the part of the physician to get him to agree to cut down or discontinue drinking. The physician could work toward establishing a contract with the patient whereby he would agree to quit drinking on his own for a month. However, the contract must stipulate that if he is not able to do this, then he will go along with a more formal evaluation.

IV. FORMAL INTERVENTION

As we have seen above, there is a whole continuum of interventions with the person who is abusing or is addicted to drugs or alcohol. Each has its place in dealing with a person who is suspected of having a problem with drug or alcohol abuse or addiction. The term *formal intervention* applies to a concept developed by Johnson in the 1960s [21]. At that time, he worked with alcoholics and was frustrated by his difficulty in getting them to grasp the effect the drinking was having on them and their families. He administered a questionnaire to 200 recovering alcoholics and found that those persons who had recovered had been led into recovery by a crisis and not by any sort of spontaneous insight. This of course fits with the concept that denial and delusion are hallmarks of the disease. As Johnson puts it

> Addicts who are ruining their lives cannot say "no" to drugs because they are incapable of comprehending what drugs are doing to them. If they are to receive the insight they must have, that insight must come from those around them through conscious, planned, and caring acts of intervention [22].

A. Key Components of an Intervention

Formal intervention should be tried either when the more simple interventions have not worked, or in some cases where it is in the judgment of the physician that the simpler interventions are not likely to work. In this case, the wall of denial can be broken through by more formal intervention. The Johnson Institute has pointed out that the most effective formal interventions involve the following five simple but extremely important steps [22].

  1. Gather together persons who are very meaningful to the drug- or alcohol-addicted person and who are concerned about his or her drug or alcohol use. These persons can be the spouse, children, other relatives, close friends, ministers, physicians, or employers, or any combination. These persons will need first-hand knowledge of incidents and behavior related to the person's chemical use such as blackouts, DWIs, loss of behavioral control, accidents, personal threats, or injury to self or others.

  2. Have those persons make written lists of specific data about the person's alcohol or drug use and its effects as well as their feeling responses. First-hand knowledge of incidents and behavior should be reported. Also changes in the person's character, behavior, and personality as observed by the concerned person can be data. They must avoid what could be gossip or second-hand information. Also, generalities should be avoided (e.g., "John we all think you use too much cocaine").

  The person reporting the data should also indicate how it makes him or her feel such as angry, embarrassed, fearful, sad, and so forth. During the actual intervention the involved persons must avoid talking down to the patient or making moral judgments. They must stick to factual reporting of incidents and behavior that caused concern. The most effective way to keep from sounding judgmental is to state how the incident made the person feel and then describe the incident. The person also needs to state his or her concern about the patient so that the patient hears that the people care and are concerned about him or her.

  3. Have the concerned persons decide upon a specific treatment plan that they expect the drug- or alcohol-dependent person to accept. Everyone must decide beforehand what type of help they want the person to get. The goal is not only to get the person to accept the help he or she needs, but to accept this help immediately upon conclusion of the intervention session.

This implies that arrangements have been made beforehand for the treatment center for evaluation and/or treatment. The bed must be obtained ahead of time and the bag packed.

In some cases, a what if clause is used. This is determined by the persons conducting the intervention ahead of time. This is used so that if the person does not accept the help offered but agrees to some lesser course of action (such as quitting on his or her own) the group can put in the what if clause. The person must be willing to get some treatment help if his or her way does not work.

4.   The people involved in the intervention must decide beforehand what they will do if the drug- or alcohol-addicted person rejects all forms of help. This is the "bottom line" consequence, or reality, of what the person will do. The spouse may have to say that they are no longer willing to continue living with the person who is using the drugs or alcohol. The employer may need to say that only if treatment is completed can the person continue to work there. It should be pointed out that not often do the involved persons need to state their bottom line because the wall of denial will be broken through prior to that time and the person will agree to get help.

5.   Meet as a group with the drug- or alcohol-addicted person and present the data and recommendations in an objective, caring, nonjudgmental manner. To be most effective the statements by these persons should include the following: expression of care and concern, specific date or period of time they were drinking or using drugs, where they were and whom they were with at the time of use, what and how much they used and for how long, description of actions and detail, description of reactions and feelings such as hurt, anger, and embarrassment, and finally concluding with "I want you to get help." It is important that the intervention session is not the time to bring out angry feelings. There will be a time for this later in the treatment setting. Those who cannot control their anger should not be part of the intervention setting.

B.   How to Prepare for an Intervention

Most often a professional counselor will be enlisted to facilitate the intervention. Trained physicians can also do this. The major tasks in preparing for an intervention are: (1) Help select and screen meaningful concerned persons for participation in the intervention process. (2) Help participants in the preintervention session to collect and prepare their data. (3) Assure that the treatment alternative has been chosen and is ready. (4) Guide the concerned persons through an intervention role play.

The characteristics of the persons who should be selected to participate are that they be directly affected by the drug or alcohol use and have some credibility and leverage with the person. They should also be in a good position to observe the effects of the drug or alcohol use on the person and on the family. This could be a physician who has noted abnormal liver function tests in his or her patient. They should also be persons whom the drug- or alcohol-addicted person likes, respects, feels close to, or is dependent on, and they should have specific leverage with the addicted person. One of the strongest forms of leverage is the employer or supervisor, since the drug- or alcohol dependent person wants to pressure his or her job. Children can also be very powerful in interventions because of their honesty.

As the concerned persons prepare the data, it is important for them to be able to come up with specific incidents in which the alcohol or drug use caused specific negative consequences. The concerned person needs to describe the behavior and not be judgmental. They also need to tie the consequences directly to the drug or alcohol use and to state their own feelings about the event they are describing. It is very important that written lists be prepared for the intervention session.

A treatment center must also be chosen ahead of time and arrangements made for the person to go directly there. This is because the person will have the wall of denial broken through at the time of the intervention, but if given a chance to reflect overnight may come up with rationalizations and other reasons not to go to treatment.

C. Case Illlustration

The following case example will illustrate many of the principles of formal intervention and the format to be followed:

Robert Smith, M.D., is a 40-year-old family physician who practices in a five-person single-specialty group in a town of 10,000, located 50 miles from a metropolitan area. His father was a physician. Dr. Smith did very well in medical school and residency and stepped into a ready-made practice when he finished residency 8 years ago. He is a very energetic physician who carries a large patient load and is active in community organizations. He is married and has two young children, ages 10 and 7.

As a colleague of his working in the same group you have been concerned how he balances his personal and professional life, but his community involvement is good for your clinic and his energetic practice style helps your clinic financially. There has been no problem with Dr. Smith's work performance, but there was an occasion during the holiday staff party in which you observed him having at least four or five drinks and then slurring his words. As a physician in the group, you are quite surprised when Dr. Smith's wife (who has come in for her annual physical) seems somewhat depressed, and when asked about this she expresses concern about her husband's drinking and cocaine use. She is also concerned regarding some financial problems they are having. She states that her husband never uses drugs or alcohol while on call, but he has taken to drinking more than a few drinks, particularly on his day off, and has used cocaine at parties when the two of them have gone to the nearby metropolitan area. She also tells you about a DWI that he had while in the first year of residency.

Two weeks later Dr. Smith asks you to do an insurance physical on him. He claims to drink only socially and not use any other drugs. His physical is normal except for mild epigastric tenderness. His chemistry panel shows an elevated GGT and his MCV is elevated. When confronted with these findings Dr. Smith denies any problem with alcohol or drugs, and claims that the GGT could be up because of some benzodiazepine he recently took to handle the stress of his financial problems. He states that he can quit drinking at any time and agrees to do so.

Two weeks later, his wife comes to your office, stating that she suspects her husband is taking large amounts of diazepam, and 2 days ago while on call appeared to be in a blackout because he did not remember delivering a baby. You decide to organize a formal intervention.

You ask Dr. Jones to facilitate the intervention. You pick a fellow physician to do this because you need someone with experience and training, and in this case, a fellow physician gives added weight. The facilitator of course will be present at the intervention as will you, as Dr. Smith's partner, the president of the clinic, Dr. Smith's wife, and both children. Before the preintervention session the facilitator will talk to each of these persons. They will be asked to write down examples of specific data to present to Dr. Smith. For example, the president of the clinic could write down, "Bob, I care a lot about you as a colleague and friend. I am concerned, however, because of your drinking. Last Christmas at the holiday party I saw you drink at least 10 drinks. You were slurring your words and making crude comments in front of the hospital administrator.

I felt embarrassed for you. If you hadn't had too much to drink this would not have happened. I want you to get some help."

The next step is to gather all of the persons who will be involved in the intervention and have the intervention role played with each person reading off their specific data. Also at this meeting, the time and place for the intervention would be set. This could be early in the morning at the hospital at the same time as a regularly scheduled meeting. When Dr. Smith arrives he would find the group present. Also at the preintervention session the evaluation or treatment center needs to be arranged and a bed obtained.

At the actual intervention the group gathers 15 min before the appointed time. Each person has his or her written data. Seating arrangements are determined with the most powerful person (clinic president) sitting directly opposite the spot that Dr. Smith will occupy. The spouse should not be either next to Dr. Smith or directly opposite. The facilitator should be between the door and Dr. Smith's assigned seat in case he makes attempts to leave. The two children will be seated next to their mother. When Dr. Smith arrives for the meeting he will be surprised, but he is told that the group has some things to say to him and he is asked please to listen and not respond until everyone has spoken. He is told that he can respond after the people are finished speaking. Then each person reads the data starting with the spouse, then you with the medical data, the clinic president, and then the children. It is not necessary in the first round to threaten the person's job. Only if the group needs to go around a second time or more does that need to be suggested. Once everyone has spoken Dr. Smith is likely to ask what the group wants him to do. It is at that point that he is told that the group wants him to get an evaluation at the treatment center in the metropolitan area and to follow through on the recommendations. He agrees to go, but just for an evaluation, and wants to delay it until next week. At this point, he is informed that his bag is packed and that a bed is waiting and that the president of the clinic will drive him there.

Most experts feel that an intervention is successful (i.e., the person agrees to the recommendations) at least 80% of the time. Even in cases in which the intervention is not successful in breaking through the patient's denial, change will occur in the system. Family members and other concerned persons can be encouraged to begin their own recovery process. Al-Anon or Alateen can provide the tools they need to be less controlled by the patient's drug or alcohol addiction. This indirect route will often allow the patient to eventually seek help.

V. INTERVENTIONS FOR PHYSICIANS

The exact incidence of drug and alcohol addiction in the medical profession is not known. Experts feel that it is at least as common as in the general population. This means that one in 10 adult male professionals who drink and one in 20 adult female professionals who drink will be alcoholic or experience a serious drinking problem [23].

For many years, the American Medical Association (AMA) has recognized the need to identify and treat the sick physician. This impetus gained momentum in 1973 when the AMA's Council on Mental Health urged physicians to assume personal responsibility for recommending treatment of a sick colleague. Since that time, all 50 state medical societies have developed programs for recognizing and aiding the impaired physician. In California, the law changed in 1980 allowing impaired physicians the opportunity to be diverted from possible medical board discipline into a statewide treatment program financed by the Board of Medical Quality Assurance. The success of that program has depended on a rapid response mechanism, an individualized treatment program, iron-clad confidentiality, and a multilevel monitoring system [24]. The success of most of these programs has been quite good [25]. A Mayo Clinic study [26] showed that 83% of physicians contrasted to 62% of the general group treated for alcoholism or drug addiction in a hospital-based inpatient program had favorable outcomes.

The way the state impaired physician programs work is that referrals to the program are accepted from colleagues, hospital and office staff, insurance carriers, licensure boards, and anyone else who is concerned about the well-being of the physician. The goal is to reach the physician before he or she hits bottom. The idea is to get help for the physician before his career has been damaged and patients have suffered.

Allegations of drug or alcohol use behavior must be investigated tactfully and confidentially. This can be done by the chairperson of the hospital's impaired physician committee or by the leader of the state medical society's impaired physician program. It is probably best to have it done by the state's medical society program to avoid questions of conflict of interest. If it is determined that a possible drug- or alcohol-addiction problem exists, then an intervention team in most states is assigned to the case.

Intervention is usually carried out by a team of two or more persons and may include a respected colleague, a physician recovering from drug and alcohol addiction, and a representative of the state medical society's impaired physician program. The team members are specially trained. As in interventions described previously, the team members need to be nonjudgmental and should emphasize advocacy. This may take the form of confrontation or a more formal intervention but, in any case, the intervention team needs carefully prepared options for treatment or follow-up.

If the physician agrees to undergo treatment he or she is asked to sign an agreement with the institution and the state program specifying the nature and terms of the treatment, rehabilitation, aftercare, and return to practice. If the impaired physician refuses treatment, the team needs to explain whatever course or measures will be taken (in most states this would take the form of notification of the state board of medical examiners or the hospital regarding privileges).

In Minnesota, a different approach has been taken. Since 1981 a group called Physicians Serving Physicians (PSP) has been organized to help physicians struggling with drug and alcohol addiction [27]. It was founded by a group of physicians recovering from drug or alcohol addiction in themselves or in a family member. It is a voluntary, self-supporting organization that provides confidential help to physicians and their concerned others whether the affected individual is a physician or a family member. The group has evolved to the point that it now handles all of the drug- and alcohol-addiction cases which are referred to the Minnesota Medical Association. Funding comes from member donations and donations from medical staffs and other organizations. It attempts to meet the needs throughout the state of Minnesota, including education and interventions for physicians and family members.

One of the things that distinguishes this group from most state impaired physician committees is that formal intervention is done for many of the cases. The executive director of the organization is a certified drug and alcohol addiction counselor. Once a situation is reported, data are collected from concerned individuals, including family members, associates, friends, and paramedical personnel. An intervention team usually including the executive director and three physician members of the group is appointed. This group then conducts a formal intervention as described previously. Once the physician enters treatment, PSP continues to support the person through assignment of a PSP "friend," weekly AA meetings, and monthly PSP meetings. There is also a reentry program which helps the individual return to practice. Only if the physician refuses help is there any mention of reporting to the state board of medical examiners.

In Minnesota, the PSP organization has been very successful, both from the point of view of organized medicine and from the point of view of recovering physicians and family members. This is clearly because of the strong sense of identification with and support of other recovering physicians.

REFERENCES

1. Coulehan, J.L., Zettler-Segal, M., Block, M. et al. Recognition of alcoholism and substance abuse in primary care patients. *Arch. Intern. Med. 147*(2):349–352 (1987).
2. Clark, W.D. Alcoholism: Blocks to diagnosis and treatment. *Am. J. Med. 71*(2):275–286 (1981).
3. Westermeyer, J. Doheny, S., and Stone, B. An assessment of hospital care for the alcoholic patient. *Alcoholism 2*(1):53–57 (1978).
4. Watson, C.G., Tilleskjor, C., Hoodecheck-Schow, E.A., Pucel, J., and Jacobs, L. Do alcoholics give valid self-reports? *J. Stud. Alcohol. 45*(4):344–348 (1984).
5. DiCicco, L., Unterberger, H., and Mack, J. Confronting denial: An alcoholic intervention strategy. *Psychiatry Ann. 8*(11):54–64 (1978).
6. Whitefield, C. Outpatient management of the alcoholic patient. *Psych Ann. 12*(4):447–458 (1982).
7. Cyr, M.G.,and Wartman, S.A. The effectiveness of routine screening questions in the detection of alcoholism. *J.A.M.A. 259*(1):51–54 (1988).
8. Mayfield, D., McLeod, G., and Hall, P. The CAGE questionnaire: validation of a new alcoholism screening instrument. *Am. J. Psychiatry 131*(10):1121–1123 (1978).
9. Selzer, M.L. The Michigan alcoholism screening test: The quest for a new diagnostic instrument. *Am. J. Psychiatry 127*(12):1653–1658 (1971).
10. Selzer, M.L., Vinokur, A., and Vam, R.L. A self administered short Michigan alcoholism screening test (SMAST). *J. Stud. Alcohol. 36*:124 (1975).
11. Pitchumoni, C.S., and Glass, G.B.J. Patterns of gastritis in alcoholics. *Biol. Gastroenterol. (Paris) 9*:11–16 (1976).
12. Rankin, J.G.D., Orrego-Matte, H., Desohenes, J., Medline, A., Findlay, J.E., and Armstrong, A.I.M. Alcoholic liver disease: The problem of diagnosis. *Alcohol. Clin. Exp. Res. 2*:327–338 (1978).
13. Brenner, B., and Selzer, M.L. Risk of causing a fatal accident associated with alcoholism, psychopathology, and stress: Further analysis of previous data. *Behav. Sci. 14*:490–495 (1969).
14. Klatsky, A.L., Friedman, G.D., Siegelaub, A.B., and Gerard, M.J. Alcohol consumption and blood pressure. Kaiser-Permanente multiphasic health examination data. *N. Engl. J. Med. 296*:1194–1200 (1977).
15. Skude, G., and Wadstein, J. Amylase, hepatic enzymes and bilirubin in serum of chronic alcoholics. *Acta Med. Scand. 201*:53–58 (1977).
16. Rosalki, S.B., and Rau, D. Serum gamma glutamyl transpeptidase activity in alcoholism. *Clin. Chim. Acta 39*:41–47 (1972).
17. Unger, K.W., and Johnson, D., Jr. Red blood cell mean corpuscular volume: a potential indicator of alcohol usage in the working population. *Am.J. Med. Sci. 267*:281–289 (1974).
18. Papoz, L., Warnet, J.M., Pequignot, G., Eschwege, E., Claude, J.R., and Schwartz, D. Alcohol consumption in a healthy population: Relationship to gamma glutamyl transferase activity and mean corpuscular volume. *J.A.M.A. 245*:1748–1751 (1981).
19. Skinner, H.A.,and Holt, S. Early intervention for alcohol problems. *J. Coll. Gen. Pract. 33*:787–791 (1983).
20. Schulz, J.E., and Mersy, D.J. Chemical dependency: What to do once you suspect it. *Postgrad. Med. 85*(5):89–91, 96 (1989).
21. Johnson, V. *I'll Quit Tomorrow*, rev. ed. New York, Harper & Row, 1980.
22. Johnson Institute: How to use intervention in your professional practice: A guide for helping professionals who work with chemical dependents and their families. Minneapolis, Johnson Institute Books, 1987.
23. Bissell, L., and Haberman, P.W. Alcoholism in the professions. New York, Oxford University Press, 1984.
24. Gualtieri, A.C., Cosentino, J.P., and Becker, J.S. The California experience with a diversion program for impaired physicians. *J.A.M.A. 249*(2):226–229 (1983).

25. Herrington, R.E., Benzer, D.G., Jacobson, G.R., and Hawkins, M.K. Treating substance use disorders among physicians. *J.A.M.A.* *247*(16):2253–2257 (1982).
26. Morse, R.M., Martin, M.A., Swenson, W.M., and Niven, R.G. Prognosis of physicians treated for alcoholism and drug dependence. *J.A.M.A.* *251*(6):743–746 (1984).
27. Vogt, P.A. Chemical Dependency-How are we dealing with it. *Hennepin Cty. Med. Soc. Bull.* *61*(2) (1989).

58

The Use of Alcoholics Anonymous and Narcotics Anonymous by the Physician in Treating Drug and Alcohol Addiction

John N. Chappel
University of Nevada School of Medicine, and Truckee Meadows Hospital, Reno, Nevada

I. INTRODUCTION

This chapter is a clinical guide for the practicing physician in the use of 12-Step programs, specifically Alcoholics Anonymous (AA) and Narcotics Anonymous (NA). A detailed history and description of these programs is covered elsewhere in this book. In most instances, the physician will be treating medical or psychiatric problems which are produced or complicated by the use of alcohol and/or other drugs. Clinical experience in most of these conditions suggests that they respond best when the patient is abstinent.

The most effective system for maintaining abstinence in alcohol-dependent individuals is AA. In a prospective study, Vaillant [Ref. 1, p. 156] found that the number of visits of AA meetings explained 28% of the variance of clinical outcome, while four prognostic items, stable psychosocial adjustment, married, employed, and never detoxified before, explained only 7% of the variance of clinical outcome. Psychotherapy of the traditional type has not helped in attaining or maintaining abstinence. In another group of college students (N = 204), selected for their good health, 26 (12.7%) became alcoholic as adults. In this group, 10 received over 100 hours of psychotherapy [Ref. 1, p. 187]. "Once recovered, several of the college sample saw their psychotherapy as having retarded recognition of their alcoholism" [Ref. 1, p. 283].

The above data illustrate the fact that the original 12-Step program, Alcoholics Anonymous, was empirically developed by a number of alcoholics, including some physicians, who had not been helped by the best efforts of medicine or psychiatry. The inability of medicine to help alcohol addicts was acknowledged by the psychiatrists Jung and Silkworth, and experienced by "Dr. Bob S.," a surgeon, and one of the cofounders of AA [2]. It took several years and many failures for the 12-Step system of long-term recovery to be developed. In this sense it can be viewed as the product of clinical research. The 12-Step program is compatible with medical and psychiatric treatment. It works best when physicians treating recovering patients are knowledgably supportive and refrain from prescribing dependence-producing or controlled medications.

Since any practicing physician can expect 10–20% of his or her patients to be alcohol or drug dependent, good medical practice requires knowledge of effective treatment approaches. For this reason, knowledge of the 12-Step programs becomes as important as knowledge of surgical, obstetrical, or other treatment approaches. The primary care physician does not need to perform the treatment, but good referral and patient support require in depth knowledge.

II. RECOVERY SUPPORTIVE MEDICAL CARE

The goal of treating alcohol and other drug addictions is recovery. This frequently used, but poorly defined, term refers to a state which is quite different from simple abstinence. This latter state, easily attained with medical help, is frequently characterized by symptoms of emotional distress referred to as a "dry drunk" or "white knuckle sobriety." Craving and drug- seeking behavior are frequent, as are irritability, defensive behavior, and multiple complaints associated with dysphoria. *Recovery* takes much longer to attain and is characterized by:

1. The ability to manage the stress of living without the support of dependence producing drugs. This ability is unusual in a society in which the use of alcohol and prescription medications for stress management is acceptable.
2. The ability to be around dependence-producing drugs without experiencing craving or engaging in drug-seeking behavior. Alcohol is the main problem owing to its ubiquity, but marijuana, cocaine, and prescription drugs are frequently encountered.

Recovery, or stable sobriety, is most commonly achieved through working a 12-Step program. This work requires time and effort, which deters many alcohol- and/or drug-addicted patients. The process can be helped greatly by recovery supportive medical care, which is characterized by the following:

1. Help resolve problems the patient experiences with recovery activities. These problems include, but are not limited to, impatience with "drunkalogues" (personal stories of alcoholics and addicts), frustration with the limitations of AA members, and dislike of the "religious" nature of AA.

2. Use short, simple instructions. In the early phases of recovery, the brain is often not working well. AA members have learned from experience to keep it simple. Physicians should do the same. Some useful statements are:

Don't drink (or use drugs)—Put a plug in the jug.
Stay in treatment.
Go to meetings.
Ask for help.
Easy does it.
Live and let live.
One day at a time.
Don't get HALT (Hungry, Angry, Lonely or Tired).
Identify, don't compare.
One is too many, a thousand not enough.

3. Encourage the patient to find a home group. Two useful purposes are served by this step. The first is that the home group provides the core of a recovery support system. The use of a telephone list and willingness to ask for help has been significantly ($p < 0.05$) associated with a good outcome [3]. The second benefit comes from taking responsibility in preparing for, participating in, and cleaning up after meetings. This introduces the patient to the experience of service.

4. Encourage the patient to find a sponsor. Sponsors are people with good recovery who help the newly recovering alcoholic or addict to work the steps and develop a program of recovery. Using a sponsor has also been significantly (p < 0.001) associated with a good outcome [3].

5. Follow the patient's step work. Each successive step usually marks a new level of growth and development for the patient. The problems frequently encountered in doing step work will be described later.

6. Expect recovery to take time. Usually 1–3 years are required for the attainment of stable recovery. The stages can be conceptualized as:

a. Unstable sobriety, when professional treatment is most needed. Initially the patient denies alcoholism or addiction and resists treatment. This is followed by a more passive compliance with treatment. The patient may pay lip service to recovery, but is very vulnerable to relapse.
b. Stabilizing sobriety occurs as the patient develops an active personal recovery program, using the tools he or she has learned in treatment. This includes working the 12 Steps and attending frequent AA/NA meetings.
c. Stable sobriety or recovery, as described above.

7. Careful prescribing to avoid dependence-producing, or scheduled, medication, which can trigger a relapse. The following sequence of prescribing is recommended:

a. Prescribe nonchemical symptom relievers. Anxiety, insomnia, somatic complaints, and other problems are common in the early months of recovery. Prescriptions can be written for exercise, relaxation, 12-Step meetings, reading, music, heat, cold, etc.
b. Prescribe disulfiram (Antabuse) for alcoholics and naltrexone (Trexan) for narcotics addicts. The use of these medications is associated with abstinence. Side effects, especially with disulfiram, are reduced with lower doses. The main problem with both these medications is the lack of a psychoactive effect on the brain, and the patient stops taking the medication.
c. Prescribe non–dependence-producing medication. This includes all nonscheduled medications. The most commonly used are nonsteroidal anti-inflammatories, sedating antihistamines, antidepressants, and buspirone (Buspar).
d. Prescribe dependence-producing medication (CII–V) carefully.
    (1) Intensify the patient's recovery plan. Write orders allowing visits from AA/NA members at any time and 12-Step meetings to be held in the patient's room. Ensure that the patient informs his or her recovery support system of the medication.
    (2) Withdraw dependence-producing medication quickly. This should be done before discharge from the hospital, if possible.
    (3) Expect craving, drug seeking, and manipulation for additional prescriptions. Do not express anger, disappointment, or other negative emotions. Curiosity and humor help maintain the physician-patient relationship. The above behaviors are normal responses when the addicted brain is reexposed to addicting agents. The patient needs help in overcoming his or her own responses.

III. THE AA/NA EXPERIENCE

One of the best descriptions of an alcoholic's experience has been written for health care professionals by Maxwell [4]. He describes the process of becoming an addict in the following terms:

1. Changes occur in perceptions of reality. There is an increasing tendency to blame others and to experience oneself as powerless.
2. A special, personal, powerful, and enduring relationship develops between the person and the drug(s). There will be resistance or even panic when separation from the drug(s) is suggested. There will also be grief over the loss when separation occurs.
3. The person thinks of himself or herself as being more acceptable when taking the drug(s). Without the drug(s) the person may experience discomfort with others and anticipate rejection, or even punishment.
4. There is a growing preoccupation with the drug(s) and anticipaton of its use. Following detoxification, the person will often feel either empty and bored, or overwhelmed with issues that have been neglected.

The above reactions are further evidence of the profound effect which alcohol and other addiction-producing drugs can have on the human brain. These effects persist long after drug use is discontinued, suggesting long-term changes in receptor sites, synaptic clefts, or neurotransmitter levels.

The 12-Step programs have developed an effective mix of activities of help the recovering alcoholic or addict maintain sobriety. Personal support is provided through relationships with other recovering people who share their experience, strength, and hope. The only requirement for membership is a desire to stop drinking or using drugs. This is often no more than a desire to stop hurting. One of the first discoveries made by "Bill W.," one of AA's cofounders, was that he could stay sober by talking to other alcoholics, even if they were drunk. It was this fact, after several months of difficult sobriety, which led him to Dr. Bob, a currently practicing alcoholic, in 1935.

As the recovering alcoholic or addict works a 12-Step program, an inner shift begins to occur. Experience with the drug has led to increases in immature defense mechanisms, such as denial, projection, minimizing, and grandiosity, all too often with associated antisocial behavior. The shift from this defensive orientation to a growth orientation is slow and unconscious. Change requires conscious effort in working a recovery program. The result is a gradual positive, even creative acceptance of reality, both internal and external. Maxwell [4] describes this process as tapping "an unsuspected inner resource." AA/NA members describe the experience as a spiritual awakening. Terms such as a personal experience of something more than self are used.

From an operational point of view, in acquiring an education in using 12-Step programs, physicians supporting a patient in the process of recovery should be able to describe the following aspects of AA and NA.

A. What Happens at AA/NA Meetings

The most unusual aspect of these meetings is the importance placed on the newcomer. Effort is made to help the new person feel welcome no matter how badly they feel or look. There are many different kinds of meetings. Discussion, speaker, step study, and *Big Book* study meetings are the most common. Patients rarely like the first meeting they attend and need encouragement from their physician to keep going. There are increasing numbers of nonsmoking meetings, which are important to physicians. Patients can also be assured that confidentiality will be observed. AA/NA members do not tell anyone who attends meetings or what is said.

B. Importance of Choosing a Home Group

The identification of a home group helps the newly recovering person develop a support system and facilitates using a telephone list. More importantly, there is an experience of responsibility with an introuction to service in helping to set up for meetings and clean up afterward.

C. Role of a Sponsor

Choosing and using a sponsor can play a powerful role in the addicted person's recovery, as has been mentioned. Some in the fellowship of AA describe a sponsor as someone who sees through you and still sees you through. A sponsor helps the newly sober "pigeon" or "baby" to slow down in the enthusiastic rush to complete the 12 Steps in 12 days. When problems arise in this relationship, the support of a knowledgable physician may be of value in helping the recovering person continue to work with their sponsor and avoid relapse.

D. Benefits and Pitfalls in Working the 12 Steps

Each step in the 12-Step program presents the newly recovering alcoholic or addict with a problem. Many choose not to apply themselves and face the distress associated with growth and personal change. Specific problems will be described later in this chapter.

E. Value of Service

Many recovering alcoholics and addicts, who have attained stable sobriety, attribute much of their success in this effort to service. The 12th Step itself provides the first experience in service, apart from helping the home group with its meetings, when the message of recovery is carried to other suffering alcoholics and addicts. Service activity can be as diverse as making home visits, going into prisons, or helping physicians and other professionals learn about the program. The benefit of service is that it helps recovering persons turn attention away from their own problems.

F. Difference Between Spiritual and Religious

Much confusion exists in this area. The 12-Step programs are not religious. They have no creed, dogma, or theology which must be learned. They are not in competition and are compatible with all known religions. Agnostics and atheists have been able to work comfortably in the program once they understand the need to acknowledge something outside themselves which can help the healing process, but which will not do anything for them that they can do for themselves. Atheist medical students and physicians understand what Paré meant when he said, "I merely dress the wound, God heals it." This is a simple acknowledgment of the fact that there are aspects of ourselves and the world which are not accessible through our five senses. The genius of the 12-Step programs is that the recovering person's experience with that healing process is left entirely up to him or her. No other person, group, or authority attempts to define or describe what it is or will be for the individual.

G. Importance of the Traditions

The 12 Traditions are less well known or understood than are the 12 Steps. They grew out of the later experience of Alcoholics Anonymous and the historical experience of similar programs. They are designed to ensure the survival of each 12-Step program. Physicians need to understand and respect the purpose of the traditions, especially anonymity and nonalliance. We are trained to expect and accept change as research opens new doors to etiology and effective treatment. It is especially tempting to try to change what appears to be a medically naive program. At best, this will be frustrating and ineffective. The mechanism for change is built into the 12-Step programs, starting with group autonomy and having many checks and balances. It is almost totally resistant, in a friendly way, to external suggestion or pressure.

H. Problems Associated with the 12-Step Programs

The problems associated with the 12-Step programs include but are not limited to the following:

1. A singleness of purpose which ignores tobacco dependence. This is probably the major cause of premature death in people with otherwise good recovery.
2. Drunkalogues may stimulate craving rather than identification with sobriety.
3. AA/NA members who express opinions which are the opposite of AA and NA. Officially, the 12-Step programs support medical care and urge their members to cooperate with their physicians' orders. There is no support for recovering members being told to stop taking disulfiram (Antabuse), lithium, or other medications.
4. Becoming "addicted" to AA/NA so that quality of life is impaired. The 12-Step programs are designed to enhance relationships, work, and other useful activities, not to replace them.

IV. THE 12 STEPS AND 12 TRADITIONS

A basic understanding of the issues involved in working the 12 Steps can help a physician provide more effective recovery supportive care. The steps themselves are on page 1257.

A. Steps 1, 2, and 3

Steps 1, 2, and 3 are the surrender steps. In admitting the need for help, the recovering person has an initial experience in humility. Acknowledging his or her limitations also helps in beginning to accept honestly reality as it is and not how it is wished or hope to be.

Barriers to these steps are denial, pride, and an unrealistic self-image. Resistance is sufficiently great that many alcoholics and addicts need to enter treatment programs in which help is provided in breaking down the barriers and working these steps.

B. Steps 4 and 5

Steps 4 and 5 are the inventory steps. This process of honest self-examination and sharing the results fits in well with psychiatric treatment. Recovering persons who have completed these steps often do very well in psychotherapy, using the experience to work on issues other than sobriety.

Barriers to these steps are guilt, shame, and grief, which can lead to depression. Physician support can do a great deal to lessen these barriers and help the recovering patient work through the pain.

C. Steps 6 and 7

Steps 6 and 7 are the character change steps. These may be the least well understood of the steps. They may also account for the striking change in personality traits which occur in some recovering persons.

The barrier to these steps is the resistance to change in character or personality which exists in all of us. The physician can encourage the recovering person to describe the aspects of character they would most like to change in as detailed a way as possible through reworking steps 4 and 5. This repeated preparation may set the stage for small but possible transformations in working Steps 6 and 7. When progress in this area occurs, especially in selfishness, self-centeredness, and other antisocial traits, it can be a great source of hope for others.

D. Steps 8 and 9

Steps 8 and 9 are the relational steps. Making amends safely in a sensitive and assertive way helps repair damaged relationships. It is hard to continue hating someone who acknowledges the wrong they have done and offers to try to repair the damage which has been done. These steps also help develop relational skills which are important in maintaining long-term relationships.

Barriers to Steps 8 and 9 are resentments, blaming, and a wish to control the behavior of other people.

E. Steps 10 and 11

Steps 10 and 11 are the maintenance steps. They involve a daily, or timely, review of the first 9 Steps, applying them to current life situations. Step 10 reviews Steps 4 through 9, whereas Step 11 reviews Steps 1 through 3. In this way, regular attention is paid to personal, relational, and spiritual health. If these steps are not being worked regularly, the physician has reason to be concerned about the quality of his or her patient's quality of recovery.

Barriers to Steps 10 and 11 include all those listed above, plus laziness and complacency.

F. Step 12

Step 12 is the service step. The obvious 12th Step is a direct visit to a still-suffering alcoholic or addict in their home or hospital room. This is usually done in pairs selected by sex, age, and background for the purpose of ease of identification by the alcoholic. Less obvious 12th-Step work includes going into jails, prisons, and treatment facilities. It also includes educating physicians and other professionals through work with the Cooperation with the Professional Community (CPC) Committee. The physician who asks for help in learning about the 12-Step programs is facilitating 12th-Step work.

Barriers to Step 12 are narcissism, shyness, and limitations of time and energy.

The *Traditions* of AA and NA have been developed to ensure the survival of these organizations and their programs. Physicians and other outsiders cannot change these Traditions, no matter how brilliant, persuasive, or well-intentioned they may be. The physician who understands and respects the Traditions will be much better able to provide effective recovery supportive medical care for his or her alcohol- or drug-dependent patients.

The Traditions are discussed on page 1258. The best short summary of the Traditions is contained in the second paragraph of the descriptions of AA printed in every issue of the *AA Grapevine*:

> The only requirement for membership is a desire to stop drinking [Tradition 3]. There are no dues or fees for AA membership; we are self supporting through our own contributions [Tradition 7]. AA is not allied with any sect, denomination, politics, organization, or institution, does not wish to engage in any controversy; neither endorses nor opposes any causes [Traditions 6 and 10]. Our primary purpose is to stay sober and help other alcoholics to achieve sobriety [Tradition 5].

The physician should understand AA's singleness of purpose. There is a temptation to expect the 12-Step programs to do more for a patient than merely stop drinking or using drugs. Such an expectation leads to frustration and discounting the real value of the programs. Like a scalpel, AA was designed for the specific purpose of attaining stable sobriety. It is inappropriate to try to use it for something else. The 12-Step programs are not like the medical profession or the health care system, even though they can be of great help to each in caring for alcohol- and drug-dependent patients.

12-Step program unity comes first in Tradition 1, so any attempts by physicians to change them will be met with a lack of response. The 12-Step programs are nonauthoritarian and nonprofessional, considering their leaders to be trusted servants (Traditions 2 and 8). The physician looking for the leaders in AA/NA will meet rotating volunteers. Each 12-Step group is autonomous and may pursue its primary purpose in any way they wish as long as they do not affect other groups of AA as a whole (Tradition 4). Some groups will do strange, perhaps even bizarre things from time to time. Although the 12-Step programs are not organized, they have developed service boards and committees which are responsible to the fellowship in providing literature and other services (Tradition 9). The best source of this help is the General Service Office of AA in New York City.

The last two traditions, 11 and 12, are sometimes a source of both confusion and distress for the physician. The distinction between attraction and promotion (Tradition 11) may be hard to make, especially for those who have come to understand educational activity, which is basically attraction, as an effective marketing tool, which can be considered to be promotion. Anonymity poses similar problems. Carrying the message to suffering alcoholics or addicts is fundamental 12-Step work. The identity of the messenger is unimportant, and may even be dangerous to the continued sobriety of the messenger if it brings him or her special attention. For this reason, AA members making 12-Step calls may be reluctant to identify themselves to the physician. Anonymity is viewed as a spiritual process in that it deemphasizes the personality of the recovering person and puts the focus on principles which are greater and more important than the person (Tradition 12). We physicians like to know our consultants and the quality of work they do. In the case of the 12-Step programs, physicians need to trust the programs and accept the inevitable variations which will occur among those sent to make 12-Step visits on patients.

Referral to a 12-Step program is best made early. Since the patient will usually resist the referral, it should be done as soon as the criteria for diagnosis are met. The referral can then be repeated by the physician as each opportunity presents itself. If the referral is based on data, there is little danger of losing the patient, especially if concern for health is emphasized. There appears to be a window of opportunity for successful referral, circumscribed by the patient's discomfort. Therefore, the issue should be raised prior to, or at the time of, detoxification. In our experience, waiting until detoxification is completed, especially in an acute care or psychiatric bed which is not on a drug- or alcohol-dependency unit, results in sufficient comfort for the patient that denial occurs, resistance increases, and referral fails.

The most successful referrals to 12-Step programs occur when direct patient contact is made with someone in recovery. This can be done efficiently by telephone from the physician's office, or by a 12-Step visit in the hospital. An immediate arrangement should be made for the patient to attent a meeting as quickly as is medically possible. The first meetings are most effective if the patient goes with a person in good recovery and has a chance to discuss his or her reactions afterward. Support and encouragement from the physician can play a critical role in helping the patient pick a temporary sponsor and begin working their own 12-Step program. Many people who attend AA drop out before making even these preliminary steps.

Alcohol- or drug-addicted patients can be encouraged to attend either AA or NA; both are effective for virtually any alcoholic or addict. Physicians are often surprised when narcotic, cocaine, or marijuana addicts do well in AA. All they need is a desire to stop drinking, which can often be developed rapidly with education or relapse experience. One reason so many addicts do well in AA is that this is the oldest and most stable of the 12-Step programs. There are more people with stable sobriety in AA than in any other program. There are also more groups in remote places and other countries. NA, while younger, is rapidly growing and has developed very effective recovering communities in many large cities.

V. DEVELOPING RECOVERY SUPPORTIVE SKILLS

Few physicians have received specific training in recovery supportive medical practice, although this situation is improving in family medicine and psychiatry residencies. The following educational process for physicians is based on several years of experience with medical students in their clinical training:

1. Call the local AA number and ask to speak to the CPC committee chair or one of the members of that committee. This step will greatly increase your chances of having a good educational and personal experience. The CPC committee is charged with the task of working with professionals and helping them become more knowledgable about AA. It is called being friends with our friends.
2. Identify yourself as a physician who is interested in learning more about the 12-Step programs. Ask for a recovery guide who will act as an instructor for you. You would like someone who has completed the 12 Steps and is working an active recovery program. Your recovery guide should also have an interest in sharing their recovery with you.
3. Meet at least four times with your recovery guide. The first time should include attendance at an AA meeting and your recovery guide's story. Then go over the schedule of local meetings to select other meetings you will attend. Pick those which meet your interests or needs. These may include Alanon, Alateen, NA, or other 12-Step meetings. Plan to attend at least four meetings. You may also have some special interests like cocaine, marijuana, or heroin addiction, overdoses, prison experience, etc. Your recovery guide can help you meet recovering people with experience in those areas. Discuss all these experiences with your recovery guide over at least three more meetings.

   The following guidelines are the ones we use for our recovery guides and may be useful to share with your recovery guide:

1. Provide basic information. Keep it simple and do not assume that the physician is experienced or knowledgable. This means that the physician may not even know what questions to ask.
2. Send the physician to the Central Office locally and recommend one or two basic brochures or brief sections of books. Base your selection on your assessment of the physician's interests and needs. Just get him or her started. Do not swamp the physician by recommending reading all of the *Big Book* or *The Twelve and Twelve*.
3. Describe the common problems people have working a 12-Step recovery program. Be willing to discuss personal experience or those of others, while preserving anonymity. Encourage questions. Describe behaviors the physician can recognize in his or her patients, both in addiction and in recovery.
4. Introduce the physician to other recovering people with experiences which would be of interest to him or her. Your goal is to meet the physician's needs to become comfortable with 12-Step programs and recovering persons. This comfort will translate into increasing knowledge and skill in helping alcoholics and addicts receive the help they need.

VI. CONCLUSIONS

Alcohol and other drug addictions pose major problems for both physicians and our society. We cannot afford to do business as usual and only treat the complications or sequelae of these disorders. The usually hidden primary disease of addiction must be treated. In this task, the 12-Step programs are a specific and valuable tool. When we work with the 12-Step programs we need to share control. Neither the programs nor their members can be ordered to carry out a specific treatment, as we are used to doing in our offices or in hospitals.

We must change our view of treatment goals. With alcohol- and drug-addicted patients, it is not enough to provide symptom relief and return them to their former dependent state of health. The goal of treatment must be recovery, which is usually a better state of health then when they were asymptomatically using alcohol or other drugs. This goal requires a change in our prescribing practices. We need to avoid addiction-producing medications and prescribe 12-Step recovery activities.

REFERENCES

1. Vaillant, G.E. *The Natural History of Alcoholism: Causes, Patterns, and Paths to Recovery.* Cambridge, Massachusetts, Harvard University Press, 1983.
2. *Alcoholics Anonymous*, 3rd ed. Alcoholics Anonymous World Services, Inc., New York, 1976.
3. Sheeren, M. The relationship between relapse and involvement in Alcoholics Anonymous. *J. Stud. Alcohol, 49*:104–106 (1988).
4. Maxwell, M.A. *The AA Experience*. New York, McGraw-Hill, 1984.

XVIII
Pharmacological Treatments

59

Alcohol Withdrawal Syndrome: Clinical Features, Pathophysiology, and Treatment

Terry K. Schultz
Walter Reed Army Medical Center, Washington, D.C.

I. INTRODUCTION

Alcohol withdrawal syndrome is a standard term of medical diagnosis. This was not always the case; validation and universal acceptance of the withdrawal syndrome are relatively recent developments.

The idea that certain seizures in the alcoholic patient are related to the withdrawal of alcohol was probably first expressed in 1852 by Huss, who drew a distinction between convulsions in epileptics who drank and convulsions that were brought about by the cessation of drinking [1]. The relationship of seizures to the cessation of drinking was also commented upon by others in the last century (see Ref. 2 for review). Nevertheless, this view failed to prevail, and Bowman and Jellinek wrote in 1941 that the withdrawal theory had been virtually discarded in the United States [3]. In Europe, this theory was also abandoned [4]. However, in 1953, Victor and Adams published impressive clinical evidence to support this concept [5]. In 1955, Isbell and coworkers replicated the observations of Victor and Adams in a carefully controlled study of chronic intoxication and withdrawal in a group of 10 volunteer subjects [6]. It is noteworthy that the manifestations of alcohol withdrawal in these subjects were very much the same as those induced by chronic intoxication and withdrawal from barbiturates as reported by Isbell et al. in 1950 [7].

In the next 2 decades that followed these clinical observations, the concept of an alcohol withdrawal syndrome was extensively confirmed by another experimental human study [8] and by a series of animal studies (see Refs. 2,9, and 10 for reviews). These clinical and experimental studies adequately answer most of the arguments that have been made against the withdrawal theory. In the past decade, rapid developments in cell biology have provided deeper insights into alcohol-induced changes at the cellular and subcellular levels, leading to a better understanding of the pathophysiology of alcohol dependence and withdrawal, and extensive reviews have recently been published [11–14].

The alcohol withdrawal syndrome, although variable in its range of signs and symptoms, is readily identifiable. Nevertheless, if is often overlooked in the general outpatient or hospital population [15,16]. Recognition of the diagnosis has important clinical implications. Its presence is certainly pivotal for the diagnosis of alcoholism and generally reflects the severity of the disease. Moreover, the clinical features of alcohol withdrawal demonstrate a major pharmacological effect of alcohol on the brain; i.e., physical dependence, a property shared with other sedative-hypnotic drugs that may be used excessively [17].

This chapter will summarize the spectrum of clinical features and current understanding of the pathophysiology of alcohol dependence and withdrawal, and discuss the implications for detoxification and protracted recovery.

II. CLINICAL FEATURES

The clinical manifestations of alcohol withdrawal show great variability in severity and duration [5,6,8,18]. It is an evolving syndrome that appears approximately 6 hr after a substantial fall in the blood alcohol level. Early symptoms may include tremulousness, malaise or weakness, hyperreflexia, mild tachycardia, increasing blood pressure, sweating, insomnia, perceptual distortions, anorexia, nausea or vomiting, anxiety, and mental depression or general irritability. These symptoms usually peak between 24 and 36 hr and may subside after 48 hr. However, hallucinations and generalized tonic-clonic seizures may also occur during this period.

A. Hallucinations

Hallucinations may ocur in 3–10% of alcoholic patients during withdrawal [19,20]. They are most commonly visual, although they may be auditory, tactile, or olfactory [21]. They are variable in duration, usually lasting only hours but may persist for weeks. Hallucinations differ from delirium tremens in that patients are rarely disoriented and they generally retain vivid recall. Since the content and intensity of these hallucinations may be similar to those seen in schizophrenia [22], a reliable history of prior alcohol use is essential. Alcoholic patients differ from schizophrenic patients in terms of age of onset, family history, and premorbid personality [23]. Nevertheless, chronic alcohol hallucinosis is sometimes mistaken for schizophrenia. Of course, dual diagnoses are sometimes present.

B. Withdrawal Seizures

Withdrawal seizures occur in 5–15% of alcoholic patients and, in the majority of cases, occur between 7 and 48 hr with a peak incidence at 24 hr after cessation of drinking [5,24]. They are generalized tonic-clonic in type and occur singly or in short bursts over a period of a few hours (usually less than 6 hr, sometimes as long as 12 hr), and rarely develop into status epilepticus. It is estimated that 30% of affected patients will go on to delirium tremens if untreated. The possibility of simultaneous withdrawal from other drugs should always be considered, especially in view of the unreliability of self-reports of drug use [25]. A serum or urine toxicology drug screen should routinely be done on admission and independent corroborative information should be obtained from family or friends of the patient whenever possible. A careful differential diagnosis should be considered, as seizures may be related to metabolic, infectious, or other neurological causes such as head trauma or idiopathic epilepsy. Focal seizures during withdrawal are unusual and deserve further evaluation to rule out space-occupying lesions or a seizure focus secondary to head trauma.

An EEG is essential, and uncomplicated alcohol withdrawal seizures generally will not show residual EEG abnormalities. Experimental studies of alcohol intoxication and withdrawal using serial EEGs [26] show that mild degrees of slowing occur during the period of intoxication. During alcohol withdrawal, sharp waves, spikes, and paroxysmal changes appear, but these changes are transient and occur only during the fifteenth to nineteenth hours of the abstinence period. This period coincides with the peak incidence of spontaneous seizures in alcoholic patients and the transient nature of the EEG abnormalities is in keeping with the brevity of the convulsive attacks. Insofar as the EEG is a record of physiological activity of the cerebral cortex, it reflects a characteristic series of changes engendered by alcohol itself—mild slowing during chronic intoxication, a rapid return to normal immediately after cessation of drinking, mild but definite dysrhythmias, or rebound phenomena, occurring in a discrete period in the withdrawal phase, and again a return to normal [26]. Except for this very transient period following alcohol withdrawal, the incidence of EEG abnormalities in patients with alcoholic epilepsy is not greater than in the normal population—in sharp contrast to patients who are indeed subject to seizures.

C. Delirium Tremens

Delirium tremens (DTs) occurs in less than 5% of patients hospitalized for alcohol withdrawal, but it is the most severe manifestation of withdrawal [5,18]. In one study, DTs lasted a mean of 56 hr, with a range of 10–150 hr [27]. It has its onset generally between 72 and 96 hr after cessation of drinking, and is a state characterized by gross tremors and agitation, disorders of sense perception, especially visual hallucinations, disorientation, confusion, and increased psychomotor and autonomic nervous system activity. Patients may also be hyperpyrexic, incontinent, and diaphoretic. As a result, they often are unable to feed themselves or take oral medications. Because of their agitation, affected patients often require restraints for their safety as well as that of the hospital staff.

Concurrent illness may be difficult to diagnose as well as treat in a patient with DTs. Recognition of hepatic encephalopathy (HE) is of special importance because both the immediate effect and the duration of action of many sedatives are increased in such patients [28]. Hepatic encephalopathy is a complex neuropsychiatric disorder that complicates hepatocellular failure regardless of its cause. The earliest signs of HE are subtle changes in behavior and intellectual function, which reflect bilateral forebrain dysfunction. Progression results in ataxia, motor impairment, and eventually the loss of consciousness. The differential diagnosis between delirium tremens and hepatic encephalopathy is important, although the conditions may coexist. Patients with DTs are typically more anxious, with a tremor that is fine and fast. Patients with HE are more obtunded, with asterixis and a slow tremor. If the diagnosis is not clear, an EEG will be helpful. Patients in withdrawal have EEGs with hyperactivity, whereas with encephalopathy the EEG shows slowing of electrical activity. An elevated ammonia level also supports the diagnosis of HE [28].

These patients pose an especially difficult problem during detoxification if they need treatment for agitation. Encephalopathy may be worsened by central nervous system depressants, especially if the drug requires hepatic metabolism. Benzodiazepines may intensify the confusion associated with HE, whereas haloperidol will more likely reduce confusion and agitation. A promising new treatment for hepatic encephalopathy is the benzodiazepine antagonist flumazenil, the use of which has demonstrated improvement in both gross behavior and EEG visual evoked response in an animal model of hepatic encephalopathy [29]. This observation supports the possibility that the gamma-aminobutyric acid–benzodiazepine receptor complex is a mediator for HE [30]. When there appears to be a paradoxical response to benzodiazepines, suspect hepatic encephalopathy.

The patients with the greatest morbidity and mortality in DTs are those with the greatest fever, tachycardia, dehydration, and with associated illnesses (pneumonia, pancreatitis, and hepatitis) [27,28]. Death most often results from cardiovascular, metabolic, or infectious complications. Therapy that prevents progression to this severe form of withdrawal is clearly indicated for all patients with evidence of the alcohol withdrawal syndrome, but it is critical for those at high risk, including those who have had severe withdrawal syndrome in the past, concomitant acute medical illness, or chronic alcohol-related disease [28]. The most recent estimates of the mortality rate for DTs are approximately 2% owing to improved supportive and pharmacological management [31].

D. Withdrawal Spectrum

Each manifestations of the alcohol withdrawal syndrome may occur more or less by itself, but more often they occur in combination, in which case they appear in a predictable sequence. Characteristically, DTs is preceded by tremulousness and transient hallucinations, and the latter symptoms may even subside considerably before the delirium becomes manifest. Similarly, when seizures and DTs occur in the same patient, the seizures invariably precede the delirium. Also, it is evident that the severity of the clinical symptoms is related to the degree and duration of drinking. The mildest degree of the syndrome, taking the form of tremulousness, anorexia, nausea, and general irritability, may occur after a few days of drinking and after a relatively short period of abstinence (e.g., after a night's sleep); the most severe form of the syndrome, i.e., DTs, occurs after many weeks or months of drinking, becoming apparent only after several days of abstinence.

III. PATHOPHYSIOLOGY OF ALCOHOL DEPENDENCE AND WITHDRAWAL

It was in 1961 that Goldstein and Goldstein [32] proposed that dependency develops as a cell or organism makes homeostatic adjustments to compensate for the primary effect of a drug. This has been a fundamental guiding principle of the neurobiological research of the addictions. Since the primary effect of alcohol is depressant to the brain, it would be expected then that neuroadaptation to chronic exposure would result in a compensatory downregulation of inhibitory and upregulation of excitatory systems. With abrupt abstinence from alcohol a maladaptive state would be unmasked, manifested by the withdrawal syndrome. Confirmatory research evidence of this pathophysiological mechanism has accumulated and will be described below.

A. Neurocellular Models

Alcohol produces a wide range of effects in the brain. Unlike most psychoactive drugs, there are no specific receptors for alcohol. Its ability to penetrate neuronal cell membranes, similar to general anesthetics, led to the assumption that its effects are mediated by its ability to alter membrane lipids in a nonspecific manner. It has become increasingly apparent, however, that some responses to alcohol depend on its interaction with specific membrane-bound proteins. It has been suggested that these proteins function as "receptive sites" for the action of alcohol [33]. As a result, earlier research emphasis on membrane lipids has shifted to include studies of neurotransmitter systems.

Neurotransmitter Systems

Gamma-aminobutyric acid receptor–chloride ionophore (GABAa). The GABAa complex is the major inhibitory neurotransmitter system in the brain. This complex has several component recognition sites, including that for GABA itself, anxiolytic/hypnotic drug recognition sites (also termed central benzodiazepine receptors), a barbiturate recognition site, a site for basic neuroproteins, a steroid recognition site, and the chloride ion channel (also a bicarbonate outflow channel) which is the final common path for these various subunits. These different recognition sites have a common function in the coregulation of the frequency and duration of chloride channel opening. The GABAa complex is the site of action of detoxification drugs which are cross-tolerant with alcohol. An experimental drug, RO 15-4513, has been shown to cause effects opposite (partial inverse agonist) to benzodiazepine by acting at the same recognition site and antagonizes the intoxicating effects of alcohol [34]. The physiological role of the benzodiazepine site is unclear.

Interestingly, alcohol metabolism induces harmane, an endogenous partial inverse agonist-like ligand [35]. Harmane is formed in the liver from acetaldehyde and tryptophan, carried on the benzodiazepine site of albumin, and crosses the blood-brain carrier. This could represent a physiological mechanism for arousal state maintenance during alcohol intake but its adaptive limits are exceeded by heavy intake.

There is considerable evidence that alcohol may also affect the GABAa receptor in a potentiating way [36,37]. Chronic exposure to alcohol appears to reduce GABAa-mediated inhibition of neurons (38) and this is a possible mechanism for alcohol withdrawal seizures.

Homeostasis of GABAa activity is dependent on other systems such as cyclic adenosine monophosphate (cAMP) second messenger systems, magnesium ions, and N-methyl-D-aspartate (NMDA) receptors, all of which are also affected by chronic exposure to alcohol, and will be discussed further below.

Adrenoceptors. Rebound overactivity of brain and peripheral noradrenergic systems occurs in alcohol withdrawal and is positively correlated with the severity of the withdrawal symptoms [39], especially hypertension, tachycardia, and general autonomic reactivity. Alpha$_2$-adrenoceptors are involved in the inhibition of this system. Alpha$_2$ adrenoceptor function has been assessed during withdrawal using the intravenous clonidine (an alpha$_2$ adrenoceptor agonist) challenge test [40], and studies of plasma norepinephrine and platelet alpha$_2$-adrenoceptor density [41]. Functional subsensitivity and receptor downregulation of alpha$_2$-adrenoceptor systems have been detected. These changes begin to return towards normal within 24 hr as the withdrawal reaction subsides. Persistence of this mechanism may have implications for the phenomenon of "kindling" [39], as well as recent evidence showing that panic disorder and generalized anxiety disorder may be more likely to follow from pathological alcohol consumption [42,43]. Subsensitivity of alpha$_2$-adrenoceptor inhibition of neuroendocrine systems may persist [40], and is discussed further below.

Glutamate, NMDA receptor, and calcium channels. As the major excitatory neurotransmitter in the brain, the amino acid glutamate serves an important role in normal brain function. In addition, excessive quantities of glutamate can cause neurotoxicity and cell death [44]. Despite the recent increase in understanding of the pharmacology of glutamate and its various receptor subtypes, knowledge of how the glutamate signal is transduced is incomplete. Its action is mediated by at least four distinct receptor systems [45]. Of these subtypes, a consensus now appears to be emerging that NMDA receptors (named for the synthetic analog that selectively activates this subtype of glutamate receptor) are a plausible neurochemical target for alcohol and may mediate some of the pharmacological effects of alcohol [46–48]. The NMDA receptor is a subtype of glutamate receptor that is involved in learning (long-term potentiation) and neuronal development, as well as in epileptiform seizure activity. Therefore, the inhibition of this receptor by alcohol may be responsible for the effects of alcohol on cognition and brain development, and the adaptive upregulation of the receptor that occurs after chronic alcohol exposure may be important in the generation of alcohol withdrawal seizures [47,49]. Treatment with NMDA during withdrawal exacerbated seizures, whereas administration of a receptor antagonist, MK-801, decreased the occurrence and severity of seizures in a dose-dependent manner. This suggests that upregulation of NMDA receptors by chronic alcohol exposure may mediate alcohol withdrawal–associated seizures.

The NMDA receptor complex is a ligand-gated ion channel that can be modulated by endogenous or exogenous substances that act at a number of distinct recognition sites on or closely associated with the receptor complex. These include binding sites for glutamate (or NMDA), glycine, magnesium ion, zinc ion, hydrogen ion, and open-channel blockers such as phencyclidine (PCP), TCP, MK-801, and dextromethorphan. Most recently it has been discovered that endogenous polyamines, including spermine and spermidine, act at a specific distinct recognition site on the receptor complex [50]. Of these separate sites alcohol appears to inhibit the ability of glycine to enhance activity of NMDA-mediated cyclic guanosine monophosphate (cGMP), a second messenger system involved in the regulation of cellular metabolism [47], an inhibitory effect of chronic alcohol more pronounced in the cerebellum. As elucidation of this receptor complex continues, it is likely that novel pharmacological strategies will emerge to prevent or counter the neurotoxic effects of this site in alcohol withdrawal.

As another consequence of alcohol exposure and excessive neuronal inhibition, depolarization-induced entry of calcium ion into central neurons is reduced. As a result, physical dependence to alcohol is associated with an adaptive upregulation of the dihydropyridine (DHP)–sensitive (L-type voltage-operated) calcium channels on excitable neurons [51]. Removal of alcohol from an organism in this adapted state causes central nervous (CNS) hyperexcitability, expressed as the physical withdrawal syndrome, as a consequence of the increase in the number of calcium channels. Dihydropyridine calcium channel antagonists can prevent alcohol withdrawal, and offer a novel approach to the therapeutic management of the withdrawal syndrome as shown by numerous animal models and recent clinical trials [11,52]. Another recent research electrophysiological report confirmed the withdrawal neuronal hyperexcitability to be secondary to the unmasking of the upregulated DHP calcium channels, plus an additional compensatory downregulated calcium ion–activated potassium conductance inhibitory system [53].

Second messenger systems: adenylate cyclase and adenosine.   Increasing evidence suggests that alcohol-induced changes in cAMP second messenger signal transduction may play a critical role in the acute and chronic effects of alcohol (see Ref. 13 for review). Although initially alcohol increases hormone- and neurotransmitter-stimulated cAMP levels in many preparations, with chronic exposure a decrease in receptor-dependent cAMP levels develops. This has been shown to be a significant marker for chronic alcoholism. Studies of lymphocytes from alcholics exhibit a fourfold decrease in adenosine receptor–stimulated cAMP levels [54,55], and membranes prepared from platelets of alcoholics also show decreased prostaglandin E_1 (PGE_1) receptor–dependent cAMP levels [56]. It has been suggested that in different areas of the brain, alcohol may interfere with different components of the adenylate cyclase (AC) system [33]. It has been shown to alter the ability of norepinephrine-like substances to bind to cortical beta-noradrenergic receptors and to activate AC activity.

Cyclic AMP, in its second messenger role, is involved in many intracellular processes, including the molecular synthesis of ribonucleic acid (RNA) and of proteins in other cell systems, and thus its proper functioning has important long-term consequences for cellular well-being. Three linked membrane components—the receptor, a stimulatory guanine nucleotide regulatory protein (referred to as G_s protein), and the catalytic unit of AC—are involved in the production of cAMP [57].

Recent evidence indicates that alcohol-induced decreases in cAMP levels appear to be due to heterologous desensitization of receptors coupled to the G_s protein [58]. This appears to be a genotropic mechanism; that is, there is a measurable decrease in messenger RNA for the alpha subunit of G_s and a consequent decrease in alpha subunit protein. Moreover, with abstinence, this mechanism is reversible after the initial 48-h withdrawal period. It has now been reported that adenosine is a critical mediator of this mechanism [59].

Adenosine is an endogenous inhibitory neuromodulator with sedative and anticonvulsant properties. The desensitization of the A_2 adenosine receptor (which is linked to G_s)

during the immediate 48-h withdrawal phase could play a role in generating alcohol withdrawal excitation or seizures [60] or contribute to kindling effects. Since xanthine substances, including theophylline and caffeine, are potent adenosine receptor antagonists, use of these drugs may increase the risk of withdrawal seizures; they should be used with caution or avoided during detoxification. It remains to be determined whether therapy directed at increasing brain A_2 adenosine receptor activity will be effective in preventing or treating the alcohol withdrawal syndrome.

Cell Membrane

The notion that alcohol may exert its acute effects in membranes derives directly from the Meyer-Overton hypothesis of anesthetic action [61]. It was proposed that alcohol's effects, such as intoxication and sedation, were the result of perturbation of neuronal membrane lipids. However, this membrane hypothesis was not corroborated until 1976 when Chin and Goldstein first demonstrated that alcohol at physiologically attainable levels dose-dependently decreases the order in brain membranes [62]. The effect seems to be related to the original membrane fluidity: The more fluid the membrane, the greater the effect. These changes in membrane fluidity can be correlated with the sedative effect of alcohol in animals. Chronic exposure to alcohol results in an adaptation within the normal membrane. This requires an alteration of various biomembrane lipids, resulting in resistance in the fluidizing effects of alcohol with uncertain functional consequences in the acute withdrawal state. Earlier studies focused on changes in bulk membrane lipids These alterations include increased cholesterol concentrations and greater saturation among the phospholipid fatty acids [63]. More recently the research focus has shifted to the membrane protein boundary lipids. Increases of acidic phospholipids, including phosphatidylserine, phosphatidylinositol, and an abnormal lipid with acidic characteristics, phosphatidylethanol, have been identified [64]. Whether acidic phospholipids are pathophysiological factors is under investigation.

Another biomembrane lipid affected by alcohol is monosialoganglioside (GM1) [65]. Gangliosides are a family of naturally occurring glycosphinogolipids that contain sialic acid, are present in abundance in neural tissue, and are probably involved in a variety of functions related to the maturation and repair of neuronal cells [66,67]. Acute exposure to alcohol is facilitated by gangliosides which increase the sensitivity of membranes to the disordering ("fluidizing") effects of alcohol [65]. With chronic exposure to alcohol, however, GM1 is decreased and takes up to 35 days to normalize [68] after cessation of alcohol. This decrease results in a reduction of the partition coefficient of anesthetics and may be an important mechanism in the increased tolerance to anesthetics in alcoholic patients. More importantly, GM1 serves an endogenous neuroprotective function by modulating the plasticity of neurons to environmental cues. It potentiates the trophic effects of nerve growth factor (NGF), thereby attentuating neurotoxic effects of NMDA [69,70], and is also essential for maintenance of forebrain cholinergic neurons [71,72]. This may be an important pathophysiological mechanism involved in such chronic consequences as protracted abstinence syndrome [73] (see Chap. 49 for review), cognitive impairments [74], and loss of cholinergic muscarinic receptors in the frontal cortex of alcohol abusers [75,76]. This may represent a future avenue of therapeutic intervention. Reversing trophic deficits or potentiating trophic effects conceivably could prevent or decrease neurotoxicity and cognitive impairment.

B. Neuroendocrine Effects and the Hypothalamic-Pituitary-Adrenal Axis

Elevated cortisol (glucocorticoid) levels, an indication of activation of the hypothalamic-pituitary-adrenal (HPA) axis, have been reported to accompany both short- and long-term consumption of alcohol and the alcohol withdrawal syndrome [77–82]. This may be a key mechanism of protracted withdrawal symptoms. Cortisol is secreted from the adrenal cortex both in a rhythmic, circadian fashion, and as part of the stress response. It is the natural human "glucocorticoid," a term coined to denote the prominent actions of this class of steroids to regulate carbohydrate metabolism and stimulate glycogen deposition. Cortisol, like other steroid hormones, acts by way of a receptor-mediated nuclear mechanism to regulate gene expression [83]. It plays a critical role in differentiation and development, in regulating metabolism, in modulating the response to many hormones and growth factors, and in adapting to stress. Physiological levels of the hormone are required for optimal function of these widely diverse responses that are mediated throughout the body, and either insufficient or excessive levels lead to disease states. In its most severe form, a pseudo–Cushing's syndrome occurs in which the physical signs of Cushing's syndrome (including truncal obesity, cutaneous striae, muscle atrophy, weakness, hypertension, diabetes, plethora, and hirsutism) are obvious, but remit spontaneously over several weeks with abstinence [84]. Pseudo–Cushing's syndrome was first identified in 1976 [85], and, like Cushing's disease, is characterized by elevated basal cortisol levels, loss of the normal diurnal variation, and failure of overnight dexamethasone suppression. The CNS characteristics of emotional instability are seen, with symptoms ranging from hypomanic behavior to depression and increased somnolence [86]. Cortisol resistance has been described in patients [87] with elevated circulating levels of cortisol but without overt signs of cortisol excess such as the stigmata of Cushing's syndrome. Corticosteroids also inhibit growth hormone secretion, and this effect has been reported to persist during prolonged abstinence [40]. A recent review of research data [88] indicates very clearly that steroid hormones, including corticosteroids, have significant modulating influences on all aspects of the serotonergic systems of the mammalian brain. One of the most striking features of the regulation of serotonergic activity by steroid hormones is the marked regional specificity of the observed effects, perhaps by modulation of different receptor subtypes in different locations in the brain through altered gene expression. Under physiological conditions, plasma corticosterone was found to be inversely correlated with serotonin levels in the amygdala and directly correlated with hypothalamic serotonin content. Effects of corticosteroid replacement on serotonin turnover appear to be region dependent. There are very strong reciprocal relationships between the serotonergic systems and the corticosteroids. Serotonin has been shown to regulate corticosteroid receptor binding in hippocampal cell cultures [89]. A preliminary study [90] implicates a role of serotonergic mechanisms in alcoholic brain syndrome and a possible useful role for serotonin reuptake inhibitors (fluvoxamine) in ameliorating memory deficits.

A recent controlled clinical study reports that alcoholics have significantly altered HPA axis functioning up to 3 weeks following the cessation of drinking, with a more subtle impairment present for greater than 6 months following abstinence [91]. These changes may be secondary to the effects of multiple episodes of withdrawal and the associated elevation in corticosteroid levels on HPA organization. Studies that have investigated CNS interaction with HPA axis functioning have suggested that limbic inhibition by glucocorticoids may be involved [92]. The hippocampus, a limbic structure particularly important for memory function and control of affective states, has been shown to be especially vulnerable to chronic exposure to alcohol [93]. The hippocampus contains specific intracellular glucocorticoid receptors and is believed to be a major target for glucocorticoid action in the brain. Long-term exposure to high concentrations of glucocorticoids has been shown to cause prominent toxic effects in the hippocampus in animal models [94]. A recent tissue culture study [95] showed that glucocorticoids potentiated the toxic effects of the glutamate receptor agonist, kainate, thereby impairing the capacity of hippocampal neurons to survive insults such as seizures. Thus, with repeated untreated alcohol withdrawals, direct damage to the hippocampus may result.

Assessment of the HPA axis may provide an opportunity to determine severity of withdrawal [77], and thereby guide the decision for pharmacotherapy. Furthermore, this may represent a pathophysiological mechanism of kindling.

C. Kindling

In the kindling paradigm, first described in an animal model by Goddard in 1967 [96], a subthreshold electrical stimulus is delivered to a local brain area once or twice a day for a duration of 1–2 sec. When first applied, the electrical stimulation results in only brief after-discharge (AD) and no behavioral alteration. Without any change in stimulation parameters, the AD gradually increases in duration and spreads from the stimulus site to increasingly distant, though synaptically related, brain regions. A progressive alteration of stimulus-induced behavior is also seen, beginning with momentary arrest of ongoing locomotion activity and proceeding through localized twitching to a major motor convulsion. It is important to note that once kindling has taken place, cessation of stimulation does not seem to result in loss of the newly established response.

In 1978, Ballenger and Post introduced the idea of kindling as an important issue to consider in alcohol withdrawal [97]. In a retrospective study, they concluded that inadequately treated withdrawals could have a cumulative effect and thereby produce future withdrawals of increased severity, a process consistent with kindling in animal models. Since this pioneering work numerous reports have added weight to their postulate [98–104].

D. Magnesium

Alcoholism is the most commonly recognized cause of disturbed magnesium balance [105]. The frequency of hypomagnesemia in alcohol withdrawal states have been noted by many investigators [2]. Approximately 25–50% of the patients hospitalized for alcohol-related problems are hypomagnesemic [105]. However, because less than 1% of the total body magnesium is present in the serum, significant deficits of magnesium can occur in the absence of any overt change in the serum magnesium concentration. That the great majority of hospitalized alcoholics are magnesium deficient, regardless of their serum magnesium concentration, has been demonstrated by the observations that alcoholic subjects retain a greater percentage of a parenterally administered magnesium load than do paired controls and that they remain in positive magnesium balance for several days following hospital admission. In alcohol withdrawal, hypomagnesemia results from deficient intake, malabsorption, excessive renal losses, and cellular uptake [105]. A strong correlation has been demonstrated between low serum magnesium, increased arterial pH, and respiratory alkalosis at the peak period of photic sensitivity (seizure risk) [2]. Many of the symptoms of alcohol withdrawal are similar to those observed in subjects with experimental magnesium deficiency and may improve with magnesium infusions. In controlled studies, administration of magnesium to patients with alcohol withdrawal symptoms abolished photomyoclonus responses within 5 min or significantly raised the threshold in all subjects [106].

Over 300 enzymes are dependent on the presence of magnesium ions for activation [107]. It is an integral part of cell membranes, and is required for membrane stability and regulation of membrane fluidity. It also regulates the permeability of membranes toward other cations, particularly calcium and potassium ions. Magnesium ion has been described as nature's physiological calcium antagonist. It exerts inhibitory control over the NMDA receptor [108,109], is essential for the rate-limiting step in G_s activation of adenylate cyclase [110,111], and increasing plasma magnesium ion concentration also dilates blood vessels and reduces hypertension [107].

In summary, magnesium ion may be involved in attenuating many of the reported neuroexcitotoxic pathophysiological mechanisms involved in alcohol withdrawal. Evidence suggests that treatment designed to improve magnesium ion homeostasis may be neuroprotective [107].

E. Summary

The pathophysiology of alcohol dependence and withdrawal can be summarized by returning to the concept of Goldstein and Goldstein: Dependency develops as a cell or organism makes homeostatic adjustments to compensate for the primary effect of a drug [32]. Now, after 3 decades of alcohol research, a comprehensive neurobiological theory is emerging to support their pioneering insight. Thus, it can be seen that alcohol acts as a nonspecific inhibitor in the brain. As a result of neuroadaptation, during withdrawal, downregulated inhibitory and upregulated excitatory processes are unmasked, resulting in excessive activation of brain functions and neurotoxicity. Better understanding of these mechanisms has led to improved detoxification protocols, and promising novel treatment approaches are under development.

IV. TREATMENT

The immediate objectives of treatment of the alcohol withdrawal syndrome are to relieve symptoms and prevent or treat concomitant medical complications or more serious forms of the syndrome such as seizures or delirium. The ultimate goal, however, is to guide the patient into a continuing and structured program of recovery.

Advances in assessment and treatment have led to a substantial decrease in morbidity and mortality [31]. With better methods of assessment and early recognition of withdrawal, improved strategies for administering drug treatment have evolved [112]. As such, treatment failure in recent years is generally a result of a delay in therapy or of the severity of concomitant illness, not alcohol withdrawal per se. Opinions vary on which medications should be used to treat alcohol withdrawal and whether detoxification should be conducted in medical or social settings. The number of variations in therapeutic approaches reflects the relatively mild nature of most withdrawal syndromes as well as the need to balance cost and efficacy. Reviews of clinical studies of alcohol withdrawal treatment published over the past 35 years reveal that most have serious deficiencies such as lack of random distribution, double-blind controls, adequate numbers of patients, or adequate assessment instruments [113,114].

A. Nonpharmacological Intervention

If careful clinical evaluation reveals only mild withdrawal symptoms, most patients do not require hospitalization and may safely respond to nonpharmacological support care [115]. Many investigators [39], however, now believe that chronic alcoholics who cannot maintain abstinence should receive pharmacotherapy to control withdrawal symptoms, thereby reducing the potential for kindling effects [91, 97–104]. A recent widely cited study [116] compared outpatient with inpatient detoxification. The researchers concluded that outpatient medical detoxification is "an effective, safe, and low-cost treatment for patients with mild-to-moderate symptoms of alcohol withdrawal." However, the data from this study indicate that inpatient detoxification was more effective than outpatient detoxification: At the 6-month follow-up those treated as inpatients reported significantly greater improvement in their drinking behavior despite having been measured as more impaired than the outpatient group at the time of admission. This point is not emphasized in the report. Whereas outpatient detoxification may be cheaper for some alcoholics, it is not clear to what extent serious comorbidities, which may be undetected outside a hospital setting, may lead to more severe and costly problems later.

An earlier uncontrolled study [20] reported success with nonpharmacological detoxification in over two-thirds of a group of ambulatory patients in mild withdrawal. The treatment consisted of screening and providing extensive social support. The investigators concluded that social detoxification offers a reduced need for medical staff, a shortened detoxification period, and no sedative interference with a patient's alertness for participating in an alcohol treatment program. In recent controlled studies, minor withdrawal symptoms and signs in 85% of emergency room patients [115] and 60% of inpatients [117] responded to supportive care in less than 6–8 hr. This supportive care included reduced sensory stimuli, maintenance of hydration, reality orientation, reassurance, nutrition, physical support, sleep or rest, and positive encouragement toward long-term rehabilitation. In addition, patient perceptions that staff seemed competent and confident about their detoxification skills are likely to relieve patient anxiety that may otherwise complicate the withdrawal syndrome.

Since supportive care is not effective for hallucinations, seizures, or arrhythmias, and since patient characteristics do not predict responsiveness to supportive care, patients in moderate-to-severe withdrawal should also receive pharmacotherapy.

B. Objective Withdrawal Severity Scales

Since 1973, starting with Gross and colleagues [118], objective quantitative scales for assessing the severity of alcohol withdrawal have been developed based on cluster analysis of subjective symptoms and physiological and behavioral parameters. Examples include the Total Severity Assessment (TSA) and its 11-item subscale called Selected Severity Assessment (SSA) [118], and its further modification referred to as the Clinical Institute Withdrawal Assessment for Alcohol (CIWA-Ar) [119]. The CIWA-Ar has been demonstrated to be a valid, reliable, and sensitive instrument to assess severity of alcohol withdrawal. It consists of nine items: nausea/vomiting, tremor, paroxysmal sweats, anxiety, agitation, tactile, auditory, and visual disturbances, and headache or fullness in the head. Each variable is rated on an 8-point anchored Likert scale (0–7). A tenth item, orientation and clouding of sensorium, is rated 0–4. The higher the score, the greater the severity of the withdrawal syndrome and the risk of seizures, confusion, and hallucinations. CIWA-Ar scores of 9 or less represent minimal or absent withdrawal for which no pharmacotherapy has been shown to be needed, 10–19 represent mild-to-moderate withdrawal, and 20 or more represent severe withdrawal [120]. These scales are helpful when monitoring the adequacy of titrating or loading doses of medications to be discussed below. One of the advantages of this standardized procedure is that the evaluators become aware of the symptoms that make up the alcohol withdrawal syndrome, thereby making it easier to assess and compare the effectiveness of treatments.

Originally developed as research tools for studying treatment efficacy, such scales are now finding clinical use. In this regard, two recent studies are worth noting. In the first, a general hospital study [121] by nursing staff using a modified version of the CIWA concluded that the scale can assist in guiding treatment and predicting patients at risk for severe alcohol withdrawal. They noted, however, that a small group of patients developed complications in spite of having had low scores or having been appropriately treated. In general, they were more seriously ill than other patients, although patients with fractured femur also seemed to be at increased risk. The scale takes approximately 5 min for a registered nurse to administer, and nurses working in all areas of the hospital readily become familiar with it. In the second, a study [122] using the CIWA-Ar scale confirmed the earlier findings on the value of this instrument in managing the alcohol withdrawal syndrome in a general hospital. The study evaluated a nursing staff training program consisting of three 1-hour didactic presentations on the pathophysiology of the alcohol withdrawal syndrome and the principles of treatment, as well as a 30-minute videotape [123] on the use of the CIWA-Ar. In evaluating the impact of this approach, using comparison patient groups before and after training, it was found that whereas 73% of patients were given drug (benzodiazepine) therapy before, only 13% of patients received drug therapy after. On the other hand, after excluding those who received no drug therapy, patients who received benzodiazepine after the training received significantly higher amounts of benzodiazepine than those who received the drug before, with the average number of hours from the first benzodiazepine dose to the last reduced from 13 to 5 hr. All patients were safely and effectively managed with decreasing CIWA-Ar scores at monitoring periods. It was concluded that staff training and use of the CIWA-Ar treatment protocol offer distinct advantages of more flexible and selective drug detoxification using symptom-triggered sedation. Both studies emphasize, however, that withdrawal severity scales should be used to complement, not replace, a thorough clinical evaluation of the patient's medical status.

C. General Measures

In addition to assessment of withdrawal severity, general principles of treatment include stabilization of vital signs and immediate treatment of life-threatening disorders such as status epilepticus and myocardial infarction; diagnosis and treatment of associated disorders; provision of a supportive and calming environment; administration of a cross-tolerant drug to reduce the severity of withdrawal; and prevention of excessive treatment and iatrogenic complications [124]. Unless persistent vomiting or diarrhea is present, frequent offers of oral fluids and not intravenous infusions are recommended [125]. Care must be taken not to overhydrate, especially in patients with head trauma and elevated intracranial pressure. Intravenous fluids may be necessary for patients with recurrent seizures, high fever, and myoglobinuria. The usual patient with severe DTs is dehydrated [28], and inadequate fluid replacement is associated with increased mortality.

Metabolic abnormalities should be corrected. Hypokalemia is seen in two-thirds of patients with DTs and may be associated with ventricular tachyarrhythmias, especially when large amounts of intravenous glucose are given to malnourished patients. Hyponatremia requires therapy only when symptomatic or severe, and must be corrected gradually to prevent precipitation of central pontine myelinolysis [126,127]. Hypomagnesemia is common in acute withdrawal and replacement therapy may help prevent or treat seizures, tremor, and arrhythmias [106]. Parenteral magnesium sulfate, 2 gm every 6 hr, in patients with normal renal function during the first 24 hr of withdrawal is helpful [106]. All patients with acute withdrawal symptoms should receive 100 mg of thiamine parenterally immediately and for the next 2 days. A caveat: Never infuse intravenous glucose prior to thiamine so as not to deplete thiamine reserves and thereby precipitate Wernicke's disease. Deficiencies of folic acid, pyridoxine, and niacin are also common and daily multivitamins should be given for several weeks [128].

D. Pharmacotherapy

The ideal drug for alcohol withdrawal should be cross-tolerant with alcohol, have sedative, anxiolytic, and anticonvulsant activity, have a rapid onset and long duration of action with a wide margin of safety, have a metabolism not dependent on liver function, and have no abuse potential.

Benzodiazepines

Although no drug meets all these requirements, almost all reviews of alcohol withdrawal treatment agree that the benzodiazepines currently offer the most advantages [18,27,113,129, 130], and are now the most commonly used drugs for alcohol detoxification. The selection of the most appropriate benzodiazepine depends on the specific clinical situation. Within this class, one can select a longer-acting or a shorter-acting drug.

Longer-acting agents: loading doses. The most widely studied and utilized benzodiazepines are the longer-acting agents diazepam and chlordiazepoxide, each effective orally or intravenously, but not intramuscularly owing to erratic absorption. Each is biotransformed to long-lived, pharmacologically active metabolites and rapid dosing results in cumulation and prolongation of effects. Diazepam and its metabolite, nordazepam, persist for relatively long periods of time with half-lives of 30–60 hr. This provides the basis for the diazepam loading detoxification procedure which has been shown to be effective [131]. In this protocol, diazepam, 20 mg every 1–2 hr, is administered until symptoms are suppressed (CIWA-Ar less than 10) or the patient becomes sedated but easily arousable. In a double-blind controlled study, patients treated with diazepam loading had a faster and greater improvement than those receiving placebo. Fifty percent responded to 60 mg of oral diazepam within 7.6 hr and most improved in less than 36 hr. More importantly, complications (seizures, hallucinations, arrhythmias) occurred exclusively in those treated with placebo, indicating that delay in therapy may be responsible for the appearance of complications in withdrawal. A recommendation of this study is that when using this procedure all patients should be loaded with at least 60 mg of diazepam. Diazepam has several advantages for treating alcohol withdrawal. Peak blood levels are reached quickly, ensuring that a large amount of the drug is available when the clinical manifestations are more severe. Because of the long half-lives of diazepam and its metabolite, a continued high drug level is maintained, permitting a withdrawal freer of cyclical variations and making additional doses unnecessary when a large enough initial dose has been given. In addition, this reduces the frequency of adverse reactions and tends to decrease drug-seeking behavior in withdrawing alcoholics. A similar regimen is effective by substituting chlordiazepoxide for diazepam. Diazepam is preferred because it is more potent and predictable, more rapidly absorbed orally, and better tolerated intravenously than chlordiazepoxide [132].

Intravenous administration of diazepam or other benzodiazpeines is recommended for patients with agitation, status epilepticus, or severe withdrawal reactions. The most serious side effects of intravenous diazepam are respiratory depression and hypotension, most often seen in patients over 65 years of age who have advanced cardiac, pulmonary, or hepatic disease. In treating alcohol withdrawal seizures, administer diazepam, 5 mg, as an IV push over 2.5 min and repeated every 5–15 min as needed to arrest seizures and to calm the patient. Intravenous diazepam has a short duration of action (15–20 min) due to tissue distribution. Therefore, additional doses are almost always necessary to control repetitive seizures and to maintain a calm state. The total dose necessary is highly variable, but is greatest in patients with DTs. In one controlled study [27] of severe DTs, the initial doses of diazepam that were required for initial calming varied unpredictably from 15 to 215 mg IV and up to 1355 mg total over a 4-day period. Combined drug therapy may be beneficial in these cases by using high potency neuroleptics (see below) for agitation and confusion, and sympatholytic drugs (see below) for autonomic hyperactivity. After the agitation, seizures, and other acute withdrawal symptoms have been controlled, oral diazepam should be given at regular intervals, and tapered gradually.

Since both diazepam and chlordiazepoxide undergo metabolic oxidation by the liver, severe liver disease can increase their half-lives by a factor of two to five [132].

Shorter-acting agents. Shorter-acting benzodiazepines without active metabolites, such as oxazepam or lorazepam, are recommended in patients with liver disease. Since both are glucuronidated, not oxidated by the liver, they may be safely administered in small divided doses. Oxazepam and lorazepam should be administered every 6 hr (oxazepam 15–60 mg, lorazepam 1–3 mg), as they both have shorter half-lives (5–10 and 10–20 hr, respectively);

tapering of either drug should begin on the second day and should be accomplished by decreasing the dose, not by increasing the interval between doses. In the event that patients cannot take oral medication, lorazepam may be preferred, since it is available in a sublingual form or in a parenteral form that is predictably absorbed intramuscularly [133]. Lorazepam has been reported to maintain seizure control longer than diazepam [134,135], and its excretion is less affected by age or renal dysfunction. Oxazepam may be safer for elderly patients because of its relatively short duration of action.

General Aspects.   The benzodiazepines produce similar side effects. Memory impairment is common [132] and may interfere with efforts toward rehabilitation during the first few days of hospitalization. Minor cardiovascular and respiratory depression may occur with high doses, although this is unusual when benzodiazepines are administered alone [132]. The striking advantage of this group of drugs is the remarkable margin of safety. Overdosage with the benzodiazepines is frequent, but serious sequelae are rare unless other drugs or alcohol are taken. Except for an additive effect with other CNS depressants, the benzodiazepines tend to have minimal pharmacokinetic interactions with other drugs, although their oxidative metabolism may be inhibited by cimetidine, disulfiram, isoniazid, and oral contraceptives. Since benzodiazepines have an additive effect with alcohol, it is important to keep in mind that the blood alcohol concentration (BAC) may take 60–90 min to peak after the last drink. Although the patient may require treatment for withdrawal prior to the BAC reaching zero, benzodiazepines should be administered with caution and close monitoring by the physician. There is no evidence supporting long-term use of benzodiazepines in alcoholics after the withdrawal symptoms are controlled. These patients are at greater risk of developing dependence on benzodiazepines and other cross-tolerant sedative hypnotics.

Carbamazepine

Carbamazepine (CBZ) has been used extensively in Scandinavia for the prevention and treatment of the alcohol withdrawal syndrome. Many animal and human studies, including four double-blind controlled clinical trials, have confirmed its effectiveness when compared with barbital, tiapride, and chlormethiazole, agents not available in the United States [130,136]. A recent U.S. double-blind controlled study [137] compared CBZ to oxazepam and concluded that CBZ is as effective and safe as benzodiazepine treatment for alcohol withdrawal. Several reviews [98,138,139] have recommended the use of CBZ to treat alcohol withdrawal states because of its specific antikindling effects in limbic structures. If kindling-like changes in limbic areas are involved with alcohol withdrawal symptoms, as has been hypothesized [39,97,98–104,138], then CBZ may have specific advantages over other agents, especially in patients with multiple attempts at alcohol withdrawal. Also, during withdrawal CBZ is therapeutic for the often-noticed heart arrhythmias [140]. A recent report [141] also recommends its use in benzodiazepine withdrawal; thus, it may be especially valuable in mixed alcohol/benzodiazepine withdrawal states. An advantage of CBZ is that it is not abused as are the benzodiazepines. A disadvantage is that it cannot be administered parenterally.

The multiple Scandinavian studies verify that optimal detoxification effects can be achieved with the following regimen: administration of doses on the first day ranges from 400 to 800 mg (in one study up to 1200 mg; usually 400 mg plus 200 mg administered on day 1). On the following 5–7 days of treatment, 400–600 mg of CBZ is administered. The goal of treatment is to establish therapeutic CBZ serum levels as fast as possible. If 400 mg of elixir is given as the first dose, protection against seizures is usually achieved within 2 hr. The second dose of CBZ on day 1 is usually 200 mg in tablet form. Thereafter, 200 mg of CBZ in tablet form is given twice a day for another 5–7 days. For many years this regimen has been used at most clinics in Scandinavia. Sometimes the daily amount of CBZ administered varies slightly: Doses up to 200 mg three times a day have been given without serious side effects and with effective anticonvulsive activity. With this regimen, CBZ blood levels increase relatively rapidly and may cause mild dose-related side effects, which are mixed with the usual withdrawal symptoms (dizziness, blurred vision, mild ataxia, etc.) and therefore are tolerated by the patient. However, CBZ may occasionally cause some severe side effects, such as hematological or dermatological reactions. In the U.S. study [137] comparing CBZ with oxazepam, CBZ, 200 mg q.i.d., was given for 7 days. The overall side effect profiles for each drug did not differ significantly. Global distress scores of the SCL-90-R indicated significantly less psychological distress for the CBZ group at the end of the study than for the oxazepam group. At this time, additional controlled studies comparing CBZ and benzodiazepines are needed before recommending CBZ use as a routine protocol.

Other Drugs

Barbiturates were frequently administered prior to the advent of benzodiazepines but are no longer routinely recommended because their therapeutic/safety index is too narrow, they cause hepatic enzyme induction, and their abuse potential is high. However, in the pregnant patient in alcohol withdrawal, phenobarbital is preferred to benzodiazepines or CBZ [142].

Paraldehyde exhibits complete cross-tolerance with alcohol and is effective in the treatment of withdrawal [27]. However, it is more toxic than benzodiazepines, parenteral administration is hazardous, it is malodorous, and it presents problems with storage stability [27].

Neuroleptics are not recommended because they do not provide anticonvulsant benefits; in fact, most lower the seizure threshold. They may have an adjunctive benefit in combination with benzodiazepines for the patient in alcohol withdrawal with agitated hallucinosis or delirium. A high-potency neuroleptic, such as haloperidol, in a dose ranging from 0.5 to 2.0 mg IM every 1–2 hr for up to five doses may be given. Usually one or two doses is sufficient to calm the patient [130].

Sympatholytic drugs (beta-adrenergic blockers and alpha$_2$-adrenergic agonists) may have an adjunctive role, but their use as a sole drug in withdrawal treatment is inappropriate, since they provide no protection against severe withdrawal states, such as hallucinations, seizures, or delirium [143]. The beta-blocker atenolol and the alpha$_2$-agonists clonidine and lofexidine attenuate symptoms of autonomic hyperactivity such as diaphoresis, tremor, tachycardia, and hypertension [143–145]. Propranolol has produced psychotoxic reactions when used during alcohol withdrawal [146] and is not recommended as an adjunctive drug.

Phenytoin, when added to treatment protocols, has not reduced the incidence of alcohol withdrawal seizures [147]. A double-blind randomized study revealed that phenytoin is no better than placebo in alcohol withdrawal [148]. Phenytoin and alcohol are not cross-tolerant. Unlike CBZ, it confers no antikindling benefit. Its routine use is not recommended for alcohol withdrawal states unless a preexisting epilepsy is present [149].

Chlormethiazole is widely used in many countries other than the United States and Canada. It is cross-tolerant to alcohol and possesses sedating, anxiolytic, and anticonvulsant activity. However, it has abuse potential and its therapeutic/safety index is lower than benzodiazepines [130].

Valproate, an anticonvulsant prescribed for simple and complex absence seizures, increases GABA levels, can be administered intravenously, and has effectively decreased alcohol withdrawal seizures in animal models, but it has not undergone rigorous clinical trials. It is associated with hepatotoxicity which is not dose related, and is not recommended at this time [136].

E. Summary

Substantial clinical improvement in morbidity and mortality has resulted from advancement in assessment instruments, better understanding of pathophysiological mechanisms, and controlled clinical studies of alcohol withdrawal treatment. Flexible and effective standardized detoxification protocols have been developed and with proper staff training are easily introduced into treatment settings.

V. FUTURE DIRECTIONS

The past 3 decades have been a period of rapid growth of knowledge about the addictions. The greatest excitement is being generated by the basic neuroscientists, who are elucidating fundamental pathophysiological addiction mechanisms at the cellular and molecular levels. In revealing the complexity of the brain-based nature of alcoholism, they have validated the disease concept and rendered moot further debate. The challenge now is to keep pace with and integrate this exponential growth of knowledge through updating our neuroscience literacy. This is a formidable but obligatory task if we are to make further inroads to understanding and preventing the widespread damage from alcoholism and other addictions to our patients and society.

REFERENCES

1. Jellinek, E.M. Classics of the alcohol literature: Magnus Huss' Alcoholismus Chronicus. *Q. J. Stud. Alcohol*, 4:85–92 (1943).
2. Victor, M. Alcohol withdrawal seizures: An overview, *Alcohol and Seizures: Basic Mechanisms and Clinical Concepts* (R. J. Porter et al., eds.), Davis, Philadelphia 1990, pp. 148–161.
3. Bowman, K.M., and Jellinek, E.M.: Alcoholic mental disorders. *Q. J. Stud. Alcohol*, 2:312–390 (1941).
4. Bleuler, E. *Textbook of Psychiatry* (authorized translation by A. A. Brill). Macmillan, New York, 1951, p. 327.
5. Victor, M., and Adams, R.D. The effect of alcohol upon the nervous system. *Res. Publ. Assoc. Res. Nerv. Ment. Dis.*, 32:526–573 (1953).
6. Isbell, H. et al. An experimental study of the etiology of "rum fits" and delirium tremens. *Q. J. Stud. Alcohol, 16*:1–33 (1955).
7. Isbell H. et al. Chronic barbiturate intoxication: An experimental study. *Arch. Neurol. Psychiatry, 64*:1 (1950).
8. Mendelson, J.H., and LaDou, J. Experimentally induced chronic intoxication and withdrawal in alcoholics. *Q. J. Stud. Alcohol*, (Suppl) 2:1–39 (1964).
9. Goldstein, D.B. The alcohol withdrawal syndrome: A view from the laboratory, *Recent Developments in Alcholism* (M. Galanter, ed.), Plenum Press, New York, 1986, pp. 231–240.
10. Emmett-Oglesby, M.W. et al. Animal models of drug withdrawal symptoms. *Psychopharmacology, 101*:292–309 (1990).
11. Koob, G.F., and Bloom, F.E. Cellular and molecular mechanisms of drug dependence. *Science 242*::715–723 (1988).
12. Charness, M.E., Simon, R.P., and Greenberg, D.A. Ethanol and the nervous system. *N. Engl. J. Med., 321*:442–454 (1989).
13. U.S. Department of Health and Human Services. Seventh Special Report to the U.S. Congress on Alcohol and Health. DHHS Pub. No. (ADM)90-1656. Washington, D.C.: Supt. of Docs., U.S. Govt. Print. Off., 1990, pp. 69–105.
14. Riederer, P., and Kopp, N. Pathophysiological aspects of alcoholism, *An Introduction to Neurotransmission in Health and Disease*. (P. Riederer, N. Kopp, and J. Pearson, eds.), Oxford University Press, 1990, pp. 321–331.
15. Moore, R.D., and Malitz, F.E. Underdiagnosis of alcoholism by residents in an ambulatory medical practice. *J. Med. Ed., 61*(1):46–52 (1986).
16. Moore, R. et al. Prevalence, detection, and treatment of alcoholism in hospitalized patients. *J.A.M.A., 261*:403–407 (1989).

17. Jaffe, J.H. Drug addiction and drug abuse, *Goodman and Gilman's The Pharmacological Basis of Therapeutics*, 8th ed. (A.G. Gilman et al., eds.), Pergamon Press, New York, 1990, pp. 522–573.

18. Naranjo, C.A., and Sellers, E.M. Clinical assessment and pharmacotherapy of the alcohol withdrawal syndrome, *Recent Developments in Alcoholism* (M. Galanter, ed.), Plenum Press, New York, 1986, pp. 265–281.

19. Gorelick, D.A., and Wilkins, J.N. Special aspects of human alcohol withdrawal. *Recent Developments in Alcoholism*. (M. Galanter, ed.), Plenum Press, New York, 1986, pp. 283–305.

20. Whitfield, C.L. et al. Detoxification of 1024 alcoholic patients without psychoactive drugs. *J.A.M.A.* *239*:1409–1410 (1978).

21. Victor, M., and Hope, J.M. The phenomenon of auditory hallucinations in chronic alcoholism. *J. Nerv. Ment. Dis.*, *126*:451–458 (1958).

22. Alpert, M., and Silvers, K.N. Perceptual characteristics distinguishing auditory hallucinations in schizophrenic and acute alcoholic psychoses. *Am. J. Psychiatry*, *127*:298–302 (1970).

23. Soyka, M. Psychopathological characteristics in alcohol hallucinosis and paranoid schizophrenia. *Acta. Psychiatr. Scand.*, *81*:255–259 (1990).

24. Victor, M., and Brausch, C. The role of abstinence in the genesis of alcoholic epilepsy. *Epilepsia*, *8*:1–20 (1967).

25. Fuller, R.K., Lee, K.K., and Gordis, E. Validity of self-report in alcoholism research: Results of a Veterans Administration Cooperative Study. *Alcohol.: Clin. Exp. Res.*, *12*:201–205 (1988).

26. Wikler, A et al. Electroencephalographic changes associated with chronic alcoholic intoxication and the alcohol abstinence syndrome. *Am. J. Psychiatry*, *43*:106–114 (1956).

27. Thompson, W.L., Johnson, A.D., and Maddrey, W.L. Diazepam and paraldehyde for treatment of severe delirium tremens: A controlled trial. *Ann. Intern. Med.*, *82*:175–180 (1975).

28. Thompson, W.L. Management of alcohol withdrawal syndromes. *Arch. Intern. Med.*, *138*:278–283 (1978).

29. Basile, A.S., Gammal, S.H., Mullen, K.D. et al. Differential responsiveness of cerebellar Purkinje neurons to GABA and benzodiazepine receptor ligands in an animal model of hepatic encephalopathy. *J. Neurosci.*, *8*:2414–2421 (1988).

30. Basile, A.S., and Gammal, S.H. Evidence for the involvement of the benzodiazepine receptor complex in hepatic encephalopathy. *Clin. Neuropharmacol.*, *11*:401–422 (1988).

31. Linnoila, M., and Martin, P.R. Benzodiazepines and alcoholism, *Benzodiazepines Divided* (M.R. Trimble, ed.), Wiley, New York, 1983, pp. 291–308.

32. Goldstein, D.B., and Goldstein, A. Possible role of enzyme inhibition and repression in drug tolerance and addiction. *Biochem. Pharmacol.*, *8*:48 (1961).

33. Tabakoff, B., and Hoffman, P.L. Biochemical pharmacology of alcohol, *Psychopharmacology: The Third Generation of Progress* (H.Y. Meltzer, ed.), Raven Press, New York 1987, pp. 1521–1526.

34. Sudak, P.D., Glowa, J.R., Crawley, J.N. et al. A selective imidazobenzodiazepine antagonist of ethanol in the rat. *Science*, *234*:1243–1247 (1986).

35. Rommelspacher,H., Damm, H., Strauss, S., et al. Ethanol induces an increase of harmane in the brain and urine of rats. *Naunyn Schmiedebergs Arch. Pharmacol.*, *327*:107–113 (1984).

36. Celentano, J.J., Gibbs, T.T., and Farb, D.H. Ethanol potentiates GABA- and glycine-induced chloride currents in chick spinal cord neurons. *Brain Res.*, *455*:377–380 (1988).

37. Ticku, M.K. Behavioral and functional studies indicate a role for GABAergic transmission in the actions of ethanol. *Alcohol Alcohol.* (Suppl),*1*:657–662 (1987).

38. Allan, A.M., and Harris, R.A. Acute and chronic ethanol treatments alter GABA receptor-operated chloride channels. *Pharmacol. Biochem. Behav.*, *27*:665–670 (1987).

39. Linnoila, M., Mefford, I., Nutt, D., et al. Alcohol withdrawal and noradrenergic function. *Ann. Intern. Med.*, *108*:875–889 (1987).

40. Nutt, D.J., Glue, P. Alpha-2 Adrenoceptor function in alcoholics. *Adv. Alcohol Subst. Abuse*, *7*:43–46 (1988).

41. Smith, A.J., Brent, P.J., Henry, D.A. et al. Plasma noradrenaline, platelet alpha-2-adrenoceptors, and functional scores during ethanol withdrawal. *Alcohol: Clin. Exp. Res.*, *14*:497–502 (1990).

42. George, D.T., Nutt, D.J., Dwyer, B.A., et al. Alcoholism and panic disorder: Is the comorbidity more than coincidence? *Acta. Psychiatr. Scand., 81*:97–107 (1990).

43. Kushner, M.G., Sher, K.J., and Beitman, B.D. The relation between alcohol problems and the anxiety disorders. *Am. J. Psychiatry,147*:685–695 (1990).

44. Choi, D.W. Glutamate neurotoxicity and diseases of the nervous system. *Neuron, 1*:623–634 (1988).

45. Watkins, J.C. The NMDA receptor concept: origins and development, *The NMDA Receptor* (J.C. Watkins and G.L. Collingridge, eds.), IRL Press, Oxford, England, 1989, pp. 1–17.

46. Lovinger, D.M., White, G., and Weight, F.F. Ethanol inhibits NMDA-activated ion currents in hippocampal neurons. *Science, 243*:1721–1724 (1989).

47. Hoffman, P.L., Rabe, C.S., Moses, F. et al. N-Methyl-D-aspartate receptors and ethanol: Inhibition of calcium flux and cyclic GMP production. *J. Neurochem., 52*:1937–1940 (1989).

48. Rabe, C.S., and Tabakoff, B. Glycine site-directed agonists reverse the actions of ethanol at the N-methyl-D-aspartate receptor. *Mol. Pharmacol. 38*:753–757 (1990).

49. Grant, K.A., and Tabakoff, B. Ethanol withdrawal seizures and the NMDA receptor complex. *Eur. J. Pharmacol., 176*:289–296 (1990).

50. Williams, K., Dawson, V.L., Romano, C., et al. Characterization of polyamines having agonist, antagonist, and inverse agonist effects at the polyamine recognition site of the NMDA receptor. *Neuron, 5*:199–208 (1990).

51. Dolin, S.J. et al. Increased dihydropyridine-sensitive calcium channels in rat brain may underlie ethanol physical dependence. *Neuropharmacology, 26*:275–279 (1987).

52. Littleton, J.M. Calcium channel activity in alcohol dependency and withdrawal seizures, *Alcohol and Seizures: Basic Mechanisms and Clinical Concepts* (R.J. Porter, R.H. Mattson, J.A. Cramer et al., eds.), Davis, Philadelphia, 1990, pp. 51–59.

53. Carlen, P., Rougier-Naquet, I., and Reynolds, J.N. Alterations of neuronal calcium and potassium currents during alcohol administration and withdrawal, *Alcohol and Seizures: Basic Mechanisms and Clinical Concepts*. (R.J. Porter, R. H. Mattson, J.A. Cramer, et al., eds.), Davis, Philadelphia, 1990, pp. 68–78.

54. Nagy, L.E., Diamond, I., and Gordon,A. Cultured lymphocytes from alcoholic subjects have altered cAMP signal transduction. *Proc. Natl. Acad. Sci. U.S.A., 85*:6973–6976 (1988).

55. Diamond, I., Wrubel, B., Estrin, W., et al. Basal and adenosine receptor stimulated levels of cAMP are reduced in lymphocytes from alcoholic patients. *Proc. Natl. Acad. Sci. U.S.A. 84*:1413–1416(1987).

56. Tabakoff, B., Hoffman, P.L., Lee J.M. et al. Differences in platelet enzyme activity between alcoholics and nonalcoholics. *N. Engl. J. Med. 318*:134–139 (1988).

57. Stadel, J.M. deLean, A., and Lefkowtiz, R.J. Molecular mechanisms of coupling in hormone receptor-adenylate cyclase systems. *Adv. Enzymol., 53*:1–43 (1982).

58. Mochly-Rosen, D., Chang, F.H., Cheever, L. et al. Chronic ethanol causes heterologous desensitization of receptors by reducing alpha$_s$ messenger RNA. *Nature, 333*:848–850 (1988).

59. Nagy, L.E., Diamond, I., Collier, K. et al. Adenosine is required for ethanol-induced heterologous desensitization. *Mol. Pharmacol., 36*:744–748 (1989).

60. Diamond, I., Mochly-Rosen, D., and Gordon, A.S. Reduced adenosine receptor activation in alcoholism: Implications for alcohol withdrawal seizures, *Alcohol and Seizures: Basic Mechanisms and Clinical Concepts* (R.J. Porter, R.H. Mattson, J.A. Cramer et al., eds.), Davis, Philadelphia, 1990, pp. 79–86.

61. Meyer, K.H. Contributions to the theory of narcosis. *Trans. Faraday Soc., 33*:1062–1068 (1937).

62. Chin, J.H., and Goldstein, D.B. Drug tolerance in biomembranes: A spin label study of the effects of ethanol. *Science, 196*:684–685 (1976).

63. Goldstein, D.B. Ethanol-induced adaptation in biological membranes. *Ann. N.Y. Acad. Sci., 492*:103–111 (1987).

64. Alling, C. The effects of alcohol on lipids in neuronal membranes, *Alcohol and Seizures: Basic Mechanisms and Clinical Concepts*. (R.J. Porter, R.H. Mattson, J.A. Cramer et al., eds.), Davis, Philadelphia, 1990, pp. 44–50.

65. Harris, R.A., Groh, G.I., Baxter, D.M. et al. Gangliosides enhance the membrane actions of ethanol and pentobarbital. *Mol. Pharmacol., 25*:410–417 (1984).

66. Toffano, G., Dal Toso, R., Facci L. et al. Gangliosides as modulators of neuronotropic interactions, *Receptor-Receptor Interactions: A new Intramembrane Integrative Mechanism* (K. Fuxe and L. F. Agnati, eds.), Plenum Press, New York 1987, pp. 54–61.

67. Hakomori, S. Bifunctional role of glycosphingolipids: Modulators for transmembrane signaling and mediators for cellular interactions. *J. Biol. Chem., 265*:18713–18716 (1990).

68. Miller, K.W., Firestone, L.L., and Forman, S.A. General anesthetic and specific effects of ethanol on acetylcholine receptors. *Ann. N.Y. Acad. Sci., 492*:71–87 (1987).

69. Facci, L., Leon, A., and Skaper, S.D. Excitatory amino acid neurotoxicity in cultured retinal neurons: Involvement of N-methyl-D-aspartate (NMDA) and non-NMDA receptors and effect of ganglioside GM1. *J. Neurosci. Res., 27*:202–210 (1990).

70. Facci, L., Leon, A., and Skaper, S.D. Hypoglycemic neurotoxicity in vitro: Involvement of excitatory amino acid receptors and attenuation by monosialoganglioside GM1. *Neuroscience, 37*:709–716 (1990).

71. Cuello, A.C., Maysinger, D., Garofalo, L. et al. Influence of gangliosides and nerve growth factor on the plasticity of forebrain cholinergic neurons, *Receptor-Receptor Interactions: A New Intramembrane Integrative Mechanism*. (K. Fuxe and L.F. Agnati, eds.), Plenum Press, New York, 1987, pp. 62–77.

72. Cuello, A.C., Garofalo, L. Kenigsberg, R.L. et al. Gangliosides potentiate in vivo and in vitro effects of nerve growth factor on central cholinergic neurons. *Proc. Natl. Acad. Sci. U.S.A., 86*:2056–2060 (1989).

73. Grant, I., Adams, K.M., and Reed, R. Intermediate duration (subacute) organic mental disorders of alcoholism, *Neuropsychiatric Correlates of Alcoholism*. (I. Grant, ed.), American Psychiatric Press Inc., Washington, D.C. pp. 38–59, 1986.

74. Tarter, R.E., and Alterman, A.I. Neuropsychological deficits in alcoholics: Etiological considerations. *J. Stud. Alcohol., 45*:1–9 (1984).

75. Freund, G., and Ballinger, W.E. Loss of cholinergic muscarinic receptors in the frontal cortex of alcohol abusers. *Alcoholism Clin. Exp. Res., 12*:630–638 (1988).

76. Janowsky, D.S., Risch, S.C., Irwin, M. et al. Behavioral hyporeactivity to physostigmine in detoxified primary alcoholics. *Am. J. Psychiatry, 146*:538–539 (1989).

77. Wilkins, J.N., and Gorelick, D.A. Clinical neuroendocrinology and neuropharmacology of alcohol withdrawal, *Recent Developments in Alcoholism*. (M. Galanter, ed.), Plenum Press, New York, 1986, pp. 241–263.

78. Mendelson, J.H., and Stein, S. Serum cortisol levels in alcoholics and nonalcoholic subjects during experimentally induced ethanol intoxication. *Psychosom Med, 28*:616–626 (1966).

79. Stokes, P.E. Adrenocortical activation in alcoholics during chronic drinking period. *Ann. N.Y. Acad. Sci., 215*:77–83 (1973).

80. Risher-Flowers, D., Adinoff, B., Ravitz, B. et al. Circadian rhythms of cortisol, during alcohol withdrawal. *Adv. Alcohol. Subst. Abuse*, 7:37–41 (1988).

81. Valimaki, M., Pelkonen, R., Harkonen, M. et al. Hormonal changes in noncirrhotic male alcoholics during ethanol withdrawal. *Alcohol Alcohol., 19*:235–242 (1984).

82. Targum, S.D., Wheadon, D.E., Chastek, C.T. et al. Dysregulation of hypothalamic-pituitary-adrenal axis function in depressed alcoholic patients. *J. Affect Disorders*, 4:347–353 (1982).

83. Feldman, D. Mechanism of action of cortisol, *Endocrinology*, (L. J. DeGroot, G.M. Besser, G. H. Cahill et al., eds.), 2nd ed. Vol. 2, Saunders, Philadelphia, 1989, pp. 557–571.

84. Van Thiel, D.H., Gavaler, J.S., and Cobb, C.F. Pseudo-Cushing syndrome and alcohol abuse, *Ethanol Tolerance and Dependence: Endocrinological Aspects*. NIAAA: ADAMHA Rockville, Maryland, U.S. Dept. of Health and Human Services, Public Health Services Monograph 13, 1983, pp. 117–126.

85. Smals, A.G., Kopppenborg, P.W. Njo, K.T. et al. Alcohol-induced Cushingoid syndrome. *Br. J. Med.*, 2:1298 (1976).

86. Haskett, R.F. Diagnostic categorization of psychiatric disturbance in Cushing's syndrome. *Am. J. Psychiatry, 142*:911–921 (1985).

87. Chrousos, G.P., Vingerhoeds, A., Brandon, D. et al. Primary cortisol resistance in man. *J. Clin. Invest., 69*:1261–1269 (1982).

88. Biegon, A. Effects of steroid hormones on the serotonergic system. *Ann. N.Y. Acad. Sci.*, *600*:427–434 (1990).

89. Mitchell, J.B. Rowe, W., Boksa, P. et al. Serotonin regulates type II corticosteroid receptor binding in hippocampal cell cultures. *J. Neurosci.*, *10*:1745–1752 (1990).

90. Stapleton, J.M., Eckardt, M.J., Martin, P. et al. Treatment of alcoholic organic brain syndrome with the serotonin reuptake inhibitor fluvoxamine: A preliminary study. *Adv. Alcohol. Subst. Abuse*, *7*:47–51 (1988).

91. Adinoff, B., Martin, P.R. Bone, G.H.A. et al. Hypothalamic-pituitary-adrenal axis functioning and cerebrospinal fluid corticotropin releasing hormone and corticotropin levels in alcoholics after recent and long-term abstinence. *Arch. Gen. Psychiatry*,*47*:325–330 (1990).

92. de Kloet, E.R. Adrenal steroids as modulators of nerve cell function. *J. Steroid Biochem.*, *20*:175–181 (1984).

93. Sapolsky, R.M., Krey, L.C. and McEwen, B.S. The neuroendocrinology of stress and aging: the glucocorticoid cascade hypothesis. *Endocrinol. Rev.* 7:284–301 (1986).

94. Sapolsky, R.M., Uno, H., Rebert, C.S. et al. Hippocampal damage associated with prolonged glucocorticoid exposure in primates. *J. Neurosci.*, *10*:2897–2902 (1990).

95. Packan, D.R., and Sapolsky, R.M. Glucocorticoid endangerment of the hippocampus: Tissue, steroid and receptor specificity. *Neuroendocrinology*, *51*:613–618 (1990).

96. Goddard, G.V. The development of epileptic seizures through brain stimulation at low intensity. *Nature*,*214*:1020–1021 (1967).

97. Ballenger, J.C., and Post, R.M. Kindling as a model for alcohol withdrawal syndromes. *Br. J. Psychiatry*, *133*:1–14 (1978).

98. Pinel, J.P.J. Alcohol withdrawal seizures: implications of kindling. *Pharmacol. Biochem. Behav.* *13*:225–231 (1980).

99. Carrington, C.D., Ellinwood, E.H., and Krishnan, R.R.: Effects of single and repeated alcohol withdrawal on kindling. *Biol. Psychiatry*, *19*:525–537 (1984).

100. Brown, M.E. Anton, R.F., Malcolm, R. et al. Alcohol detoxification and withdrawal seizures: Clinical support for a kindling hypothesis. *Biol. Psychiatry*, *23*:507–514 (1988).

101. Syapin, P.F., and Alkana, R.L. Chronic ethanol exposure increases peripheral-type benzodiazepine receptors in brain. *Eur. J. Pharmacol.*, *147*:101–109 (1988).

102. Maier, D.M., and Pohorecky, L.A. The effect of repeated withdrawal episodes on subsequent withdrawal severity in ethanol-treated rats. *Alcohol Depend.* 23:103–110 (1989).

103. McCown, T.J., and Breese, G.R. Multiple withdrawals from chronic ethanol "kindles" inferior collicular seizure activity: Evidence for kindling of seizures associated with alcoholism. *Alcohol: Clin. Exp. Res.*, *14*:394–399 (1990).

104. Lechtenberg, R., and Worner, T.M., Seizure risk with recurrent alcohol detoxification. *Arch. Neurol.*, *47*:535–538 (1990).

105. Pitts, T.O., and Van Thiel, D.H. Disorders of divalent ions and vitamin D metabolism in chronic alcoholism, *Recent Developments in Alcoholism*. Vol. 4 (M. Galanter, ed.), Plenum Press, New York, 1986, pp. 364–367.

106. Wolfe, S.M., and Victor, M. The physiological basis of the alcohol withdrawal syndrome, *Recent Advances in Studies in Alcoholism*. (N.K. Mello and J.H. Mendelson, eds.), U.S. Government Printing Office, Washington, D.C. 1971, p. 188.

107. Vink, R., McIntosh, T.K., and Faden, A.I. Magnesium in central nervous system trauma, *Neuroscience Year* (G. Adelman, ed.), Supplement 1 to the Encyclopedia of Neuroscience. Birkhauser, Boston, 1989, pp. 93–94.

108. Lodge, D., Jones, M., and Fletcher, E. Non-competitive antagonists of N-methyl-D-aspartate, *The NMDA Receptor* (J.C. Watkins and G.L. Collingridge, eds.), IRL Press, Oxford, England, 1989, pp. 38–39.

109. Sacaan, A.I., and Johnson, K.M., Competitive inhibition of magnesium-induced [^{3}H]N-(1-[Thienyl]cyclohexyl)piperidine binding by arcaine: Evidence for a shared spermidine-magnesium binding site. *Mol. Pharmacol.*, *38*:705–710 (1990).

110. Premont, R.T., and Iyengar, R. Adenylyl cyclase and its regulation by G$_s$, *G Proteins* (R. Iyengar and L. Birnbaumer, eds.), Academic Press, San Diego, 1990, pp. 147–78.

111. Fillenz, M. *Noradrenergic Neurons*. Cambridge University Press, Cambridge, England 1990, pp. 61–65.
112. Naranjo, C.A., and Sellers, E.M. Clinical assessment and pharmacotherapy of the alcohol withdrawal syndrome, *Recent Developments in Alcoholism* (M. Galanter, ed.), Plenum Press, New York, 1986, pp. 265–281.
113. Moskowitz, G., Chaimers, T.C. Sacks, H.S. et al. Deficiencies of clinical trials of alcohol withdrawal. *Alcohol: Clin. Exp. Res., 7*:42–46 (1983).
114. Gallant, D.M. How can alcoholism treatment be improved? *Alcohol Health & Research World, 13*:328–333 (1990).
115. Naranjo, C.A., Sellers, E.M., Harrison, M., et al. Nonpharmacologic interventions in the treatment of acute alcohol withdrawal. *Clin. Pharmacol. Ther., 34*:214–219 (1983).
116. Hayashida, M., Alterman, A.I., McLellan, A.T. et al. Comparative effectiveness and costs of inpatient and outpatient detoxification of patients with mild-to-moderate alcohol withdrawal syndrome. *N. Engl. J. Med., 320*:358–365 (1989).
117. Sellers, E.M., Naranjo, C.A., Harrison, M. et al. Oral diazepam loading: Simplified treatment of alcohol withdrawal. *Clin. Pharmacol. Ther., 34*:822–826 (1983).
118. Gross, M.M., Lewis, E., and Nagarajan, M. An improved quantitation system for assessing the acute alcoholic psychoses and related states (TSA and SSA), *Advances in Experimental Medicine and Biology*. Vol. 35. Alcohol Intoxication and Withdrawal: Experimental Studies (M.M. Gross, ed.)., Plenum Press, New York, 1973, pp. 365–376.
119. Shaw, J.M., Kolesar, G.S., Sellers, E.M. et al. Development of optimal treatment tactics for alcohol withdrawal. I. Assessment and effectiveness of supportive care. *J. Clin. Psychopharmacol., 1*:383–387 (1981).
120. Sellers, E.M., and Kalant, H. Alcohol withdrawal and delirium tremens, *Encyclopedic Handbook of Alcoholism* (E.M. Pattison and E. Kaufman, eds.), Gardner Press, New York, 1982, pp.147–166.
121. Foy, A., March, S.M., and Drinkwater, V. Use of an objective clinical scale in the assessment and management of alcohol withdrawal in a large general hospital. *Alcohol: Clin. Exp. Res., 12*:360–364 (1988).
122. Wartenberg, A.A., Nirenberg, T.D., Liepman, M.R. et al. Detoxification of alcoholics: Improving care by symptom-triggered sedation. *Alcohol: Clin. Exp. Res., 14*:71–75 (1990).
123. *Alcohol Withdrawal Syndrome: Introduction, Assessment and Treatment*. Addiction Research Foundation, Toronto, 1986.
124. Morris, J.C.,and Victor, M. Alcohol withdrawal seizures. *Emerg. Med. Clin. North Am., 5*:827–839 (1987).
125. Mander, A.J., Young, A. Merrick, M.V. et al. Fluid balance, vasopressin and withdrawal symptoms during detoxification from alcohol. *Drug and Alcohol Depend. 24*:233–237 (1989).
126. Norenberg, M.D., Leslie, K.O., and Robertson, A.S. Association between rise in serum sodium and central pontine myelinolysis. *Ann. Neurol., 11*:128–135 (1982).
127. Ayus, J.C. Krothapalli, R.K. and Arieff, A.I.: Treatment of symptomatic hyponatremia and its relation to brain damage: A prospective study. *N. Engl. J. Med., 317*:1190–1195 (1987).
128. Morgan, M.Y. Alcohol and nutrition. *Br. Med. Bull., 38*:21–29 (1982).
129. Nutt, D., Adinoff, B., and Linnoila, M. Benzodiazepines in the treatment of alcoholism, *Recent Developments in Alcoholism* (M. Galanter, ed.) Plenum Press, New York 1989, pp. 283–313.
130. Guthrie, S.K. The treatment of alcohol withdrawal. *Pharmacotherapy, 9*:131–143 (1989).
131. Sellers, E.M., Naranjo, C.A., Harrison, M. et al. Oral diazepam loading: Simplified treatment of alcohol withdrawal. *Clin. Pharmacol. Ther., 34*:822–826 (1983).
132. Rall, T.W. Hypnotics and sedatives; ethanol, *Goodman and Gilman's The Pharmacological Basis of Therapeutics*. 8th ed. (A.G. Gilman et al., eds.), Pegamon Press, New York, 1990, pp. 345–382.
133. Greenblatt, D.J. et al. Clinical pharmacokinetics of the newer benzodiazepines. *Clin. Pharmacokinet., 8*:233–252 (1983).
134. Walker, J.E., Homan, R.W., Vasko, R.M. et al. Lorazepam in status epilepticus. *Ann. Neurol., 6*:207–213 (1979).

135. Crawford, T.O., Mitchell, W.G., and Snodgrass, S.R. Lorazepam in childhood status epilepticus and serial seizures: Effectiveness and tachyphylaxis. *Neurology, 37*:190–195 (1987).

136. Sternebring, B. Treatment of alcohol withdrawal seizures with carbamazepine and valproate, *Alcohol and Seizures: Basic Mechanisms and Clinical Concepts* (R.J. Porter, R.H. Mattson, J.A. Cramer et al., eds.), Davis, Philadelphia, 1990, pp. 315–320.

137. Malcolm, R. Ballenger, J.C., Sturgic, E.T. et al. Double-blind controlled trial comparing carbamazepine to oxazepam treatment of alcohol withdrawal. *Am. J. Psychiatry, 146*:617–621 (1989).

138. Ballenger, J.C., and Post, R.M. Carbamazepine in alcohol withdrawal syndromes and schizophrenic psychosis. *Psychopharmacol. Bull., 20*:572–584 (1984).

139. Butler, D., and Messiha, F: Alcohol withdrawal and carbamazepine. *Alcohol, 3*:113–129 (1986).

140. Corday, E. et al. Antiarrhythmic properties of carbamazepine. *Geriatrics, 26*:78–81 (1971).

141. Ries, R, Roy-Byrne, P., Ward, N. et al. Carbamazepine treatment for benzodiazepine withdrawal. *Am. J. Psychiatry,146*:536–537 (1989).

142. Aminoff, M. Maternal neurologic disorders, *Maternal-Fetal Medicine* (R. Creasy and R. Resnik, eds.), Saunders, Philadelphia, 1984, pp.1005–1010.

143. Robinson, B.J., Robinson, G.M. Maling, T.J.B. et al. Is clonidine useful in the treatment of alcohol withdrawal? *Alcohol: Clin. Exp. Res., 13*:95–98 (1989).

144. Kraus, M., Gottlieb, L., Horwitz, R. et al. Randomized clinical trial of atenolol in patients with alcohol withdrawal. *N. Engl. J. Med., 313*:905–909 (1985).

145. Cushman, P. Forbes, R., Lerner, W. et al: Alcohol withdrawal syndromes: Clinical management with lofexidine. *Alcohol: Clin. Exp. Res., 9*:103–108 (1985).

146. Bogin, T.M., Nostrant, T.T., and Young, M.I.: Propranolol for the treatment of the alcoholic hangover. *Am. J. Drug Alcohol Abuse, 13*:175–180 (1987).

147. Simon, R.P. Alcohol and seizures. *N. Engl. J. Med., 319*:715–716 (1988).

148. Alldredge, B.K., Lowenstein, D.H., and Simon, R.P. A placebo-controlled trial of intravenous diphenylhydantoin for the short-term treatment of alcohol withdrawal seizures. *Am. J. Med., 87*:645–648 (1989).

149. Alldredge, B.K., and Simon, R.P. Treatment of alcohol withdrawal seizures with phenytoin, *Alcohol and Seizures: Basic Mechanisms and Clinical Concepts*, (R.J. Porter, R.H. Mattson, J.A. Cramer, et al., eds), Davis, Philadelphia, pp. 290–297 (1990).

60

Update on Methadone Maintenance

George E. Woody and Charles P. O'Brien
Philadelphia Veterans Affairs Medical Center, and University of Pennsylvania, Philadelphia, Pennsylvania

I. INTRODUCTION

Narcotic substitution therapy, of which methadone maintenance is the most prominent example, was first introduced by Dole and Nyswander (1965). Methadone very quickly came into wide use for the treatment of opioid dependence and it has continued to be one of the most commonly used treatments. Much additional investigative work has been done since methadone maintenance began, and this work has been conducted in diverse areas. These include evaluation of treatment outcome; descriptive studies of the behavioral and psychiatric disorders seen in methadone-maintained addicts; evaluation of ancillary treatments that may improve outcome, particularly those treatments that affect the psychiatric disorders of methadone-maintained patients; development of instruments to measure the spectrum of problems seen in opioid addicts; studies of the value of matching specific types of patients to specific ancillary treatments; testing the efficacy of maintenance drugs other than methadone; reviewing the outcome of patients treated with high versus low methadone doses; studying various methods of methadone detoxification; and evaluating the effects of opioid dependence and methadone treatment in neonates.

Most of this work has been aimed at evaluation and refinement of the original concept and technique of narcotic substitution therapy. This chapter will briefly describe work that has been done in each of these areas.

II. EVALUATION OF OUTCOME

A number of large-scale studies have been conducted to reexamine the original positive findings regarding the efficacy of methadone maintenance. Maintenance treatment for opioid dependence has always been controversial, with both proponents and critics. Part of this ambivalence may be inherent within the maintenance concept itself, which substitutes a legally prescribed narcotic for an illicitly obtained and self-administered one. By doing so, one chooses to deliver a treatment that maintains, rather than discontinues, the problematic narcotic use. This approach differs from that seen in many other areas of medicine in which immediate attempts are made to do something to reverse the underlying symptoms of the disease, such as the surgical removal of an inflamed appendix. The rationale for the maintenance approach has been that if narcotic substitution is delivered with proper controls and appropriate supportive services, the addict or patient will do better than he or she would have done if maintenance treatment had not been used. It is important to note that methadone treatment programs have developed in environments in which illicit opiates or opioids are easily available. Opioid addicts who are not on methadone generally have little difficulty obtaining narcotics, provided they can pay for them. The methadone programs claim to provide a positive alternative for addicts within this type of environment. One of the major accomplishments over the last several years has been to reexamine this basic concept.

The most systematic and comprehensive reexamination is found in a review that was carried out recently by the National Institute of Drug Abuse (NIDA). This agency sponsored a series of meetings that summarized and critiqued many aspects of methadone treatment, including outcome (Cooper et al., 1983). Several large-scale studies were available for inclusions in this review, particularly those of Sells (1979) and McLellan et al. (1982). These studies were supportive of the initial positive findings of Dole and Nyswander (1965), which were that methadone-treated patients showed significant gains when compared with addicts not in treatment. These gains were seen in reductions of illicit drug use, reductions in crime, and increased rates of employment. Substantial reductions in criminal activity by maintenance patients was further documented by the findings of Ball et al. (1983), who studied treated and untreated addicts in Baltimore and Philadelphia. Addicts who were in methadone treatment reported significant reductions in criminal activity compared with those reported during comparable time periods prior to treatment. Comprehensive arrest, penal, hospital, and other institutional data were also available to verify the interview reports.

All these studies are somewhat "soft" in that many rely on historical controls or on patient self-reports. Independent measures such as police records, urine test results, or documentation of employment are available in some studies (Ball et al., 1983) but not in others. We know of only two studies that were prospective and used random assignment. The first (Dole et al., 1969) was weakened somewhat by the use of a relatively narrow (but important) range of outcome measures (relapse, employment, and crime) and by the lack of description of psychosocial treatments that were (or were not) available to the control (nonmethadone) group. However, the results of this prospective study were overwhelmingly in favor of the methadone group (Dole et al., 1969). A second controlled prospective study took place in Hong Kong (Newman and Whitehill, 1979). One hundred heroin addicted volunteers were randomly assigned to either methadone or placebo. All received a broad range of supportive services. After 32 weeks, only 10% of the controls remained in treatment, whereas 76% of the methadone group continued. The rate of convictions for criminal activity was more than twice as great in the control patients. The impressive thing about these studies is that they *all* found that methadone treatment was effective. Thus, we cannot escape concluding that a substantial amount of data are now available that indicate that methadone maintenance is an effective treatment when administered to patients who are chronic narcotic addicts, who are actively addicted, and who are living in an environment in which narcotics are readily available. No evidence is available that maintenance is a steppingstone toward permanent discontinuation of narcotic addiction, however. Rather than curing addiction, methadone maintenance appears to provide control over its adverse personal and social consequences. No work is available that measures the level of physiological dependence on opioids prior to methadone treatment and then relates this to dose and outcome. Methadone treatment outcome data derive from approved programs that are periodically inspected for compliance with the U.S. Food and Drug Administration (FDA) requirements for maintenance treatment. The FDA mandates current physiological dependence plus other characteristics that signify long-term addiction, but the regulations do not define criteria that quantify degrees of dependence. The only study even remotely evaluating outcome as it relates to degrees of physiological dependence is that of McLellan et al. (1983), who showed that the amount of drugs used and the length of the drug dependence did not relate to treatment outcome. Thus, information on this point is very sketchy, but the limited data available point to features other than levels of physiological dependence as major determinants of outcome.

III. BEHAVIORAL AND PSYCHIATRIC DISORDERS OF ADDICTS

Another area that was studied and reviewed is that concerning the psychiatric and behavioral problems seen in opiate addicts, both while in and out of treatment. Both medical and lay personnel have noted that opioid addicts often display serious behavioral and psychiatric problems. The successful management of these problems is of great importance to both the addict and the community. Failure on the part of a treatment program to successfully control their patients' behavioral disorders has sometimes resulted in community pressure to close the program, and in some cases this pressure has achieved its intended result. An inability to treat the psychiatric disorders of the addict or patient has contributed to poor treatment response and sometimes premature termination from therapy.

A. Behavioral Disorders

A second NIDA review (Grabowski et al., 1984) described some of the behavioral problems demonstrated by addicts and ways to manage them. Most participants in this review felt that many of these problems originate from drug-seeking behavior that is, of course, a characteristic of the addiction syndrome. Such problems include fabricating stories to obtain controlled substances, buying or selling illicit drugs, attempting to falsify urine samples to avoid loss of take-home methadone doses, or attempting to divert methadone at the pharmacy window.

A serious problem reported by many programs was loitering. The most common motive for loitering appeared to be social contact, but a considerable amount of drug dealing was also observed to take place (Hunt et al., 1984). Persistent loitering was felt to serve as a nidus for the development of other behavioral problems such as arguments or fights. Loitering was also noted to be frightening to people who happened to be in the vicinity of the program and who were not familiar with the personalities and lifestyles of addicts. Threats, disruptive behavior, fighting, or even carrying weapons were reported occasionally. These problems were thought to be related to the addiction itself, to personality disorders or other psychiatric problems, or to socioenvironmental circumstances. Participants in the NIDA conference (Grabowski et al., 1984), which reviewed these problems, were in reasonably good agreement in feeling that a combination of support and structure involving specified rules that include suspension of those who display serious behavioral problems was essential for effective control of these disorders.

B. Psychiatric Disorders

A number of studies were reviewed that described the types of psychiatric problems seen in opiate addicts. These studies found that almost every psychiatric illness that can occur in nonaddicts also occurs in addicts. The most thorough evaluation of psychiatric disorders in addicts was that done by Rounsaville et al. (1982b). A sample of 533 opiate addicts was given a thorough and careful psychiatric evaluation as part of a comprehensive diagnostic study. Depression was the most commonly diagnosed illness among addicts, with about 60% of the sample having had some form of depression at least once. The next most common problem was alcoholism, followed by antisocial personality disorder and anxiety disorders. Occurring with a much lower frequency were schizophrenia, other types of personality disorders, mania, and hypomania. Eighty-five percent of the patient sample were found to have had a psychiatric disorder in addition to opiate dependence at some time in their lives. Not included in this study but also seen regularly are acute situational reactions that involve intense but transient feelings of anger, anxiety, or depression; psychiatric disorders complicated by medical conditions such as hepatitis; and illnesses or injuries that produce chronic pain such as pancreatitis, sickle cell anemia, or trauma resulting in nerve root irritation. Rounsaville et al. (1982b) also studied untreated addicts and found them to have types of psychiatric illnesses similar to patients who were in treatment and in relatively similar proportions. The major difference between treated and nontreated addicts was that the latter group was less likely to have a current psychiatric illness. This finding can be interpreted as indicating that concurrent psychiatric illness serves as a motivator to seek treatment.

C. Depression

Special attention was given to depression, which was found to be the most commonly diagnosed psychiatric disorder in opiate addicts. The course of the depression seen in methadone-maintained patients was also studied by Rounsaville et al. (1982a). It was found that a substantial reduction in symptoms of depression occurred within the first month of methadone treatment. However, the amount of depression that remained, even after this initial improvement, was substantially greater than that observed in nonaddicted controls. These researchers also found that the depressions seen, although usually diagnosed as major depressive disorder, were of mild to moderate intensity and were usually not of the severely retarded or psychotic levels that are commonly seen on psychiatric inpatient units. Another finding that emerged from this study was that those addicts who remained depressed beyond the initial 1-month period usually improved within 6 months, even without specific antidepressant treatment. It was also found that some patients who were not initially depressed at program intake became depressed at some later point.

These findings, when taken together, painted the following picture of the depressions experienced by addicts: (1) they usually fit the criteria for major depressive disorder, although other types of depression are also seen; (2) they are very common at program intake but often improve within the first month of treatment; (3) they are of mild to moderate intensity; (4) they usually improve without specific antidepressant treatment; however, recovery may take 4–6 months or longer; (5) they tend to recur; and (6) they are often precipitated by situational factors such as the loss of important relationships, arrest, or job difficulties.

IV. TREATMENTS FOR ADDICTS WITH PSYCHIATRIC DISORDERS

Studies were also conducted that examined the efficacy of treatments for methadone-maintained addicts who have specific psychiatric disorders, such as depression. These studies included examinations of pharmacotherapy and psychotherapy.

A. Tricyclic Antidepressants

Four controlled studies have provided evidence that doxepin is an effective drug for methadone-maintained addicts who are clinically depressed (McBride et al., 1982; Titievsky et al., 1982;

Woody et al. 1975, 1982). Doxepin was found to reduce the signs and symptoms of depression more quickly than occurred when the depression was not treated by specific antidepressant medication. The benefits seen appeared to be similar to those obtained with doxepin in depressed patients who are not addicts in that it accelerated the usual course of recovery.

Few other antidepressants have been studied; however, the less-sedating tricyclics desipramine and imipramine have been tried and they do not appear to be generally useful (Kleber et al., 1983; Woody et al., 1982). Thus, the mechanism for the improvement seen with doxepin may relate to its antianxiety properties as much as its antidepressant effects. However, practically speaking, doxepin has been found to be a useful adjunctive therapy for the more refractory depressions seen in methadone-maintained addicts. These depressions are those that have endogenous signs and symptoms such as anorexia, insomnia, psychomotor retardation or agitation, and suicidal thoughts. Beck Depression Inventory (Beck, 1972) scores would be in the range of 15–20 or more, and patients tried on a tricyclic would be those who have not responded to counseling or other psychological treatments.

The treatment recommendation that emerges from the studies of depressive illness and of doxepin as an antidepressant treatment is as follows: Many of the depressions seen in addicts are transitory and are best left to improve without additional antidepressant therapy. However, those depressions that last longer than 2–4 weeks may be improved upon by adding doxepin, imipramine, or desipraine have been studied in these patients. Tricyclics other than doxepin may work. Amitriptyline has been observed to be abused by methadone-maintained addicts, in the same manner as diazepam, and should be used with great caution or not at all (Cohen et al., 1978). We are not aware of reports describing abuse of doxepin, and we have not seen it clinically.

B. Psychotherapy

Other work studied the efficacy of professional psychotherapy with nonpsychotic addicts when added to routine counseling services in a methadone program. Two major studies were completed in this area and their results varied. One showed no difference in outcome when interpersonal psychotherapy was added to drug counseling in a full-service methadone treatment program (Rounsaville et al., 1983). This study, although well-designed, did not succeed in engaging many patients in the psychotherapy, and it also had a high drop-out rate. The recruitment methods used suggested that some patients who did participate were probably unusually resistant to treatment, since they were referred to the research project as a last resort prior to being discharged from the program for showing little improvement.

A second study of psychotherapy had a higher recruitment rate, fewer dropouts, and a larger total number of subjects (Woody et al., 1983). This study provided good evidence that professional psychotherapists can provide additional benefits to those obtained with paraprofessional drug counselors. The treatments used are described in detail elsewhere (Woody et al., 1983). One of the most interesting findings from this work emerged when outcome was assessed for patients classified as low, mid, or high severity on the basis of the number and intensity of their psychiatric symptoms as rated by standard assessments such as the Beck Depression Inventory (Beck, 1972) or the SCL-90 (Derogatis, 1970). Low-severity patients made considerable and approximately equal progress with the additional psychotherapy or with counseling alone. Mid-severity patients had better outcomes with the additional psychotherapy than with counseling alone, but counseling was associated with numerous significant improvements. High-severity patients made little progress with counseling alone, but made considerable progress if they had the additional psychotherapy.

Patients with only antisocial personality disorder showed little response to the additional therapy, but others, especially those with depression, had a good response. It was also found that there was considerable variation in outcome among therapists, with some achieving consistently better outcomes than others (Luborsky et al., 1985). Those therapists who had the best results were noted as having the best doctor patient relationships and also as being the most successful in conforming to the specifications of their particular school of therapy.

The overall results of these studies, and of other similar but less comprehensive ones (Abrams, 1979; Connett, 1980; LaRosa et al., 1974; Resnick at al., 1980; Stanton and Todd, 1982; Willett, 1973), indicate that professional psychotherapy can probably make a valuable contribution to ongoing treatment services, particularly if it is targeted to that segment of the nonpsychotic addict population with moderate to high levels of psychiatric symptoms. The therapy program is not always simple to apply to this population (Rounsaville et al., 1983; Stanton and Todd, 1982; Woody et al., 1983) and must be well integrated into the overall drug rehabilitation program. It must also employ skilled therapists who relate well to opioid addicts. Few programs are using professional psychotherapists at this time. Our impression is that available services could be improved, especially for the most disturbed patients, by the selective use of skilled psychotherapists who have an interest in working with opiate-addicted individuals.

C. Other Psychotropic Medications

The last 10 years have also seen the use of psychotropic drugs other than tricylic antidepressants for addicts with psychiatric disorders. Ciccone et al. (1980) and Kleber (1983) reviewed evidence for the efficacy of these psychotropic medications, including antianxiety agents, lithium, and disulfiram. These reviews indicated that each of these medicines may be helpful for addicts with the specific disorder for which the drugs have been found helpful in other, nonaddict populations. Kleber (1983) advised a conservative approach to using benzodiazepines. Many clinicians have noted that diazepam and also quite possibly alprazolam (R. Millman, personal communication, 1985) have a significant abuse potential with this population and should be prescribed sparingly or not at all.

Disulfiram (Antabuse) has been found to be useful in opiate addicts who are also alcoholics. Up to 25% of patients on methadone programs have been reported to have drinking problems. While these problems can frequently be controlled by behavioral means such as breathalizer testing, disulfiram may be indicated. Liebson et al. (1973) found the rewarding effects of methadone to compliment the use of disulfiram in a small successful study. A large Veterans Administration collaborative study (Ling et al., 1983), however, found that the placebo-control method worked poorly for disulfiram comparison. The patients tended to test with alcohol to determine whether they were receiving placebo. While the VA investigators found no disulfiram–placebo differences in the methadone-maintained patients, the drinking problems in both groups showed improvement, probably owing to the structure imposed by the disulfiram study. The investigators concluded that willingness to accept disulfiram was significant in the beneficial effects observed and that there was no evidence of adverse interaction between methadone and disulfiram.

V. MEASURING THE PROBLEMS SEEN IN OPIOID ADDICTS

Other work focused on documenting and measuring the types of problems seen in methadone-maintained addicts and on matching patients to treatments. This work was made possible by the development of the Addiction Severity Index (ASI) by McLellan et al. (1080a). The ASI is a structured, 40-min, clinical research interview designed to assess problem severity in seven areas commonly affected by addiction: medical, legal, drug, alcohol, employment, family, and psychiatric. In each of these areas, objective questions are asked that measure the number, extent, and duration of problem symptoms in the patient's lifetime and in the past 30 days. The patient also supplies a subjective report of the recent severity and importance of the symptoms within the problem areas. Severity is operationally defined on all ASI scales as the number, duration, frequency, and intensity of symptoms in that specific area. Severity is rated by a trained technician from a patient's answers to questions regarding the lifetime and recent (past 30 days) experience of problem symptoms. The interviewer assimilates the two types of information to produce seven global ratings reflecting problem severity in each area. The patient's answers form the baseline against which subsequent follow-up interviews can be used to assess improvement. These 10-point (0–9) ratings have been shown to provide reliable and valid general estimates of problem severity for both alcoholics and drug addicts.

VI. PATIENT–PROGRAM MATCHING

Patient–program matching is a concept that could produce considerable progress in methadone treatment. The heterogeneity of methadone patients, as described earlier, provides ample justification for studies of patient–program matching. In addition there appears to be tremendous variability among methadone programs themselves, occasionally in regard to dose policies (high dose vs low dose), but particularly in regard to the ancillary services that are available, the quality of treatment facilities, and the levels of discipline imposed. Some programs have very little physician coverage, whereas others have one or more physicians actively involved in the treatment program. Counseling services, psychotherapy, social work, vocational counseling, and other aspects of drug rehabilitation services are similarly unevenly distributed among programs. Some states require paraprofessional drug counselors to pass an examination and others appear to have no competency standards. Thus, the variability among programs adds another dimension to patient–program matching.

Very little work has been done in this important area. Some of the treatment-outcome studies mentioned in this chapter (antidepressant drugs, psychotherapy, disulfiram, contingency contracting) represent attempts to match patients to treatments. McLellan and his colleagues have completed several studies of patient–program matching. Follow-up studies done using the ASI showed that patients with different symptom profiles showed different responses to residential versus outpatient treatments. For example, patients with significant sedative abuse or those with a highly unstable living arrangement appeared to do better in a residential program than in an outpatient methadone program. Generally, patients with significant amounts of psychiatric symptoms and those with stimulant abuse did better in methadone maintenance than in residential drug-free programs (McLellan et al., 1980b, 1983). This probably occurred because these more disturbed patients need support and medication. Psychotropic drugs are usually not prescribed in a residential drug rehabilitation program and treatment may involve confrontation and stress. Methadone itself may have psychotropic effects and methadone programs tend to utilize supportive therapy and ancillary psychotropic medications in addiction to methadone. These studies also found that a global rating of psychiatric severity was a good predictor of outcome in both residential and outpatient programs (McLellan et al., 1983). Patients with low levels of psychiatric symptoms did reasonably well in either outpatient or inpatient programs. Patients with mid-levels of psychiatric symptoms did better than patients with high levels and the patients with high ratings of psychiatric symptoms did not do well in either outpatient or inpatient programs. Matching of patients to programs appeared to be most helpful for those with mid-level psychiatric symptoms and least necessary for low-severity patients.

Another earlier attempt in the area of patient–program matching was that formulated by Goldstein (1976) regarding a sequential drug treatment strategy in which first methadone, then Levo-alpha-acetyl methadol (LAAM), and finally naltrexone are used in a progression from daily street opiate use to successful abstinence. We have not seen this progression to occur with any regularity either in the literature or in our experience. The psychiatric, social, and learned aspects of opioid dependence appear to be much stronger determinants of outcome then the pharmacological ones that are implicit in this theory. However, the efficacy of such a pharmacological progression, perhaps combined with psychosocial treatments, remains to be studied.

VII. TESTING THE EFFICACY OF MAINTENANCE DRUGS OTHER THAN METHADONE

A. LAAM

Other work was done to evaluate new drugs that may be used in place of methadone for narcotic substitution therapy. The most promising of these was LAAM. LAAM has pharmacological effects similar to methadone, but with LAAM their onset is slower and their duration is longer. One dose of LAAM can suppress opioid withdrawal symptoms for 48–72 hr. LAAM appears to have no serious toxicity when used properly; however, some patients report an increase in psychomotor activity while on LAAM, possibly due to its having greater stimulant effects than methadone (Ling et al., 1980). The major advantage of LAAM is that patients need come to clinic only three times per week. This is especially beneficial for those who must travel long distances or who have long hours or irregular work schedules. It is also desirable from a public health standpoint because its use almost eliminates the problems caused when patients sell or otherwise improperly use methadone that is dispensed to consume outside the clinic. Studies done to date show that treatment results for those who remain on LAAM compared favorably with those obtained with methadone, although LAAM's slower onset probably contributes to the higher initial drop-out rates seen when LAAM is compared with methadone (Ling et al., 1980). LAAM is still classified as an investigational drug by the FDA largely because it has had no commercial sponsor to shepherd it through the approval procedures. If it is eventually approved for general use, treatment programs would be in a position to offer most patients either LAAM treatment three times per week or daily methadone. This policy could lead to a marked improvement in the safety of methadone by practically eliminating the diversion of take-home methadone to illicit street users.

B. Propoxyphene

Propoxyphene napsylate, a drug with weak narcotic effects, was also tested for efficacy as a maintenance drug. Propoxyphene can suppress abstinence symptoms in patients who have low levels of physical dependence, and open clinical trials showed that some addicts could be maintained on propoxyphene (Tennant, 1974). However, double-blind studies comparing low doses of methadone (maximum 36 mg/day) with high doses of propoxyphene (maximum 1200 mg/day in divided doses) showed that propoxyphene was not nearly as effective as methadone (Woody et al., 1981). Drop-out rates and street drug use was considerably higher in patients maintained on propoxyphene than in those treated with methadone. The results of these studies were instrumental in propoxyphene being judged inappropriate for use as a maintenance treatment.

VIII. BEHAVIORAL TREATMENTS TO IMPROVE OUTCOME

Attention was also focused on behavioral treatments, especially as they apply to patients who demonstrate a poor response to methadone therapy. One serious problem that occurs with some maintenance patients is persistent drug use in spite of methadone doses that are more than sufficient to suppress withdrawal symptoms, and that also provide some degree of cross tolerance to injected opioids, thus reducing or eliminating the "reward" of using street opioids. Patients who continue to use opiates in spite of being treated with adequate doses of methadone are often not keeping regular counseling appointments and usually show little initiative to engage in constructive activities such as school or work. In these cases, some recommend raising the methadone dose to the highest allowable levels (80–100 mg/day). Sometimes this process is combined with a treatment contract that states that the patient must accomplish certain behaviors within a specified period of time or face suspension from the program (Bigelow et al., 1984). Goals to be achieved can include drug-free urine specimens, keeping all counseling appointments, and demonstrating proof that job-seeking behavior is occurring. Selectivity in choosing patients for contracts is important, as is choosing realistic goals. A recent study shows that 50–60% of carefully selected patients who were given a treatment contract succeeded by achieving the specified goals within the alloted time (Dolan et al., 1985). Those who fail a contract can be offered the option of transferring to another methadone program or of entering another treatment modality, such as a therapeutic community or narcotic antagonist (naltrexone) treatment.

IX. HIGH- VERSUS LOW-DOSE METHADONE TREATMENT

The last several years saw a partial resolution of the debate over whether patients need high methadone doses (more than 60 mg) or whether they will do just as well on lower doses (50 mg or less). Several studies explored this question and the conclusion was that patients can do well on any dose, that there are many variables that influence outcome, but that patients on high doses generally use fewer drugs and tend to do better than those on low doses (McGlothlin and Anglin, 1981). Thus, dose can be important, but for most patients it is only one of many variables that influence outcome.

X. DETOXIFICATION FROM METHADONE

Another series of studies examined detoxification from methadone maintenance. Several areas were explored. One group of investigations examined the proportion of detoxified addicts who remained abstinent. Stimmel et al. (1977) followed up 335 persons who were successfully detoxified from methadone maintenance for as long as 6 years. Of the 269 persons located, 35% were narcotic free, 58% had returned to narcotic use, and 8% were either jailed or deceased. This study concluded that while abstinence after narcotic dependence is possible, it is not a realistic goal for all. Premature detoxification was associated with a high relapse rate. Trained staff were able to identify those candidates who were most likely to succeed, although the exact criteria for identification were not specified. Kleber (1977) described similar findings and also found that successful withdrawal is possible, but only for a small proportion of patients.

Senay et al. (1977) studied rate of methadone withdrawal as a determinant of successful detoxification. One hundred twenty-seven successfully maintained addicts were randomly assigned to four treatment groups and it was found that patients who were detoxified at the rate of 3% per week were more likely to successfully detoxify then those who were reduced by 10% per week. Other studies demonstrated that clonidine, a nonopioid α-adrenergic agonist already approved for use as an antihypertensive drug, can suppress the autonomic symptoms of opiate withdrawal (Gold et al., 1978). Patients treated with clonidine can obtain significant relief from withdrawal symptoms; however, tolerance develops to the effect in 7–10 days. Many programs now use clonidine as an adjunct to routine services during detoxification. A comprehensive review on clonidine has been written by Ginzberg (1983).

The conclusions one draws from all the work on detoxification are as follows: some patients can be successfully detoxified, but candidates should be carefully selected by trained staff as those most likely and able to achieve success; premature detoxification can be harmful; a slow decrease (3% per week or less) will provide the best chance for success in an outpatient methadone detoxification program; and clonidine can be a useful short-term aid to detoxification.

XI. OPIOIDS AND PREGNANCY

Opioid-dependent women have been found to have increased rates of miscarriage and to give birth to children of reduced birth weight. Furthermore, children born to opioid-dependent women often, but not always, experience narcotic withdrawal symptoms shortly after birth. The neonatal mortality rate for the opioid exposed fetus is between 3 and 4.5%, with the majority of complications being related to low birth weight. The causes for this relationship are not exactly clear, but they probably relate to poor nutrition, fetal anoxia produced by changes in placental blood flow when the mother experiences the opiate withdrawal syndrome, and a direct effect of the opioid drug on the developing fetus.

These problems appear to be reduced by methadone maintenance. However, if maintenance is used to maintain pregnant addicts, it should be given only to those who are unlikely to successfully detoxify and it should be given in the lowest possible effective dose. The incidence of withdrawal symptoms seen in newborns is probably reduced by lower methadone doses. Neonatal withdrawal, when it occurs, can be treated with paregoric or phenobarbital.

Detoxification is not advised prior to 14 weeks gestation because of the potential risk of inducing abortion. Detoxification also should not be performed after the thirty-second week of pregnancy because of possible withdrawal-induced fetal stress.

Most patients who are maintained during pregnancy are controlled on 20–35 mg of methadone per day. Methadone-maintained women have often been found to complain of increasing withdrawal symptoms as pregnancy progresses. This is probable due to the pregnancy producing an increased extracellular fluid space with a consequent lowering of plasma methadone levels. These symptoms should be treated with elevation of the oral dose sufficient to suppress the withdrawal symptoms. These findings are discussed in detail by Kaltenbach and Finnegan (1984).

Wapner and Finnegan (1981) reviewed five longitudinal studies that evaluated methadone-exposed infants throughout the first 2 years of life. The results of these studies suggested that no long-term developmental sequelae are directly associated with methadone exposure in utero. Although differences were often found between methadone-exposed infants and comparison infants, developmental scores for the methadone-exposed infants were well within the normal range. Follow-up data at age 14 of those exposed to methadone in utero revealed no significant differences in cognitive performance between methadone-exposed and comparison children, although scores for both groups were in the low normal range (Wapner and Finnegan, 1981).

The question regarding whether there are permanent developmental sequelae associated with in utero methadone exposure has not been conclusively resolved at this time. The number of follow-up studies in small, and most encompass only the first 2 years of life. Although the findings are relatively consistent in finding no serious problems, a general consensus regarding their interpretation has not emerged owing to the relatively small amount of data currently available. Work is currently being done in this area; thus, future years should see more information on these important issues.

REFERENCES

Abrams, J. (1979). A cognitive behavioral versus nondirective group treatment program for opioid addicted persons: An adjunct to methadone maintenance, *Int. J. Addict., 14*:503–511.

Ball, J.C., Shaffer, J.W., and Nurco, D.N. (1983). The day to day criminality of heroin addicts in Baltimore—A study in the continuity of offense rates, *Drug Alcohol Depend., 12*:119–142.

Beck, A.T., and Beck, A.W. (1972). Screening depressed patients in family practice, *Postgrad. Med. 52*:81–85.

Bigelow, B.E., Stitzer, M.D., and Leibsan, I. The role of behavioral contingency management in drug abuse treatment, *Behavioral Intervention Techniques in Drug Abuse Treatment* (J. Grabowski, M.L. Stitzer, J. Henningfield, eds.). NIDA Research Monograph Series NO. 46, Rockville, Maryland, 1984, pp. 36–52.

Ciccone, P.E., O'Brien, C.P., and Khatami, M. (1980). Psychotropic agents in opiate addiction: A brief review, *Int. J. Addict., 15*(4):449–513.

Cohen, M., Hanbury, R., and Stimmel, B. (1978). Abuse of amitriptyline, *J.A.M.A., 240*:1372–1373.

Connett, G. (1980). Comparison of progress of patients with professional and paraprofessional counselors in a methadone maintenance program. *Int. J. Addict., 15*:585–589.

Cooper, J.R., Alterman, F., Brown, B.J., and Czechowicz, D. (eds.). *Research on the Treatment of Narcotic Addiction*, U.S. Government Printing Office, Rockville, Maryland, 1983.

Derogatis, L.R. (1970). Dimensions of outpatient neurotic pathology: Comparison of a clinical vs. an empirical assessment, *J. Consult. Clin. Psychol., 34*(2):164–171.

Dolan, M.P., Black, J.L., Penk, W.E., Robinowitz, R., and Deford, H.A. (1985). Contracting for treatment termination to reduce drug use among methadone maintenance treatment failures, *J. Consult. Clin. Psychol., 53*(4):549–551.

Dole, V.P., and Nyswander, M.E. (1965). A medical treatment for diacetylmorphine (heroin) addiction, *J.A.M.A., 193*(8):646–650.

Dole, V.P., Robinson, J.W., Orraca, J., Towns, E., Seargy, P., and Caine, E. (1969). Methadone treatment of randomly selected criminal addicts, *N. Engl. J. Med., 280*:1372–1375.

Ginzberg, H. Use of clonidine or lofexidine to detoxify from methadone maintenance or other opioid dependencies, *Research on the Treatment of Narcotic Addiction* (J.R. Cooper, F. Altman, B.J. Brown, and D. Czechowicz, eds.). U.S. Government Printing Office, Rockville, Maryland, 1983, pp. 174–224.

Gold, M.S., Redmond, D.E., and Kleber, H.D. (1978). Clonidine blocks acute opiate withdrawal symptoms, *Lancet, 2*:599–602.

Goldstein, A. (1976). Heroin addiction, sequential treatment employing pharmacological supports, *Arch. Gen. Psychiatry, 33*:353–358.

Grabowski, J., Stitzer, M., and Henningfield, J.E. (eds.). *Behavioral Intervention Techniques in Drug Abuse Treatment*, NIDA Research Monograph Series No. 46, U.S. Government Printing Office, Rockville, Maryland, 1984.

Hunt, D., Lipton, D.S., Goldsmith, D.S., and Strug, D.L. Problems in methadone treatment: The influence of reference groups, *Behavioral Intervention Techniques in Drug Abuse Treatment* (J. Grabowski, M.L. Stitzer, and J.E. Henningfield, eds.). NIDA Research Monograph Series No. 46, U.S. Government Printing Office, Rockville, Maryland, 1984, pp. 8–22.

Kaltenbach, K., and Finnegan, L.P. (1984). Developmental outcome of children born to methadone maintained women: A review of longitudinal studies, *Neurobehav. Toxicol. Teratol. 6*:271–275.

Kleber, H.D. (1977). Detoxification from methadone maintenance: The state of the art, *Int. J. Addict., 12*:807–820.

Kleber, H.D. Concomitant use of methadone with other psychoactive drugs in the treatment of opiate addicts with other *DSM-III* diagnoses, *Research on the Treatment of Narcotic Addiction* (J.R. Cooper, F. Altman, G.S. Brown, and D. Czechowicz, eds.). U.S. Government Printing Office, Rockville, Maryland, 1983, pp. 119–149.

Kleber, H.D., Weissman, M., Rounsaville, B., Wilber, C., and Prusoff, B. (1983). Imipramine as treatment for depression in methadone treated addicts. *Arch. Gen. Psychiatry, 40*:649–653.

LaRosa, J.C., Lipsius, J.H., and LaRosa, J.H. (1974). Experiences with a combination of group therapy and methadone maintenance in the treatment of heroin addiction, *Int. J. Addict., 9*:605–617.

Liebson, I., Bigelow, G., and Flamer, R. (1973). Alcoholism among methadone patients: A specific treatment method, *Am. J. Psychiatry, 130*:483–485.

Ling, W., Klett, J., and Gillis, R. (1980). A cooperative clinical study of methadyl acetate, *Arch. Gen. Psychiatry, 37*:908–911.

Ling, W., Weiss, D.G., and Charuvastra, C.V. (1983). Use of disulfiram for alcoholics in methadone maintenance programs, *Arch. Gen. Psychiatry, 40*:851–854.

Luborsky, L., McLellan, A.T., Woody, G.E., O'Brien, C.P., and Auerbach, A. (1985). Therapist success and its determinants, *Arch. Gen. Psychiatry, 42*:602–611.

McBride, D.C., Westie, K.S., and Goldstein, B.J. The alleviation of depression in a population of narcotic users, *Final Report to the National Institute of Drug Abuse*, 1982.

McGlothlin, W.H., and Anglin, D. (1981). Long-term follow-up of clients of high- and low-dose methadone programs, *Arch. Gen. Psychiatry, 38*:1055–1063.

McLellan, A.T., Luborsky, L., Woody, G.E., and O'Brien, C.P. (1980a). Improved diagnostic instrument for substance abuse patient: The addiction severity index, *J. Nerv. Ment. Dis., 168*:26–33.

McLellan, A.T., Druley, K.A., O'Brien, C.P., and Kron, R. (1980b). Matching substance abuse patients to appropriate treatments, *Drug Alcohol Depend., 3*:189–195.

McLellan, A.T., Luborsky, L., O'Brien, C.P., Woody, G.E., and Druley, K.A. (1982). Is treatment for substance abuse effective? *J.A.M.A., 247*:1423–1428.

McLellan, A.T., Luborsky, L., Woody, G.E., Druley, K.A., and O'Brien, C.P. (1983). Predicting response to alcohol and drug abuse treatments: Role of psychiatric severity, *Arch. Gen. Psychiatry, 40*:620–625.

McLellan, A.T., Childress, A.R., Griffith, J., and Woody, G.E. (1984). The psychiatrically severe drug abuse patient: Methadone maintenance or therapeutic community? *Am. J. Drug Alcohol Abuse, 10*:77–95.

Newman, R.G., and Whitehill, W.B., 1979, Double-blind comparisons of methadone and placebo maintenance treatments of narcotic addicts in Hong Kong, *Lancet, 8141*:485–488.

Resnick, R.B., Washton, A.M., Stone-Washton, N., et al. Psychotherapy and naltrexone in opioid dependence, *Problems of Drug Dependence, 1980* (L.S. Harris, ed.). NIDA research monograph 34, DHHS publication (ADM) 81–1058. U.S. Dept. of Health and Human Services, National Institute of Drug Abuse, Rockville, Maryland, 1980, pp. 109–115.

Rounsaville, B.J., and Kleber, H.D. (1985). Untreated opiate addicts: How do they differ from those seeking treatment? *Arch. Gen. Psychiatry, 42*:1072–1077.

Rounsaville, B.J., Weissman, M.M., Crits-Christoph, K., Wilber, C., and Kleber, H.D. (1982a). Diagnosis and symptoms of depressions in opiate addicts, *Arch. Gen. Psychiatry, 39*:151–156.

Rounsaville, B.J., Weissman, M.M., Kleber, H.D., and Wilber, C.H. (1982b). The heterogeneity of psychiatric diagnosis in treated opiate addicts, *Arch. Gen. Psychiatry, 39*:161–166.

Rounsaville, B.J., Glazer, W., Wilber, C.H., Weissman, M.M., and Kleber, H.D., 1983, Short-term interpersonal psychotherapy in methadone-maintained opiate addicts, *Arch. Gen. Psychiatry, 40*:630–636.

Sells, S.B. Treatment effectiveness, *Handbook on Drug Abuse* (R.L. Dupont, A. Goldstein, and J. O'Donnell, eds.), National Institute of Drug Abuse, Rockville, Maryland, 1979, pp. 105–118.

Senay, S.C., Dorus, W., Goldberg, F., and Thornton, W. (1977). Withdrawal from methadone maintenance. Rate of withdrawal and expectation, *Arch. Gen. Psychiatry, 34*:361–367.

Stanton, M.D., Todd, T. (eds.) *The Family Therapy of Drug Abuse and Addiction*, New York, Guilford Press, 1982.

Stimmel, B., Goldberg, J., Rotkopf, E., and Cohen, M. (1977). Ability to remain abstinent after methadone detoxification, *J.A.M.A., 237*:1216–1220.

Tennant, F.S. (1974). Propoxyphene napsylate (Darvon-N) treatment of heroin addicts, *J. Natl. Med. Assoc., 66*:23–24.

Titievsky, J. Guillermo, S., and Barranco, M. (1982). Doxepin as adjunctive for depressed methadone maintenance patients: A double-blind study, *J. Clin. Psychiatry, 39*:151–156.

Wapner, R.J., and Finnegan, L.P. (1981). Perinatal aspects of psychotropic drug abuse, *Perinatal Med., 20*:384–417.

Woody, G.E., O'Brien, C.P., and Rickels, K. (1975). Depression and anxiety in heroin addicts: A placebo-controlled study of doxepin in combination with methadone, *Am. J. Psychiatry, 132*:4,447–450.

Woody, G.E., Mintz, J., Tennant, F., O'Brien, C.P., McLellan, A.T., and Marcovici, M., (1981). Propoxyphene for maintenance treatment, *Arch. Gen. Psychiatry, 38*:898–900.

Woody, G.E., O'Brien, C.P., McLellan, A.T., Marcovici, M., and Evans, B. (1982). The use of antidepressants with methadone in depressed maintenance patients, *Ann. N.Y. Acad. Sci., 1982*:120–127.

Woody, G.E., Luborsky, L., McLellan, A.T., O'Brien, C.P., Beck, A.T., Blaine, J., Hermer, I., and Hole, A. (1983). Psychotherapy for opiate addicts. Does it help? *Arch. Gen. Psychiatry, 40*:639–645.

Woody, G.E., McLellan, A.T., Luborsky, L., O'Brien, C.P. (1984). Severity of psychiatric symptoms of a predictor of benefits from psychotherapy: The Veterans Administration–Penn Study, *Am. J. Psychiatry, 141*:1172–1177.

61

Opioid Detoxification and Maintenance with Blocking Agents

Arthur Margolin and Thomas R. Kosten
Yale University School of Medicine, New Haven, Connecticut

I. INTRODUCTION

Chronic opioid addiction is a complex phenomenon involving physiological, behavioral, psychological, and environmental factors, and its treatment optimally includes intervention into many of these interacting factors simultaneously. Pharmacotherapy with opioid blockers constitutes an important intervention into physiological factors sustaining addiction, and is supported by simultaneous intervention into other contributory factors. Tools in the clinician's armamentarium today include medications with varying degrees of opioid-blocking and opioid agonist properties, from pure blockers, such as naltrexone, to pure agonists, such as methadone. In this chapter, we will discuss the theory and clinical use of agents for opioid detoxification procedures—procedures which must be completed before administration of pure blockers can be started. Because practicing clinicians utilize a variety of conceptual frameworks for making clinical judgments—scientific and intuitive—we have attempted in this chapter to elucidate frameworks supported by empirical research that we hope will be applicable to their needs. We begin by outlining a multiphasic view of detoxification; we then discuss the physiology of opioid addiction and detoxification from a homeostatic perspective; finally, we discuss the use of opioid antagonists and partial agonists during various phases of the opioid detoxification process. In the appendix, we have included a brief procedural manual for the detoxification procedures discussed in the chapter.

II. TRIPARTITE MODEL OF OPIOID ADDICTION

The treatment of opioid addiction takes place with respect to and ultimately seeks to reverse opioid tolerance and withdrawal symptoms. Given the continuity of underlying physiological and psychological processes, this statement implies that no rigid boundaries exist between detoxification and prior or successive phases in the addiction process. Because of the variable and extended clinical time course of the detoxification procedure, we think it is useful to conceive of the detoxification process as being flanked by, and interlocking with, two adjacent phases: an antecedent phase (addiction) and a consequent phase (aftercare).

addiction → detoxification → aftercare

In the addiction phase, the structure of the addiction is established—the biochemical characteristics of the abused opioid interacts with the individual addict's physiology, psychology, and environment to produce that form of maladaptive behavior we label *drug addiction*. Detoxification initiates the restructuring of these factors—most immediately by removing the biochemical component of the addiction. In the aftercare stage, the consequences of biochemical alterations for both physiological and psychological systems are dealt with, and an attempt is made to help the patient establish a drug-free lifestyle. Unfortunately, for many patients, the trajectory is circular rather than linear, as they relapse back into the addiction phase after detoxification and maintenance [1].

Each phase partially determines input values for the successive stage: the characteristics of the opioid from which the patient is being detoxified is a partial determinant of the choice of the detoxification procedure, which in turn partially determines optimal conditions of maintenance and aftercare. The detoxification process may thus be regarded as creating a specific trajectory for a specific patient through this tripartile landscape. This suggests that the patient's needs and resources in the aftercare phase should already be a consideration in choosing a detoxification procedure. The clinician, for example, may decide to manipulate certain characteristics of the addiction phase by transferring the patient to an opioid agonist or partial agonist which exhibits certain desirable withdrawal characteristics relative to the chosen detoxification approach.

Because the time course of detoxification to recovery is highly variable among patients, and because the many factors, psychosocial and physiological, affected by opioid addiction normalize at different rates, we think it is clinically useful to draw a distinction between the externally administered, temporally invariant, detoxification *procedure*, and the internally enduring, patient-dependent, detoxification *process*. The procedure may take as few as 3–4 days; the process, insofar as it is a consequence of processes in progress before the procedure is initiated, may be thought of as beginning prior to the detoxification procedure, and terminates not with the end of the formal procedure, but when the psychophysiological processes altered by chronic opioid administration have been normalized. This may take months or, in some cases, years. This extended normalization process may underlie the protracted abstinence syndrome, which we will discuss in a later section.

III. HOMEOSTATIC PERSPECTIVE

Given the variable and perhaps extended time course of what we have termed the detoxification process, it is useful to have a framework which functions both as model for empirical research in opioid addiction, and as a framework for the clinician treating opioid addicts. The homeostatic framework constitutes a useful model for both domains of activity, clinical and basic research [2]. In general, the homeostatic framework views physiological functioning as a way of maintaining "stability in the face of variability" [3]. Variability usually takes the form of external disturbances acting on a system, causing it to deviate from a its "normal" value—its reference point. The mechanism by which stability is maintained usually includes compensatory adjustments to counteract the disturbance, returning the system to the range of the reference point—the familiar negative feedback loop [4–6]. In opioid addiction, the chronic use of opioids constitutes a disturbance, most conspicuously to neurophysiological systems, and these systems respond with compensatory adjustments that oppose the effects of opioid administration [7]. In this framework, pharmacological tolerance is a manifestation of successful adaptation of the system to the opioids. With tolerance, the dose of morphine originally needed for a response is no longer effective in producing this response; e.g., euphoria. The disturbance has been successfully countered, but usually at some cost. Withdrawal symptoms result from these adaptive changes. The control loops go out of reference range in the absence of the opioids whose effects they oppose. In subsequent sections, we will examine some hypotheses concerning mechanisms of neural adaptation to opioids as they relate to opioid withdrawal and its treatment.

The clinician treating drug addicts must daily make clinical judgments concerning medical action in complex psychophysiological systems whose defining characteristics at many different levels of structure are never fully known. In the absence of definitive data defining a given patient's condition, the homeostatic framework constitutes a heuristically useful perspective to guide clinical thinking. The perspective from which the treatment of opioid addiction may be profitably viewed is simply stated but, we think, potentially richly comprehensive: Chronic opioid use transforms numerous subsystems within the addict owing to compensatory physiological adjustments; the treatment process induces recompensation of these subsystems over time in the absence of opioids. If we include under "subsystems" domains within which significant factors relevant to opioid addiction have been found—physiological, psychological, and interpersonal—the complex implications of this simple framework are immediately apparent. In this chapter, we will examine some of the implications of this homeostatic framework as a way of addressing the converging, but not always identical, concerns of the medical practitioner and the medical researcher.

IV. THREE PHASES OF ADDICTION: HOMEOSTATIC CONSIDERATIONS AND THE USE OF BLOCKING AGENTS

A. Phase I: Addiction

Although addictive behavior is a function of both positive and negative reinforcement systems [8], withdrawal from opioids is associated with negative reinforcement alone—the need to take the drug to ameliorate discomfort. Researchers and clinicians concerned with detoxification procedures have thus focused on addiction from the standpoint of the effects of chronic administration of opioids on those areas of the brain that are principally activated in negative reinforcement and withdrawal. Experiments with rodents have implicated the periaqueductal gray area in the brainstem as having a primary role in opioid physical dependence [9–13]. The treatment of opioid dependence in humans has been based in part upon research conducted on primates investigating the locus coeruleus, a brainstem nucleus located near the periaqueductal gray in the anterior pons [14]. Because there is evidence that the brain's noradrenergic system has an important role in opioid withdrawal [15], studies of opioid regulation of the noradrenergic system have concentrated on the locus coeruleus, which possesses a high density of opioid receptors, and which provides over 90% of the noradrenergic innervation of the cerebral cortex [16,17]. In the primate there is evidence that excitation of the locus coeruleus mediates anxiety, fear, and panic responses that characterize withdrawal from opioids [15]. These responses may constitute significant impediments to a patient's willingness to discontinue opioid abuse [18].

Opioids exert their affects upon locus coeruleus neurons through neuromodulation [19]. Neuromodulation by opioids does not seem to occur through changes in opioid receptors or ion channels directly, but rather through intracellular second messenger systems, perhaps involving G proteins and cyclic adenosine monophasphate (cAMP) [20,21]. Current evidence suggests that opioids act through second-messenger systems to decrease the rate of firing of neurons in the locus coeruleus, and therefore activity-dependant release of norepinephrine in the brain [17].

A possible mechanism of this inhibition is consistent with the following summary outline of intracellular events [7]: Opioids occupy mu opioid receptors which regulate adenylate cyclase, an enzyme which participates in the formation of cAMP; the occupation of the receptor by the opioid molecule suppresses adenylate cyclase activity, through a G protein link to the mu receptor, causing a reduction in cAMP levels and reducing protein phosphorylation. The reduction in protein phosphorylation in turn causes potassium channels to open, increasing inflow of potassium, which hyperpolarizes the neuron, and inhibits neuronal firing. (Readers interested in a comprehensive discussion of the second-messenger theory of opioid action may consult Nestler [17]). Because there is evidence that this compensatory upregulation of adenylate cyclase in the locus coeruleus may be in part responsible for withdrawal symptoms [7,22], it is not unreasonable to speculate that the treatment of these symptoms produced by the hyperactivity of the locus coeruleus may be crucial to a successful detoxification [15].

B. Phase II: Detoxification

A drug addict who presents for treatment has typically been abusing opioids illegally for 5–8 years [23]. Entry into treatment has important consequences not only for the addict, but also for the community of which he or she is a member, as the illicit acquisition of drugs is replaced with an institutionally controlled treatment [24]. Detoxification may be viewed as a transitional phase, of either a short or long duration, during which time the patient normalizes physiologically in the absence of opioids. As already noted, chronic opioid use can be regarded as a disturbance in feedback loops which maintain homeostatic values in systems regulated by endogenous opioids. In withdrawal, the compensatory adjustments to exogenous opioids transforms values in brain regions implicated in negative reinforcement, leading to hyperactive states in the absence of opioids. Fortunately, states produced by opioid withdrawal do not create life-threatening divergences from normal homeostatic processes, as may happen, for example, after abrupt termination of benzodiazepines.

Since opioid receptors exist throughout the body [25], many systems are disregulated by the withdrawal of opioids, producing a variety of dysphoric symptoms over varying time courses, in addition to the aforementioned fear and anxiety. These may include disturbances in thermal regulation, gastrointestinal distress, and sleep and appetite disturbances [26,27]. Detoxification procedures will optimally reduce the subjective distress attendant to disregulation, and also will promote the rapid normalization of homeostatic processes.

As we stated above, the hyperactivity of the opioid-adapted locus coeruleus in the absence of opioids has been implicated in mediating anxiety symptoms of withdrawal. A possible sequence of events leading to the hyperactivation of the locus coeruleus has been developed based on research on rodents and primates [15,17]. Suppression of adenylate cyclase by exogenous opioids elicits a compensatory cellular upregulation of this enzyme, as outlined in the previous section. When the opioid is cleared from the receptor, the compensatory upregulation of adenylate cyclase is no longer brought into set-point range by the opioid's suppressive effects. As a consequence, levels of adenylate cyclase rise, and this causes, through subsequent increases in cAMP, increased rates of protein phosphorylation, which in turn causes the closing of potassium channels. This change in ionic conductance of the neuron puts it into a depolarized state, causing it to go into a state of excitability, with resultant rapid firing [7]. The effects of this hyperexcitability in locus coeruleus neurons is tantamount to an intense, protracted activation of anxiety systems. Needless to say, the patient experiences this activation as extremely distressing. Thus, there have been attempts to develop detoxification procedures that satisfy two main desiderata: (1) dampen the excitation in locus coeruleus neurons caused by the absence of opioids, and (2) compress the time course of the normalization procedure to sustain the patient's motivation to stop using drugs.

If the goal of treatment is detoxification and induction onto naltrexone, then the physician has two general courses of action: (1) long-term detoxification by slow taper from a stabilizing opioid, and (2) rapid detoxification utilizing blocking agents. The choice of a particular procedure for a given patient is a complex decision based as much on physiological as on motivational considerations. One important consideration is the patient's ability to withstand the distress of withdrawal. One study found that the best predictor of failure in outpatient detoxification was a high level of psychological symptoms, such as elevated levels of anxiety or depression, determined before initiation of detoxification [28]. Failure to complete the detoxification may have been related to the inability of the patient to tolerate withdrawal symptoms. Recent developments in opioid treatment research have given the clinician the option to choose between slow or rapid detoxification procedures, and thus to match the rate of opioid reduction to the needs and resources of the patient.

Slow Detoxification

The usual course of a slow detoxification is an incremental decrease in the administration of a long-acting opioid, usually methadone. This slow detoxification consists of tapering the dose 20% a day for inpatients, for a 1- to 2-week long procedure, or 5% a day for outpatients in a detoxification lasting as long as 6 months. In either procedure, the patient will experience low-level withdrawal symptoms such as sleep and mood disturbances, [29] which, in addition to psychological factors, may precipitate relapse. While inpatient rates of successful detoxification may be over 80%, the success rate in outpatient detoxifications from methadone, as determined by completion of the procedure and successful naloxone challenge test, is about 40% [30]. However, relapse rates at 3 months after inpatient or outpatient detoxifications alone are as high as 80% [31].

One advantage of the long-term or extended detoxification is that the patient's body normalizes in small increments, each of which is relatively painless [32]. However, there are some disadvantages in this approach: The addict's motivation may waver, and there is increased risk of relapse during the slow taper itself. In order to address limitations of the slow detoxification procedures, two of its parameters have come under particular scrutiny: amelioration of the withdrawal symptoms and shortening of the procedures's duration. Amelioration of the dysphoric experiences of the detoxification procedure has obvious benefits—the fear of intense withdrawal distress which constitutes a primary reason for some patient's reluctance to undergo detoxification would be assuaged. In addition, a shorter detoxification procedure may have the advantage of being commensurate with a addict's motivational levels, which tend to deteriorate within several days. Hence, it may be crucial to the success of any detoxification to address the issue of matching the pace of the detoxification procedure to the patient's need to get it over with quickly, and also the pace at which he or she can create a new identity as an ex-addict. If the patient's resources are sufficient, an overall strategy would be to detoxify the patient rapidly, and follow this with naltrexone maintenance therapy. This procedure also has the significant advantage of being applicable to outpatient settings.

Rapid Detoxification Procedures

Rapid detoxification procedures build on two principles: (1) rapid clearing of opioids from cells, and (2) treatment of consequent systemic disregulation. Restoration of "normal" activity of opioid-regulation neurons is accelerated by the use of opioid antagonists, primarily naltrexone; and treatment of the precipitated symptoms is effected through alpha$_2$-adrenergic agonists such as clonidine.

Opioid Blockers

Opioid antagonists compete with opioid agonists at opioid receptor sites, but antagonists have a higher affinity for these sites and, therefore, precipitate withdrawal [25]. Opioid antagonists can reverse opioid agonist effects within 5 min, but since this will produce severe withdrawal symptoms, they are not clinically useful except in the acute treatment of opioid overdose. The two opioid antagonists most widely used are naltrexone and naloxone. Naltrexone has a greater usefulness in outpatient settings because it is administered orally; naloxone is administered intravenously. They are competitive, not irreversible antagonists. Hence, they can by "overridden" by a high enough dose of opioid agonist. Manipulations of the opiod molecule have given rise to substances with varying degrees of antagonist activity at different opioid receptor sites. Some antagonists, such as nalorphine, block the mu receptor responsible for euphoria, but are agonists at other receptors such that they produce hallucinations and other dysphoric effects. Naltrexone and naloxone are the antagonists most frequently used in opioid addiction treatment because they possess antagonist action equally at all opioid receptors.

Clonidine-Naltrexone Detoxification

Because the locus coeruleus has been implicated in producing withdrawal symptoms, the alpha$_2$ agonist, clonidine, is used to suppress the opioid-dependent hyperactivity by direct inhibition. Initial studies of the use of clonidine in opioid addiction [33] were followed by double-blind, placebo-controlled studies showing clonidine to be more effective than placebo, and as effective as a 20-day methadone taper in alleviating the symptoms of methadone withdrawal [34]. However, the use of clonidine in outpatient detoxification was found to be less successful than the 80–90% success rate of inpatient studies. Moreover, numerous studies showed that clonidine failed to substantially shorten the time required for withdrawal. This is especially problematic in the outpatient setting, in which a long duration of mild withdrawal symptoms may create conditions in which patients are liable to resume opioid use. Blachley et al. [35] found that the pure opioid antagonist naloxone given parenterally to opioid-dependent patients precipitated withdrawal and shortened the withdrawal period to 1 or 2 days. They noted that the intensity of this precipitated withdrawal decreased with successive doses of naloxone over the 2 days of treatment. Other groups who have tried this technique [36,37], however, were not able to satisfactorily ameliorate the intensified withdrawal symptoms with symptomatic medication.

Because clonidine has been noted to ameliorate naloxone-induced morphine withdrawal [38], Riordan and Kleber [39] combined clonidine and naloxone therapy to successfully withdraw three heroin users and one methadone patient over a 4-day period. Charney et al. [40,41] subsequently used clonidine and naltexone in combination to provide a safe, effective, and rapid withdrawal for patients maintained on methadone. Thirty-eight of 40 (95%) patients completely withdrew from opioids over the 4- or 5-day period. Combination clonidine and naltrexone therapy has also proven effective in the outpatient setting. Over a 5-day period, Kleber et al. [34] successfully withdrew 12 of 14 (86%) heroin users while simultaneously initiating naltrexone therapy. These studies demonstrated that combination clonidine and naltrexone therapy speeds the time course of opioid withdrawal without increasing symptomatology, and suggests that recovery from physical dependency on opioids might be accelerated by the introduction of an opioid antagonist [34,40,41]. Failure of earlier outpatient clonidine detoxification procedures to match inpatient success rates may have been largely due to the greater temptation and opportunity to cope with residual withdrawal discomfort through illicit opioid use. The addition of naltrexone therapy prevented this recourse by introducing opioid blockade early in therapy. The addition of the opioid blocker allowed success rates for outpatient clonidine plus naltrexone detoxifications to approach that of in-patient clonidine detoxifications.

A possible mechanism of the rapid normalization of the opioid system with naltrexone-clonidine has been modeled within the second-messenger system previously discussed [7]: The administration of an opioid antagonist may increase the number of opioid receptors, which in turn recompensates for the augmentation of adenylate cyclase levels produced as a compensatory response in the opioid addiction. The entire system is thus "reset," with increased numbers of opioid receptors and increased levels of adenylate cyclase activity. Endogenous opioids such as beta endorphin would then be able to sufficiently drive the system to produce a "normalized" state in the locus coeruleus. Studies have shown that in primates maintained on daily doses of methadone [42], opioid dependence and endpoint withdrawal symptoms are substantially reduced with single doses of naloxone every third day while opioid agonist effects of the maintenance opioid are still in evidence. This finding is consistent with the hypothesis that the antagonist resets the opioid system, preventing or reversing the development of agonist dependence [43].

Partial Agonists

In behavioral terms, a drug is defined as an antagonist for a given opioid if it produces withdrawal in an animal maintained on that substance. The study of the behavioral effects of opioid drugs have given rise to a class of drugs, partial agonists, that seem to possess paradoxical properties. Partial agonists will precipitate abstinence in addicts who are opioid dependent and will produce opioidlike effects in subjects who are not opioid dependent [44]. In addition, they will suppress withdrawal symptoms in persons who have a low level of addiction. The dose-response curve of a partial agonist is less steep than that of a pure agonist, and its agonist effects show a ceiling effect [44].

A partial agonist which has increasingly drawn the interest of drug addiction researchers is buprenorphine. Buprenorphine differs from methadone, an opioid agonist, in exhibiting reduced agonist activity with increasing doses, and in having a less severe withdrawal syndrome after chronic use [45]. It is reported to produce a generalized feeling of contentment rather than euphoria or a "rush" [46]. Buprenorphine exhibits agonist properties at lower doses, and at increasing doses antagonist properties increase. In its agonist activity, buprenorphine has been found to be 100 times more potent than morphine [44], but as a partial agonist, its agonist action shows a ceiling effect and declines with increased dose until at relatively high doses it antagonizes its own analgesic properties.

Use of Buprenorphine.

Stabilization. Patients on heroin or methadone can be transferred to buprenorphine by substituting 2–4 mg of buprenorphine for 20–30 mg of methadone, or the usual dose of "street" heroin. At this rate, the patient should experience minimal withdrawal symptoms, even though buprenorphine may act as an opioid antagonist at doses as low as 8 mg. Depending on the needs of the patient, a transfer onto buprenorphine can be regarded as a partial detoxification, as a new maintenance agent, or as a prelude to a further complete detoxification. In the context of detoxification, this transfer may be considered stabilization of the opioid addict.

Several 1-month "detoxification" trials have been done with buprenorphine. One study randomized heroin addicts to tapering doses of either methadone or buprenorphine and found substantial dropout from both groups as the dose of medication was lowered [47]. The dropout rate was extensive in the buprenorphine group below 2 mg daily sublingually. Another study by our group at Yale used a stable dose of 2–8 mg of buprenorphine for a month, followed by abrupt discontinuation [48]. Discontinuation of buprenorphine elicited far fewer withdrawal symptoms than discontinuation of methadone [49]. Outpatient retention was much higher with this stable dose—70% retention to the end of the trial. Illicit opioid use declined to 22%

during the month for the patients who remained in treatment. In addition to a decline in illicit opioid use, patients in this study showed a substantial (eight- to 10-fold) reduction in cocaine abuse. Abuse of cocaine occurs in approximately 65% of opioid abusers and has not been well controlled by methadone maintenance treatment [50]. However, evidence suggests that cocaine abuse in methadone-maintained patients may be substantially reduced by switching them over to buprenorphine treatment [51,52].

Advantages of buprenorphine include an abuse potential less than that of heroin or methadone, and a relatively symptom-free detoxification to a drug-free state after sustained treatment. Buprenorphine also seems to discourage "speedballing" (combining cocaine and heroin) [53]. There are no data as yet on the long-term effects of maintaining patients on buprenorphine, so the extent to which it can be considered a prospective drug for the addiction phase is not clear. At present, several studies are underway at Yale and other institutions comparing the effectiveness of buprenorphine to methadone in a maintenance program.

Detoxification with buprenorphine. Buprenorphine's dual agonist/antagonist properties suggested its use as a transitional agent between pure agonists, such as methadone, and pure antagonists, such as naltrexone, to forge a relatively "seamless" detoxification procedure. The rationale behind its use is that when buprenorphine is given to a heroin addict or a patient maintained on methadone, it will precipiate minimal or no withdrawal symptoms, and thus allow for a tolerable transition onto this partial agonist. Over a month's time buprenorphine's antagonist action would reset the opioid system, as previously discussed, thus reducing or eliminating precipitation of severe withdrawal symptoms by the opioid antagonist naltrexone and allowing for a smooth transition onto naltrexone maintenance therapy.

Several studies have shown that the first transition from illegal heroin use or methadone maintenance to buprenorphine can be satisfactorily conducted. Kosten et al. [49] inducted 10 opioid-addicted patients onto buprenorphine within 24 h of their last opioid administration at three different sublingual dosages: 2, 3, and 4 mg. Patients exhibited minimal withdrawal symptoms. The patients remained on fixed dosages of buprenorphine for 30 days before receiving a naltrexone or placebo challenge. Two other studies have also reported switching opioid-dependent patients to buprenorphine with minimal withdrawal symptoms [46,54].

A recent study at Yale showed that the second transition from buprenorphine to naltrexone can also be satisfactorily conducted [55]. Methadone patients stabilized for a month on buprenorphine at 3 mg sublingual daily were given high-dose intravenous naloxone (0.5 mg/kg) to precipitate withdrawal. The withdrawal syndrome was less intense than that produced by even 10-fold lower doses of naltrexone (0.05 mg/kg) in methadone-maintained patients. Naltrexone maintenance can be rapidly initiated after the naloxone precipitated withdrawal without precipitating further withdrawal symptoms. These findings are consistent with a resetting of the opioid system by buprenorphine's antagonist activity before entry into the study all of the patients were demonstrably dependent on pure opioid agonists. The most severe withdrawal symptoms in this three-phase detoxification procedure, including muscle aches and some anxiety, occurred in the transition from the partial agonist buprenorphine to the competitive antagonist naloxone. These precipitated symptoms reduced satisfaction and compliance with the procedure, but pretreatment with clonidine or a similar agent has been found to ameliorate the severity of this transition and improve its clinical utility (unpublished data).

C. Phase III: Aftercare

In the detoxification stage, many of the systems disregulated by opioid use have only ostensibly returned to normal. After detoxification it may take up to 6 months, and in some cases longer, for physiological values to stabilize. These may include measures of weight, sleep, basal metabolic rate, temperature, and respiration rates [27]. With specific relevance to withdrawal symptoms, Guitart and Nestler [16] have advanced the hypothesis, within the second-messenger model previously outlined, that chronic opioid exposure may lead to an increase in protein phosphorylation in locus coeruleus neurons by two mechanisms: an increase in the total amounts of specific phosphoproteins; or by an increase in the phosphorylation states of constant amounts of other phosphoproteins. They suggest that these two mechanisms could normalize during detoxification at different rates, with alterations in phosphorylation states recovering much more rapidly than changes in total amount. The former may be involved in immediate opioid withdrawal, and the latter in symptoms of protracted withdrawal. The condition in which multiple values disregulated by chronic opioid administration take several months or more to stabilize after detoxification has been hypothesized to be a contributory factor in a condition termed the protracted abstinence syndrome. No large-scale studies have yet been conducted to statistically quantify this syndrome in detoxified addicts, although Martin's studies form the 1960s provide benchmark data [26,27].

It has been found that addicts who have post-detoxification psychosocial support available to them, especially the support of family members [56–59], do better after detoxification than do addicts undergoing a purely pharmacological procedure. In the phase following detoxification, intensive support is necessary because the addict may be in at least triple jeopardy for relapse. Physiologically, the patient may be undergoing a protracted abstinence syndrome, with values not stabilizing for months after the formal detoxification was completed. Psychologically, the patient may be susceptible to conditioned drug cues for several years into abstinence. These cues may cause a conditioned withdrawal response [60], or a conditioned euphoria response [61]. Both responses may induce drug-craving, which may in turn initiate drug-seeking behavior [62–64]. Lastly, the clinical staff may regard the addict as "officially detoxified," and the possibility that several systems may continue to be disregulated for some time after the detoxification procedure has concluded may be ignored. Neither patient not staff may realize the need for continued psychological and pharmacological support. It is to counteract these possible misunderstandings and misconceptions that we earlier urged the informal distinction between the (external) detoxification procedures, and the usually much longer (internal) detoxification processes. The patient, the patient's family, and the clinical staff, could well operate under the assumption that the detoxification process will extend well into the aftercare stage, and that helping the patient to overcome the many residual effects of his addiction—physiological and psychological—constitute some of the fundamental tasks after the detoxification procedure is formally concluded.

Naltrexone in Aftercare Phase

There is evidence that craving for opioids diminishes under conditions of drug unavailability [65]. By rendering the patient unable to experience the euphorogenic effects of the drug, naltrexone's opioid-blocking action has the effect of making the drug psychologically unavailable to the patient, thus rendering even an environment of drug access tantamount to one of drug unavailability. In the case in which drug taking is resumed, naltrexone maintenance may be viewed as a quasi-naturalistic extinction paradigm, insofar as drug craving and drug use are not reinforced by drug effect (euphoria) owing to the naltrexone blockade. However, taking naltrexone presupposes a level of motivation on the patient's part at least commensurate with rendering himself or herself unable to experience the eurphorogenic effects of opioids for the following 24–36 h. The best results from naltrexone maintenance have therefore been in the context of family support [66], psychotherapy support, and external limits on behavior [57,67], all of which sustain and enhance the patient's motivation to continue naltrexone maintenance.

Maintenance on naltrexone has not shown serious side effects, although it does increase adrenocorticotropia hormone (ACTH) levels and levels of other hormones as well as affecting the endogenous opioid system [30]. One consideration in the implementation of a long-acting naltrexone delivery system has been the potential impairment of the patient's endogenous opioid system during severe stress, for example, an automobile accident. However, patients have been maintained on naltrexone for 2–3 years without serious side effects. Those side effects that have been reported include headaches, gastrointestinal distress, and potential hepatotoxicity [30].

Much of the preceding discussion presupposes a model in which the continued use of drugs is motivated by a need to reduce the physiological distress of opioid withdrawal. Drug use, however, has also been linked to the need to reduce non–drug-related psychological distress, such as anxiety and depression [68]. It has been suggested that opioid use ameliorates social isolation [69]. Yet there is no evidence that naltrexone reduces the intensity of these negative psychological states. In addition, there is increasing evidence that drug addiction is mediated by a positive reinforcement system, centered in the medial forebrain bundle, which links the medial basal forebrain to the ventral tegmental area of the midbrain [70], anatomically and functionally distinct from the site of the negative reinforcing system in the brainstem [8]. The positive reinforcement system generates approach behavior based on incentive motivation independent of the reduction of needs, drives, or dysphoric states. Research into positive and negative reinforcement systems points to drug-seeking behavior as governed by fundamental motivational systems which are protected by evolution because of their intrinsic survival functions. Animal studies suggest that the "artificial" drug activation of the reward system, a system which has evolved for adaptive functioning when activated by "natural" reinforcers such as food, sex, and love, may constitute a profoundly and "unnaturally" powerful stimulation that evolution has not equipped mammals to deal with. We note that this powerful activation of the reward system by addictive drugs exerts such profound control over behavior that we would not expect such treatment tactics as naltrexone administration together with admonishments and adjurations to by themselves have much of an effect on drug-seeking behavior.

A basic treatment strategy for patients in aftercare should be the development of adaptive rewards whose attainment is incompatible with drug use. This establishes avoidance behavior with respect to drugs, and approach behavior toward non–drug-related objects, people, and contexts. However, it is often difficult to create for drug-addicted individuals, particularly inner-city addicts, conditions of life which favor the activation of the reward system in contexts other than drug use. The development of family support systems, rewarding employment, and a sustained sense of self-esteem are not usually attainable in short-term treatments. Nor is the inner strength necessary for coping with adversity readily constituted. Thus, with naltrexone we can block the effects of opioids, but we cannot—and would not—pharmacologically abolish the need for comfort, love, self-worth, novelty, and even "fun," which, when chronically unavailable, may become incarnated in the form of an all too readily available drug. In this chapter, we have attempted to show that opioid antagonists and partial agonists have an important potential for creating a variety of treatment contexts in which these "natural" positive reinforcers can, over time, be individually developed.

ACKNOWLEDGMENTS

Supported by the National Institute on Drug Abuse, Grants P50-DA04050, R18-DA06190, 5T32-DA7238 and KO2-DA00112 (TRK).

REFERENCES

1. Dehmael, S., Klett, F., and Buhringer, G. (1986). Description and first results of an outpatient drug-free treatment program for opiate dependents, *Treating Addictive Behaviors* (W.E. Miller and N. Heather, eds.). New York, Plenum Press, p. 263.
2. Guyton, A.C. *Textbook of Medical Physiology*, Philadelphia, Saunders, 1986.
3. Marken, R.S. (1988). The nature of behavior: Control as fact and theory, *Behav. Sci., 33*:196–206.
4. Cannon, W.B. (1929). Organization for physiological homeostatis, *Physiol. Rev., 9*:399–431.
5. Weiner, N. *Cybernetics, or Control and Communication in the Animal and the Machine*, New York, MIT Press & Wiley.
6. Powers, W.T. (1973). *Behavior: The Control of Perception*. New York, Alpine de Gruyter.
7. Kosten, T.R. (1990). Neurobiology of Abused Drugs, *J. Nerv. Ment. Dis. 178*(4):217–227.
8. Wise, R.A. (1988). The neurobiology of craving: Implications for the understanding and treatment of addiction, *J. Abnorm. Psychol., 97*:118–132.
9. Bozarth, M.A., and Wise, R.A. (1981). Intracranial self-administration of morphine into the ventral tegmental area of rats, *Life Sci., 28*:551–555.
10. Bozarth, M.A., and Wise, R.A. (1982). Localization of the reward-relevant opiate receptors, *Problems of Drug Dependence, 1982* (L.S. Harris, ed.). Rockville, Maryland, National Institute of Drug Abuse, p. 171.
11. Bozarth, M.A., and Wise, R.A. (1984). Anatomically distinct opiate receptor fields mediate reward and physical dependence, *Science, 224*:516–517.
12. Wei, E.T., Loh, H.H., and Way, E.L. (1973). Brain sites of precipitated abstinence in morphine-dependent rats, *J. Pharmacol. Exp. Ther., 185*:108–115.
13. Wei, E.T., Sigel, S., and Way, E.L. (1975). Regional sensitivity of the rat brain to the inhibitory effects of morphine on wet shake behavior, *J. Pharmacol. Exp. Ther., 193*:56–63.
14. Foote, S.L., Bloom, F.E., and Aston-Jones, G. (1983). Nucleus locus coeruleus: New evidence of anatomical and physiological specificity, *Physiol. Rev., 63*:844–914.
15. Redmond, D.E., Jr., and Krystal, J.H. (1984). Multiple mechanisms of withdrawal from opioid drugs, *Ann. Rev. Neurosci., 7*:443–478.
16. Guitart, X., and Nestler, E.J. (1989). Identification of morphine- and cyclic AMP-regulated phosphoproteins (MARPPs) in the locus coeruleus and other regions of rat brain: Regulations by acute and chronic morphine, *J. Neursci., 9*(12):4371–4387.
17. Nestler, E.J. (in press). Opiate withdrawal and the rat locus coeruleus: Behavioral, electrophysiological, and biochemical correlates, *J. Neurosci.,*
18. Milby, J.B., Gurwitch, R.H., Wiebe, D.J., Ling, W., McLellan, T., and Woody, G.E. (1986). Prevalence and diagnostic reliability of methadone maintenance detoxification fear, *Am. J. Psychiatry, 143*(6):739–743.
19. Loh, H.H., Tao, P.-L., and Smith, A.P. (1988). Invited review: Role receptor regulation in opioid tolerance mechanisms, *Synapse, 2*:457–462.
20. Christie, M.J., Williams, J.T., and North, R.A. (1987). Cellular mechanisms of opioid tolerance: Studies in single brain neurons, *Mol. Pharmacol., 32*:633–638.
21. Nestler, E.J., Terwilliger, R., Erdos, J.J., Dulman, R.S., and Tallman, J.F. (1989). Regulation by chronic morphine of G-proteins in the rat locus coerlueus, *Brain. Res., 476*–230–239.
22. Charney, D.S., Redmond, D.E., and Galloway, M.P. (1984). Naltrexone precipitated withdrawal in methadone addicted human subjects: Evidence for noradrenergic hyperactivity, *Life Sci., 35*:1263–1272.
23. Robins, L.N. Addicts' careers, *Handbook on Drug Abuse* (R.I. Dupont, A. Goldstein, J. O'Donnell, and B. Brown, eds.). Rockville, Maryland, National Institute of Drug Abuse, 1979.
24. Kosten, T.R., Kleber, H.D., and Kreek, M.J. (in press). Arresting the spread of aids: Pharmacotherapy for intravenous heroin addiction, *Sci. Am.,*
25. Jaffe, J.H., and Martin, W.R. Opioid analgesics and antagonists *The Pharmacological Basis of Therapeutics* (7th ed.) (A.G. Goodman and L.S. Gilman, eds.). New York, Macmillan, 1985, pp. 491–531.

26. Martin, W.R., Wikler, A., Endes, C.G., and Pescor, F.T. (1963). Tolerance to and ophysical dependence on morphine in rats, *Psychopharmacology, 4*:247–260.

27. Martin, W.R., and Jasinski, D.R. (1969). Physiological parameters of morphine dependence in man—tolerance, early abstinence, protracted withdrawal, *J. Psychiatr. Res., 7*:9–17.

28. Rounsaville, B.J., Kosten, T.R., and Kleber, H.D. (1985). Success and failure at outpatient opioid detoxification. Evaluating the process of clonidine- and methadone-assisted withdrawal, *J. Nerv. Ment. Dis., 173*:103–110.

29. Jaffe, J.H. Pharmacological agents in treatment of drug dependence *Psychopharmacology: The Third Generation of Progress* (H.Y. Meltzer, ed.). New York, Raven Press, 1987, pp. 1605–1616.

30. Kleber, H.D. (1985). Naltrexone, *J. Subst. Abuse Treat., 2*:117–122.

31. Sells, S.B. Follow-up and Treatment Outcome, *Substance Abuse: Clinical Problems and Perspectives*, (J.H. Lowinson and P. Ruiz, eds.). Baltimore, Williams & Wilkins, 1981, p. 783.

32. Kreek, M.J. Multiple drug abuse patterns and medical consequences, *Psychopharmacology: The Third Generation Of Progress* (H.Y. Meltzer, ed.). New York, Raven Press, 1987, p. 1597.

33. Gold, M.S., Redmond, D.E., and Kleber, H.D. (1978). Clonidine for opiate withdrawal, *Lancet, 1*:929–930.

34. Kleber, H.D., Topazian, M., Gaspari, J., Riordan, C.E., and Kosten, T.R. (1987). Clonidine and naltrexone in the outpatient treatment of heroin withdrawal, *Am. J. Drug. Alcohol Abuse, 13*:1–17.

35. Blachly, P., Casey, D., Marcel, L., and Denney, D. Rapid detoxification from heroin and methadone using naltrexone, *Developments in the Field of Drug Abuse* (E. Senay, V. Shutey, and H. Alkesne, eds.). Rochester, Vermont, Schenkman, 1975, p. 327.

36. Kurland, A.A., and McCabe, L. (1976). Rapid detoxification of the narcotic addict with naloxone hydrochloride: A preliminary report, *Clin. Pharmacol., 16*:66–75.

37. Resnick, R.B., Kentenbaum, R.S., and Washton, A. (1977). Naloxone-precipitated withdrawal: A method for rapid induction onto naltrexone, *Clin. Pharmacol. Ther., 21*:409–413.

38. Meyer, D.R., and Sparber, S.B. (1976). Clonidine antagonized body weight loss and other symptoms used to measure withdrawal in morphine-pellated rates given naloxone, *Pharmacologist, 18*:236.

39. Riordan, C.E., and Kleber, H.D. (1980). Rapid opiate detoxification with clonidine and naltrexone, *Lancet, 2*:1079–1080.

40. Charney, D.S., Riordan, C.E., and Kleber, H.D. (1982). Clonidine and naltrexone: A safe, effective, and rapid treatment of abrupt withdrawal from methadone therapy, *Arch. Gen. Psychiatry, 39*:1327–1332.

41. Charney, D.S., Heninger, G.R., and Kleber, H.D. (1986). The combined use of clonidine and naltrexone as a rapid, safe, and effective treatment of abrupt withdrawal from methadone, *Am. J. of Psychiatry, 143*:831–837.

42. Krystal, J.S., Heninger, G.R., and Walker, M.W. (in press). Intermittent naxolone attenuates the development of dependence on methodone in rhesus monkeys, *Eur. J. Pharmacol.,*

43. Jacob, J.J.C., Michaud, G.M., and Trembley, E.C. (1979). Mixed agonist-antagonist opiates and physical dependence, *Br. J. Clin. Pharmacol., 7*:291s–296s.

44. Martin, W.R. (1979). History and development of mixed opioid agonists, partial agonists and antagonists, *Br. J. Clin. Pharmacol., 7*:273S–279S.

45. Lewis, J.W. (1985). Buprenorphine, *Drug Alcohol Depend., 14*:363–372.

46. Jasinski, D.R., Pevnick, J.S., and Griffith, J.D. (1978). Human pharmacology and abuse potential of the analgesic buprenorphine, *Arch. Gen. Psychiatry, 35*:510–516.

47. Bickel, W.K., Stitzer, M.L., Bigelow, G.E., Liebson, I.A., Jasinski, D.R., and Johnson, R.E. (1988). A clinical trial of buprenophine comparison with methadone in the detoxification of heroin addicts, *Clin. Pharmacol. Rev., 43*:72–78.

48. Kosten, T.R., Kleber, H.D. (1988). Buprenorphine detoxification for opioid dependence: A pilot study, *Life Sci., 42*:635–641.

49. Kosten, T.R. (in press). New approaches for rapid detoxification and induction onto naltrexone, *Adv. Alcohol. Subst. Abuse.*

50. Kosten, T.R., Rounsaville, B.J., and Kleber, H.D. (1986). A 2.5-year follow-up treatment retention and reentry among opioid addicts, *J. Subst. Abuse Treat., 3*:181–189.
51. Kosten, T.R., Kleber, H.D., and Morgan, C. (1989). Treatment of cocaine abuse with buprenorphine, *Biol. Psychiatry, 26*:637–639.
52. Kosten, T.R., Krystal, J.H., Charney, D.S., Price, L.H., Morgan, C.H., and Kleber, H.D. Opioid antagonist challenges in buprenorphine maintained patients, *Drug Alcohol Depend., 25*:73–78, 1990.
53. Kosten, T.R. Current Pharmacotherapies for opioid dependence, *Psychopharmacol. Bull., 26*:69–74, 1990.
54. Jasinski, D.R., Boren, J.J., Henningfield, J.E., et al. (1984). Progress report from the NIDA Addiction Research Center, Baltimore, Maryland (L.S. Harris, ed.) *Problems of Drug Dependence 1983*, National Institute of Drug Abuse, Research Monograph 49, Rockville, Maryland, pp. 69–76.
55. Kosten, T.R., Krystal, J.H., Charney, D.S., Price, L.H., Morgan, C.H., and Kleber, H.D. (1989). Rapid detoxification from opioid dependence, *Am. J. Psychiatry, 146*(10):1349.
56. Anton, R.F., Hogan, I., and Jalali, G. (1981). Multiple family therapy and naltrexone in the treatment of opioid dependence, *Drug Alcohol Depend., 8*:157–168.
57. Kleber, H.D., and Kosten, T.R. (1984). Naltrexone induction: Psychologic and pharmacologic strategies, *J. Clin. Psychiatry, 45*:29–38.
58. Kleber, H.D. (1986). The role of the family in the clinical use of naltrexone, *Subst. Abuse Bull., 2*(1):1–6.
59. Murphy, P.N., Bentall, R.P., and Owens, R.G. (1989). The experience of opioid abstinence: The relevance of motivation and history, *Br. J. Addict., 84*:673–679.
60. Wikler, A. (1980). *Opioid Dependence: Mechanisms and Treatment*. New York, Plenum Press.
61. Stewart, J., de Wit, H., and Eikelboom, R. (1984). Role of unconditioned and conditioned drug effects in the self-administration of opiates and stimulants, *Psychiatry Rev., 91*(2):251–268.
62. Baker, T.B., Morse, E., and Sherman, J.E. The motivation to use drugs: A psychobiological analysis of urges, *Nebraska Symposium on Motivation: Alcohol and Addictive Behaviors* (P.C. Rivers, ed.). University of Nebraska Press, Lincoln, Nebraska, 1986, pp. 257–323.
63. Niaura, R.S., Rohsenow, D.J., Binkoff, J.A., Monti, P.M., Pedraza, M., and Abrams, D.B. (1988). Relevance of cue reactivity to understanding alcohol and smoking relapse, *J. Abnorm. Psychol., 97*:133–152.
64. Tiffany, S.T. (1990). A cognitive model of drug urges and drug-use behavior: Role of automatic and nonautomatic processes, *Psychol. Bull., 97*:147–168.
65. Meyer, R.B., and Mirin, S.M. A psychology of craving: Implications of behavioral research, *Substance Abuse: Clinical Problems and Perspectives* (J.H. Lowinson and P. Ruiz, eds.). Baltimore, Williams & Wilkins, 1981, p. 57.
66. Kosten, T.R., Jalali, B., Hogan, I., and Kleber, H. (1983). Family denial as a prognostic factor in opiate addict treatment outcome, *J. Nerv. Ment. Dis., 171*(10):611–616.
67. McLellan, A.T., Woody, G.E., Luborsky, L., and Coehl, L. (1988). Is the counselor an "active ingredient" in substance abuse rehabilitation? An examination of treatment success among our counselors, *J. Nerv. Ment. Dis. 176*(7):423–430.
68. Khantzian, E.J. (1985). The self-medication hypothesis addictive disorders: focus on heroin and cocaine dependence, *Am. J. Psychiatry, 142*:1259–1264.
69. Panksepp, J., Herman, B., Conner, R., Bishop, P., and Scott, J.P. (1978). The biology of social attachments: Opiates alleviate separation distress, *Biol. Psychiatry, 13*(5):607–618.
70. Wise, R.A. The brain and reward, *The Neuropharmacological Basis of Reward* (J.M. Liebman and S.J. Cooper, eds.). New York Oxford Science, 1989, p. 377.

APPENDIX

A. Treatment Protocols

The following schedules assume that detoxification procedures will begin at 8:30 a.m. The duration of successive phases can be adjusted for different starting times. In addition to the protocols described below, a short-acting benzodiazepine (oxacepam, 15–30 mg, every 6 h) can be administered to control muscle cramps and insomnia during detoxification. As with the other drugs used, only enough oxazepam should be dispensed to meet the needs of the patient until the next regularly scheduled visit.

Clonidine Detoxification

This procedure is designed to take place over a 10-day period.

1. Day 1: clonidine, 0.2 mg p.o. at 9:00 a.m. Blood pressure to be checked every 15 min for 1 hour, then every 30 min for an additional hour. Patients should be discharged with enough clonidine to take up to a total of 0.8 mg (0.2 mg every 6 hours) or less, as needed. Oxazepam can be dispensed 15–30 mg every 6 hours as needed (maximum dose of 90 mg/24 h).
2. Days 2–9: Patients should be seen daily. Clonidine can be administered (if appropriate) at 8:30 a.m., and vital signs should be monitored until at least 10:30 a.m. Appropriate medications (clonidine and oxazepam) should be dispensed according to the patient's withdrawal symptoms and blood pressure toleration, with the blood pressure cut off being 85/55 mm Hg with minimal orthostatic changes. Over several days after days 5–7 the clonidine should be tapered appropriately.
3. Days 10–12: initiation of naltrexone maintenance: Patients who have been opioid free (as determined by history and urine toxicology) will be started on naltrexone (25 mg day 9; 50 mg on subsequent days, if appropriate) while withdrawal symptoms are monitored.

Patients undergoing this detoxification procedure will have completed detoxification by day 12.

Clonidine-Naltrexone Detoxification

This procedure is designed to take place over a 3- to 4-day period. Patients undergoing this detoxification will spend an entire day in the medical facility for observation of withdrawal symptoms on day 1 and on day 2, if necessary. This requirement reflects the fact that withdrawal is induced by administration of naltrexone. Visits on subsequent days (days 3–4) are generally brief.

1. Day 1
    a. Clonidine: 0.2 mg p.o. at 9:00 a.m. and every 4 h for a daily total of up to 1.0 mg. Blood pressure should be checked every 15 min for 1 h, then every 30 min for the next 6 h.
    b. Oxazepam: 15–30 mg p.o. at 9:00 a.m., 15–30 mg orally every 6 h as needed, for a maximum daily total of 90 mg. Increased initial dosage is needed to control the muscle cramps induced by naltrexone.
    c. Naltrexone: 12.5 mg p.o. at 10:0 a.m.
2. Day 2: similar to day 1, except 25 mg of naltrexone should be administered.
3. Days 3–4: similar to days 1 and 2, except that 50 mg of naltrexone is administered. <?> Clonidine and oxazepam tapering should begin so that they are discontinued by day 5.

By day 4, patients will be on blocking doses of naltrexone and ready to be followed on a naltrexone maintenance program.

Buprenorphine Detoxification (experimental, need IND [investigational new drug] from FDA)

This procedure is designed to take place over a 10 to 12-day period of time. This includes a 7-day buprenorphine induction phase, in which patients are started and maintained on buprenorphine, 3 mg sublingually for 1 week. This allows patients a 7-day period to be free of i.v. opioid use. This is followed by naloxone-precipitated withdrawal on day 8 followed by naltrexone induction.

1. Days 1–8: Buprenorphine: 3 mg sublingually at 9:00 a.m. (IND is needed, since the usual dose is 0.2–0.3 mg subcutaneously).
2. Day 9: Patients who are opioid free for 3 days and who have a negative urine toxicology for opioids on day 8 will proceed onto the following schedule.
    a.   9:30 a.m.: clonidine, 0.2 mg orally.
    b.   10:00 .am.: naloxone, 35 mg i.v. (an IND is needed, since the usual dose is about 0.4 mg.)
    c.   10:00 a.m.–12:00 p.m.: vital signs taken every 15 min; patient observed for withdrawal symptoms.
    d.   2:00 p.m.: naltrexone, 12.5 mg orally.
    e.   oxazepam, 15–30 mg orally every 6 h if needed up to a maximum of 90 mg.
3. Day 10: naltrexone can be increased to 25 mg beginning in the morning. Patients should be monitored for withdrawal symptoms for 2 h, and sent home with tapered doses of clonidine and oxazepam, if needed.
4. Days 11–12: naltrexone can be increased to 50 mg/day. Clonidine and oxazepam doses should be tapered to 0.

Patients undergoing this detoxification procedure will have completed it by day 12.

62

Pharmacotherapeutic Interventions for Cocaine Addiction

Thomas R. Kosten
Yale University School of Medicine, New Haven, Connecticut

I. INTRODUCTION

Cocaine addiction has become a major public health problem in the United States, with over 20 million abusers (Adams and Durell, 1984). With a problem of this magnitude, most psychiatrists, mental health professionals, and even general medical practitioners can expect to be confronted with these patients. Because the treatment of drug-addicted patients is frequently conducted by subspecialists, many specialized techniques and conceptual models of treatment may be unfamiliar to general mental health practitioners. These techniques include purely psychological treatments for helping cocaine addicts, but these psychological treatments have some limitations with the more severe intravenous and free-base cocaine addicts of the 1980s and 1990s (Carroll et al., 1987; Kleber and Gawin, 1986). Thus, new pharmacological treatments have been developed as adjuncts, and specific, manual-guided psychotherapies based on interpersonal psychotherapy and Marlatt's relapse prevention program have also been integrated with these pharmacological approaches to cocaine addiction (Rounsaville et al., 1985). This chapter will attempt to place these psychotherapies and medications in a practical clinical context that deals with the heterogeneity of patients in a typical clinical practice.

Cocaine addiction pharmacotherapies have included desipramine and lithium to reduce long-term relapse and bromocriptine and amantadine to reduce acute cocaine craving. These pharmacological adjuncts to cocaine addiction treatment are beginning to be widely used, and critical issues have arisen in their proper use. The issues include whom to treat with medications, when to treat and for how long, what are cocaine abuse pharmacotherapies, where or which settings are best suited for the initiation and maintenance of treatments, and how to match patients to specific treatments. These five major issues in matching cocaine addicts to appropriate treatments are shown in Table 1, along with several key items to be

Adapted from *Journal of Nervous and Mental Disease, 177*(7):379–387, 1989. Copyright by Williams and Wilkins. Reprinted by permission.

Table 1 Issues in Matching Patients to Treatments

Issue	Determining factors
Whom to treat	Neuroadaptation—high-intensity users (e.g., free-basers)
	Psychiatric vulnerability—concurrent affective disorders
	Medical risk—cardiac disease, pulmonary dysfunction
When to treat	Precipitants
	Recovery phases—crash, withdrawal, extinction
	Relapse potential
What treatments	Acute vs chronic
	Psychiatric or medical comorbidity
	Other drug abuse
Where to treat	Inpatient
	Outpatient maintenance
How to match	Abuse severity—route and amount used
	Recovery phase
	Comorbidity

considered in addressing each issue. The subsequent sections will develop these items in discussing each issue.

II. WHOM TO TREAT

Among the large number of cocaine addicts, who is an appropriate candidate for pharmacological adjuncts? In addressing this question, the reasons that a "recreational" cocaine user becomes dependent on cocaine and seeks treatment may dictate important aspects of the treatment approach. Three general categories of patients are recognized as appropriate for pharmacological interventions: those who have developed neuroadaptation to heavy cocaine use, those who have psychiatric vulnerability, and those who have substantial medical risks from continued cocaine use.

The first category includes cocaine users who switch to the high-intensity routes of cocaine administration—intravenous or free-base smoking—and then markedly increase their quantity and frequency of cocaine use. This high-intensity transition may lead to neuroadaptation or functional brain changes in various neurotransmitter systems (e.g., dopamine or serotonin) (Gold et al., 1985; Spyraki et al., 1982; Wise, 1984). Although the details of this neuroadaptation model are incomplete, much useful information has been drawn from animal studies of cocaine self-administration and from the neurochemical changes that are induced by cocaine in animals (Spyraki et al., 1982; Wise, 1984). When animals are repeatedly administered cocaine, dopaminergic receptors are changed and develop increased sensitivity (Taylor et al., 1979). This neurochemical change may be related to the substantial prolactin changes that have been observed in human cocaine abusers (Gawin and Kleber, 1985).* Prolactin is particularly interesting, because it is regulated by dopamine, and brain dopaminergic pathways are thought to underlie some of the reinforcing actions of cocaine (Buckman and Peake, 1978; Wise, 1984). Further evidence for actual structural brain changes induced by cocaine in heavy human users has been presented in studies using magnetic resonance

---

* I. Extein, W.Z. Potter, M.S. Gold, et al. Persistent neurochemical deficit in cocaine abuse. Paper presented at the 140th Meeting of the American Psychiatric Association, Chicago, IL, May 10–15, 1987.

imaging.* In these studies, small areas of cortical damage have been described, suggesting that neuroadaptation during chronic cocaine addiction may be part of a process by the brain to control damage from cocaine use. Abnormalities have also been noted in neuropsychological testing of heavy cocaine addicts, again suggesting some damage or derangement in brain functioning, although specific anatomical or neurochemical localization is not possible with these tests (Siegel, 1984). Thus, high-intensity cocaine use may induce brain changes that may require biological interventions to reverse and to halt the cocaine addiction. One example of such a change that can be reversed by a pharmacological treatment in animals is the supersensitivity of dopaminergic receptors induced by cocaine. This supersensitivity can be reversed by tricyclic antidepressants, and in the animal studies this reversal is associated with improvement in cocaine-induced behavioral deficits (Kokkinidis et al., 1980).

The second category includes patients with psychiatric vulnerabilities. These patients come to treatment with lesser amounts of cocaine use and lower-intensity routes of administration. Compared with addicts without psychiatric comorbidity, our cocaine addicts with concurrent psychiatric disorders such as depression use significantly less cocaine and are more likely to use it intranasally (Gawin and Kleber, in press). In studies of treatment-seeking cocaine addicts, the rates of pscyhiatric disorders have been substantial, including both affective and personality disorders (Kleber and Gawin, 1984; Weiss et al., 1986). Depression has been the most common disorder, with up to 35 % of the cocaine abusers being currently depressed, but interesting subgroups of patients with relatively rare disorders such as adult attention deficit disorder (ADD) have also been observed. It is tempting to speculate that these patients with concurrent disorders may use cocaine to self-medicate. They would find this solution inadequate relatively rapidly and then seek treatment focusing on the cocaine, but also needing help with the underlying disorder. In terms of a biological model, these patients would already by vulnerable to brain derangement by chronic cocaine use. In contrast to the above "recreational" users, they would experience cocaine-induced disruption earlier and with the lower-intensity administration route (e.g., intranasal) and with lesser amounts of cocaine. The inadequancy of cocaine for ameliorating depression has been shown by Post et al. (1974), and the possibility of cocaine inducing further depression has been strongly suggested (Gawin and Kleber, 1986; Kosten et al., 1987b). In addition to depression, paranoid psychoses may be precipitated by cocaine, and patients may acutely need pharmacological treatment (Castellani et al., 1985). Whether these psychotic patients have an underlying psychiatric vulnerability or this is purely a pharmacologicla effect of cocaine has been difficult to determine in a general way, but some patients have clear underlying disorders and are sensitive to surprisingly small doses of cocaine (McLellan et al., 1979). Moreover, a large group of psychiatrically vulnerable cocaine addicts may be in need of pharmacological treatments for somewhat different reasons than the recreational users who go through a transition to high-intensity use.

The third category includes patients with significant medical risks from continued cocaine addiction. Within this category are the intravenous cocaine addicts who share needles and are thereby at risk of developing acquired immune deficiency syndrome (AIDS). Aggressive interventions are justified in trying to halt their cocaine addiction, because of both the individual and public health risks of their particular route of cocaine administration (Des Jarlais et al., 1985; Kosten et al., 1987a).

Another group of patients to be considered are those who have sustained major medical illnesses due to cocaine. Again the intravenous user who develops endocarditis is one

---

*F.H. Gawin and R. Byck. Magnetic resonance imaging in chronic cocaine abusers: A preliminary report. Paper presented at the American College of Neuropsychopharmacology, 1984.

example because continued intravenous use could lead to acute heart valve failure and rapid death (Cherabin, 1967). The myocardial damage that has been described with cocaine may also be an indication for pharmacological interventions with affected addicts (Cregler and Mark, 1986; Gay, 1982). When considering pharmacological treatment of these medically ill patients, the risks from the medications themselves need careful assessment. Some of the treatment options can themselves have risks of cardiac toxicity, and if the patient combines cocaine with the treatment medication the further risks are largely unknown, but are potentially fatal (Ritchie and Greene, 1985). Well-informed clinical judgment on the risks and benefits to each patient is clearly needed.

A more difficult clinical decision in this category of medical risk indications involves pregnancy. Most physicians are quite uneasy about prescribing any medication to women during pregnancy, and the pharmacological management of drug addiction has a very limited place during pregnancy. Because significant neonatal problems have been described with cocaine-addicted mothers, pharmacological approaches to cocaine addiction treatment in pregnancy could compound these problems if the mother continued to use cocaine while taking a treatment medication (Chasnoff et al., 1986). Thus, pharmacological management should generally be avoided. However, for opiate-addicted pregnant women, methadone maintenance has been recommended (Finnegan et al., 1972). Many of the heroin-addicted women seeking treatment during pregnancy are also addicted to cocaine in combination, called a "speedball" by the addicts (Kosten et al., 1986). For these cocaine addicts with concurrent opiate addiction, methadone maintenance should be considered for several reasons. First, methadone is a well-established treatment for the opiate addict. Second, by having the pregnant women in treatment, the provider can work with her on the cocaine addiction using psychological approaches. Third, prenatal care can be arranged through the methadone program. Overall, management of the cocaine-addicted pregnant women is a very difficult problem, and residential treatment should be strongly encouraged to remove access to all illicit drugs.

III. WHEN TO TREAT

A second critical issue for cocaine addiction pharmacotherapy is when to initiate treatment and, as a corollary, when to stop the medications. There are five important points in addressing this issue, as shown in Table 2. First are phases in the recovery process from cocaine addiction. Second are precipitants of seeking treatment and of decreases in cocaine use. Third are the psychosocial problems associated with increases in cocaine use. Fourth is the central role of depression in cocaine addiction, and fifth is relapse potential as a determinant of pharmacotherapy duration.

Recovery from cocaine addiction can be conceptualized as evolving over a three-phase process. These phases have been identified by our group as the crash, withdrawal, and extinction phases (Gawin and Kleber, 1986). The symptoms that occur during each of these phases may respond best to different pharmacological strategies. During the crash phase, lasting from only a few hours to 4 days, the symptom picture may be dominated by sleep and show no indication for medications. In other cases, significant paranoia and agitation may require the use of neuroleptics (Castellani et al., 1985). When these patients become suicidal, hospitalization may be required. During the withdrawal phase, lasting from 2 to 10 weeks, the potential for relapse is higher, and pharmacological adjuncts to treatment are most clearly indicated in those addicts who have previously relapsed in nonpharmacological treatment regimens. The symptom pattern can closely resemble a depressive disorder with intense craving for cocaine (Gawin and Kleber, 1986). This intense craving may simply lead to impulsive use, but can also be associated with significant anticipatory anxiety when patients reenter settings in which they previously used cocaine. Unfortunately, because these

Table 2 When to Start and Stop Medications

Precipitants of seeking treatment
  Arrest or other legal pressure
  Acute medical emergency, overdose
  Family or social pressure
  Multiple relapses in self-treatment
Phases of recovery
  Crash (2–18 h): paranoid, suicidal
  Withdrawal (2–10 weeks): anxious, depressed
  Extinction (3–12 months): conditioned craving cues
Associated psychosocial problems
  Resolution of legal problems
  Medical stabilization
  Family and other social supports
  Employment and future income
  Addiction to another drug concurrent with cocaine
Psychiatric comorbidity in some addicts
  Depression and suicidality
  Underlying cyclothymia
  Antisocial personality disorder
Relapse potential and stopping medications
  Stabilization in psychotherapy
  Control of any concurrent drug addiction

settings frequently include places of employment and recreation, their avoidance may require major life disruptions. In the severe cases of cocaine addiction, the required level of "disruption" may be 4–8 weeks of inpatient hospitalization. In these cases, extensive planning is then needed for aftercare, when patients will reenter the settings associated with their cocaine addiction.

During the extinction phase, lasting from 3 to 12 months, relapse to cocaine use becomes more closely tied to a limited number of environmental cues that stimulate cocaine craving, and craving is not a pervasive aspect of the abuser's daily life. At this phase of recovery it would be very unusual to initiate any new medication, and the question is when to stop any medications that have been started during the previous two phases of recovery. The type of patient being treated is an important determinant of when to stop medications, inasmuch as the underlying problems of patients in the psychiatric vulnerability category may require more extended treatment than would be possible for patients in the neuroadaptation category.

The precipitants of seeking treatment and of decreases in cocaine use were addressed by our group in a recent 2.5-year follow-up of cocaine addicts (Kosten et al., in press). Because these were primarily heavy intravenous users who frequently used opiates concurrently, their severe problems may not be evident among recreational cocaine users who snort cocaine on weekends. However, less severe recreational users are probably also not candidates for pharmacological interventions. In our sample, we broke the 30-month follow-up period into five 6-month blocks and compared the 6 months before, during, and after the index events of either starting or stopping cocaine-addicted behavior. In the 6 months just before stopping cocaine-addicted behavior addiction, these addicts had substantially increased medical and legal problems, suggesting that these problems motivated them to decrease their use (Kosten et al., in press). The legal problems included arrests for crimes against property and persons. Clearly, the criminal justice system can make some impact on cocaine addiction, inasmuch as none of these addicts went to jail for more than a few days, and almost all of them substantially reduced or stopped their cocaine use for the next 6 months. The medical problems made an impact on a somewhat different subgroup of these addicts who were usually not arrested for crimes; instead, they suffered from major medical complicationsof their cocaine use. Because these were primarily intravenous users, abscesses and systematic infection were common and some had developed symptoms of AIDS. Free-base users are not without major medical complications, however, as illustrated by several famous users who were burned in free-base explosions and by recent reports of lung damage in free-base smokers (Weiss et al., 1981). Thus, cocaine addicts tend to seek treatment after experiencing substantial legal or medical problems, and these medical problems must be carefully considered before initiating pharmacological interventions for their cocaine addiction.

The problems associated with increased use of cocaine were also examined in our 2.5-year follow-up (Kosten et al., 1987a, 1988a, in press). When cocaine abuse increased from occasional (one to four times per month) to more intensive use (up to six times a day), problems accumulated in a wide range of areas. Legal and medical problems, which led to treatment seeking, clearly rose, and other areas such as employment, family, and psychological problems got worse. Cocaine addiction was not a circumscribed habit with little impact on lifestyle; instead, its use pervaded the lives of these addicts and wrought many other problems. Because of the massive psychosocial problems associated with escalating cocaine addiction, the risks of pharmacological interventions must be carefully weighed, but frequently are considered relatively low.

The central role of depression in cocaine addiction is demonstrated not only by the striking resemblance of the cocaine withdrawal syndrome to a depressive disorder, but also by our finding that depressive disorders were the only disorders that predicted increased cocaine use over our 2.5-year follow-up (Kleber and Gawin, 1984; Kosten et al., 1987a; Weiss et al., 1986). The concept of self-medication for affective disorderes with cocaine is a reasonable speculation suggesting some specific utility for antidepressants in cocaine addiction treatment. Because depression predicts subsequent cocaine addiction, then pharmacological treatment of this depression may indeed be an important preventive strategy with those at risk for cocaine addiction.

Relapse potential determines the duration of pharmacotherapy, and this potential for relapse will vary by the category of patient, the phase of recovery, concurrent psychotherapeutic progress, and the precipitants of seeking treatment. The psychiatric vulnerability category of patient and to some extent the medical-risk patient will probably need more extended treatment than the current treatment trials of 1–3 months (Gawin and Kleber, 1984; Giannini et al., 1986; Kosten et al., 1987b; Tennant and Sagherian, 1987).* For those two categories of patients, extending medication maintenance during the extinction phase of recovery to 6 months or more would be reasonable. For the earlier phases of recovery (e.g., crash and withdrawal), the duration of medication maintenance is closely related to the type of medication being used. As an example, if a neuroleptic such as chlorpromazine is started owing to psychotic symptoms during the crash, its continuation should be carefully reassessed daily over the first 2 weeks of treatment. Because chronic treatment with these agents can produce tardive dyskinesias, their use should be kept to a minimum in patients without schizophrenia or related psychotic disorders (Task Force on Late Neurological Effects of Antipsychotic Drugs, 1980).

---

*C. O'Brien. Controlled studies of pharmacological and behavioral treatments of cocaine dependence. Paper presented at the North American Conference on Cocaine Abuse. Washington, DC. September 16, 1987.

An interesting suggestion has been made with patients who became repeatedly paranoid and threatening with cocaine use (Gawin, 1986a). Neuroleptics were given to several of these patients, and they were instructed to take the medication just before using cocaine in order to prevent violent behavior. It is obviously difficult to implement such a strategy while trying to encourage abstinence from cocaine, but "slips" are not uncommon during the early weeks of treatment, and prevention of disastrous outcomes from a slip is an important consideration. As a second example during the withdrawal phase, a patient might be started on amantadine for several weeks and then have this discontinued with substitution of some other medication or development of a behavior-modification program. The final determinants of when to stop medication are related to the precipitants that either led to or were associated with seeking treatment. Resolution of the medical, legal, or psychosocial problems precipitating treatment must occur before establishing a schedule for stopping an effective pharmacological treatment. Without this resolution, relapse is almost certain.

Resolution of these various problems will depend on the psychotherapeutic relationship developed during any pharmacotherapy. The concurrent psychotherapeutic progress made during treatment with medications is critical to cocaine abstinence either while taking or after stopping medications. Obviously, the simplest arrangement to assure that psychotherapy is complementary and not antagonistic is for the same person to supply the medication and to conduct the psychotherapy; then the medications are likely to be given in the most supportive, yet controlled, atmosphere. However, treatment increasingly is designed as a cooperative effort between a physician prescribing medications and a nonphysican psychotherapist or counselor, and the nonphysician must cultivate in the patient an attitude that supports medication treatment. In a nonsupportive or rejecting atmosphere, the patient may use pharmacotherapy as an excuse for continued addiction and even report increased craving while using medications. In some cases, this induction of craving may indeed occur, such as with methylphenidate in several patients (Kleber and Gawin, 1986), but cocaine craving is not induced by the other medications covered in this overview and would be a very rare complication. The usual issue is a conflict in therapeutic approaches between the medicating physician and the psychotherapist. Medications can be useful adjuncts, but no psychosocial or psychological problem is going to be resolved by a "magic bullet."

While this is not a review of psychotherapeutic approaches to cocaine addiction treatment, approaches must be adopted that are not antagonistic to medication use (Carroll et al., 1987). Any approach that rejects medications as "drugs to treat drugs" is not a compatible adjunct, and this category may unfortunately include some types of self-support groups. Traditional drug counseling can have a major role in coping with the frequent social problems that occur concurrently with cocaine addiction, and a limit-setting type of confrontational style of treatment including urine monitoring has worked well with our cocaine addicts. Drug counselling around concurrent alcohol and opioid use may be particularly effective, if the cocaine addiction is also addressed (Kosten et al., 1987b). In general, progress in psychotherapy or drug counseling can be used as an indication that the patient is ready to discontinue medications, assuming that he or she has remained abstinent from cocaine for several weeks to months. The first weeks after stopping medications should include careful monitoring for relapse by the psychotherapist or counselor, with restarting of the medication, if a relapse or a "slip" occurs. Without real progress in psychotherapy, the patient is unlikely not only to resist effectively cocaine use after stopping the medications, but also to remain compliant with the medications for any sustained period of abstinence. In summary, stopping any effective medication must be considered a trial in a patient with a chronic relapsing disorder such as cocaine addiction, and a good psychotherapeutic relationship will enable the clinician to restart this medication, if needed.

IV. WHAT ARE COCAINE ADDICTION THERAPIES?

The pharmacological treatment of cocaine addiction posits a neurochemical substrate underlying both chronic high-intensity periods of abuse (binges) and the "crash" following these high-intensity use periods (Gawin and Kleber, 1986; Gold et al., 1985; Spyraki et al., 1982; Taylor et al., 1979; Wise, 1984). A number of parallels have been drawn between the intracranial self-stimulation model of cocaine use in animals and the high-intensity human abuse of cocaine by free-base smokers and intravenous users (Gawin and Kleber, 1984, 1986; Gold et al., 1985). The neurochemical alterations induced by chronic cocaine use in animals, including dopaminergic receptor supersensitivity, may also occur in humans and may respond to agents that reduce receptor sensitivity, such as tricyclic antidepressants (Gawin and Kleber, 1984, 1986; Taylor et al., 1979). Other hypotheses have been that dopamine depletion occurs during chronic cocaine use and that either the amino acid precursor—tyrosine—or a direct dopamine agonist (e.g., bromocriptine or L-dopa) would ameliorate the cocaine crash (Gold et al., 1985; Tennant, 1985; Tennant and Sagherian, 1987). Based on these neuroadaptation models, several studies have sought general agents that may reverse cocaine-induced brain changes and thereby possess anticraving properties, block cocaine euphoria, or decrease cocaine crash and withdrawal symptoms.

A. Acute vs Chronic Agents

Two classes of cocaine treatment agents have evolved during the last few years—acute and chronic agents. These various agents are listed in Table 3. Within the group of acute agents, a division can be made between those used primarily during severe crash symptoms and those anticraving agents used for early withdrawal symptom relief. During the crash, neuroleptics may be useful for psychotic symptoms, although two caveats need consideration. First, in cocaine "overdoses," an agitated state associated with hyperthymia has been described and, when in this state, neuroleptics may worsen the condition and even lead to death by heightening the hyperthymia (Kosten and Kleber, 1987, 1988; Mittleman and Wetli, 1984). Second, recent animal data have shown that various neuroleptics may differentially affect mesolimbic dopamine receptors thought to be involved in cocaine's actions (Thierry et al., 1986). Thus, haloperidol, which is at one extreme in this dichotomy, and fluphenazine, which is at the other extreme, may have very different efficacies in the treatment of these crash symptoms. No controlled human work has been done yet on this question. Other agents that are commonly used by cocaine addicts themselves during the crash are benzodiazepines. While a widely abused benzodiazepine such as diazepam would be a poor choice to administer, other agents such as oxazepam have shown less addiction potential and might be considered for several days of use after a heavy cocaine binge (Owen and Tyrer, 1983; Woody et al., 1975). This use of oxazepam for acute symptom relief may be an important strategy to engage a cocaine addict in further drug addiction treatment.

The second division of acute anticraving agents may be particularly useful in ameliorating early withdrawal symptoms after cocaine binges, because these agents appear to have their onset of action within a day of starting (Dackis et al., 1987; Gawin and Kleber, 1986; Giannini and Baumgartel, 1987; Khantzian et al., 1984; Kleber and Gawin, 1986; Kosten et al., 1988b; Morgan et al., in press; Rosen et al., 1986; Tennant and Sagherian, 1987). These agents include amantadine, bromocriptine, L-dopa, and methylphenidate. No adequate, long-term, placebo-controlled, double-blind studies have been done with any of these agents, but their acute efficacy has been suggested in several single-dose, placebo crossover trials (Dackis et al., 1987; Giannini and Baumgartel, 1987; Tennant and Sagherian, 1987). Several trials

Table 3 Types of Pharmacotherapy for Cocaine Addiction

Acute agents	Chronic agents
anticraving activity	general prevention of relapse
amantadine	desipramine
bromocriptine	imipramine
L-dopa	trazedone/serotonergic agents
crash symptom relief	comorbid psychiatric disorders
neuroleptics (e.g., chlorpromazine)	lithium
benzodiazepines (e.g., oxazepam)	methylphenidate or pemoline

have examined amantadine at 200–300 mg daily and found that it reduces craving and use for several days to 3 weeks (Morgan et al., in press; Tennant, in press; Tennant and Sagherian, 1987). Four trials have examined bromocriptine at dosages varying from 0.125 to 0.6 mg three times daily, but have had contradictory results on efficacy owing mostly to dropout due to side effects (Dackis et al., 1987; Giannini and Baumgartel, 1987; Kosten et al., 1988b; Tennant and Sagherian, 1987). Two open studies of L-dopa and methylphenidate have shown short-term (2-week) reductions in cocaine craving (Khantzian et al., 1984; Rosen et al., 1986).

The "chronic" agents have a delayed onset of action in reducing cocaine craving. Desipramine would be typical of this class, and its onset of action is usually delayed for 10–20 days. A rationale for use of these drugs has been that they reduce dopaminergic receptor sensitivity and thereby reverse the cocaine-induced supersensitivity (DeWitt and Wise, 1977; Gawin and Kleber, 1984; Roberts and Koob, 1982; Taylor et al., 1979; Wise 1984). The most carefully controlled studies have been done with these chronic agents. With desipramine, several research groups have reported open and double-blind trials involving more than 150 patients (Gawin and Kleber, 1984; Giannini et al., 1986; Kosten et al., 1987b; Tennant, 1984).* ** These trials have shown significant decreases in cocaine use and craving. One low-dose, short-term trial could not show any difference between placebo and desipramine (Tennant, 1984). The trials by Gawin and Kleber (1984) and by Giannini et al. (1986) have involved "pure" cocaine abusers, whereas those of Kosten et al. (1987b) and O'Brien* have involved methadone-maintained cocaine abusers. In these trials, desipramine has been relatively free of side effects and patients have shown good compliance after an initial dropout rate of 25–30% during the first 2 weeks of treatment. This dropout rate may be due to the relatively delayed onset of desipramine's action, and there may be an important role for the "acute" agents in reducing this dropout rate. Other chronic agents have been suggested in pilot work including imipramine, doxepin, and trazadone (Gawin, 1986b; Rowbotham et al., 1984),† but the results of controlled trials with these agents have not appeared. In future treatment of cocaine addicts, a sequential use of acute and chronic agents may evolve to minimize symptoms and maximize compliance.

---

*C. O'Brien. Controlled studies of pharmacological and behavioral treatments of cocaine dependence. Paper presented at the North American Conference on Cocaine Abuse, Washington, DC. September 16, 1987.

**F.H. Gawin, R. Byck, and H.D. Kleber. Double-blind comparison of desipraine and placebo in chronic cocaine abusers. Paper presented at the 24th meeting of the American College of Neuropharmacology, Kaanapali, Hawaii. December 9–13, 1985.

†J. Rosecan. The treatment of cocaine abuse with imipramine, L-tyrosine, and L-tryptophan. Paper presented at the VII World Congress of Psychiatry, Vienna, Austria. July 14–19, 1983.

B. Role of Comorbid Psychopathology

Other work has examined specific diagnostic subpopulations of cocaine addicts in whom cocaine may be used for self-medication. These studies focus on the category of patients with psychiatric vulnerability. Drug addicts often regulate painful feelings by drug use, and these cocaine-addicted patients have significant comorbid psychopathology, particularly depression (Gawin and Kleber, 1984; Kleber and Gawin, 1984; Kosten et al., 1987a; Rounsaville et al., 1982; Weiss et al., 1986). Cocaine addicts may self-medicate three types of axis I (DSM-III-R; *Diagnostic and Statistical Manual of Mental Disorders*. 3rd edition revised. American Psychiatric Association, Washington, DC., 1987) disorders: ADD, major depressive disorder, and cyclothymia or bipolar disorder. Moderate dosages of stimulant medication have been reported as effective in treating cocaine addicts with ADD (Khantzian et al., 1984), although these medications are generally abused by non-ADD cocaine users. Cocaine addicts with cyclothymia have had a good response to lithium, although this medication has been ineffective in our preliminary work with cocaine addicts who do not have this diagnosis (Kleber and Gawin, 1986). Earlier studies suggested that lithium blocked cocaine euphoria, but more recent controlled studies and our clinical trial have not supported this earlier suggestion (Cronson and Flemenbaum, 1978; Kleber and Gawin, 1986; Mandell and Knapp, 1976). Finally, depressed cocaine addicts have responded well to desipramine in terms of reduced cocaine use and craving as well as improved depressive symptoms (Kleber and Gawin, 1986; Kosten et al., 1987b). As indicated above, desipramine may also be useful as a general agent to reduce cocaine use.

C. Concurrent Drug and Alcohol Addiction

Cocaine addicts are a heterogeneous group not only in their reasons for using and response to cocaine, but also in their combining cocaine with other drugs. Particularly among the more severe addicts, concurrent alcoholism or opiate addiction is common, and treatment of this concurrent addiction needs attention (Kleber and Gawin, 1984; Kosten et al., 1987a; Rounsaville et al., 1982; Weiss et al., 1986). In a recently completed survey of almost 300 cocaine users specifically excluding concurrent opiate abusers, we found that 70% of the cocaine users were alcoholics (Rounsaville and Carroll, in press). Only about 30% of these alcoholics were primary alcoholics; that is, their alcoholism preceded their cocaine abuse. When we examined this finding in more detail, most of the alcoholics (70% of that 70%) reported that they only used alcohol to ameliorate the crash symptoms from cocaine use. Thus, when they stopped their cocaine use, they also stopped their alcohol abuse. For the remaining 21% (30% of that 70%) of cocaine addicts, however, alcohol was a major problem that needs treatment. A number of nonpharmacological treatments are available for alcoholism and these are clearly indicated, but consideration should also be given to concurrent use of disulfiram, an alcohol "antagonist" that produces an aversive response when alcohol is used (Heath et al., 1965). Although this is not the first-line treatment of choice, it is an important option for this population and can be used in combination with pharmacological agents targeted for the cocaine addict.

Among the intravenous cocaine addicts, heroin is frequently used in combination to make a speedball (Kosten et al., 1986). Well over 50% of our opiate addicts also use cocaine, and the trend to use cocaine with opiates has had an alarming increase since the late 1970s (Hubbard et al., 1983; Kaul and Davidow, 1981; Kosten et al., 1986, 1987a). Concurrent treatment with naltrexone, an orally active opiate antagonist, or methadone maintenance should be considered in these intravenous cocaine addicts. The pressure from the spread of AIDS by intravenous drug addicts makes this treatment mandate even more acute, and the need for innovative pharmacological as well as psychological approaches is pressing. Detoxification alone or followed by drug-free outpatient treatment has been very ineffective with this population, and pharmacological management seems to be critical (Kosten et al., 1987a; Simpson and Sells, 1974).

V. WHERE IS TREATMENT OCCURRING?

Much of cocaine addiction treatment deals with prevention of relapse and is necessarily an outpatient program. While hospitalized, important pharmacological approaches can be used to prevent suicide or to control psychosis as well as to ameliorate withdrawal symptoms after the crash symptoms subside, but aftercare will be critical. Inpatient settings may be very useful for initiating treatment with medications such as amantadine, bromocriptine, and desipramine, because the risks of cocaine interacting with treatment medications are minimized. These medications may then be continued with an aftercare program focusing on relapse prevention. When starting medications with outpatient cocaine addicts, care must be taken to warn the patient of potential interactions between cocaine and the treatment medication. As an example, because tricyclic antidepressants are catecholamine reuptake blockers, high blood pressure could result from the release of epinephrine by cocaine combined with the reuptake blockade by the tricyclic (Fischman et al., 1976). Later in treatment this potential interaction is less likely, because the tricyclics will decrease the sensitivity of the postsynaptic adrenergic receptors (Charney et al., 1981). Thus, inpatient induction onto the various types of anticraving agents for cocaine addiction provides a very safe protocol that will minimize potential medical complications. However, outpatient induction onto cocaine addiction treatment is widely practiced and has not been associated with any major medical complications.

VI. HOW TO MATCH PATIENTS TO TREATMENTS

As more pharmacological treatments for cocaine addiction have been proposed and developed, an important question is not only who is appropriate for pharmacotherapy, but also what type of pharmacotherapy is appropriate. How does one match patients to appropriate treatments? The criteria for determining good candidates for pharmacological interventions include the severity of abuse, psychiatric vulnerability, medical risk factors, and prior treatment failure with nonpharmacological approaches. These criteria have been reviewed above in detail. The question of patient-treatment matching is an active concern of many researchers in drug addiction, as well as general psychiatry (Luborsky and McLellan, 1978; McLellan et al., 1980). Although some matching studies have been done in the treatment of alcoholism and opiate dependence, the treatment of cocaine abuse is too young to have any studies providing guidelines. Some guidelines can be derived from the combination of phases of recovery, comorbid psychiatric disorders, and concurrent drug addiction. In the previous sections, some specific medications have been suggested for particular types of patients, such as methylphenidate for adult ADD patients, and psychiatric vulnerability may suggest particular choices such as this. Similarly, the phase of recovery in which a patient seeks treatment will suggest particular medications such as amantadine during the acute withdrawal phase and desipramine during the later withdrawal and extinction phases. Concurrent drug and alcohol addiction may suggest the addition of naltrexone, methadone, or disulfiram to cocaine anticraving agents. Some medications that might be selected for patients in the neuroadaptation or psychiatric vulnerability categories by each phase of recovery are suggested in Table 4. The different phases offer several choices in medications, and during the crash and extinction phases some specificity in medication choice may be considered for the two types of

Table 4 Medications Selection by Patient Type and Recovery Phase

Recovery phase	Patient type	
	neuroadaptation	psychiatric vulnerability[a]
Crash	Benzodiazepines	Neuroleptics (psychotic)
Withdrawal	Amantadine	Amantadine
	Bromocriptine	Bromocriptine
	L-Dopa	L-Dopa
Extinction	Desipramine	Lithium (bipolar)
	Imipramine	Methylphenidate (ADD)
	Trazadone	Desipramine (depressed)

[a]Parentheses indicate specific types of comorbid psychiatric disorders suggested for each medication.

patient. The specific types of comorbid psychiatric disorders suggested for each medication are shown in Table 4.

In matching patients to medications, the clinician should consider the ratio of risks to benefits for the individual patient, including the possibility that medications may worsen the drug addict's problems. The first risk to consider is related to medical complications from either the medications themselves or from interactions with cocaine during slips or relapses. Cardiac risks are the most significant, and ECGs should be routinely done (Cregler and Mark, 1986; Gay, 1982). Conduction difficulties such as heart block are of concern with the use of tricyclics, for example. Because the risk of hepatotoxicity has been suggested from animal studies of cocaine administration as well as from the use of medications such as tricyclics, liver function tests should be performed before starting any medications (Rauckman et al., 1982; Ritchie and Greene, 1985). The transaminases (e.g., serum glutamic pyruvic transaminase) have been the most sensitive indicators of hepatotoxicity. Typical guidelines for using liver function tests with drug and alcohol addicts have been that any elevation three times above normal should be a contraindication to pharmacological management (Kreek et al., 1972). In the range from two to three times elevation, medications must be carefully justified and liver function tests repeated within 2–3 weeks. If at the repeat testing the liver functions are still elevated beyond twice the upper limit of normal, then discontinuation of the medication is indicated.

Other potential problems are related to the psychosocial aspects of pharmacotherapy. These problems may stem from addiction to the treatment medication itself. In our early work with methylphenidate, we found that antisocial cocaine addicts without childhood ADD would simply abuse this medication (Kleber and Gawin, 1986; Khantzian, 1983).* Thus, the role of stimulant substitution for cocaine addiction treatment seems quite limited, and if used injudiciously this substitution may worsen a drug addict's problems. More subtle interactions with potentially efficacious medications can also occur. It has been suggested that relief of aversive early withdrawal symptoms by medications such as bromocriptine or amantadine may encourage cocaine addiction by removing those aversive aspects of cocaine use. Related to this speculation is our 2.5-year follow-up finding that patients in methadone maintenance had more severe cocaine addiction problems than did patients who got detoxification alone (Kosten et al., 1987a). One interpretation of this finding was that because most intravenous cocaine addicts prefer mixing opiates such as heroin or methadone with the cocaine

---

*I. Extein, W.Z. Potter, M.S. Gold, et al. Persistent neurochemical deficit in cocaine abuse. Paper presented at the 140th Meeting of the American Psychiatric Association, Chicago, IL. May 10–15, 1987.

(i.e., speedballs), having a steady dose of the methadone made the cocaine crash and withdrawal significantly less dysphoric (Kleber and Gawin, 1986; Kosten et al., 1986). In this way, some of our best treatments for opiate or cocaine addiction may facilitate cocaine addiction in poorly motivated patients. As in any effective treatment, a commitment to stopping the drug addiction must be made by the patient, and without this committment treatment may inadvertently facilitate further addiction.

In developing pharmacological treatment programs, a psychotherapeutic approach must be established that will reinforce compliance with medications. It is most critical for success that the psychotherapy not be set up in opposition to the pharmacotherapy, because medication compliance is particularly important in drug addiction treatment settings. The tone of enforced compliance in drug abuse treatment is set at least in part by an association with legal systems who refer patients and by the regimented quality of methadone maintenance programs. Urine toxicology screens are a routine part of most drug addiction treatment, and rules of acceptable behavior are commonly reinforced in programs by threats of administrative termination or return to the criminal justice system (Kosten et al., 1982). These somewhat coercive or policing tactics to reinforce limit setting are not a typical part of outpatient psychiatric treatment, but behavior modification treatments have used reinforcement for a variety of behaviors that might include medication ingestion. In general, a synergism between the pharmacotherapy and psychotherapy is needed, and the proper balance of limit setting and more open supportive treatment must be developed for each patient to optimize the match with a combined psychopharmacological approach.

A well-matched patient may flow through a sequential treatment approach in which treatment is not static, but shifts as his or her needs change. As a general pattern of sequential treatment, the patient may be treated first with a neuroleptic or benzodiazepine during the crash and perhaps may need hospitalization. This may be followed by discontinuation of these crash medications and initiation of amantadine to cope with early withdrawal symptoms. In addition, desipramine may be started along with the amantadine. The rationale is that amantadine will provide early relief of withdrawal symptoms, whereas desipramine will provide more sustained anticraving actions, but may take 10 to 14 days to be fully effective. Thus, at about 2–3 weeks after starting both desipramine and amantadine, the amantadine could be stopped and the desipramine continued. Later discontinuation of desipramine would be individually determined, but we generally consider discontinuation when 3–4 months of abstinence from cocaine has been attained unless a major affective disorder suggests a longer period of antidepressant maintenance.

VII. CONCLUSIONS

In summary, some guidelines are evolving for patient-treatment matching in the pharmacological management of cocaine addiction. Although limited research data are available, initial clinical trials for cocaine addiction have suggested that desipramine can effectively reduce cocaine use and craving in outpatients. Because it has some delay in its onset of action, patient dropout during the first 2 weeks of treatment has been a problem. However, other work with amantadine suggests some promise for this medication as an agent that will acutely decrease craving and use of cocaine. Other agents have shown promise with specific subgroups of patients; however, in every treatment program, medication compliance is a major issue that needs to be addressed through a comprehensive psychotherapeutic approach that strives to optimize the match of patient to treatment. In the future, important contributions will be made to the interaction of particular psychotherapeutic approaches along with pharmacotherapy, as well as to the general issue of patient-treatment matching for cocaine addiction.

ACKNOWLEDGMENT

This work was supported by a Research Scientist Development Award from the National Institute on Drug Abuse DA00112, Center Grants P50-DA04050, RO1-DA04505, and RO1-DA04029.

REFERENCES

Adams, E.H., and Durell, J. (1984). Cocaine: A growing public health problem. *Natl. Inst. Drug Abuse Res. Monog., 50*:9–14.

Buckman, M.T., and Peake, G.T. (1978). Dynamic evaluation of prolactin secretion with perphenazine in normal and hyperprolactinemic subjects. *Hormones Metab. Res., 10*:400–408.

Carroll, K.M., Keller, D.S., Fenton, F.R., and Gawin, R.H. (1987). Psychotherapy for cocaine abusers. In D. Addle (ed.), *The Cocaine Crisis*. Plenum Press, New York.

Castellani, S., Petrie, W.M., and Ellinwood, E.H. (1985). Drug-induced psychosis: Neurobiology mechanisms. In A.I. Alterman (ed.), *Substance Abuse and Psychopathology*. Plenum Press, New York, pp. 173–210.

Charney, D.S., Menkes, D.B., and Heninger, G.R. (1981). Receptor sensitivity and the mechanism of action of antidepressant treatment. *Arch. Gen. Psychiatry, 38*:1160–1180.

Chasnoff, I.J., Burns, E.J., Schnoll, S.H., and Burns, K.A. (1986). Effects of cocaine on pregnancy outcome. In L.S. Harris (ed.). *Proceedings, Problems of Drug Dependence, 1985*. Rockville, Maryland, National Institute on Drug Abuse.

Cherabin, C.E. (1967). The medical sequelae of narcotic addiction. *Ann. Intern. Med., 67*:23–30.

Cregler, L.L., and Mark, H. (1986). Medical complications of cocaine abuse. *N. Engl. J. Med., 315*:1495–1500.

Cronson, A.J., and Flemenbaum, A. (1978). Antagonism of cocaine highs by lithium. *Am. J. Psychiatry, 135*:856–857.

Dackis, C.A., Gold, M.S., Sweeney, D.R. et al. (1987). Single-dose bromocriptine reverses cocaine craving. *Psychiatry Res., 20*:261–264.

Des Jarlais, D.C., Friedman, S.R., and Hopkins, W. (1985). Risk reduction for the acquired immunodeficiency syndrome among intravenous drug users. *Ann. Intern. Med. 103*:755–759.

DeWitt, H., and Wise, R.A. (1977). A bloackade of cocaine reinforcement in rats with the dopamine blocker pimozide but not with the noradrenergic blockers phentolamine or phenoxybenzamine. *Can. J. Psychol., 31*:195–203.

Finnegan, L.P., Connaughton, J.F., Emich, J.P., and Wieland, W.F. (1972). Comprehensive care of the pregnant addict and its effect on maternal and infant outcome. *Contemp. Drug Problems, 1*:795–810.

Fischman, M.W., Schuster, C.R., Resnekov, I. et al. (1976). Cardiovascular and subject effects of intravenous cocaine administration in humans. *Arch. Gen. Psychiatry, 10*:535–546.

Gawin, F.H. (1986a). Neuroleptic reduction of cocaine induced paranoia but not euphoria? *Psychopharmacology, 90*:142–143.

Gawin, F.H. (1986b). New uses of antidepressants in cocaine abuse. *Psychosomatics, 27*:24–29.

Gawin, F.H., Kleber, H.D. (1984). Cocaine abuse treatments: An open pilot trial with lithium and desipramine. *Arch. Gen. Psychiatry, 41*:903–910.

Gawin, F.H., and Kleber, H.D. (1985). Neuroendocrine findings in chronic cocaine abusers. *Br. J. Psychiatry, 147*:569–573.

Gawin, F.H., and Kleber, H.D. (1986). Abstinence symptomatology and psychiatric diagnosis in chronic cocaine abusers. *Arch. Gen. Psychiatry, 43*:107–113.

Gawin, F.H., and Kleber, H.D. (in press). Cocaine abuse in a treatment population: Patterns and diagnostic distinctions. *Natl. Inst. Drug Abuse Res. Monogr. Ser.*

Gay, G.R. (1982). Clinical management of acute and chronic cocaine poisoning. *Ann. Emerg. Med., 11*:562–572.

Giannini, A.J., and Baumgartel, P.D. (1987). Bromocriptine therapy in cocaine withdrawal. *J. Clin. Pharmacol., 27*:267–270.

Giannini, A.J., Malone, D.A., and Giannini, M.C. et al. (1986). Treatment of depression in chronic cocaine and phencyclidine abuse with desipramine. *J. Clin. Pharmacol., 26*:211–214.

Gold, M.S., Washton, A.M., and Dackis, C.A. (1985). Cocaine abuse: Neurochemistry, phenomenology, and treatment. *Natl. Inst. Drug Abuse Res. Monogr. Ser., 61*:130–150.

Heath, R.G., Nesselhof, W., Bishop, M.P. et al. (1965). Behavioral and metabolic changes associated with administration of tetraethylthiuram disulfide (Antabuse). *Dis. Nerv. Syst., 29*:99–105.

Hubbard, R.L., Allison, M., Bray, R.M. et al. (1983). An overview of client characteristics, treatment services, and during treatment outcomes for outpatient methadone clinics in the treatment outcome prospective study (TOPS). In J.R. Cooper, F. Altman, B.S. Brown, and D. Czechowicz (Eds.), *Research on the Treatment of Narcotic Addiction: State of the Art*. Rockville, Maryland, National Institute on Drug Abuse, pp. 714–747.

Kaul, B., and Davidow, B. (1981). Drug abuse patterns of patients on methadone maintenance treatment in New York City. *Am. J. Drug Alcohol Abuse, 8*:17–25.

Khantzian, E.J. (1983). Extreme case of cocaine dependence and marked improvement with methylphenidate treatment. *Am. J. Psychiatry, 140*:784–785.

Khantzian, E.J., Gawin, F.H., Riordan, C., and Kleber, H.D. (1984). Methylphenidate treatment of cocaine dependence: A preliminary report. *J. Subst. Abuse Iss., 1*:107–112.

Kleber, H.D., and Gawin, F.H. (1984). Cocaine abuse: A review of current and experiment treatment. *J. Clin. Psychiatry, 45*(12, sec 2):18–23.

Kleber, H.D., and Gawin, F.H. (1986). Psychopharmacological trials in cocaine abuse treatment. *Am. J. Drug Alcohol Abuse, 12*:235–246.

Kokkinidis, L., Zacharko, R.M., and Predy, P.A. (1980). Post-amphetamine depression of self-stimulation responding from the substantia nigra: Reversal by tricylic antidepressants. *Pharmacol. Biochem. Behav., 13*:379–383.

Kosten, T.R., and Kleber, H.D. (1987). Sudden death in cocaine abusers: Relation to neuroleptic malignant syndrome. *Lancet, 1*:1198–1199.

Kosten, T.R., and Kleber, H.D. (1988). Rapid death during cocaine abuse: Variant of the neuroleptic malignant syndrome? *Am. J. Drug Alcohol Abuse, 14*:335–346.

Kosten, T.R., Astrachan, B.M., Riordan, C., and Kleber, H.D. (1982). The organization of a methadone maintenance program. *J. Drug Iss. Fall., 333–342.*

Kosten, T.R., Rounsaville, B.J., Gawin, F.H., and Kleber, H.D. (1986). Cocaine abuse among opioid addicts: Demographic and diagnostic characteristics. *Am. J. Drug and Alcohol Abuse, 12*:1–16.

Kosten, T.R., Rounsaville, B.J., and Kleber, H.D. (1987a). A 2.5 year follow-up of cocaine use among opioid addicts. *Arch. Gen. Psychiatry, 44*:281–284.

Kosten, T.R., Schumann, B., Wright, D. et al. (1987b). A pilot study using desipramine for cocaine abusing methadone maintenance patients. *J. Clin. Psychiatry, 48*:442–444.

Kosten, T.R., Rounsaville, B.J., and Kleber, H.D. (1988a). Antecedents and consequences of cocaine abuse among opioid addicts: A 2.5 year follow-up. *J. Nerv. Ment. Dis., 176*:176–181.

Kosten, T.R., Schumann, B., and Wright, D. (1988b). Bromocriptine treatment of cocaine abuse in methadone maintained patients (letter). *Am. J. Psychiatry, 145*:381–382.

Kosten, T.R., Rounsaville, B.J., and Kleber, H.D. (in press). A 2.5 year follow-up of abstinence and relapse to cocaine abuse in opioid addicts. In L.S. Harris (Ed.), *Proceedings, Committee on Problems of Drug Dependence.*

Kreek, M.J., Dodes, L., Kanes, S. et al. (1972). Long term methadone maintenance therapy: Effects on liver function. *Ann. Intern. Med., 77*:598–602.

Luborsky, L., and McLellan, A.T. (1978). Surprising inability to predict the outcomes of drug abuse treatments. *Am. J. Drug Alcohol Abuse, 5*:387–398.

Mandell, A.J., and Knapp, S. (1976). Neurobiological antagonism of cocaine by lithium. In E.H. Ellinwood, and M.M. Kilby (Eds.), *Cocaine and Other Stimulants*. Plenum Press, New York, pp. 187–200.

McLellan, A.T., Woody, G.E., and O'Brien, C.P. (1979). Development of psychiatric illness in drug abusers: Possible role of drug preference. *N. Engl. J. Med., 301*:1310–1314.

McLellan, A.T., O'Brien, C.P., Krow, P. et al. (1980). Matching substance abuse patients to appropriate treatments. *Drug Alcohol Depend., 5*:189–195.

Mittleman, R., and Wetli, C.V. (1984). Death caused by recreational cocaine use. *J.A.M.A.*, *252*:1889–1892.

Morgan, C.H., Kosten, T.R., Gawin, F.H., and Kleber, H.D. (in press). A pilot trial of amantadine for cocaine abuse. In L.S. Harris (Ed.), *Proceedings, Committee on Problems of Drug Dependence, 1987.*

Owen, R.T., and Tyrer, P. (1983). Benzodiazepine dependence: A review of the evidence. *Drugs, 25*:385–398.

Post, R.M., Kotin, J., and Goodwin, F.K. (1974). The effects of cocaine on depressed patients. *Am. J. Psychiatry, 131*:511–517.

Rauckman, E.J., Rosen, G.M., Cavagnano, J. (1982). Norcocaine nitroxide: A potential hepatotoxic metabolite of cocaine. *Mol Pharmacol., 21*:458–462.

Ritchie, J.M., and Greene, N.M. (1985). Local anesthetics. In A.G. Gilman, L.S. Goodman, T.W. Rall, and F. Murad (Eds.), *The Pharmacological Basis of Therapeutics.* 6th ed. Macmillan, New York, pp. 302–321.

Roberts, D.C.S., and Koob, G. (1982). Disruption of cocaine self-stimulation following 6-hydroxydopamine lesions of the ventral tegmental area in rats. *Pharmacol. Biochem. Behav., 17*:901–904.

Rosen, H., Flemenbaum, A., Slater, V.L. (1986). Clinical trial of carbidopa-L-dopa combination for cocaine abuse. *Am. J. Psychiatry, 143*:1493.

Rounsaville, B.J., and Carroll, K. (in press). Psychiatric disorders in cocaine abusers. *Natl. Inst. Drug Abuse Res. Monogr. Ser.*

Rounsaville, B.J., Weissman, M.M., Kleber, H.D., and Wilbur, C. (1982). Heterogeneity of psychiatric diagnosis in treated opiate addicts. *Arch. Gen. Psychiatry, 39*:151–156.

Rounsaville, B.J., Gawin, F.H., and Kleber, H.D. (1985). Interpersonal psychotherapy adapted for ambulatory cocaine abusers. *Am. J. Drug Alcohol Abuse, 11*:171–192.

Rowbotham, M., Jones, R.T., Benowitz, N., and Jacob, P. (1984). Trazodone-oral cocaine interactions. *Arch. Gen. Psychiatry, 41*:895–899.

Siegel, R. (1984). Changing patterns of cocaine use: Longitudinal observations, consequences, and treatment. *Natl. Inst. Drug Abuse Res. Monogr. Ser., 50*:92–110.

Simpson, D.D., and Sells, S.B. (1974). Patterns of multiple drug abuse: 1969–1971. *Int. J. Addict., 9*:301–314.

Spyraki, C., Fibiger, H.C., and Phillips, A.C. (1982). Cocaine-induced place preference conditioning: Lack of effects of neuroleptics and 6-hydroxydopamine lesions. *Brain Res., 253*:195–203.

Task Force on Late Neurological Effects of Antipsychotic Drugs (1980). Tardive dyskinesia: Summary of a task force report of the American Psychiatric Association. *Am. J. Psychiatry, 137*:1163–1172.

Taylor, D.L., Ho, B.T., and Fagan, J.D. (1979). Increased dopamine receptor binding in rat brain by repeated cocaine injection. *Commun. Psychopharmacol., 3*:137–142.

Tennant, F.S., Jr. (1984). Double-blind comparison of desipramine and placebo in withdrawal from cocaine dependence. *Natl. Inst. Drug Abuse Res. Mongr. Ser., 55*:159–163.

Tennant, F.S., Jr. (1985). Effect of cocaine dependence on plasma phenylalanine and tyrosine levels and on urinary MHPG excretion. *Am. J. Psychiatry, 142*:1200–1201.

Tennant, F.S., Jr. (in press). Pharmacological management of cocaine withdrawal. *Proceedings, Committee on Problems of Drug Dependence, 1987.*

Tennant, F.S., Jr., and Sagherian, A.A. (1987). Double-blind comparison of amantadine and bromocriptine for ambulatory withdrawal from cocaine dependence. *Arch. Intern. Med., 147*:109–112.

Thierry, A.M., LeDouarin, C., Penit, J. et al. (1986). Variation in the ability of neuroleptics to block the inhibitory influence of dopaminergic neurons in the activity of cells in the rat prefrontal cortex. *Brain Res. Bull., 16*:155–160.

Weiss, R.D., Goldenheim, P.D., Mirin, S.M. et al. (1981). Pulmonary dysfunction in cocaine smokers. *Am. J. Psychiatry, 138*:110–112.

Weiss, R.D., Mirin, S.M., Michael, J.L., Sollogub, A.C. (1986). Psychopathology in chronic cocaine abusers. *Am. J. Drug Alcohol Abuse, 12*:17–29.

Wise, R. (1984). Neural mechanisms of the reinforcing action of cocaine. *Natl. Inst. Drug Abuse Res. Monogr. Ser., 50*:15–53.

Woody, G.E., O'Brien, C.P., and Greenstein, R. (1975). Misuse and abuse of diazepam: An increasingly common medical problem. *Int. J. Addict., 10*:843–848.

XIX
Treatment Outcome

63

Drug and Alcohol Addiction Treatment Outcome

Patricia Ann Harrison*, Norman G. Hoffmann†, and Susan G. Streed
Ramsey Clinic, St. Paul, Minnesota

I. INTRODUCTION

Issues surrounding outcome of drug and alcohol addiction treatment are varied and complex. Results from outcome studies are dependent upon a host of variables: patient psychosocial backgrounds and alcohol and drug use histories; treatment modality, length, intensity, staffing, philosophy, format, and techniques; patient living environment, availability of supportive resources, and preponderance of detrimental influences following treatment; sample selection; sample attrition associated with nonconsent and losses to follow-up; measures of follow-up functioning; and methodological issues such as validity and reliability of patient self-report, and accuracy in data collection, analysis, and interpretation [1–6].

Alcohol- and drug-use patterns as well as the definition and recognition of what constitutes alcohol- and drug-use problems or addictions are interrelated with societal and cultural promotion, tolerance, or constraints around the use of alcohol or drugs [7–8]. Even within societies or cultures, varied levels or patterns may be accepted or proscribed for different subgroups, such as those identified by age, gender, or occupation. Some attitudes shift dramatically over time; others remain relatively constant. To simplify our discussion of treatment outcome, we shall concentrate our discussion on private treatment programs within the United States. Even setting this arbitrary limit, however, cannot ensure homogeneity of patient or program samples. Quite the contrary, patient populations vary widely and have changed a great deal even within the last 20 years, influenced most dramatically by the increase in illicit drug use in the United States and the onset of both drug and alcohol use by younger and younger segments of the population [9–11]. Treatment also underwent dramatic improvements during recent decades, most notably the expansion of efforts to increase family programming, and the development of aftercare, or recovery maintenance components of treatment [12].

Current affiliations:
*Minnesota Department of Human Services Chemical Dependency Division, St. Paul, Minnesota.
†CATOR/New Standards, Inc., St. Paul, Minnesota.

II. INPATIENT VERSUS OUTPATIENT TREATMENT: CLARIFYING THE ISSUES

A. Why Compare Inpatient and Outpatient Treatment?

There are two key reasons to study the efficacy of inpatient and outpatient treatment. The first is to assure that each individual receives the type of treatment most likely to arrest his or her illness. The second is to reduce the costs of drug and alcohol dependency treatment whenever possible, without sacrificing effectiveness.

Cost of treatment is a key motivator for determining the relative efficacy of treatment modalities in an era of diminishing health care dollars [13–16]. Room and board charges and the additional staffing (e.g., round-the-clock nursing care) required in residential settings make inpatient treatment much more costly than outpatient treatment for the same duration. Inpatient treatment may also involve other costs for the patient, such as time lost on the job or placement of children in foster care. Yet when treatment is effective, much of the cost is often recouped in terms of future benefits to the individual and the family and significant others as well as to society. Cost offsets are realized through reduction in medical care utilization, improved family functioning necessitating fewer social services, less drug- and alcohol-related criminal activity and violence, and improved vocational functioning [17–25]. However, it is reasonable to question the justification for more expensive treatment options unless they are comparatively more effective than less expensive options as determined by higher success rates for a given population, or unless they can serve a population less likely to benefit from less costly treatment.

B. Program Differences

Inpatient programs can differ from outpatient programs in level of care, content, format, or context. The most obvious differences, of course, are level of care and context, with residential treatment offering more intensive observation, programming, and structure in a secure environment. Many private treatment programs in the United States, regardless of context, are more similar than dissimilar in content and format. Many reflect the so-called Minnesota model of treatment [12,26], which is grounded in the philosophy and recovery program of Alcoholics Anonymous. Total abstinence from all mood-altering drugs is the goal of treatment. Lecture and group sessions are the primary components of the rehabilitative format.

Although the basic subject material presented to patients is very similar at most facilities, inpatient programs can offer a higher intensity of treatment because of increased staff-patient contact time [27]. Programming in residential settings may extend up to 12 h a day, 7 days a week. Inpatients also have opportunities for extended peer contact at meals, with roommates, and during unstructured times, and staff have increased time to observe patients [27]. In contrast, outpatient programs are usually limited to 60–120 h of staff-patient contact time over a 4- to 8-week period, and there is comparatively little unstructured time for informal peer contact.

In addition to program differences, other differences related to context distinguish inpatient treatment from outpatient treatment. Participation in an inpatient treatment program constitutes a major disruption in a person's life, much like a lengthy hospitalization for a physical or mental illness. A person leaves the home environment, the work environment, the social sphere, the neighborhood, and community, giving up daily routines and responsibilities, to reside in a foreign environment structured to provide almost exclusive emphasis on the recovery process. Personal and telephone contact with persons outside the treatment center may be strictly limited. Outside of family treatment sessions, even contact with significant others may be restricted. Theoretically, inpatients are removed and protected, as much as possible, from the stresses and strains of daily life: family, work, friends, interpersonal, occupational, and environmental concerns [27]. Perhaps most significantly, inpatients do not have access to alcohol or drugs within their protected environment, and when they leave treatment, they have experienced several weeks of enforced abstinence. They then must transfer their learning to dissimilar situations, facing a reentry phase which may pose difficulties not experienced by outpatients.

In contrast to inpatients, outpatients continue to function in their everyday environment, maintaining for the most part their daily routines and responsibilities. Treatment does not constitute "getting away," but may in fact add several hours of structured time to a day already filled with family responsibilities and/or employment demands. Outpatients must continue to confront existing interpersonal and environmental stressors while they devote week nights to rehabilitative sessions. Outpatients have continuing and unrestricted access to alcohol and drugs during their weeks in treatment, and for them abstinence during treatment results from their own capacity and willingness to refrain from substance use. When outpatients successfully complete treatment, they have several weeks of "practice" and unenforced sobriety behind them to bolster their resolve to remain abstinent.

C. Assumptions Governing Placement

Several key assumptions have traditionally guided placement decisions. One assumption seems to be a clear outgrowth of the medical model of treatment: The more seriously ill a person is, the more likely it is that he or she requires hospitalization. The corollary for drug and alcohol dependency is that the more serious the drug and alcohol abuse or dependence, the more appropriate intensive residential treatment. A second assumption relates to frequency of drug and alcohol use. Greater frequency of use is assumed to denote greater severity of illness. In practice, daily use is considered a strong indicator of the need for inpatient treatment. It is likewise assumed that daily users will have a more difficult time than less-frequent users with voluntary abstinence in an uncontrolled environment. A third assumption is that persons with drug- and alcohol-use problems cannot be treated for those problems while they continue to use these substances. This assumption leads to the conclusion that treatment can be effective only if it occurs during a period of abstinence. This assumption interacts with another: Some people have the capacity to refrain from the use of alcohol and other drugs and others do not. Obviously, these two assumptions play a key role in clinical recommendations for treatment placement. A final assumption operative in treatment placement decisions is that concomitant problems in other life areas increase the importance of supervised, residential treatment.

D. Placement Guidelines

The assumptions outlined above are considered along with individual factors and pragmatic concerns leading to eventual treatment placement. It would be misleading to suggest that treatment placement is based solely on a clinical assessment of the severity of drug and alcohol dependency. The following outline is based on discussions with clinicians and a review of treatment placement guidelines [28]. Although not an exhaustive list, it details clinical factors and other considerations weighed in the inpatient versus outpatient decision-making process.

Drug or Alcohol Use

Frequency of use. Daily use is considered an indication for inpatient treatment; less frequent use points to outpatient treatment.

Use of multiple drugs. Multiple drug use is usually assumed to be an indicator of greater problem severity and an indication for inpatient treatment.

Severity and number of consequences of drug abuse. Harmful consequences are taken into consideration in clinical assessment. Serious consequences, especially if recent and related to interpersonal loss (separation, divorce) or vocational deterioration (job loss), may be used as indicators of the need for inpatient treatment. Evidence of few or relatively minor consequences may lead to a recommendation for outpatient treatment.

Recent use and likelihood of withdrawal symptoms. A history of withdrawal symptoms is associated with problem severity and is frequently used to justify inpatient care. Hospitalization to provide medical supervision of withdrawal may be deemed appropriate. The absence of a dependence syndrome may lead to a recommendation for outpatient treatment.

History of previous treatment. Prior treatment with relapse, especially in the absence of periods of sustained abstinence, usually results in a recommendation for inpatient treatment.

Physical Illness

Presence of a chronic illness. A disorder such as diabetes or high blood pressure may lead to a recommendation for inpatient treatment in order to provide medical monitoring and management of symptoms, especially during alcohol or drug withdrawal.

Physical disability. Inpatient care may be recommended for persons with disabilities, especially those which affect mobility and make travel to outpatient treatment a hardship.

Emotional Disturbance

Depression. Depressive symptoms are often associated with alcohol use, drug use, and withdrawal, making clinicians cautious because of associated risks of suicide. Inpatient care may be recommended to provide an opportunity for increased observation and evaluation.

History of psychiatric disorder. Persons with a history of psychiatric disorder, especially those on psychotropic medication, may be referred to inpatient treatment for stabilization.

Other emotional disturbance. Persons exhibiting high levels of anxiety or other distress during evaluation may be judged likely to benefit from a structured environment.

Environmental Factors

Drug and alcohol use by significant others and peers. Clinicians may refer to inpatient treatment those persons in home or peer environments in which drug and alcohol use is widespread.

Family violence. When violence exists in the home environment, the drug or alcohol abuser may be referred to inpatient treatment to provide at least temporary protection from this additional stressor.

Disruptive interpersonal relationships. Persons experiencing disruptive relationships with significant others are often referred to inpatient treatment. Persons with key interpersonal relationships intact who can receive support from these sources, are often referred to outpatient treatment.

Social support networks. The absence of supportive resources may indicate a need for the increased structure and support provided by residential care.

Family Responsibilities

Care of children. Persons who are primary caretakers of children and who cannot or are unwilling to relinquish this responsibility to others may be referred to outpatient treatment, even in the face of strong clinical indications for inpatient treatment.

Care of spouse or parents. Persons who provide physical care to an ailing or disabled spouse or parent may refuse inpatient treatment.

Vocational Considerations

Employment. A person may express a strong preference, or need, to continue working while involved in treatment.

School. A student may be unwilling to drop out of school to participate in inpatient treatment.

Referral Source Pressures

Court. In some cases, the court mandates treatment placement.

Employee assistance program (EAP) counselors. In some cases, EAP counselors indicate a strong preference of treatment type for their employees.

Availability of Treatment Type

Program availability. In some localities, only one treatment program is available; therefore, there is no choice.

Program location. Outpatient treatment is an option only when within a reasonable commuting distance of a person's home and when transportation is available.

Third-Party Payment

Insurance coverage may provide more complete reimbursement for one modality than another (e.g., 100% of inpatient care and 80% of outpatient care).

HMO. Health maintenance organizations can dictate the type of treatment their participants receive.

Government assistance. Regulations for Medicare and Medicaid patients may dictate eligibility for treatment cost reimbursement to the provider, restricting the options available for patients on government assistance.

Patient Preference

Patient refusal. A patient may refuse the option recommended by a clinical assessor because of family or job concerns or for other reasons. Patients refusing one type of treatment may be accepted into another.

As this outline suggests, the placement process is a complex interplay among clinical assessment, administrative regulations, and personal and pragmatic considerations. The ultimate decision proceeds from an assessment of drug- and alcohol-use involvement, physical and emotional health, and environmental stress. The clinical recommendation is mediated by pragmatic concerns such as eligibility for third-party reimbursement, distance of residence from the treatment site, and the patient's personal preference. The clarification of issues involved in the treatment placement process is integral to the analyses of differences in inpatient and outpatient population characteristics and the interpretation of differences in measures of treatment outcome [29].

III. DIFFERENCES BETWEEN INPATIENT AND OUTPATIENT POPULATIONS

A. General Characteristics of Treatment Populations

In private alcohol and drug addiction treatment centers, inpatient populations can be distinguished from outpatient populations by the severity of their alcohol and drug involvement, and by the extent of coexisting emotional, social, and vocational problems [29–35].

One common error in the interpretation of outcome study results is the comparison of inpatient and outpatient recovery or improvement rates even though the inpatient and outpatient populations are very dissimilar with respect to characteristics which may influence outcomes. It cannot be assumed that if recovery rates for two treatment populations are similar then the treatments must be similarly effective. Unless random assignment of patients is utilized in a study design, a selection bias typically results from the patients' referral or self-selection into inpatient or outpatient modalities. In addition, even if random assignment is made, researchers must restrict which patients are permitted in the study sample; the most severely and the least severely affected are usually excluded. Finally, randomization does not guarantee that no initial differences existed in group assignment.

Studies that carefully analyze and describe the characteristics of patients admitted to treatment consistently report that inpatients are more impaired by drug and alcohol abuse and tend to manifest less social stability than outpatients [29,31–35]. In most studies, inpatients are older than outpatients, less likely to be married, and less likely to be employed. They also typically manifest more serious medical and psychiatric problems.

In a study of inpatients and outpatients at the Hazelden Foundation in Minnesota [34], for example, inpatients exhibited a greater number of symptoms associated with severe alcoholism and physiological dependence than outpatients, including higher levels of use, tremors, morning drinking, periods of continuous intoxication, and decreased tolerance. Inpatients reported higher rates of hospitalization associated with alcohol use than outpatients. Inpatients also had higher levels of psychopathology as evidenced by greater depression, anxiety, bizarre thoughts and behavior, and somatic complaints. Inpatients also reported more social alienation than outpatients. Another Minnesota study also found inpatients to be older, more likely to drink daily, and to exhibit more severe symptoms of alcohol and drug dependence [29].

A Toronto study reflected similar differences between inpatient and outpatient treatment populations [33]. Inpatients were drinking more, and more frequently, than outpatients. Inpatients evidenced more loss of control and compulsive drinking behavior, were more likely to experience withdrawal symptoms, reported more problems related to their drinking, and exhibited greater social maladaptation than outpatients. Inpatients had higher levels of depression, anxiety, and somatic complaints, and neuropsychological testing revealed greater evidence of cognitive disorders, including memory lapses, confusion, and difficulties with abstract reasoning and coordination. Inpatients also exhibited greater impulsivity and recklessness than outpatients.

A study of 44 alcoholism treatment centers across the country concluded that inpatients had more alcoholism symptoms than outpatients, and a lower socioeconomic status at intake into treatment [32]. Two earlier studies, one in Michigan [31] and one in Connecticut [30], both describe inpatient populations that displayed less evidence of social integration than outpatients and more impairment related to alcoholism.

In summary, studies that compare intake characteristics of inpatients and outpatients consistently report among inpatients a higher prevalence of factors generally associated with a poorer prognosis. In spite of initial differences showing inpatients to be sicker than outpatients, nonrandomized studies consistently show no differences in outcome at follow-up [36]. But similar recovery rates for inpatients and outpatients do not prove that the treatments they receive are equally effective. Similar outcomes for the two groups may mean merely that less impaired drug and alcohol abusers respond to outpatient treatment about as well as more impaired drug and alcohol abusers respond to inpatient treatment. No conclusions about the relative efficacy of the treatments can be drawn from such studies, unless patient subgroups are matched for intake characteristics and analyses conducted for interactions between patient variables and treatment type. None of the studies reviewed reported such an analysis.

Random assignment to treatment type would obviously address this selection bias. However, ethical and pragmatic considerations to such experimental procedures can be insurmountable [29]. Furthermore, the range of severity of addiction and coexisting disorders may have to be restricted so severely as to limit the validity of the findings. Some researchers have drawn conclusions regarding the relative efficacy of inpatient versus outpatient treatment based on a limited number of controlled studies [14], all of which report relatively poor outcomes. These conclusions have been soundly challenged, however; there are serious problems with their definitions of treatment modality, outcome measures, and other methodological issues, making any conclusions with respect to such comparisons premature [27].

B. CATOR as a Treatment Outcome Auditor

CATOR (Comprehensive Assessment and Treatment Outcome Research) was founded out of the growing concern for documentation of treatment effectiveness. Seven programs in the Minneapolis–St. Paul metropolitan area collaborated to design data-collection instruments and study procedures [20]. In time, other programs entered the fee-for-service registry system. After 10 years CATOR had collected intake data on more than 50,000 adults from 80 programs in 29 states, and 6000 adolescents from 28 programs in 15 states.

Treatment programs in the CATOR registry use standardized data-collection instruments to collect information on each admission at intake and discharge. Each patient fills out a detailed background questionnaire. Patients are asked for consent to follow-up, and approximately 90% of the patients agree to interviews after treatment [20,25].

All individual patient data are, of course, confidential. Treatment center data are also confidential; only the designated official at each participating treatment program receives reports on the program. As part of their contract with CATOR, participating programs agree that their data can be aggregated and analyzed for the purpose of general treatment population and outcome studies. It is this compilation of vast amounts of data over time, from a variety of sources, with centralized follow-up procedures and exact standards for data analysis that lend credibility to CATOR findings. The following analyses, based on CATOR data, illustrate the nature and extent of differences between inpatient and outpatient populations.

Demographic Characteristics

Some demographic characteristics are remarkably similar for the two populations. Males outnumber females almost three to one in both settings (73 vs 27%), and identical proportions in each sample are married. Inpatient programs, however, have a greater proportion of patients over age 50, whereas outpatient programs have a greater proportion of patients under age 30. Inpatients have less formal education than outpatients. They are also less likely to be employed, a difference not accounted for by the greater proportion of retired inpatients.

Drug- and Alcohol-Use Histories

Inpatients are more likely to be daily drinkers than outpatients, and they are also more likely to use other drugs on a frequent basis. Although inpatients are, on average, older than outpatients, and thus entered adolescence and adulthood before alcohol and drug use were commonplace among the young, more inpatients began drinking and using drugs before age 14 than outpatients.

Although the average symptom count related to alcohol dependence for inpatients and outpatients is similar (10.5 vs 10.6), there are some differences in their manifestation of alcohol-related problems. More inpatients than outpatients report binge drinking (staying drunk for at least 2 days), drinking despite medical complications, preoccupation with drinking, drinking to combat a hangover or withdrawal symptoms, and delirium tremens, all signs typically associated with chronic addiction and physical dependence. In contrast, more outpatients than inpatients report blackouts, unusual or erratic behavior while under the influence, drinking more than planned, and neglect of responsibilities, which may result from episodic intoxication rather than physical dependence. A much higher proportion of outpatients cite a recent driving-while-intoxicated (DWI) arrest as the immediate impetus for their entering treatment, which supports the claim that outpatients are coping with behavioral consequences

Table 1 Inpatient-Outpatient Comparison of Demographic Characteristics

	Inpatients (N = 9199) (%)	Outpatients (N = 1042) (%)
Sex		
male	73	73
female	27	27
Age		
under 20	6	3
20–29	33	41
30–39	34	36
40–49	14	14
50–59	7	4
60–69	4	1
70 and older	2	<1
Race		
Asian	<1	<1
black	18	4
Hispanic	4	2
native American	3	3
white	73	89
biracial	<1	<1
other	2	2
Education		
no diploma	23	17
high school/GED	53	54
2-year degree	13	17
college graduate	8	9
postgraduate	3	3
Employment status at admission		
full time	61	70
part time	8	11
none, by choice	10	6
unemployed	19	12
missing data	2	1
Personal income		
less than $10,000	29	32
$10,001–$20,000	26	28
$20,001–$30,000	19	18
$30,001–$50,000	11	12
over $50,000	4	5
does not say	11	5
Family income		
less than $10,000	13	18
$10,001–$20,000	18	20
$20,001–$30,000	18	18
$30,001–$50,000	19	21
over $50,000	13	11
does not say	19	12

(continued)

Table 1 *(continued)*

	Inpatients (N = 9199) (%)	Outpatients (N = 1042) (%)
Medical care coverage		
Medicare	8	2
Medicaid	6	9
Blue Cross/Blue Shield	22	18
private/group insurance	50	33
HMO	4	5
self-pay	6	22
other	9	12

of their use, whereas inpatients are confronting continuous use and severe medical complications.

Although mean alcohol symptom counts are similar for inpatients and outpatients, mean symptom counts for illicit drugs clearly set inpatients apart. Although the difference related to marijuana use is relatively small (3.2 vs 2.8), the average symptom counts for cocaine (4.4 vs 2.4) and all other drugs combined (3.0 vs 1.5) illustrate the much greater drug-use severity among inpatients. Inpatients are also 1.5 times as likely as outpatients to have a history of intravenous drug use.

Vocational Impairment

Job-related impairment is another area in which differences between inpatients and outpatients are measurable. Although interpersonal and performance problems are only slightly more common among employed inpatients than employed outpatients, employed inpatients are much more likely to report problems with being late and missing work altogether. Reported frequencies of working under the influence of alcohol or other drugs reflects these differences. Inpatients are more than twice as likely as outpatients to report working under the influence almost every day, and more also report being impaired at work at least once a week.

Emotional and Behavioral Problems

Inpatients are more likely than outpatients to have been in drug and alcohol dependency treatment before; overall their histories suggest a greater range of difficulties. More inpatients than outpatients report a history of depression. Multiple depressive episodes are more common among inpatients, and among the depressed in both groups, inpatients experience more symptoms. More inpatients have also attempted suicide. Previous psychiatric or psychological treatment histories support the differences seen in self-reported levels of distress. More inpatients than outpatients have histories of treatment for depression and for other emotional disorders. Histories of antisocial behavior during childhood are also more common among inpatients. Although more outpatients report recent arrests for DWI and other driving violations, more inpatients report recent arrests for criminal offenses.

Medical Care History

Recent use of medical care is also much higher among inpatients, and the differentials are greater than can be accounted for by their older age. Inpatients were much more likely than outpatients to have been hospitalized during the previous year for detoxification, alcohol, or drug treatment, psychiatric care, and medical illnesses or injuries. They also had more psychiatric and medical emergencies. They were receiving more outpatient psychiatric and medical care as well.

Table 2 Inpatient-Outpatient Drug Use Frequency

	Inpatients (N = 9199) (%)	Outpatients (N = 1042) (%)
Alcohol		
daily	32	21
weekly[a]	69	67
monthly[a]	82	83
Marijuana		
daily	14	10
weekly	27	21
monthly	38	31
Cocaine		
daily	10	3
weekly	26	11
monthly	36	19
Other stimulants		
weekly	6	5
monthly	12	9
Barbiturates/sedatives		
weekly	6	2
monthly	10	4
Tranquilizers		
weekly	9	3
monthly	15	5
Painkillers		
weekly	6	3
monthly	11	6
Opiates		
weekly	6	1
monthly	7	2
Hallucinogens		
weekly	2	1
monthly	5	2

[a]Frequency percentages are cumulative; weekly use includes daily use; monthly use includes weekly and daily use.

Table 3 Inpatient-Outpatient Comparison of Addiction Symptoms (% of Patients Reporting Symptoms)

	Alcohol		Marijuana		Cocaine		Other Drugs	
	IP (%)	OP (%)	IP (%)	OP (%)	IP (%)	OP (%)	IP (%)	OP (%)
Blackouts	66	72	9	8	11	5	12	5
Binges	45	40	16	15	29	17	15	9
Unusual behavior	67	77	15	14	28	15	18	11
Unplanned use	69	78	23	22	34	21	18	9
Medicate physical pain	43	39	19	17	12	5	18	9
Medicate emotional pain	70	75	29	25	30	16	20	11

(continued)

Table 3   *(Continued)*

	Alcohol		Marijuana		Cocaine		Other Drugs	
	IP (%)	OP (%)	IP (%)	OP (%)	IP (%)	OP (%)	IP (%)	OP (%)
Injury under the influence	38	38	7	5	8	3	9	4
Ignore medical illness	34	25	9	6	14	7	10	4
Family objections	72	75	27	24	32	17	20	11
Job absenteeism	51	53	15	9	26	13	15	8
Neglect of children	24	26	6	6	11	6	7	4
Neglect of responsibilities	64	71	21	20	32	18	19	10
Physical violence	50	54	8	6	13	7	11	6
Preoccupation	62	57	30	24	32	17	18	8
Scheduling around use	48	46	20	16	25	12	13	5
Tolerance	47	50	17	14	21	13	14	7
Shakes	46	42	5	3	14	9	12	7
Use to combat hang-over/withdrawal	51	44	17	17	16	10	15	7
Inability to stop use	59	59	18	15	30	15	17	8
Need in order to keep going	44	37	15	13	23	12	19	10

Abbreviations: IP, inpatient; OP, outpatient.

Table 4   Inpatient-Outpatient Comparison of Job Impairment

	Inpatient (%)	Outpatient (%)
On-the-job difficulties for past-year employees		
problems with coworkers	19	18
problems with supervisors	28	24
problems completing work	20	17
problems doing quality work	24	22
making mistakes	27	24
missing work	46	29
being late	39	27
getting injured	10	7
Frequency of working under the influence of alcohol and/or drugs		
almost every day	25	12
1 to 3 times a week	21	15
1 to 3 times a month	13	14
less than once a month	14	16
never	27	44

IV. INPATIENT TREATMENT OUTCOME

The inpatient sample is based on data aggregated from 19 treatment centers in 13 states between 1986 and 1988. Of the 6042 patients admitted to treatment at these centers during the study period, 84% completed their treatment programs.

A. Inpatient Treatment Completion versus Noncompletion

Treatment completion is the first step toward successful recovery. In order to determine which patients are at highest risk for noncompletion, patients who left treatment against staff advice or who were discharged for noncompliance with the treatment regimen were compared with completers.

Women and men are equally likely to complete inpatient treatment. Marital status is also not a predictor of treatment completion. Age is of marginal significance as a predictor, with younger patients only slightly more likely than older patients to leave treatment early. With respect to race or ethnicity, Hispanics are less likely to complete treatment than whites, blacks, or other minority patients. Other factors may be confounding this finding. An obvious explanation is the possibility of a language barrier for Hispanics rather than ethnicity itself. Drug-use patterns, socioeconomic factors, and geographic area of residence are also confounded with race and ethnicity in the United States, making suspect any findings in which ethnicity emerges as a statistical predictor.

Socioeconomic and social stability factors are significantly related to inpatient treatment completion. Patients who did not complete high school, those receiving welfare or disability assistance, those who are unemployed at admission, and those with low incomes are more likely to drop out of treatment than other patients. Obviously, there is a great deal of overlap among these characteristics. A history of antisocial or criminal behavior also increases the likelihood of treatment dropout. One of the highest dropout rates for a subgroup, for example, was seen among patients who reported two or more arrests (other than traffic violations) during the year before admission to treatment.

There were also some differences in treatment completion rates based on an analysis of drug-use patterns. Patients with serious consequences from drugs other than alcohol, marijuana, and cocaine had a higher dropout rate than patients not involved with these substances. At the other end of the severity-of-use spectrum, patients with minimal symptoms who denied regular use were also more likely to leave treatment early. This latter group of dropouts probably included some questionable admissions as well as patients with more serious problems who were denying the extent of their problems; this low-severity group accounted for fewer than 10% of the early terminations from inpatient treatment. The following discussion is limited to treatment completers in order to examine treatment effectiveness.

B. Treatment Completer Sample Bias

Any factor which accounts for attrition in a study sample can inject sample bias [3–5]. For this study sample of 5078 inpatient treatment completers, 12% refused to consent to follow-up interviews. An analysis comparing consenters with nonconsenters identified few factors associated with nonconsent.

Fewer Hispanics (80%) and blacks (84%) consent to follow-up than whites (92%) or other minority patients (94%). These findings may, however, be an artifact of consent procedures in different settings; that is, a treatment center or centers with a low consent rate that happened to have a high proportion of black and Hispanic patients could account for this finding. To study this possibility, the consent rate was examined within a large, urban treatment center with high proportions of ethnic minority patients; no significant ethnic

Table 5 Inpatient-Outpatient Comparison of Comorbidity

	Males		Females	
	Inpatient (%)	Outpatient (%)	Inpatient (%)	Outpatient (%)
Psychiatric history				
history of depressive episode	52	44	68	59
suicide attempt	15	10	33	26
treatment for depression	20	14	41	29
treatment for other emotional				
disorder	15	9	26	20
Past year medical care				
hospital/detoxification	18	9	20	9
hospital/alcohol-drug/treatment	20	9	21	14
hospital/psychiatric care	5	2	10	5
hospital/medical care	24	15	26	16
emergency room/psychiatric care	3	2	6	5
emergency room/medical care	35	27	34	26
outpatient/alcohol-drug treatment	15	12	16	16
outpatient/psychiatric care	8	6	17	14
outpatient/medical care[a]	42	39	45	46

[a]Excluding routine examinations.

difference was seen. This supports the hypothesis that facility, rather than racial or ethnic differences, is largely responsible for the observed variations in consent.

Sex, age, and marital status do not predict consent with the single exception that patients separated from their spouses (but not divorced) are somewhat more likely to refuse consent. The consent rate shows a very slight, but statistically significant, decline as income level increases. A similar trend exists for education level, but the relationship is not statistically significant. City dwellers are slightly less likely to grant follow-up consent than town or rural area residents. A related finding is that patients involved only with alcohol and/or marijuana have higher consent rates than those involved with cocaine and other drugs. Patients who deny drug- and alcohol-abuse problems also have lower consent rates. Although several factors have been identified that are statistically associated with refusal to grant consent for follow-up, the overall effect of consent bias is very slight. For one thing, only 12% of all treatment completers refuse to participate in the follow-up study, and even when consent rates are lower for identified subgroups of patients, differences are typically only a few percentage points, limiting the overall effect on the total sample.

In contrast, contact bias accounts for most of the attrition in this sample, and therefore has a greater effect on the generalizability of outcome findings than consent bias. Of the 4436 inpatients with CATOR *History* questionnaires who agreed to participate in the follow-up study, both 6- and 12-month interviews were conducted with the patient for 43%. Responses from significant others were excluded from the outcome analysis. Most demographic factors are significant predictors of contact. Sex, age, race, marital status, employment status, education level, income level, and geographic area of residence are all associated with contact status. A smaller proportion of men than women are contacted, along with fewer younger than older patients. Fewer minority patients are contacted than whites. Single, separated, and divorced patients have lower contact rates than married or widowed patients.

Patients with less formal education have lower contact rates than those with more. Contact rates are lower for patients receiving welfare assistance, disability assistance, and those who were unemployed at admission than for the treatment completer sample as a whole.

Table 6 Inpatient-Outpatient Comparison of Recent Arrests

	Males		Females	
	Inpatient (%)	Outpatient (%)	Inpatient (%)	Outpatient (%)
Any arrest past year	34	48	20	24
Jail overnight past year	23	31	11	9
Specific past year arrests				
DWI/DUI	17	35	9	14
other traffic violation	12	13	6	7
disorderly conduct	6	5	3	2
assault or battery	4	4	2	1
theft/robbery/burglary	4	3	3	3
possession of drugs	5	4	3	1

City dwellers are less likely to be interviewed than patients residing in towns or rural areas. This finding is related, in all likelihood, to a combination of geographic stability and drug-use patterns. Higher levels of cocaine and other drug use are found in urban areas, and such drug use is also predictive of failure to contact.

Another key consideration with respect to sample bias is the disproportionate number of patients with histories of antisocial behavior lost to follow-up. Childhood antisocial histories as well as recent arrest histories are significant predictors of noncontact. In fact, a recent arrest for a criminal offense is the most significant predictor of noncontact identified in the contact bias analysis. Within the group of arrested inpatients, the contact rate declines as the number of arrests increases.

The effect of contact bias in this inpatient follow-up study is to create more favorable treatment outcome results. This is consistent with other research showing that nonresponders, while not necessarily treatment failures, tend to be doing more poorly than responders [3,37]. Nevertheless, despite the number of characteristics that distinguish noncontacted patients from contacted patients, the number of patients affected by these contact predictors is fairly small because such characteristics tend to cluster among patients. In fact, an analysis of 29 risk factors revealed that the overlap between contacts and noncontacts in terms of number of risk factors exceeds 80%. In other words, for four out of five patients, contact may be more a function of chance than of risk. There is evidence from other studies as well that noncontacts do not necessarily constitute a poorer prognosis group [38].

As will be discussed later, many of the factors associated with noncontact are also predictive of increased likelihood of relapse. It must be concluded, then, that the majority of inpatient treatment completers for whom complete 1-year outcome data are not available are faring at least somewhat worse than the minority described in this report. An attempt to measure the effect of sample bias by extrapolating results to the patients lost to follow-up is included in the discussion section of this chapter.

C. Inpatient 1-Year Outcome Findings

Abstinence Rate

Of the selected sample of 1918 inpatient treatment completers who were interviewed at 6 and 12 months after discharge, 72% remained abstinent from alcohol and other drugs for the first 6 months after treatment, and 63% were abstinent for the entire first year. Early success is a strong predictor of continued success: seven out of eight patients who did not return to alcohol or other drug use during the first 6 months after treatment were sober or drug free the entire year. Other research has also documented that the highest risk for relapse occurs during the first 6 months following treatment [24,25,39].

Examination beyond a simple success/failure dichotomy reveals that most inpatients (87%) are abstinent at least 6 months (not necessarily consecutively) out of the first 12 months after treatment. The month-by-month breakdown also shows that three-fourths of the patients are either totally abstinent or report only a brief relapse or relapses affecting only 1 or 2 months out of the year. This way of viewing results illustrates that very few inpatients who complete treatment return to regular continuous use, the pattern that afflicted most of them before admission. Other researchers have also noted this predominance of brief relapse periods [39].

Pretreatment Correlates of Abstinence/Relapse Among Inpatients

Demographic and Socioeconomic Factors.   Contrary to persistent myths about treatment outcome, women are more likely than men to be abstinent 1 year after treatment. That women do at least as well as men after treatment has, in fact, been a consistent finding [40,41]. Age and marital status are the most statistically significant demographic characteristics predictive of recovery status. There is a clear and consistent relationship between age and abstinence: The older the patient, the greater the likelihood of successful recovery. Married and widowed patients have a better prognosis than separated or divorced parents, who in turn have a better prognosis than single patients. Marriage is typically cited as a favorable factor in outcome studies [42]. Fewer high school dropouts report abstinence than their counterparts. Full-time employees fare only slightly better than the unemployed (63 vs 60%), with part-time employees and those who choose not to work faring better than either of these two groups (68%). This finding contrasts with most research identifying employee status as a strong predictor of outcome [42], but it may be that unemployment cannot be equated with unemployability in this predominantly middle-class sample; the unemployed among other study populations may represent the more advanced "skid row" alcoholics more commonly found in publicly funded programs. There appears to be a slight, though nonsignificant, trend for personal income to be associated with recovery, with prognosis improving as income rises; this trend is not seen with family or household income. These descriptors are of limited usefulness because at least one patient in 10 does not provide income information. Ethnicity does not significantly predict outcome.

Drug- and Alcohol-use History Factors.   An examination of drug- and alcohol-use variables also finds key recovery predictors. Illicit drug use is associated with much poorer treatment outcomes than alcohol use only. A history of intravenous drug use lowers the prognosis even further. Because substance choice plays such a key role in treatment outcome, a more detailed discussion of this issue is warranted.

If patients admitted to drug and alcohol dependency treatment could easily be classified in mutually exclusive drug choice categories, comparisons based on drug choice would be simplified. The reality is much more complex than the theoretical ideal, however. For purposes of analysis, a drug choice variable was computed based on frequency of use during the year before admission and lifetime symptoms associated with a specific substance or substance category. To restrict questions to a reasonable number, the CATOR *History* questionnaire asked about 20 drug-specific symptoms or use consequences only for alcohol, marijuana, and cocaine. Another drug category lumped together symptoms associated with the use of opiates, tranquilizers, stimulants, painkillers, barbiturates or sedatives, and hallucinogens.

To meet drug-abuse criteria for this study, a patient had to acknowledge regular use (at least once a month) of the drug or drug category for the preceding year as well as three or more lifetime consequences related to use. The breakdown of patients by drug-abuse category is presented in Table 7. Of the inpatients in the follow-up sample, 7% deny either regular use or more than two consequences of use for any one drug; this number comprises the denies-substance-abuse group. The largest category comprises patients who acknowledge only alcohol abuse (48% of the sample); although 81% of the patients meet study criteria for alcohol abuse, only 48% are in the alcohol abuse only group. In other words, 40% of the patients who met criteria for alcoholism also met criteria for at least one other drug. Even though three symptoms was used as the cutoff qualification, most patients who met criteria for alcohol abuse were much more severely affected by their drinking; in fact, more than three-fourths of the alcohol abusers had at least 10 symptoms.

Since marijuana is generally considered rather benign in comparison to other drugs, this drug choice hierarchy next considered marijuana abusers. Although 25% of the follow-up sample meet criteria for marijuana abuse, only 9% abuse marijuana but no other illicit or prescription drug. Most of the patients in the marijuana abuse group also abuse alcohol.

The next drug choice category requires more explanation. Already categorized at this point are all patients who meet study criteria for abuse of only alcohol and/or marijuana. This other drug abuse category includes patients who acknowledge monthly use of any drug other than alcohol, marijuana, or cocaine, and also acknowledge three or more harmful consequences not associated with alcohol, marijuana, or cocaine use. (Cocaine abuse automatically moved patients into the final classification category). This other drug abuse group comprises 11% of the follow-up sample. The majority of patients in the other drug abuse category also abuse alcohol and one-third also abuse marijuana. The other drug abusers report varied patterns of substances used. Roughly 40% of this group take tranquilizers at least once a week; painkillers, barbiturates or sedatives, and stimulants (other than cocaine) are each taken weekly by approximately one-fourth of the other drug abusers. The typical patient in this group, then, is a regular user of drugs from one or two categories in addition to alcohol and perhaps marijuana. Symptom counts are high, too: two-thirds of the patients who meet criteria for other drug abuse report at least 10 consequences.

The final drug choice classification group comprises patients who meet study criteria for cocaine abuse, irrespective of abuse of any other substance; 24% of the follow-up sample are cocaine abusers. More than two-thirds of the cocaine abusers have at least 10 symptoms. Cocaine abusers are typically multiple drug abusers; only one cocaine abuser out of seven meets study criteria only for cocaine abuse. Three-fourths of cocaine abusers also abuse alcohol, one-half also abuse marijuana, and one-fourth abuse other drugs.

Table 7 Inpatient Treatment Completers 1-Year Outcome by Drug Choice

Total sample	N = 1918	Abstinence rate (%)
		63
Substance abuse based on monthly use and 3+ consequences[a]		
denies substance abuse	142	70
alcohol abuse only	914	71
marijuana abuse (with or without alcohol abuse)	179	52
other drug abuse (with or without alcohol and marijuana but excluding cocaine)	218	62
cocaine abuse (irrespective of any other substance abuse)	465	50

[a]Chi square p value < 0.0001.

Table 7 also illustrates the predictive value of this drug choice classification scheme. The 1-year abstinence rate for alcohol-only abusers is 71%, for marijuana abusers 52%, for other drug abusers 62%, and for cocaine abusers 50%. Because the generalizability of these treatment outcome findings is open to challenge, these figures are most useful in terms of their relative rather than their absolute value. The comparative outcomes related to drug choice classification hold up even when the drug choice categories are controlled for sex and for age.

The relatively poor outcome for cocaine abusers compared with alcohol-only abusers comes as no surprise to treatment professionals. The comparatively poor outcome of marijuana abusers may be unexpected, however. This finding has been consistently documented in CATOR outcome studies [43], and cannot be explained away by age. Even among patients in their 20s and 30s, the age groups with the highest rates of marijuana abuse, marijuana abusers have significantly lower 1-year abstinence rates than alcohol-only abusers. The relatively low symptom count among marijuana abusers may contribute to an illusion of less associated harm (fewer than half report 10 or more symptoms in contrast to three-quarters of alcohol abusers and over two-thirds of cocaine abusers). Patients who are not convinced that marijuana use is harmful may not be motivated to alter this behavior.

Outcome differences related to substance choice cannot automatically be attributed to differences in pharmacological effects. There may be differences in patient characteristics associated with drug choice. For instance, in an adolescent sample, drug choice was significantly associated with a history of sexual abuse [44,45]. Although this relationship was not documented in the adult sample, it illustrates how patient factors may obscure the role of drug effects in the recovery process. Illicit drug use is also associated with a history of antisocial behavior, and antisocial behavior during childhood as well as recent arrest lowers the likelihood of successful recovery. Intravenous drug use is an even more potent predictor of outcome than drug choice. A history of previous treatment also lowers the likelihood of successful outcome.

Treatment and Posttreatment Correlates of Abstinence/Relapse Among Inpatients

Family Participation in Treatment. Most treatment programs promote or even require the involvement of significant others in the patient's treatment process, based on the recognition that drug dependency is a family illness and that family members may be enabling the patient's substance abuse [46]. More than four patients out of five in this treatment follow-up sample had family members or significant others involved in their treatment. In some cases, however, significant others refused to participate (8%), and in a small number of cases the patient refused to have family members involved (2%). For other patients (5%), no significant other was identified or available to participate.

Patients without family involvement were somewhat more likely to relapse than patients with family program participation. The poorest outcomes were associated with the group for whom the family refused to become involved. In contrast, patients without available significant others and those who refused to have anyone involved had outcomes much more similar to patients with family involvement. These results raise an important issue with respect to mandated significant other involvement. Only a small number of patients in this sample refused family involvement, so it may be premature to draw recommendations from these results. However, similarity of this group's prognosis to that of patients with family involvement suggests the possibility that patient refusal may sometimes be a healthy decision, and that mandated family participation may be detrimental to resistant patients. For example, patients confronting physical or sexual abuse within their families may do better with distance from family members.

Program Aftercare. Approximately three out of four inpatients in this follow-up sample reported some involvement in a formal aftercare program sponsored by the treatment center.

It cannot be determined from the data collected whether nonparticipation was a matter of personal choice, schedule or transportation problems, or program unavailability. However, since many inpatient programs treat clients from diverse geographic areas, it is known that at least a proportion of the nonattenders did not reside close enough to the treatment facility to continue in aftercare. Excluding the nonparticipants, a strong relationship can be seen between length of aftercare involvement and abstinence. Inpatients involved in aftercare for the full year after treatment had an 84% abstinence rate compared with 72% for those involved 6–11 months, and 54% for those involved less than 6 months. This empirical support for the importance of aftercare programs is consistent with other research [2,47–50].

Alcoholics Anonymous (AA) and Other Peer Support Groups.   One of the most consistent findings in CATOR treatment outcome studies over the past 10 years is the significant relationship between support group involvement after treatment and recovery status [24,25,43]. Other studies support these findings [51–54]. Almost half of the patients in this follow-up sample attended AA or other support groups meetings every week; their 1-year abstinence rate was much higher than that for monthly attenders, infrequent attenders, those who never attended at all, and those who stopped attending.

Few patients were involved in other peer support groups who did not also attend AA. Only 2% of the total inpatient sample were involved with another kind of support group who were not also regularly attending AA. However, the available evidence suggests that it is frequent and consistent participation rather than the specific kind of group that increases the prognosis for successful recovery.

Patients' Perceptions of Recovery Impediments.   At the end of the 12-month interview, patients are asked about certain factors which may have contributed to their drinking or drug use or which may have made recovery difficult. Relapsed patients were asked to indicate whether each factor had contributed to their starting to use and abstinent patients were asked to indicate whether each factor had made it hard to avoid using.

The impediment to recovery cited most frequently by both relapsed and abstinent inpatients is emotional distress, such as boredom, anger, loneliness, or depression. Family stress and relationship problems are also among the commonly mentioned impediments to recovery. Emotional problems and family problems have been associated with relapse in other studies as well [50,55–57], with at least one study finding a depressed or anxious mood the most common reason given for relapse [39].

The largest absolute differences between abstinent and relapsed patients are seen for craving alcohol or drugs and for not really wanting to quit; these differences are most striking even though relapsed patients clearly have more difficulties in all areas than abstinent

Table 8 Inpatient Treatment Completers 1-Year Outcome by Peer Support Group Participation

Total Sample	N = 1918	Abstinence rate (%) 63
Any peer support group attendance (AA or other)[a]		
did not attend	519	51
stopped attending	186	41
once a month or less	136	54
several times a month	115	62
weekly	943	76

[a]Chi square p value < 0.0001.

Table 9 Inpatient Treatment Completers Patients' Perceptions of Recovery Impediments

Perceived impediments to recovery	Abstinent patients N = 1211 (%)	Relapsed patients N = 707 (%)
Marital or relationship problems[a]	24	40
Stress from family problems[a]	27	42
Financial problems[a]	21	35
Boredom, anger, loneliness, or depression[a]	33	59
Craving alcohol or drugs[a]	17	46
Not really wanting to quit[a]	7	36
Belief that you're not chemically dependent[a]	10	25

[a]Chi square p value < 0.0001.

patients. Another noteworthy finding is that one out of four relapsed patients and one out of 10 abstinent patients still have difficulties accepting that they are drug dependent, which suggests that the treatment process was unsuccessful in breaking through problem denial.

These differences between abstinent and relapsed patients suggest possibilities for improving treatment outcome. They also raise an intriguing question, however, about which comes first: distress or relapse. To address this question, additional analyses were performed comparing inpatients who were abstinent both the first and the second 6 months after treatment with inpatients who were abstinent during the first 6 months but who relapsed during the second 6 months. These findings clearly show that abstinent patients reporting difficulties in the first follow-up interval were much more likely than those without these problems to suffer a subsequent relapse. Because significantly higher rates of boredom, craving, and difficulty associated with people using alcohol or drugs are seen among abstinent patients who subsequently relapse, the association between problems and relapse cannot be dismissed as merely an attempt on the part of these patients to rationalize their return to drug or alcohol use. These results offer strong support for relapse-prevention efforts which incorporate comprehensive plans for relapse prevention. Relapse prevention and aftercare programs that focus only on a limited number of these issues will fail to address the needs of patients experiencing other impediments to recovery. Further improvements in this area may be a key step toward improving patient outcomes.

Other Measures of Treatment Impact

Health Care Comparison. The hospitalization rates for inpatients during the year after treatment are much lower than during the year before treatment. The hospitalization rate for illness or injury declines by half (hospitalizations related to pregnancy or childbirth are excluded from health care analyses). Although the psychiatric hospitalization rate is much lower overall, the proportional decline is similar. Not surprisingly, hospitalizations required for detoxification show the most dramatic decline: a 75% reduction.

The use of an emergency room for health care also declines following treatment. Before treatment, one-third of the patients reported an emergency room visit related to illness or injury compared with a 23% rate following treatment. Rates of psychiatric emergency room

Table 10 Inpatient Treatment Completers Health Care Before and After Treatment

| | (N = 1918) | |
Health care	Year before treatment (%)	Year after treatment (%)
Hospitalizations		
medical		
0	78	89
1	15	7
2 or more	7	4
psychiatric		
0	95	98
1	4	1
2 or more	1	1
detoxification		
0	84	97
1	12	3
2 or more	4	<1
Emergency room visits		
medical		
0	67	77
1	21	17
2 or more	12	6
psychiatric		
0	96	99
1	3	1
2 or more	1	<1

visits, like psychiatric hospitalizations, are much smaller than those related to illness or injury, but they also show a similar rate of decline.

In contrast to hospitalization and emergency care, outpatient care is relatively unchanged following inpatient treatment. In fact, where differences are notable, they are in the direction of increases following treatment. The most marked difference in this area is the increase in patients reporting at least nine outpatient psychiatric care visits.

It is sometimes argued that posttreatment reductions in health care utilization merely reflect a statistical artifact known as regression to the mean. This is the tendency for abnormally high values to revert to more normal values over time. There is no doubt that for many patients, physical and emotional health has deteriorated with drug abuse, and a health crisis may in fact precipitate seeking treatment. Yet the dramatic reductions seen in this study cannot be attributed solely to regression to the mean. Neither regression to the mean nor transitory effects of ancillary health care during treatment account for observed differences [58]. Other studies have also documented similar reductions in posttreatment health care utilization [17,18,20,21]. Posttreatment hospitalizations and emergency care are both significantly associated with relapse, proving that successful treatment can reduce other health care requirements. The overall hospitalization rate after treatment for relapsed patients is 21% compared with 11% for abstinent patients; the emergency room use rate is 30% compared with 21% for abstinent patients.

Legal Problems and Motor Vehicle Accidents.   The number of patients reporting a motor vehicle accident in which they were the driver is reduced by half during the year following treatment. The arrest rate for DWI offense and other moving traffic violations also decreases following treatment, with the most significant decline seen in multiple arrests. The criminal arrest rate also declines after treatment. Major changes in criminal behavior following treatment have also been reported in other studies [19].

Posttreatment arrests, whether for traffic violations or criminal offenses, are significantly associated with relapse. Whereas only 9% of abstinent patients report traffic arrests following treatment, 16% of relapsed patients are arrested for traffic violations. The arrest rate for criminal offenses after treatment is 1% for abstinent patients and 7% for relapsed patients. There is also a significant relationship between posttreatment motor vehicle accidents and relapse. Only 7% of abstinent patients report a motor vehicle accident after treatment compared with 13% of relapsed patients. This evidence strongly argues in support of treatment effectiveness in reducing traffic accidents and criminal involvement among drug- and alcohol-dependent adults.

Job Problems.   In other to conduct pretreatment-posttreatment comparisons of job problems, the comparison sample was restricted to those patients who were employed full time for the 12-month periods before and after treatment. This inclusion criterion eliminates the potential influence of varying lengths of employment on job experiences. Of the 1918 patients in the follow-up sample, 754 met this qualification.

Job problems reported before treatment were very common. Two out of five patients reported problems with absenteeism and tardiness. One-third were making mistakes on the job, and one-fourth each noted difficulties in completing assigned tasks or difficulties with a boss or supervisor. In addition, almost one out of 10 was injured on the job during the year before treatment. The very high prevalence of job problems is not surprising in light of reported levels of working under the influence of alcohol or drugs. Two out of five patients acknowledged that they were working under the influence at least once a week (half of these almost every day). Only one-third of these employed patients stated that they were never under the influence at work during the year before treatment.

Consistent with other research [19], dramatic reductions are seen in job absenteeism and tardiness, making mistakes, and problems completing work. Interpersonal problems are also

Table 11 Inpatient Treatment Completers Legal Problems Before and After Treatment

	(N = 1918)	
Legal problem	Year before treatment (%)	Year after treatment (%)
Motor vehicle accidents		
0	80	91
1	15	7
2 or more	5	2
Traffic violation arrests		
0	81	88
1	12	9
2 or more	7	3
Criminal offense arrests		
0	90	97
1	7	2
2 or more	3	1

Table 12 Inpatient Treatment Completers Job Problems for Patients Employed Full Time During the Year Before and the Year After Treatment

	(N = 754)	
Job problem	Year before treatment (%)	Year after treatment (%)
Difficulties with boss or supervisor	24	14
Completing work	23	5
Making mistakes	32	6
Being absent	42	5
Being late	39	7
On-the-job injury	9	5
Frequency of working under the influence of alcohol/drugs		
almost every day	21	<1
1–3 times a week	19	<1
1–3 times a month	14	1
less than once a month	14	1
never	32	97

	For a 30-day period		
Number of days absent from work	Before admission to treatment (%)	Before the 6-month interview (%)	Before 12-month interview (%)
0	46	76	79
1	15	13	11
2	13	5	5
3 or more	26	6	5

reported less frequently, although the difference in this area is less marked than in other areas. The rate reporting on-the-job injury is cut in half after treatment.

Even patients who report a relapse following treatment are very unlikely to report that using affects their job. Only 4% of the employee follow-up sample report any working under the influence during the year after treatment (compared with 67% reporting at least occasional impairment before treatment).

Actual days of absenteeism were measured only for 30-day intervals because of the difficulty in recalling over longer intervals. More than half the employee sample reported at least 1 day absent during the month preceding admission to treatment. In contrast, only one-fourth reported any absenteeism for the month preceding the 6-month contact, and even fewer reported absenteeism for the month preceding the 12-month contact. Multiple or prolonged absences show an even greater posttreatment decline.

D. Summary of Inpatient Findings

A 1-year alcohol and drug dependency treatment outcome study of inpatients entered in the CATOR registry provides significant information about the correlates of successful recovery. The sample, based on patient discharges from 19 centers in 13 states between 1986 and 1988, includes a selection of patients diverse in terms of demographic and socioeconomic factors, personal experiences, and drug use histories.

Of the 1918 patients in the follow-up sample, 63% reported total abstinence for the year after treatment, and an additional 24% reported at least 6 months of abstinence out of 12. Most relapses occurred during the first 6-month interval; 88% of patients who were abstinent the first 6 months maintained this status for the full year.

Women had better outcomes than men, older patients had better outcomes than younger ones, and married patients had better outcomes than those not married. Patients abusing drugs other than alcohol had much poorer outcomes than those abusing alcohol only, and this finding held up even when drug choice was controlled for sex and age of patients. Intravenous drug use was an important predictor of relapse, as was a history of antisocial behavior.

Family participation in treatment increased the likelihood of successful recovery. An even stronger relationship to outcome was seen for patient participation in an aftercare program, and for weekly attendance at peer support group meetings.

Both relapsed and abstinent patients cited impediments to recovery, but they were much more common among relapsers. Emotional distress, relationship difficulties and family problems, financial difficulties, craving, and being around others who use alcohol and drugs are all seen as making the commitment to abstinence more difficult. There is clear evidence also that increased difficulty in these areas is predictive of later relapse.

Comparisons of pretreatment and posttreatment measures of patient functioning revealed a decreased need for expensive health care services, such as hospitalization and emergency room care. The motor vehicle accident rate, traffic arrest rate, and criminal offense arrest rate all showed posttreatment declines. On-the-job problems also decreased dramatically following treatment. Posttreatment difficulties were disporportionately higher among patients who had returned to drug use than among patients who remained abstinent, documenting that successful treatment can have an impact in many areas that improves the quality of life for patients themselves (along with their families and communities) as well as reduces the high economic costs associated with alcohol and drug abuse in our society. Cost offsets for drug dependency treatment are substantial and of broad scope; they are also directly related to the recovery rate.

V. OUTPATIENT TREATMENT OUTCOME

A. Outpatient Treatment Completion versus Noncompletion

The outpatient follow-up sample is based on 914 patient discharges between 1986 and 1988.

The treatment completion rate for outpatients in this study (75%) is lower than that for inpatients (84%). Nevertheless, the outpatient completion rate is in stark contrast to reports of attrition in excess of 50% [16].

A comparison of treatment completers with noncompleters found men and women equally likely to complete outpatient treatment. Married men had a higher completion rate than unmarried men, but no relationship was found between marital status and outpatient treatment completion for women. White patients were somewhat more likely than minority patients to complete treatment, but the relatively small size of the minority patient sample (101 patients) limits generalizability. In addition, socioeconomic factors and drug-use histories are confounding variables; this sample is too small to tease these apart.

Age is related to outpatient treatment completion, much more so than for inpatient treatment. The relationship is linear with younger patients more likely to drop out than older patients. Socioeconomic and social stability factors are also related to outpatient treatment completion just as they are for inpatient treatment completion. Outpatients who did not complete high school, those who were unemployed at admission to treatment, and those with low incomes were more likely to drop out of treatment. A history of recent criminal behavior is also a significant predictor of dropout, another predictor which parallels inpatient findings.

Several factors are predictive for women but not for men. Childhood antisocial behavior, chronic dysphoria, and physical or sexual abuse histories all lower the likelihood of outpatient treatment completion for women.

Overall, drug-use patterns have little predictive value with respect to outpatient treatment completion. In fact, findings in the regard are strikingly consistent with those seen for inpatients. The only drug-use history variable examined that lowered the likelihood of treatment completion was the severity of use consequences associated with drugs other than alcohol, marijuana, or cocaine.

B. Treatment Completer Sample Bias

Since the purpose of this study is to examine treatment effectiveness, the remaining discussion will be limited to treatment completers. Of the 914 outpatient treatment completers discharged during the study period, 91% consented to follow-up. Of these 828 patients, both the 6-month and 12-month interviews were conducted with 359 patients, and one or both contacts were unsuccessful for 469 patients. The follow-up sample represents only 39% of the original sample of treatment completers, limiting the generalizability of the findings. As with the inpatient sample, in which the attrition rate was comparable, analyses were conducted to determine the nature and extent of sample bias.

The only factors found associated with nonconsent were ethnic minority status and daily use of two or more drugs. Contact, or lack thereof, contributed a greater potential for bias. Ethnic minority patients were less likely to be contacted, although the difference between white and minority patients was not statistically significant because of the relatively small sample. Other factors were statistically significant and paralleled contact bias identified for the inpatient sample; proportionately fewer men than women were contacted along with fewer younger than older patients, and fewer high school dropouts. Whereas marital status, employment status, and income level were predictive of contact for inpatients, they did not predict contact in this outpatient sample.

A disporportionate number of outpatients with histories of childhood antisocial behavior and recent arrests are lost to follow-up. There is also a trend for illicit drug use to lower likelihood of contact. These patterns are identical to those seen in the inpatient sample, and confirm the conclusion that the evidence of contact bias seen here would suggest that patients lost to follow-up are faring somewhat worse after treatment, on the whole, than those interviewed for this study. A closer examination of characteristics associated with contact bias among outpatients, however, reveals that the contacted group and noncontacted group are far more similar than dissimilar. In fact, the extent of overlap between the two groups is 85% in terms of proportions with the same number of identified contact predictors. It is reasonable to conclude then that chance plays a greater role in successful contact than prognostic factors for this outpatient sample. There is empirical support elsewhere for such an interpretation [38].

C. Outpatient 1-Year Outcome Findings

Abstinence Rate

Of the selected sample of 359 outpatient treatment completers who were interviewed at 6 and 12 months after discharge, 83% remained abstinent from alcohol and other drugs for the first 6 months after treatment, and 75% were abstinent for the full year. Early success is a strong predictor of continued success: nine out of 10 patients who did not return to substance use during the first 6 months after treatment were drug free the entire year. The 1-year abstinence rate for outpatients is considerably higher than that seen for inpatients in the CATOR registry (75 vs 63%). The higher rate of successful outcomes is consistent with earlier CATOR studies [23] and with the more favorable prognosis projected for outpatients in terms of greater social stability and lesser drug involvement and symptom severity.

Pretreatment Correlates of Abstinence/Relapse Among Outpatients

Demographic and Socioeconomic Factors.   Consistent with findings on inpatients, two demographic characteristics are predictive of recovery status in outpatient analyses. Age and marital status are associated with a greater likelihood of abstinence. Outpatients in their 40s or older have a greater likelihood of successful recovery than those under age 40, and married and widowed patients have a better prognosis than divorced, separated, or single patients. Women are as likely as men to be abstinent 1 year after outpatient treatment. Ethnicity, education, income, and employment do not predict outpatient outcome. However, since minority patients, high school dropouts, and unemployed and low-income patients are more likely to leave treatment early and are more often lost to follow-up, sample bias may challenge the validity of these findings.

Drug- and Alcohol-use History Factors.   Examination of drug- and alcohol-use variables for outpatients reveals a key recovery predictor: illicit drug use, most notably cocaine, is associated with much poorer treatment outcomes than alcohol use only. A history of intravenous drug use also lowers the prognosis, although the number of intravenous drug users in outpatient treatment is small.

The drug choice variable described in the inpatient study was used for this analysis as well. The largest category in the drug choice hierarchy comprises patients who acknowledge only alcohol abuse (56% of the sample). Ten percent abuse marijuana but no other illicit or prescription drug. Patients in the marijuana abuse group typically also abuse alcohol. The other drug abuse group comprises only 7% of the follow-up sample. The typical patient in this group is a regular user of other drugs in addition to alcohol and perhaps marijuana. The final drug choice classification group comprises the 13% of the follow-up sample who are cocaine abusers. Cocaine abusers are typically multiple substance abusers.

The 1-year abstinence rate for alcohol-only abusers is 80%, for marijuana abusers 74%, for other drug abusers 64%, and for cocaine abusers 58%. Because the generalizability of these treatment outcome findings is open to challenge, these figures are most useful in terms of their relative rather than their absolute value. The poorer outcomes associated with illicit drug use hold up even when use consequences are not as severe as those seen in inpatient populations.

Treatment and Posttreatment Correlates of Abstinence/Relapse Among Outpatients

Family Participation in Treatment.   Over two-thirds (70%) of the patients in this treatment follow-up sample had family members or significant others involved in their treatment. In some cases, however, significant others refused to participate (7%), and in a small number of cases (5%) the patient refused to have family members involved. For 19% of the patients, no significant other was identified or available to participate. Family involvement is less common for outpatients than inpatients. In contrast to inpatient results, family involvement is not a significant predictor of outcome for this sample of outpatients.

Program Aftercare.   Approximately four out of five patients in the outpatient follow-up sample reported some involvement in a formal aftercare program sponsored by the treatment center. It cannot be determined from the analyses conducted whether nonparticipation was a matter of personal choice, schedule or transportation problems, or program unavailability.

Outpatients have a higher rate of aftercare participation than inpatients; this is not surprising, since outpatients attend programs within commuting distance, whereas some inpatients attend programs far from home. As with inpatients, a clear relationship can be seen between length of aftercare involvement and abstinence. Patients involved in aftercare for the full year after treatment had a 94% abstinence rate compared with 72% for those involved less than a full year and 68% for those not involved at all.

Alcoholics Anonymous and Other Peer Support Groups.   Over half (55%) of the patients in this follow-up sample attended AA or other support group meetings on a weekly basis, a slightly higher rate than that for inpatients (49%). Their 1-year abstinence rate (87%) was higher than that for less frequent attenders (76%) or those who stopped attending or never attended at all (55%).

Patients' Perceptions of Recovery Impediments.   Many more relapsed than abstinent outpatients report emotional distress (boredom, anger, loneliness, depression), not wanting to quit, and not believing that they are drug or alcohol dependent as impediments to recovery. Craving is reported by twice as many relapsed as abstinent patients; even so, almost two-thirds of relapsed outpatients do not acknowledge craving as a problem, suggesting that craving is overemphasized as a contributor to relapse. Patients' failure to recognize their addiction and their unwillingness to give up alcohol or drugs may demand greater attention during aftercare planning.

Other Measures of Treatment Impact

Health Care Comparison.   The hospitalization rate for outpatients during the year after treatment is much lower than that during the year before treatment. The hospitalization rate for illness or injury declines by more than half, from 17 to 6% (hospitalizations related to pregnancy or childbirth are excluded from health care analyses). Hospitalizations required for detoxification also decline (7–2%).

The use of an emergency room for health care also decreases following treatment, although the decrease is small. Before treatment, one-fourth (24%) of the patients reported an emergency room visit related to illness or injury compared with 20% following treatment. In contrast

Table 13 Outpatient Treatment Completers Patients' Perceptions of Recovery Impediments

Perceived impediments to recovery	Abstinent patients N = 270 (%)	Relapsed patients N = 89 (%)
Marital or relationship problems[a]	23	38
Stress from family problems	30	36
Financial problems	25	37
Boredom, anger, loneliness, or depression[b]	29	54
Craving alcohol or drugs[c]	19	38
Not really wanting to quit[b]	4	37
Belief that you're not drug dependent[b]	8	24

[a]Chi square p value < 0.05.
[b]Chi square p value < 0.0001.
[c]Chi square p value < 0.01.

to hospitalization and emergency care, outpatient health care is relatively unchanged following treatment.

Legal Problems.   The number of outpatients reporting a motor vehicle accident in which they were the driver is reduced by nearly two-thirds during the year following treatment. The arrest rate for DWI offenses and other moving traffic violations also decreases by two-thirds following treatment (27–9%), with the most notable decline seen in multiple arrests. The criminal arrest rate also declines after treatment. Whereas almost one patient out of 10 was arrested during the year before treatment, only 1% report an arrest following treatment.

Job Problems.   In order to conduct pretreatment-posttreatment comparisons of job problems, the comparison sample was restricted to those patients who were employed full time during the 12-month periods before and after treatment. This inclusion criterion eliminates the potential influence of varying lengths of employment on job experiences. Of the 359 patients in the follow-up sample, 177 met this qualification.

Job problems reported before treatment were very common. Almost one-fourth of these patients reported problems with supervisors, making mistakes on the job, and tardiness. One-fifth reported absenteeism. In addition, almost one out of 10 was injured on the job during the year before treatment. This high prevalence of job problems is not surprising in light of reported levels of working under the influence of alcohol or drugs. One out of five employed patients acknowledged that they were working under the influence at least once a week (half of these almost every day). However, half of these employed patients stated that they were never under the influence at work during the year before treatment.

Dramatic reductions are seen in job absenteeism and tardiness, making mistakes, and problems completing work. Interpersonal problems are also reported less frequently, although the difference in this area is less marked than in other areas. The rate reporting on-the-job injury is cut in half after treatment.

Even patients who report a relapse following treatment are very unlikely to report that using affects their job. Only 2% of the employee follow-up sample report any working under the influence during the year after treatment (compared with 48% reporting at least occasional impairment before treatment).

Actual days of absenteeism were measured only for 30-day intervals because of the

Table 14 Outpatient Treatment Completers Legal Problems Before and After Treatment

	(N = 359)	
Legal problem	Year before treatment (%)	Year after treatment (%)
Motor vehicle accidents		
0	83	92
1	13	6
2 or more	4	2
Traffic violation arrests		
0	74	89
1	17	10
2 or more	9	1
Criminal offense arrests		
0	90	99
1	8	1
2 or more	2	0

Table 15 Outpatient Treatment Completers Job Problems for Patients Employed Full Time During the Year Before and the Year After Treatment

	(N = 177)	
Job problem	Year before treatment (%)	Year after treatment (%)
Difficulties with boss or supervisor	23	11
Completing work	12	3
Making mistakes	22	1
Being absent	20	4
Being late	22	4
On-the-job injury	9	4
Frequency of working under the influence of alcohol/drugs		
almost every day	11	1
1–3 times a week	11	0
1–3 times a month	9	0
less than once a month	17	1
never	52	98

	For a 30-day period		
Number of days absent from work	Before admission to treatment (%)	Before the 6-month interview (%)	Before 12-month interview (%)
0	70	78	82
1	12	15	10
2	4	3	3
3 or more	14	4	5

difficulty in recalling over longer intervals. Thirty percent of the employee sample reported at least 1 day absent during the month preceding admission to treatment. In contrast, 22% reported any absenteeism for the month preceding the 6-month contact, and only 18% reported absenteeism for the month preceding the 12-month contact. Multiple or prolonged absences show the greatest posttreatment decline.

D. Summary of Outpatient Findings

A 1-year outcome study of alcohol and drug dependency outpatients entered in the CATOR registry provides information about the correlates of successful recovery. Of the 359 patients in the follow-up sample, 75% reported total abstinence for the year after treatment. Most relapses occurred during the first 6 months after treatment; nine out of 10 patients who were abstinent the first 6 months maintained this status for the full year.

Older patients had better outcomes than younger ones, and married patients had better outcomes than those not married. Patients abusing drugs other than alcohol had much poorer outcomes than those abusing alcohol only. Participation in an aftercare program and weekly attendance at peer support group meetings were predictive of successful recovery. More relapsed than abstinent patients cited impediments to recovery. Emotional distress, relationship difficulties and family problems, financial difficulties, and craving are all seen as making the commitment to abstinence more difficult. Relapsed patients were much less likely to believe they were drug dependent and many were not sure they wanted to quit.

Comparisons of pretreatment and posttreatment measures of patient functioning revealed a decreased need for expensive health care services. The motor vehicle accident rate, traffic arrest rate, and criminal offense arrest rate all showed posttreatment declines. On-the-job problems also decreased dramatically following treatment. CATOR studies consistently find that posttreatment difficulties are disproportionately higher among patients who return to drug and alcohol use than among patients who remain abstinent, documenting that successful treatment can have an impact in many areas.

VI. DISCUSSION

A. Outcome Findings in Context

One-year abstinence rates for inpatients (63%) and outpatients (75%) treated at private treatment centers suggest that these treatment programs are quite successful at achieving their primary goal. Because these findings can be challenged with respect to their generalizability, further discussion of this issue is warranted. In order to provide an appropriate context in which to evaluate these results, we will address three key points: population characteristics, sample attrition and generalizability, and the validity of patient self-report.

Population Characteristics

Some critics of treatment effectiveness cite high relapse rates to argue against efficacy. Indeed, numerous studies can be found to justify skepticism about costly investments in treatment, with relapse rates ranging from 67 to 100% over periods ranging from 6 months to 2 years [59–63]. Yet a careful examination of studies reporting on such poor outcomes highlights population and program differences. The populations are comprised predominantly of chronic alcoholics or drug addicts with histories of social instability and treatment recidivism. With recent emphasis on earlier intervention for drug abuse, treatment populations currently include larger proportions of less-affected patients than found in programs in past decades. Treatments described in earlier studies often fall far short of what is considered state-of-the art in the private sector.

Consistent with the findings reported here, studies on similar populations tend to show abstinence rates in excess of 50% for 1 year [23–25,39,64–71]. It is most likely true that the greatest proportion of treatment outcome variance is attributable to patient characteristics rather than program characteristics. The possibility that better programs can produce better outcomes cannot be dismissed, however, simply because research has not yet reached the level of sophistication to document such differences.

Sample Attrition and Generalizability

Since it is generally assumed that nonparticipants in follow-up studies have poorer outcomes than participants, we developed a procedure to address the attrition in our outcome samples. Since the outcome results were based on only a minority of treatment completers in both inpatient and outpatient samples (approximately 40%), there is obviously a great deal of room for sample bias. We identified a series of 29 patient characteristics or history variables that had differential predictive value in terms of posttreatment abstinence for contacted patients. These variables were primarily related to social stability (socioeconomic factors and antisocial histories) and the severity of addiction. A composite variable was then constructed counting the number of such characteristics associated with each patient. Abstinence rates were determined for contacted patients in the inpatient and outpatient samples according to number of identified relapse predictors. Not surprisingly, there was a strong linear relationship between the number of risk factors and the associated abstinence rate. For instance, among inpatients, the few with no risk factors were all abstinent compared with only one-third of those with 15 or more risk factors. These associated abstinence rates were then applied to subgroups of patients in the respective inpatient and outpatient noncontact samples matched for total number of risk factors.

As expected, noncontacted patients were projected to have poorer outcomes than contacted patients. However, the differences were quite small. Noncontacted inpatients have a projected abstinence rate of 58% (compared with 63% for contacted inpatients), resulting in an estimate of 60% for the entire inpatient treatment completer sample. Noncontacted outpatients have a projected abstinence rate of 72% (compared with 75% for contacted outpatients), resulting in an estimate of 74% for the entire outpatient treatment completer sample.

The finding that this method of extrapolating observed results to entire samples reduces recovery rates by only a few percentage points runs counter to generally held assumptions of doomsday predictions for patients not successfully followed. The explanation lies in the extent of overlap of risk factors between contacted and noncontacted samples (covering 82% of inpatients and 86% of outpatients). Since only a very small proportion of patients in each sample differs in terms of number of risk factors, even the large differential observed for abstinence rate from low risk to high risk has a small effect overall on the outcome results for the whole sample.

One caution must be highlighted with respect to this method for extrapolating results. It assumes that the only differences between contacted and noncontacted patients are those that existed at admission and were identified in our analyses. There may in fact be other differences, particularly in posttreatment characteristics or environment that affect recovery which are not subject to measurement by this method. Therefore, it cannot be ruled out that noncontacted patients are faring worse than projected. A final consideration, of course, is that these projections refer only to treatment completers, and it is reasonable to expect that noncompleters are much more likely to resume drug or alcohol use, if they stopped at all.

Validity of Patient Self-Report

The truthfulness of patient responses in drug dependency outcome studies is constantly challenged [68]. For example, an article in *Science* states that "self-reports of drinking behavior are notoriously unreliable" (p. 20) [16]. The unquestioned acceptance of this viewpoint results in part from evidence of denial as a facet of chemical dependency, and in part from a long-standing and widespread perception of alcoholics and addicts as morally defective [69,70]. The weight of empirical evidence, however, suggests just the opposite. When respondents are guaranteed confidentiality, when questions are clear and objective, that is, behaviorally oriented, and when the interviewer is not personally invested in the outcome, respondents tend to give honest answers [69,71–74].

In our own attempt to quantify the extent of patient underreporting of drug use after treatment, we found that 87% of patient reports of abstinence were corroborated during a separate interview with a significant other [43]. If we apply this factor to the 60% abstinence rate we extrapolated for the inpatient sample and the 74% rate for the outpatient sample, we arrive at 1-year abstinence rates of 52% for inpatients and 64% for outpatients. Thus, even with the application of statistical techniques to take into account potential sample bias and patient overreporting of abstinence, recovery estimates clearly substantiate treatment effectiveness for a diverse aggregate of private treatment programs in the United States.

B. Recommendations

Clearly, treatment is responding very well to many patients' needs. Yet improvement is needed in some areas. More needs to be learned about why some patients drop out of treatment and what can be done to retain them. Special needs of particular subgroups of patients must be considered, particularly people with weak or nonexistent social and economic resources. Patients with less formal education also demand further consideration. People who may have dropped out of high school because they could not learn well in traditional settings or by traditional methods may find themselves facing similar frustrations with lectures and "chalk talks" in treatment. Treatment professionals need to take care that the treatment process not further stigmatize or shame undereducated or illiterate patients who seek help for alcohol and drug problems.

Treatment may also have to incorporate changes to respond to the increasing numbers of patients abusing illicit drugs. Models developed for alcoholics do not appear to be as effective for drug abusers, and it would be irresponsible to attribute differential outcomes solely to patient characteristics. Two key points come to mind. Younger patients, those most likely to be involved with drugs, began substance use at earlier ages than older patients. They may then demand more habilitative services rather than rehabilitative services. Also, whereas many alcoholics can give up alcohol but retain at least some of their social support networks, many drug users must literally change worlds when they dissociate themselves from drug subcultures. This transition may be particularly challenging for young patients still seeking an identity.

Clearly, the strong relationship between participation in aftercare programs and peer support groups substantiates the need for increased attention, and possibly increased financial support, for such recovery maintenance systems. Further research is needed to determine why some patients do not avail themselves of posttreatment recovery resources, and how supportive services can be tailored more to their liking. Services must be sensitive to the needs of particular groups such as people of color, lesbians and gay men, illicit drug users, people with human immunodeficiency virus (HIV) infections, single parents, young adults, and abuse victims. They must be affordable, conveniently located, and attempt to accommodate varying schedules. Increasing the attractiveness and accessibility of long-term supportive services would improve patient outcomes.

ACKNOWLEDGMENTS

Outcome findings are based on data provided by: HCA Las Encinas Hospital, Pasadena, California; Glenbeigh of Tampa, Florida; Commencement Center, Athens, Georgia; Columbus Hospital, Chicago, and Hopedale Hall, Hopedale, Illinois; Forest City Treatment Center, Forest City, Marian Health Center and St. Luke's Gordon Recovery Centers, Sioux City, Iowa; St. Joseph Medical Center, Wichita, Kansas; Charter Ridge Hospital, Lexington, Kentucky; HCA De Paul Hospital, New Orleans, and HCA Parkland Hospital, Baton Rouge, Louisiana; New Beginnings, Salisbury, Maryland; Fountain Lake Treatment Center, Albert Lea, New Beginnings, Waverly, St. Mary's/Riverside Medical Center, Minneapolis, and St. Paul–Ramsey Medical Center, St. Paul, Minnesota; Smithers Alcohol Treatment Center and Stuyvesant Square/Doctors Hospital, New York, New York; Glenbeigh Hospitals Cleveland and Rock Creek, Talbot Hall/St. Anthony's Medical Center, Columbus, Ohio; Saint Francis Hospital, Tulsa, Oklahoma; Vanderbilt University Medical Center North, Nashville, Tennessee; HCA Sun Valley Regional Hospital, El Paso, Texas; Medical Center Hospital of Vermont, South Burlington, Vermont; Lakeside-Milam Recovery Centers, Buthell, Washington; St. Francis Monastery, La Crosse, Tellurian Community, Inc., Madison, Theda Clark Clinic, Green Bay, and Theda Clark Hospital, Neenah, Wisconsin.

Data base management provided by Michael G. Luxenberg, Ph.D., President, Professional Data Analysts, Minneapolis. Computer support provided by Academic Computing Services at the University of Minnesota, Minneapolis.

REFERENCES

1. Pattison, E.M., Coe, R., Doerr, H.O. (1973). Population variation among alcoholism treatment facilities. *Int. J. Addict., 8*:199-229.
2. Costello, R.M. (1975). Alcoholism treatment and evaluation. In search of methods. II. Collation of two-year follow-up studies. *Int. J. Addict., 10*:857-867.
3. Vannicelli, M., Pfau, B., and Ryback, R.S. (1976). Data attrition in follow-up studies of alcoholics. *J. Stud. Alcohol, 37*:1325-1330.
4. Emrick, C.D., and Hansen, J. (1983). Assertions regarding effectiveness of treatment for alcoholism. Fact or fantasy. *Am. Psychol., 38*:1078-1088.
5. Nathan, P.E., and Skinstad, A. (1987). Outcomes of treatment for alcohol problems: Current methods, problems, and results. *J. Consult. Clin. Psychol., 55*:332-340.
6. Nace, E.P. (1989). The natural history of alcoholism versus treatment effectiveness: Methodological problems. *Am. J. Drug Alcohol Abuse, 15*:55-60.
7. Kissin, B., and Hanson, M. (1982). The bio-psycho-social perspective in alcoholism. *Alcoholism Clin. Psychiatry* (J. Solomon, ed.). New York, Plenum Press.
8. Zucker, R.A., and Gomberg, E.S.L. (1986). Etiology of alcoholism reconsidered. The case for a biopsychosocial process. *Am. Psychol., 41*:783-793.
9. Johnston, L.D. (1985). The etiology and prevention of substance use. What can we learn from recent historical changes?, *Etiology of Drug Abuse: Implications for Prevention* (C.L. Jones and R.J. Battjes, eds.). National Institute of Drug Abuse Research Monograph 56, Department of Health and Human Services Publication No. (ADM) 85-1335. Rockville, Maryland.
10. Harrison, P.A. (1989). Women in treatment: Changing over time. *Int. J. Addict., 24*:655-673.
11. Johnston, L.D., O'Malley, P.M., and Bachman, J.G. (1989). *Drug Use, Drinking and Smoking: National Survey Results from High School, College, and Young Adult Populations 1975-1988.* Department of Health and Human Services Publication No. (ADM) 89-1638, U.S. Government Printing Office, Washington, D.C.
12. Kirn, T.F. (1986). Advances in understanding of alcoholism initiate evolution in treatment programs. *J.A.M.A., 256*:1405-1412.
13. Annis, H.M. (1986). Is inpatient rehabilitation of the alcoholic cost effective? Con position. *Adv. Alcohol Subst. Abuse, 5*:175-190.
14. Miller, W.R., and Hester, R.K. (1986). Inpatient alcoholism treatment: Who benefits? *Am. Psycholog., 41*:794-805.
15. Gordis, E. (1987). Accessible and affordable health care for alcoholism and related problems: Strategy for cost containment. *J. Stud. Alcohol, 48*:579-585.
16. Holden, C. (1987). Is alcoholism treatment effective? *Science, 236*:20-22.
17. Jones, K.R., and Vischi, T.R. (1979). Impact of alcohol, drug abuse, and mental health treatment on medical care utilization: A review of the research literature. *Med. Care, 17(Suppl.)*:1-82.
18. Holder, H.D., and Hallan, J.B. (1981). Medical care and alcoholism treatment costs and utilization: A five-year analysis of the California pilot project to provide health insurance coverage for alcoholism. Chapel Hill, North Carolina, H-2, Inc.
19. McLellan, A.T., Luborsky, L., O'Brien, C.P., Woody, G.E., and Druley, K.A. (1982). Is treatment for substance abuse effective? *J.A.M.A., 247*:1423-1428.
20. Hoffmann, N.G., Harrison, P.A., and Belille, C.A. (1984). Multidimensional impact of treatment for substance abuse. *Adv. Alcoholism Subst. Abuse, 3*:83-94.
21. Holder, H.D., Blose, J.G., and Gasiorowski, M.J. (1985). *Alcoholism Treatment Impact on Total Health Care Utilization and Costs: A Four-Year Longitudinal Analysis of the Federal Employees Health Benefit Program with Aetna Life Insurance Company.* Chapel Hill, North Carolina, H-2, Inc.

22. Lessard, R.J., Harrison, P.A., and Hoffmann, N.G. (1985). Cost and benefits of chemical dependency treatment. *Minn. Med., 68*:449–451.
23. Harrison, P.A., and Hoffmann, N.G. (1988). *CATOR Report. Adult outpatient treatment: Perspectives on admission and outcome*. St. Paul, Minnesota, Ramsey Clinic.
24. Hoffmann, N.G., and Harrison, P.A. (1988). *CATOR Report. Treatment outcome: Adult inpatients two years later*. St. Paul, Minnesota, Ramsey Clinic.
25. Harrison, P.A., and Hoffmann, N.G. (1989). *CATOR Report. Adult inpatient completers one year later*. St. Paul, Minnesota, Ramsey Clinic.
26. Laundergan, J.C. (1982). *Easy Does It*. Center City, Minnesota, Hazelden Foundation.
27. Nace, E.P. (1990). Inpatient treatment of alcoholism: A necessary part of the therapeutic armamentarium. *Psychiatr. Hosp., 21*:9–12.
28. Hoffmann, N.G., Halikas, J.A., and Mee-Lee, D. (1987). *Cleveland Admission, Discharge, and Transfer Criteria*. Cleveland, Ohio, Greater Cleveland Hospital Association.
29. Harrison, P.A., Hoffmann, N.G., Gibbs, L., Hollister, C.D., and Luxenberg, M.G. (1988). Determinants of chemical dependency treatment placement: Clinical, economic, and logistic factors. *Psychotherapy, 25*:356–364.
30. Straus, R., and Bacon, S.D. (1951). Alcoholism and social stability. A study of occupational integration in 2,023 male clinic patients. *Q. J. Stud. Alcohol., 31*:972–974.
31. Prothro, W.B. (1963). Inpatient versus outpatient alcoholism rehabilitation. *J. Mich. St. Med. Soc., 62*:1004–1007.
32. Armor, D.J., Polich, J.M., and Stambul, H.B. (1978). *Alcoholism Treatment*, New York, Wiley.
33. Skinner, H.A. (1981). Comparison of clients assigned to inpatient and outpatient treatment for alcoholism and drug addiction. *Br. J. Psychiatry, 138*:312–320.
34. Spicer, J., Nyberg, L.R., and McKenna, T.R. (1981). *Apples and Oranges*. Center City, Minnesota, Hazelden Foundation.
35. Evenson, R.C., Reese, P.J., and Holland, R.A. (1982). Measuring the severity of symptoms in outpatient alcoholics. *J. Stud. Alcohol, 43*:839–842.
36. Cole, S.G., Lehman, W.E., Cole, E.A., and Jones, A. (1981). Inpatient versus outpatient treatment of alcohol and drug abusers. *Am. J. Drug Alcohol Abuse, 8*:329–345.
37. Moos, R., and Bliss, F. (1978). Difficulty of follow-up and outcome of alcoholism treatment. *J. Stud. Alcohol, 39*:473–490.
38. LaPorte, D.J., McLellan, A.T., Erdlen, F.R., and Parente, R.J. (1981). Treatment outcome as a function of follow-up difficulty in substance abusers. *J. Consult. Clin. Psychol., 49*:112–119.
39. Pickens, R.W., Hatsukami, D.K., Spicer, J.W., and Svikis, D.S. (1985). Relapse by alcohol abusers. *Alcoholism Clin. Exp. Res., 9*:244–247.
40. Beyer, J.M., and Trice, H.M. (1981). A retrospective study of similarities and differences between men and women employees in a job-based alcoholism program from 1965 to 1977. *J. Drug Iss., 11*:233–265.
41. Lyons, J.P., Welte, J.N., Brown, J., Sokolow, L., and Hynes, G. (1982). Variation in alcoholism treatment orientation: Differential impact upon specific subpopulations. *Alcoholism Clin. Exp. Res., 6*:333–343.
42. Gibbs, L., and Flanagan, J. (1977). Prognostic indicators of alcoholism treatment outcome. *Int. J. Addict., 12*:1097–1141.
43. Hoffmann, N.G., and Harrison, P.A. (1986). *CATOR Report. Findings two years after treatment*. St. Paul, Minnesota, Ramsey Clinic.
44. Harrison, P.A., Hoffmann, N.G., and Edwall, G.E. (1989). Differential drug use patterns among sexually abused adolescent girls in treatment for chemical dependency. *Int. J. Addict., 24*:499–514.
45. Harrison, P.A., Hoffmann, N.G., and Edwall, G.E. (1989). Sexual abuse correlates: Similarities between male and female adolescents in chemical dependency treatment. *J. Adolesc. Res., 4*:385–399.
46. *Sixth Special Report to the U.S. Congress on Alcohol and Health* (1987). Department of Health and Human Services, Publication No. (ADM) 87-1519. U.S. Government Printing Office, Washington, D.C.

47. Costello, R.M. (1980). Alcoholism aftercare and outcome: Cross-lagged panel and path analyses. *Br. J. Addict.*, *75*:49–53.

48. Ahles, T.A., Schlundt, D.G., Prue, D.M., and Rychtarik, R.G. (1983). Impact of aftercare arrangements on the maintenance of treatment success in abusive drinkers. *Addict. Behav.*, *8*:53–58.

49. Walker, R.D., Donovan, D.M., Kivlahan, D.R., and O'Leary, M.R. (1983). Length of stay, neuropsychological performance, and aftercare: Influences on alcohol treatment outcome. *J. Consult. Clin. Psychol.*, *51*:900–911.

50. Svanum, S., and McAdoo, W.G. (1989). Predicting rapid relapse following treatment for chemical dependence: A matched-subjects design. *J. Consult. Clin. Psychol.*, *57*:222–226.

51. Farris-Kurtz, L. (1981). Time in residential care and participation in Alcoholics Anonymous as predictors of continued sobriety. *Psychol. Rep.*, *48*:633–634.

52. Pettinati, H.M., Sugerman, A.A., DiDonato, N., and Maurer, H.S. (1982). The natural history of alcoholism over four years after treatment. *J. Stud. Alcohol*, *43*:201–215.

53. Hoffmann, N.G., Harrison, P.A., and Belille, C.A. (1983). Alcoholics Anonymous after treatment: Attendance and abstinence. *Int. J. Addict.*, *18*:311–318.

54. Vaillant, G.E., Clark, W., Cyrus, C., Milofsky, E.S., Kopp, J., Wulsin, V.W., and Mogielnicki, N.P. (1983). Prospective study of alcoholism treatment. Eight-year follow-up. *Am. J. Med.*, *75*:455–563.

55. Orford, J., Oppenheimer, E., Egert, S., Hensman, C., and Guthrie, S. (1976). The cohesiveness of alcoholism-complicated marriages and its influence on treatment outcome. *Br. J. Psychiatry*, *128*:318–319.

56. Finney, J.W., Moos, R.H., and Mewborn, C.R. (1980). Posttreatment experiences and treatment outcome of alcoholic patients six months and two years after hospitalization. *J. Consult. Clin. Psychol.*, *48*:17–29.

57. Vanicelli, M., Gingerich, S., and Ryback, R. (1983). Family problems related to the treatment and outcome of alcoholic patients. *Br. J. Addict.*, *78*:193–204.

58. Hoffmann, N.G., Rode, S., and Fulkerson, J. (1990). Medical care utilization before and after alcoholism treatment for the elderly. *Southwestern: J. Aging Southwest*, *6*:142–148.

59. Mosher, V., Davis, J., Mulligun, D., and Iber, F.L. (1975). Comparison of outcome in a 9-day and 30-day alcohol treatment program. *J. Stud. Alcohol*, *36*:1277–1281.

60. Orford, J., Oppenheimer, E., and Edwards, G. (1976). Abstinence or control: The outcome for excessive drinkers two years after consultation. *Behav. Res. Ther.*, *14*:409–418.

61. Wilson, A., White, J., and Lange, D.E. (1978). Outcome evaluation of a hospital-based alcoholism treatment programme. *Br. J. Addict.*, *73*:39–45.

62. McLachlan, J.F., and Stein, R.L. (1982). Evaluation of a day clinic for alcoholics. *J. Stud. Alcohol*, *43*:261–272.

63. Fink, E.B., Longabaugh, R., McCrady, B.M., Stout, R.L., Beattie, M., Authelet, A.R., and McNeil, D. (1985). Effectiveness of alcoholism treatment in partial versus inpatient settings, twenty-four month outcomes. *Addict. Behav.*, *10*:235–248.

64. Patton, M. (1979). *Validity and Reliability of Hazelden Treatment Follow-up Data*. Center City, Minnesota, Hazelden Foundation.

65. Laundergan, J.C. (1982). *The Outcome of Treatment: A Comparative Study of Patients 25 Years Old and Younger and 26 Years and Older Admitted to Hazelden in 1979*. Center City, Minnesota, Hazelden Foundation.

66. Neuberger, O.W., Miller, S.I., Schmitz, R.E., Matarazzo, J.D., Pratt, H., and Hasha, N. (1982). Replicable abstinence rates in an alcoholism treatment program. *J.A.M.A.*, *248*:960–963.

67. Weins, A.N., and Menustik, C.E. (1983). Treatment outcome and patient characteristics in an aversion therapy program for alcoholism. *Am. Psychol.*, *38*:1089–1096.

68. Watson, C.G., Tilleskjor, C., Hoodecheck-Schow, E.A., Pucel, J., and Jacobs, L. (1984). Do alcoholics give valid self-reports? *J. Stud. Alcohol*, *45*:344–348.

69. Sobell, L.C., and Sobell, M.B. (1986). Can we do without alcohol abusers' self-reports? *Behav. Ther.*, *9*:141–146.

70. Hoffmann, N.G., and Harrison, P.A. (1989) Relapse: Conceptual and methodological issues. *J. Chem. Depend. Treat.*, *2*:27–51.

71. Freedberg, E.J., and Johnston, W.E. (1980). Validity and reliability of alcoholics' self-reports and use of alcohol submitted before and after treatment. *Psychol. Rep., 46*:999–1005.

72. Polich, J.M. (1982). The validity of self-reports in alcoholism research. *Addict. Behav., 7*:123–132.

73. Maisto, S.A., Sobell, L.C., and Sobell, M.B. (1982–83). Corroboration of drug abusers' self-reports through the use of multiple data sources. *Am. J. Drug Alcohol Abuse, 9*:301–308.

74. Verinis, J.S. (1983). Agreement between alcoholics and relatives when reporting follow-up status. *Int. J. Addict., 18*:891–894.

XX

Outpatient Treatment

64

History and Theory of a Treatment for Drug and Alcohol Addiction

George A. Mann
St. Mary's Hospital, Minneapolis, Minnesota

I. INTRODUCTION

It is important to understand the evolution leading to the development of the modern methods of treatment for alcoholism and drug addiction. The current "treatment industry," as it is seen today, was launched in the late 1960s and early 1970s. Prior to that time, the entire concept and approach to rehabilitation was very different than it is in most treatment centers today. There is a fairly long history to the drug maintenance modality, as seen in the methadone maintenance programs that go back to the 1950s or even earlier. That approach has little to do with the current approach to rehabilitation.

Following World War II, American medicine underwent a substantial evolution in surgery, the treatment of infectious diseases, the management of chronic disease, and the pharmacological management of major psychiatric illnesses. During the 1950s and 1960s, the entire issue of alcohol and drug addiction was largely ignored by organized medicine. There was a widely accepted belief that these problems were merely symptoms of underlying psychiatric problems and were best treated by discovering the underlying problem and applying the appropriate therapy. Alcoholism and drug addiction were not considered to be primary problems, but rather were always secondary to something else.

During this period, individuals who were mostly recovering alcoholics reacted to this lack of what they considered to be appropriate and effective care. They began to experiment with the development of an innovative system of treatment which was entirely separate from organized medicine. This system was based on the premise that alcoholism was a primary disease rather than a symptom of some other problem. During this time, there was no clearly identifiable therapy available for alcoholism in the various divisions of most American general or psychiatric hospitals. Typically, hospitals did not even have an admitting diagnosis for alcoholism. Health care insurance policies provided no coverage for the problem. Consequently, alcoholics could only receive needed care in a hospital under a surreptitious diagnosis, or waited until the disease had reached its later stages and physical complications developed.

Certainly, alcoholism and drug addiction were being treated in these hospitals, but not under that diagnosis. Alcoholics were admitted under a variety of diagnoses: depression, personality disorders, cirrhosis, pancreatitis, gastroenteritis, organic brain syndrome, alcohol toxicity, and just plain old flu! It is difficult to find reliable data reflecting the effectiveness of therapy during those years, but it is commonly known that success was unlikely. During this same time, a number of public hospitals developed inpatient detoxification protocols. These detoxification units managed the detoxification and related acute medical emergencies. The full extent of the responsibility of physicians and hospitals was considered complete after the detoxification protocols were completed. The advent of the benzodiazepines greatly simplified the detoxification process while reducing mortality and morbidity. In some hospitals, this attitude and belief is very much alive and well in 1990. An additional problem, at that time, was a sociocultural attitude that in order for an adult to be considered "normal" they should be able to drink alcohol! Consequently, much therapeutic time and energy were spent on developing therapies based on "teaching" alcoholics how to drink socially. The theory was that if the alcoholic could be taught to use alcohol as a social beverage, the problem of alcoholism would disappear. The fact that none of these efforts produced the desired results did not deter health care professionals from continuing this myopic pursuit. Some went so far as to actually publish faulty data in order to support and advance this cultural belief.

While organized medicine involved itself in these nonproductive activities, the nonmedical treatment system grew and flourished. It grew in its capacity to treat patients, but more importantly it grew in therapeutic effectiveness. This nonmedical approach held that alcoholism was a primary disorder, and therefore the logical approach was to institute an abstinence-based approach to rehabilitation. This pragmatic approach believed alcohol consumption was the basic problem, and the complete elimination of this drug from the life of the patient was a reasonable and achievable goal. Places like the Hazelden Foundation in Minnesota and Chit Chat in Pennsylvania are examples of this early pioneering. They borrowed heavily from the 12 Steps and practices of Alcoholics Anonymous (AA), which was established in 1935.

These pioneers integrated the basic philosophy of AA into inpatient programs. A standard program and a uniform therapeutic approach was offered for all patients. It was inexpensive, and compared to what was being offered by organized medicine, quite effective. This approach received wide support from the AA community, who received the graduates of these programs into their welcoming arms and supplied them with on-going support mainly of AA activities and group support. A system of educational sessions developed which taught patients the "nature" of alcoholism and introduced them to the 12 Steps of the AA program. There was also a program of suggested reading material developed. It was used as the basis for daily discussion groups. They also developed a longitudinal aftercare support and follow-up system that was community based and incorporated into the existing AA framework.

During the middle and late 1960s, a number of private hospitals recognized that alcoholism was a serious problem in their communities and decided to attempt to develop services that would directly address this problem. They began to recognize that many of their medical, surgical, and psychiatric beds were being utilized by alcoholics, who presented themselves with a wide variety of problems. The hospitals realized that while they were treating the complications of alcoholism they were capable of doing little to address the basic problem.

After a period of investigation and study, the decision was made to attempt to develop a new modality of treatment which would maintain the medical model but would borrow heavily from the existing nonmedical model. This of course called for a radical change in philosophy and clinical approach to alcoholism. There had been a disease theory of alcoholism concept in existence for some time. E. M. Jellinek M.D., had developed a progressive paradigm based on clinical signs and symptoms of alcoholism which was of great value in the early development of the natural course of this disease. Both the World Health Organization (WHO) and the American Medical Association (AMA) had embraced this theory much earlier (during the 1950s). An immediate controversy began in these hospitals between those who fought to continue the traditional medical position and those desiring to move therapy into a new era. In many hospitals, this controversy continues even today! Finally, the decision was made by a few hospitals to allow limited space and resources for the development of this radical new approach to the problem.

The intent of this system was to maintain and enhance the traditional medical expertise in physiology, pathology, and pharmacology. Internal medicine and psychiatry were envisioned to play an important clinical role in these programs. Some programs were organized under one of these two departments and came under their management structure. It was important that these programs became a part of the medical staff and departmental committee structure. This would allow the normal check and balance mechanisms to function.

There were four major changes integral to this system:

1. The intent of therapy was to attempt to instill a level of insight in the patient which would provide sufficient motivation for the acceptance of the concept of life-long abstinence from alcohol and all other mood-altering drugs.
2. The diagnosis and treatment of serious medical and psychiatric problems—obstacles to the maintenance of abstinence.
3. The involvement of the patient's family and other significant persons as a regular part of the clinical program.
4. A prolonged system of aftercare and follow-up with in-depth involvement of community self-help organizations (i.e., AA) as well as hospital-based support groups.

The theory of treatment as it continued to evolve in the 1970s and 1980s consisted of a set of beliefs and skills that came directly out of traditional medical and psychiatric disciplines. These were integrated with the accumulated knowledge of Alcoholics Anonymous and the nonmedical treatment programs existing at that time. The theory was fundamentally based on the disease theory of alcoholism. For the first time alcoholism was addressed as a primary disease. It was obvious that alcoholics were prone to develop a wide range of medical and psychiatric problems secondary to their alcoholism that needed to be diagnosed and treated. If these secondary problems were not appropriately handled, the outlook for successful treatment (prolonged abstinence and sobriety) were dim. It was this capacity for treating these complicating problems that distinguished these early hospital-based programs from the nonmedical programs.

During these early years, the drug explosion hit America. Prior to the Vietnam War and the counter-culture movement, alcohol was traditionally the most common addictive drug used in the United States. For decades there had been relatively small populations of heroin addicts, prescription drug addicts, and even fewer marijuana users. Following the 1960s and 1970s, however, the addictive drug picture dramatically changed. Alcohol was no longer the drug of choice for great numbers of patients being admitted for care. Therapists were dealing with issues and substances and accompanying lifestyles with which they had little or no experience. Treatment programs saw an influx of patients and drugs very different from the typical alcoholic population they had been accustomed to. It was unknown whether the approaches, lexicon, and therapy that had been effective with the alcoholic population would be useful with this new group of patients.

Many changes in language, terminology, and therapy techniques had to be made. For example, the term *Alcoholic Treatment Program* no longer described the purpose of the program. The term *chemical dependency* was adopted as a substitute. This title seemed to best describe what the programs were treating. Since that time, this term had effectively replaced the previous terminology. It should be noted, however, that the old standby alcohol has never been really replaced by any of the popular drugs. More commonly, these individuals present themselves with multiple drug problems, one of which is usually alcohol. The drug-using population tends to be very avant-garde in its drugs of choice. Consequently, the popular drug of today, whether its "crack" cocaine or amphetamine "ice," will rather quickly be replaced. So while the drug repertoire may change rapidly, alcohol remains a common denominator.

While this innovation in treatment was occurring, (1970–1980) tremendous progress was also being made in basic science research on the addictive process. NIAAA (National Institute of Alcohol Abuse and Alcoholism), NIH (National Institute of Health), NIDA (National Institute of Drug Abuse) as well as various universities devoted a considerable amount of their research energies into expanding our knowledge base of the mechanisms involved in alcoholism and drug addiction. One area that has been particularly outstanding has been the work done in the genetic transmission of alcoholism. These discoveries as well as the work in neurophysiology regarding the functions of the various neurotransmitters has literally revolutionized our understanding of alcoholism and drug addiction. These discoveries have obviously had dramatic effects on the entire therapeutic and philosophical approach to these problems. The disease theory as described in the 1950s and 1960s had a great deal of validity, but left significant gaps in the understanding of etiology, transmission, and basic pathology. The work done during the past 2.5 decades has filled in many of these gaps. The theory of treatment has, therefore, had to be a dynamic process, constantly being updated and revised as these new discoveries were reported and published. As a result, treatment programs have become more sophisticated. They are more effectively integrated with the various scientific disciplines. As advances were made, treatment programs gradually developed standards of care through the interdisciplinary mechanisms of hospital and medical staff committees as well as the Joint Commission for Hospital Accreditation. This organization was helpful in this process by developing objective national criteria by which to measure and judge these services. By the mid 1980s, most accredited programs had evolved into the following service units. It is important to remember that in all of these, the underlying concept was the basic medical model joined to the disease theory of alcoholism and drug addiction.

II. DETOXIFICATION

The entire attitude regarding detoxification has changed during the past 20 years. Formerly, it was seen as an endpoint of treatment by itself. The medical responsibility was to treat the toxic state, manage existing medical complications, and discharge the patient. Consequently, the regimens developed for detoxification reflected this attitude. They tended to be dramatic and very vigorous. The general rule was to treat very aggressively. There may have been some aversive conditioning benefit to this whether intended or not. Later the advent of the benzodiazepines made it possible to detoxify fairly rapidly and simply. Many of the detoxification complications seen in the previous protocols were avoided.

Detoxification is now seen simply as a prelude to therapy for the basic problem. It is an opportunity for the physician to recognize the problem, diagnose, and recommend appropriate therapy. It is widely recognized today that to detoxify a patient without appropriate follow-up is detrimental to the ultimate patient welfare, as it allows the addictive process to continue without providing appropriate therapy. These programs of detoxification without access to treatment have evolved into the classic "revolving door" model of care. These programs spend very large sums of public money without reduction of the basic problem. They permit and even encourage the progression from acute alcoholism to chronic alcoholism with all of its attendant social and medical problems. They are the last remnant of the former philosophy of detoxification as an isolated therapy rather than a necessary prelude to treatment of the alcoholism.

The current epidemic of illegal drugs reflects altered national drug-using behavior and has changed issues of detoxification. Much of the problem has shifted from the detoxification services to the emergency room. While emergency rooms have always been involved with the initial assessment and triage of alcoholics and drug addicts, they now face an entirely new set of problems. There are more difficulties involved in both the diagnosis of the problems and the increased mortality seen with some of the newer drugs. The individual who was acutely intoxicated with alcohol was a fairly clear-cut diagnostic problem. People present themselves today with a history (probably inaccurate) of a full "buffet" of drugs whose pharmacology and interactions make timely and accurate assessment much more difficult. It is, therefore, essential that emergency room personnel be trained and oriented to the issues of drug addiction, including pharmacology, physiology, detoxification, diagnosis, and intervention.

III. EVALUATION/ASSESSMENT

The area of the greatest development and sophistication during the past 20 years has been in the process of evaluation and assessment of the alcoholic and drug addict. In the past, there were many patients treated for medical and/or psychiatric problems when the primary diagnosis was alcoholism or drug addiction. This mistreatment allowed the basic problems to progress without appropriate treatment until they reached late-stage disease. When the correct diagnosis was finally made, it was frequently too late for rehabilitation; hence, the high morbidity and mortality rates we have traditionally seen in these problems.

Not many years ago the diagnosis of alcoholism was almost entirely dependent upon evidence of physical addiction. So long as the patient did not show evidence of tremors, delirium, seizures, and other physical signs most physicians were reluctant to make the diagnosis. Even the identification of cirrhosis, pancreatitis, or neuropathy did not necessarily result in the diagnosis of alcoholism.

During the past 2 decades, a much more accurate diagnostic methadology has been developed and accepted. This system is based both on behavior patterns and the physical complications of late-stage disease. A great advantage exists in the diagnostic interplay of behavioral and medical indices: early diagnosis. The former tendency to late-stage diagnosis has been responsible for much of the medical pessimism regarding appropriate treatment, treatment outcome, and high rates of recidivism.

The evaluation/assessment services in the treatment program must be able to accurately diagnose alcoholism and drug addiction based on standardized signs and symptoms. The evaluation staff must be well acquainted with the revised third edition of the American Psychiatric Association's *Diagnostic and Statistical Manual of Mental Disorders*, 1987 (DSM-III-R) as well as other recently developed diagnostic criteria. This diagnostic process uses the patient's physical history, laboratory studies, psychometric testing, and alcohol and drug history. The psychosocial history and corroborating third-party data from family, employer, and others are also used as diagnostic indicators. It is important to be able to distinguish between alcoholism, alcohol abuse, situational drinking, drug addiction, social drug use, and drug abuse. These differential diagnoses become critically important when making recommendations for care.

The individuals involved in the evaluation/assessment process are typically physicians, nurses, alcohol/drug counselors, social workers, and psychologists. The development of this team into an integrated, functioning unit is critical in producing the final diagnosis and recommendations. This team is responsible for identifying any secondary problems or issues that will effect the treatment outcome or recommendations. These problems will include secondary medical problems such as cardiovascular disease, diabetes, liver or pancreatic disease, etc. They also include a wide range of psychiatric and psychological issues. In addition, there are frequently social issues involving the family, employer, legal system, and finances that will directly impact the patient's motivation and treatment outcome. A well-functioning assessment team will identify problems, prioritize them, and make a final diagnosis. Recommendations for appropriate treatment of the primary problem as well as the secondary ones are offered to the patient.

This entire process is absolutely essential to effective treatment. It is dangerous if this process is either ignored or done in a superficial manner. The development of this evaluation/assessment process has been one of the most important developments in the entire treatment field.

IV. PRIMARY TREATMENT

The entire treatment process is based on the following principles:

1. Treatment does not "cure" the disease—the expectation is that by instituting an achievable method of abstinence the disease will be put into remission.
2. All therapeutic efforts are directed at helping the patient reach a level of motivation that will enable him or her to commit to this abstinence program.
3. An educational program is developed to assist the patient in becoming familiar with the addictive process, insight into compulsive behaviors, medical complications, emotional insight, and maintenance of physical, mental, and spiritual health.
4. The patient's family and other significant persons are included in the therapeutic process with the understanding that recovery does not occur in a vacuum, but rather in interpersonal relationships.
5. The patient is indoctrinated into the Alcoholics Anonymous program and instructed as to the content and application of the 12 Steps of the program.
6. Group and individual therapy are directed at self-understanding and acceptance with emphasis on how alcohol and/or drugs have affected their lives.
7. There is insistence on participation in a longitudinal support and follow-up program based on the belief that as in the management of all chronic disease processes, maintenance is critically important to the ultimate outcome of any therapy. This follow-up usually consists of on-going support provided by the treatment facility as well as participation in community self-help groups such as AA, Narcotics Anonymous (NA), Opiates Anonymous (OA), etc.

There has been much discussion regarding the effectiveness of this approach. During the past 20 years, papers have been published questioning treatment outcomes. Most of these papers have done studies on populations of late-stage alcoholics who were desocialized and had serious medical complications. This population traditionally does very poorly regardless of the treatment approach. Norman Hoffmann, Ph.D. and the CATOR group in St. Paul, Minnesota, have done some of the best follow up studies measuring long term outcomes. They have particularily good methadology and nonbiased conclusions. The very negative, fatalistic position taken by some authors does nothing to further the development of realistic, effective treatment systems. The current system of care certainly has flaws and deficiencies, which is why diligent efforts must continue to advance both treatment techniques and improved outcomes. What exists today is significantly different from what was considered state of the art 10 years ago. It is a far more sophisticated, objectified discipline.

The two activities that make up the bulk of the primary treatment experience are the educational component and the group/individual therapy sessions. The therapy is built around these basic therapeutic goals:

To have the patient gain insight into the extent and consequences in their lives of their alcohol and drug use.

To become aware of the defense mechanisms employed to facilitate their continued alcohol and drug use.

To recognize and admit to themselves that they indeed are alcoholic and addicted to drugs.

To recognize the extent of their emotional and spiritual impairment.

To examine their relationships and see how they have been adversely affected by their use of alcohol and drugs.

To develop strategies which will prevent them from returning to the use of these alcohol and drugs in the future.

In order to attain these goals there are several hours of group therapy daily. The groups are lead by qualified, experienced therapists who are well acquainted with the special problems presented by the alcoholic and drug-addicted patient. It is important for the therapist to constantly stress the fact that alcohol and drug use is the primary problem and that the patients must become responsible for their behavior and the resulting problems. Without this point being stressed again and again the patients will not take the responsibility for their recovery. Patients are encouraged to both support and challenge one another on these basic points.

It is also important that problems of family dynamics, employment problems, legal changes, and sexuality issues be addressed. These problems may not be resolved during the primary treatment phase, but certainly are subjects that must be addressed during the aftercare/follow-up phase of treatment. A grave mistake is to confuse patients with these problems rather than focusing on the primary problem of alcoholism/drug addiction.

When serious medical or psychiatric problems are identified in the primary treatment phase, it is important that appropriate therapy be instituted as soon as possible. The symptoms and dysfunction accompanying these complications will act as a barrier to recovery. In the past, life-threatening problems such as severe hypertension when not addressed has led to increased mortality figures. The high incidence of cardiopulmonary, gastrointestinal, neoplastic, and metabolic diseases in this population calls for diagnostic and therapeutic vigilance on the part of all health care professionals. The medical problems encountered in the drug-addicted population are changing. The increased rates of morbidity and mortality accompanying these changes are a matter of great concern. The incidence of psychiatric disease, particularly monophasic depression, is high in this population regardless of the addictive drug used.

The following is a list of titles of the educational sessions provided by a local treatment program. It should be noted that the patient population is exposed to several educational sessions daily. The material in these lectures covers a wide range of topics aimed at helping the patients gain insight into themselves and their problems.

The Experience of Intoxication
Change
Other Chemicals
Chemical Dependency and the Family
Family Violence
Seniors and Prescription Drugs
Disease of Alcoholism

Chemical Dependency and Health
Intimacy and Addiction
Staying Sober, Keeping Straight
Leisure Time
Seniors and Alcohol Abuse
Recovery and Relationships
Relapse
Pot
AA and Recovery
Recovery from Cocaine Addiction
Stages of Addiction
Sex and Drugs—The Intimate Connection
Cocaine—Prognosis
Sex, Drugs, and AIDS
Pathology of Alcoholism
Alcoholism and the Family

This is not a complete list of all the topics covered, but is an overall view of the scope of educational topics covered during the patient's stay in primary treatment. If the underlying goal of therapy is motivation, these subjects contain the tools necessary to translate motivation into productive changes.

V. FAMILY THERAPY

The patient's family must play a signficant role in the therapeutic process. When the patient leaves the treatment facility, he or she most likely will interact and react to the family dynamics he or she experiences. Much of the guilt, anger, and remorse experienced by these patients is directed at their families of origin as well as their spouses and children. These issues must be addressed while the patient is in primary treatment if any positive therapeutic results are expected. Consequently, the patient's family is invited and encouraged to involve themselves with the family therapy offered by the treatment facility.

This invitation is frequently resisted by patient and family alike. The interfamily relationships are generally quite strained and often damaged by the time the patient arrives at the treatment facility. The family generally has little insight and no understanding of the problems and issues facing the patient. They are angry, disappointed, guilty, anxious, and need help in how to handle these distressing emotions. Consequently, the typical family is filled with stress and chaos, which it deals with in destructive ways. The goal of family involvement is aimed at the expression and resolution of these feelings and the development of an attitude of mutual support in the family. Obviously this is not possible in all cases, but it is important for the patient and family to at least have an opportunity to listen to the concerns and problems of the other.

It is generally agreed that to treat the patient as an isolated entity almost guarantees that the therapeutic response will be poor. Another important factor is the simple fact that most patients do not tell their therapists the truth! Frequently it is not until the family comes in that the full extent of the patient's alcohol and drug-use and behavior are revealed. These revelations are critical in order to gain a complete understanding of the patients and their problems. Patients frequently paint a very negative picture of the family members, who obviously have "caused" all of their problems. When the true picture is revealed to the therapist and the patient's group, proper insight and realistic therapy goals can be established.

VI. AFTERCARE

An understanding in the early therapy was that alcoholism or drug addiction is a chronic disease, characterized by remissions and exacerbations. The goal of therapy then was to extend the remission periods for as long as possible while reducing the likelihood of an exacerbation or relapse. What was needed was to have a system that would identify a relapse quickly and administer appropriate therapy. It was clear that these goals would be best accomplished by the development of an after–follow-up–support system. This system would assist the patient in solidifying the gains made in primary treatment. It helped patients find new ways to cope with the pressures and stresses they would face upon returning to their families, jobs, and social situations. The system also identified signs and symptoms of an imminent relapse and provided the necessary steps to eliminate it.

These ambitious goals were met through the development of ongoing weekly support groups that the patient attended on a weekly basis. The patients would attend these accompanied by their spouses or the persons they were closest to. They are encouraged to attend these sessions for at least 12 months. They were instructed also to attend at least one weekly meeting of AA, NA, or some other appropriate 12-Step recovery self-help group in the community. Patients were routinely referred to specific therapists to address the other problems that were identified during primary treatment. These might be marital or parenting problems, financial or employment problems, sexual issues, legal problems, or whatever other problems that could lead to a relapse or behavior problems. Patients with medical or psychiatric problems were instructed to maintain regular contact with their physician and to adhere to prescribed medication schedules. This entire schema is developed by a negotiation process between the patient and an aftercare therapist. The entire aftercare plan is completed and agreed to prior to discharge from primary treatment.

The patients who complete primary treatment and follow their aftercare plan are those who do best in long-term follow-up studies. Those who do not follow through with the aftercare recommendations do poorly. There is a very clear cause and effect relationship to longitudinal abstinence and these factors. There are other factors that enter into long-term recovery, but these two are pivotal. The aftercare developments that have occurred during the past 10 years have done more to effect recovery statistics than anything else. When commitment to aftercare is lacking either on the part of the patient or the treatment facility, the recovery figures quickly deteriorate.

VII. CONCLUSIONS

It must be clear to the reader at this point that there really is no theory of treatment. That is, no theory was developed and then tested on a patient population. What has occurred is that two quite separate concepts and approaches to the issue of addiction came together and found congruent grounds on which the positive aspects of each were integrated to form a unified philosophic and pragmatic whole. The breakthroughs in basic research of the past 20 years have supplemented the earlier concepts and have been incorporated into the entire process.

This evolution is by no means complete. Recent work in the identification of biological markers, genetic coding, and new concepts concerning the specific metabolic processes will be incorporated into the treatment disciplines.

There was a basic shift in emphasis and approach which in itself was amazingly simple. It was the understanding that addiction to alcohol or drugs and the reluctant problems were a therapeutic entity unto themselves. There was no need to embellish the problem, but rather to address the problem head on. There was (and in some quarters, still is) an approach that attributes alcoholism to such factors as

Depression
Anger
Family conflicts
Anxiety
Loss of job
Divorce

It seemed that there always needed to be a primary cause more basic than the alcoholism. A classic statement made by alcoholics is, "I get drunk on sunny days; I get drunk on cloudy days; I get drunk at funerals; I get drunk at weddings; I get drunk when I get fired; I get drunk when I receive a promotion; I get drunk when I'm angry; I get drunk when I'm happy." The events of each day are sufficient reason to drink or take drugs.

It was the acceptance of this basic kind of addictive drive that is behind the development of the emerging system for the treatment of the addictive disorders. When therapists focus their attention on the central issue, the *use* of alcohol and/or drugs progress can be made. When their efforts are deflected or diluted by focusing on other issues and problems, the therapeutic results are generally poor. As we have seen, these complicating problems do need attention, but the initial primary goal must be to halt the use of the damaging drugs.

As our nation faces increasingly serious problems from drug use and addiction, it is imperitive that cooperation continue between the basic biological sciences and the clinical practitioners of treatment. There are new problems facing health care which are included in addictive problems of the 1990s. Among these are the birth defects and other health problems of newborns which are directly linked to drug and alcohol use of biological parents. Recent work showing the effects of paternal alcohol use are of interest. The problems of the acquired immune deficiency syndrome (AIDS) in the addicted population is also of growing concern. This population is proving to be the most resistant to efforts aimed at prophylactic lifestyle changes. Current efforts aimed at law enforcement and drug interdiction can only be partially useful in developing the public health policies that will be critically important in the next decade. The ultimate answer must be a combined program of effective prevention programs and adequate treatment of the addicted population. The outcome of treatment must be improved by the use of the tools and methods being explored in our basic science laboratories. Although treatment modalities for alcoholism and drug addiction have improved substantially in the past 25 years, the system is lacking the necessary basic science information needed for the future.

SELECTED READING

Ahles, T.A., Schlundt, D.G., Prue, D.M., and Rychtarik, R.G. (1983). Impact of after arrangements on the maintenance of treatment success in abusive drinkers. *Addict. Behav.*, 8:53–58.

Alford, G.S. (1980). Alcoholics Anonymous: An empirical outcome study. *Addict. Behav.*, 5:359–370.

Anderson, D.J. (1979). *Delivery of essential services to alcoholics through the continuum of care.* Cancer Res., 39:2855–2858, 1979.

Baekland, F., Lundwall, L., and Kissen, B. Methods for the treatment of chronic alcoholism: A critical appraisal, *Research Advances in Alcohol and Drug Problems*, Vol. 2 (J.F. Gibbons, Y. Israel, O. Kaland, R.E. Popham, W. Schmidt, and R.G. Smart, eds.). New York, Wiley, 1975, pp. 247–327.

Bandura, A. (1978). Reflections on self-efficacy. *Adv. Behav. Res. Ther.*, 1:237–269.

Beglieter, H. *Accelerating Progress in Research and Practice*. Presented at the National Conference on Alcohol Abuse and Alcoholism Addressing the Human, Social, and Economic Costs to the Nation, Washington, D.C., November, 1987.

Brown, S.A. (1985). Reinforcement expectancies and alcoholism treatment: Outcome after a one-year follow-up. *J. Stud. Alcohol, 46*:304–308.

Comp Care Corporation, Care Unit. *Evaluation of Treatment Outcome*. Irvine, California, Comprehensive Care Corporation, 1988.

Costello, R.M. (1980). Alcoholism aftercare and outcome: Cross-lagged panel and path analyses. *Br. J. Addict., 75*:49–53.

Donovan, D.M.A., and Chaney, E.F. Alcoholic relapse prevention and intervention: Models and methods, *Relapse Prevention*. (G.A. Marlatt and J.R. Gordon, eds.). New York, Guilford Press, 1985.

Emrick, C.D. (1974). A review of psychologically oriented treatment of alcoholism: I. The use and interrelationships of outcome criteria and drinking behavior following treatment. *Q. J. Stud. Alcohol., 35*:523–549.

Emrick, D.D. Thoughts on treatment evaluation methodology, *Future Directions in Alcohol Abuse Treatment Research* (B.S. McCrady, N.E. Noel, and T.D. Nirenbert, eds.). National Institute of AAA Research Monograph No. 15. U.S. Department of Health and Human Services, Publication No. (ADM) 85-1322, Washington, D.C., U.S. Government Printing Office, 1985.

Gorski, T.T., and Miller, M. *Counseling for Relapse Prevention*. Independence, Missouri, Herald House–Independence Press, 1982.

Gregson, R.A.M., and Taylor, G.M. (1977). Prediction of relapse in men alcoholics. *J. Stud. Alcohol, 38*:1749–1760.

Harrison, P.A., and Hoffman, N.G. *Chemical Dependency Inpatients and Outpatients: Intake Characteristics and Treatment Outcome*. Report to the State of Minnesota Department of Human Services Chemical Dependency Program Division, January, 1986.

Harrison, P.A., and Hoffman, N.G. *CATOR 1987 Report/Adolescent Residential Treatment: Intake and Followup Findings*. St. Paul, Minnesota, Ramsey Clinic, 1987.

Hoffman, N.G., Harrison, P.A., and Belille, C.A. (1983). Alcoholics Anonymous after treatment: Attendance and abstinence. *Int. J. Addict., 18*:311–318.

Kleber, H.B., and Gawin, F.H. (1984). Cocaine abuse: A review of current and experimental treatments, *Cocaine: Pharmacology, Effects and Treatment of Abuse*. (O. Grabowski, ed.). National Institute of Drug Abuse Research Monograph No. 50.

Laundergan, O. *Easy Does It—Alcoholism Treatment Outcomes. Hazelden and the Minnesota Model*. Center City, Minnesota, Hazelden Foundation, 1986.

Litman, G.K. Relapse in alcoholism: Traditional and current approaches, *Alcoholism Treatment in Transition* (G. Edwards and M. Grant, eds.). London, Croom Helm, 1980.

Macdonald, J.G. (1987). Predictors of treatment outcome for alcoholic women. *Int. J. Addict., 22*:235–248.

Maisto, S.A., and McCollam, J.B. (1980). The use of multiple measures of life health to assess alcohol treatment outcome: A review and critique, *Evaluating Alcohol and Drug Abuse Treatment Effectiveness: Recent Advances* (L.D. Sobell, M.B. Sobell, and E. Ward, eds.). New York, Pergamon Press, 1980.

Marlatt, G.A. (1983). The controlled drinking controversy: A commentary. *Am. Psychol., 38*:1097–1110.

McCrady, D.S., and Sher, K. Treatment variables, *Future Directions in Alcohol Abuse Treatment Research*. (B.S. McCrady, N.E. Noel, and T.D. Nirenberg, eds.). National Institute of Drug Abuse Research Monograph No. 15 U.S. Department of Health and Human Services, Publication No. (ADM) 85-1322, Washington, D.C., U.S. Government Printing Office, 1985.

Miller, W.R., and Hester, R.K. (1986). Inpatient alcoholism treatment: Who benefits? *Am. Psychol., 41*:794–805.

Miller, William R., and Hesterm Reid K. The effectiveness of alcoholism treatment—what the research reveals, *Treating Addictive Behaviors, Processes of Change* (W.E. Miller and N. Heather, eds.). New York, Clemon Press, 1986.

National Council on Alcoholism Criteria Committee (1972). Criteria for the diagnosis of alcoholism. *Am. J. Psychiatry, 129*:127–135.

National Conference of Commissioners on Uniform State Laws: Uniform Alcoholism and Intoxication Treatment Act, Eightieth Annual Conference, Vail, Colorado, 1978.

Pattison, E.M. New directions in alcoholism treatment goals, *Future Directions in Alcohol Abuse Treatment Research* (B.S. McCrady, N.E. Noel and T.D. Nirenberg, eds.). National Institute on Drug Abuse Research Monograph No. 15. U.S. Department of Health and Human Services, Publication No. (ADM) 85-1322, Washington, D.C. U.S. Government Printing Office, 1985.

Patton, M.Q. *The Outcomes of Treatment: A Study of Patients Admitted to Hazelden in 1976.* Center City, Minnesolta, Hazelden Foundation, 1970.

Propping, P., Kruger, J., and Mark, N. (1981). Genetic predisposition to alcoholism: An EEG study in alcoholics and relatives. *Hum. Genet., 59*:51–59.

Sandahl, C. (1984). Determinants of relapse among alcoholics: A cross-cultural replication study. *Int. J. Addict., 19*:833–848.

Schaefer, H.H., Sobell, M.G., and Sobell, L.C. (1972). Follow up of hospitalized alcoholics given self-confrontation experience by video tape. *Behav. Ther., 3*:283–285.

Schuckit, M.A. (1987). Biological vulnerability of alcoholism. *J. Consult. Clin. Psychol., 55*:301–309.

Schuckit, M.A., Li, T.K., Cloninger, C.R., and Deitrich, R.A. (1985). University of California, Davis–Conference: Genetics of alcoholism. *Alcoholism Clin. Exp. Res., 9*:475–492.

Schuckit, M.A., and Calahan, D. Evaluation of alcoholism treatment programs, *Alcohol and Alcohol Problems: New Thinking and New Directions.* (W.J. Finstead, J.J. Ross, and M. Keller, eds.). Cambridge, Massachusetts, Ballinger, 1976.

Schuckit, M.A., Schwei, M.G., and Gold, E. (1986). Prediction of outcome in inpatient alcoholics. *J. Stud. Alcohol, 47*:151–155.

Sobell, M.B., and Sobell, L.C. (1973). Individualized behavior therapy for alcoholics. *Behav. Ther., 4*:49–72.

Spicer, J., and Barnett, P. *Hospital-Based Chemical Dependency Treatment: A Model for Outcome Evaluation.* Center City, Minnesota, Hazelden Foundation, 1980.

Vaillant, G.E. *The Natural History of Alcoholism—Causes, Patterns and Paths to Recovery.* Cambridge, Massachusetts, Harvard University Press, 1983.

Vannicelli, M., Gingerich, S., and Ryback, R. (1983). Family problems related to the treatment and outcome of alcoholic patients. *Br. J. Addict., 78*:193–204.

Wallace, J. Working the preferred defense structure of the recovering alcoholic, *Practical Approaches to Alcoholism Psychotherapy*, 2nd ed. (S. Zimber, J. Wallace and S. Blume, eds.). New York, Plenum Press, 1985.

Zimberg, S., Wallace, J., and Blume, S. (eds.). *Practical Approaches to Alcoholism Psychotherapy.* New York, Plenum Press, 1978, p. 3.

65

Outpatient Treatment of Drug and Alcohol Addiction

James Cocores
Fair Oaks Hospital, Summit, New Jersey

I. INTRODUCTION

Self-help groups such as Alcoholics Anonymous (AA) [1] began flourishing throughout the country in the late 1930s prior to the advent of inpatient rehabilitation programs [2]. Once introduced, inpatient drug and alcohol addiction treatment centers traditionally admitted severe heroin or alcohol abusers for treatment only after advanced mental, social, and physical consequences had evolved. Inpatient drug and alcohol addiction treatment was reserved for the most difficult and extreme cases because of insufficient bed availability. But even today the ability to receive professional treatment is a function of availability and cost [3]. Individuals in need of professional treatment for their drug and alcohol problems frequently have to be admitted to facilities in distant locals than they reside. Dependents resistant to inpatient treatment and hesitant to participate in self-help groups might seek treatment in the private sector. Private clinicians often are not experienced in drug and alcohol addiction treatment and may take a predominantly psychiatric approach which may view drug or alcohol addiction as a symptom rather than a separate disorder requiring a specialized treatment plan [4]. Regular urine drug screening is rarely done to confirm abstinence during individual therapy. Drug and alcohol addiction is usually minimized by the addict participating in individual therapy only. The addict frequently manipulates the therapist and therapy topics away from drug and alcohol addiction issues. Incomplete drug and alcohol addiction treatment is often rendered when individual treatment is the only treatment modality used.

Inpatient programs designed to treat the family members of alcohol or drug dependents exist but are scarce. Inpatient drug and alcohol facilities often have family treatment [5], but too often the services rendered are sparse and infrequent. Although education is important, emphasis is often placed on drug and alcohol addiction issues rather than the problems experienced by the family members directly. Although a large network of family self-help groups such as Tough Love, Families Anonymous, and Al-Anon [6] exist throughout the country, family members initially contemplating treatment for themselves prefer professional-guided individual or group therapy. Family treatment is discussed in Chapter 46.

Structured outpatient drug and alcohol programs were developed to make treatment less costly and more available to individuals in earlier stages of the disease [7]. Like inpatients, participants in intensive outpatinet programs are involved in frequent and comprehensive alcohol and drug treatment. Unlike inpatients, outpatients continue their daily involvement at work and at home. Therefore, patients are better able to practice newly learned coping and problem-solving skills on a daily basis with peers and family members. Although inpatient treatment is required for some (especially dependents with concurrent major psychiatric or medical problems), many more people can benefit from the in vivo treatment offered on an outpatient basis.

Treatment of drug and alcohol addicts and their family members requires careful planning tailored to the patient. A variety of treatment approaches should be available and applied appropriately to each patient depending on their history and needs. The treatment approach offered by most inpatient rehabilitation centers can be made available on an outpatient basis. Some outpatient treatment models are outlined below. But it is important to first consider the assessment process prior to presenting some types and levels of outpatient treatment.

II. OUTPATIENT ASSESSMENT

An essential prerequisite for involvement in an outpatient drug and alcohol treatment program is a thorough evaluation and assessment. The evaluation must not only probe drug and alcohol addiction history and prior treatment attempts, but also must include a medical history and physical, drug and alcohol addiction withdrawal physical examination, psychiatric assessment, and psychosocial evaluation prior to admission. The hospital emergency room is the setting most often used for the evaluation process. But evaluations can also be conducted in a free-standing clinic that has easy access to a hospital for transfer when needed.

In free-standing clinics, calls are first carefully screened for appropriateness. Because patients and family members usually make their first contact for help via telephone, individuals collecting intake information must be knowledgeable about medicine, psychology, and addiction. The very key intake persons are supervised by a medical doctor. Most patients that call are ambivalent about the need for drug abuse treatment. Therefore, intake personnel must be confident, knowledgeable, firm, and pleasant. The successful intake person rapidly gathers pertinent medical information. In the interest of time, safety, and accuracy, data collection is focused on drug and alcohol use both qualitatively and quantitatively over the previous few months. Daily opiate, benzodiazepine, or alcohol abusers are often referred for inpatient detoxification following consultation and confirmation by a medical doctor. Many patients will negotiate toward outpatient detoxification. The hazards, unreliability, and poor outcome of outpatient detoxification should be explained in order to further encourage compliance with the initial treatment plan. Patients who do not give a history which clearly warrants inpatient detoxification may be scheduled for an outpatient assessment where the determination can be assessed with more precision. The need for medical detoxification is a major contraindication for involvement in outpatient treatment programs. Following detoxification, the patient may require continued inpatient rehabilitation. The detoxified patient may also be referred to a structured outpatient treatment program following detoxification when 24-h drug and alcohol addiction rehabilitation is not required.

Previous treatment attempts are useful to know about at the time of the initial phone call. Multiple prior outpatient drug abuse treatment attempts may warrant referral to a inpatient drug and alcohol addiction treatment unit or a dual diagnosis treatment center [4]. Never before–treated drug and alcohol addicts should begin on an outpatient basis when appropriate. Even individuals who have been unable to abstain from drugs and alcohol for extended periods of time following multiple inpatient rehabilitation efforts can benefit from an outpatient trial.

Current physical problems and medications are important to know about at the time of initial contact. Some presciption medications may be dependence-prone drugs, which should always be avoided in drug and alcohol addicts. For example, a barbiturate containing medication used for migraine headaches should be replaced by a medication that is not habit forming. Use of a beta blocker or amitriptyline are examples of medical alternatives. Too often patients are admitted for detoxification and treatment of opiate dependence following extended abuse of pain relievers. These individuals classically have a high tolerance to most other opiate-type prescription pain relievers. Nonaddiction-prone medical alternatives must be made available (i.e., nonsteroidal anti-inflammatory agents) along with physiotherapy or other non-pharmacological problems associated with drug and alcohol addiction are best managed initially in a hospital setting.

A history of major psychiatric illness is an important piece of information to detect during the initial conversation. Alcohol or drug abusers presenting with active major psychiatric illnesses are best treated in an outpatient drug and alcohol addiction clinic only after the psychiatric crisis has been stabilized. Such cases should be referred to more appropriate dual diagnosis facilities, local inpatient treatment facilities, or an emergency room. The intake person must master the skills practiced by persons working suicide prevention helplines and other crisis intervention and resource hotlines. An appointment for a thorough assessment is made after the initial screening process is complete.

The assessment counselor obtains a detailed psychosocial, psychiatric, and drug and alcohol addiction history, which typically takes about 2 h. The physician and the assessment counselor then determines the most appropriate treatment for the drug and alcohol addict and their family member(s). If inpatient detoxification and rehabilitation is required, then the referral is made and facilitated. If detoxification only is needed, then the patient begins an outpatient program when medically stable. If the patient is in psychiatric crisis, then the crisis is stabilized, and then the need for drug and alcohol addiction treatment is assessed. In most cases, drug and alcohol addicts begin outpatient treatment shortly after the initial assessment if they are not in need of medical detoxification, acutely psychotic, suicidal, or homocidal. Outlined in Table 1 are some of the outpatient treatment models we have found useful in our clinics over the past decade.

III. OUTPATIENT ADOLESCENT DRUG AND ALCOHOL TREATMENT

A. Early Intervention Programs

It is often difficult to evaluate and validate the extent of an individuals drug- and alcohol-use history even after an intensive and thorough evaluation. This is especially common when evaluating early adolescent drug and alcohol users. Frequently, a parent or teacher discovers a piece of evidence suggestive of illicit drug use and the student is referred for an evaluation.

Table 1 Outpatient Treatment Models

Inpatient	vs	Outpatient
Medical detoxification		Medical clearance
Suicidal or homocidal		Stabilized psychiatric problems
Acute psychiatric problems		
Unable to abstain from drugs and alcohol for more than 1 week		Unsuccessful at individual or infrequent group therapy
Prior unsuccessful outpatient attempts		Unsuccessful with self-help groups alone

There may sometimes be insufficient drug and alcohol abuse history to warrant inpatient or outpatient treatment. What can be done when there is enough data to raise suspicion and concern but not enough to warrant formal treatment? Early intervention programs (EIPs) are an excellent alternate approach when alcohol or drug use is suspected but inpatient or structured outpatient rehabilitation are not indicated. Although early intervention programs exist for adults, they are usually less practical because adults more regularly have evolved past the early experimentation phase of the disease.

Early intervention programs allow individuals to learn about drug and alcohol abuse without the categorization and stigmatization of drug or alcohol addiction. This approach can be as nonthreatening as any other class the student may attend. But because their potential to develop a drug or alcohol addiction may be higher than nonexperimentors, a period of drug and alcohol abstinence needs to be documented and enforced with biweekly random comprehensive urine drug screens.

Patients who enter an EIP are assumed not to have a drug or alcohol addiction, and therefore education is emphasized. The EIP patients learn about progression, tolerance, and the disease concept of drug and alcohol addiction [8]. They are introduced to self-help groups, such as Narcotics Anonymous [9], and learn about the possible detriments which may arise with continued drug use [10]. Most importantly, they are taught about the insidious and usually unnoticed evolutionary process that begins with carefree experimentation and results in drug or alcohol addiction.

The structure of an EIP consists of 4- to 8-month evaluation, education, and therapy period. Involvement consists of one group therapy plus a 45-min individual session each week. A multifamily group meets twice a month. Biweekly supervised urine drug screens are obtained to help ensure abstinence. One urine sample is obtained when they attend the clinic and another is supervised by a family member. Family conferences are scheduled two times during the length of the program. Parents are also involved in a parents' 2-h education and support group weekly during the program. Parents also benefit by attending family-oriented self-help meetings [11].

The EIP programs offer solutions to most of the previously ignored potential problems that often follow experimental or "early" drug or alcohol abuse. After the adolescent and their significant others complete an EIP, one of the following recommendations are usually made:

No need for further intervention. The patient has completed the program with minimal resistance and good attendance. Urine drug screens were negative, confirming drug and alcohol abstinence. Education may serve sufficiently to deter progression of the disease. As a minimum, the EIP serves as an educational experience not only about drugs and alcohol, but also improves communication skills. Students are also exposed to individual and group therapies.

Another primary problem may be discovered during the EIP. A partial seizure disorder, disorder of impulse control, major depression, or a domestic violence problem may become apparent and a referral is made.

A more serious drug or alcohol abuse problem is realized than was initially suspected. Here a series of positive urine drug screens, or additional drug and alcohol abuse history warrants referral to a more intensive level of treatment.

A drug or alcohol addiction is coupled with a major psychiatric problem which requires a specialized treatment referral such as an inpatient dual diagnosis treatment unit.

Evidence is accrued suggestive of a drug or alcohol addiction and/or psychiatric problem in a family member or significant other. Assessment and referral for appropriate treatment may follow.

An EIP is an excellent way of delivering a thorough and complete evaluation to persons suspected of alcohol or drug experimentation or abuse.

B. Adolescent Day Patient Rehabilitation

Severe and advanced cases of adolescent drug or alcohol addiction usually warrant inpatient rehabilitation. But inpatient treatment beds are limited and reserved for the more advanced, usually dualy diagnosed, adolescent drug and alcohol addictions. The lack of sufficient quality inpatient adolescent treatment centers leave the majority of young abusers in need of rehabilitation without recourse. A neophyte may not be referred for treatment of any type in hope of spontaneous remission. Adolescent day patient programs (ADPs) was designed to accommodate a previously overlooked population of adolescent drug and alcohol abusers. Like the EIPs, the ADPs make drug and alcohol treatment available to persons earlier in the disease process in the hope of arresting further consequences of the disease and avoiding inpatient treatment.

Exclusion Criteria for Adolescent Day Programs

Not in need of medical detoxification. Candidates must not show signs of alcohol or drug withdrawal to the extent requiring inpatient detoxification. Medical clearance is required.

An actively suicidal patient is a psychiatric emergency, and as such must be managed immediately in an emergency room or crisis center. Suicidality is not always best addressed on an inpatient basis. For example, in cases of borderline personality disorder and other illnesses regularly associated with suicidal ideation in which inpatient treatment could further deteriorate the condition, stabilization of the psychiatric disorder is a prerequisite to ADP admission. Suicidal patients who are expected to benefit from inpatient treatment should be referred even if the suicidality is considered to result directly from the drug and alcohol addiction.

Homicidal gestures or verbalization are futilely difficult to manage on an outpatient basis. Adolescents with a history of runaway behavior are also relatively poor treatment risks and often do not comply with the outpatient treatment plan. Untreated cases of disorder of impulse control is but another relative contraindications to an ADP.

Advantages of Adolescent Day Patient Programs

Structured and intensive substance abuse rehabilitation on an outpatient basis. Patients participate in a geographically local outpatient rehabilitation that offers a therapy schedule comparable to inpatient rehabilitation.

Individualized instruction occurs daily so that school is not interrupted. The amount of tutor time required each day varies from state to state. Because treatment does not involve losing school class time, is closer to home, and is less costly than inpatient treatment, more drug and alcohol addicts are likely to enter rehabilitation earlier on in the evolution of their chemical dependence.

A work-study situation can also be arranged. That is, the student attends school in the morning and 2-day drug and alcohol groups at the treatment center in the afternoon.

An ADP provides treatment in a more practical and realistic setting. Because inpatient treatment is confining and geographically distant, the treatment rendered may be affected. An ADP is better integrated into the drug and alcohol addict's usual lifestyle and, therefore, more condusive to the development of more effective problem-solving skills. School and family problems are addressed daily and as they arise. Solutions can be practiced by patients when they see their family members later on in the day.

Adolescent Day Patient Program Schedule

Phase one of treatment is the most intense and comprehensive rehabilitation stage. Patients
   attend therapy sessions Monday through Friday from 9 a.m. until 3 p.m. Most patients
   achieve treatment plan goals of the first phase in 8–12 weeks. Each day patient participates
   in the following treatment modalities:

> Group therapy
> Individual counseling
> Individualized instruction
> 12-Step–oriented rehabilitation
> Alcohol and drug education

Successful achievement of treatment plan goals are met prior to transition to phase two,
and commonly consist of:

Integration and regular attendance at local self-help meetings
Good attendance
Abstinence from all drugs and forms of alcohol with confirmatory urine drug screens
Understanding the disease concept of drug and alcohol addiction and how it has and may
   continue to affect aspects of their own life
Relapse prevention techniques
Stress management
Good exercise and nutrition practices
A willingness to correct character defects which are incompatible with continued abstinence
Willingness to improve family and school relations
Compliance with recommendations for additional psychiatric, medical, or neurological assess-
   ment and referral

Phase two consists of components and goals previously listed but meets less frequently
at a biweekly rate. Patients are expected to begin increasing their weekly attendance at local
self-help meetings during this phase. The primary goal of phase two is to ease, supervise,
and troubleshoot the transition back to a more complete home life, school, the community,
and phase three. Phase two usually has served its purpose in 2 weeks.

Phase three meets one evening each week for about 8 months. Relapse prevention is
emphasized during the first half of phase three. Continued reinforcement of self-help meeting
attendance is the rule. Urine monitoring may be more discretionary during phase three, and
could vary from no weekly urine to three collections. A parent may supervise the urine at
home in cases in which numerous weekly urines are desirable. This is usually the exception
rather than the rule because by phase three the therapist is familiar with the patient and is
likely to address the behavioral relapse or "slip" that often precedes relapse to alcohol or
other drugs. The latter portion of phase three focuses less on relapse prevention and stresses
repair of character defects and improving problem-solving capabilities. Simple day to day
coping mechanisms are addressed throughout phase three. For example, the apparently simple decision of how to spend the New Year's eve can be cause of justifiable alarm in a recovering adolescent drug or alcohol addict. This warrants group discussion, as it pertains to many
other group members who may not have realized the potential problems. Continued involvement in self-help groups is the rule throughout phase three.

C. Adolescent Aftercare Treatment

Aftercare admission requirements usually consist of completing an inpatient drug or alcohol
treatment program or upon the completion of a structured outpatient treatment program like
the one outlined above. This phase of treatment has also been termed growth group or

relapse prevention group. Although these later terms are more descriptive, they do not describe the multifaceted goals of aftercare. For example, aftercare treatment not only emphasizes relapse prevention and self-improvement, but also comprises progress toward eliminating character defects, improving communication skills, practicing honesty, repairing weakened family and school ties, developing a new drug-free peer group, involvement in local Alcoholics Anonymous and Narcotics Anonymous groups, and most importantly practicing better problem-solving skills each day [12].

Aftercare treatment usually is conducted on a weekly basis. Groups are held in the evening or late afternoon, making it more convenient for students and their parents. If urine drug screens are desirable during the aftercare phase of treatment, then one urine sample can be obtained at the weekly aftercare meeting and an additional one can be obtained during the week by a parent or guardian. Aftercare treatment varies and depends on the treatment facility and the patient. Length of aftercare often ranges from 6 months to 2 years. Most aftercare programs are about 1 year in length.

D. Adolescent Dual Diagnosis Recognition and Treatment

A significant number of adolescent drug- and alcohol-addicted patients also have a coexisting major psychiatric disorder. It is virtually impossible to identify dually diagnosed patients prior to a 1-month drug and alcohol abstinence period because drug or alcohol toxic effects regularly mimic the symptoms of many psychiatric disorders. For example, cocaine toxicity may mimic attention deficit disorder [13] or bipolar disorder [14]. The longer the evaluation period, the higher the probability of accurate identification of the dually diagnosed adolescent. It is for this reason that inpatient, outpatient, and aftercare drug and alcohol addiction treatment staff must be trained in the identification and treatment of the dually diagnosed adolescent.

IV. ADULT OUTPATIENT DRUG AND ALCOHOL ADDICTION TREATMENT

A. Recovery-Sensitive Individual Counseling

Individual therapy with drug and alcohol addicts can be an essential adjunct to structured outpatient drug abuse treatment. Individual therapy, drug abuse aftercare, and self-help group attendance are common recommendations upon discharge from inpatient treatment centers. Individual therapy along with self-help group attendance can even be an effective initial approach to the management of drug and alcohol addiction, providing urine drug screens are obtained. Whatever the setting, individual therapists can be invaluable in treatment planning because of the large array of coexisting problems that can satellite the drug and alcohol abuser like incest, rape, postraumatic stress disorder, marital problems, and borderline personality disorder, to name a few. An open relationship should exist between the private therapist and the drug abuse treatment staff so that their respective efforts work in unison.

B. Adult Evening Treatment

The adult evening rehabilitation program was designed with the employed drug and alcohol addict in mind. Traditionally, higher-functioning dependent people who had not suffered severe consequences but sought professional assistance were offered no help, once a week individual counseling, or inpatient treatment. Besides the usual reasons, many drug and alcohol addicts postpone treatment because infrequent individual counseling is easily manipulated and lacks structure, or inpatient care is viewed as excessive. Structured evening programs offer assistance to a large population of previously untreated addicts. Usually evening program candidates are experiencing mild difficulties at work as a result of drug and alcohol addiction. Marital problems are often present, but not usually irreparable. Minor drug and alcohol addiction–related legal incidences are also common in this population of patients. Rarely do major psychiatric problems coexist in this population, which probably parallels the general higher level of functioning shared by patients admitted to a structured evening adult program. Some evening program participants have suffered no significant consequences and simply want help to stop using alcohol or drugs because their own efforts alone have failed.

The format of adult evening programs vary. A common model is as follows. Patients attend two groups therapy sessions from 6:30 to 10:00 p.m. each Monday, Tuesday, Thursday, and Friday evenings for 6–8 weeks. Biweekly random supervised comprehensive urine drug screens are obtained during the first two phases of treatment. Patients are encouraged to attend a self-help meeting on Wednesday evening, Saturday, and Sunday. Patients attend the evening program twice each week for an additional 2 weeks (phase two). A primary goal of phase two, as with adolescents, is to gradually ease into less supervised and structured free time in order to minimize relapse. Individuals in phase two offer hope and support to new patients entering phase one. Patients in phase three attend one session per week for about 9 months. Phase three reinforces relapse prevention in day to day activities, and personal growth with respect to improved communication skills, and self-improvement of character defects. Most patients are well integrated into self-help groups and have self-help sponsors during phase three of treatment.

C. Adult Day Treatment

Admissions to day outpatient rehabilitation programs usually lie between inpatient and evening program candidates with regard to severity of illness. Day programs make available a level of treatment which surpasses the evening program, but is shy of 24-h treatment. Day program schedules typically consist of three groups per day, 5 days each week for about 8 weeks. A vocational component is necessary as most day patient program participants are unemployed. Dual diagnosis is frequently encountered because day patients have a lower level of functioning as compared to evening participants. Day drug treatment programs must, therefore, have dual diagnosis identification and treatment capabilities. This requires specialized treatment staff and additional inservices on dual diagnosis topics.

One of the treatment goals that marks transition to the aftercare phase of treatment is securing employment. Aftercare meets weekly (two sessions per evening) for about 1 year. Patients begin attending additional self-help meetings, and recovery-sensitive individual therapy after the initial daily phase of drug treatment is complete.

D. Dual Diagnosis Capabilities

Outpatient drug treatment is incomplete without dual diagnosis capabilities. The outpatient alcohol and drug clinical staff must be experienced and have ongoing training in the diagnosis and treatment of psychiatric disorders in drug-dependent individuals. Although most of the psychiatric symptoms inevitably present in active abusers gradually improve with drug abstinence, there exists a minority of drug dependents who also have a coexisting major psychiatric disorder requiring psychopharmacological treatment. Multiple relapse is the rule when both disorders are not treated simultaneously.

Dual diagnosis patients can be identified only after a careful evaluation by a specialized clinical staff and a period of drug and alcohol abstinence. The treatment of a psychiatric disorder in drug and alcohol addicts must be carefully coordinated with the addiction treatment. Drug and alcohol addiction should never be viewed as a byproduct of a psychiatric disorder. If it is presented this way, the drug and alcohol abuser will avoid the responsibility of remaining abstinent and participating in the rehabilitative process. Medication used to treat the psychiatric illness should not be interpreted as a solution to the drug or alcohol addiction. Physicians treating the psychiatric disorder must be sufficiently sophisticated regarding drug and alcohol addiction treatment to avoid undermining the rehabilitative process. Addiction-prone medications should be avoided when treating the dually diagnosed patient. For example, cocaine addicts with a concurrent incapacitating anxiety disorder may be treated with a tricyclic antidepressant rather than the benzodiazepine alprazolam [15]. Even less addiction-prone medicines should be discouraged where possible. For example, it is prudent to recommend a non–alcohol containing antitussive for acute coryza.

V. DRUG SCREENING

Urine drug screening in outpatient treatment is analogous to the protection from drug and alcohol use provided by the walls of an inpatient facility. Urine drug screens are often used even on inpatient drug and alcohol units to document and monitor abstinence [16]. Urine drug screens are essential in the outpatient treatment of drug and alcohol addiction. Breath analyzers should be available for alcohol detection. Patients are likely to drop out of treatment or use drugs and alcohol while attending treatment without the appropriate use of urine drug screens.

The ideal situation would involve obtaining a comprehensive urine drug screen each day. This is not only impractical and unnecessary, but also very costly. On the other hand, obtaining one urine drug screen per week is worthless because drugs like cocaine (benzoylecgonine) go undetected after a few days [17]. That is, it is very possible to use cocaine following the weekly urine drug screen and the cocaine use will go undetected by the next urine screen. A good compromise is obtaining urine drug screens a minimum of two times each week during the initial phase of treatment.

Many patients and even clinicians are resistant to the idea of urine drug screens. The majority of patients eventually find security and safety in the fact that their urine are being monitored for a variety of drugs and alcohol. Many patients offer how other outpatient programs "Didn't help me because I used while going there . . . they didn't even take urines." Therapists complain about the difficult task of fostering a therapeutic alliance, promoting honesty, and at the same time supporting urine drug screening. This can be a trying dilemma solved only by the knowledge and wisdom furnished by drug and alcohol treatment experience.

Urine drug screens must be supervised by trained personnel. An unsupervised urine screen is of little clinical value. Drug and alcohol abusers have been known to add water, bleach, and a whole host of other adulterants to urine in the hope of negating a potentially positive urine sample. Knowledge of urine specific gravity is useful, but it does not replace supervising urine collection. Another technique involves either purchasing or otherwise obtaining a drug- or alcohol-free, or "clean," urine sample before going to a clinic and then switching samples. A more crafty technique involves filling a nasal spray bottle with urine that is presumed to be drug and alcohol free. The spray bottle is kept close to the body in undergarments so the sample is warm and the spray bottle can be used in a way that mimics the sound of urination.

Urine drug and alcohol screens should also be obtained on a random schedule. The clinical utility of drug screens is decreased further if the drug or alcohol addict is faced with a predictable schedule (e.g., each Monday and Friday). A varying weekly schedule is far less predictable and more useful.

VI. CONCLUSIONS

The trend away from institutionalization of psychiatric patients continues because many patients have benefited from outpatient care. An initial countermeasure to institutionalization was the establishment of community mental health centers. This trend was further refined by the development of partial hospitalization programs [4]. Partial hospitalization programs provide the kind of quality and comprehensive psychiatric treatment to outpatients that was previously available only on an inpatient basis. In much the same way, it has become apparent that many people can be clinically managed for alcohol and drug addiction in a structured outpatient setting. The alcohol and drug addiction treatment process [18] previously available only in an inpatient facility can now be delivered in a local outpatient setting as patients continue employment and improve family relations.

REFERENCES

1. *Alcoholics Anonymous* (1976). 3rd ed. New York, Alcoholics Anonymous World Services, Inc.
2. Stuckey, R.F., and Harrison, J. (1982). The alcohol rehabilitation treatment center, *Encyclopedic Handbook of Alcoholism* (E. Patterson and E. Kaufman, eds.). New York, Gardiner Press, p. 865.
3. Cocores, J.A., Slaby, A.E., and Gold, M.S. (1989). *Outpatient Alcohol and Drug Rehabilitation*. Presented at 20th Annual Meeting of the American Medical Society on Alcoholism & Other Drug Dependencies, Inc., Atlanta, Georgia, 8:23.
4. Cocores, J.A. (1990). Treatment of the dually diagnosed adult drug user, *Dual Diangosis Patients* (A.E. Slaby and M.S. Gold, eds.). New York, Marcel Dekker, p. 211.
5. Cocores, J.A. (1987). Co-addiction: A silent epidemic, *Fair Oaks Hosp. Lett.*, 5(2):5.
6. *First Steps: Al-Anon 35 years of beginnings* (1986). New York, Al-Anon Family Group Headquarters, Inc., p. 8.
7. Cocores, J.A. and Gold, M.S. (1989). Recognition and crisis intervention treatment with cocaine abusers, *Crisis Intervention Handbook* (A.R. Roberts, ed.). Pacific Grove, California, Wadsworth, p. 118.
8. Jellinek, E.M. (1960). *The Disease Concept of Alcoholism*. New Haven, Connecticut, Hillhouse Press, p. 139.
9. *Narcotics Anonymous* (1984). World Service Office, Inc., Van Nuys, California, p. 55.
10. Miller, N.S., Gold, M.S., Cocores, J.A., and Pottash, A.C. (1988). Alcohol dependence and its medical consequences. *N.Y. St. J. Medi.*, 88:467.
11. Cocores, J.A. (1988). New Treatment for co-addiction disorder, *Psychiatr. Times May*:13.
12. Cocores, J.A. (1990). *800 Cocaine Guide to Recovery*. New York, Villard Books, p. 118.
13. Cocores, J.A., Davies, R.K., Mueller, P.S., and Gold, M.S. (1987). Cocaine abuse and adult attention deficit disorder, *J. Clin. Psychiatry*, 48(9):376.
14. Cocores, J.A., Patel,, M.D., Gold, M.S., and Pottash, A.C. (1987). Cocaine abuse, attention deficit disorder, and bipolar disorder, *J. Nerv. Ment. Dis.*, 175(7):431.
15. *Physicians Desk Reference* (1989). Oradell, New Jersey, Medical Economics Company Inc., p. 2190.
16. Gold, M.S., and Estroff, T.W. (1985). The comprehensive evaluation of cocaine and opiate abusers, *Handbook of Psychiatric Diagnostic Procedures* (R.C.W. Hall and T.P. Beresford, eds.). New York, Spectrum, p. 213.
17. Gawin, F.H., Kleber, H.D., Byck, R., et al. (1989). Desipramine facilitation of initial cocaine abstinence, *Arch. Gen. Psychiatry*, 46:117.
18. Miller, N.S. (1987). A primer of the treatment process for alcoholism and drug addiction, *Fair Oaks Hosp. Lett.*, 5(7):30.

66

Office Practice in Drug and Alcohol Addiction

Marc Galanter
New York University School of Medicine, New York, New York

I. INTRODUCTION

All too often, practitioners are left without specific approaches to the management of alcohol and drug addiction. Yet it is important that the clinician have access to an effective format for rehabilitation for these patients, since traditional individual therapy techniques may have limited impact on addictive illness [1,2]. A treatment approach will be outlined here to achieve an optimal outcome based on the use of a social support network as an integral part of individual office therapy.

II. INDICATIONS FOR THE NETWORK TECHNIQUE

The network approach can be useful in addressing a broad range of addicted patients characterized by the following clinical hallmarks of addictive illness. When addicts initiate consumption of their addictive agent, be it alcohol, cocaine, opiates, or depressant drugs, they frequently cannot limit that consumption to a reasonable and predictable level; this phenomenon has been termed loss of control by clinicians who treat alcohol- or drug-dependent persons [3]. Also, addicts consistently demonstrate relapse to the agent of addiction; that is, they have attempted to stop using the drug for varying periods of time, but have returned to it despite a specific intent to avoid it. To aid in diagnosis, particularly in the face of denial, it is of singular importance to have historical information from the patient's family and friends. They provide patterns of drinking and insight into the social consequences of the patient's addiction problem.

This treatment approach is not necessary for those abusers who can, in fact, learn to set limits on their abuse; their abuse may be treated as a behavioral symptom in a more

---

This chapter is based on material published by the author in *Psychiatric Annuals* (1989) and *Advances in Alcohol and Substance Abuse* (1986).

traditional psychotherapeutic fashion. Nor is it directed at those patients for whom the addictive pattern is most unmanageable, such as alcoholics with unusual destabilizing circumstances such as homelessness, severe character pathology or psychosis, or cocaine addicts who binge almost continuously. These patients may need special supportive care such as inpatient detoxification or long-term residential treatment.

In reviewing this material the reader should focus on those aspects of the treatment outlined here which are at variance with his or her usual therapeutic approach. While it is essential to rely on acquired clinical judgment and experience, it is equally important with the alcoholic to be prepared to depart from the usual mode of psychotherapeutic treatment. For example, activity rather than passivity is essential when a problem of drug exposure is suggested; the concept of therapist and patient enclosed in an inviolable envelope must be modified; immediate circumstances which may expose the patient to alcohol or drug use must take precedence over issues of long-term understanding and insight. These principles are applicable within the technique outlined here. Other approaches, too, such as the use of multiple family groups [4], may incorporate some of these principles.

III. THE INITIAL ENCOUNTERS: STARTING A SOCIAL NETWORK

The patient should be asked to bring his spouse or a close friend to the first session. Alcoholic patients often do not like certain things they hear when they first come for treatment and may deny or rationalize even if they have voluntarily sought help. Because of their denial of the problem, a significant other is essential to both history taking and to implementing a viable treatment plan. A close relation can often cut through the denial in the way that an unfamiliar therapist cannot, and can therefore be invaluable in setting a standard of realism in dealing with the addiction.

Some patients make clear that they wish to come to the initial session on their own. This is often associated with their desire to preserve the option of continued drug abuse and is born out of the fear that an alliance will be established independent of them to prevent this. While a delay may be tolerated for a session or two, there should be no ambiguity at the outset that effective treatment can only be undertaken on the basis of a therapeutic alliance built around the alcohol issue which includes the support of significant others, and that it is expected that a network of close friends and/or relations will be brought in within a session or two, at the most.

The weight of clinical experience supports the view that, as a general principle, abstinence is the most practical goal to propose to the addicted person for his or her rehabilitation [5–7]. For abstinence to be expected, however, the therapist should assure the provision of necessary social supports for the patient. Let us consider how a long-term support network is initiated for this purpose, beginning with availability of the therapist, significant others, and a self-help group.

In the first place, the therapist should be available for consultation on the phone, and should indicate to the patient that he or she wants to be called if problems arise. This makes the therapist's commitment clear, and sets the tone for a team effort. It begins to undercut one reason for relapse, the patient's sense that he or she will be on his or her own if a situation becomes unmanageable. The astute therapist, though, will assure that he or she does not spend excessive time at the telephone or in emergency sessions. A support network should be developed which can handle the majority of problems involved in day to day assistance to the patient. This will generally leave the therapist only to respond to occasional questions of interpreting the terms of the understanding between the therapist, the patient, and support network members. If there is question about the ability of the patient and network to manage the period between the initial sessions, the first few scheduled sessions may be arranged at intervals of only 1–3 days. In any case, frequent appointments should be scheduled at the outset if a pharmacological detoxification with benzodiazepines is indicated, so that the patient need never manage more than a few days' medication at a time.

What is most essential, though, is that the network be forged into a working group to provide necessary support for the patient between the initial sessions. Membership ranges from one to several persons close to the patient. Larger networks have been utilized by Speck [8] in treating schizophrenic patients. Contacts between network members at this stage typically include telephone calls (at the therapist's or patient's initiative), dinner arrangements, and social encounters, and should be preplanned to a fair extent during the joint session. These encounters are most often undertaken at the time when alcohol or drug use is likely to occur. In planning together, however, it should be made clear to network members that relatively little unusual effort will be required for the long term: After the patient is stabilized, their participation will come to little more than attendance at infrequent meetings with the patient and therapist. This is reassuring to those network members who are unable to make a major time commitment to the patient as well as to those patients who do not want to be placed in a dependent position.

Composition of the network will be crucial in determining the balance of the therapy. This is not without problems, and the therapist must think in a strategic fashion of the interactions which may take place among network members. The following case illustrates the nature of their task.

A 25-year-old graduate student had been addicted to cocaine since high school, in part drawing funds from his affluent family, who lived in a remote city. At two points in the process of establishing his support network, the reactions of his live-in girlfriend, who worked with us from the outset, were particularly important. Both he and she agreed to bring in his 19-year-old sister, a freshman at a nearby college. He then mentioned a "friend" of his, a woman whom he had apparently found attractive even though there was no history of an overt romantic involvement. The expression on his girlfriend's face suggested that she did not like this idea, although she offered no rationale for excluding this potential rival. The idea of having to rely for assistance solely on two women who might see each other as competitors, however, was unappealing. I, therefore, tactfully discouraged the idea of the "friend," and we moved on to evaluating the patient's uncle, whom he initially preferred to exclude despite the fact that his girlfriend thought him appropriate. It later turned out (as I had expected) that the uncle was perceived as a potentially disapproving representative of the parental generation. I encouraged the patient to accept the uncle as a network member nonetheless, so as to round out the range of relationships with the group, and did spell out my rationale for this inclusion. In matter of fact, the uncle turned out to be caring and supportive, particularly after he was helped to understand the nature of the addictive process.

IV. DEFINING THE NETWORK'S TASK

As conceived here, the therapist's relationship to the network is like that of a task-oriented team leader rather than that of a family therapist oriented toward insight. The network is established to implement a straightforward task—that of aiding the therapist to sustain the patient's abstinence. It must be directed with the same clarity of purpose that a task force is directed in any effective organization. Competing and alternative goals must be suppressed, or at least prevented from interfering with the primary task.

Unlike family members involved in traditional family therapy, network members are not led to expect symptom relief or self-realization for themselves. This prevents the development of competing goals for the network's meetings. It also assures the members protection from having their own motives scrutinized, and thereby supports their continuing involvement without the threat of an assult on their psychological defenses. Since network members have—kindly—volunteered to participate, their motives must not be impugned. Their constructive behavior should be commended. It is useful to acknowledge appreciation for the contribution they are making to the therapy. There is always a counterproductive tendency on their part to minimize the value of their contribution.

The network must, therefore, be structured as an effective working group with good morale. This is not always easy:

> A 45-year-old single woman served as an executive in a large family-held business— except when her alcohol problem led her into protracted binges. Her father, brother, and sister were prepared to banish her from the business, but decided first to seek consultation. Because they had initiated the contact, they were included in the initial network, and indeed were very helpful in stabilizing the patient. Unfortunately, however, the father was a domineering figure who intruded in all aspects of the business, evoking angry outbursts from his children. The children typically reacted with petulance, provoking him in return. The situation came to a head when 2 months into the treatment both the patient's siblings angrily petitioned me to exclude the father from the network. This presented a problem because the father's control over the business made his involvement important to securing the patient's compliance. The patient's relapse was still a real possibility. This potentially coercive role, however, was an issue that the group could not easily deal with. I decided to support the father's membership in the group, pointing out the constructive role he had played in getting the therapy started. It seemed necessary to support the earnestness of his concern for his daughter rather than the children's dismay at their father's (very real) obstinacy. It was clear to me that the father could not deal with a situation in which he was not accorded sufficient respect, and that there was no real place in this network for addressing the father's character pathology directly. The hubbub did, in fact, quiet down with time. The children became less provocative themselves, as the group responded to my pleas for civil behavior.

The following guidelines should be made clear from the first, so that network members can collaborate in implementing their respective roles in working with the patient. Above all, they should be conveyed by example. The correction of misapprehensions about these norms should be given a high priority; similarly, violations of these guidelines are discussed as soon as detected, and in a supportive manner.

1. The purpose of the network is to help the patient maintain his or her abstinence; unrelated benefits for other members are not pursued in network sessions, either by the patient, network members, or the therapist.
2. Information relevant to the patient's abstinence or slips into drug use will be promptly reported to the therapist and to other network members.
3. Supportiveness for the patient is primary. Members should help him or her to deal with problems he or she confronts regarding abstinence, but not be critical of difficulties in achieving a recovery.
4. If a slip is detected by a network member, the patient will be offered assistance, but the member will not impose a course of action without consultation with the therapist.
5. The nature of confidentiality is important. The patient's own exchanges with the therapist which are unrelated to drug problems are kept in confidence. Information revealed by network members to the therapist, however, will be brought up in the group if relevant.

V. USE OF 12-STEP PROGRAMS

The use of 12-step modalities modeled on the principles of Alcoholics Anonymous (AA) is desirable whenever possible. For the alcoholic, certainly, participation in Alcoholics Anonymous is strongly encouraged. Groups such as Narcotics Anonymous, Pills Anonymous, and Cocaine Anonymous are modeled after AA, and play a similarly useful role for drug abusers. One approach is to tell the patient that he or she is expected to attend at least two such meetings a week for at least 1 month so as to become familiar with the program. If after a month, he or she is quite reluctant to continue, and other aspects of the treatment are going well, nonparticipation may have to be accepted. This may be done with the contingency that the patient return if a slip occurs.

Some patients are more easily convinced to attend AA meetings. Others may be less compliant. The therapist should mobilize the support network as appropriate in order to continue pressure for the patient's involvement with AA for a reasonable trial. It may take a considerable period of time, but ultimately a patient may experience something of a conversion, wherein he or she adopts the group ethos and expresses a deep commitment to abstinence, a measure of commitment rarely observed in patients who experience psychotherapy alone. When this occurs, the therapist may assume a more passive role in monitoring the patient's abstinence, and keep an eye on his or her ongoing involvement in AA. Nonetheless, the therapist will continue to address interpersonal issues, such as marital conflict, and may apply specific techniques such as cognitive therapy and confrontation.

VI. USE OF DISULFIRAM

For the alcoholic, disulfiram may be of marginal use in assuring abstinence when used in a traditional counseling context [9], but it becomes much more valuable when carefully integrated into work with the patient and network, particularly, when taken under observation. It is a good idea to use the initial telephone contact to engage the patient's agreement to be abstinent from alcohol for the day immediately prior to the first session. The therapist then has the option of prescribing or administering disulfiram at that time. For a patient who is in earnest about seeking assistance for alcoholism, this is often not difficult, if some time is spent on the phone making plans to avoid a drinking context during that period. If it is not feasible to undertake this on the phone, it may be addressed in the first session. Such planning with the patient will almost always involve organizing time with significant others, and therefore serves as a basis for developing the patient's support network.

The administration of disulfiram under observation is a treatment option which is easily adapted to work with social networks. A patient who takes disulfiram cannot drink; a patient who agrees to be observed by a reasonable party while taking disulfiram will not miss his dose without the observer's knowing. This may take a measure of persuasion and, above all, the therapist's commitment that such an approach can be reasonable and helpful. It should not, however, be seen as an alternative to the patient's own initiative in assuming continued abstinence.

Disulfiram is typically initiated with a dose of 500 mg, and then 250 mg daily. It is taken every morning, when the urge to drink is generally least. Particulars of administration in the context of treatment should be reviewed [9].

As noted previously, individual therapists have traditionally seen the abuser as a patient with a poor prognosis. This is largely because in the context of traditional psychotherapy, there are no behavioral controls to prevent the recurrence of drug use, and resources are not available for behavioral intervention if a recurrence takes place—which it usually does. A system of impediments to the emergence of relapse, resting heavily on the actual or symbolic role of the network, must therefore be established. The therapist must have assistance in addressing any minor episode of drinking so that this ever-present problem does not lead to an unmanageable relapse or an unsuccessful termination of therapy.

How can the support network be used to deal with recurrences of drug use when, in fact, the patient's prior association with these same persons did not prevent him or her from using alcohol or drugs? The following example illustrates how this may be done. In this case, a specific format was defined with the network to monitor a patient's compliance with a disulfiram regimen.

A 33-year-old public relations executive had moved to New York from a remote city 3 years before coming to treatment. She had no long-standing close relationships in the city, a circumstance not uncommon for a single alcoholic in a setting removed from her origins. She presented with a 10-year history of heavy drinking, which had increased in severity since her arrival, no doubt associated with her social isolation. Although she consumed a bottle of wine each night and additional hard liquor, she was able to get to work regularly. Six months before the outset of treatment she attended AA meetings for 2 weeks and had been abstinent during that time. She had then relapsed, though, and became disillusioned with the possibility of maintaining abstinence.

At the outset of treatment, it was necessary to reassure her that prior relapse was in large part a function of not having established sufficient outside supports (including more sound relationship within AA), and having seen herself as failed after only one slip. There was, however, basis for real concern as to whether she would do any better now if the same formula were reinstituted in the absence of sufficient, reliable supports, which she did not seem to have. Together we came upon the idea of bringing in an old friend whom she saw occasionally, and whom she felt she could trust. We made the following arrangement with her friend. The patient came to sessions twice a week. She would see her friend once each weekend. On each of these thrice-weekly occasions, she would be observed taking disulfiram, so that even if she missed a daily dose in between, it would not be possible for her to resume drinking on a regular basis undetected. The interpersonal support inherent in this arrangement, bolstered by conjoint meetings with her and her friend, also allowed her to return to AA with a sense of confidence in her ability to maintain abstinence.

VII. FREQUENCY OF CONTACTS

At the outset of therapy, it is important to see the patient with the group on a weekly basis for at least the first month. Unstable circumstances demand more frequent contacts with the network. Sessions can be tapered off biweekly, and then monthly intervals after a time.

In order to sustain the continuing commitment of the group, particularly that between the therapist and the network members, network sessions should be held every 3 months or so for the duration of the individual therapy. Once the patient has stabilized, the meetings tend less to address day to day issues. They may begin with a recounting by the patient of the drug situation. Reflections on the patient's progress and goals, or sometimes on relations between the network members, may then be discussed. In any case, it is essential that network members contact the therapist if they are concerned about the patient's possible use of alcohol or drugs, and that the therapist contact the network members if he or she becomes concerned over a potential relapse.

VIII. INTRUSIVE MEASURES

Certain circumstances may necessitate further incursions on the patient's autonomy, so as to assure compliance with treatment. This is particularly true when the patient has begun treatment reluctantly, as with overt pressure from family or employer, or when the possibility of relapse will have grave consequences. Options include the possibility of financial constraints, a spouse's moving out, and urine monitoring. These, of course, can only be undertaken with the patient's agreement, based on the fact that greater or more immediate loss is being averted. Such steps may also provide greater certitude against relapse to all concerned, including an uneasy therapist and family.

> A 35-year-old man had used heroin intranasally for 2 years and then intravenously for 8 months. He had previously used other drugs. He was stealing money from the family business where he worked. The patient underwent ambulatory detoxification, but relapsed to heroin use, and finally underwent a hospitalization that lasted 5 weeks. He was then referred to me upon discharge, and was to continue with meetings of Narcotics Anonymous. His network consisted of his mother and his wife, and the following family members involved in the family business: his father, his younger sister and brother, and his uncle. His family was very concerned about allowing him to get involved in the business. We, therefore, agreed to do two things, so that he might be included with less concern on everyone's part. The patient agreed to have his urine spot checked on a regular basis, and he and I, along with the network, discussed his financial circumstances in the firm, clarifying what consequences might emerge should he return to active addiction. An informal, but explicit, agreement was reached in this matter, thereby helping the patient understand the constraints under which he was operating, and leaving the family more comfortable about his returning to work. Since this agreement was undertaken with the network, it became a part of the treatment plan.

IX. ADAPTING INDIVIDUAL THERAPY TO THE NETWORK TREATMENT

As noted above, network sessions are scheduled on a weekly basis at the outset of treatment. This is likely to compromise the number of individual contacts. Indeed, if sessions are held once a week, the patient may not be seen individually for a period of time. This may be perceived as a deprivation by the patient unless the individual therapy is presented as an opportunity for further growth *predicated* on achieving stable abstinence assured through work with the network.

When the individual therapy does begin, the traditional objectives of therapy must be ordered so as to accomodate the goals of the alcohol and drug addiction treatment. For insight-oriented therapy, clarification of unconscious motivations is a primary objective; for supportive therapy, the bolstering of established constructive defenses is primary. In the therapeutic context which we are describing, however, the following objectives are given precedence.

Of first importance is the need to address exposure to alcohol and drug addiction, or exposure to cues which might precipitate alcohol or drug use [10]. Both patient and therapist should be sensitive to this matter and explore these situations as they arise. Second, a stable social context in an appropriate social environment—one conducive to abstinence with minimal disruption of life circumstances—should be supported. Considerations of minor disruptions in place of residence, friends, or job need not be a primary issue for the patient with a character disorder or neurosis, but they cannot go untended here. For a considerable period of time the alcohol and drug addict is highly vulnerable to exacerbations of the addictive illness and must be viewed with the considerable caution, in some respect, as one treats the recently compensated psychotic.

Finally, after attending to these priorities, psychological conflicts which the patient must resolve relative to his or her own growth are considered. As the therapy continues, these come to assume a more prominent role. In the earlier phases, they are likely to directly reflect issues associated with previous drug use. Later, however, as the issue of addiction becomes less compelling from day to day, the context of the treatment will come increasingly to resemble the traditional psychotherapeutic context. Given the optimism generated by an initial success over the addictive process, the patient will be in an excellent position to move forward in therapy with a positive view of his future.

REFERENCES

1. Vaillant, G.E. Dangers of psychotherapy in the treatment of alcoholism, *Dynamic Approaches to the Understanding and Treatment of Alcoholism* (M.H. Bean and N.E. Zinberg, eds.). New York, Free Press, 1981, pp. 36–54.
2. Hayman, M. Current attitudes to alcoholism of psychiatrists in Southern California. *Am. J. Psychiatry, 112*:484–493 (1956).
3. Jellinek, E.M. *The Disease Concept of Alcoholism.* New Haven, Connecticut, Hillhouse Press, 1963.
4. Gallant, D.M., Rich, A., Bey, E., and Terranova, L. Group psychotherapy with married couples: A successful technique in New Orleans Alcoholism Clinic patients. *J. La. St. Med. Soc., 122*:41–44 (1970).
5. Helzer, J.E., Robins, L.N., Taylor, J.R., et al. The extent of long-term drinking among alcoholics discharged from medical and psychiatric facilities. *N. Engl. J. Med., 312*:1678–1682 (1985).
6. Gitlow, S.E., and Peyser, H.S. (eds.). *Alcoholism: A Practical Treatment Guide.* New York, Grune & Stratton, 1980.
7. Pattison, E.M. Non-abstinent drinking goals in the treatment of alcoholism: A clinical typology. *Arch. Gen. Psychiatry, 33*:923–930 (1976).
8. Speck, R. Psychotherapy of the social network of a schizophrenic family. *Fam. Process, 6*:208 (1967).
9. Fuller, R., Branchey, L., Brightwell, D.R., et al. Disulfiram treatment of alcoholism. A Veterans Administration Cooperative Study. *J.A.M.A., 256*:1449–1455 (1986).
10. Galanter, M. Psychotherapy for alcohol and drug abuse: an approach based on learning theory. *J. Psychiatr. Treat. Eval., 5*:551–556 (1983).

XXI

Inpatient Treatment

67

Inpatient Treatment of Drug and Alcohol Addiction

Charles A. Dackis
Hampton Hospital, Westampton, New Jersey

Mark S. Gold
Fair Oaks Hospital, Summit, New Jersey, and Delray Beach, Florida

I. INTRODUCTION

The treatment of alcoholics and drug addicts often requires hospitalization before abstinence can be assured and medical, psychiatric, and rehabilitative therapies successfully instituted. The outcome of hospitalization frequently determines whether the patient achieves long-term recovery or even survival. Drug and alcohol rehabilitation differs greatly from standard psychiatric treatment in its emphasis on self-help groups, a directive philosophy, and behavioral approaches. Specialized treatment units are, therefore, optimal in providing care for alcoholics and drug addicts and treatment on standard psychiatric units is difficult, even though a vast number of such individuals have concomitant psychiatric illness. These patients are best treated with a skillful coordination of psychiatric and rehabilitative approaches. This chapter will outline the essential aspects of inpatient treatment of addiction with an emphasis on psychiatric and medical aspects of care.

II. THE NATURE OF ADDICTION

Effective treatment of alcoholism and drug addiction must be based on an understanding of addiction's nature and dynamics. Euphoria and craving are the major forces of addiction and alternate repeatedly in what has been termed the cycle of addiction. These reinforcers must be addressed before any treatment approach can be viable. The power of the euphoria produced by cocaine is illustrated by its self-administration by monkeys to the point of death [1]. Craving is a negative reinforcer that appears to derive from the same neuronal systems involved in the natural drive states of hunger, thirst, and libido [2]. Craving can, therefore, be conceptualized as an acquired natural drive possessing equivalent or even greater power than natural drive states. Craving and euphoria alternate repeatedly and eventually become entrenched as the line is crossed into addiction. Progressive dyscontrol over intake results and hazards of addiction are increasingly tolerated.

The gradual process of progression is hidden from the addict through the defenses of denial, minimization, and rationalization. A major task of treatment is to confront these defenses and make the patient cognizant of his or her lack of control. Only then will the addict be willing to counter the forces of euphoria and craving through the arduous process of recovery. At any time along the way, one indiscretion can reactivate the cycle of addiction, leading to rapidly to recidivism. Therein lies the challenge of treatment and the insidious tenacity of addiction. The inpatient phase of treatment, when indicated, is the most powerful means of breaking the cycle of addiction long enough to address denial, orient addicts to their precarious situation, and proceed with medical and psychiatric stabilization.

III. WHETHER TO HOSPITALIZE

Clinical indications for hospitalization represent an area of some dispute in the fields of medicine and drug rehabilitation. Intense pressure from third-party payers to limit or omit inpatient insurance coverage for drug addiction and alcoholism has played an increasing role in the clinician's options. Many patients that were once hospitalized are now treated in structured outpatient settings. This shift toward outpatient treatment has changed the clinical mixture of inpatient units to include patients that are much more ill from a psychiatric and medical perspective. Drug and alcohol units must now be proficient in the evaluation and treatment of coexisting psychiatric disorders.

Psychiatric illness with suicidality, homocidality, or grossly disorganized mental status obviously requires hositalization. Some patients with incapacitating anxiety or depression might require inpatient stabilization before being capable of benefiting from outpatient rehabilitation. Addicts with serious medical complications such as drug overdose, abstinence syndromes, and many diseases resulting from their addiction require hosptialization for proper medical evaluation and stabilization. Severe addiction is a life-threatening situation. When patients begin to risk lethal overdose or continue drug use in the face of serious medical disorders such as seizures, cardiac disease, acquired immune deficiency syndrome (AIDS), and hepatitis, hospitalization is indicated.

Unsuccessful outpatient treatment is generally considered to be an indication for hospitalization, although insincere or half-hearted attempts may be repeated successfully. Since many addicts are pressured to seek treatment by their family, friends, employer, or law enforcement agencies and may not actually wish to be abstinent, internal motivation is often lacking. Intravenous drug addicts respond poorly to outpatient treatment and are particularly vulnerable to medical illness and overdose. For this reason, and owing to the present threat of AIDS, these individuals are best treated initially in the hospital. Drug dealers have great difficulty establishing abstinence as outpatients, as do other patients with easy access to drugs or immersed in the drug environment. Finally, patients adverse to treatment but externally motivated by legal, family, or job pressure may require intensive inpatient rehabilitation before internal motivation can be cultivated.

IV. THE INPATIENT UNIT

At the onset of treatment, the alcoholic and drug addict must be thoroughly evaluated from a medical perspective owing to the risk of medical complications. Psychiatric complications are also prevalent and should be properly evaluated and treated. Drug intoxification, drug withdrawal, medical disorders, and psychiatric complications are best identified with a systematic, integrated, and structured approach that begins the moment the patient enters the hospital. This approach has been previously discussed [3] and its essentials are outlined below.

Drug addicts and alcoholics are optimally treated on specialized units with multidisciplinary staff versed in all aspects of addiction. A crucial aspect of treatment involves exposure to self-help groups based on Alcoholics Anonymous (AA) and Narcotics Anonymous (NA) philosophy. Staff members undergoing personal recovery are extremely useful because they can self-disclose and relate more directly to the inpatients. Typically staffed with psychiatrists, nurses, certified addiction counselors (CACs), social workers, psychologists, creative therapists, and mental health associates, the unit should deliver care in an integrated multidisciplinary team approach. Although the CAC is typically responsible to lead groups and teach AA/NA philosophy, all staff members should be familiar with the rehabilitative approach and the CAC should be knowledgeable about psychiatric disorders. In this way, the psychiatric and rehabilitative therapies can be coordinated and splitting between the two minimized.

Regimented unit rules, procedures, and precautions are necessary on an alcohol and drug addiction unit because addicts are out of control and practiced in the art of deception. Failure to address their manipulative and deceptive nature will convey naivete about addiction, and negatively impact the therapeutic alliance. A locked or carefully supervised unit should limit drug access as well as impulsive departures from the hospital. Luggage must absolutely be inspected and a body search conducted immediately on admission, since a certain percentage of patients will arrive with hidden drugs. Vital signs are monitored closely and a physical examination is performed immediately to assess intoxication and withdrawal signs. A psychiatric evaluation should be conducted to assess mental status, especially suicidality, psychosis, and delirium. A supervised urine sample for drug analysis is obtained *prior* to medication administration. Visitors must be judiciously screened, since they may bring drugs into the unit or provoke craving in other patients if they are intoxicated.

The patient should be oriented to unit rules and held responsible for compliance. The violation of certain rules (drug use, sexual acting out) may constitute grounds for discharge. Adherence to unit rules is an important measure of the addict's motivation, and deviations should be confronted. Addicts habitually lie, manipulate, and conceal their activities. The staff should, therefore, be alert to inconsistencies and be able to confront "addict behavior." This is best done when there are daily treatment plan meetings of the multidisciplinary staff in which information from interviews, unit behavior, past records, and family input can be communicated and integrated.

V. MEDICAL EVALUATION AND STABILIZATION

A medical history, review of systems, and physical examination are conducted by the admitting physician. The physical examination must obviously evaluate the possibility of intoxication, overdose, and withdrawal. The physician should be familiar with opiate, sedative-hypnotic, and stimulant overdose syndromes [3–5] as well as with drug and alcohol abstinence symptoms. Attention to objective measures such as vital signs, reflexes, pupil size, and diaphoresis is more reliable than subjective patient complaints.

The physical examination should also evaluate diseases related to the drugs abused and routes of administration. Needle track marks may be present on the arms of intravenous users and unusual sites of injection such as the jugular or femoral veins should be inspected and auscultated for bruits. The nasal septum may show signs of necrosis or perforation. Hepatomegaly, spider angiomas, and jaundice may be present with liver disease. Skin lesions, cachexia, or generalized lymphadenopathy should raise the level of suspicion for AIDS. The admitting physician must, therefore, be familiar with the physical stigmata of these medical disorders that are associated with drug and alcohol addiction.

Laboratory tests provide further objective information. A routine medical screening should be ordered on admission to identify medical complications. Covert use of cocaine, benzodiazepines, and opiates identified by urine monitoring will illuminate detoxification and identify lying at the onset of treatment. The urine collection should be supervised, analyzed for specific gravity, and assayed by reliable means such as radioimmunoassay or gas chromatography mass spectrometry [6]. Plasma testing should be ordered to identify drug intoxication. Hepatitis and HIV (human immunodeficiency virus) testing is imperative in high-risk individuals for diagnostic information and the protection of other patients and staff.

A. Detoxification

Detoxification has been reviewed elsewhere [7,8] but certain points warrant additional emphasis. The clinician should always rely on objective measures when assessing withdrawal and maintain a high level of suspicion for medication-seeking behavior. Initial therapeutic alliances are dramatically affected by the way detoxification (read taking over the addict's drug supply) is managed. Lack of expertise that leads to unnecessary discomfort or overmedication will damage the therapeutic alliance, interfere with trust formation, and jeopardize the patient's medical condition. Skillful detoxification sets the stage for successful rehabilitation. Covert alcohol and sedative-hypnotic withdrawal is very common, can develop into a medical emergency if untreated, and should never be overlooked. In particular, urine evaluation and family interviews shouldbe performed to uncover sedative dependence. Benzodiazepine, barbiturate, and methadone detoxification may take several weeks and is complicated by slow release of drug from fat stores. Small daily reductions must, therefore, be pursued and assessed over several days, since the effects of these drugs are delayed. Opiate detoxification with clonidine is preferable to methadone because of its relative lack of drug euphoria [9]. Finally, with mixed dependence, it is usually preferable to detoxify one agent at a time.

B. Medical Complications

Medical complications of drug and alcohol addiction have been previously reviewed [3], and largely comprise tissue damage caused by drugs and their contaminants, direct pharmacological actions, and pathology related to the route of administration. Examples of tissue damage are liver toxicity resulting from alcohol exposure and damage to retinal capillary beds from the intravenous injection of microscopic talc particles found in pulverized pills. A direct pharmacological action leading to medical problems is that of cocaine-induced arrhythmia. Pernicious complications related to route of administration include hepatitis [10] and AIDS [11]. The following paragraphs outline some of the more common medical conditions encountered by clinicians treating addicts in the hospital.

Medical complications arising from the route of administration are most common with intravenous addicts. Covert intravenous use should be suspected in opiate and stimulant addicts. Pulmonary and cardiac infections resulting from intravenous drug administration include pneumonia, septic emboli, abscesses, mycotic aneurysms, and endocarditis. Renal failure may result from antigen-antibody complex deposits in patients with hepatitis or endocarditis [12], or from hepatic failure. Hepatitis B is easily acquired among addicts because it can be transmitted in minute amounts of blood and other body fluids [10]. Antigen and antibody measurements for hepatitis A and B are often positive in addicts without past needle use owing to their association with intravenous users. Hepatitis precautions are necessary for patients at risk until the results of the antigen test is available. Patients should eat on disposable trays with disposable utensils, and their linens, towels, and clothes should be washed separately. Transmission via saliva, sputum, urine, feces, blood, and seminal or vaginal fluid must be avoided. Patients unable or unwilling to follow these instructions require confrontation and special supervision.

AIDS in drug addicts can be acquired through needle sharing (which is still common) and sexual relationships with addicts or carriers. Lifestyle factors as well as route of administration place addicts at risk for exposure the AIDS virus. AIDS may comprise a variety of medical conditions, including *Pneumocystis carinii* pneumonia, disseminated herpes simplex, mycobacterial infections, lymphadenopathy, Kaposi's sarcoma, and dementia [11]. Extreme care must be taken to avoid transmission of this fatal disease to other patients and staff members. Universal precautions are probably sufficient in patients with definite or suspected HIV positiveness, although transmission of the HIV virus has not been thoroughly research. Patients who have recently learn they are HIV positive may be suicidal and should be carefully evaluated. These individuals are also at high risk of acute recidivism and should be supported and retained in the hospital until their crisis subsides.

Other forms of administration are more benign than intravenous use, although "skin-popping" can introduce similar infections. Intranasal use of cocaine causes tissue necrosis secondary to vasoconstriction, leading to perforation of the nasal septum and chronic sinusitis. Intrapulmonary use with marijuana can produce emphysema, whereas "free-basing" cocaine or smoking "crack" cocaine and its adulterants damages the alveolar surface.

Direct pharmacological effects of drugs comprise most overdose and abstinence syndromes [3,13]. For instance, opiates and barbiturates depress central respiratory centers pharmacologically. Central stimulants cause cardiac arrhythmias, myocardial infarction, hypertension, and hyperthermia [14]. Cocaine produces severe vasoconstriction that leads to organ strangulation, including the brain, heart, and bowel, and even spontaneous abortions due to inadequate blood supply. Cocaine also produces hyperprolactinemia in some patients [15], leading to infertility and impotence [16], whereas marijuana and opiates inhibit testosterone and reduce the libido [17].

Alcohol is most likely to cause direct toxic effects on tissue, in part because of its lack of specific receptor action and its use in much greater molar quantities than other drugs. Toxic effects include cirrhosis, dementia, peripheral neuropathy, cardiomyopathy, peptic ulcer disease, pancreatitis, and birth defects. Alcoholism also progresses at a slower rate than opiate and stimulant addictions, and hospitalized alcoholics are usually older than their drug-addicted counterparts, partially accounting for their increased prevalence of medical conditions.

Drug and alcohol addiction is associated with numerous medical disorders that should be accurately diagnosed and treated. The causal relationship between substance abuse and the medical disease should be clearly explained to the patient and family and may reduce initial resistance to treatment. Surprisingly, fear of illness or death alone is seldom sufficient to motivate prolonged abstinence. Medical stabilization, including treatment of overdose and withdrawal, is therefore only the first step in the overall treatment of the addict and must be followed by vigorous rehabilitation.

VI. PSYCHIATRIC EVALUATION AND STABILIZATION

The psychiatric evaluation of drug addicts is an essential part of their treatment, since psychopathology poses a direct threat to recovery. Psychiatric symptoms may be entirely secondary to addiction, or result from the self-medication of an underlying psychiatric disorder. In this latter case, addictive patterns may eventually become entrenched and develop into an autonomous addiction. When psychiatric and addictive illnesses coexist, recovery can be difficult and a skillful coordination of psychiatric and drug rehabilitative treatment is necessary.

Psychiatric disorders can only be diagnosed reliably after intoxification and withdrawal symptoms have abated. Even at this point, protracted psychiatric syndromes may be seen.

For this reason, a "washout" period of about 2 weeks without pharmacotherapy should be allowed, when clinically feasible, with attention directed toward the spontaneous diminution of psychiatric symptoms.

In addition to confounding effects of drug intoxication, withdrawal, and protracted withdrawal states, the drug addict mentality often interferes with the psychiatric evaluation. Addicts are often reluctant or unable to describe psychiatric symptoms. Patients abusing a myriad of unknown or contaminated street drugs are often surprisingly resistant to psychotropics and may minimize psychiatric symptoms. Others may exaggerate psychiatric symptoms to minimize their addiction or receive more medications. Sequential psychiatric assessments must, therefore, be performed with great reliance on behavioral observations and objective informants.

The initial mental status examination may be confounded by intoxication or withdrawal effects and should be repeated. The psychiatric history should focus on psychopathology occurring during periods of abstinence or prior to drug abuse because periods of active use are of limited help in distinguishing psychiatric illness from drug-induced disorders. Family informants are very helpful in corroborating past periods of drug abstinence and psychiatric symptom constellations. Positive psychiatric family histories increase the likelihood of an independent psychiatric disorder.

As mentioned, psychiatric treatment in drug addicts must be carefully coordinated with drug rehabilitation. Addiction should not be viewed as merely secondary to psychiatric illness or the addict will avoid responsibility for recovery and deny the drug's euphoric reinforcement. Similarly, psychiatric treatment should not be sabotaged by drug counselors and other recovering staff. This is especially important when medications are necessary. Except for detoxification, addictive agents should be avoided entirely. This obvious guideline is often violated, particularly with the prescribing of benzodiazepines [18]. Even with nonaddictive psychotropics, there should be a true need for pharmacotherapy that outweighs its interference with rehabilitation. It is the physician's role as unit chief to understand psychiatric and rehabilitative approaches, and integrate these often divergent therapies.

A. Mood Disorders

Depression is a frequent complaint of recently hospitalized drug addicts and alcoholics. Situational conditions such as interpersonal deterioration, divorce, loss of employment and even incarceration often exist at the time of hospitalization and certainly contribute to depression. Depression may also result from affective illness, or protracted withdrawal from drugs and alcohol. For instance, opiate addicts have high rates of depression, which may result from alterations of brain endorphin or noradenergic systems [19]. These syndromes are often very persistent, but they respond to antidepressant medications. Depressed alcoholics, on the other hand, seldom require antidepressants because their depressive syndromes tend to remit spontaneously within days of their last drink [20]. Cocaine addicts experience withdrawal (or "crash") that includes anergia, hypersomnia, psychomotor retardation, depressed mood, and irritability, which generally resolves wihtin a period of hours. The clinician should, therefore, be familiar with the time course, severity, and character of divergent affective syndromes that are secondary to specific drugs of addiction.

Persistent depressive symptoms are usually indicative of underlying affective illness. Although currently unpopular, research findings indicate that neuroendocrine testing is helpful in distinguishing primary from secondary depressions. The dexamethasone suppression test (DST) is diagnostically reliable in the evaluation of major depression when conducted 2 weeks after detoxification of alcoholics [21] and opiate addicts [22]. The TRH test is not specific for major depression in alcoholics [21] or cocaine addicts [23]. It is well established that depressed addicts have high rates of recidivism [24]. It is, therefore, crucial that persistent symptoms of depression be properly diagnosed and treated.

Self-medication of depression as a basis for addiction is a very popular but probably overrated concept. Freud theorized that depressed individuals self-medicate with cocaine [25], but later research found that this drug actually exacerbates depression [26]. Indeed, most drugs of abuse produce withdrawal syndromes that involve dysphoria and depression. It is our experience that depression is much more likely to result from drugs and alcohol than to serve as a cause of addiction.

Antidepressant therapy should be vigorously pursued once major depression has been diagnosed. In general, antidepressants with a large degree of anticholineric activity are best avoided due to their mild potential for abuse. Antidepressants that block dopamine reuptake are also probably unsuitable, since this neurochemical effect is the primary mechanism of action of cocaine and amphetamine. Patients should be educated about psychotropic medications, especially that they do not produce euphoria or dependence. A meeting with the essential family members and patient is useful to clarify diagnostic and treatment issues and circumvent family resistance.

Acute mania must be distinguished from intoxication states with cocaine [27], amphetamine, phencyclidine [28], and hallucinogens [29]. This can be accomplished by observing physical signs [3] while awaiting the results of blood analysis. Elevated and irritable mood may continue for several days after the cessation of phencyclidine (PCP) intoxication [28]. With central stimulants, there should be a discernible improvement over hours to days as the drug is metabolized and eliminated. Sedative-hypnotics, alcohol, and opiate withdrawal could resemble mania, but these are usually differentiated easily by their characteristic physical signs [3]. Manic symptoms that persist without improvement are usually found only in bipolar disorders. Past manic or depressive episodes during periods of clearly documented drug abstinence are confirmatory of this diagnosis, as is a positive family history of affective disorder. There is often an extensive and obvious history of bipolar disorder with treatment failures due to lithium noncompliance and active addiction.

It is a common error to misdiagnose addiction in manic patients. These individuals typically exhibit impaired judgment and over use drugs/alcohol in order to control their mood. For this reason, drug taking occurring only during manic episodes does not qualify as true addiction. Conversely, if abuse is present during depressed and euthymic periods, the patient is probably an addict and usually requires rehabilitative treatment. It is obvious that continued drug and alcohol addiction in a bipolar patient destabilizes mood and interferes with lithium efficacy. The fact that neither bipolar disorder nor addiction can be effectively treated without stabilization of both renders manic addicts very difficult and challenging to treat.

B. Anxiety Disorders

Anxiety is always found in hospitalized drug addicts and can result from family turmoil, employment difficulties, functional deterioration, and even drug craving. Since drug addicts use drugs to alleviate anxiety, it is understandable that anxiety is experienced after access to drugs has been eliminated. Abstinence syndromes involve anxiety and should not be confused with independent anxiety disorders. Similarly, intoxication with cocaine, marijuana, hallucinogens, and phencyclidine produces anxiety and panic symptoms. Anxiety caused by addiction should, therefore, be distinguished from independent anxiety disorders, which may lead to self-medication with drugs, especially sedative-hypnotics, alcohol, and opiates.

It is often very difficult to evaluate anxiety in sedative-dependent patients. Barbiturates, benzodiazepines, and glutethimide usually require a prolonged detoxification during which anxiety may be a cardinal symptom of withdrawal. Physical withdrawal signs, including hypertension, tremor, diaphoresis, tachycardia, and hyperreflexia, may be helpful in this evaluation. However, until the completion of detoxification the issue may remain clouded. Detoxification from sedatives may require several weeks and must be done gradually. Adjunctive treatment with beta blockers can potentiate the agent used for detoxification and reduce anxiety symptoms.

Drug addicts with anxiety, especially panic disorders, should be properly stabilized on nonaddictive medications to avoid recidivism in the pursuit of symptom relief. Patients with a social phobia tend to avoid rehabilitation groups and usually benefit dramatically from beta blockers. A common mistake is to prescribe benzodiazpines for anxiety or panic disorders [18]. Addicts typically use benzodiazepines addictively or revert to their drug of choice after benzodiazepine administration. Since many physicians still prescribe benzodiazepines to addicts, patients must understand that it is *their* responsibility to abstain from addictive drugs. Of course, in most cases, addicts manipulate physicians to prescribe substances of addiction, and often utilize several physicians at a time. Unless anxiety is debilitating or interferes directly with recovery, it is best to be conservative and avoid pharmacotherapy. In fact, anxiety is a hallmark of early recovery from addiction and should not be overdiagnosed. Before meaningful abstinence is possible, drug addicts must learn to experience unpleasant feelings without artificial means of anxiety regulation.

C. Psychotic Disorders

Drug-induced psychosis can usually be identified by physical examination [3], careful history, and plasma or urine testing. Central stimulants, phencyclidine, marijuana, and hallucinogens are frequent offenders, especially when consumed by the intrapulmonary route. Recent experience with addicts smoking crack and "ice" (methamphetamine) includes increased emergency room visits for psychotic episodes and a dramatic increase in violence and homicide. Drug-induced psychosis usually remits once the acute intoxication state has resolves, although PCP psychosis can last days to weeks [28]. Psychotic symptoms may also be found in alcohol or sedative withdrawal [30,31], and detoxification should be completed before a final diagnosis is made.

Certain medical complications of addiction may also produce psychosis. Temporal lobe epilepsy (TLE) can generate psychotic symptoms [32] and may manifest when the seizure threshold is diminished by alcohol and sedative withdrawal or stimulant intoxication. Epilepsy may also be theoretically produced by stimulants through the process of kindling [33]. Temporal lobe epilepsy is best evaluated by electroencephalograph (EEG) utilizing the sleep-deprived EEG with nasopharangeal leads or 24-h EEG telemetry. Addicts may also have an increased incidence of seizures due to head trauma during intoxication.

Drug addicts are often at increased risk of exposure to the AIDS, which can reportedly lead to psychosis and dementia [34]. Viral antibodies in the plasma or cerebral spinal fluid can be measured when viral encephalography is suspected and HIV testing, as mentioned, is often an essential part of the addict's evaluation. Neuropsychological testing may also be useful when brain dysfunction is suspected. Given the vast number of medical causes for psychosis in drug addicts, it stands to reason that psychotic symptoms be observed for spontaneous remission before the institution of neuroleptics.

The persistence of psychotic symptoms beyond 3 days of drug abstinence is rarely attributable to intoxication (except with PCP) and is much more typical of schizophrenia, mania, or other psychiatric and medical causes of psychosis. In these cases, the clinician should inquire about past psychotic episodes during periods of drug abstinence and family history of psychosis in order to assess a possible psychiatric etiology.

Schizophrenia is not usually difficult to diagnose in drug addicts unless seen as the first break. More typically, there is an extensive and obvious history of chronic psychosis with multiple hospitalizations and numerous neuroleptic trials. Schizophrenic patients with a drug addiction are extremely difficult to treat with present societal resources. They usually have great difficulty interacting in self-help groups that demand intact social skills, and may even decompensate with standard rehabilitative approaches. Once decompensated, their vulnerability to craving is diminished and recidivism to drug addiction is almost inevitable. Similarly, in the face of drug addiction, neuroleptics are either discontinued or ineffective. A structured, psychiatrically oriented residential treatment for these patients is often necessary but seldom available. State psychiatric institutes seldom address addiction adequately, even though drug and alcohol addiction is rampant in these facilities. Outpatient resources are even more limited owing to poor funding and extensive supervision requirements of these patients.

VII. TREATMENT OF ADDICTION

The purpose of inpatient treatment is to provide a safe period of abstinence while medical and psychiatric conditions are stabilized and rehabilitative therapies are begun. Effective inpatient care should pave the way for self-help group involvement, which is ultimately the mainstay of recovery. It is the responsibility of the staff to provide guidance to establish a caring and motivated peer group on the inpatient unit that functions as a therapeutic community. Cynical, oppositional, and subversive patients should be confronted aggressively by staff and peers. Negative attitudes are important to confront because they adversely affect the therapeutic community and nearly always precede relapse in outpatients. For this reason, patients should be accountable to their peers and the staff for their attitudes as well as their behavior. They are expected to be honest and open minded, to attend and participate in meetings, and to follow rules and assist each other through caring support and confrontation. In particular, patients must cease their active resistance to treatment, and "give up control" of their treatment plan. This involves receptiveness to feedback and a willingness to follow suggestions and adhere entirely to aftercare recommendations. Inpatient treatment should focus primarily on group meetings that espouse the AA and NA philosophy and prepare the addict for outpatient recovery meetings.

Individual therapy is an important adjunct in inpatient rehabilitation, but it must facilitate self-help group work and be consistent with the AA/NA philosophy. Individual therapists should be knowledgeable of this philosophy and avoid undermining rehabilitation or confusing the patient. For instance, it is not as important why the addict uses drugs or alcohol as it is how he or she will cease use the substances. Furthermore, the major "reasons" why addicts use drugs are the reinforcers of craving and euphoria. The therapist should understand and convey that the resolution of psychological conflict is important, but is neither sufficient therapy for addiction nor the major task of inpatient hospitalization. The essential task at hand is rather to end the cycle of addiction and establish a commitment to outpatient rehabilitation. In patients with coexisting psychiatric disorders, the therapist should explore the address resistance to psychiatric treatment. Psychotherapy is also useful in addressing the numerous lifestyle issues and adjustments that arise during early recovery.

Family therapy addresses pathological family dynamics that serve to perpetuate addiction or obstruct recovery. Pathological family patterns, also termed *enabling*, are always present to some extent in the families of drug addicts. Families learn to compensate for the addict's dysfunction as the insidious progression of addiction develops. This process is usually so gradual that it remains unnoticed and even overt manipulation is often unrecognized until pointed out in family treatment. For this reason, pathological family dynamics should be specifically identified and addressed. An initial meeting with the family identifies essential family patterns and engages significant family members in treatment. It is often useful to have family members rehearse and discuss how the addict's addiction has affected them personally. This procedure, similar to family interventions done prior to admission, can be extremely powerful. Families should learn to set limits with the patient and must communicate how they will respond to recidivism. Subsequent family or multiple family meetings serve to educate, improve communication, change pathological dynamics, and plan discharge living arrangements.

Education is a crucial component of rehabilitation and should be provided to patients and families with an emphasis on AA and NA principles and the disease concept of addiction. This view emphasizes the disease of addiction and avoids judgmental and moralistic outlooks. Addicts should understand that they have a disease and are responsible for treatment, but that they are not bad people. In fact, low self-esteem is usually an impediment to recovery. Certain dogmatic and directive principles should also be conveyed. Patients must completely abstain from their drug of choice *and* avoid all other addictive agents, including marijuana and alcohol. Addicted friends, places, or situations that stimulate drug urges should be actively avoided. Patients should understand that their inability to control drug use is a permanent vulnerability that does not resolve even after long periods of abstinence. Controlled or recreational drug use is every addict's fantasy, but should be recognized as a form of denial that leads directly to recidivism. Patients should be generally suspicious of their own motives and thoughts, since their desire for drugs will manifest covertly. Owing to the ever-present threat of relapse, addiction is best viewed as treatable but not curable, necessitating continued involvement in outpatient self-help groups and reliance on other individuals for direction.

Progress and attitude in treatment should be monitored daily on the inpatient unit to determine the treatment plan and establish a reasonable discharge date. The degree of motivation, honesty, and willingness to follow specific aftercare recommendations are useful indicators of progress and prognosis. Patients who are persistently resistant have a destructive impact on the inpatient unit and may not be ready to work in recovery. Once medically and psychiatrically stabilized, these patients should be evaluated for discharge if they continue to exert a negative influence on the peer group. Otherwise the therapeutic community will be less effective and the recidivism rate for other patients may increase. An individual's progress in treatment is best determined by the entire treatment team and peer feedback.

VIII. CONCLUSIONS

Hospitalization is indicated under certain circumstances to break the cycle of active addiction and provide a setting in which medical and psychiatric complications can be stabilized. Medical stabilization is the first objective of hospitalization and involves treating intoxication and withdrawal states as well as numerous complications of drug and alcohol addiction and the addiction lifestyle. Familiarity with the evaluation and treatment of medical and psychiatric complications of addiction is, therefore, crucial in the planning of any comprehensive inpatient treatment. Indeed, the presence of a psychiatric disorder interferes with rehabilitation and sometimes accounts for past treatment failures. It is also imperative that the principles of drug rehabilitation and the self-help group approach be integrated into the treatment plan from the moment of admission. The addict must eventually return to the outside world and his or her recovery is usually dependent on regular participation in outpatient AA and NA self-help groups. Inpatient rehabilitation should, therefore, prepare for this eventuality by exposing drug addicts and alcoholics to the principles of AA and NA and the power of self-help groups.

REFERENCES

1. Deneau, G.A., Yanagita, T., and Seevers, M.H. (1969). Self-administration of psychoactive substances by the monkey. *Psychopharmacologia, 16*:30–48.
2. Wise, R.A., and Bozarth, M.A. (1987). A psychomotor stimulant theory of addiction. *Psychol. Rev., 94*:469–492.
3. Dackis, C.A., Gold, M.S., and Estroff, T.W. (1989). Inpatient Treatment of Addiction, *Treatments of Psychiatric Disorders: A Task Force Report of the American Psychiatric Association*, Washington, D.C., APA Press, pp. 1359–1379.
4. Gay, G.R. (1982). Clinical management of acute and toxic cocaine poisoning. *Ann. Emerg. Med., 11*:562–572.
5. Goldfrank, L., and Bresnitz, E. (1978). Toxicologic emergencies: opioids. *Hosp. Physician, 10*:26.
6. Gold, M.S., and Dackis, C.A. (1986). Role of the laboratory in the evaluation of suspected drug abuse. *J. Clin. Psychiatry, 47*:17–23.
7. Smith, D.E., Landry, M.J., and Wesson, D.R. (1989). Barbiturate, sedative and hypnotic agents, *Treatments of Psychiatric Disorders: A Task Force Report of the American Psychiatric Association*, Washington, D.C., APA Press, pp. 1294–1308.
8. Jaffe, J.H., and Kleber, H.D. (1989). Opioids: General issues and detoxification, *Treatments of Psychiatric Disorders: A Task Force Report of the American Psychiatric Association*, Washington, D.C., APA Press, pp. 1294–1308.
9. Gold, M.S., and Dackis, C.A. (1984). New insights and treatments: Opiate withdrawal and cocaine addiction. *Clin. Therapeut., 7*(1):6–21.
10. Krugman, S. (1982). The newly licensed hepatitis B vaccine. *J.A.M.A., 247*:2012–2015.
11. Justice, A.C., Feinstein, A.R., and Wells, C.K. (1989). A new prognostic staging system for the acquired immunodeficiency syndrome. *N. Engl. J. Med., 320*:1388–1392.
12. Gutman, R.A., Striker, G.E., and Gilliland, B.C. (1972). The immune complex glomerulonephritis of bacterial endocarditis. *Medicine, 51*:1–23.
13. Wetli, C.V., and Wright, R.K. (1979). Death caused by recreational cocaine use. *J.A.M.A., 241*:2519–2522.
14. Shukla, D. (1982). Intracranial hemorrhage associated with amphetamine use. *Neurology, 32*:917–918.
15. Dackis, C.A., Gold, M.S., Estroff, T.W., et al. (1984). Hyperprolactinemia in cocaine abuse. *Soc. Neurosci. Abst., 10*:1099.
16. Cocoras, J.A., Dackis, C.A., and Gold, M.S. (1986). Sexual dysfunction secondary to cocaine abuse in two patients. *J. Clin. Psychiatry, 47*:384–385.
17. Kolodny, R.C., Masers, W.H., Kolodner, R.M., et al. (1974). Depression of plasma testosterone levels after chronic intensive marijuana use. *N. Engl. J. Med., 290*:872–874.
18. Annitto, W.A. and Dackis, C.A. (1990). Use of benzodiazepines by alcoholics. (letter) *Am. J. Psychiatry, 147*:128–129.
19. Dackis, C.A., and Gold, M.S. (1984). Depression in opiate addicts, *Substance Abuse and Psychopathology* (S.M. Mirin, ed.). Washington, D.C., APA Press, pp. 19–40.
20. Dackis, C.A., Pottash, A.L.C., Gold, M.S., and Sweeney, D.R. (1986). Evaluating depression in alcoholics. *Psychiatry Res., 17*:105–109.
21. Dackis, C.A., Bailey, J., Pottash, A.L.C., Stuckey, R.F., Extein, I.L., and Gold, M.S. (1984). Specificity of the DST and TRH test for major depression in alcoholics. *Am. J. Psychiatry, 141*:680–682.
22. Dackis, C.A., Pottash, A.L.C., Gold, M.S., et al. (1984). The dexamethasone suppression test for major depression in opiate addicts. *Am. J. Psychiatry, 141*:810–811.
23. Dackis, C.A., Estroff, T.W., Sweeney, D.R., Pottash, A.L.C., and Gold, M.S. (1985). Specificity of the TRH test for major depression in patients with severe cocaine abuse. *Am. J. Psychiatry, 142*:1097–1099.
24. Rounsaville, B.J., Weissman, M.M., Crits-Christoph, K., et al. (1982). Diagnosis and symptoms of depression in opiate addicts. *Arch. Gen. Psychiatry, 39*:151–156.
25. Byck, R. (1974). *Cocaine Papers: Sigmund Freud*. New York, Stonehill, p. 64.

26. Post, R.M., Kotin, J., and Goodwin, F.R. (1974). The effects of cocaine of depressed patients. *Am. J. Psychiatry, 131*:511–517.

27. Siegel, R.K. (1978). Cocaine hallucinations. *Am. J. Psychiatry, 135*:309–314.

28. Allen, R.M., and Young, S.J. (1978). Phencyclidine-induced psychosis. *Am. J. Psychiatry, 135*(9):1081–1083.

29. Hollister, L.E. (1984). Effects of hallucinogens in humans, *Hallucinogens: Neurochemical, Behavioral, and Clinical Prespectives* (B.L. Jacobs, ed.). New York, Raven Press, pp. 19–34.

30. MacKinnon, G.L., and Parker, W.A. (1982). Benzodiazepine withdrawal syndrome: A literature review and evaluation. *Am. J. Drug Alcohol Abuse, 9*:19–33.

31. Schopf, J. (1983). Withdrawal phenomena after long-term administration of benzodiazepines. A review of recent investigations. *J. Pharmacopsychol., 16*:1–8.

32. Rivinus, T.M. (1982). Psychiatric effects of anticonvulsants regimens. *J. Clin. Psychopharmacol., 2*(3):165–192.

33. Post, R.M., Kopanda, R.T., and Black, K.E. (1976). Progressive effects of cocaine on behavior and central amine metabolism in the rhesus monkey: relationship to kindling and psychosis. *Biol. Psychiatry., 11*:403–419.

34. Faulstich, M.E. (1987). Psychiatric aspects of AIDS. *Am. J. Psychiatry, 144*:551–556.

68

Hospital Treatment of Eating Disorders with Drug and Alcohol Addiction

Lynne Hoffman and Katherine Halmi
Cornell University Medical College, The New York Hospital–Cornell Medical Center, White Plains, New York

I. INTRODUCTION

Over the past few years, a significant body of data has accumulated suggesting a link between eating disorders and addictive disorders. This link was originally suggested by the observation that certain behaviors characteristic of people with eating disorders are similar to those seen in drug addicts and other dependent states. These behaviors include "loss of control" over the substance, preoccupation with the substance, use of the substance to cope with stress or negative feelings, a tendency to keep the behavior secretive and the continuation of the behavior in the face of negative social and occupational consequences (summarized by Hatsukami et al. 1982; Szmukler and Tantam, 1984). Other theoretical considerations also suggest that the two illnesses are connected. Jonas and Gold (1987) treated eight bulimics with the long-acting opioid antagonist naltrexone and noted highly significant reductions in the number of binge-free days, purge-free days, and duration of binging. They proposed that in bulimia an individual's binge eating may be maintained by an autoaddiction to endogenous opioids. They further suggest that "multiple addictions may arise because behavioral and psychological factors which occur as the result of one addiction increase the chance that another addiction develops, or because an innate addictive diathesis predisposes individuals to become addicted to one or more substances, either endogenous or exogenous." Brisnan and Siegel (1984) reviewed the literature on the psychodynamics of drug addiction and bulimia. They suggest that both illnesses result from developmental deficits in ego structure, and that both drugs and bulimic eating patterns serve as pathological attempts to minimize the impact of ego deficits and compensate for one's sense of incompleteness. At this time, the evidence substantiating the relationship between these disorders falls into three categories.

1. Several studies to date have shown that the eating-disordered population has a higher incidence of drug or alcohol addiction than the population at large. In a controlled study using DSM-III (*Diagnostic and Statistical Manual of Mental Disorders*, 3rd ed. American Psychiatric Association, 1980) diagnostic criteria, Hudson et al. (1987) found their bulimic

population had a lifetime prevalence of drug or alcohol addiction of 49%, compared to 21% of depressed controls and 11% of nonpsychiatric controls. Similarly, Mitchell et al. (1985) reported that 34.4% of 275 bulimics met DSM-III criteria for a history of drug or alcohol addiction. Several other studies substantiate a higher incidence of drug addiction in individuals with eating disorders, both anorexia and bulimia, with the coincidence rate of these disorders running between 18 and 50% (Beary et al., 1986; Hatsukami et al., 1984; Pyle et al., 1983). Other studies using the opposite approach started with a population of drug addicts and found their prevalence of eating disorders to be greatly increased compared to the general population. Jonas and Gold (1986) and Jonas et al. (1987) administered a structured telephone interview to 259 callers to the National Cocaine Hotline who met DSM-III criteria for cocaine abuse. They found that 32% of this population met DSM-III criteria for either anorexia nervosa, bulimia nervosa, or both. Lacey and Mourelli (1986) interviewed 27 alcoholic women, and found that 40% of them gave a history consistent with a past or present diagnosis of bulimia. Similarly, Beary et al. (1986) reported that 30% of alcoholic women in an inpatient drug rehabilitation program met criteria for bulimia or anorexia.

2. A number of studies have examined the family histories of individuals with eating disorders, and found an increased incidence of drug and alcohol dependence in the first-degree relatives of individuals with bulimia and anorexia. Bulik (1987a, 1987b) administered a battery of structured interviews to 35 bulimics, and found that the most frequently occurring psychopathology in at least one of their first-degree relatives was alcoholism (48.6%), and that that relationship held true even when the bulimic subject had no drug addiction. Pyle et al. (1983) reported that 50% of their bulimic population indicated alcoholism in at least one first-degree relative, and that 21% reported that their fathers were alcoholic. Claydon (1987) identified a group of college students who were children of alcoholics, and found that they were more than twice as likely to report an eating disorder as controls; this was particularly evident in the male subjects. Many other studies substantiate an increase in drug and alcohol addiction in the families of those with eating disorders (Beary et al., 1986; Halmi and Loney, 1973).

3. Some investigators have tried to link drug and alcohol addicts to those with eating disorders on the basis of their psychological profiles. Although the results of these studies are less clear-cut, they suggest some interesting parallels between the two groups, and raise many questions for future research. Hatsukami et al. (1982) compared the Minnesota Multiphasic Personality Inventory (MMPI) scores of 52 bulimics with those of 120 females in treatment for drug or alcohol abuse. Although there were differences between the two groups within subscales, they found similar mean MMPI profiles and a similar distribution of MMPI codetypes. Filstead et al. (1988) studied inpatients undergoing concurrent treatment for both drug addiction and an eating disorder, who met DSM-III criteria for both types of illness. Using self-reports they found some similarities in the intensity of specific high-risk situations as represented by questionnaire subscale scores for both of the problem behaviors. Again, there were also important differences in the risk situations for these two illnesses, and the interpretation of the data is further complicated by the lack of comparison data between individuals with either an eating disorder or a drug addiction, but not both. Jansen et al. (1989) found that "restrained eaters," like addicts, scored high on a standard sensation-seeking scale, and habituated faster to neutral stimuli than did controls. They hypothesized that rapid habituation may result in sensation-seeking behavior which is manifested as excessive consumption of either food or drugs, and that the restrictive behavior represents an attempt to effect some control over these impulses. While these data are provocative and suggest a neurophysiological link between eating disorders and alcoholism, they also need to be interpreted with considerable caution. The subjects were a subclinical population who did not meet DSM-III criteria for any eating disorder, but rather scored

high on a restraint scale which consisted of 10 items measuring attitudes toward eating, frequency of dieting, and weight fluctuations, and thus may not necessarily reflect the true eating-disordered population.

The remainder of this chapter will be devoted to a description of a behaviorally oriented inpatient program for the treatment of eating disorders, and a comparison of it to traditional 12-Step programs. It has been noted previously that the usual treatment strategies for eating disorders and drug addiction share many commonalities, including the need for education about the health consequences of the disorder, a combination of behavioral, dynamic, and cognitive approaches, the nature of the recovery process as central to treatment, the importance of family involvement, and the role of hospitalization as an intensive experience that optimally serves as a powerful first step in a long-term recovery process (reviewed by Zweben, 1987). Owing to the many similarities between the eating-disordered and drug-addicted populations, and their degree of symptom overlap, it is reasonable to expect that strategies useful in treating one group may be effective when applied to the other.

II. EATING DISORDER PROGRAM

The eating disorder program treats both anorectics and bulimics. Although the overall orientation of the ward is strongly behavioral, we have a multidimensional approach to treatment which utilizes a variety of therapeutic modalities and strategies.

A. Initial Phase

Evaluation

The initial evaluation is the same for all patients. It includes a full medical and psychiatric history and family evaluation. Laboratory data are collected on all patients within 24 h of admission, and the following tests are routinely run: electrolytes, BUN, Cr, FBS, thyroid and liver function tests, vitamin B_{12} and folate, cholesterol, amylase, CBC with differential, urine analysis, and EKG. Every week during their hospital stay patients have their electrolytes, CBC, and amylase measured. Within 48 h of admission patients are assigned a target weight and a 5-lb acceptable weight range. Depending on how far they are from their target weight, they may not be informed of their goal immediately.

Feeding and Weight Gain

Anorectics more than 5 lb from their target weight are placed on six equal feedings of Sustacal/day and continue on this liquid diet until they reach their goal. The amount of Sustacal initially used is determined using the Mayo normogram, and is calculated as the number of calories required to maintain their weight, plus 50% for weight gain. The quantity of Sustacal is increased as required to maintain a weight gain of 3–4 lb/week. If the Sustacal is refused, a nasogastric tube is inserted daily and the patient fed in that manner (even highly resistant patients are rarely able to tolerate the discomfort and perceived embarrassment of a nasogastric tube for more than a few days). Normal-weight bulimics are initially fed from prearranged trays for the first part of their hospital stay, with no control over their food selection. The purpose of the trays is to help individuals visualize three appropriately sized meals/day, and initiate the development of normal eating behavior. Access to food is restricted to mealtimes and supervised snacks.

During this period and for some time later, purging behavior is controlled with a response prevention technique. All patients, regardless of their progress in the program, remain in a day room under staff supervision for 1 h after each meal. Patients are initially restricted to commodes in their bedrooms which they may only use at specified times of the day, inputs and outputs are closely monitored and measured, and showers are supervised. These measures generally successfully inhibit most patients from vomiting. Additionally, amylase levels are measured each week, since hyperamylasemia is a fairly reliable marker for ongoing vomiting in the absence of other pathology. Stool examinations are necessary to monitor for ongoing laxative abuse. Weights are measured every morning after voiding and before the first meal. Initially weight gain, and not eating behavior, is the reinforced variable until patients show they are able to maintain a normal weight.

Activities

During the initial phase of the hospitalization patients' activities are highly limited. Anorectics remain on the unit until they reach target weight except for the adolescents, who are allowed off to attend the hospital school. Bulimics remain on the unit for a minimum of 3 weeks. During this period both telephone calls and visits are limited. The goal is to help patients begin thinking about their behavior and problems and start to develop a sense of discipline and control.

Therapy

Although progress through the hospital program is based on a behavioral model, a variety of therapeutic techniques are employed from the outset of hospitalization. All patients receive individual psychotherapy which is insight-oriented when appropriate. Cognitive therapy, aimed at getting patients to challenge and re-evaluate their distorted beliefs and body perceptions, is commonly used (for a review of the use of this approach with this population, see Garner and Bemis, 1984). All patients attend at least three different groups/week. These include an adult or adolescent group in which age-appropriate interpersonal issues are the focus, a discharge group which looks at aftercare planning and concerns, and an eating disorders group which examines ongoing difficulties with food, eating behavior, and body perception. Family counseling is considered an essential component of the hospital program and commences immediately after admission. Since many of our patients are unemployed, or pursuing a career that is not suitable or feasible for them, they generally receive a complete vocational assessment during their hospital stay. Finally, milieu therapy and peer interactions are central to the treatment program and are fostered through community meetings and patient government.

B. Second Phase

Meals

During the second phase patients gradually gain control over their food intake. Once they reach their target weight, anorectics (like bulimics) spend 3–4 weeks eating from prearranged trays. The daily calories are calculated to be enough to maintain their new weight plus 30% for activity. Patients then begin to choose their own foods, one meal each week. Once they are choosing all their own foods and successfully maintaining their weight, they gradually progress to situations in which they eat off the unit with their families, alone, and in a variety of social situations. On any day that the patient's weight falls below range he or she is restricted to the unit. If this occurs frequently, the patient may be placed back on trays, or even Sustacal if necessary. All such decisions are made at a weekly team meeting (which includes representation by the therapeutic staff, nursing and social work), and are always presented as a team decision. This strategy minimizes struggles between patients and individual staff members. At this point, progress on the unit becomes contingent on appropriate eating behavior as well as weight maintenance.

Privileges and Activities

As the patients slowly gain control and mastery over eating situations, they also acquire privileges and responsibilities in other spheres. These include increased telephone calls and visitation rights, free use of the bathroom and showers, more passes off the hospital grounds, and increased status within the hospital system. Again, these decisions are all made in the setting of the team meeting.

Discharge Planning

Aftercare arrangements are tailored to fit the needs of the individual, and designed to provide an optimum setting for maintaining and building on the progress made in the hospital. It is often recommended that patients not return to their former living situation because of conflicts that existed there. In such cases, a supervised living situation such as a halfway house can provide an effective transition to independent living. For adolescents, a residential treatment facility will often serve the same purpose. Adult patients often benefit from a period of day hospitalization after discharge, especially for those whose employment histories had been erratic, or who were in unsuitable jobs. This approach helps patients structure their lives outside the hospital, provides them with support, and prevents them from being immediately overwhelmed following discharge. Continued psychotherapy is essential for all patients. It provides them with an opportunity to continue the gains made in self understanding that began in the hospital, and also serves as another source of support following discharge. Additionally, many patients benefit from either group or family therapy.

C. The Drug-Addicted and Eating-Disordered Population

There are no specific changes in this protocol for patients who enter with a drug or alcohol addiction. Initially they are encouraged to focus only on their eating disorder. If a detoxification is necessary it is provided, although we strongly prefer this to occur on a specialized unit prior to admission to our ward. Patients have no access to their drug of choice; thus abstinence is enforced. Once their status is increased, addicted patients are encouraged to attend Alcoholics Anonymous (AA) meetings within the hospital. When they start to go out on passes, urine samples are randomly sent for drug screens and their progress in the program then becomes contingent on continued abstinence as well as weight maintenance and appropriate eating behavior. Many of these patients do go on to drug and alcohol rehabilitation programs after discharge from our unit. However, a certain subgroup feel that the sense of discipline and control they attain from completing the eating disorder protocol, combined with the fairly lengthy period of abstinence from drug use that our hospitalization entails (average length of stay on our unit is 4 months), and their introduction to AA through the hospital, may substitute for a formal drug rehabilitation program. At this time, we do not have any data comparing these two groups with respect to their long-term outcome.

III. COMPARISON TO 12-STEP PROGRAMS

Below are listed the traditional 12 Steps which form the cornerstone of Alcoholics Anonymous and the basis for most inpatient drug rehabilitation programs.

1. We admitted we were powerless over alcohol and that our lives had become unmanageable.
2. We came to believe that a power greater than ourselves could restore us to sanity.
3. We made a decision to turn our will and our lives over to the care of God as we understood him.

4. We made a searching and fearless moral inventory of ourselves.

5. We admitted to God, to ourselves and to another human being the exact nature of our wrongs.

6. We were entirely ready to have God remove all these defects of character.

7. We humbly asked him to remove our shortcomings.

8. We made a list of all persons we have harmed and became willing to make amends to them all.

9. We made direct amends to such people whenever possible, except when to do so would injure them or others.

10. We continued to take personal inventory and when we were wrong, promptly admitted it.

11. We sought through prayer and meditation to improve our conscious contact with God as we understood him, praying only for knowledge of his will for us and the power to carry that out.

12. Having had a spiritual awakening as a result of these steps we tried to carry the message to alcoholics to practice these principles in all our affairs. (Alcoholics Anonymous, 1955)

The eating disorders unit does not explicitly utilize a 12-Step program as part of its inpatient protocol. However, philosophically and in practice there is considerable overlap in goals, which are outlined below, as well as the important differences.

The major distinction between the eating disorders protocol and traditional 12-Step programs is the absence of a requirement for any formal recognition of, or reliance on, a higher power. We do, however, strongly encourage our patients to draw support from the therapy staff, stable relatives, and friends. We also encourage them to put their trust in the program and the process of change they are undergoing. These concepts are similar to the broad interpretations applied to the idea of a higher power in traditional 12-Step programs.

The first of the 12 Steps is also one of the cornerstones of the eating disorders program. It is often very difficult for our patients to acknowledge that their illness, either bulimia or anorexia, is no longer under their control, but rather is controlling their lives. They deny the impact of the illness on their interpersonal relationships, vocational achievements, and general level of functioning. Cutting through this denial is essential for the individual to succeed. Admitting that they are out of control is the first step in regaining control of their lives.

As outlined earlier in this chapter, our program works by the slow acquisition of rights and privileges as one demonstrates the ability and willingness to control their eating and behave responsibly. This sense of personal responsibility and growth (which echoes the language of Steps 4, 5, 8, 9, and 10) is considered crucial to success in the program. It is recognized that this process only begins during the hospital stay and must continue in psychotherapy afterwards. Within our treatment setting this sense of responsibility is fostered by a confrontational approach to group and individual therapy, and during family sessions, all of which force the patients to examine the impact of their behaviors on the other people in their lives as well as themselves.

Thus, although the eating disorders program does not formally incorporate a 12-Step program into its structure, the goals are often comparable. This is particularly evident in the need to cut through the patient's denial of the effects of their illness, and to foster a sense of personal responsibility.

IV. CONCLUSIONS

Clinicians are advised to approach eating-disordered patients with a high degree of suspicion for the coexistence of drug addictions, and to appreciate that the risk for developing an addictive disorder increases when the bulimic or anorectic behavior is brought under control.

Inpatient treatment of the eating-disordered individual utilizes a multidimensional approach in the setting of a behaviorally oriented ward milieu. This includes cognitive and insight-oriented psychotherapies (both individual and group), appropriate medical management of these disorders, and family counseling throughout the hospital stay. Whenever possible, drug and alcohol detoxification should occur first on a specialized unit, followed by transfer to the eating disorders unit. The aftercare program varies according to the needs of the individual, and may include a drug rehabilitation program, a supervised living situation together with a day hospital program, or a residential treatment facility for the adolescent patient. Ongoing psychotherapy, individual and/or group, is considered essential in achieving a long-term remission of the eating disorder. It is hoped that as the nature of the link between eating disorders and drug addictions is clarified, treatment strategies appropriate for both these illnesses will become increasingly available.

REFERENCES

Alcoholics Anonymous. 2nd ed. New York, Alcoholics Anonymous Publishing Company, 1955, pp. 59.

Beary, M.D., Lacey, J.H., and Merry, J. Alcoholism and eating disorders in women of fertile age. *Br. J. Addict., 81*:685–689 (1986).

Brisnan, J., and Siegel, M. Bulimia and alcoholism: Two sides of the same coin? *J. Subst. Abuse Treat., 1*:113–118 (1984).

Bulik, C.M. Alcohol use and depression in women with bulimia. *Am. J. Drug Alcohol Abuse, 13*(3):343–355 (1987a).

Bulik, C.M. Drug and alcohol abuse by bulimic women and their families. *Am. J. Psychiatry, 144*(12):1604–1606 (1987b).

Claydon, P. Self-reported alcohol, drug, and eating-disorder problems among male and female collegiate children of alcoholics. *J. Am. Coll. Health, 36*:111–116 (1987).

Filstead, W.J., Parrella, D.P., and Ebbitt, J. High risk situations for engaging in substance abuse and binge-eating behaviors. *J. Stud. Alcohol, 49*(2):136–141 (1988).

Garner, D.M., and Bemis, K.M. Cognitive therapy for anorexia nervosa, *Handbook of Psychotherapy for Anorexia Nervosa and Bulimia* (D.M. Garner and P.E. Garfinkel, eds.). New York, Guilford Press, 1984, pp. 107–146.

Halmi, K.A., and Loney, J., Family alcoholism in anorexia nervosa. *Br. J. Psychiatry, 123*:53–54 (1973).

Hatsukami, D., Owen, P., Pyle, R., and Mitchell, J. Similarities and differences on the MMPI between women with bulimia and women with alcohol or drug abuse problems. *Addict. Behav., 7*(4):435–439 (1982).

Hatsukami, D., Eckert, E., Mitchell, J.E., and Pyle, R., Affective disorder and substance abuse in women with bulimia. *Psychol. Med., 14*:701–704 (1984).

Hudson, J.I., Pope, H.G., Yurgelun-Todd, D., Jonas, J.M., and Frankenburg, F.R. A controlled study of lifetime prevalence of affective disorder and other psychiatric disorders in bulimic outpatients. *Am. J. Psychiatry, 144*:1283–1287 (1987).

Jansen, A., Klaver, J., Merckelbach, H., and van den Hout, M. Restrained eaters are rapidly habituating sensation seekers. *Behav. Res. Ther., 27*(3):247–252 (1989).

Jonas, J.M., and Gold, M.S. Cocaine abuse and eating disorders. *Lancet, 1*:390–391 (1986).

Jonas, J.M., and Gold, M.S. Naltrexone treatment of bulimia: Clinical and theoretical findings linking eating disorders and substance abuse. *Adv. Alcohol Subst. Abuse, 7*(1):29–37 (1987).

Jonas, J.M., Gold, M.S., Sweeney, D., and Pottash, A.L.C. Eating disorders and cocaine abuse: A survey of 259 cocaine abusers. *J. Clin. Psychiatry, 48*(2):47–50 (1987).

Lacey, J.H., and Mourelli, E. Bulimic alcoholics: Some features of a clinical subgroup. *Br. J. Addict., 81*:389–393 (1986).

Mitchell, J.E., Hatsukami, D., Eckert, E.D., and Pyle, R.L. Characteristics of 275 patients with bulimia. *Am. J. Psychiatry, 142*:482–485 (1985).

Pyle, R.L., Mitchell, J.E., and Eckert, E.D. Bulimia: A report of 34 cases. *J. Clin. Psychiatry, 42*:60–64 (1983).

Szmukler, G.I., and Tantam, D. Anorexia nervosa: Starvation dependence. *Br. J. Med. Psychol., 57*:303–310 (1984).

Zweben, J.E. Eating disorders and substance abuse. *J. Psychoactive Drugs, 19*(2):181–192 (1987).

XXII
Long-Term Treatment

69

12-Step Programs in Recovery from Drug and Alcohol Addiction

Jerome E. Schulz
University of California, San Francisco, California

I. INTRODUCTION

This chapter will discuss several support groups available to help people recover from the disease of drug and alcohol addiction. There are millions of people worldwide who are living fuller and more complete lives because of their involvement in support groups. The prototpye of these groups, and the one with the longest history, is Alcoholics Anonymous (AA), which was started in 1935. The discussion of support groups will emphasize AA and its 12 Steps of Recovery. Several other programs, including Al-Anon, Alateen, Narcotics Anonymous, and Adult Children of Alcoholics, will also be described. Only support groups with a 12-Step philosophy will be discussed.

Support groups can help people in several ways [1,2]. First, support groups can break the feeling of uniqueness and isolation which people with drug and alcohol addiction and others close to them often experience. When patients go to a support group, they frequently report they do not feel so alone for the first time in their lives; finally someone else understands what they have been feeling for so many years. Thus, the "terminal uniqueness" and isolation is broken down. Another major benefit of support groups is to educate patients about the disease of drug and alcohol addiction. By hearing other people share what they have experienced and learned in their recovery, patients can gain insight into their own problems and potential solutions to those problems. Next, support groups can benefit patients by showing them there is hope for recovery. By going to meetings and associating with people in recovery, they can see that recovery has been possible for others no matter how bad the situation. They also see that recovery can be a wonderful positive joyful experience. Support groups can also help teach the person basic socialization skills. Many alcoholics and drug addicts become isolated and self-focused. The association with recovery groups helps the patient relearn (or sometimes learn for the first time) basic group and socialization skills. The support groups understand this need and give newcomers unconditional loving support as they struggle in early recovery. Another major way that support groups help is in providing a reality base for patients in recovery. When people think they are unique and begin to isolate themselves, they have no source of feedback on what they are doing and the potential consequences of their behavior. The "anatomy of a slip" (drinking again for the alcoholic) can be described in the following way [3].

Stinking Thinking → Isolation → Slip

In AA terms, "stinking thinking" is the result of many years of faulty reasoning and thinking. Stinking thinking is accepted (in 12-Step support groups) as being very common in both active and recovering alcoholics and drug addicts. If people isolate themselves, the stinking thinking becomes their only reality base. The next step is to start thinking the drug or alcohol problem is not that great and one drink will not hurt. This can lead to a slip or using chemicals again. The support group plays an integral role in stopping this pattern before the slip occurs. The group can caringly point out errors in the newcomer's (and frequently the oldtimer's as well) thinking and behavior in a way that is nonjudgmental and caring and able to be heard by members. Support groups can also help when people experience setbacks which are inevitable in recovery. The members of the group can share how they have dealt with similar problems in their recovery without going back to using drugs or alcohol. A final positive aspect of support groups is to help people fill the time which is freed up in recovery when they stop drinking and using drugs. This can be a major problem for people in early recovery who have spent most of their time in the past drinking or using drugs. The simple act of going to a meeting provides a positive way for people to constructively use the excess time.

II. ALCOHOLICS ANONYMOUS

A. History

Alcoholics Anonymous was started in 1935 by a stockbroker ("Bill W.") and a physician ("Dr. Bob"). Bill Wilson was an alcoholic who had sobered up in early 1935. He had become involved with a religious group called the Oxford Movement, and through this movement he had been able to achieve a brief period of sobriety. While on a business trip to Akron, Ohio, Bill W. once again had failed in a business venture. His thoughts turned to drinking to relieve his pain. In an attempt to overcome the urge to drink, he contacted a local member of the Oxford Movement and asked for the name of an alcoholic in the area who might need help. He was given the name of Dr. Bob, and he arranged a "brief" meeting that was to last only 15 min. That meeting lasted several hours and marked the beginning of Alcoholics Anonymous. The two continued to meet for the next few days, and Bill actually stayed in Akron for several months. During this time, he and Dr. Bob tried to reach out to other alcoholics, and they began to formulate the basic philosophy of Alcoholics Anonymous. Thus, one of the basic principles of AA was established—one alcoholic reaching out to another alcoholic could help himself or herself stay sober.

The initial growth of AA was slow and painful for Bill W. and Dr. Bob. Although they had many ideas about how to start the organization and to foster AA's growth, for many years very few people were exposed to AA's concepts. Although in the early years the AA program was closely tied to the Oxford Movement, its founders came to feel that this association restricted the effectiveness of AA. In response, they wrote *Alcoholics Anonymous* (the Big Book) [4]. In writing this book they broke off from the Oxford Movement and established AA for alcoholics only. Growth continued slowly until the *Saturday Evening Post* published an article [5] by Jack Alexander in 1941. Because of the popularity and widespread circulation of this magazine, millions were exposed to AA for the first time. Many newspapers and magazines all over the country picked up this article and disseminated the information about AA. Within a very short time, the number of people in AA rose dramatically and AA was on its way.

B. Overview and Philosophy

Alcoholics Anonymous has helped millions of people afflicted with the disease of alcoholism achieve sobriety. The preamble of Alcoholics Anonymous [6], which is frequently read at the beginning of AA meetings, points out many of the important facts about AA and how AA works:

> *Alcoholics Anonymous is a fellowship of men and women who share their experience, strength and hope with each other that they may solve their common problem and help others to recover from alcoholism.
>
> The only requirement for membership is a desire to stop drinking. There are no dues or fees for AA membership; we are self-supporting through our own contributions.
>
> AA is not allied with any sect, denomination, politics, organizations or institution; does not wish to engage in any controversy; neither endorses nor opposes any causes.
>
> Our primary purpose is stay sober and help other alcoholics to achieve sobriety.

Alcoholics Anonymous is a spiritual program based on 12 Steps and 12 Traditions.

12 Steps †

1. We admitted we were powerless over alcohol—that our lives had become unmanageable.
2. Came to believe that a Power greater than ourselves could restore us to sanity.
3. Made a decision to turn our will and our lives over to the care of God as we understand Him.
4. Made a searching and fearless moral inventory of ourselves.
5. Admitted to God, to ourselves, and to another human being the exact nature of our wrongs.
6. Were entirely ready to have God remove all these defects of character.
7. Humbly asked Him to remove our shortcomings.
8. Made a list of all persons we had harmed, and became willing to make amends to them all.
9. Made direct amends to such people wherever possible, except when to do so would injure them or others.
10. Continued to take personal inventory and when we were wrong promptly admitted it.
11. Sought through prayer and meditation to improve our conscious contact with God as we understood Him praying only for knowledge of His will for us and the power to carry that out.
12. Having had a spiritual experience (awakening) as the result of these steps, we tried to carry this message to alcoholics, and to practice these principles in all our affairs.

The 12 Steps are the principal basis of AA and the backbone of recovery for AA members. It is important to point out that AA is a spiritual program and not religious. As the preamble states, AA "is not allied with any sect or denomination." One of the problems patients may have with AA is that they feel it is a religious organization. AA literature points out that "God" is not used in a religious sense and is not connected to any religious belief. The concept is one of a higher power that is a source of strength to the alcoholic. The higher power can be the AA group that the person attends or any other higher power outside of themselves.

---

*Reprinted by permission of Grapevine.
†Reprinted by permission of Alcoholics Anonymous World Services, Inc.

There are many atheists and agnostics in AA, and this can be helpful to tell patients who are reluctant to go to AA because of their discomfort with God. The Big Book has an entire chapter titled "We agnostics" to help people overcome this obstacle.

The 12 Steps have been applied effectively to many other problems in life such as gambling, sex, and emotional and eating disorders. They offer the alcoholic a simple (but not necessarily easy) way to change his or her life so that alcohol is no longer an obsession or requirement to survive. The 12 Steps require a willingness to look at onself and change the things that prevent one from being a healthy caring human being who can live harmoniously with others.

12 Traditions*

1. Our common welfare should come first; personal recovery depends on AA unity.
2. For our group purpose there is but one ultimate authority—a loving God as He may express Himself in our group conscience. Our leaders are but trusted servants; they do not govern.
3. The only requirement for AA membership is a desire to stop drinking.
4. Each group should be autonomous except in matters affecting other groups or AA as a whole.
5. Each group has but one primary purpose—to carry its message to the alcoholic who still suffers.
6. An AA group ought never endorse, finance, or lend the AA name to any related facility or outside enterprise, lest problems of money, property and prestige divert us from our primary purpose.
7. Every AA group ought to be fully self-supporting, declining outside contributions.
8. Alcoholics Anonymous should remain forever nonprofessional, but our service centers may employ special workers.
9. AA, as such, ought never be organized; but we may create service boards or committees directly responsible to those they serve.
10. Alcoholics Anonymous has no opinion on outside issues; hence, the AA name ought never be drawn into public controversy.
11. Our public relations policy is based on attraction rather than promotion; we need always maintain personal anonymity at the level of press, radio, and films.
12. Anonymity is the spiritual foundation of all our traditions, ever reminding us to place principles before personalities.

The 12 Traditions are the guidelines that help Alcoholics Anonymous function smoothly. There are more than 73,000 AA groups with more than 1.5 million members [7] worldwide guided by the 12 Traditions. Yet no one individual or group is in charge. The General Service Office (GSO) in New York works as a clearinghouse for AA information and publications. It is under the direction of the General Service Board, which is made up of both alcoholics and nonalcoholics. Neither the Office or the Board has any authority over AA members or groups. Both the Office and the Board are responsible to the AA groups and report annually to the General Services Conference. The Conference includes members selected by the groups in the United States and Canada. This large loosely structured leaderless system works because AA closely adheres to the 12 Traditions.

Membership in AA is very easy to obtain. Basically all a person has to do is show up at a meeting and according to the third tradition of AA "have a desire to stop drinking."

---

*Reprinted by permission of Alcoholics Anonymous World Services, Inc.

There is no formal sign up or application form. Many groups will have a phone list of the group members so individuals can phone each other for support and help between meetings. Being on the phone list is strictly optional.

C. Meetings

The two main types of AA meetings are open and closed. Anyone may attend an open meeting. Closed meetings are restricted to alcoholics only. AA meetings usually start with the Serenity Prayer (which will be described later) and each person then introduces himself or herself by saying, "Hi I'm ——— and I'm an alcoholic." Many groups have a brief business meeting which takes less than 10 min. At open meetings, a speaker usually gives the classic AA talk about how it was, what happened, and how it is now. Speakers frequently talk for up to an hour, and almost never use notes or scripts. AA speakers feel this helps them "talk from the heart and not the head."

If asked, some closed groups will allow physicians and clergy who are not alcoholics to observe a closed meeting. They do this to help the professional better understand what happens at AA meetings. There are several different types of closed AA meetings. Some discuss one of the 12 Steps each week with one member sharing what the Step means to him or her. The group members then share what the Step means to them, or they can talk about anything that is of concern to them that week. Members can also choose to pass if they do not want to share anything. Frequently, people will be afraid to go to AA meetings because they do not want to talk or share. This is easily remedied in a meeting by simply saying, "I pass." Closed meetings can also be discussion meetings during which a specific topic is discussed such as resentments, fear, or anger. Some meetings will discuss the Big Book (*Alcoholics Anonymous*), which is the bible in AA. The Big Book was written in 1939 by Bill W. and the other founders of AA. It discusses the basic concepts and philosophy of AA, and includes a section in which the early members of AA tell their stories. An important part of the Big Book, which is often read at the beginning of AA meetings, is a portion of chapter 5, which is entitled "How It Works." The 12 Steps are presented in "How It Works." The 12 Steps are also discussed in *Twelve Steps and Twelve Traditions* [8] (the 12 by 12), which is another important book in AA. Some meetings will read about and discuss one of the Steps or Traditions from the 12 by 12 each week.

Generally, AA meetings last 1 h, and most meetings close with the Lord's Prayer. Frequently, after a meeting the members will continue to socialize (commonly by going for coffee). This gives the group a chance to continue to talk about the meeting topic or to just socialize. It is also gives the newcomer a chance to get to know the members on a more personal basis and to experience their humanness.

D. Types of Groups

As AA has grown, a wide variety of special groups have developed. The groups can be classified by the type of meeting they conduct, as described above, or they can be classified by who attends the meeting. It is very important to know this when working with patients who say they cannot find a meeting with anyone like themselves. In most larger metropolitan areas, there are special meetings for diverse groups. With one-third of AA's membership being women, women's groups have become very popular. There are also young peoples' meetings and senior citizens' meetings. In many areas, there are also AA meetings for gays and lesbians.

Nonsmoking AA meetings are also becoming very common. Many large groups will split into smaller groups, after the initial opening, for smokers and nonsmokers. There are also some groups that are totally nonsmoking. There are also special meetings for blacks and hispanics. In many areas, there are special meetings for professionals such as nurses, physicians, lawyers, and clergy.

D. Sponsorship

One of the basic concepts in Alcoholics Anonymous is sponsorship. When someone comes into AA, he or she is urged to get a sponsor. Often groups will appoint a temporary sponsor for newcomers. The purpose of a sponsor is to help the newcomer early in recovery and to be a personal contact who the person can call, especially when he or she is thinking about drinking or having problems (which is almost always for newcomers). The sponsor is someone of the same sex and who has been in AA for a longer period of time. Frequently, the person will talk with his or her sponsor between meetings and meet with them for breakfast, lunch, or dinner to talk about how things are going. The sponsor becomes a mentor and role model for the newcomer, and is an example of how the AA program works.

E. Anniversaries

There are several rituals in AA to support people who have reached various milestones in recovery. Many groups will give out "chips" to newcomers attending their first AA meeting (a red poker chip). This is to help them remember to stay sober one day at a time. The chip is to be put in the same pocket as the money for alcohol, so that whenever they are tempted to drink, they will see the chip and have a reminder of the need to stay sober for just that day. After they have been sober for 1 month, they turn in the red chip for a white chip, which is a celebration that they have been sober for that period of time. After 4 months of sobriety, they get a blue chip to signify their continuing sobriety and commitment to recovery.

Many groups give out medallions instead of chips. The medallion usually has the Serenity Prayer on one side and something about AA on the other side, with a number signifying the sober and straight time the person has achieved. Medallions are given out at 3, 6, and 9 months, and then every year. The yearly anniversary is a special time for people in recovery, and may even be celebrated with a cake and party.

As a physician, a very important date to be aware of for recovering alcoholics is their dry date. This is the first day that they did not use alcohol or other mood-altering drugs. This date can be put on the problem list with the patient's diagnosis of alcoholism, so that when an anniversary comes up the physician can congratulate the patient on his or her continued recovery.

F. AA Slogans

AA has many slogans and sayings that are frequently repeated at meetings and when one alcoholic talks to another alcoholic. The slogans may seem simple or corny to an outsider, but several studies have shown that alcoholics suffer permanent cognitive learning deficits because of their chronic alcohol intake. These simple, often repeated slogans may be a very basic way to overcome these deficits. One of the oldest slogans in AA is "One day at a time." This slogan emphasizes one of the basic philosophies of AA—the alcoholic has to be concerned only with today. This is applied particularly to drinking, and means that he or she may go on a roaring drunk tomorrow, but he or she needs to stay sober just today. Alcoholics also project all kinds of fears and irrational concerns about what may happen tomorrow, next week, or in the next 100 years. This simple slogan helps them live in the present.

Another frequently heard slogan is "Easy does it." Alcoholics early in recovery tend to want to get everything resolved right away. All of the problems that have come up in their lives because of their alcohol use should somehow be resolved the minute they become sober. They will frequently want to go on diets, start exercising, and quit smoking along with resolving all their personal conflicts immediately after they sober up. Needless to say, this approach usually fails and can precipitate a relapse. By taking things easy and not trying to do everything at once, they will not become frustrated, and thus have less chance of drinking.

The spiritual aspect of AA is emphasized by the slogan "Let go and let God." Most alcoholics have tried desperately to control their drinking in the past, and this can frequently spill over into controlling other areas in their lives. This can continue into sobriety. This slogan helps them realize that there is a higher power ("God as we understand Him") that can run things if they can just let go.

Another favorite slogan is "Keep it simple." Alcoholics have a knack for complicating things, and this slogan helps overcome this problem. The slogan is also applicable to working the AA program. In simple terms, what is recommended is to not drink, go to meetings, read the Big Book, work the Steps, and reach out to other suffering alcoholics (doing 12th-Step work).

An acronym used by AA is HOW, which stands for *h*onesty, *o*penness and *w*illingness. The Steps of AA require members to be honest with themselves, their higher power, and people around them. For many alcoholics, this is the first time in their lives (or in years) that they have been truly honest. Openness helps alcoholics overcome their narrow-minded attitudes and their lack of ability to share what they are feeling. They are encouraged to "open" their minds to new ideas and to share what they are really feeling and experiencing in their lives. This means they need to stop putting up the "front" they worked so hard at developing when they were drinking. The willingness involves being willing to look at their old destructive ways and trying to change.

HALT is an acronym which warns alcoholics not to get to *h*ungry, *a*ngry, *l*onely, or *t*ired. An excess of any of these feelings can lead to a slip. "First things first" emphasizes that an alcoholic must always remember that staying sober is their most important priority.

By becoming familiar with these slogans, the physician can use them in caring for his or her alcoholic patients. When recovering alcoholics are having difficulties, these simple slogans can frequently redirect their thinking and make them less likely to use alcohol or any other drug to overcome their frustration. The physician's commitment to the patient's recovery is obvious when the physician knows enough about AA to use the slogans.

The simple suggestion by the physician that the patient go to extra AA meetings in stressful times can also be life saving for the alcoholic.

G. Serenity Prayer

The Serenity Prayer is a basic AA prayer. The Serenity Prayer provides a simple solution to so many of the frustrations that alcoholics (and for that matter everyone) experience in life.

> God grant me the serenity to accept the things I can not change, the courage to change the things that I can and the wisdom to know the difference.

Almost all AA meetings will either open or close with this simple prayer, and alcoholics will use this prayer many times during the day to help them deal with frustrating and stressful situations.

H. How to Refer a Patient to AA

AA can be a valuable resource for physicians in helping their alcoholic patients. In a 1987 AA membership survey [9], only 7% of newcomers reported coming to meetings through a physician's referral. A referral to AA can help the patient begin to see the devastating effects of alcohol on his or her life and the need to change that pattern. There are several ways you can refer patients to AA. In most larger cities (and even many small ones), there is a listed telephone number for AA. By calling the number, AA will have volunteer members contact the patient and they will share their stories with the patient, emphasizing that things can get better. The hope is that the patient will identify with the stories and be willing to attend an AA meeting. If you use this method, it is essential that you obtain the patient's permission and make the call while he or she is in your office. Merely giving the patient the number of AA will almost always result in nothing happening.

Another method of referring patients to AA is to have a list of AA members in your practice who are willing to do 12th-Step calls. These patients are also an excellent resource to help you better understand AA. Some physicians will take patients to AA meetings themselves. If they are not an alcoholic, they can frequently find a closed meeting that is willing to allow them to do this, or they can take the patient to an open AA meeting. Although this is time consuming, it will show the patient just how important you think AA is for his or her recovery program. By calling the local AA office (frequently referred to as Intergroup), the physician can usually get an up-to-date list of all the AA meetings in your area. This will usually include a brief description of the type of meeting and whether it is a special-interest group. A summary of these suggestions (from AA) is in Table 1 [10].

Most drug and alcohol addiction treatment programs have a strong AA component, and will strongly encourage patients to attend AA as a regular part of their aftercare program.

I. Patient Objections to AA [11]

1. "I don't believe in all that God stuff." This is a common objection of people to AA. The AA program is a spiritual program that is not allied with any religion and does not require the members to believe in anything except a higher power ("God as we understand Him"). There are many atheists and agnostics in AA

2. "I don't like to talk in a group." There is no requirement to talk at an AA meeting. Just say "pass" if you do not want to talk.

3. "I can't stand all the smoke." Almost all areas now have nonsmoking meetings available or large groups will split into smoking and nonsmoking discussion groups.

4. "I don't have a way to get there." By calling the local AA number, transportation can almost always be arranged for an interested newcomer.

5. "I don't want anyone to know about my drinking." Anonymity is one of the basic concepts of AA. What is said in a meeting stays there and no AA member has the right to break the anonymity of another AA member.

6. "I can't stay sober." The third tradition of AA clearly states "The only requirement for AA membership is a desire to stop drinking." Many oldtimers spent a long time going to meetings before they were able to stay sober and they understand the plight of the newcomer.

J. Danger Signs in AA Members

Prior to a relapse, AA members may show certain danger signs. The first of these is an unwillingness to share how their program is going. This may be a sign that the patient has decreased the frequency of meeting attendance or may not be attending AA at all! Another measure you can use to assess the quality of the patient's sobriety to ask when he or she last had any contact with his or her sponsor. Balking at this question (or if it has been a long time) can be a sign of isolation and an impending slip. If patients stop going to meetings, they begin to exhibit what is called the dry drunk syndrome. When this happens, the patient becomes irritable and short tempered, with very little patience. This is commonly seen when alcoholics are not drinking and not going to AA meetings regularly. They loose their reality base and get back to stinking thinking, which frequently includes resentments and a multitude of other feelings that can lead to drinking again to relieve the pain.

Table 1 Suggestions to the Physician

1. If you think your patient is an alcoholic, tell him or her.
2. Tell the patient he or she is suffering from an illness, not a moral weakness.
3. Tell the patient alcoholism is progressive and can only get worse if the alcoholic continues to drink.
4. Tell the patient alcoholism is a treatable disease.
5. Try to get the patient to admit his or her troubles are caused by drinking, not the other way around.
6. Tell the patient where help is available—clinics, detoxification units, therapy groups, etc.
7. Tell the patient about AA.
8. Go to an AA meeting yourself to see how it works.
9. Get a local AA meeting list.
10. Get to know some AA members for referral purposes.

K. Some Things AA is Not [12]

There are several things that AA emphasizes that it is not. AA does not solicit members. AA will only reach out to people who ask for help. AA does not keep any records of membership (although some AA groups will provide phone lists as described previously). AA also does not engage in or do any research. AA does not try to control or follow up on its members in formal ways. AA does not have any hospitals and does not make any medical or psychological diagnoses. It is up to each individual member to decide if he or she is an alcoholic. AA as a whole does not provide housing, food, clothes, jobs, or money to newcomers (although individual members may do this). AA is also self-supporting through its own members' contributions; therefore, it does not accept money from any outside sources.

L. Can AA Help?

Alcoholics Anonymous has over 50 years of experience helping alcoholics who in the past were considered hopeless. Exactly how AA works is a mystery. That it does work is a fact. Medicine may be able someday to understand how AA works, but for now it is important that physicians understand that it does work. Physicians need to know how to use AA effectively to help alcoholics recover from the disease of alcoholism. By knowing about AA in your community and knowing a few simple concepts of AA, you can be an invaluable resource to your alcoholic patients.

III. NARCOTICS ANONYMOUS

"We cannot change the nature of the addict or addiction. We can help to change the old lie 'Once an addict, always an addict,' by striving to make recovery more available. God, help us to remember this difference." [13]

This is the basic premise upon which Narcotics Anonymous is built. Narcotics Anonymous (NA) was started at the U.S. Public Health Service Hospital in Lexington, Kentucky, in 1947 [14]. NA spread to New York City in 1948 through Dan Carlson, who had been treated as a patient at Lexington. In 1953, a group of AA members, who were also addicts, started an NA group in Sun Valley, California. This group was the seed from which NA grew. This group emphasized the need for NA to closely follow the 12 Steps and 12 Traditions of AA. NA started because of the discomfort many narcotics and drug addicts felt when attending AA meetings (at times even resentment by the AA members). At NA meetings, members are able to share their particular problems related to drugs other than alcohol. The only differences in the Steps are in Step 1, which in NA states, "We admitted we were powerless over our *addiction*, that our lives had become unmanageable," and the 12th Step, which states, "Having had a spiritual awakening as the result of these steps, we tried to carry the message to *addicts* and to practice these principles in all our affairs." By changing from a specific substance (alcohol) to addiction, NA was able to include all drugs. This was a very important distinction for NA.

NA believes that addiction is a disease that is progressive and life long, and involves more than the use of drugs. Recovery is based on abstinence from all mood-altering drugs, including alcohol. Addiction leads to the "triangle of self-obsession." [15]. The triangle is described as resentment, anger, and fear. Resentment is the addict's way of dealing with the past. Anger is the way of dealing with the present. Fear is the feeling associated with the future. Through the 12 Steps, the addict is encouraged to change these character defects to acceptance of the past, love in the present, and faith in the future. Addiction is also defined by what it is not [16].

1. Addiction is not freedom.
2. Addiction is not personal growth.
3. Addiction is not good will.
4. Addiction is not a way of life.

The goals of the addict in recovery then become freedom, goodwill, creative action, and personal growth. There are certain characteristics of addicts in early recovery which are unique because the drugs they use are illegal. Manipulation and suspicion are very common traits in the recovering addict. Other group members can help newcomers identify these problems in themselves and give them helpful suggestions about how to overcome them. The goal of recovery is not just to abstain from mood-altering drugs—it is to live life in a way in which mood-altering drugs are no longer needed to find positive feelings. By associating with other people in recovery, the addict is able to see the many benefits of being "straight and clean."

A. Structure and Meetings

The structure of NA is almost identical to AA. The basic unit is the group. Groups have area service boards and also a World Services Office which reports to a 15-member World Service Board of Trustees. Two-thirds of the members of this Board are recovering addicts with at least 5 years of abstinence. Five nonaddicts are also on the Board. The World Services Office works as the information center for NA.

The meetings of NA are similar to those of AA, and are generally either discussion, Step, or speaker meetings. Sponsorship [17] is also an integral part of the NA program, and all newcomers are urged to get a sponsor. Many of the AA slogans and sayings are also used in NA.

B. Literature

NA has a "Big Book" entitled *Narcotics Anonymous* [18], which outlines the principles of NA, and also has the personal stories of early NA members. One of the many excellent pamphlets published by NA is *Welcome to Narcotics Anonymous*. This pamphlet outlines the principles of NA and explains to the newcomer how things can get better. This is an excellent resource for physicians to have available for their patients who are interested in NA. The pamphlet states: "Our message is simple: We have found a way to live without using drugs and we are happy to share it with anyone for whom drugs are a problem." *Staying Clean on the Outside* is an excellent resource to give patients when they are leaving a treatment program or hospital after being treated for their addiction. For people in communities with no NA group, the World Services Office provides an NA Group Starter Kit, which describes how to start an NA group.

C. Referral to NA

Referral to NA can be done in the same way as to AA. It may be harder to identify NA members in your practice, and there may not be as many. NA will frequently have a listed phone number which you can use to help addicts contact NA. Many treatment centers will also have lists of NA meetings available in your area. If none of these resources are available, the World Services Office in Van Nuys, California (P.O. Box 9999), can provide you with help and a wealth of information about NA.

D. Cocaine Anonymous

With the national epidemic of cocaine addiction surfacing in the last 10 years, Cocaine Anonymous groups have started in many metropolitan areas across the country. These groups are based on the 12 Steps, and are open to anyone suffering from addiction to cocaine. Many cocaine addicts also attend either Narcotics Anonymous or Alcoholics Anonymous meetings because they can find people with longer periods of being drug free, and frequently they are also addicted to other drugs or alcohol.

IV. FAMILY SUPPORT GROUPS

If we estimate there are 20 million alcoholics in this country, and for every alcoholic four other people are affected, then there are approximately 80 million people affected by alcoholism in some way. This estimate is very close to the findings of a Gallup poll which showed that 24% of people interviewed said they had been affected by an alcoholic in some way in their lives [19].

As the field of drug and alcohol addiction has become more sophisticated, it has been realized that the disease of alcoholism and drug addiction is indeed a family disease. Everyone in the family is affected—not just the identified alcoholic or drug-addicted patient. With this understanding, support groups for the family members of alcoholics have started and grown rapidly. These support groups all emphasize that even if the person who is drug-dependent continues to use drugs, the family members can get help. The emphasis is on helping the individual family member, not the drug-addicted person.

A. Al-Anon

The oldest family program is Al-Anon, which was started by Lois Wilson (Bill Wilson's wife). Early in the history of AA, the wives would frequently accompany their husbands to AA meetings. While the men were having their meeting, the wives would get together to talk and support each other. Many of these groups tried to follow the 12 Steps and to apply them to their lives as their husbands were doing. They began to see that they too were affected by the alcoholism in the family, and they needed help and support in their recovery. In 1950, 87 of these family groups asked AA to publish their meetings in the AA directory. Because the meetings were not for alcoholics, AA refused to do this. Lois Wilson and several other oldtimers decided to unify the groups and start their own Central Service Center. Out of this unification process came the first Al-Anon literature and *Purposes and Suggestions for Al-Anon Family Groups*. Focusing on themselves and not the alcoholic was the major theme of the work. This simple philosophy was earth shattering in its meaning and application to people who had previously spent most of their energy and time concentrating on the alcoholic. The growth of Al-Anon, like AA, was very slow in the beginning until an article appeared in the *Saturday Evening Post* in the late 1950s. In 1962, Ann Landers published information about Al-Anon in her daily newspaper column. This one article spurred over 4000 letters to the Al-Anon headquarters. A later article brought 10,000 letters to the office, and a reprint of that article brought in another 11,000 letters. Al-Anon was on its way! In 1978, Al-Anon opened a World Services Office in New York City.

Basic Concepts of Al-Anon

Al-Anon is a spiritual (not religious) program based on the 12 Steps of AA. The steps are exactly the same except for the 12th Step, which states: "Having had a spiritual awakening as the result of these Steps, we tried to carry this message to *others*, and to practice these principles in all our affairs." There are two main ideas stressed by Al-Anon [20]. The first is that alcoholism is a disease. This is pointed out very clearly in the Al-Anon Preamble, which is read before most Al-Anon meetings.

> *The Al-Anon Family Groups are a fellowship of relatives and friends of alcoholics who share there experience, strength and hope in order to solve their common problems. We believe alcoholism is a family illness and that changed attitudes can aid recovery.

A person does not choose to have a disease and no one can cause a person to have a disease. Acting in a certain way or doing certain things will not change the disease in the alcoholic. The second major idea emphasizes that the program is for the person, not the alcoholic. This concept is emphasized in the Al-Anon welcome.

> *We welcome you to the [name of the group] and hope you will find in this fellowship the help and friendship we have been privileged to enjoy.
>
> We who live, or who have lived, with the problem of alcoholism understand as perhaps few others can. We, too, were lonely and frustrated, but in Al-Anon we discover that no situation is really hopeless, and that it is possible for us to find contentment, and even happiness, whether the alcoholic is still drinking or not.
>
> We urge you to try our program. It has helped many of us find solutions that lead to serenity. So much depends on our own attitudes, and as we learn to place our problem in its true perspective, we find it loses its power to dominate our thoughts and our lives.

The Al-Anon program teaches the person to look at what she or he can do to feel better about herself or himself and to "let go" of the alcoholic while still caring. This concept is sometimes referred to as "tough love." An important part of tough love is to stop *enabling* the alcoholic. This means the person needs to let the alcoholic be responsible for the consequences of his or her drinking and alcoholism. Al-Anon has described this concept in a pamphlet called *Detachment* [21]. It states that detachment is a tool of recovery for the families in Al-Anon to help them help themselves. They encourage people to "let go of our obsession with another's behavior and begin to lead happier and more manageable lives." Al-Anon helps them learn:

> Not to suffer because of the action or reactions of other people;
> Not to allow ourselves to be used or abused in the interest of another's recovery;
> Not to do for others what they should do for themselves;
> Not to manipulate situations so others will eat, go to bed, get up, pay bills, etc'
> Not to cover up another's mistakes or misdeeds;
> Not to create a crisis;
> Not to prevent a crisis if it is in the natural course of events.

---

*Reprinted by permission of Al–Anon Family Group Headquarters, Inc.

Newcomers often come into Al-Anon with resentments and anger which have never been acknowledged. Al-Anon helps them view the alcoholic as someone with a disease rather than someone who is "trying to get them." The first step points out that they are powerless over alcohol and that their lives are unmanageable. This means they have no control over the alcoholic. The second and third steps help the person reach outside herself or himself for help from a higher power. This letting go of the control and trusting a higher power are basic concepts of the Al-Anon program.

Membership and Meetings

The third tradition of Al-Anon states, "The only requirement for membership is that there be a problem of alcoholism in a relative or friend." There are over 15,000 Al-Anon groups in the United States and Canada. Al-Anon meetings usually start with the Serenity Prayer, the preamble, and the welcome, and are followed by introductions. There are speaker, discussion, and Step meetings. The meetings emphasize sharing, support, and encouragement to work on oneself. They usually last for 1 h and have a standard closing:

> *The opinions expressed here were strictly those of the persons who gave them. Take what you like and leave the rest. A few special words to those of you who haven't been with us long: Whatever your problems, there are those among us who have had them too. If you try to keep an open mind, you will find help. You will come to realize that there is no situation too difficult to be bettered and no unhappiness too great to be lessened. We aren't perfect. The welcome we give you may not show the warmth we have in our hearts for you. After a while, you'll discover that though you may not like all of us, you'll love us in a very special way—the same way we already love you.

The leader then emphasizes that everything said in the meeting is considered confidential and, "What's said here stays here." Frequently, there is a social time after the meeting for further support and sharing.

Al-Anon Literature

In 1966, Al-Anon published *Al-Anon Family Groups* [22], which is equivalent to the Big Book in AA. This book sets down the basic principles of Al-Anon and tells the stories of the founders. There is also a book of *Al-Anon's Twelve Steps and Twelve Traditions* [23], which discusses the Steps and Traditions from an Al-Anon perspective. *One Day at a Time in Al-Anon* [24] is a daily mediation guide book which many members read to give themselves inspiration and guidance. Al-Anon also publishes over 50 pamphlets which deal with special topics such as men in Al-Anon, denial, alcoholism as a family disease, and adult children of alcoholics. These pamphlets are available from Al-Anon Family Group Headquarters, Inc. P.O. Box 862, Midtown Station, New York, NY 10018-0862, or your local Al-Anon office.

Referral to Al-Anon

In many cities, Al-Anon has a listed phone number. If this is not the case, frequently the AA office will supply you with the locations and times of Al-Anon meetings. The more physicians know about Al-Anon, the better they are able to help refer patients in need to Al-Anon. An excellent way to find out about Al-Anon is to talk with members of Al-Anon about their experiences with the program and to attend a local meeting. In your practice, it is also helpful to have a list of Al-Anon members who are willing to take people to Al-Anon meetings and to do 12th-Step work. It is important for the physician to emphasize that it takes time to get comfortable with Al-Anon and to recommend that the patient attend a minimum of six meetings before deciding if Al-Anon is for her or him. As with AA, sponsorship is a strong component of Al-Anon.

---

*Reprinted by permission of Al–Anon Family Group Headquarters, Inc.

Alateen

Alateen is a separate program of Al-Anon Family Groups. It was started by a teenager in California in 1957. This program is specifically for teenagers, and follows the Al-Anon Steps and Traditions. Every Alateen group has an active adult member of Al-Anon who serves as a sponsor for the group. The sponsor provides guidance and stability to the group and helps the group stay focused on the 12 Steps and 12 Traditions. A key to being a good sponsor is to guide without dominating. The group can have a group inventory and decide to get a new sponsor, if the relationship is not working out. Alateen meetings frequently meet at the same place as Al-Anon but in a different room. Many schools also have Alateen meetings. A referral to Alateen can be made through the local Al-Anon office.

Alateen has its own literature especially directed to the teenager. In *Hope for Children of Alcoholics—Alateen* [25], there is a chapter devoted to explaining alcoholism in terms teenagers can understand. Alcoholics are described as being anyone, and not necessarily "skid row bums." One section discusses why alcoholics drink, with an explanation about obsession, addiction, and compulsion. The symptoms of alcoholism and the family disease concept are also explained, with an emphasis on denial, anger, anxiety, and the feeling that the teenagers are "caught in the middle." As in Al-Anon, the alcoholic is described as being sick and not able to control his or her alcohol intake or reactions. The book also talks about the slogans and explains each slogan. Another chapter in the book has personal stories to help the teenager feel he or she is not alone. At the end of the book, there is a detailed explanation about how to start and organize an Alateen group. A special page labeled "Remember" encourages the groups to focus on the common problem of alcoholism and not to gossip, waste time, be impatient, become bossy, or talk about what happens in the group outside of the group. As the members become older, they are encouraged to join Al-Anon to continue their recovery.

B. Adult Children of Alcoholics

Over the past 10 years, a new movement has developed in recovery groups in alcohol addiction. This movement has been identified as Adult Children of Alcoholics (ACA, ACOA, or COA). The number of new members and new groups in Adult Children of Alcoholics has risen rapidly. As early as 1960, researchers began looking at adults who had been raised in alcoholic homes, and tried to identify common characteristics among these individuals. Books published as a result of this research [26,27] were the impetus for starting support groups for this population (by some estimates as many as 30–40 million). This movement grew rapidly, and it did not have the advantage of time to develop and mature as did AA and Al-Anon. Many separate groups began developing support systems for these people. There was a movement within Al-Anon itself to have special meetings for adult children of alcoholics. Groups such as the National Association for Children of Alcoholics were also started. There was a lack of clarity in what the groups should and should not do, and many new groups had no one who had any real time in the program to help provide guidance and direction. Some of these groups became more therapy groups than support groups. Heavy confrontation was often used rather than a reliance on the 12 Steps and 12 Traditions. Although these problems still exist in some groups, most ACA groups have matured and now offer excellent support for adult children of alcoholics.

Characteristics of Adult Children of Alcoholics

Adult children of alcoholics have certain common characteristics. One common characteristic is a need to control [28], and when faced with stressful life situations, adult children of alcoholics frequently try to increase their control of the situation even when this is totally impossible. Denial, dishonesty, secretiveness, and suppression of feelings are characteristics commonly seen in alcoholic families. Janet Woititz has described the characteristics of adult children of alcoholics as follows [29]:

1. Adult children of alcoholics guess at what normal behavior is.
2. Adult children of alcoholics have difficulty following a project through from beginning to end.
3. Adult children of alcoholics lie when it would be just as easy to tell the truth.
4. Adult children of alcoholics judge themselves without mercy.
5. Adult children of alcoholics have difficulty having fun.
6. Adult children of alcoholics take themselves very seriously.
7. Adult children of alcoholics have difficulty with intimate relationships.
8. Adult children of alcoholics overreact to change over which they have no control.
9. Adult children of alcoholics constantly need approval and affirmation.
10. Adult children of alcoholics usually feel that they are different from other people.
11. Adult children of alcoholics are super responsible or super irresponsible.
12. Adult children of alcoholics are extremely loyal even in the face of evidence that the loyalty is undeserved.
13. Adult children of alcoholics are impulsive. They tend to lock themselves into a course of action without giving serious consideration to alternative behaviors or possible consequences. This impulsivity leads to confusion, self-loathing, and loss of control over their environment. In addition, they spend an excessive amount of energy cleaning up the mess.

If physicians are aware of these common characteristics, they can look for them in patients and identify adult children of alcoholics in their practices. These patients will frequently have large charts with frequent visits. Until they are identified as adult children of alcoholics, they can be frustrating for the physician to care for.

Meetings and Referral

Once the problem has been identified, the physician can be instrumental in helping the patient start a program of recovery by referring the patient to Adult Children of Alcoholics. It is essential that the physician be familiar with the group that he or she refers the patient to. The group should have some history and experience, and have members who have been involved in other 12-Step programs. The group should have the 12 Steps as the basis of its philosophy. Good groups offer the person support and caring while understanding the pain the person is in when the issues of being an adult child of an alcoholic start surfacing. The group should not allow "cross-talk" [30]. This is defined as confrontation or interruptions of the person who is sharing. The meeting must be felt to be "safe" by the newcomer (and oldtimer for that matter). By listening (they do not have to say anything if they do not want to), the newcomer can hear other people tell their stories and identify with those stories. For the first time in many of their lives, they do not feel so alone and unique in what they are feeling. The purpose of ACA groups [30] is

> to shelter and support newcomers in confronting denial; to comfort those mourning their early loss of security, trust and love; and to teach the skills for re-parenting themselves with gentleness, humor, love and respect.

Most Adult Children of Alcoholic meetings last 1.5 h. They usually start with the Serenity Prayer and a welcome. The 12 Steps, the problem (which describes what happens when you are raised in an alcoholic home) and the solution (which describes what ACA recommends for recovery) are also frequently read. At some meetings, the characteristics are read. Then a member will talk about a Step or characteristic and how it effects his or her life. Each member of the group then has the opportunity to share his or her feelings about the topic or talk about any other concerns he or she may have. As with the other 12-Step programs, the meeting usually closes with a prayer (the Lord's Prayer). Members are encouraged to socialize after the meeting and frequently go for coffee.

Newcomers are encouraged to attend six meetings to help them become comfortable with the group and develop the trust that is essential to recovery. Sponsors are also an important part of ACA, and newcomers are encouraged to get a sponsor. Most groups have phone lists and encourage members to call each other for support. As with AA and Al-Anon, an important part of recovery in ACA is reaching out to others and trying to help them. ACA members are willing to take people to meetings, and can be a helpful resource for physicians.

Many therapists have adult children of alcoholic therapy groups. These are quite different from the groups described above. They are lead by a therapist who has experience and training in the concepts of adult children of alcoholics. Confrontation and feedback are frequently given in these groups to help the patients break through the denial and minimization of the consequences of being raised in an alcoholic home. This type of group requires a skilled therapist to direct the group and provide support to the patients when they are starting to give up control and to open up (which can be absolutely terrifying for an adult child of an alcoholic). A therapy group can be effective in helping the patient identify and recover from the wounds of living in an alcoholic home, and should be used in conjunction with a firm base in a 12-Step ACA group. Therapy groups can show the patient that conflict can be worked out in a healthy manner, which is different from the destructive methods commonly used in alcoholic homes.

When you have a patient who you feel is an adult child of an alcoholic, remember that alcoholism is an inherited disease. The *patient* is at high risk for becoming an alcoholic. The physician needs to screen these patients and refer them if there is any suspicion of an alcohol problem. Also remember that although these patients may appear to be emotionally stable, they are often fragile under the external shell, which they so effectively construct. They need to be treated with care, understanding, and gentleness by the physician.

REFERENCES

1. Bassin, A. (1975). Psychology in action, *Am. Psychol., 30*(6):695–696.
2. Canavan, D. (1983). Impaired Physicians Program-Support Groups. *J. Med. Soc. N.J., 80*(11):953–954.
3. Anonymous AA Member (1983). AA Meeting, Atlanta, Georgia.
4. *Alcoholics Anonymous* (1976). Alcoholics Anonymous World Services, Inc., New York City.
5. Alexander, J. (1941). Alcoholics Anonymous, *Sat. Evening Post, 213*:9–12.
6. Anonymous. *Grapevine*. Alcoholics Anonymous World Services, Inc., New York.
7. Anonymous (1987). *AA Membership Survey*. Alcoholics Anonymous World Services, Inc., New York.
8. Anonymous (1952). *Twelve Steps and Twelve Traditions*. Alcoholics Anonymous World Services, Inc., New York.
9. Anonymous (1987). *AA Membership Survey*. Alcoholics Anonymous World Services, Inc., New York.
10. Anonymous (1975). Ten tips from Alcoholics Anonymous for family doctors, *Med. Times, 103*(6):74–76.
11. Anonymous (1982). *AA as a Resource for the Medical Profession*, Alcoholics Anonymous World Services, Inc., New York.
12. Anonymous (1972). *A Brief Guide to Alcoholics Anonymous*. Alcoholics Anonymous World Services, Inc., New York.

13. Anonymous (1983). *Narcotics Anonymous*. World Services Office, Inc., Van Nuys, California.

14. Peyrot, M. (1985). Narcotics Anonymous: Its history, structure, and approach, *Int. J. Addict.,* *20*(10):1509–1522.

15. Anonymous (1983). *The Triangle of Self-Obsession*. Narcotics Anonymous World Services Office, Inc., Van Nuys, California.

16. Anonymous (1984). *Another Look*. Narcotics Anonymous World Services Office, Inc., Van Nuys, California.

17. Anonymous (1983). *Sponsorship*. Narcotics Anonymous World Services Office, Inc., Van Nuys, California.

18. Anonymous (1982). *Narcotics Anonymous*. Narcotics Anonymous World Services Office, Inc., Van Nuys, California.

19. Robertson, N. (1988). *Getting Better Inside Alcoholics Anonymous*. Fawcett Crest Book/Ballantine Books, New York.

20. Anthony M. (1977). Al-Anon, *J.A.M.A., 238*(10):1062–1063.

21. Anonymous (1979). *Detachment*. Al-Anon Family Group Headquarters, Inc., New York.

22. Anonymous (1966). *Al-Anon Family Groups*. Al-Anon Family Group Headquarters, New York.

23. Anonymous (1981). *Al-Anons Twelve Steps & Twelve Traditions*, Al-Anon Family Group Headquarters, Inc., New York.

24. Anonymous (1973). *One Day at a Time in Al-Anon*, Al-Anon Family Group Headquarters, Inc., New York.

25. Anonymous (1973). *Alateen—Hope for Children of Alcoholics*. Al-Anon Family Group Headquarters, Inc., New York.

26. Wegscheider, S. (1981). *Another Chance*. Palo Alto: Science and Behavior Books, Palo Alto, California.

27. Black, C. (1982). *It Will Never Happen To Me!* M.A.C. Printing and Publishing Division, Denver, Colorado.

28. Cermak, T., and Rosenfeld, A. (1987). Therapeutic considerations with adult children of alcoholics. *Adv. Alcohol Subst. Abuse, 6*(4):17–32.

29. Woititz, J. (1983). *Adult Children of Alcoholics*. Health Communications, Pompano Beach, Florida.

30. Jacobson, S. (1987). The 12-Step program and group therapy for adult children of alcoholics. *J. Psychoactive Drug, 19*(3):253–255.

XXIII

**Interactions Between Drugs/Alcohol
and Brain/Behavior**

70

A Review of the Interactions in Psychiatric Syndromes and Drug and Alcohol Addiction

Norman S. Miller
Cornell University Medical College, The New York Hospital–Cornell Medical Center, White Plains, New York

I. INTRODUCTION

Psychiatric syndromes are linked to alcohol and drug addiction (1) because there is a high rate for both categories of disorders, the two are likely to occur together by chance alone [1–3]; (2) the clinical severity can be greater when the two categories of disorders appear together; clinicians and researchers are more likely to identify either or both of them [4–7]; and (3) intoxication and withdrawal from alcohol and drugs can produce psychiatric symptoms and syndromes [5,6,8,9].

Two major populations are ordinarily studied to determine the prevalence rates of psychiatric syndromes in alcohol and drug addiction; the general population and patient populations [1,4,5,10]. The prevalence rates for both categories of disorders is high in general and patient populations; consequently the two major categories of disorders occur together by chance alone in both types of populations [12,13]. Predictably, the prevalence rates for comorbidity is greater in patient populations than the general population. The increase in severity in the psychopathology from the co-occurrence of both categories of disorders attracts the attention of clinicians and researchers [14,15].

Of primary importance is that there is unequivocal evidence that psychoactive drugs and alcohol can produce psychiatric syndromes through several pharmacological mechanisms: (1) Stimulant intoxication can cause symptoms of mania; i.e., euphoria, hyperactivity and delusions, and of anxiety similar to obsessive compulsive disorder, panic disorder, phobias, and generalized anxiety disorder [16–19]. (2) Stimulant withdrawal and repeated depressant intoxication can cause severe and incapacitating depression that is indistinguishable from the syndrome of major depression [20,21]. (3) Depressant withdrawal can produce anxiety syndromes similar to stimulant intoxication acutely, and may produce less severe symptoms of anxiety during a protracted abstinence syndrome [7,22–24]. (4) Stimulant intoxication as with amphetamines and cocaine and depressant withdrawal as with alcohol can produce a syndrome of auditory hallucinations and paranoid delusions that can resemble schizophrenia [20,25,26].

In spite of many reports of psychiatric syndromes linked to the use of drugs and alcohol, few studies examine the "interaction" between alcohol and drug addiction and psychiatric syndromes under controlled conditions. Frequently, a self-medication hypothesis is assumed to explain drug and alcohol use and addiction, and few studies emphasize the role of addictive behaviors in drug and alcohol use. Furthermore, subject to considerable methodological error is the practice of using a cross-sectional and/or retrospective analysis of psychiatric syndromes in drug- and alcohol-addicted patient populations or drug and alcohol use in psychiatric patient populations [27,28]. Unfortunately, a prolonged period of observation during detoxification from alcohol and drug addiction/use in either population is not utilized to study the "clearance" or "persistence" of psychiatric syndromes during abstinence [29,30].

II. GENERAL POPULATION

The recent Epidemiologic Catchment Area (ECA) study performed in the general population provides prevalence rates of diagnostic categories for alcohol and drug addiction and other psychiatric disorders in five major cities in the United States (St. Louis, Missouri, Los Angeles, California, Durham, North Carolina, Baltimore, Maryland and New Haven, Connecticut). For the first time in a major prevalence study of alcohol and addiction in the general population, actual diagnoses were obtained in a structured interview using DSM-III (*Diagnostic and Statistical Manual of Mental Disorders*, American Psychiatric Association, Washington, D.C., 1980) criteria. Previous large-scale studies on prevalence of alcohol and drug addiction in nonpatient populations were based on estimates of the disorders according to index criteria; i.e., consumption rates, medical illness, and chart reviews [10,11].

A. Alcohol and Drug Addiction and Psychiatric Disorders

The combined five-site ECA data for lifetime disorders revealed that alcohol addiction was the most common diagnosis at 13.7% of the general population. Phobias was the second most common psychiatric diagnosis at 12.8%, followed by drug abuse and addiction at 6.9%, by depression at 5.1%, and antisocial personality disorder at 2.5%. Of importance is that alcoholism was a common disorder in comparison to other psychiatric disorders. Phobias, as would be expected, represent a pervasive disorder in the community, yet second to alcoholism. Drug abuse and addiction were also frequent disorders, after phobias. Other psychiatric disorders had prevalence rates that were similar to those reported by other studies in nonalcoholics in the general population [10].

As might be expected, the findings in the ECA study for the prevalence rates of major DSM-III disorders indicate that psychiatric disorders associated with alcohol and drug addiction are common. One-third of the total population in the ECA sample met lifetime criteria for one of the psychiatric diagnoses, and one-third of those with one diagnosis had a second psychiatric diagnosis. Among those with the DSM-III diagnosis of alcoholism, almost half (47%) had a second psychiatric diagnosis. The study did not assign causality or attempt to make primary and secondary etiological distinctions in diagnostic categories [10,11].

The lifetime prevalence rates for psychiatric disorders were higher among those with alcoholism than those without alcoholism in the general population. When the prevalence rates of additional psychiatric disorders in alcoholics were compared to those in nonalcoholics, surprisingly, alcoholic women (28%) were more likely to have an additional diagnosis of drug abuse or addiction than men (18.2%). The use of prescription medication among women accounted for a substantial amount of the drug use. As expected from previous inpatient studies, both female and male alcoholics had considerably greater prevalence of drug abuse or addiction than female (3.3%) and male (4.0%) nonalcoholics. The multiple drug-addicted alcoholic is an increasingly common finding among patients, particularly younger alcoholics [10,11].

Both alcoholic and nonalcoholic men (14.6 and 1.3%, respectively) were more often diagnosed as having antisocial personalities than women (10.1 and 0.4%, respectively) as is generally recognized in both general and patient populations. The higher prevalance of antisocial personality disorder among both male and female alcoholics is also well documented [3,4,9]. Phobic disorders were also distinctly more common among female (33.1%) than male (13.5%) alcoholics, being greater than in either female (16.2%) or male (7.9%) nonalcoholics as well. These findings regarding phobic disorders among alcoholics have also been substantiated in patient populations (as will be discussed).

Depression/dysthymia were clearly more common among alcoholic females (23.4%), considerably greater than in male alcoholics (8.0%) and in both female (8.2%) and male (3.3%) nonalcoholics. These findings are comparable to other studies of patient populations where depression is more common among female alcoholics [31]. The weaker association of depression with alcoholism in the ECA data, particularly for men, may represent the bias away from more severely affected alcoholics who seek treatment because of depression complicating the alcoholism. The temporal sequence of onset of alcohol addiction and depression found in the ECA study was the following: in men, alcoholism preceded the onset of depression in the majority (78%), whereas in women, depression was the antecedent diagnosis in 66% of the cases [10,11].

Panic disorder was increased among female alcoholics 7.9 to 1.8% and among male alcoholics 2.1 to 0.5% over nonalcoholics, but the numbers of those affected were small. Somatization disorder and mania were both increased severalfold in male and female alcoholics over nonalcoholics, although, again, the numbers of those affected were small [10,11].

B. Alcohol and Drug Addiction

The lifetime prevalence rates for alcohol addiction among those with a diagnosis of drug addiction reveal high rates in the ECA study. In those who were addicted to tetrahydrocannabinol (THC) as the only drug, 36% were alcoholic. Among the other drug-addicted diagnoses, the rate of alcohol addiction for the following drugs was respectively 71% for barbiturates, 62% for amphetamines, 64% for hallucinogens, 84% for cocaine, and 67% for opioids [10,11].

C. Alcohol Addiction

The lifetime prevalence rates for alcohol addiction according to age, sex, and race and the age of onset of alcoholism was determined at the time of interview. The lifetime prevalence for alcohol dependence in the total general population was 13.7%, 23.8% in men and 4.6% in women, but alcohol and drug addiction appeared to be rising rapidly among women at the time of the study. The prevalence was greater among those under 45 years old than those above; almost 40% was diagnosable between ages 15 and 19, and the proportion of cases that were diagnosable by age 30 was 80%. At all ages, men had an earlier onset of alcohol addiction than women; mean ages at age of interview in years for male vs female: 17.8 vs 18.4 [18–29], 24.2 vs 27.3 [30–59], 31.0 vs 40.6 (60+) [10,11].

III. PATIENT POPULATIONS

Many studies of patient populations, including inpatients and outpatients, have assessed the prevalence of the co-occurrence of psychiatric syndromes disorders with alcohol and drug addiction. These studies are biased toward a more severely affected patient, representing those who may have sought treatment because of psychiatric symptoms associated with alcohol and drug addiction or vice versa. Clinicians are more likely to be responsible for diagnosing and treating this population of patients. Researchers are more likely to identify these patients with both categories of disorders [1–8].

A. Medical and Psychiatric Populations

Many studies have found a prevalence of alcohol and drug addiction between 25–50% for general medical populations [32], more for inpatient than outpatients, and between 50–75% for general psychiatric populations, also more for inpatients [33–35]. According to these studies, the concurrent diagnoses of alcohol *and* drug addiction is common in all of these populations. The common psychiatric syndromes cited are depression, anxiety, personality disorders, and schizophrenic disorders [36–38].

Studies indicate further that these patients with multiple drug and alcohol addiction and psychiatric disorders have an overall poorer prognosis. The patients with comorbid disorders tend to be younger, more often male, and have poorer medication compliance. In addition, they are nearly twice as likely to be rehospitalized during 1-year follow-up. Alcohol and multiple drug addiction appear to add the problems of disruptive, disinhibited, and noncompliant behaviors in cases of chronic mental illness [39–41].

B. Multiple Drug and Alcohol Addiction

The prevalence of multiple drug and addiction that includes alcohol is very high for the contemporary drug addicts being admitted for inpatient and outpatient treatment [14,42]. In large-scale studies of inpatient populations of adult and adolescent alcoholics and drug addicts in various treatment facilities, the number of cocaine addicts with the diagnosis of alcohol addiction was in the 70–90% range. Similar studies of methadone and heroin addicts show rates of alcohol addiction between 50 and 75%. Approximately 80–90% of hospitalized cannabis addicts are dependent on alcohol [43,44].

Over 80% of alcoholics in treatment populations are addicted to at least one other drug, usually more than one. A triad of alcohol, marijuana, and cocaine addiction is a regular occurrence among the alcoholics currently being admitted to inpatient and outpatient facilities. According to studies, the younger alcoholic begins using alcohol in the early teenage years, around 13–15 years old, and progresses to the addictive use of alcohol by 15–16 years old. A year or 2 after the onset of alcohol use and dependence, other drugs are tried and often used addictively; these include tobacco, marijuana, and cocaine, followed by hallucinogens (PCP), benzodiazepines, and barbiturates in frequency. Cigarette smoking is particularly troublesome because, unlike some other drug use which may wax and wane, the use of tobacco often remains persistent well into adulthood, with its particular, well-known complications. The pattern of cocaine use has changed dramatically and continues to do so to the present day, most remarkably characterized by a progressively earlier age of onset of use and pattern of addictive use. The skillful marketing techniques for the initially cheaper form of cocaine, "crack," have lured younger individuals to addictive use [43,44].

IV. AFFECTIVE SYNDROMES/DISORDER AND ALCOHOL AND DRUG DEPENDENCE

A. Prevalence

The prevalence rates of affective syndromes/disorders in alcoholism and drug addiction reported are highly variable within a wide range. According to studies done under various conditions, the lifetime prevalence rates for depression among alcoholics are from 5 to 98% in general and patient populations [31,45].

For comparison to affective disorders not associated with alcoholism, a survey of the rate of affective disorders in five communities in the United States demonstrated a lifetime risk for bipolar disorder of approximately 1.2%, a lifetime risk of major depression of 4.4% (with rates significantly higher for women than men), and rates of dysthymia of 3.1% [31].

B. Methodological Considerations

The methodological considerations pertaining to studies of affective syndromes/disorders and alcohol and drug use/addiction include the following:

1. Inpatient vs outpatient populations vs the general population. Most of the investigations involve the use of inpatients, which generally yields high rates of affective symptoms because of the more severely affected population, up to 59% [43,44,46,47]. Therefore, most prevalence rates for depression among alcoholics are based on a severely affected population which may not represent the true frequency in the native state. The ECA (Epidemiological Catchment Area) data supports this notion by the finding that rates for affective disorder among alcoholics in the general population is similar to the rates for affective disorders in the general population [10,11].

2. The prevalence rates for affective syndromes/disorder in drug addiction are similar to those for alcoholics. Several studies have documented significant and, at times, long-lasting residual affective symptoms from both sedative and stimulant drugs. The drugs may be prescription or illicit drugs, however, often used addictively [48,49].

3. Severity of intoxication and addictive use as well as time after drinking and drug use is often disparate from study-to-study. Weissman found that 59% of alcoholics interviewed shortly after their last drink had a depressive syndrome with symptom patterns similar to major depression [31]. Other studies have found similarly high prevalence rates for depression among recently intoxicated or detoxified alcoholics. Many studies clearly demonstrate that the depressive syndrome diminishes rapidly over days in the majority of the alcoholics and drug addicts, and persists in only a small minority [44,46,47,50,51].

4. Age and sex. studies have clearly shown that cognitive deficits (including dementia syndromes), and to a lesser extent depression, are correlated with advancing age [52]. The older alcoholics are more likely to show cognitive deficits and depressive mood than younger alcoholics. Some of these studies are substantiated with radiographic studies, showing greater cerebral atrophy in the older alcoholics [53]. Women alcoholics tend to show a greater prevalence of affective symptoms and disorders than their male counterparts. Women who are addicted to drugs also show a significant rate of depression [10,31].

5. The instruments used to diagnose depression in alcoholics and drug addicts are important sources of methodological variance. There are differences in sensitivity and specificity across the various objective and subjective tests used to measure depression. The DSM-III diagnosis by clinical interview and the Hamilton Depression Scale show higher sensitivity and specificity than the Beck Depression Inventory and the Depression Scale of the Minnesota Multiphasic Personality Inventory. However, all measures do show high rates and improvements of depression among alcoholics and drug addicts with abstinence [54,55].

6. Course of alcoholism vs affective disorder. Although the signs and symptoms of depressions occurring with alcohol and drug intoxication are similar on cross-sectional analysis to major depressive disorders, the sociodemography, family histories, and early life course of problems in the depressed alcoholics more closely resemble those observed for alcoholics than for those with major depression [56,57].

7. Vaillant has shown that a retrospective analysis of the course of alcoholism yields significant error. In his prospective studies, Vaillant has found that premorbid personality and psychiatric diagnosis do not contribute significantly to the etiology of alcoholism. He concluded that the illusions based on retrospective studies are derived from the consequences of alcoholism; i.e., depression and anxiety are assigned incorrectly as etiological. The cross-sectional and retrospective analyses may lead to falsely high rates of diagnoses of affective and anxiety disorders because of the pharmacological effects of alcohol- and drug-induced affective and anxiety states [5-9,58,59].

C. Alcohol and Drug and Affective Symptoms

Schuckit reviewed the relationship between alcoholism and drug addiction and affective disorders and delineated five possible types of interactions. (1) Alcohol (drugs) can cause depressive symptoms in anyone; (2) signs of transient, serious depression can follow prolonged drinking (drug use); (3) drinking (drug use) can escalate during primary affective episodes in some patients, typically in mania; (4) depressive symptoms from alcohol and drug use occur coincidentally in other psychiatric disorders; and (5) a small proportion of patients have independent alcoholism and affective disorder [5-7].

Administration of low to moderate doses (three to five drinks) of alcohol produce sadness and irritability under controlled experimental conditions in normal, healthy subjects. Similar alcohol administration in healthy women produce mood disruptions that can still be measured the day after the experiment. Other investigators have studied the intake of higher doses over longer periods of time and have found elevations in depression rating scale scores and clinical pictures that resemble major depressive episodes [50,51].

Schuckit has found that depressive symptoms occur in 98% of the alcoholics at some time in their life histories, and one-third meet criteria for persistent depressions interfering with functioning over a period of 2 or more weeks. After 2-4 weeks of regular alcohol intake, 5-10% of male and 15% female alcoholics may show evidence of severe depression [5-7].

Studies clearly demonstrate the development of depression following acute and chronic stimulant use. Data exist to show that mood disturbances are commonly associated with cannabis intoxication [59]. The co-occurrence of depressive symptoms is high in individuals on methadone maintenance, and with opiate intoxication and withdrawal. Rounsaville et al. (1986) found that 90% of 533 patients (opiate addicts) met research diagnostic criteria (RDC) for some psychiatric syndrome at some time during their lifetime. Diagnoses included major depression in 74%, alcoholism in 34%, and antisocial personality in 27% [60],

Khantzian and Treece (1985) found in 133 narcotic addicts that 60% met criteria for an affective disorder by DSM-III criteria [46]. Others have also found high rates of affective disorders among cocaine addicts with 50% of 30 outpatients and 70 inpatients meeting DSM-III criteria for affective disorders [24,61,62].

D. Family and Genetic Evidence

Schuckit found that sons of alcoholics and controls had no differences in clinical scores and diagnoses in affective disturbances [63]. Goodwin demonstrated no marked increase for depressive syndromes in adopted sons of alcoholics (daughters of alcoholics showed an increased rate of depressive symptoms only when raised by the alcoholic) [64]. Cadoret and Valliant have reported no increased rate of depressive disorders in adolescents and adults who later developed alcoholism [58,65].

According to a recent and comprehensive review of alcoholism and affective disorders, the two disorders were found to be genetically independent [66]. One of the few findings that might be to the contrary is by Winokur, who reported a higher prevalence of alcoholism in men and affective disorders in women in families with affective disorders (depressive spectrum disorder) [67].

V. ANXIETY SYNDROMES/DISORDERS AND ALCOHOL AND DRUG ADDICTION

A. Prevalence

Anxiety disorders are also highly linked to alcohol and drug addiction disorders. However, as with affective syndromes, most studies have examined the prevalence of anxiety syndromes using cross-sectional and retrospective analyses and in the active state of alcohol and drug addiction and/or closely following active alcohol and drug use in the early period of detoxification [44]. The rates for phobic states, particularly, agoraphobia, are relatively high in comparison to other psychiatric disorders [10,11].

Winokur and Holemon, using criteria similar to that of DSM-III panic disorder, found that five (16%) of 31 patients showed signs of excessive drinking at the time of the interview [68]. Similarly, Woodruff et al. found that nine (15%) of 61 anxiety disorder patients in a psychiatric clinic had alcoholism [69]. Mullaney and Trippett reported that one-third of their inpatient alcoholic population had clinically disabling agoraphobia or social phobia [70]. Hesselbrock et al. found a lifetime history of phobia in 27% and panic disorder in 10% of a hospitalized alcoholic population. In his sample, alcohol abuse occurred subsequent to panic disorder in 63% of the men and 50% of the women [37].

Small and Stockwell et al. reported that 32 out of 40 male alcoholic inpatients had agoraphobia, social phobia, or both when last drinking. The more severely phobic males were also found to be the most addictive to alcohol, and those with no phobias were the least alcohol addictive [71]. In other similar studies, Stockwell and Small et al. found in a retrospective study that periods of heavy drinking and addiction to alcohol were associated with an exacerbation of agoraphobia and social phobias. Subsequent periods of abstinence were associated with substantial improvements in these phobic anxiety states [72].

In other studies of alcoholics admitted for detoxification, 19 of 84 (22.6%) subjects met DSM-III criteria for one or more anxiety disorders [73]. In a group of 48 inpatient alcoholics diagnosed by SADS-L, approximately 44% were suffering from phobias [74]. In a large retrospective study, 173 acutely abstinent patients were screened for phobias and avoidant personality disorder; over half (51.4%) met criteria for agoraphobia (8.5%), social phobia (7.8%), and avoidant personality disorder (35.1%). More than 70% in each diagnostic category were men [75].

B. Alcohol and Drug and Anxiety Symptoms

The mechanism responsible for the generation of the anxiety by alcohol and drugs involve the autonomic nervous system as alcohol and drug intoxication and withdrawal is characterized by the discharge of the sympathetic nervous system. The release of catecholamines by the adrenergic neurons produces excitatory responses of signs and symptoms that are similar to those present in the anxiety disorders. The sympathetic nervous system is implicated in anxiety disorders as the "biological basis" of the panic attack. Of interest is that the lactate infusion test precipitates panic attacks in alcoholics as well as in those with an apparent vulnerability to panic attacks [76]. Also, chronic alcoholics tend to have high lactate blood levels during periods of intoxication, suggesting further that chronic alcohol intake is etiological in the production of anxiety [48].

Cocaine stimulates the sympathetic nervous system during intoxication by enhancing the effects of the catecholamines on the postsynaptic neurons. Cocaine administration, particularly in chronic use, produces intense anxiety and other physiological manifestations of anxiety. Suspiciousness and phobic fears and paranoid delusions are common in acute and chronic cocaine intoxication [17,18].

The consumption of stimulants and depressants can intensify symptoms of preexisting major psychiatric disorders. Many patients actually refrain from using these drugs and alcohol to avoid a worsening of their anxiety disorder. In many instances, abstinence from alcohol and drugs will result in an amelioration or elimination of many of the symptoms of anxiety, including panic attacks, phobias, generalized anxiety, and obsessive compulsive disorders. It may take days, weeks, or months before the many autonomic and electrophysiological changes from alcohol and drugs revert to normal [6,7,23].

Finally, when data are generated before the onset of severe alcohol and drug problems or beyond the syndrome, little evidence of elevated rates of major anxiety syndrome is present [77].

C. Family and Genetic Evidence

There is little evidence to support a significantly elevated rate of independent anxiety disorders in alcoholics and drug addicts. Schuckit compared the anxiety scores and diagnoses of anxiety disorders on 200, 18- to 25-year-old sons of alcoholics with scores from 200 controls and found no increased prevalence of either anxiety symptoms or disorders in the group at high risk for developing alcoholism [63]. Also, all known adoption studies of children of alcoholics have failed to demonstrate an increased risk for major anxiety disorders [64]. Additionally, when alcoholic twin pairs are followed over time, it is only the heavy drinking twin who shows anxiety symptoms [64].

Studies have found an elevated rate of alcoholism among close relatives of individuals with panic disorders. However, these studies were derived from data in interviews with the alcoholic subjects and not confirmed with corroborated interviews with family members [77]. Finally, long-term studies of the general population revealed no increased rate of preexisting anxiety syndromes in those who later developed alcoholism with severe abstinence syndromes compared to those who did not [5,7,58].

VI. THE INTERACTION OF ADDICTIVE DISORDERS AND PSYCHIATRIC SYNDROMES

A. Exclusionary Criteria

The emphasis in the terminology for the diagnostic categories used to describe alcoholism (drug addiction) have changed in the revision of the DSM-III (DSM-III-R) [78]. The behaviors of addiction to alcohol and drugs have remained at the core of the diagnostic criteria whether the terms are substance, alcohol, or drug abuse or dependence [78]. An addiction is a preoccupation with acquiring drugs or alcohol, compulsivity (use in spite of adverse consequences), and a pattern of relapse after abstinence [78]. Six of the nine criteria of the dependence syndrome in DSM-III-R represent the behaviors of addiction; and three criteria represent pharmacological tolerance and dependence. Because a diagnosis of substance addiction may be made with any three criteria, the diagnosis of the dependence syndrome is possible without tolerance and dependence or without addictive behaviors, unfortunately. Although the changes in diagnostic labels have led to conceptual and practical confusion, drug addiction/alcoholism/alcohol/drug abuse or dependence has remained an independent disorder [79].

There are several Axis I diagnoses in DSM-III-R that require alcohol and drug use diagnoses to be excluded before another diagnosis can be made. These diagnoses refer to schizophrenia, somatization disorder, residual phase, cyclothymia, panic disorder, insomnia, hypersomnia, generalized anxiety, obsessive-compulsive disorder, Tourette's disorder, chronic motor or vocal motor disorder, transient kids disorder, and intermittent explosive, psychogenic amnesia. Also, organic factors, including specific mention of intoxication and withdrawal from drugs or alcohol, are to be excluded for symptoms related to schizophrenia, delusional (paranoid disorder), brief reactive psychosis, schizophreniform disorder, schizoaffective disorder, atypical psychosis, manic episodes, dysthymia, psychogenic fugue, dream anxiety disorder, sleep-terror disorder, sleep walking disorder, alcohol-related blackout, or cannabis dependence. There are also categories with general exclusions for any Axis I disorder [78].

Perhaps the most compelling reasons to give exclusionary status to the alcohol and drug diagnosis is for purposes of prognosis and treatment. The psychiatric syndromes induced by alcohol and drugs will closely follow the course of an addictive disorder, i.e., the psychiatric symptom will lessen or resolve with abstinence over days, weeks, and perhaps months in protracted withdrawal. A number of diagnostic neuroendocrine tests have documented abnormalities that normalize with continued abstinence from alcohol and drugs [80,81]. The treatments that are effective usually will reflect the etiology and prognosis of the alcohol- and drug-induced disorders. Proper treatment of any disorder is essential for efficacy and to avoid unnecessary and harmful treatments. Because clinical diagnosis is principally used to designate prognosis and treatment, the need to make precise diagnostic assessments is clear [5-7,55,56,80,81].

B. Self-Medication Hypothesis

Evidence

The evidence for a self-medication hypothesis as an etiology or genesis of addictive use of alcohol and drugs is lacking. The self-medication hypothesis states that alcohol and drug use and addiction occur because of an underlying or other causative disorder [82,83]. This assumption is often made as a part of retrospective diagnosis of psychiatric disorders. Because of the limitations inherent in retrospective methodology and a combination of state dependent learning during the intoxication and withdrawal states, denial arising from addictive use, and cognitive impairments from alcohol and drug use, the retrospective analysis of alcohol and drug use and its relation to independent psychiatric symptomatology is subject to large error [84,85]. The self-medication hypothesis is based on the belief that the alcohol and drugs are used to "treat" or ameliorate distressing symptoms associated with other psychiatric disorders. There are no available objective studies in the literature which support this common interpretation that psychiatric disorders are responsible for sustaining addictive use. Self-medication with alcohol and drugs in addictive patterns to relieve distressing psychiatric symptoms has not been documented by controlled studies, and, therefore, remains an hypothesis.

Some reports have suggested that during addictive use, self-medication may occur to neutralize the adverse effects of pharmacological intoxication and withdrawal from drugs and alcohol [61]. However, the etiological role of withdrawal in continued drug and alcohol addictive use is limited because only a period of abstinence will relieve the withdrawal effects, whereas further alcohol and drug use often serves to aggravate them [29,85,86]. Furthermore, an explanation remains lacking for relapse after a prolonged period of abstinence when no withdrawal effects are discernible [79].

C. Motivated Use vs Addictive Use

Central to the concept of self-medication is perception of what motivates normal or nonaddictive use of alcohol and drugs. There is little evidence that the motivation for nonaddictive use of alcohol and drugs is the same as for their addictive use. Motivated use of alcohol and drugs is a poorly documented approach to explain addictive behavior bcause what may motivate normal use such as elation or sadness may discourage alcohol and drug use in the pathological state of these moods [58]. Finally, there is no evidence that motivated use sustains addictive use.

The experimental studies that have been performed under controlled conditions in humans and animals examining the role of mood states in addictive disorders contradict the self-medication hypothesis. Mayfield studied the "interaction" between alcohol and affect/mood. He selected three groups of subjects, depressed alcoholics, depressed nonalcoholics, and nondepressed nonalcoholics and measured their mood and affective responses to ingested alcohol. The results were unexpected and contrary to the long-held belief that alcoholics drank to feel better; but supportive of the motivation behind "normal" or nonaddictive use of alcohol. The depressed nonalcoholic experienced the greatest improvement in mood and affect followed by the nondepressed, nonalcoholics (normals) and the least benefit provided to depressed alcoholics. The depressed alcoholics appear to drink in spite of the alcohol-induced depression [85].

Tamerin and Mendelson examined chronic alcoholics under laboratory conditions and found that their self-reports during intoxication contradicted their experiences in the abstinent state. Although the alcoholics claimed that drinking made them feel more relaxed and less depressed, anxiety and depression appeared and worsened with increasing intoxication during the experiment under controlled conditions of amount and interval of alcohol dosing. Anxiety and depression resulted from chronic inebriation contrary to reports by the alcoholics that preexisting anxiety and depression were relieved by drinking. Concomitantly, suicidal thinking appeared during intoxication, and resolved with abstinence, and was often denied in the sober state [51].

D. Interactions Between Drinking and Depression

Mayfield also performed a prospective and retrospective study of cyclic manic depressives. He followed 59 patients over 2 years and examined 41 cases in a review of records. Excessive drinking was noted in 20% of the patients with cyclic affective disorder. One-half of the patients who drank had a change in drinking during an episode of affective disorder, mostly in the manic state. Some relationships between excessive drinking and depressive episodes was noted in one-third of the depressive groups, and the majority either reduced or did not change their drinking behavior. Overall, alcohol consumption was positively and consistently related to elation in mania and was negatively and inconsistently related to depression [84,87]. Mayfield concluded that to "feel good" did not appear to be the explanation for why alcoholics drink.

Pauleikhoff examined almost 900 "cyclic depressives" and found only two cases of excessive drinking restricted to depression [88]. Campanella and Fossi reported four out of five alcoholics ceased drinking during depressive episodes [89]. Mayfield's interpretation of his study and the others was similar to Pitts and Winokur, who started that in mania excessive drinking occurs together with other evidences of euphoria, overactivity, and poor judgment [90].

E. Cocaine and Psychiatric Symptoms

The psychiatric symptoms induced by cocaine are well-documented pharmacological effects in studies and surveys. Cocaine effects have been examined under laboratory conditions in studies involving humans. In one study, intravenous cocaine was administered to cocaine addicts who reported sensations of euphoria followed by paranoia and depression [16]. In another study, cocaine addicts who inhaled cocaine reported paranoia [17]. In a National Institute of Drug Abuse (NIDA)–sponsored survey, depression and suicidal thoughts were among the most common psychiatric symptoms followed by paranoia.

In animal studies, cocaine is self-administered in spite of serious and fatally adversive consequences. Under conditions of unlimited supply, monkeys and rats continue to self-administer by pressing a bar to receive injections of cocaine to the endpoint of convulsions, inanition, exhaustion, and death [91]. The pursuit of cocaine and not some underlying psychological factors appeared to motivate this addictive cocaine use. The animals, as in addicted humans, pursue some pharmacological effects of cocaine yet to be fuly elucidated, although studies to date suggest involvement of the reward center in the hypothalamus [92]. Other theories incorporate the drive states in association with cocaine to produce an autonomous urge for cocaine as in other drives such as eating and sex [93].

F. Addiction Syndrome and Psychiatric Syndromes

Edwards affirmed in his studies that "loss of control" was central to the criteria to the dependence syndrome that was endorsed by the World Health Organization and later incorporated by Rounsaville in DSM-III-R. Loss of control over drug and alcohol use is pervasive to the criteria in the dependence syndrome in DSM-III-R [94]. Characteristic of the six of the nine criteria for preoccupation, compulsive use, and relapse is the persistent and uncontrollable pursuit and use of drugs and alcohol [106]. No data exist that show the loss of control is generated by another underlying psychological condition or psychiatric disorder [94]. As self-medication implies a volitional attempt to ameliorate an intolerable state, it cannot explain the uncontrolled continued use in spite of a worsening of psychiatric symptoms, often beyond any original severity [79]. Finally, clearance or amelioration of the psychiatric syndromes with abstinence from the offending, addictive pharmacological agents is inconsistent with an active medicating effect [5–7,79,95–100].

REFERENCES

1. Pepper, B., Kirshner, M.C., and Ryglewicz, H. (1981). The young adult chronic patient: Overview of a population. *Hosp. Commun. Psychiatry, 32*(7):463–469.
2. Kofoed, L., Kania, J., Walsh, T., and Atkinson, R.M. (1986). Outpatient treatment of patients with substance abuse and coexisting psychiatric disorders. *Am. J. Psychiatry, 143*(7):867–872.
3. Schwartz, S.R., and Goldfinger, S.M. (1981). The new chronic patient: Clinical characteristics of an emerging subgroup. *Hosp. Commun. Psychiatry, 32*(7):473–474.
4. Hekimian, L.J., and Gershon, S. (1968). Characteristics of drug abusers admitted to a psychiatric hospital. *J.A.M.A., 205*(3):75–80.
5. Schuckit, M. (1985). Clinical implications of primary diagnostic groups among alcoholics. *Arch. Gen. Psychiatry, 42*:1043–1049.
6. Schuckit, M.A. (1982). The history of psychotic symptoms in alcoholics. *J. Clin. Psychiatry, 43*(2):53–57.
7. Schuckit, M.A. (1988). Dual diagnosis: Psychiatric pictures among substance abusers. *Drug Abuse Alcoholism Newslett.*, Vista Hill Foundation, March.

8. Kosten, T., and Kleber, H. (1988). Differential diagnosis of psychiatric comorbidity in substance abusers. *J. Subst. Abuse Treat., 5*:201–206.
9. Powell, B.J., Penick, E.C., Othmer, E., Bingham, S.F., and Rice, A. (1982). Prevalence of additional psychiatric syndromes among male alcoholics. *J. Clin. Psychiatry, 43*(10):404–407.
10. Helzer, J.E., and Przybeck, T.R. (1988). The co-occurrence of alcoholism with other psychiatric disorders in the general population and its impact on treatment. *J. Stud. Alcohol, 49*(3):219–224.
11. Robins, L.N., Helzer, J.E., Przybeck, T.R., and Regier, D.A. (1988). Alcohol disorders in the community: A report from the epidemiological catchment area, *Alcoholism: Origins and Outcome.* (R. Rose and J. Barrett, eds.), Raven Press, New York, pp. 15–28.
12. Safer, D.J. (1987). Substance abuse by young adult chronic patients. *Hosp. Commun. Psychiatry, 38*(5):511–514.
13. Brown, V.B., Ridgely, M.S., Pepper, B., Levine, I.S., and Ryglewicz, H. (1989). The dual crises: Mental illness and substance abuse, present and future directions. *Am. Psychologist,* 565–569.
14. McLellan, A.T. (1983). Predicting response to alcohol and drug abuse treatments: Role of psychiatric severity. *Arch. Gen. Psychiatry, 40*:620–625.
15. Osher, F.C., and Kofoed, L.L. (1989). Treatment for patients with psychiatric and psychoactive substance abuse disorders. *Hosp. Commun. Psychiatry, 40*(10):1025–1030.
16. Sherer, M.A. (1988). Intravenous cocaine: Psychiatric effect, biological mechanism. *Biol. Psychiatry, 24*:865–885.
17. Siegal, R.K. (1984). Cocaine smoking disorders: Diagnosis and treatment. *Psychiatr. Ann., 14*(10):728–732.
18. Miller, N.S., Gold, M.S., and Mahler, J.C. (1990). A study of violent behaviors associated with cocaine use: Theoretical and pharmacological implications. *Ann. Clin. Psychiatry, 2*(1):67–71.
19. Powell, J., Penick, E.C., Othmer, E., Bingham, S.F., and Rice, A.S. (1982). Prevalence of additional psychiatric syndromes among male alcoholics. *J. Clin. Psychiatry, 43*:404–407.
20. Gawin, F.H., and Ellinwood, E.H. (1988). Cocaine and other stimulants: Actions, abuse and treatment. *N. Engl. J. Med., 318*:1173–1182.
21. Miller, N.S., Millman, R.B., and Gold, M.S. (1989). Amphetamines: Pharmacology, abuse and addiction. *Adv. Alcohol. Subst. Abuse, 8*(2):53–69.
22. Harvey, S.C. (1985). Hypnotics and sedatives, *The Pharmacological Basis of Therapeutics*, 7th ed. (A.G. Gilman, L.S. Goodman, T.W. Rall, and F. Murad, eds.). Macmillan, New York, pp. 339–371.
23. Roeloffs, S.M., and Dikkenberg, G.M. (1987). Hyperventilation and anxiety: Alcohol withdrawal symptoms decreasing with prolonged abstinence. *Alcohol, 4*:215–220.
24. Gawin, F.H., and Kleber, H.D. (1986). Abstinence symptomatology and psychiatric diagnosis in cocaine abusers: Clinical observations. *Arch. Gen. Psychiatry, 43*:107–113.
25. Post, R.M., Kotin, J., and Goodwin, F.K. (1974). The effects of cocaine on depressed patients. *Am. J. Psychiatry, 131*(5):511–517.
26. Ellinwood, E.H. (1967). Amphetamine psychoses: I. Description of the individuals and process. *J. Nerv. Ment. Dis., 144*:273–283.
27. Lewis, C., et al. (1983). Diagnostic interactions: Alcoholism and antisocial personality. *J. Nerv. Ment. Dis., 171*(2):105–113.
28. Nace, E., Saxon, J., and Shore, N. (1983). A comparison of borderline and non-borderline alcoholic patients. *Arch. Gen. Psychiatry, 40*:54–56.
29. Schuckit, M.A. (1979). Alcoholism and affective disorder: Diagnostic confusion, *Alcoholism and Affective Disorders* (D.W. Goodwin and C.K. Erickson, eds.) SP Medical and Scientific Books, New York, pp. 9–19.
30. Schuckit, M. (1973). Alcoholism and sociopathy diagnostic confusion. *Q. J. Stud. Alcohol., 34*:157–164.
31. Weissman, M., and Myers, T. (1980). Clinical depression in alcoholism. *Am. J. Psychiatry, 137*(3):372–373.
32. Curtis, J.L., Millman, E.J., Mariakutty, J., Charles, J., and Bajwa, W.K. (1986). Prevalence rates for alcoholism, associated depression and dementia on the Harlem Hospital Medicine and Surgery Services. *Adv. Alcohol. Subst. Abuse, 69*(1):45–64.

33. Lyons, J.S., and McGovern, M.P. (1989). Use of mental health services by dually diagnosed patients. *Hosp. Commun. Psychiatry, 40*(10):1067–1069.
34. Drake, R.E., and Wallach, M.A. (1989). Substance abuse among the chronic mentally ill. *Hosp. Commun. Psychiatry, 40*(10):1041–1045.
35. Meyers, J.K., Weissman, M.M., Tischler, G.L., and Holzer, C.E. (1984). Six-month prevalence of psychiatric disorders in three communities. *Arch. Gen. Psychiatry, 41*:959–967.
36. Lehman, A.F., Myers, C.P., and Corty, E. (1989). Assessment and classification of patints with psychiatric and substance abuse syndromes. *Hosp. Commun. Psychiatry, 40*(10):1019–1025.
37. Hesselbrock, M.N., Meyer, R.E., and Keener, J.J. (1985). Psychopathology of hospitalized alcoholics. *Arch. Gen. Psychiatry, 42*:1050–1055.
38. Hellman, J. (1981). Alcohol abuse and the borderline patient. *Psychiatry, 44*:307–317.
39. Kay, S.R., Kalanthara, M., and Meinzer, A.E. (1989). Diagnostic and behavioral characteristics of psychiatric patients who abuse substances. *Hosp. Commun. Psychiatry, 40*(10):1062–1064.
40. Ananth, J., Vondewald, S. Kamal, M., Brodsky, A., Ganial, R., and Miller, M. Missed diagnoses of substance abuse in psychiatric patients. *Hosp. Commun. Psychiatry, 40*(10):297–299.
41. McCarrick, A.K., Manderscherd, R.W., and Bertolucci, D.E. (1985). Correlates of acting-out behaviors among young adult chronic patients. *Hosp. Commun. Psychiatry, 36*(8):848–853.
42. Blankenfield, A. (1986). Psychiatric symptoms in alcohol dependence: Diagnostic and treatment implications. *J. Subst. Abuse Treat., 3*:275–278.
43. Miller, N.S., and Mirin, S.M. (1989). Multiple drug use in alcoholics: Practical and theoretical implications. *Psychiatr. Ann., 19*(5):248–255.
44. Miller, N.S., Gold, M.S., Belkin, B.M., and Klahr, A.L. (1989). Family history and diagnosis of alcohol dependence in cocaine dependence. *Psychiatr. Res., 29*:113–121.
45. Liepman, M.R., Nirenberg, T.D., Porges, R.E., and Wartenberg, A.A. (1987). Depression associated with substance abuse, *Presentations of Depression* (O.G. Cameron, ed.). Wiley, New York.
46. Dackis, C.A., Gold, M.S., Pottash, A.L.C., and Sweeney, D.R. (1986). Evaluating depression in alcoholics. *Psychiatr. Res., 17*:105–109.
47. Dorus, W., Kennedy, J., Gibbons, R.D., and Ravi, S. (1987). Symptoms of diagnosis of depression in alcoholics. *Alcoholism: Clin. Exp. Res., 11*(2):1150–1154.
48. Goodwin, D.W., and Guze, S.B. (1989). *Psychiatric Diagnosis*. Oxford University Press, New York.
49. Kranzler, H.R., and Liebowitz, N.R. (1988). Anxiety and depression in substance abuse: Clinical implications. *Med. Clin. North Am., 72*:867–885.
50. Mayfield, D.G., and Montgomery, D. (1972). Alcoholism, alcohol intoxication, and suicide attempts. *Arch. Gen. Psychiatry, 27*:349–353.
51. Tamerin, J.S., and Mendelson, J.H. (1969). The psychodynamics of chronic inebriation: Observations of alcoholics during the process of drinking in an experimental group setting. *Am. J. Psychiatry, 125*:886.
52. Parsons, O.A., and Leber, W.R. (1981). The relationship between cognitive dysfunction and brain damage in alcoholics: Causal, interaction or epiphenomenal. *Alcoholism: Clin. Exp. Res., 5*(2):326–343.
53. Cala, L.A., and Mastaglia, F.L. (1981). Computerized tomography in chronic alcoholics. *Alcoholism: Clin. Exp. Res., 5*(2):283–294.
54. Pettinati, H.M., Sugerman, A.A., and Maurer, H.S. (1982). Four year MMPI changes in abstinent and drinking alcoholics. *Alcoholism: Clin. Exp. Res., 6*(4):487–494.
55. Willenbring, M.L. (1986). Measurement of depression in alcoholics. *J. Stud. Alcohol, 47*(5):367–372.
56. Galanter, M., Castaneda, R., and Ferman, J. (1988). Substance abuse among general psychiatric patients. *Am. J. Drug Alcohol Abuse, 14*(2):211–235.
57. Woodruff, R.A., Guze, S.B., Clayton, P.J., et al. (1973). Alcoholism and depression. *Arch. Gen. Psychiatry, 28*:97–100.
58. Vaillant, G.E., and Milofsky, E.P. (1982). The etiology of alcoholism: A prospective viewpoint. *Am. Psychol., 37*(5):494–503.

59. Tunving, K. (1985). Psychiatric effects of cannabis use. *Acta Psychiatri., Scand., 72*:209–217.

60. Rounsaville, B.J., Weissman, M.M., Kleber, H. et al. (1982). Heterogeneity of psychiatric diagnosis in treated opiate addicts. *Arch. Gen. Psychiatry, 39*:161–166.

61. Mirin, S.M., Weiss, R.D. (1986). Psychopathology in chronic cocaine abusers. *Am. J. Drug Alcohol Abuse, 12*(1/2):17–29.

62. Weiss, R.D., Mirin, S.M., Michael, J.L., et al. (1986). Psychopathology in chronic cocaine abusers. *Am. J. Drug Alcohol Abuse, 12*:17–19.

63. Schuckit, M.A., and Sweeney, S. (1987). Substance use and mental health problems among sons of alcoholics and controls. *J. Stud. Alcohol, 48*(6):528–534.

64. Goodwin, D.W. (1985). Alcoholism and genetics: The sins of our fathers. *Arch. Gen. Psychiatry, 42*:171–174.

65. Cadoret, R., and Winokur, G. Depression in alcoholism. *Ann. N.Y. Acad. Sci., 233*:34–39.

66. Schuckit, M.A. (1986). Genetic and clinical implications of alcoholism and affective disorders. *Am. J. Psychiatry, 143*(2):140–147.

67. Winokur, G., Rimmer, J., and Reich, T. (1971). Alcoholism IV: Is there more than one type of alcoholism? *Br. J. Psychiatry, 118*:525–531.

68. Winokur, G., and Holeman, E. (1963). Clinical and sexual aspects. *Acta Psychiatr. Scand., 39*:384–412.

69. Woodruff, R.A., Guze, S.B., and Clayton, P.J. (1972). Anxiety neurosis: Clinical and psychiatric outpatients. *Compr. Psychiatry, 13*:165–170.

70. Mullaney, J.A., and Trippett, C.J. (1979). Alcohol dependence and phobias. Clinical description and relevance. *Br. J. Psychiatry, 135*:565–573.

71. Small, P., Stockwell, T., Canter, S., and Hodgson, R. (1984). Alcohol dependence and phobic anxiety states. I. A prevalence study. *Br. J. Psychiatry, 144*:53–57.

72. Stockwell, T., Small, P., Hodgson, R., and Canter, S. (1984). Alcohol dependence and phobic states. II. A retrospective study. *Br. J. Psychiatry, 144*:58–63.

73. Weiss, K.J., and Rosenberg, D.J. (1985). Prevalence of anxiety disorder among alcoholics. *J. Clin. Psychiatry, 46*:3–5.

74. Bowen, R.C., Cipwnyk, D., D'Arcy, C., and Keegan, D. Alcoholism, anxiety disorders and agoraphobia. *Alcoholism: Clin. Exp. Res., 8*(1):48–50.

75. Stavynski, A., Lamontagne, Y., Lavallee, Y-J. (1986). Clinical phobias and avoidant personality disorder among alcoholics admitted to an alcoholism rehabilitation setting. *Can. J. Psychiatry, 31*:714–719.

76. Sheehan, D.V., Carr, D.B., Fishman, S.M., Walsh, M.M., and Peltier-Saxe, D. (1985). Lactate infusion in anxiety research: Its evolution and practice. *J. Clin. Psychiatry, 46*:158–165.

77. Munjack, D.J., and Moss, H.B. (1981). Affective disorder and alcoholism in families of agoraphobics. *Arch. Gen. Psychiatry, 38*:869–871.

78. *Diagnostic and Statistical Manual of Mental Disorders*, 3rd ed., Revised. American Psychiatric Association, Washington, D.C., 1987.

79. Miller, N.S., and Gold, M.S. (1989). Suggestions for changes in DSM-III-R criteria for substance use disorders. *Am. J. Drug Alcohol Abuse, 15*(2):223–230.

80. Willenbring, M.L., Morley, J.E., Niewoehner, C.B., Heilman, R.O., Carlson, C.H., and Shafer, R.B. (1984). Adrenocortical hyperactivity in newly admitted alcoholics: Prevalence, course and associated variables. *Psychoneuroendocrinology, 9*(4):415–422.

81. Giannini, A.J., Malone, D.A., Louiselle, R.H., and Price, W.A. (1987). Blunting of TSH response to TRH in chronic cocaine and phencyclidine abusers. *J. Clin. Psychiatry, 48*:1.

82. Khantzian, K.J. (1985). The self-medication hypothesis of addictive disorders: Focus on heroin and cocaine dependence. *Am. J. Psychiatry, 142*(11):1259–1264.

83. Wurmser, L. (1974). Psychoanalytic considerations of the etiology of compulsive drug use. *J. Am. Psychoanal. Assoc., 22*:820–843.

84. Mayfield, D.G. (1979). Alcohol and affect: Experimental studies, *Alcoholism and Affective Disorders* (1979). (D.W. Goodwin, and C.K. Erickson, eds.). SP Medical and Scientific Books, New York, pp. 99–107.

85. Mayfield, D.G., and Coleman, L.L. (1968). Alcohol use and affective disorder. *Dis. Nerv. Sys.*, 29:467–474.

86. Dorus, W., and Senay, E.C. (1980). Depression demographic dimensions and drug abuse. *Am. J. Psychiatry, 137*:699–704.

87. Mayfield, D., and Allen, D. (1967). Alcohol and affect: A psychopharmacological study. *Am. J. Psychiatry, 123*:1346–1351.

88. Pauleikoff, B. (1953). Uber die Seltenbeit von alkoholabuses bein zyklothyn depressiven. *Nervenavzt, 24*:445–448.

89. Campanella, G., and Fosse, E. (1967). Considerazioni sui rapporti fra alcoolismo e manifestazioni depressive. *Rass. Stud. Psychiatry, 52*:617–632.

90. Pitts, F.N., and Winokur, G. (1966). Affective disorder—Vol. VII: *Alcoholism and affective disorder. J. Psychiatry Res.*, 4:37–50.

91. Aigner, T.G., and Balster, R.L. (1978). Choice behavior in rhesus monkeys: Cocaine versus food. *Science, 201*:534–535.

92. Dackis, C.A., and Gold, M.S. (1985). New concepts in cocaine addiction: The dopamine depletion hypothesis. *Neurosci. Biobehav. Rev.*, 9(3):469–477.

93. Miller, N.S., Dackis, C.A., and Gold, M.S. (1987). The relationship of addiction, tolerance and dependence to alcohol and drugs: A neurochemical approach. *J. Subst. Abuse Treat.*, 4:197–207.

94. Edwards, G., and Gross, M.M. (1976). Alcohol dependence: Provisional description of a clinical syndrome. *Br. Med. J.*, 1:1058–1061.

95. Dackis, C.A., and Gold, M.S. (1983). Opiate addiction and depression—cause or effect. *Drug Alcohol Depend.*, 11:105–109.

96. Frances, R.T., Franklin, J., and Flaven, D.K. (1986). Suicide and alcoholism. *Ann. N.Y. Acad. Sci.*, 487:316–326.

97. Crowley, T.J., Chesluk, D., Pitts, S., and Hart, R. (1974). Drug and alcohol abuse among psychiatric admissions. *Arch. Gen. Psychiatry, 30*:13–20.

98. Cummings, C.P., Prokop, C.K., and Cosgrove, R. (1985). Dysphoria: The cause or the result of addiction? *Psychiatr. Hosp., 16*(13):131–134.

99. Kofoed, L., et al. (1986). Outpatient treatment of patients with substance abuse and coexisting psychiatric disorders. *Am. J. Psychiatry, 143*(7):867–872.

100. Kaufman, E. (1989). The psychotherapy of dually diagnosed patients. *J. Subst. Abuse Treat.*, 6:9–18.

Index

O

Q

X

About the Editor

NORMAN S. MILLER is Assistant Professor of Psychiatry at Cornell University Medical College and formerly Director of the Alcohol and Drug Treatment Services at New York Hospital–Cornell University Medical Center, White Plains, New York. Previously he was Medical Director of the Alcohol and Drug Treatment Unit at Fair Oaks Hospital in Summit, New Jersey. Dr. Miller is a member of the American Society of Addiction Medicine, American Academy of Psychiatrists in Alcoholism and Addictions, American Psychiatric Association, Society of Biological Psychiatry, Research Society on Alcoholism, International Society for Biomedical Research on Alcoholism, and American Academy of Clinical Psychiatrists among others. Dr. Miller received the A.B. degree (1966) from the University of Michigan, Ann Arbor, and M.D. degree (1974) from Howard University, Washington, D.C.; he did his residency training in psychiatry at the Johns Hopkins Hospital, Baltimore, Maryland, and in neurology and fellowship training in Clinical Pharmacology at the University of Minnesota.